KT-473-046

THE PRINCIPLES AND PRACTICE OF MEDICINE

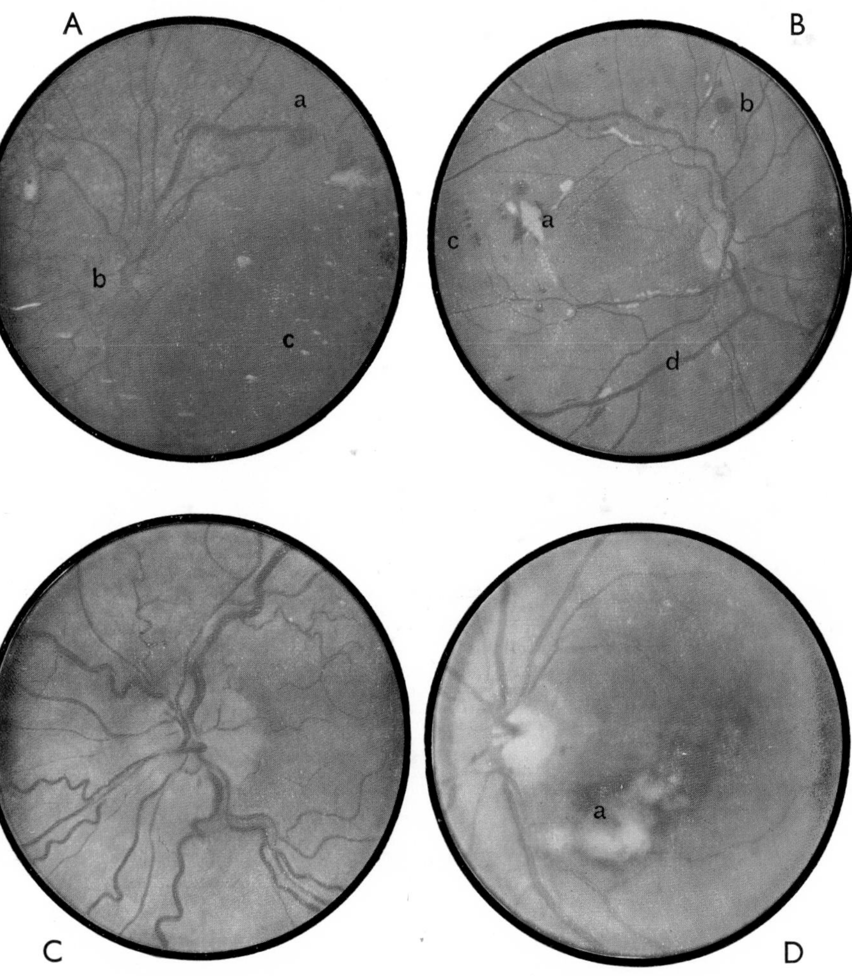

PLATE I

A. Diabetic retinopathy. a. Loops or coils in large veins; b. new vessels on disc, c. subhyaloid haemorrhage.

B. Diabetic retinopathy. a. Exudates; b. dot haemorrhages; c. microaneurysms; d. congested veins.

C. Papilloedema.

D. Thrombosis of lower temporal branch of the central retinal artery. a. Haemorrhage and exudates.

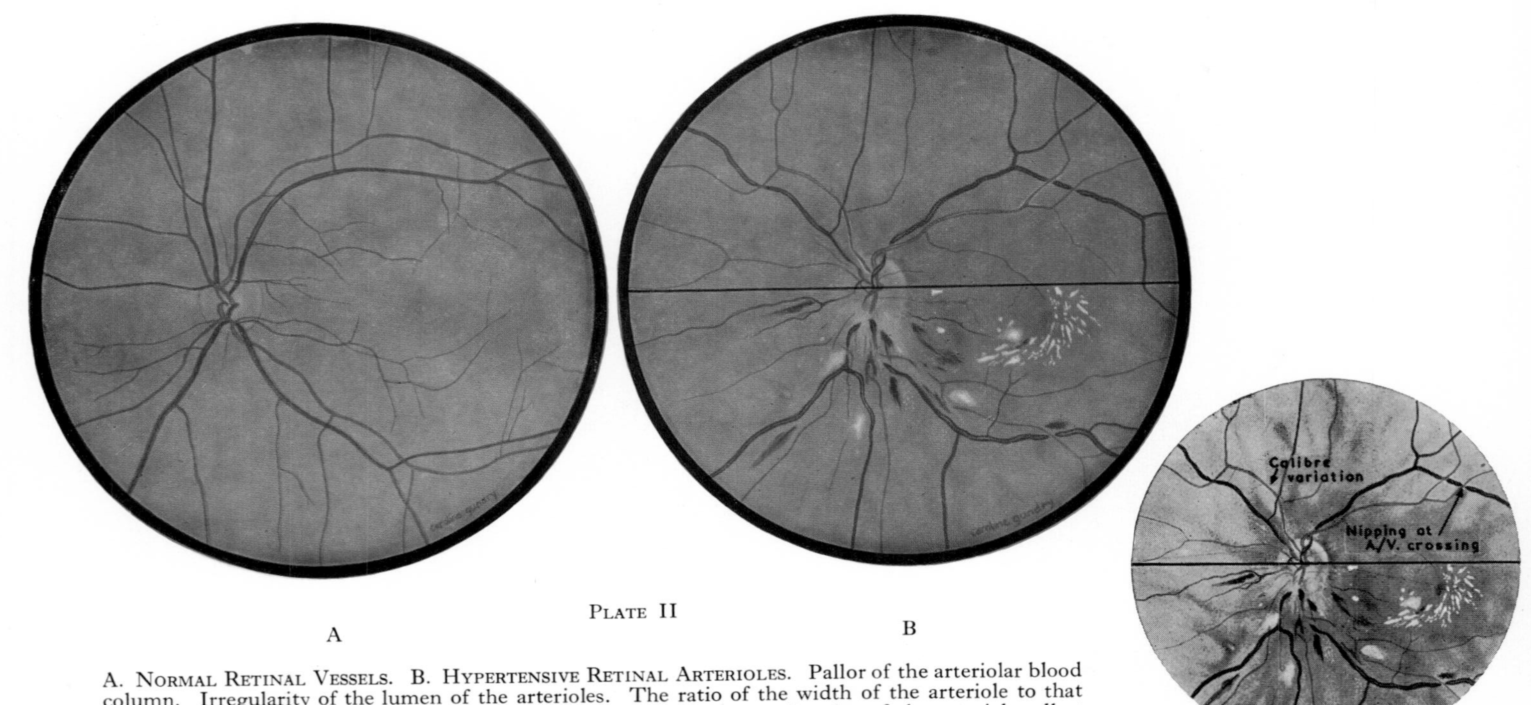

PLATE II

A. NORMAL RETINAL VESSELS. B. HYPERTENSIVE RETINAL ARTERIOLES. Pallor of the arteriolar blood column. Irregularity of the lumen of the arterioles. The ratio of the width of the arteriole to that of its companion vein is 3/6. Nipping at arterio-venous crossings. Opacity of the arterial wall at arterio-venous crossings. Light reflex broader or more prominent than is normal. C. KEY TO B.

(By Permission of the Department of Ophthalmology, University of Edinburgh.)

[*Facing Title*

THE PRINCIPLES AND PRACTICE OF MEDICINE

A Textbook for Students and Doctors

By

SIR STANLEY DAVIDSON

B.A.Cantab., M.D., F.R.C.P.Edin., F.R.C.P.Lond., M.D.Oslo, LL.D., F.R.S.Edin.

Extra Physician to H.M. the Queen in Scotland
Professor of Medicine and Clinical Medicine
University of Edinburgh 1938-1959
Physician-in-Charge, Royal Infirmary, Edinburgh, 1938-1959
Regius Professor of Medicine, University of Aberdeen, 1930-1938

and

Past and Present Members of the Staff of
The Department of Medicine,
University of Edinburgh
and Associated Clinical Units

NINTH EDITION

REPRINT

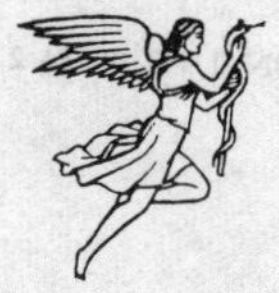

E. & S. LIVINGSTONE LTD
EDINBURGH & LONDON
1971

First Edition	1952
Reprinted	1953
Second Edition	1954
Reprinted	1955
Third Edition	1956
Reprinted	1957
Fourth Edition	1958
Reprinted	1959
Fifth Edition	1960
Reprinted	1961
Sixth Edition	1962
Reprinted	1963
Seventh Edition	1964
Reprinted	1965
First E L B S Edition published	1965
Eighth Edition	1966
Reprinted	1968
Second E L B S Edition published	1967
Ninth Edition	1968
Third E L B S Edition published	1968
Ninth Edition Reprinted	1969
Reprinted	1970
Reprinted	1971

ISBN 0 443 00584 2

Printed in Great Britain by
T. & A. Constable Ltd., Edinburgh.

PREFACE TO THE NINTH EDITION

THE phenomenal sales of this textbook, first published in 1952 and now in its ninth edition, still continue to exceed all expectations. This has necessitated no less than nine editions and eight large reprints during the past 16 years. The Editor and all concerned with its publication are convinced that the policy on which all previous editions were based is a sound one. Accordingly this policy, which is fully explained in the preface to the fifth edition has been maintained in the hope that the ninth edition will prove as acceptable as its predecessors. The preface to the fifth edition is again recorded for the benefit of new readers.

Each section has been carefully revised and brought up to date. Considerable additions have been made, especially to the sections on Nutritional Disorders, Diseases of the Pancreas and Diseases of the Liver and Biliary Tract. Dr. Richmond is now a joint contributor to the section on hepatic diseases with Dr. Robson, while Dr. Joyce Baird has taken the place of the Editor as co-author of the section on Diabetes Mellitus.

The section on Psychological Medicine has been rewritten and expanded by Professor G. M. Carstairs. This change has been prompted by the fact that with the introduction of the new psychotropic drugs many patients suffering from organic or functional psychoses are now treated in their homes by their family doctors. Such patients are also encountered in the medical and surgical wards of general hospitals. Patients with neurotic and psychosomatic symptoms are even more frequently seen in everyday medical practice and every practitioner now needs to have more familiarity with the psychoses and psychoneuroses and their appropriate treatment than was formerly the case.

A separate supplement dealing with tropical diseases, for students and doctors working in India, Asia, Africa and South America, first published in 1964 has been very well received. Brigadier Baird is now a joint author with Dr. Wright of the section on Tropical Diseases and Helminthic Infections. Because of the difficulty of obtaining adequate amounts of foreign currency to pay for imports from abroad, including medical literature, a large paperback edition, combining both *The Principles and Practice of Medicine* and the *Tropical Diseases* supplement, has had large sales in many underdeveloped countries at a greatly reduced price.

Having scrutinised with the greatest care every paragraph of the ninth edition and having contributed subject matter to nearly every section of this book, I must accept the main responsibility for any criticisms which may be evoked as to its educational and clinical value. By careful editing it has been possible to reduce slightly the size of the ninth edition despite a considerable expansion of the section on Psychological Medicine.

The production of a very large number of copies has enabled the publishers to market the book at a very modest price which differs little from that charged five years ago.

It is with great pleasure that I acknowledge the help I have received from friends and colleagues in the Edinburgh Medical School and elsewhere at home and abroad. I am particularly grateful to Drs. Andrew Doig and John Richmond, to my contributors and publishers and to Mrs. Mona Wilson on whom the chief burden of secretarial work continues to fall.

STANLEY DAVIDSON.

Edinburgh 1968.

PREFACE TO THE FIFTH EDITION

WITHIN the short period of eight years five editions and four large reprints of this textbook have been published. In addition the book has been translated into Spanish for sale in Spain and in particular South America, and as we go to press requests for translations have come in from other sources. It seems reasonable to assume, from the phenomenal demands reported by booksellers in the British Commonwealth, the United States of America and other parts of the world, that the style, composition and presentation of material have met with the approval of large numbers of students and doctors, and that the general policy governing the selection of material for description and discussion in the previous editions should be maintained.

This policy, as clearly stated in the preface to the First Edition, is as follows. 'It was also decided that no attempt should be made to describe every rare disease or syndrome, but to devote most of the space available to those disorders most commonly encountered in practice. The selection of the rarer diseases for inclusion and the amount of space devoted to them was based principally on their cultural interest or their educational value as examples of applied anatomy or physiology.' In addition, although such diseases as diphtheria, typhoid fever and rabies are rarely encountered in Great Britain, and the incidence of tuberculosis, syphilis and their complications has fallen greatly in recent years, nevertheless such diseases are still of great importance in many parts of Asia, Africa and South America where this book is very widely read. It was also decided that each section of the book should start with a discussion of the anatomy and physiology of the system concerned, in order to encourage a rational approach to an understanding of symptomatology and treatment, and should end with a review of the measures available for the prevention of disease.

It is indeed gratifying to have had the privilege of preparing so many editions in such a short space of time. While this has been a considerable strain on the editor and contributors it has enabled them to keep each edition abreast with the rapid advances in medical knowledge which are continually being made.

As a result of new material in almost every section, the size of this book has been increased by 45 pages. This increase would have been even greater if every chapter had not been carefully reviewed with the object of deleting any material that was redundant or out of date.

The contributors are drawn from past and present Staff of the Department of Medicine of the University of Edinburgh and its associated clinical units. Furthermore, in each edition every section has been carefully reviewed not only by the editor but by one or more of the other contributors to this book. It is my belief that one of the main reasons for the success of this textbook is the close co-operation existing between the contributors and myself in its production. As a result it has been possible to achieve the balanced style and composition which are said to characterise the work of a single author, and at the same time to reflect the diversity and depth of knowledge and experience which can only be contributed by a team of physicians.

The belief of the editor and the publishers that the sale of the Fifth Edition will be of the same magnitude as that of previous editions has encouraged them to print an even larger number of copies to avoid an increase in the published price.

Having scrutinised with the greatest care every paragraph with regard to content, style and clarity of expression, and having contributed subject matter to a greater or lesser extent to practically every chapter of the book, I must accept the main responsibility for the production of the Fifth Edition of this textbook and for any criticisms which may be evoked as to its educational and clinical value.

It is a great pleasure to acknowledge the help received from my colleagues who contributed so much of the contents of the book and assisted in the editing and correcting of proofs.

I should like to take this opportunity of thanking those teachers of Medicine in many parts of the world who have recommended this textbook to their students.

I am also greatly indebted for helpful advice to certain distinguished medical men who are not on the staff of the Department of Medicine, and particularly to Professor John McMichael of the Postgraduate Medical School of London.

The production of this book has meant a great increase of secretarial work and I wish to express my thanks especially to Mrs. Mona Wilson on whom the chief burden fell. Finally, it is a pleasure to acknowledge the help and kindness I have received from the publishers.

STANLEY DAVIDSON.

Edinburgh 1960.

LIST OF CONTRIBUTORS

BAIRD, J. P., M.D., F.R.C.P.Edin., F.R.C.P.Lond. *Consulting Physician to the British Army. Formerly Professor of Military Medicine of the Royal Army Medical College and the Royal College of Physicians, London.*
Tropical Diseases and Helminthic Infections.

BAIRD, Joyce D., M.A., M.B., Ch.B.Aberd. *Hon. Lecturer, Department of Medicine (Western General Hospital), Edinburgh.*
Diabetes Mellitus.

CARD, W. I., M.D., F.R.C.P.Edin., F.R.C.P.Lond. *Professor of Medicine in Relation to Mathematics and Computing, University of Glasgow.*
Diseases of the Digestive System.

CARSTAIRS, G. M., M.D., F.R.C.P.Edin., D.P.M. *Professor of Psychological Medicine, University of Edinburgh. Hon. Consultant, Royal Edinburgh Hospital and Royal Infirmary, Edinburgh. Director of the Medical Research Council Unit for Research on the Epidemiology of Psychiatric Illness.*
Psychological Medicine.

DAVIDSON, Sir Stanley, B.A.Cantab., M.D., F.R.C.P.Edin., F.R.C.P.Lond., M.D.Oslo, LL.D., F.R.S.Edin. *Professor Emeritus, University of Edinburgh.*
Nutritional Disorders, including Obesity.

DUTHIE, J. J. R., M.B., Ch.B., F.R.C.P.Edin. *Professor of Medicine (Northern General Hospital), University of Edinburgh. Hon. Consultant Physician, Northern General Hospital. Physician-in-charge, Rheumatic Diseases Unit, Northern General Hospital, Edinburgh.*
Chronic Rheumatic Diseases.

FRENCH, E. B., B.A., M.B., B.Chir.Cantab., F.R.C.P.Edin., F.R.C.P.Lond. *Reader in Medicine, University of Edinburgh. Hon. Consultant Physician, Western General Hospital, Edinburgh.*
Infection and Disease.
Infectious Diseases.
Diseases of the Kidney and Urinary System.

GIRDWOOD, R. H., M.D., Ph.D., F.R.C.P.Edin., F.R.C.P.Lond., F.C.Path. *Professor of Therapeutics, University of Edinburgh. Hon. Consultant Physician, Royal Infirmary, Edinburgh.*
Disorders of the Blood.

GRANT, I. W. B., M.B., Ch.B., F.R.C.P.Edin. *Consultant Physician, Respiratory Diseases Unit, Northern General Hospital, Edinburgh.*
Diseases of the Respiratory System.

HARRIS, E. A., M.D.L'pool, Ph.D.Edin., M.R.C.P.Lond., M.R.A.C.P. *Consultant Physician, Respiratory Diseases Unit, Northern General Hospital, Edinburgh.*
Diseases of the Respiratory System.

INNES, James, M.D., F.RC.P.Edin. *Senior Lecturer in Medicine, University of Edinburgh. Consultant Physician, Royal Infirmary, Edinburgh.*
Disorders of the Blood.
Diseases of the Pancreas.

MACLEOD, J. G., M.B., Ch.B., F.R.C.P.Edin. *Senior Lecturer in Medicine (Western General Hospital), University of Edinburgh. Consultant Physician, Western General Hospital, Royal Edinburgh Hospital.*
Infectious Diseases.
Chemotherapy of Infections.

MATTHEW, Henry, M.B., Ch.B., F.R.C.P.Edin. *Consultant Physician, Royal Infirmary. Physician-in-charge, Poisoning Treatment Centre. Director, Scottish Poisons Information Bureau.*
Acute Poisoning.

RICHMOND, John, M.D., F.R.C.P.Edin., M.R.C.P.Lond. *Reader in Medicine, University of Edinburgh. Hon. Consultant Physician, Royal Infirmary, Edinburgh.*
Genetics in Relation to Medicine.
Diseases of the Liver and Biliary Tract.

ROBSON, J. S., M.D., F.R.C.P.Edin. *Reader in Medicine, University of Edinburgh. Hon. Consultant Physician, Royal Infirmary, Edinburgh.*
Diseases of the Kidney and Urinary System.
Disturbances in Water and Electrolyte Balance
and in Hydrogen Ion Concentration.
Diseases of the Liver and Biliary Tract.

SIMPSON, J. A., M.D., F.R.C.P.Edin., F.R.C.P.Lond., F.R.C.P.Glasg. *Professor of Neurology, University of Glasgow, Senior Neurologist, Institute of Neurological Sciences, Royal and Western Infirmaries, Glasgow.*
Diseases of the Nervous System.

SIRCUS, W., Ph.D., M.D., F.R.C.P.Edin., F.R.C.P.Lond. *Senior Lecturer in Medicine (Western General Hospital), University of Edinburgh. Hon. Physician-in-charge, Gastro-intestinal Unit, Western General Hospital, Edinburgh.*
Diseases of the Pancreas.

STRONG, J. A., M.B.E., M.A., M.D.Dubl., F.R.C.P.Edin., F.R.C.P. Lond. *Professor of Medicine (Western General Hospital), University of Edinburgh. Hon. Consultant Physician, Western General Hospital, Edinburgh.*
Diseases of the Endocrine System, including Diabetes Mellitus.

TURNER, R. W. D., O.B.E., M.A., M.D.Cantab., F.R.C.P.Edin., F.R.C.P.Lond. *Reader in Medicine, University of Edinburgh. Hon. Consultant Physician, Western General Hospital. Physician-in-charge, Cardiac Department, Western General Hospital, Edinburgh.*
Diseases of the Cardiovascular System.

WRIGHT, F. J., M.A., M.D.Cantab., F.R.C.P.Edin., F.R.C.P.Lond. D.T.M.&H. *Senior Lecturer in Diseases of Tropical Climates, University of Edinburgh. Hon. Consultant Physician-in-charge, Tropical Diseases Unit, City Hospital, Edinburgh.*
Tropical Diseases and Helminthic Infections.

CONTENTS

INFECTION AND DISEASE

THE life and health of human beings, animals and plants is constantly threatened by invasion by parasites of all kinds, especially by micro-organisms. During the last century numerous micro-organisms have been identified and studied, their modes of spread have been recognised, and various effective methods of prevention and treatment have been discovered. Consequently many of the infections which used to be the major cause of death both in peace and war have almost vanished and their lethal effects have been greatly reduced. Infections still, however, play a large part in the production of disease and are responsible for much absenteeism at school and at work. Prophylaxis cannot be effective without full knowledge of the sources and spread of infection and of the factors which determine the resistance of the host and the virulence of the parasite.

SOURCES OF INFECTION

1. **Human sources**

(*a*) **Patients** in the incubation period or during the course or convalescent stage of an infection.

(*b*) **Carriers**

Healthy carriers are persons in good health who harbour pathogens such as *Strep. pyogenes*, *Staph. pyogenes*, *C. diphtheriae* or *N. meningitidis*.

Convalescent carriers are persons who harbour the causal organism, sometimes for many years, after clinical recovery from a disease, e.g. typhoid bacilli have been recovered from a carrier 25 years after an attack of typhoid fever.

(c) **Autoinfection.** From the time that the foetus enters the maternal birth canal, all individuals tend to accumulate a similar symbiotic flora, among which are many potential pathogens. Various factors which lead to autoinfection are recognised. A general lowering of resistance enables micro-organisms such as the virus of herpes simplex or the fungus of thrush to gain a foothold. Antibiotic therapy, which interferes with ecological conditions, may lead to overgrowth of resistant bacteria and cause disease such as staphylococcal enteritis. If organisms are transferred to an unaccustomed site, then infection may ensue. Thus haemolytic streptococci, derived from the upper respiratory tract, may cause cellulitis in wounds, *Streptococcus viridans* may enter the blood stream from the mouth and cause subacute bacterial endocarditis, while *Esch. coli* may pass up the female urethra and infect the urinary tract.

2. **Animal Reservoirs.** Diseases of animals which may be acquired by man include psittacosis, acute lymphocytic choriomeningitis, Q fever, bovine tuberculosis, leptospirosis and helminth infections in which the organism enters the body through one of the natural routes. Others spread by bites of various animal vectors are listed in Table 1 on p. 4.

3. **Soil.** The organisms causing tetanus, gas gangrene and botulism are normally found in cultivated soil.

SPREAD OF INFECTION

1. Airborne

(a) *Droplet.* During talking, organisms present in the nose, throat or mouth are expelled in minute droplets of moisture and projected for several feet. The more violent expirations which accompany sneezing project numerous droplets, and coughing similarly disseminates organisms from the bronchial tree. Thus it is important to teach the public not to spit, and to cover the mouth or nose with a clean handkerchief during coughing or sneezing. Nurses and doctors should wear suitable masks during operations, the dressing of wounds and attendance on infants in hospitals.

(b) *Dust.* When infected droplets dry, a protective layer of protein enables organisms to survive and remain airborne for a long time. These along with other particles derived from contaminated clothing, handkerchiefs, bedclothes, carpets and floors of buildings may be inhaled or may infect wounds. This mode of spread is especially important in streptoccocal and staphylococcal infections in hospital.

Spread of infection is airborne in diseases of the throat and respiratory tract, in meningococcal meningitis and in many of the common infectious diseases of childhood. The risks of infection can be reduced by the provision of ample fresh air, sunlight and good ventilation in all buildings. In hospitals and institutions there must be an adequate distance between beds; dust should be removed by vacuum cleaner or damp mopping; bedclothes should be made of material which can be boiled.

2. **Ingestion.** Contamination of food and drink by human faeces is responsible for diseases which are apt to occur epidemically. These include the enteric fevers, dysenteries, cholera, some types of food poisoning and infections carried by enteroviruses such as poliomyelitis and infective hepatitis. Examples of sources of contamination are:

(*a*) The soiled hands of workers employed in the preparation and distribution of food and milk.
(*b*) Soiled lavatory chains, door handles and public towels contaminating the hands.
(*c*) The faulty disposal of sewage.
(*d*) Flies.

3. **Direct Invasion.** Examples of invasion of the skin, conjunctiva or mucous membranes either directly or through an abrasion are:

(*a*) Skin diseases, e.g. impetigo contagiosa, erysipelas, fungal infections, scabies.
(*b*) Conjunctivitis due to various causes.
(*c*) Venereal diseases—syphilis, gonorrhoea and lymphogranuloma venereum.
(*d*) Hookworm, schistosomiasis, leptospirosis.
(*e*) Urinary tract infection through catheterisation.

4. **Contamination of Wounds.** Airborne organisms may infect wounds, particularly during the changing of

dressings, as already mentioned. Dirt and soil, especially from well manured ground, may contain the spores of tetanus and gas gangrene.

5. **Inoculation.** The medical and allied professions may introduce infections through imperfect sterilisation of instruments, or by tranfusion of blood, plasma or serum. The most common of these is homologous serum jaundice (p. 1011), and even with the utmost care in the selection of donors, the disease follows at least one in a thousand transfusions, and the mortality rate in the older age groups is high. Organisms may also be inoculated through the skin by insect or animal vectors, as indicated in Table I.

TABLE 1

Insect and Animal Vectors

Disease	Type of Organism	Vector	Reservoir
Yellow fever	Virus	Mosquito	Man, monkeys
Rabies	Virus	Dog, jackal, etc.	Same species
Typhus fever	Rickettsia	Louse	Man
Scrub typhus	Rickettsia	Mite	Small rodents
Murine typhus	Rickettsia	Flea	Rat
Plague	Bacterium	Flea	Rat and other rodents
Relapsing fever (1)	Spirochaete	Louse	Man
Relapsing fever (2)	Spirochaete	Tick	Rodents
Rat-bite fever	Spirochaete	Rat	Rat
Malaria	Protozoon	Mosquito	Man, monkeys
African sleeping sickness	Protozoon	Tsetse fly	Man, antelopes, etc.
Kala azar	Protozoon	Sandfly	Man, dog.
Filariasis	Nematode	Mosquito	Man

INCUBATION PERIOD. This refers to the time which elapses between the entry into the body of the infective agent and the appearance of symptoms or signs of disease. Its duration varies with the infection, e.g. diphtheria one to four days, measles about 10 days, infective hepatitis one month, homologous serum jaundice three months, leprosy one to several years.

DEFENCE OF THE HUMAN HOST

The First Line of Defence is principally mechanical and depends upon the integrity of the skin and mucous membranes. For instance the respiratory tract is protected from inhaled particles by the hairs of the vestibule of the nose, the moist turbinates and nasal septum, and by the sharp alterations in direction to which the air current is subjected in its passage to and from the alveoli. Most particles come into contact with and stick to the tenacious mucus covering the respiratory tract and are then brought up by ciliary action and expelled from the mouth and nose or swallowed. Cilia are paralysed and damaged by tobacco smoke and atmospheric pollution. An additional protective feature is the continuous flow of secretions, which in the case of bile and gastric juice may also have an antibacterial action. Some organisms can penetrate the skin or mucous membranes without any pre-existing breach of surface (p. 3).

Second Line of Defence. When there has been a breach in the first line of defence by a pathogenic organism, a series of protective reactions occur, which can be grouped as cellular, humoral and mechanical.

Cellular defence. Various leucocytes and tissue cells take an active part in the general and local response to infection. The neutrophil polymorphonuclear leucocytes, the monocytes of the blood and the cells of the reticulo-endothelial system are phagocytic. The plasma cells and lymphocytes produce antibodies. The role of the eosinophil cells which increase in number in helminthic infections, in allergic reactions and during convalescence from acute infections is unknown. Phagocytosis by leucocytes has been shown to be more efficient in the presence of specific antibody.

Humoral defence. The inoculation or absorption of foreign protein (antigen) stimulates the production of chemically specific globulin (antibody), which can be detected in the serum (antiserum). The antibody combines with the antigen and neutralises any effects which the latter might have on the body. After the injection of an antigen, it is approximately one week before antibodies can be detected in the serum. During the course of viral infections, antibodies develop and may be detectable in the serum in some cases for the rest of the patient's life. There is evidence that antiviral antibody is important in prophylaxis, but it does not appear to play a dominant role in recovery. A substance called interferon has been isolated from cells grown in tissue culture infected with virus. This substance inhibits the growth of virus *in vitro*, but so far this discovery has not led to advances in treatment.

Mechanical defence. In many infections a mechanical barrier forms against the spread of infection, e.g. the fibrin from the acute inflammatory reaction of a pyogenic infection, or the fibrous tissue around a tuberculous focus or a hydatid cyst. It should be remembered however that some organisms elaborate substances which weaken this defensive barrier, e.g. β-haemolytic streptococci may produce a fibrinolysin which dissolves fibrin, or hyaluronidase, a substance which enables the organisms or their products to spread more rapidly through the tissues.

The nature of the responses of the body and their intensity depend upon the type of infecting agent, its quantity and its virulence. Viral infections tend to excite a local lymphocytic reaction and a polymorph leucopenia with relative lymphocytosis in the blood, e.g. infective hepatitis, measles, mumps. Rarely there is an initial polymorph leucocytosis, e.g. acute anterior poliomyelitis. Worm infections are frequently associated with an eosinophilia. When the infection is bacterial, the character of the ensuing reaction will depend mainly on the type of infecting agent. Pyogenic organisms (staphylococci, streptococci, pneumococci, meningococci, gonococci and *Esch. coli*) give rise to an acute local inflammation with the outpouring of neutrophil polymorphonuclear leucocytes, serum and fibrin and a general reaction of abrupt onset with pyrexia and polymorph leucocytosis. Typhoid and paratyphoid infections cause a local monocyte response, a polymorph leucopenia and a gradual increase of fever over several days. Whooping-cough induces a lymphocytosis. Tuberculosis and leprosy are more chronic infections, with a local reaction of lymphocytes and reticulo-endothelial cells; fever is less marked or may be absent.

The course of an infection depends upon the patient's psychological, physical and nutritional state. An absence of fever and leucocytosis in pneumococcal pneumonia, for instance, indicates a poor response and a bad prognosis. This is especially liable to occur in elderly or alcoholic subjects. It has long been recognised that the mental attitude of the patient towards his affliction can affect his power of recovery. The doctor's ability to give confidence to the patient and the relatives is a very important part of treatment. Though the mechanism of this effect of the mind is not clear, it is known that the activity of the endocrine glands and the autonomic nervous system is to some extent controlled by psychological factors through the influence of the higher centres upon the hypothalamus. That the endocrine glands may play an important role in the defence mechanism is suggested by the increased susceptibility to and mortality from infection in diabetes mellitus and in Addison's disease, and by the powerful influence of corticosteroids for good or ill in allergic and inflammatory states.

Susceptibility of Host to Infection. Many animal species and the various races of mankind differ in their susceptibility to infection by a variety of organisms. Negroes whose red cells contain haemoglobin S or are deficient in glucose 6-phosphate dehydrogenase are relatively immune to malaria (p. 632). Man and the guinea-pig may be infected by human or bovine strains of the tubercle bacillus, but are unaffected by the avian strain. Rabbits are very susceptible to experimental infection with the bovine strain, though they seldom if ever contract tuberculosis naturally. Birds on the other hand are susceptible only to the avian variety. When measles was first introduced by traders into the Fiji Islands there was a very high mortality rate at all ages.

An unfavourable environment may decrease resistance to the infection. For instance anthrax, a serious disease in cattle and man, does not effect the normal hen, even when large doses of the organism are injected. If, however, the hen is exposed to low temperatures, inoculation of anthrax bacilli may produce a fatal disease. Similarly if man is harbouring a pathogenic organism, exposure to cold and damp may precipitate disease.

Infants during their first six months of life are rarely susceptible to many of the common infectious fevers owing to an immunity derived from the mother.

Virulence of Micro-organisms. If bacteria and viruses grow under adverse conditions a loss of virulence may occur. In many instances this can be shown to be associated with a partial loss in antigenicity and with a loss of the capsule in capsulated organisms. Conversely, organisms grown in ideal circumstances may become more virulent. It has been suggested that this may happen as an organism passes from one person to another in the course of an epidemic.

The capacity of an organism to produce disease after penetration of the tissues of the host may depend upon special conditions for growth. Thus suitable anaerobic conditions are necessary for the development of tetanus spores, which may lie dormant in normal tissues for years.

Acquired Drug Resistance. In many instances drug resistance in bacteria arises by spontaneous mutation; in others it results from the transfer of genetic material from a resistant to a susceptible organism. Not only may treatment of the individual with chemotherapy prove ineffective, but such organisms may then pass to a previously uninfected patient and cause disease which will not respond to chemotherapy. For instance the gonococcus was susceptible to sulphonamides when these drugs were first introduced. After several years, resistant strains became so numerous that gonorrhoea was resuming its previous severity until the discovery of penicillin and now this drug is sometimes ineffective. Of even greater importance are staphylococci, many strains of which were at one time susceptible to penicillin and to various antibiotics but which have now become resistant to the action of many chemotherapeutic agents. Resistant strains of tubercle bacilli also develop readily unless the instructions given on p. 425 are followed.

It is the duty of every doctor to try to prevent the development of resistant strains of bacteria by giving therapeutically effective doses of a drug and it is unwise to continue treatment which is not having the anticipated effect without careful consideration of the reasons for failure. Antimicrobial agents must not be used for colds or other viral infections, not only because such treatment is ineffective but also because resistant bacteria may develop and because of the risk of superinfection (p. 65).

Prevention of Infection. The elimination of a disease by finding, treating or isolating the human and animal reservoirs of infection is an ideal which should be vigorously pursued and it has met with success in the campaigns against many diseases including smallpox, diphtheria, malaria and tuberculosis. Infections spread by faecal contamination have been largely eliminated by sanitary measures.

Autoinfection may be reduced by good personal hygiene and by the use of chlorhexophane incorporated in soap or cream. Infection from the mouth during dental extractions must be prevented in patients with valvular heart disease by prophylactic penicillin. Infection arising from operations on the alimentary tract may be minimised by appropriate pre-operative 'sterilisation' of the gut by chemotherapy. The probability of patients and known carriers acting as a source of infection can be reduced by isolation. Dependent upon the nature of the infection it may also be necessary to disinfect or destroy the surgical dressings, sputum or excreta, to sterilise the clothing and utensils of patients or carriers, and to take special precautions against the liability of spread by those attendant upon the patient and by those concerned with the handling of food.

In addition, those individuals who have been in contact with serious and highly infectious diseases like smallpox are placed in quarantine. The term is derived from the original period of 40 days compulsory isolation of ships after leaving a port where certain infectious diseases were raging. The duration of quarantine has come to be two days more than the maximum known incubation period of the disease in question. For the common infectious fevers of childhood a period of observation has replaced quarantine.

From the viewpoint of the individual, apart from encouraging the maintenance of general health by good food, fresh air and exercise, adequate sleep and good housing conditions, certain specific steps may be taken to increase resistance to infection.

(*a*) ACTIVE IMMUNISATION. The production of antibodies may be stimulated by the injection of a suitable antigen. Some infections do not confer lasting immunity to further attacks by similar organisms, e.g. pyogenic infections, pneumonia, influenza. Other infections are followed by an almost complete and lifelong immunity. It is in members of the latter group that active immunisation has been found to be effective in preventing or modifying the severity of infection. The practical difficulty is to prepare antigenically effective, yet relatively non-toxic material for inoculation.

In Great Britain parents should be advised to have their children immunised against whooping-cough, diphtheria, tetanus, smallpox and poliomyelitis. Expectant mothers should be immunised against poliomyelitis. When indicated, active immunisation may also be given against tuberculosis, enteric fevers, cholera, plague, typhus, yellow fever and rabies. Immunisation against measles has also been introduced recently and may soon be in general use. At present the following schedule is recommended.

Schedule of Vaccination

Age	Visits	Vaccine	Intervals
3 to 6 months	3	Three administrations of D.T.P.+O.P.V.	Not less than four weeks
1 to 2 years	1	Booster D.P.T.+O.P.V.	Not less than four weeks
	1	Smallpox vaccination	
First year at school	1	Booster D.T.+O.P.V.	
8 to 12 years	1	Booster D.T.+O.P.V.	
12 years	1	B.C.G. for the Tuberculin negative	

D.T.P.=Diphtheria, tetanus, pertussis ('triple') vaccine.
O.P.V.=Oral poliomyelitis vaccine.
D.T.=Diphtheria, tetanus vaccine.

(*b*) Passive Immunisation. An injection of specific antiserum will produce immunity for about six weeks only and should be followed by active immunisation with the appropriate antigen. The most common example of the use of antiserum is in protection against tetanus, but there are others. For instance, diphtheria occurring in a school may be prevented from spreading by injecting susceptible (Schick positive) children with anti-diphtheritic serum. Antitetanic and antidiphtheritic sera are prepared from the horse, and their injection induces the production of antibodies against horse serum. Subsequent injections of serum are therefore not only likely to be ineffective, but are also prone to cause sensitivity reactions (p. 37). Some viral infections, notably measles, may also be prevented in exposed persons by the injection of human immunoglobin. Again the immunity is temporary. Human serum itself is not used owing to the possibility of transmitting the virus of homologous serum jaundice, a risk which is eliminated by the use of immunoglobin.

Defective Defence. The outcome of an infection depends *inter alia* upon the numbers, type, virulence and portal of entry of the infecting agent in addition to the efficiency of the defensive mechanisms of the host which have been outlined above. The latter may break down at any point. Agranulocytosis, lymphopenia, leukaemia and lymphadenoma may each depress the cellular defence. Antibody formation is impaired in congenital and acquired hypogammaglobulinaemia and in dysgammaglobulinaemia (e.g. in multiple myelomatosis). The mechanical barrier which walls off an infection such as the fibrosis around a tuberculous lesion in the lung may in some cases make the tubercle bacillus less accessible to chemotherapy and thus perpetuate the infection. Indeed a tuberculous cavity may facilitate the growth of other organisms ranging from virulent staphylococci to the saprophytic aspergilli.

An ill-defined lowering of resistance to infection is observed in alcoholics, drug addicts, malnourished patients, those under treatment with adrenocorticosteroids or suffering from the nephrotic syndrome, reticulosis or other debilitating disease. Such patients are prone to a variety of infections, including unusual ones such as systemic candidiasis and torulosis.

Finally a local predisposition to infection may be determined by ischaemia or a foreign body in the tissue, while obstruction to the outflow of any secretion sooner or later leads to retrograde infection. Examples are parotitis, sinusitis, lung abscess, bronchiectasis, cholangitis and pyelonephritis.

EPIDEMICS

A study of the onset and the distribution and incidence of cases in an epidemic helps to trace the source of infection.

Epidemics of explosive onset affecting relatively large numbers of a given community are likely to arise from the ingestion of infected food, milk or water. After the initial outbreak, case to case infection may occur and this may give rise to a secondary epidemic wave. The time of appearance of this wave will vary according to the incubation period of the disease.

Epidemics of gradual onset, rising to a peak and then slowly declining are commonly due to airborne spread. Many such epidemics have a seasonal incidence, and some show a rhythm over a period of years, e.g. measles, which is endemic in Great

Britain at all times, but appears in epidemic form every two or three years. Epidemics occur when there is an accumulation of a sufficient number of susceptible people.

Influenza provides a particularly interesting field of study owing to its liability to spread in pandemic form throughout the world. An attack confers immunity to the responsible virus for about two years. Of three distinct viruses (A, B and C) virus A especially has undergone mutation to form subtypes to which the whole population may be susceptible, as was the case in the 1957 pandemic of Asian (A_2) influenza. Influenza also occurs in some animals. The mortality is largely dependent upon secondary bacterial invasion.

Clinical Features of Infections. Symptoms common to most febrile infections are malaise (a feeling of ill-health), anorexia (loss of appetite), lassitude and headache. 'Hot and cold' feelings, chilliness or shivering are frequently described and are due to vasoconstriction in the skin associated with a rising temperature. Deep seated aching in the back and limbs is common in viral infections. In addition to these general complaints, many infectious diseases cause specific or localising clinical features which may be of diagnostic value.

The rapidity of the onset of symptoms may also be characteristic. Pneumococcal pneumonia for instance has in most cases an abrupt onset. Special complaints are rigor (severe shivering), dry cough, pain in one side of the chest on inspiration or coughing, and the appearance of herpes on the lips. These points strongly suggest the diagnosis of pneumonia even before a physical examination has been made. Indeed in the early stages abnormal signs in the chest may not be detectable, and the diagnosis will depend upon the history and the general appearance of the patient. Typhoid fever on the other hand starts so insidiously that patients may continue with their normal occupation for a few days before seeking advice.

The following signs are common to most infections.

Pyrexia. Normal body temperature shows a diurnal variation of about 1° C. (1·5° F.), being lowest in the early morning and highest in the afternoon. The upper limits are 37·2° C. (99° F.) in the rectum, 37° C. (98·4° F.) in the mouth and 36·7° C. (98° F.) in the axilla. Pyrexia may be defined as an increase in the diurnal variation of more than 1° C. (1·5° F.) or a rise above the maximum normal temperatures just mentioned.

The rate of rise and fall of fever may be of diagnostic value. A rigor raises body temperature rapidly in spite of every indication that the patient feels cold. Heat production is increased by muscular contractions and heat loss is decreased by constriction of the skin vessels. Rigors are common in pneumococcal pneumonia, acute pyelonephritis, septicaemia, and malaria. Subsidence of pyrexia may be rapid by 'crisis' within 24 hours as in pneumococcal pneumonia, or slow by 'lysis' over several days as was typical in typhoid fever before the introduction of chloramphenicol. Enough has already been said to indicate that a properly recorded temperature chart may sometimes be an invaluable diagnostic aid.

Types of Pyrexia

1. *Continued.* The temperature remains at a constant level above normal, the diurnal variation being not more than 1° C. (1·5° F.), as in pneumococcal pneumonia.

2. *Remittent.* The temperature varies more than 1° C. (1·5 °F.), but even at its lowest remains above normal. This is the most common type of fever.

3. *Intermittent.* The temperature rises, but returns to normal some time during the day, as in vivax malaria.

4. *Hectic.* There is a big swing in temperature. It may rise 3° C. (5° F.) during the night, but returns to normal in the morning. The fall is accompanied by sweating. This occurs in septicaemia and advanced tuberculosis.

Causes of fever other than infection include exercise, a hot bath, the injection of pyrogens, sensitivity to foods and drugs, severe anaemia, venous thrombosis, pulmonary or myocardial infarction, connective tissue disorders, malignant growth, especially when associated with necrosis or generalised dissemination, Hodgkin's disease, pontine haemorrhage. An apparent rise in body temperature is produced not infrequently in malingerers.

SWEATING. At the height of the fever the skin is hot, flushed and dry. Sweating occurs as the temperature subsides. In rheumatic fever sweating is prominent throughout. Profuse perspiration may lead to a sweat rash (sudamina) consisting of numerous minute vesicles.

CARDIOVASCULAR SIGNS. The heart rate is increased. There is a slight rise in the systolic and fall in the diastolic blood pressure.

The result is a rapid pulse of large amplitude which is often described as bounding. For every 0·5° C. (1° F.) rise in temperature an increase of about 10 beats per minute in the pulse rate may be anticipated. Exceptions to this general rule are acute tuberculosis, scarlet fever and acute rheumatic carditis in which it is faster, and enteric fever, viral infections and often meningitis in which it is slower than expected from the height of the temperature.

RESPIRATORY SIGNS. The respiratory rate is increased by fever in proportion to the pulse. The normal ratio of 4 : 1 is maintained except with acute infections of the respiratory tract in which this ratio is reduced to 3 : 1 or 2 : 1.

ALIMENTARY SIGNS. The tongue is furred and dry. Foul crusts (sordes), consisting of bacteria, food and dried saliva, may collect around the teeth and on the lips. Appetite is poor; there may be nausea, vomiting and constipation.

URINARY SIGNS. The urine is scanty and concentrated, i.e. with high specific gravity, owing to loss of fluid by sweating. There is often a brick-red urate deposit. Proteinuria is frequently present, but it disappears on recovery from the fever without any residual renal damage.

BLOOD CHANGES. The alterations which may occur in the circulating leucocytes are indicated on p. 6. In chronic infections normochromic or hypochromic anaemia may develop.

Diagnosis of Infectious Disease. A knowledge of infections prevailing in the locality may be an invaluable guide to diagnosis, e.g. when mumps is prevalent the occurrence without apparent cause of acute epididymo-orchitis in an adult may be attributed to mumps with some confidence, a diagnosis which could not be made on clinical evidence alone. Mild or atypical cases of fever may be correctly diagnosed on similar grounds, e.g. infectious hepatitis without jaundice occurring in a person who has been in contact with that disease. It is wise to enquire about contacts among the family, friends and workmates. Persons following certain occupations may be unduly exposed to infection, e.g. leptospirosis (p. 1011) occurs in coal miners, sewer-workers, fish cleaners; anthrax occurs in tanners and in handlers of imported bone meal.

Residence abroad within the previous year or two raises the possibility of malaria, amoebic abscess of the liver or other exotic disease. A recent history of laparotomy or of obscure abdominal pain should suggest the possibility of subphrenic or intrahepatic abscess.

In many fevers a diagnosis beyond all reasonable doubt may be made on clinical grounds, e.g. measles, chickenpox, mumps, rheumatic fever. In others there may be doubt about the identity of the causal organism and demonstration of its presence is essential for diagnosis. Other considerations such as the tracing of a carrier may make it desirable to ascertain the precise strain of organism present.

Identification of Organisms. Infecting agents may be identified by direct examination, by culture and by animal inoculation. The following are examples.

(1) *Direct examination. Treponema pallidum* by dark ground illumination of serum from a chancre; *N. gonorrhoeae* or *N. meningitidis* by microscopical examination of pus obtained from a urethral discharge or cerebrospinal fluid respectively, stained by Gram's method; *Myco. tuberculosis* from sputum, stained by Ziehl-Neelsen's method; malaria by examination of a stained blood smear; various organisms by microscopic examination of biopsy specimens such as inclusion bodies from the vesicles of variola or varicella, *Myco. leprae* in scrapings from the nose or skin in leprosy or Leishman-Donovan bodies in the bone marrow in kala azar.

(2) *Culture. C. diphtheriae* from a throat swab, *S. typhi* from blood, *Esch. coli* from urine, *Strep. pneumoniae* from sputum, dysentery bacilli from faeces. Many viruses may be grown in tissue culture.

(3) *Animal Inoculation. Myco. tuberculosis* or *Leptospirae icterohaemorrhagiae* by inoculation of a guinea-pig.

Diagnosis of Infection by the Measurement of Specific Antibodies in the Patient's Serum. When direct evidence of an infecting agent is unobtainable, the cause of an infection may be inferred from the presence of specific antibodies in the patient's serum. Antibodies formed in response to an infection are not present in significant amounts until at least a week after the onset of symptoms. The demonstration of antibodies is often of value in establishing the diagnosis of salmonella infections, typhus, brucellosis, leptospiral infections, syphilis, glandular fever, toxoplasmosis and chronic gonococcal infections. The clinical value of the test for the individual patient is limited in viral infections by the fact that recovery has often occurred before a positive result has been obtained.

Pyrexia of Unknown Origin

Most cases of fever are due to infection and often the disease can be diagnosed by clinical examination alone. In other instances a suspected diagnosis may require confirmation by haematological examination, radiological examination, bacteriological investigation of blood or other body fluids, discharges or excreta, or detection of specific antibodies in the serum may have to be undertaken before the diagnostic problems can be solved. Occasionally the cause of a febrile illness remains uncertain in spite of such investigations and such a case is categorised as P.U.O. In order to establish the diagnosis the following measures should be undertaken:

1. Take the history again; a symptom may have been overlooked or misinterpreted or new complaints may have developed.
2. Repeat the physical examination of the patient; new signs may have appeared while others could have been missed or their significance not appreciated. The throat and ears of children in particular should be inspected again.
3. Examine the urine repeatedly for protein, white and red blood cells and micro-organisms.
4. Inspect the whole series of temperature charts from time to time for evidence of some characteristic appearance such as the undulations seen in some cases of reticulosis (Pel-Ebstein fever).
5. Review the results of laboratory investigations, thoroughly scrutinise any radiographs again and repeat such examinations as may seem necessary.

If the diagnosis is still uncertain, further tests will be required. These will be indicated by any new information obtained as a result of the clinical reassessment. It should be borne in mind that most cases of undiagnosed fever are due to some common disorder with an unusual presentation. In the absence of clues, investigations should be planned in accordance with the most probable causes of P.U.O. taking into account the age and sex of the patient and the country in which the patient lives. In Great Britain the more common causes of P.U.O. can be grouped as follows:

1. **Tumours.** Hodgkin's disease and other reticuloses especially, but also carcinoma of the lung, kidney, stomach and other sites with or without metastases.
2. **Infections.** Tuberculosis; brucellosis; subacute infective endocarditis; infections in the biliary tract; hepatic, subphrenic, abdominal, pelvic or prostatic abscess; pyelonephritis.
3. **Connective Tissue Disorders.** Disseminated lupus erythematosus; polyarteritis nodosa; giant cell arteritis; dermatomyositis.
4. **Fever due to Hypersensitivity to a Drug.** The following diagnostic investigations appropriate to these different groups may be required:

1. *Tumours.* Radiological examination of chest (P.A. and lateral) and of abdomen; pyelography; faecal occult blood tests; radiological studies of the alimentary tract; biopsy of liver, lymph nodes, bone marrow or any suspicious local lesion; laparotomy.
2. *Infections.* Blood cultures or special serological tests; skin sensitivity tests; abdominal radiography in the erect and recumbent position; pyelography, cholecystography, cholangiography; biopsy of liver.
3. *Connective Tissue Disorders.* Blood examination for L.E. cells; total eosinophil count; serum protein electrophoresis; rheumatoid and antinuclear factors in serum; biopsy of superficial arteries, skin, muscle, kidney.

Having decided on the most hopeful line of investigation, it is a good policy to start with the simplest and least hazardous test. By reviewing the probabilities in the light of previous examinations and directing further investigations accordingly, the patient will be spared as far as possible the discomfort and dangers of unnecessary procedures.

Mysterious fevers, particularly in patients who have some knowledge of medicine or nursing, may be due to deceit. Doubts should be raised if the skin of a supposedly febrile patient does not feel hot or if the general health does not deteriorate in spite of persistent fever. The occurrence of some bizarre symptom or sign may arouse suspicion that the temperature is being falsified. There are both subtle and simple techniques for doing this. The latter include holding the thermometer close to a hot water bottle or other source of heat, dipping it into a hot drink, applying friction to the bulb, or shaking it in a retrograde manner.

If the diagnosis remains obscure another opinion should be obtained from an experienced physician, as reconsideration of the evidence by an unbiased observer may throw new light on the position.

When a diagnosis still cannot be established and the patient's condition is deteriorating, various remedies, e.g. antibiotics, may be tried empirically in the hope of influencing the course of the disease. A therapeutic trial should not be regarded as a satisfactory diagnostic test.

Treatment

1. GENERAL. *Rest.* The patient should be put to rest in bed and protected from cold in a well-ventilated room. Attention to detail makes for the greater comfort and well-being of the patient. The practitioner should be satisfied that the position of the light is suitable for reading, and as soon as the patient is fit enough, books, magazines, handwork and a wireless or television set should be provided. The room should be kept clean and tidy and if possible brightened by pictures or some fresh flowers.

It is the doctor's duty also to satisfy himself that due attention is being given to special points in nursing:—adequate washing and changing of linen; tepid sponging for the relief of high fever; care of the mouth and the prevention of suppurative parotitis; care of the skin and the prevention of bedsores over pressure points; the prevention of the spread of infection and the disposal of infected excreta.

Fluid. Fluid intake sufficient to give a urinary output of at least 1,500 ml. daily should be ensured. Patients left to themselves may be too ill, weak or apathetic to drink even average quantities; yet a greater fluid intake is desirable since sweating increases extra-renal water loss, and the raised metabolic rate of fever requires a higher urinary output than normal to excrete the waste products of catabolism.

Food. Patients may be allowed whatever they fancy, but in a thin patient it is important to maintain a high caloric intake to prevent wasting, especially if the illness is likely to be prolonged. Anorexia is a feature of most infections and so it is usually wise to advise a light diet (Diet No. 1, p. 1284).

Sleep. Insomnia should be prevented by ensuring that the bedclothes are comfortably straightened and by giving a hot drink or two tablets of aspirin last thing at night. When necessary, hypnotics such as chloral hydrate or barbiturates may be administered. It should be borne in mind that if cough or pain is responsible for sleeplessness, suitable symptomatic measures must be taken.

2. Symptomatic. Symptoms requiring special treatment must be considered for each individual case. Pain may be eased by the application of a counterirritant such as heat, by the use of analgesics such as aspirin, phenacetin and codeine or if necessary by morphine. Cough may require linctus methadone (N.F.) for its relief, particularly at night. Itching, sweating, constipation or diarrhoea may also require attention.

3. Chemotherapy. See Chapter 3.

4. Use of Specific Antisera. Theoretically the toxaemia of an infectious disease should be neutralised by injecting a suitable antiserum. In practice this has been found to be successful in only a limited number of infections. Antisera are of value in those diseases in which an exotoxin is present, e.g. in diphtheria, tetanus, gas gangrene and botulism. With the advent of sulphonamides and the antibiotics, other antibacterial sera are no longer used, but with the emergence of drug resistant strains, it is possible that antisera or immunoglobulin may once again prove to be of value.

Prognosis in Infections. Some diseases have shown a spontaneous decline in severity within living memory, e.g. scarlet fever. Infections also vary in their intensity from one epidemic to another, depending upon the resistance of the population at risk, the virulence of the parasite and the presence of secondary invaders, e.g. the 1918-19 influenza pandemic destroyed more lives in a few months than did the First World War in four years.

The prognosis of infections due to bacteria, spirochaetes and protozoa has also been entirely changed by the discovery of curative drugs. The outlook depends largely upon giving the right drug in adequate dosage and at the earliest possible stage of the illness. In contrast the prognosis of viral infections has been little altered by the introduction of antibiotics apart from the benefits which may be derived from the treatment of secondary bacterial infections.

However, there are some recent instances of specific antiviral chemotherapy. The local application of IUDR (5-iodo-2′-deoxyuridine) is effective in the treatment of herpetic ulcers of the cornea. N-methylisatin β-thiosemicarbazone (Methisazone) has been shown to prevent the development of smallpox in close contacts.

ALLERGY

By means of the defence mechanisms mentioned above, a state of immunity or complete insensitivity to reinfection develops at least temporarily. Sometimes however renewed exposure causes a reaction which is totally different from that occurring in a primary infection. The word 'allergy' (altered reaction) was coined by von Pirquet in 1906 to denote this different reaction, based especially upon the changes in the degree of skin sensitivity to tuberculin which he observed during the various phases of tuberculosis. In the previously uninfected person there is no skin reaction to tuberculin, but two or more weeks after infection by tubercle bacilli or the inoculation of BCG (p. 431), the Mantoux test becomes positive. In other words everyone infected by tuberculosis becomes allergic to tuberculin. This altered reaction is correlated in man with a greatly increased resistance to infection, while in reinfected animals it has been shown that the dissemination of tubercle bacilli from a site of inoculation is much delayed. Although the development of an inflammatory reaction in response to the injection of a substance which has no effect upon a normal person can scarcely be claimed as an advantage, on the whole the assets of allergy in tuberculosis appear to exceed the liabilities. The conflict between the protective power of immunity and the potentially damaging effect of the closely related sensitivity led to the introduction of the term 'allergy' for the latter. In the allergic disorders on the other hand, tissue damage is entirely the result of sensitisation. This is not necessarily due to bacteria; in fact sensitisation to many chemical substances of varying complexity is even more common. Moreover, only a minority of persons become allergic to such substances in spite of repeated exposure. For example few of those who inhale pollen spores during the appropriate season develop hay fever. This difference may depend upon whether or not the antigen can penetrate the first line of defence.

The nature of allergic reactions is not fully understood, but their development appears to be due to an imperfection in the mechanism of immunity; the fundamental process involves a combination of antigen with specific antibody on or within tissue cells. The passive transfer test (Prausnitz-Küstner or P.K. reaction) provides an illustration of this process. Antibodies can be demonstrated by injecting a small amount of the allergic patient's serum into the skin of a non-sensitive person; after an interval of at least 24 hours the causative antigen is injected into the same site and an urticarial reaction appears immediately. In contrast, no such reaction occurs if the antigen is injected into adjacent skin. This effect was first demonstrated in 1921 when Dr. Küstner who was allergic to cooked fish, conferred his sensitivity upon a small test area of the skin of Dr. Prausnitz who was not allergic to fish. The P.K. reaction is positive in diseases presenting with the immediate types of allergy like urticaria or hay fever in which the response appears within minutes of exposure to the allergen. It is negative in delayed types of allergy like the tuberculin reaction in which passive transfer can only be effected by cells or cell extracts.

Recent work in clarifying the roles of the different immunoglobulins in immunity and allergy has shown that these proteins comprise three main groups which are classified in ascending order of molecular size as follows: Ig G or γ G is produced by plasma cells and is concerned with resistance to infection; it is transferred across the placenta and is responsible for the immunity of the baby during the first few months of life. Ig A or γ A is produced by plasma cells and is found in tears, saliva and intestinal secretions in addition to the serum; it is probably important as a protective antibody.

Ig M or γ M is produced by specialised lymphocytes and is concerned in the Wassermann and other heterophile antibody reactions; it forms the specific antibody in response to the injection of typhoid O antigen and is responsible for cold agglutinins. Additional subtypes of immunoglobulins are being defined.

Allergic reactions cause cell damage. The antigen-antibody reaction of normal immunity produces no such effect. The abnormality may lie in a congenital defect in the tissues concerned (since allergy is frequently inherited), or to aberrant antibody production. The features of the allergic reaction are largely due to the release locally or into the blood stream of one or more of several pharmacologically active substances.

A single allergen may cause reactions at several sites; thus a patient allergic to egg protein may suffer a local reaction in the gut and also an attack of asthma or urticaria when the absorbed allergen is carried by the blood to the lungs and skin. Ingested proteins do not usually enter the blood stream unchanged, for they are normally split in the gut into their component polypeptides and amino acids which after absorption have no allergenic properties. But sometimes small amounts of protein may be absorbed unchanged; allergic manifestations may then occur.

The routes by which inanimate allergens may reach the patient's tissues are similar to those described for infections. These are through the skin (contact dermatitis), by ingestion (food allergy, p. 980), by inhalation (asthma, p. 340) or by inoculation (insect bites, serum sickness). The resulting reactions may appear as a skin eruption (urticaria, eczema, angioneurotic oedema), as abdominal symptoms (vomiting, diarrhoea, abdominal colic), or commonly as respiratory symptoms (hay fever, bronchial asthma).

Allergic diseases may be acute, e.g. angioneurotic oedema, or chronic, e.g. eczema; they may be trivial as in mild urticaria due to eating strawberries or so serious as to result in sudden death (anaphylactic shock p. 26). The mechanism underlying this severe form is illustrated by the following experiment. A guinea-pig is made sensitive to the serum of another animal by the injection of a single minute dose of the serum. This produces a specific antibody but on an inadequate scale. After an interval of at least 10 days, a second but larger dose of the serum is given, which results in profound and often fatal collapse of the animal. Repeated daily injections have no such effect. Anaphylaxis in man occurs soon after the injection of antiserum or a drug to which sensitivity has developed in consequence of previous treatment.

Clinical disorders due to allergy are extremely common and at least 1 in 10 persons in Britain suffers at some time from asthma, vasomotor rhinorrhoea, eczema, angioneurotic oedema, urticaria or intestinal allergy. These apparently dissimilar conditions have many points in common. Thus there is a strong hereditary tendency and a frequent coincidence of two or more of these reactions in the same patient. The basic causes, appropriate lines of investigation, the pathology, treatment and prognosis are all very similar. The average clinical course is of long periods of normal health interrupted by occasional or frequent acute relapses. The attacks may be precipitated by one or more exogenous factors and it is well recognised that emotion and nervous tension may augment the tendency to an allergic state. Though the exogenous allergens are often proteins, other substances, including many drugs become antigenic by linking with body proteins.

It has for a long time been known that in acute allergic disorders a histamine-like substance is released as a result of contact between allergen and antibody located within or on sensitised tissue cells. It is now recognised not only that histamine itself is released, but that several other substances such as acetylcholine, 5-hydroxytryptamine (5-HT), SRS-A (the slow reacting substance of anaphylaxis) and bradykinin are also sometimes concerned. In this connection it is worthy of note that the juice of the stinging nettle (*Urtica dioica*), from which is derived the name urticaria, contains histamine, 5-HT and acetylcholine. It is also known that histamine is released by pressure on the skin in dermatographia, that 5-HT is secreted by the tumours in the carcinoid syndrome in which asthma may be a feature, and that acetylcholine liberated at the autonomic nerve endings is a link between the mind and the skin lesions in patients subject to emotionally induced urticaria. Furthermore urticaria may result from other physical factors such as heat, cold and light. It is apparent from these illustrations that syndromes occur which are clinically identical with familiar allergic disorders, but which do not appear to require the interaction of antigen and antibody for their production. Urticaria is of course also commonly due to allergy to food or drugs and an allergen can sometimes be incriminated as a cause of bronchial asthma. Intermediary effector substances also are involved; histamine is concerned with both types of reaction while in asthma it has been demonstrated that SRS-A is released when antigen and antibody come into contact in the bronchial tree and is important as a cause of bronchial constriction.

The pathology of the allergic diseases is closely allied to acute and chronic inflammatory reactions. In the immediate or acute reacting types of allergy which have just been discussed from the point of view of pathogenesis, there is capillary dilatation, increased capillary permeability and oedema, surrounded by erythema due to reflex arteriolar dilatation. Hypersecretion occurs when mucous membranes are involved, and smooth muscle of the bronchi and gut contracts when the respiratory and alimentary systems are affected. The appearance of eosinophil cells, both locally and in increased numbers in the blood stream is a characteristic feature commonly present in the immediate types of allergy and seldom seen in other disorders. If an explanation for the presence of these cells could be provided, it might prove a valuable clue to the better understanding of these diseases, but at present the function of the eosinophil cell is uncertain.

Treatment of individual allergic disorders is dealt with in the appropriate chapters of this book. The value of some of the measures is however relevant to the present discussion of the allergic state.

Antihistamines are commonly effective in urticaria and hay fever, but are of little use in eczema or bronchial asthma. One of the reasons for the latter is the presence of SRS-A, but it is also known from *in vitro* experiments on human bronchi that a very much higher concentration of mepyramine maleate is required to inhibit the histamine released by an allergic reaction compared with a similar amount of histamine applied externally. This unfortunate fact is not perhaps so remarkable as the failure of antihistamines to affect the stimulation of acid gastric secretion by subcutaneously injected histamine (p. 897).

Vasoconstrictor substances, particularly adrenaline and isoprenaline, are of great value in the emergency treatment of urticaria and may be life saving in their effect upon angioneurotic oedema and bronchial asthma.

Aminophylline is especially valuable in relaxing bronchospasm Neither aminophylline nor adrenaline will relieve the distress of asthma when plugging of the bronchi by viscid mucus is the main causes of the dyspnoea.

Adrenocorticosteroids are of particular value in asthma and eczema, but have little or no effect on urticaria and angioneurotic oedema. Owing to their undesirable and even dangerous side-effects, their use should be restricted to patients in whom all other measures have failed.

Salicylates have a place as inhibitors of the inflammatory reaction (e.g. rheumatic fever) and it is of interest also that aspirin specifically antagonises the bronchoconstrictor action of bradykinin in the guinea-pig. Salicylates may however precipitate attacks of urticaria or bronchial asthma in some patients.

It is important to remember that aggravating factors such as infection and states of emotional tension often require treatment. The abnormal condition of the skin in eczema and of the nasal or bronchial mucosa in allergy of the respiratory tract predisposes to secondary infection. In bronchial asthma in particular it is agreed by most clinicians, and indeed volunteered by many of the patients, that worry, anxiety, excitement or other psychological factors may precipitate attacks. The means by which the state of mind can influence the physical condition of the bronchial tree is a problem yet to be solved, but it is encouraging that the mechanism of one type of emotionally induced urticaria is at least partly understood (cholinergic urticaria, p. 23).

Prevention and control of the allergic state should be attempted by identifying the allergen so that the patient may, if possible, avoid coming into contact with it. Unfortunately in asthma and food allergy it is often impossible to recognise the allergen and desensitisation is rarely so successful. If the cause cannot be found or contact with it is unavoidable, then symptomatic treatment with the drugs already mentioned must be employed. When the allergen is known, as in hay fever, and symptomatic treatment is not satisfactory, then a long course of subcutaneous injections of increasing doses of the specific pollen may be given. This results in a high titre of serum antibodies which block the access of the natural allergen to the sensitised cells. Alternatively two or three injections of depot vaccine, freshly prepared, may be given annually for the prevention of hay fever. For this purpose an active emulsion of pollens is injected from a specially designed syringe in such a way that the pollen is positioned in the middle of a quantity of inactive emulsion which comprises the first part of the injection.

There are many other diseases in which allergy may be implicated, but they show little or no clinical affinity with the group mentioned above. Examples are rheumatoid disease, bacterial allergy represented by acute nephritis and rheumatic fever, and rare disorders such as haemolytic anaemia.

Anaphylactic Shock

The clinical features vary with different animal species. In man there is usually sudden severe and sometimes fatal circulatory collapse. The hypotension may be accompanied by giant urticaria and acute bronchial asthma.

Treatment. Urgent measures are required to prevent death. The patient should be laid down with the feet raised. Clothing at the neck should be loosened and a free airway ensured, and if the heart has stopped beating, cardiopulmonary resuscitation (p. 180) must be started immediately. An injection of 1·0 ml. adrenaline, 1 : 1000 solution, should be given intramuscularly, but if the sensitising substance has been injected subcutaneously or intramuscularly then the adrenaline solution should be injected into the same site. Mepyramine maleate 50 mg. and hydrocortisone hemisuccinate 100 mg. should be given intravenously at once, and repeated after quarter of an hour if necessary. Severe hypotension and shock should be treated with noradrenaline or metaraminol (p. 222).

E. B. French.

Books recommended:

Burnet, Sir Macfarlane (1962). *The Natural History of Infectious Disease*, 3rd ed. London: Cambridge University Press.

Gell, P. G. H. & Coombs, R. R. A. (1963). *Clinical Aspects of Immunology*. Oxford: Blackwell.

INFECTIOUS DISEASES

(*Contagious or Communicable Diseases*)

DISEASES due to infection are of great importance because of their prevalence throughout the world. This is especially the case in tropical countries where insect-borne diseases are common and in underdeveloped communities with low standards of hygiene and nutrition. Although their incidence and ill-effects have been markedly decreased over the last half-century by efficient public health measures and, more recently, by the development of specific methods of treatment, infections are still a major cause of time lost at school and at work.

The wide range of diseases due to infection is indicated by considering the main groups of organisms responsible—bacteria, spirochaetes, fungi, protozoa, metazoa, rickettsiae and viruses, in all of which great strides have been made in prevention. The bacteria may be subdivided into two main categories according to their staining properties, gram-positive and gram-negative. Examples of the former are pneumococci, streptococci, staphylococci, diphtheria bacilli and the clostridia. Tubercle bacilli, though weakly gram-positive, are better demonstrated by the Ziehl-Neelsen method. Examples of gram-negative bacteria are the neisseriae causing meningococcal meningitis and gonorrhoea, the haemophili causing respiratory infections, the brucellae causing undulant fever and the intestinal bacilli causing such diseases as typhoid fever, bacillary dysentery and urinary tract infections. Syphilis, Weil's disease and yaws are important examples of spirochaetal infections, and ringworm and thrush of fungal infections. Diseases due to protozoa, metazoa and rickettsiae are mainly encountered in the tropics; thus protozoa cause malaria, amoebic dysentery, sleeping sickness and kala azar; metazoal diseases include helminthic infections with roundworms, tapeworms, and flukes. The rickettsiae are intermediate in character between bacteria and viruses and when transmitted to man the most important disease they cause is typhus fever. Most of these infections can now be successfully treated by chemotherapy, whereas, in striking contrast, effective specific therapeutic measures are not yet available for diseases caused by viruses. Important examples of the latter are chickenpox, smallpox, mumps, measles and German measles; respiratory illness such as the common cold, pharyngitis and influenza; diseases of the nervous system such as poliomyelitis, choriomeningitis and herpes zoster; and liver disorders such as infective hepatitis and yellow fever. The problem of chemotherapy is to kill the virus without damaging the host cell on which it is so intimately dependent. The prevention of viral diseases by the use of prophylactic vaccines, which has been employed for over 150 years in the case of smallpox, has also been successfully accomplished in rabies, yellow fever, poliomyelitis and measles. Several viral infections may be prevented temporarily by passive immunisation. Control over viral infections is in fact comparable to the position of bacterial infection prior to the revolution in chemotherapy which began with the introduction of sulphonamides in 1935.

Although it is generally agreed that there is no sharp dividing line between 'infectious' and 'infective' disease, it is customary to use the former term with the restricted meaning of indicating only those highly communicable or contagious diseases which are preferably not treated in the wards of a general hospital but in a special hospital, 'The Infectious Diseases Hospital', or at home if the patient can be effectively isolated and given adequate medical and nursing care. Because of the ease with which these diseases are transmitted a knowledge of their incubation periods is of importance to practitioners who have the responsibility of supervising contacts. The incubation period may be short (1-7 days) as in diphtheritic, streptococcal and staphylococcal infections, of medium duration (7-14 days) as in typhoid fever, measles, smallpox and whooping-cough, or long (14-21 days) as in chickenpox, German measles and mumps. Some common or important infective diseases are described in this chapter, while others involving one system predominantly, and diseases of the tropics are dealt with elsewhere in this book.

TYPHOID AND PARATYPHOID FEVERS

(*The Enteric Fevers*)

In many countries where sanitation is primitive, enteric fevers are an important cause of illness. In Britain and other highly developed countries they are relatively rare. Nevertheless comparatively recent outbreaks of typhoid fever in Zermatt and in Aberdeen clearly indicate the need for students and doctors to appreciate the importance of early diagnosis and effective control of the enteric fevers. In addition the decision to describe typhoid fever in considerable detail is based on the belief that this disease exemplifies many features of great educational interest. It illustrates the diagnostic value of the temperature chart, of comparing the pulse rate with the temperature, of doing a leucocyte count and of taking blood for culture early in the course of an undiagnosed fever. It indicates the importance of searching for enlargement of the spleen when septicaemia is suspected, and of recognising the appearance of rashes and knowing about their location and duration. It also shows how a knowledge of pathology will enable the doctor to appreciate the nature and time of onset of complications.

Finally, typhoid fever illustrates excellently the important part played by modern sanitation in reducing the incidence of disease and the prophylactic value of active immunisation by vaccines.

Aetiology. Typhoid and paratyphoid fever are diseases with a world-wide distribution which occur endemically wherever sanitation is poor and the water supply is liable to be contaminated by human excreta. In such regions flies may also transmit the disease. In Britain, where the water supply is generally satisfactory, it is usually spread by carriers through the contamination of food, milk or water; infected shell fish are occasionally responsible for an outbreak. The bacilli may live in the gall-bladder for months or years after clinical recovery and pass intermittently in the stools. They belong to the Salmonella group of bacteria; *S. typhi* and *S. paratyphi B* are the organisms encountered in Britain.

In the initial stage there is a septicaemia, which explains the non-specific symptoms at the outset and the great variety of complications. After a few days the organisms become localised mainly in the lymphoid tissue of the small intestine. The typical lesion is in the Peyer's patches which become swollen and may ulcerate. The ulcers may heal, or they may perforate or bleed. The neighbouring lymph nodes become inflamed and the spleen commonly shows enlargement.

The incubation period of typhoid fever is usually about 10-14 days; that of paratyphoid is somewhat shorter. The diseases are notifiable. Quarantine is not necessary, but contacts are kept under surveillance for three weeks.

Clinical Features. (1) *Typhoid Fever.* The onset of typhoid fever is insidious and often the patient may walk about for three or four days before being forced to take to bed. The temperature rises in a step-ladder fashion over the first four or five days, being higher at night than in the morning. During this time there is a vague feeling of malaise, with increasing headache, drowsiness and aching in the limbs. There may be some cough and epistaxis is not uncommon; constipation is usually present. The pulse is often slower than would be expected from the height of the temperature. A leucopenia is a highly characteristic finding. At the end of the first week the typical rash may appear on the upper abdomen and on the back as sparse slightly raised, rose-red spots which fade on pressure. After two or three days they disappear, to be succeeded sometimes by fresh crops of spots. About the 7th to 10th day of illness the spleen becomes palpable. It is soft and seldom extends more than one or two finger breadths below the costal margin. Often about this time constipation is succeeded by looseness of the stools (pea-soup stools), and abdominal distension and tenderness in the right iliac fossa is noted. Bronchitis may develop and there may be some delirium. By the end of the second week the patient may be profoundly ill unless the disease is modified by antibiotic treatment. In the third week the patient becomes increasingly ill from toxaemia and may pass into coma and die. The prognosis may also suddenly become more grave at this stage due to haemorrhage from or perforation of the ulcerated Peyer's patches. In those who recover the temperature falls by lysis, the appetite returns, distension disappears, and strength improves. After an initial recovery a recrudescence of the disease may occur. Many of the points mentioned above are illustrated in the accompanying chart (Fig. 1).

(2) *Paratyphoid Fever.* The most common variety in Britain is due to *S. paratyphi B.* The course tends to be shorter and milder than that of typhoid fever but the onset is often more abrupt with acute enteritis. The rash may be more abundant and the intestinal complications less frequent.

Complications of the Enteric Fevers. The dangerous complications of typhoid and paratyphoid fevers are those of haemorrhage and perforation which occur at the end of the second week or during the third week of the illness. The bleeding may be sudden and very severe. The features of shock suggesting that a haemorrhage has occurred are described on p. 910. Perforation usually occurs from ulcers near the ileo-caecal valve. The features of perforation in typhoid fever do not differ from those of a

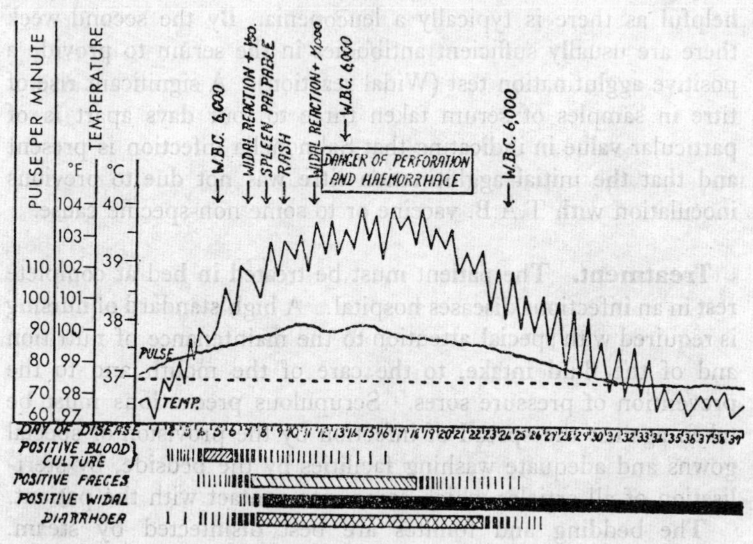

CHART ILLUSTRATING THE TYPICAL FEATURES IN A SEVERE CASE OF TYPHOID FEVER AS SEEN PRIOR TO THE INTRODUCTION OF CHLORAMPHENICOL THERAPY.

FIG. 1

perforated peptic ulcer in regard to suddenness of onset or the general symptoms of peritonitis, except that shoulder-tip pain is uncommon and insufficient gas escapes into the peritoneal cavity to cause obliteration of liver dullness. Apart from these two main complications, almost any viscus or system can become involved as a result of the septicaemia which is present during the first week of the illness. Pneumonia, thrombophlebitis, myocarditis, myositis, arthritis, periostitis, osteomyelitis, meningitis and cholecystitis are all recognised complications.

Diagnosis. In the first week of the disease the diagnosis may be very difficult as in this invasive stage of septicaemia the symptoms are those of a generalised infection without localising features. In a suspected case, blood should always be taken for culture. This is by far the most important diagnostic method, particularly during the first week of the disease. During this period the organism may or may not be grown from the stool or urine using selective media. These excreta become more heavily infected during the second and third weeks. A white blood count may be helpful as there is typically a leucopenia. By the second week there are usually sufficient antibodies in the serum to provide a positive agglutination test (Widal reaction). A significant rise of titre in samples of serum taken three to four days apart is of particular value in indicating that Salmonella infection is present and that the initial agglutination titre was not due to previous inoculation with T.A.B. vaccine or to some non-specific cause.

Treatment. The patient must be treated in bed at complete rest in an infectious diseases hospital. A high standard of nursing is required with special attention to the maintenance of nutrition and of the fluid intake, to the care of the mouth and to the prevention of pressure sores. Scrupulous precautions must be taken against the spread of infection by the provision of special gowns and adequate washing facilities by the bedside, by sterilisation of all articles which come into contact with the patient.

The bedding and fomites are best disinfected by steam. Faeces and urine can be disposed of directly into a water closet when a modern sewage disposal system is in operation.

Chloramphenicol (p. 81) has completely altered the prognosis in typhoid fever. There is usually a dramatic improvement about 48 hours after chloramphenicol has been administered. The dose for an adult is 2 g. daily for a fortnight. Ampicillin (p. 73) is also effective in typhoid fever but chloramphenicol is to be preferred for the treatment of the acute infection. Even with effective chemotherapy there is still a danger of complications, of recrudescence of the disease and of the development of a carrier state. For at least three weeks the patient must be kept under careful supervision while healing of the bowel takes place. For the first few days a semi-fluid diet should be given (Diet 1, p. 1284), followed by the low roughage diet, Diet 2. A second course of chemotherapy must be given in the event of a relapse and it usually produces good results. The chronic carrier should be treated with ampicillin for at least a month, as chloramphenicol has proved ineffective in these circumstances and its prolonged use is undesirable. In some cases cholecystectomy may be necessary. The treatment of haemorrhage is described on p. 911. Prior to the introduction of chloramphenicol the treatment of perforation was by immediate recourse to surgery, which carried a high mortality in the seriously ill. Such patients can be treated conservatively while chloramphenicol is continued, but advice from a surgeon should be sought. The patient should be considered as infective until six consecutive stools are found to be negative on bacteriological examination.

Prophylaxis. Those who propose to travel or live in countries where enteric infections are endemic should be inoculated with T.A.B., a vaccine composed of killed *S. typhi* and *paratyphi A* and *B* which provides a considerable degree of immunity for approximately two years. An intradermal injection of 0·2 ml. is given and repeated 10 days later. There is practically no general reaction and less local reaction than with subcutaneous administration.

DIPHTHERIA

By 1946 diphtheria, which was formerly a common and lethal disease in Britain, became so rare as a result of prophylactic inoculation that many doctors have never seen a case. In 1936 there were 397 deaths from this cause in Scotland, whereas in 1963 there was not even a single case of diphtheria. In many parts of Asia and Africa diphtheria is still an important cause of illness. It is essential that doctors should press for prophylactic inoculation, for complacency due to the virtual disappearance of diphtheria is resulting in a falling rate of immunisation, and the disease has reappeared in small epidemics. Both for practical reasons and as an illustration of some general principles, this disease is described at considerable length. The immediate treatment of the disease is of such vital importance to the patient that the doctor must always bear the condition in mind when examining a patient who complains of a sore throat. A description of the local lesion provides an opportunity for a discussion of the differential diagnosis of conditions causing a sore throat. In addition diphtheria, being an example of disease caused through the absorption of toxin from a localised infection, illustrates the use of modified toxin (toxoid) as an antigen, and the value of antitoxin and the dangers of injecting horse serum for treatment.

Infection with *Corynebacterium diphtheriae* occurs most commonly in the upper respiratory tract and sore throat is frequently the presenting feature. The disease is usually spread by droplet infection from cases or carriers. The organisms remain localised at the site of infection and the serious consequences result from the absorption of a soluble exotoxin which damages the heart muscle and the nervous system. The mortality in an epidemic is proportional to the virulence of the infecting organism, which varies greatly from strain to strain. Sometimes culture of a throat swab yields organisms which are morphologically and culturally identical with *C. diphtheriae* and yet are found to be avirulent on guinea-pig inoculation. Persons susceptible to diphtheria can be detected by the appearance of an inflammatory reaction in response to the intradermal injection of 0·2 ml. of standard toxin. This is the Schick test and the result should be read after five to seven days.

The infection may occur rarely on the conjunctiva or the genital tract, or it may complicate wounds, abrasions or diseases of the skin. For example, it was a relatively frequent complication of sores during the Second World War in the Near and Far East.

The disease is notifiable. The average incubation period is two to four days. Quarantine is not necessary. Cases are isolated until clinical recovery is complete and until cultures from three consecutive nose and throat swabs, taken at intervals of not less than two days, are negative.

Clinical Features. The tonsils and the fauces are most often the site of the infection, and next in frequency is the nose. Occasionally the pharynx, larynx or trachea are affected without obvious infection of the fauces. The onset is gradual over one or two days, with malaise, headache, anorexia, mild pyrexia and sore throat. In some cases the sore throat may be inconspicuous. The diagnostic feature is the pearl-grey elevated membrane of variable extent with a well-defined edge and surrounded by a zone of inflammation. The membrane is comparatively firm and is adherent. It can be swabbed off only with difficulty in contrast to the ease with which the purulent exudate of streptococcal tonsillitis can be removed. On occasion the membrane may be dirty-grey or even black due to admixture with blood. There may be swelling of the neck and tender enlargement of the lymph nodes. In the mildest infections, especially in the presence of a high degree of immunity, membrane may never appear and the fauces are merely slightly injected. In these circumstances, diagnosis cannot be made clinically but depends upon obtaining a positive culture from a throat swab. Anterior nasal diphtheria is invariably mild, but the disease is important from the point of view of the spread of infection. The chief feature is nasal discharge, which is thin and serous at first, but is frequently blood-stained. A similar discharge may result from the presence of a foreign body in the nose.

In addition to the local signs, tachycardia develops in association with a soft compressible pulse, the blood pressure falls and the heart sounds become faint. The gravity of the prognosis is proportional to the extent of these changes. Sudden heart failure is responsible for most of the fatalities, and it is associated with degenerative changes in the myocardium which result from the action of diphtheritic toxin. There is no permanent damage to the heart.

Involvement of the nervous system sometimes occurs, and after faucial diphtheria it usually commences with palatal palsy on about the tenth day of the illness. The voice assumes a nasal quality, while regurgitation of fluids through the nose and sluggishness of palatal movements may be observed. Paralysis of accommodation soon follows and may be inferred from the patient's complaint of difficulty in reading small print. Such paralysis may occur irrespective of the site of infection. In myopes it may pass unnoticed.

A week or two later, though somewhat rarely, the symptoms and signs of multiple neuritis may develop. Recovery from such neuritis is always ultimately complete. In exceptional cases paralysis of the diaphragm and respiratory muscles may necessitate the use of a mechanical respirator.

Complications. In addition to the cardiac and neurological complications, mention must be made of diphtheritic involvement of the larynx which may result in stridor or in respiratory obstruction. The latter is more frequent at an age when the air passages are small, and immediate tracheostomy may be necessary. Occasionally bronchopneumonia or pulmonary collapse may result from the inhalation of membrane which has become detached.

Diagnosis. It must be emphasised that the clinical diagnosis in many cases of diphtheria may present considerable difficulties owing to the mildness of the disease resulting from the immunisation of a high proportion of the population. The disease must be considered in the differential diagnosis of any condition giving rise to sore throat and more especially if in addition there is a membrane, exudate or deposit on the mucous membranes of the throat and nose. The following conditions should be borne in mind:

(1) *Streptococcal tonsillitis*, in which the onset is abrupt and the initial constitutional disturbance often severe. There is widespread inflammation of the throat, whereas the exudate, usually follicular but occasionally confluent, is always limited to the tonsils. It is yellowish-white in colour and is easily wiped off with a swab. *Strep. pyogenes* may be isolated on culture.

(2) *Vincent's angina*, in which an ulceromembranous lesion, often spreading from the gums, is present. The breath smells more unpleasant than in diphtheria. Constitutional disturbance is absent or slight, there is often a coincidental painful marginal gingivitis and the presence of spirochaetes and fusiform bacilli may be demonstrated in a stained smear.

(3) *Glandular fever* is frequently associated with an inflamed throat accompanied by exudate. The lymph nodes in many situations are often moderately enlarged, and the spleen may be palpable. Sooner or later the characteristic blood changes appear, and the Paul-Bunnell test may become positive (p. 646).

(4) *Agranulocytosis*, *aplastic anaemia* or *acute leukaemia*, in any of which ulceration may occur in the throat, can be diagnosed by the characteristic blood changes (pp. 643, 638, 647).

(5) *Thrush*, due to infection by the fungus, *Candida albicans*, gives rise to white deposits adherent to the buccal mucosa, palate and tonsils. There is little inflammation surrounding the lesions. When the disease is extensive and some of the patches are confluent, it may be distinguished from diphtheria by the white colour, by the presence of multiple outlying patches which resemble milk curds, and by the absence of cervical lymphadenitis or constitutional disturbance. Microscopic examination shows

the presence of budding yeast-like growths and mycelial threads.

Treatment. Upon making a clinical diagnosis of diphtheria, the case should be notified to the Medical Officer of Health and sent urgently to a hospital for infectious diseases. If immediate hospital admission is impracticable or delayed, refined antitoxic serum should be injected intramuscularly without awaiting the bacteriological report on a throat swab. Every moment of delay increases the danger to the patient, because toxin, once fixed to the tissues, can no longer be neutralised by antitoxin. However, horse serum, in which antitoxin is contained, being a foreign protein, is liable to cause undesirable reactions. Firstly, there may be an immediate anaphylactic reaction with dyspnoea, pallor and collapse or even death. Secondly, after 7-12 days so-called serum sickness, with fever, urticaria and joint pains may occur, as a rule in the absence of any previous history of inoculation of horse serum. If there is such a history, the symptoms commonly appear earlier, i.e. in three or four days. As anaphylaxis is potentially lethal, two questions must be asked before an injection of horse serum is given to any patient for any purpose:

1. Has the patient ever received horse serum before?
2. Is there any personal or family history of asthma, hay fever, infantile eczema or food allergy?

If the answer to both questions is 'No' the full dose of antitoxin may be given intramuscularly (I.M.) and the patient observed for half an hour. There is no danger of anaphylaxis after this period.

If the answer to question 1 is 'Yes' then a trial dose of 0·2 ml. of serum is injected subcutaneously and the patient observed for half an hour and then the full dose given I.M. If a mild reaction occurs after the test dose, 0·2 ml. should be given subcutaneously at half-hourly intervals until the whole dose has been given. In the event of a more severe reaction a smaller dose should be given and preceded by an intramuscular injection of 50 mg. of mepyramine maleate.

If the answer to question 2 is 'Yes' *special care* must be taken. A dose of 0·2 ml. of serum diluted 1 : 10 is injected subcutaneously. If no reaction occurs after half an hour, 0·2 ml. of undiluted serum is given. In the absence of a reaction during the next half-hour, the full dose may be given I.M. When a reaction does occur after either test dose in an allergic subject, rapid desensitisation must be undertaken with extreme caution. In all cases a sterile syringe and an effective (i.e. colourless) solution of adrenaline must be close at hand to deal with any immediate type of reaction. The treatment of anaphylactic shock is discussed on p. 26.

In a very severe case the risk of anaphylactic shock is outweighed by the mortal danger of diphtheritic toxaemia and up to 100,000 units of antitoxin should be injected intravenously if the test dose has given rise to no symptoms. For cases of moderate severity 16,000-32,000 units I.M. will suffice, and for mild cases 4,000-8,000 units. After the use of horse serum, active immunisation against tetanus should be given for the reasons stated on page 11.

Phenoxymethylpenicillin or erythromycin should be administered for five days to eliminate *C. diphtheriae*.

Complete rest is essential for at least three weeks owing to the danger of cardiac and circulatory failure. This period must be lengthened if there is evidence of myocardial involvement. After a moderate attack, judged by the clinical state, the patient may be fit for discharge in six or seven weeks. After severe attacks, patients may not be fit for three months, while those who have had polyneuritis may take six to nine months to recover.

Prophylaxis. The liability of allergic subjects to a severe reaction emphasises the great importance of recommending active immunisation at an early age against both diphtheria and tetanus. Active immunisation should be given in accordance with the instructions on p. 11.

If a case of diphtheria occurs in a closed community, such as a school, a daily examination of the throat of all contacts should be made during the incubation period and swabs taken for the detection of carriers and potential cases. Those with positive throat swabs or with the slightest suspicion of clinical diphtheria should be isolated and given penicillin and an intramuscular injection of 2,000 units of antitoxin. All contacts should also be advised to have a booster dose of toxoid or active immunisation, depending on the history of previous inoculations.

Cases, convalescents and healthy carriers are isolated until three successive throat swabs taken at intervals of not less than two days are negative on culture.

SCARLET FEVER
(*Scarlatina*)

Haemolytic streptococcal infection in man results in features which vary with the invasiveness of the organism, with its capacity to produce toxins causing systemic and other effects, with the site of infection and with the reaction of the host to the infection. If the resistance to infection is low and the invasive properties of the haemolytic streptococcus high a rapidly spreading erysipelas, cellulitis or septicaemia may result. The severity of the systemic effect will vary with the capacity of the organism to produce toxins. In particular, the haemolytic streptococcus may produce a specific exotoxin responsible for an erythematous skin reaction. In some persons erythema does not appear because the erythrogenic toxin is neutralised by specific antibodies produced as a result of previous haemolytic streptococcal infection. When the infection is associated with a rash the syndrome is known as scarlet fever. Susceptibility to scarlet fever can be demonstrated by the production in 12-18 hours of an area of erythema in response to the intradermal injection of small quantities of the erythrogenic toxin. This is the Dick test which is only of academic interest as a negative test indicates only the presence of circulating antibody to the erythrogenic toxin and in no way implies immunity to haemolytic streptococcal infection.

Haemolytic streptococci may be classified by precipitin tests (Lancefield) into thirteen groups. The majority of strains causing significant infection in man belong to group A. These may be further subdivided by agglutination tests (Griffith) into over forty types. The same type of streptococcus may produce in one person acute tonsillitis, in another scarlet fever and in a third erysipelas.

Prior to the discovery of the sulphonamides, streptococcal infection frequently caused very serious disease. Apart from the development of effective chemotherapeutic control, however, streptococcal infections have been undergoing a spontaneous decline in their severity. Although scarlet fever is at present a mild disease, it may not necessarily remain so, as fluctuations in its severity have been recorded for the past two or three hundred years.

The primary site of infection in scarlet fever is usually the pharynx or the tonsils but the disease may follow haemolytic streptococcal infection in other situations, e.g. in the genital tract after childbirth resulting in 'puerperal' scarlet fever or in wounds resulting in 'surgical' scarlet fever. It is transmitted by airborne infection, or more rarely by milk or ice-cream contaminated by streptococci. The disease is notifiable. The incubation period is about two to four days. Quarantine is not necessary.

Clinical Features. Scarlet fever occurs most commonly in children from three to ten years of age. It has a sudden onset and the more severe cases present with a sore throat, shivering, headache, and vomiting. There is inflammation of the fauces; the tonsils are enlarged and may be covered with a follicular exudate which occasionally becomes confluent. The exudate may be distinguished from the membrane seen in diphtheria by its yellow appearance and the ease with which it is wiped off. There is tender enlargement of the tonsillar lymph nodes. The rash, which usually appears first behind the ears on the second day, rapidly becomes a generalised punctate erythema. It is most intense in the flexures of the arms and legs. The face is not affected by the rash, though it is usually flushed due to fever, and the region round the mouth is pale. The tongue is initially furred but shows prominent red papillae, an appearance known as the 'white strawberry' tongue. In two or three days the fur peels leaving the 'red strawberry' tongue. The rash fades in about one week and is succeeded by desquamation of the skin.

Complications. The complications are less common than formerly as a result of the mild form of the disease and the introduction of effective chemotherapy. Extension of infection along the Eustachian tubes may lead to acute suppurative otitis media. Cervical adenitis and upper respiratory tract infections such as rhinitis and sinusitis also occur. Rheumatic fever and acute nephritis are rare sequelae which develop two or three weeks after the onset of the illness and are due to hypersensitivity.

Diagnosis. *Infectious mononucleosis* (p. 645), *measles* (p. 51), and *German measles* (p. 53) may sometimes be mistaken for scarlet fever. Rashes resulting from *sensitivity to a drug* are more commonly encountered in adults than in children and may differ from scarlet fever in their persistence and distribution. In scarlet fever a profuse growth of haemolytic streptococci can usually be obtained from a throat swab.

Treatment. The treatment of scarlet fever is the same as for streptococcal sore throat. Most cases respond rapidly to phenoxymethylpenicillin in doses of 250 mg. six-hourly for seven days.

Prophylaxis. An institutional epidemic calls for chemoprophylaxis with penicillin which has superseded both active and passive immunisation.

ERYSIPELAS

Erysipelas is an acute local haemolytic streptococcal infection of the skin. It occurs in both sexes and at all ages. The incubation period is about two to four days. The disease is notifiable. A quarantine period is not necessary.

Clinical Features. The onset is abrupt with local heat and pain in the infected region of the skin together with a general systemic upset. There is a rapidly spreading red patch of inflamed skin with much underlying oedema of the subcutaneous tissues. The edge of the patch is palpably raised and clearly defined. As the oedema subsides vesicles and bullae appear in the central part of the affected area. The face is involved in at least 80 per cent. of all cases of erysipelas as a result of the spread of streptococcal infection from the nose or throat.

Treatment. Erysipelas is usually brought under complete control within 48 hours of treatment with penicillin; hence the prognosis is now excellent for a disease which used to be very serious.

STAPHYLOCOCCAL INFECTIONS

Staphylococcus pyogenes is the main pathogen of this species and it is responsible for a variety of suppurative conditions in man such as boils, carbuncles, perinephric abscess, osteomyelitis, pneumonia, necrotising entero-colitis and septicaemia with pyaemic abscesses. The organism may also contaminate food and produce a heat-labile toxin which, if ingested, causes acute vomiting and diarrhoea.

The infection is derived from a human source. Commonly this

is the nose, perineum or fingers of a carrier. Not infrequently the patient is a carrier and autoinfection occurs. The widespread use of antibiotics and sulphonamides has led to the emergence of strains of staphylococci which are resistant to many antibacterial agents. Such strains are commonly encountered in staphylococcal infections acquired in hospital. It is the duty of every nurse, doctor, medical student and hospital worker to take all possible precautions against the spread of infection.

Necrotising entero-colitis is usually the result of the unrestricted growth of drug-resistant staphylococci in the gut following the virtual elimination of the other intestinal flora during oral chemotherapy. The illness is sometimes so severe as to resemble cholera in the severity of the diarrhoea and the ensuing dehydration and collapse.

Patients with staphylococcal infections should be nursed with full barrier precautions against the spread of infection. The choice of antibiotic depends to some extent on whether the infection has been acquired inside or outside hospital. In the latter case the organism will probably be sensitive to benzylpenicillin and the tetracyclines. If the therapeutic response is not satisfactory within 48 hours, then sensitivity tests should be carried out by a bacteriologist. Since the majority of staphylococcal infections acquired in hospital are resistant to the commonly used antibiotics, the organism should be submitted to sensitivity tests from the outset. If the patient is seriously ill treatment should be commenced with cloxacillin (p. 73). If the staphylococcus proves to be sensitive to benzylpenicillin this antibiotic can then be substituted, a change which will be no less effective and which will substantially reduce the expense of treatment. If the patient is hypersensitive to the penicillins, either erythromycin (p. 77), lincomycin (p. 82), fucidin (p. 82) or cephaloridine (p. 84) may be used, depending on the sensitivity of the organism and the severity of the illness.

WHOOPING-COUGH

(*Pertussis*)

Whooping-cough is a highly infectious disease of the respiratory tract caused by *Bordetella pertussis*. It is spread by droplet infection. Clinical diagnosis in the early and most infectious stage is virtually impossible so that epidemics are common. However, the incidence and severity of the disease have been decreasing over the last few years since the institution of more effective prophylactic measures. The disease is notifiable. The incubation period is 7-14 days to the catarrhal stage. A quarantine period is not necessary. Whooping-cough occurs at all ages but approximately 90 per cent. of cases are children under 5 years of age.

Clinical Features. The first stage of whooping-cough consists of a highly infectious upper respiratory catarrh lasting about one week during which conjunctivitis, rhinitis and an unproductive cough are present. The distinctive paroxysmal stage follows and is characterised by severe bouts of coughing. The number of such paroxysms in 24 hours varies from an occasional attack to 40 or 50 and they are always more severe at night. Each paroxysm consists of a succession of short sharp coughs, gathering in speed and duration and ending in a deep inspiration during which the characteristic whoop may be heard. The occurrence of the whoop depends upon coincidental spasm of the glottis. During these paroxysms, the face becomes congested and cyanosed, and the tongue is protruded to such an extent that ulceration of the frenum may occur from trauma by the lower teeth. The last paroxysm of a series frequently ends with the expectoration of tenacious mucus and in vomiting. The physical signs in the chest are those of bronchitis. The paroxysmal stage lasts from one to several weeks and it is followed by the stage of convalescence during which the cough becomes less frequent and the sputum less tenacious. After the illness there is usually a lasting immunity. Second atypical attacks are sometimes seen in adults who, although not seriously ill, may be greatly distressed by the spasmodic coughing.

Complications. The most important complications of whooping-cough are bronchopneumonia and segmental or lobar collapse which may be followed by bronchiectasis. Convulsions are of grave significance especially if they are frequent. Subconjunctival or periorbital haemorrhage, ulceration of the frenum of the tongue, and prolapse of the rectum, which are not infrequent, are relatively unimportant results of the stress of coughing. The mortality is greatest in the first year of life.

Diagnosis. The diagnosis of whooping-cough is very difficult in the catarrhal stage when the disease is most infectious. It can be confirmed in the laboratory by the isolation of *Bordetella pertussis* from per-nasal swabs (taken from the posterior wall of the nasopharynx on small swabs passed along the floor of the nose) or less frequently from cough-plates containing Bordet's medium. Examination of the blood shows a lymphocytosis which, however, may not develop until the disease is well established. The diagnosis is easy in the paroxysmal stage when the whoop has developed, but by this time the danger of transmission of infection has largely disappeared.

Treatment. The tetracyclines reduce the severity of the infection if taken during the catarrhal stage. Palatable suspensions of tetracycline containing 100 mg. per ml. are available. One ml. b.d. would suffice for a child aged 5 years and weighing about 20 kg. (3 st.) The milder case need not be kept in bed, and is better out of doors. A cough suppressant such as linctus methadone may be helpful in controlling the severity of paroxysms. When the illness is of long duration and vomiting is frequent, patient skilled nursing will be required to maintain the nutrition, especially in infants and young children. Feeds are usually accepted and retained if they are given immediately after the vomiting which frequently follows a paroxysm of coughing.

Prophylaxis. Active immunisation should be given in accordance with the instructions on p. 11. It is important that the patient should be segregated as early as possible. Contacts should be isolated on the first sign of catarrhal symptoms and per-nasal swabs taken.

CHICKENPOX

(*Varicella*)

Chickenpox is a viral infection which spreads by droplets from the upper respiratory tract, by contamination from the discharge from ruptured lesions of the skin or through contact with a patient with herpes zoster. Herpes zoster appears to be due to a latent infection with chickenpox virus which is reactivated by some specific cause. It may be accompanied by a varicelliform rash. Chicken-pox is highly infectious and chiefly affects children under

10 years of age. Most children are little incommoded by this disease but, as often happens with viral infections, adults may develop a more severe illness. Second attacks are very rare. The disease is not notifiable. The incubation period is about a fortnight. A quarantine period is not necessary.

Clinical Features. Constitutional symptoms are usually brief and mild, and the first sign of the disease is often the appearance of the rash. Lesions are sometimes present on the palate before the characteristic rash appears on the trunk on the second day of the illness. Then the face and finally the limbs are involved. The spots reach their maximum density upon the trunk, and are more sparse on the periphery of the limbs. The axillae should be inspected as this region is almost invariably affected, while in smallpox the reverse is true (Fig. 2). Macules appear first and within a few hours the lesions become papular and then vesicular. The vesicles are unilocular, very superficial, thin-walled and surrounded by a wide zone of erythema. The shape is elliptical rather than spherical. Within 24 hours the lesions become pustular. The vesicles and pustules are so fragile that they may be ruptured by the chafing of garments. Damage from scratching is also frequent, since itching may be troublesome. Whether or not the pustules rupture, they dry up in a few days to form scabs. The spots appear in crops, so that lesions at all stages of development are seen in any area at the same time. The course of the disease is usually uneventful.

Complications. Secondary infection of the lesions in the mouth and upon the skin by staphylococci and streptococci is the only common complication. Encephalomyelitis may occur (p. 1186). Concomitant herpes zoster is unusual.

Diagnosis. Although the typical case of chickenpox presents no diagnostic problem it is important to remember that great difficulty may be encountered in cases of modified smallpox and variola minor. When the rash has fully developed, however, the peripheral distribution of the lesions in smallpox is preserved. Serious consideration of the possibility of smallpox must be given to apparent cases of chickenpox occurring in patients who have just returned from an endemic area or at times when an outbreak of smallpox is known to be present. Typical variola major may be distinguished by certain features which contrast with those of chickenpox. In smallpox

(*a*) there is a prodromal illness of two to four days;
(*b*) the density of the lesions is greatest at the periphery, the rash is relatively profuse on convex and exposed surfaces, and the axillae are not affected (Fig. 2);
(*c*) the spots are deep-set, multilocular, circular lesions and are present predominantly at a single stage of development.

Treatment. No treatment is required in the majority of cases. Itching may be relieved by an antihistamine drug taken orally. At the first sign of secondary infection a local antiseptic should be applied to the skin, e.g. chlorhexidine (Hibitane). If bacterial infection progresses, an appropriate antibiotic should be prescribed.

Spread of infection can be prevented by isolation of the patient and the sterilisation of all soiled articles, but the disease is so mild that in domiciliary practice these precautions are not normally required. The patient is no longer infectious after the vesicles have dried up.

SMALLPOX

(*Variola*)

The virus of variola major (severe or 'classical' smallpox) causes a serious and highly infectious disease which spreads by droplet infection from the respiratory tract or by contamination with material from the skin lesions. There are also two variants of this virus (1) variola minor virus causes a much milder disease, which is similar in its clinical features and mode of spread, but is seldom fatal; (2) vaccinia virus (cowpox) is seldom the cause of systemic disease, and cannot be spread readily from one person to another. Immune antibodies to all these viruses are developed in response to infection by any one of them, though vaccinia gives rise to a less permanent immunity than an attack of variola. Smallpox has been eliminated from Britain, where it was at one time a terrible scourge, but sporadic cases and even epidemics result from the introduction of the disease from abroad, and there is increased liability for this to occur since air travel has removed the

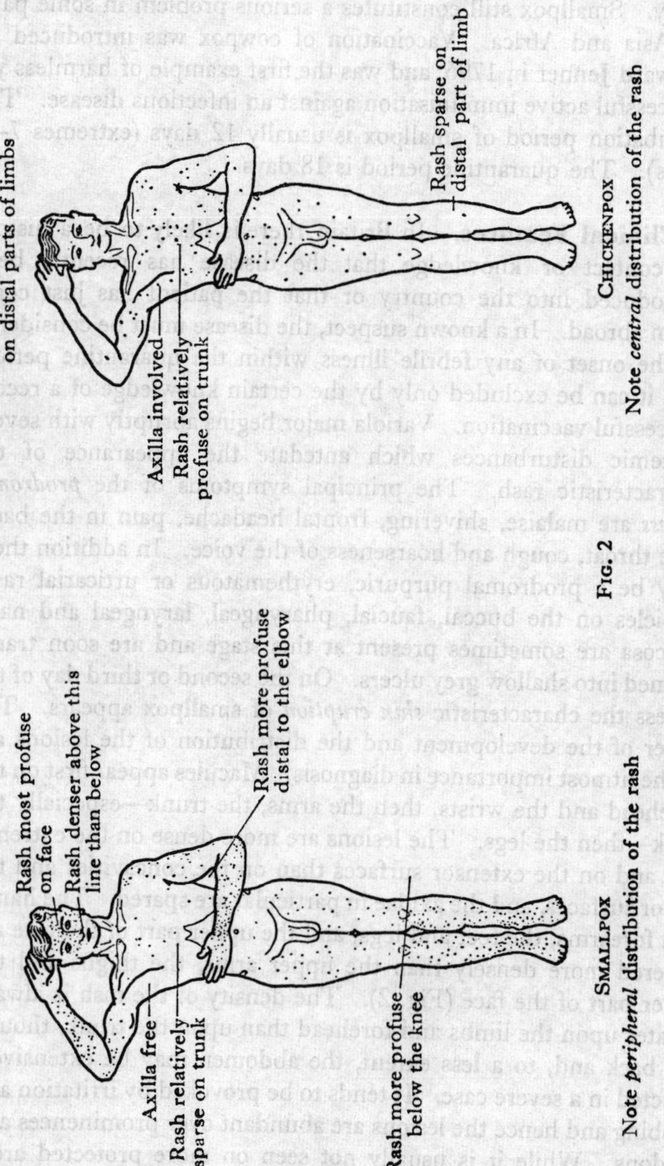

Fig. 2

Smallpox
Note *peripheral* distribution of the rash

Chickenpox
Note *central* distribution of the rash

(Harries & Mitman: 'Clinical Practice in Infectious Diseases')

time barrier of a long sea voyage. On the slightest suspicion of smallpox the Medical Officer of Health should be notified immediately. Smallpox still constitutes a serious problem in some parts of Asia and Africa. Vaccination of cowpox was introduced by Edward Jenner in 1796, and was the first example of harmless yet successful active immunisation against an infectious disease. The incubation period of smallpox is usually 12 days (extremes 7-16 days). The quarantine period is 18 days.

Clinical Features. In Britain there is likely to be a history of contact or knowledge that the disease has recently been introduced into the country or that the patient has just come from abroad. In a known suspect, the disease must be considered at the onset of any febrile illness within the quarantine period, and it can be excluded only by the certain knowledge of a recent successful vaccination. Variola major begins abruptly with severe systemic disturbances which antedate the appearance of the characteristic rash. The principal symptoms of the *prodroma illness* are malaise, shivering, frontal headache, pain in the back' sore throat, cough and hoarseness of the voice. In addition there may be a prodromal purpuric, erythematous or urticarial rash. Vesicles on the buccal, faucial, pharyngeal, laryngeal and nasal mucosa are sometimes present at this stage and are soon transformed into shallow grey ulcers. On the second or third day of the illness the characteristic *skin eruption* of smallpox appears. The order of the development and the distribution of the lesions are of the utmost importance in diagnosis. Macules appear first on the forehead and the wrists, then the arms, the trunk—especially the back—then the legs. The lesions are more dense on the extremities and on the extensor surfaces than on the concavities and the flexor surfaces, and the axillae in particular are spared. The hands and forearms, the feet and legs, and the upper part of the face are covered more densely than the upper arms, the thighs and the lower part of the face (Fig. 2). The density of the rash is always greater upon the limbs and forehead than upon the trunk, though the back and, to a less extent, the abdomen may be extensively affected in a severe case. It tends to be provoked by irritation and rubbing and hence the lesions are abundant over prominences and tendons. While it is usually not seen on more protected areas such as the antecubital fossae and axillae, it can be profuse in the skin folds of a fat baby's axilla. The rash develops in a regular sequence. Macules turn to deep-set, dark-pink papules in a matter of hours. The final appearance of papules may take two or three days. The conversion of papules to vesicles then commences with those lesions which were first to appear, and the whole process may take a further 24 hours. The vesicles feel hard and are not easily ruptured, for they are deep-set and multilocular. The outline of the lesions is circular. After about two days the vesicular stage merges into the pustular stage. The pustules are surrounded by a zone of erythema at first, but this gradually disappears. During the ensuing eight or nine days the pustules gradually dry up to form dark brown or almost black scabs. These separate after several days leaving pitted scars or 'pocks'.

After the initial fever and the outbreak of the rash, the patient improves and the temperature, which falls, may even be normal for a short period. During the pustular stage, however, the temperature rises again and the patient becomes extremely toxic. This recrudescence of severe illness is probably due to invasion of the skin lesions by bacteria, usually staphylococci or streptococci. The patient is in a miserable state, for in addition to feeling exceedingly ill, there is oedema of the skin and ulceration of the conjunctivae, mouth, throat, larynx and trachea, and a concomitant pneumonia is common.

Complications. Heart failure and peripheral circulatory failure may result from toxaemia. Secondary bacterial invasion of the ulcerated respiratory tract gives rise to bronchitis and bronchopneumonia. There may be delirium or convulsions, and encephalomyelitis may occur. Lesions of the conjunctiva may lead to corneal ulcer and impairment or loss of vision.

Diagnosis. A typical case of smallpox presents little diagnostic difficulty, especially when the patient has come recently from abroad or if an epidemic is present.

It is essential, however, to emphasise the fact that the diagnosis of variola minor, and particularly of variola major developing in a patient who is partially immune owing to previous vaccination (modified smallpox) may present the greatest difficulties.

In variola minor or in modified smallpox the prodromal illness is less severe and the secondary fever is slight or absent. The rash may be sparse and considerably modified in many of its features, but the distribution of the lesions is precisely that of smallpox. The trivial nature of the illness in some of these cases may result in the disease being entirely overlooked. The recognition of these infections is clearly of the utmost importance from the point of view of public health. Modified smallpox gives rise to secondary cases of variola major, whereas variola minor breeds true. The Medical Officer of Health must be informed immediately any suspicion of smallpox arises. Laboratory investigations must be used to confirm the diagnosis when the clinical features are dubious. Four procedures are available. These are (1) microscopical examination of a smear of fluid obtained from a skin lesion for evidence of inclusion bodies. Several reference laboratories are now able to carry out these examinations by electron microscopy, enabling a rapid and specific diagnosis to be made; (2) culture of the virus by inoculation of material into the chorio-allantoic membrane of a hen's egg; (3) complement fixation tests; (4) agar gel diffusion plate. The chief differential diagnosis is from chickenpox, and the points of distinction have already been mentioned on p. 45. Apparent cases of chickenpox appearing during an outbreak of smallpox, or occurring in patients who have recently arrived from regions in which smallpox is endemic should be scrutinised with the utmost care for the possibility of modified smallpox.

Treatment. General nursing care, by attendants who have been recently vaccinated, is the essence of treatment. The prevention of secondary infection by special care in the hygiene of the mouth and of the skin is of importance; when infection occurs appropriate antibacterial therapy must be employed. When the last scab has been shed the patient is no longer infectious.

Prophylaxis. Efficient prophylactic vaccination, the isolation of cases, and the placing of contacts in quarantine have been shown to control and eventually eliminate smallpox.

Vaccination is compulsory before travelling to an endemic area. Active immunisation should be given in accordance with the instructions on p. 11. Except for contacts during an epidemic, it is contraindicated in the presence of active skin diseases, especially infantile eczema, owing to the probable development of generalised vaccinia, which may be fatal. Should generalised vaccinia occur, the outlook can be greatly improved by the injection of human immunoglobulin.

Thiosemicarbazones, such as methisazone, have proved to be effective in preventing the disease in close contacts. It should be given as early as possible in the incubation period in a dose of 3 g. twice daily for four days. The main side effects of nausea and vomiting can be largely avoided by giving the drug after meals. The reintroduction of the disease into the British Isles by sea or by air has been largely prevented by the vigilance of port health authorities.

MEASLES
(*Morbilli*)

Measles is a viral disease which spreads by droplet infection. One attack confers a high degree of immunity. Most people suffer from measles in childhood, and a mother who has had the disease confers passive immunity on her infant for the first six months of life. The infection is generalised, but the clinical evidence of it is mainly found in the respiratory tract, the skin, the mouth and the conjunctivae. Measles is prevalent during the first 6 months of the year with a peak incidence in March. The disease is notifiable in England but not in Scotland. The incubation period is about 10 days to the commencement of the catarrhal stage. A quarantine period is not necessary.

Clinical Features

Catarrhal stage. Measles commences in much the same way as a common cold. There is an acute febrile onset, with nasal catarrh, sneezing, redness of the conjunctivae, some swelling of the eyelids and watering of the eyes. In addition a short cough, hoarseness of the voice due to laryngitis, and photophobia usually appear by the second day. During the catarrhal stage, which lasts for three or four days before the appearance of the specific rash, a diagnosis of measles may be made from the presence of Koplik's spots on the mucous membrane of the mouth. These are very small white spots, often compared with grains of salt, surrounded by a narrow zone of inflammation. They are best seen in daylight. Though often numerous on the inside of the cheeks, they may be sparse and confined to the region around the opening of the parotid duct. The disease is highly infectious during the catarrhal stage.

Exanthematous stage. After three or four days of the catarrhal stage, the diagnostic Koplik's spots disappear while the dark red macular or maculo-papular skin rash develops. The rash is first seen at the back of the ears and at the junction of the forehead and the hair. Within a few hours there is invasion of the whole skin area, and there is usually some accentuation of fever. As the spots rapidly become more numerous they fuse to form the characteristic blotchy appearance of measles. The face is ordinarily the most densely covered area. When the rash is fully erupted, it tends to deepen in colour and then fade into a faint brown staining. Finally there is a fine, branny desquamation of the skin. The malaise and the fever subside as the rash fades.

Complications. Secondary infection by haemolytic streptococci or pneumococci is responsible for the most common and serious complications, namely otitis media and bronchopneumonia which are particularly dangerous in the first 18 months of life. persistent conjunctivitis may be followed by corneal ulceration which, if neglected, may result in impairment or loss of vision. Stomatitis, gastroenteritis, appendicitis and encephalomyelitis may also occur.

Diagnosis. Considerable difficulty may arise in those cases in which a prodromal rash indistinguishable from *scarlet fever* develops in the catarrhal stage. However, in measles Koplik's spots are present and the eyes have the appearance of those of a child that has recently been crying. The differential diagnosis from *German measles* is discussed on p. 54. It is important to remember that *drug rashes* are common and may simulate closely the eruptions of measles, German measles or scarlet fever.

Treatment. The patient should be isolated if possible and excluded from school for 14 days from the appearance of the rash. Nursing on a verandah or in a well-ventilated room reduces the chances of secondary respiratory infection. Bacterial complications should be treated promptly with an appropriate antibiotic such as penicillin. Contacts should be examined daily for the first sign of infection.

Prophylaxis.

ACTIVE IMMUNISATION. In 1968 the Ministry of Health recommended that vaccination, using one injection of live attenuated measles virus, should be offered to children over one year old who have not had the disease. Vaccination may be followed by a mild febrile disturbance.

Passive Immunisation. Human immunoglobulin is recommended for the prevention or attentuation of measles, particularly for contacts under 18 months of age and for debilitated children. Injections should be given intramuscularly within five days after exposure in the dosage advised by the Ministry of Health (Table 2).

Table 2

Available for	*Usual Dosage*
(1) Control of hospital and institutional outbreaks.	*Prevention*
	3 years and over 750 mg.
(2) Persons suffering from intercurrent illness or living in a poor environment for whom an attack of measles would be dangerous.	1-2 years . 500 mg.
	Under 1 year . 250 mg.
	Attenuation
	All ages . 250 mg.
(3) Children under 3 years of age.	

GERMAN MEASLES

(*Rubella*)

Rubella is a viral disease which spreads by droplet infection. One attack confers a high degree of immunity. The disease tends to affect older children, adolescents and young adults and it spreads less readily than measles. It occurs mainly in the spring and summer months. The disease in children is trivial. In adults the illness may be more severe, but of short duration and of little importance except when it develops in a woman during the first three to four months of pregnancy. In such cases the child may be born with a congenital malformation such as a cardiac or mental defect, cataract or deafness. The disease is not notifiable. The incubation period is usually about 18 days. A quarantine period is not necessary.

Clinical Features. Mild constitutional symptoms are accompanied by nasal catarrh and conjunctivitis. There may be some stiffness of the neck, and the development of slightly tender and enlarged posterior cervical lymph nodes is usual. In young children, the rash, which ordinarily appears on the second day, may be the first indication of the disease. The spots are pink macules which appear first behind the ears and on the forehead. The rash spreads rapidly, first to the trunk and then to the limbs. There may be generalised enlargement of the lymph nodes, in addition to those in the neck. The whole illness is over in two or three days, and the rash fades without any staining or peeling of the skin.

Complications. Complications are very rare. Encephalomyelitis, thrombocytopenic purpura and polyarthritis may occur, and complete recovery is the rule.

Diagnosis. The disease may be distinguished from *measles* by its trivial nature, its brief duration, the pink colour of the rash, the absence of Koplik's spots and the presence of enlargement of cervical lymph nodes. The morphology of the rash of German measles may vary from one epidemic to another. Sometimes there is a close resemblance to the punctate erythema of *scarlet fever*, but in rubella the circumoral region is not spared. *Glandular fever* is another disease which should be considered in the differential diagnosis (p. 645). *Rashes due to drugs* may have a similar appearance and since they commonly occur, enquiry should always be made in regard to the taking of medicines.

The diagnosis can be confirmed by isolation of the virus or by demonstration of specific antibodies.

Treatment. None is required. In the present state of knowledge the development of the disease in children is to be encouraged so that women are immune and men are no longer a possible source of infection. Isolation of cases or contacts is justified only when it is necessary to protect a previously unaffected woman during the first three or four months of pregnancy. Women who have been exposed to infection during this time may be protected by the intramuscular injection of human immunoglobulin, but this may fail to protect the foetus.

MUMPS

(*Epidemic Parotitis*)

Mumps is caused by a virus which spreads by droplet infection and affects mainly children of school age and young adults. The virus has a predilection for certain gland tissues. The common site of infection is one or both parotid glands, but sometimes there is involvement of the submandibular or sublingual salivary glands, the testicle, the pancreas or ovary alone or in combination. Encephalomyelitis is rare, but examination of the cerebrospinal fluid early in the course of mumps frequently shows an increase in lymphocytes. The infectivity rate is not very high. Most cases occur in the spring. The disease is not notifiable. The incubation period is about 18 days. A quarantine period is not necessary: contacts should be watched for the first sign of disease from the 12th to the 28th day after exposure.

Clinical Features. Constitutional disturbance is slight or moderate, and may be present for several days before any specific symptom is present. During this time it may be possible to suspect mumps by observing inflammatory swelling round the orifice of the parotid duct. More often the diagnosis is not evident until there is painful spasm of the jaw muscles on attempting to open the mouth and tender swelling of one or both parotid glands appears. Indeed, parotid swelling alone is often the first feature. Mumps should also be considered when a patient suffers from acute inflammation of a submandibular gland or of a testicle for which there is no local cause. Obscure abdominal pain may also rarely be due to pancreatitis or oöphoritis. Acute lymphocytic meningitis is another mode of presentation. If such conditions are due to mumps, they are accompanied by a lymphocytosis. It is also of great diagnostic value in such obscure cases to know that mumps is epidemic in the district at the time.

The swollen glands subside in a few days, and may be succeeded by swelling of a previously unaffected gland. Orchitis occurs at puberty or in early manhood and is usually on one side only, but if it is bilateral, sterility may be a sequel.

Diagnosis. Most cases of mumps can be diagnosed on clinical grounds alone. A compliment fixation test can establish the diagnosis as early as the sixth day from the onset of symptoms, and is of value in atypical cases.

Treatment. Oral hygiene is important when the mouth is very dry due to lack of saliva. Difficulty in opening the mouth may necessitate feeding through a straw. Apart from the relief of symptoms as they appear, no other treatment is necessary. Orchitis can be relieved by the administration of prednisolone for a few days without apparent danger of dissemination of infection. Cases of mumps should be isolated until the gland last affected has subsided.

TETANUS

(*Lockjaw*)

This disease results from infection with *Clostridium tetani*, which exists as a commensal in the gut of man and domestic animals and is found in cultivated soils. Infection enters the body through wounds, which in civilian practice are usually trivial, such as penetrating injuries from a splinter, a nail in the boot, or a garden fork, or septic infections such as dirty abrasions or a whitlow. The disease is thus most commonly found in agricultural workers and gardeners.

In circumstances unfavourable to the growth of the organism, spores are formed and these may remain dormant for years. Spores germinate and bacilli multiply only in the anaerobic conditions which occur in areas of tissue necrosis or if the oxygen tension is low as a result of the presence of other organisms, particularly aerobic ones. The bacilli remain localised but produce an exotoxin with an affinity for motor nerve endings and motor nerve cells. Involvement of the former by direct spread causes local tetanus. The anterior horn cells are affected after the exotoxin has passed into the blood stream and their involvement results in rigidity and convulsions. Symptoms first appear from two days to several weeks after injury—the shorter the incubation period, the more severe the attacks and the outcome may well be fatal with an incubation period of only a few days.

Clinical Manifestations. Much the most important early symptom is trismus—a painless spasm of the masseter muscles which causes difficulty in opening the mouth and in masticating.

This tonic rigidity spreads to involve in turn the muscles of the face, neck and trunk. Contraction of the frontalis and the muscles at the angles of the mouth gives rise to the 'risus sardonicus'. There is rigidity of the muscles of the neck and trunk of varying degree. The back is usually slightly arched and the boarb-like abdominal wall resembles that seen a few hours after the perforation of a peptic ulcer, but there is little tenderness. In the more severe cases sudden violent spasms lasting for a few seconds to three or four minutes may be induced by diverse stimuli such as moving the patient, knocking the bed or making a noise. These reflex convulsions are painful, exhausting and of very serious significance, especially if they appear soon after the onset of symptoms. They gradually increase in frequency and severity for about one week and the patient may die from exhaustion, from asphyxia or from aspiration pneumonia. In less severe cases reflex convulsions may not commence for about a week after the first sign of rigidity and in very mild infections they may never appear.

Rarely the only manifestation of the disease may be *local tetanus* —stiffness or spasm of the muscles near the infected wound—and the prognosis is good if treatment is commenced at this stage. If local tetanus follows wounds of the head and neck, the resulting irritation or paralysis of cranial nerves may resemble tuberculous meningitis or polioencephalitis and in cases of doubt the cerebrospinal fluid should be examined; in tetanus it is normal. Lumbar puncture should be avoided except in cases of real doubt.

The diagnosis is made on clinical grounds. It is rarely possible to isolate the infecting organism from the original locus of entry. Spasm of the masseters due to alveolar abscess, septic throat or other causes is painful, in contradistinction to tetanus.

Treatment. Treatment should be begun as soon as possible and because of the technical difficulties and the seriousness of the complications, this should be undertaken in hospital. The essentials are as follows:—

1. Prevention of Further Absorption of Toxin from the Wound. A single intravenous injection of immune serum containing 20,000 international units of antitoxin should be given immediately the diagnosis is suspected. If the patient is allergic or has received a previous injection of ATS, ovine anti-tetanus serum or human immunoglobulin anti-tetanus can now be

obtained. The wound requires to be thoroughly cleaned and drained if there is evidence of necrotic tissue, foreign body or sepsis. Surgery should not be undertaken until one hour after the injection of antitoxin. Benzylpenicillin should be administered in doses of 500,000 units twice daily as it is effective against *Cl. tetani*.

2. Control of Reflex Spasms

(*a*) *General measures*. The patient should lie in a quiet darkened room on a flat comfortable bed, with the bedclothes supported by a cradle. A notice should be put outside the door requesting quietness from those who pass or enter. All necessary manipulation of the patient should be done as gently as possible and with due warning, for it is unexpected stimuli which are particularly liable to provoke reflex spasms. Expert nursing is of supreme importance.

(*b*) *Sedatives and antispasmodics*. In mild cases when trismus is not so severe as to prevent feeding, spasms may be prevented by large doses of phenobarbitone. This can be supplemented with, or replaced by, chlorpromazine, 50 mg. four-hourly. In more severe cases thiopentone will be required, e.g. 0·5-1 g. being added to each 500 ml. of intravenous fluid. In really critical cases curare, which paralyses the neuromuscular junctions, should be given intravenously, but only if an experienced anaesthetist is available as respiration may have to be maintained by tracheostomy and intermittent positive pressure respiration. The aim of such heroic measures is to control spasms which are terrifying, exhausting and occasionally fatal from asphyxia.

3. Prevention of Intercurrent Infection. One of the great risks is pneumonia due to the patient's inability to cough up bronchial secretions. Penicillin, which has been given daily from the onset may act as a prophylactic against pneumonia, but in the event of its failure, another antibiotic, based on sputum culture, should be prescribed.

4. Maintenance of Strength and of Fluid Intake. Sufficient food and fluids are of vital importance to enable the patient to survive an ordeal which may be prolonged and violent. In milder cases it may be possible for the patient to swallow fluids or even to tolerate a stomach tube left *in situ*. If oral treatment is impossible, intravenous feeding should be commenced without delay.

Prophylaxis. Active immunisation should be given in accordance with the instructions on p. 10.

Contaminated injuries must be treated by the removal of all debris and non-viable tissue. The immediate danger of tetanus can be greatly reduced by the injection of a large dose of a long acting preparation of penicillin. When the risk of tetanus is judged to be great, further protection may be given by a subcutaneous injection of 1,500 international units of tetanus antitoxin, after taking the precautions described on p. 37. All patients should in addition be given an injection of adsorbed tetanus toxoid. Previously unprotected patients should be persuaded to take further injections at six weeks and three months.

BRUCELLOSIS

(*Undulant fever: Malta fever; Abortus fever*)

Undulant fever is a septicaemia caused in Britain by *Brucella abortus* which is spread to man by the ingestion of raw milk from infected cattle. It is also an occupational hazard of veterinary surgeons, laboratory personnel, slaughter-house workers and others. In Malta, the disease is due to *Br. melitensis* and is transmitted by infected goat's milk. In the U.S.A. and the Far East *Br. suis* acquired from pigs may be the causative organism. The disease is not notifiable. The incubation period is about three weeks.

Clinical Features. The disease commences as a blood stream infection and the clinical manifestations are gradual in onset and variable. The symptoms in order of frequency are sweating, weakness, headache, anorexia, pains in limbs and back, constipation, rigors, cough, sore throat, and joint pains. The spleen is palpable in about 20 per cent. of cases and a variable rash occurs in about 10 per cent. The temperature characteristically shows undulations, during which febrile and afebrile periods alternate. In other cases the pyrexia may be continuous and sweating may be profuse. Untreated, the disease may last for a few days or continue for many months, and in the latter case the patient often becomes extremely depressed or irritable. Neutropenia and lymphocytosis usually occur in the more severe case. Subacute arthritis of one or more joints may develop. The spine is often the site affected and occasionally radiological changes due to osteomyelitis of a vertebra can be demonstrated. The diagnosis of undulant fever can usually be confirmed by blood culture or by agglutination tests. Other conditions causing prolonged fever must be considered in differential diagnosis (p. 16).

Treatment. Tetracycline 250 mg. six-hourly is usually effective in the early uncomplicated case, but for the chronic or relapsing disease the triple combination of tetracycline (1 g. daily), streptomycin (1 g. daily) and sulphadimidine (4 g. daily) is indicated for a period of two or three weeks.

Prophylaxis. Undulant fever can largely be prevented by the boiling or pasteurisation of all milk used for human consumption, as *Br. abortus* is readily destroyed by heat. It is difficult to eradicate the disease in cattle because herds readily become reinfected. In practice, active immunisation of young animals is the most effective measure.

VENEREAL DISEASE

Venereal diseases are almost invariably contracted during coitus with an infected person. Gonorrhoea and other forms of urethritis are common in Britain, but syphilis is relatively rare. Following the introduction of effective treatment with antibiotics the incidence of these diseases greatly decreased from 1946 to 1955. Since then it has increased for a variety of reasons.

GONORRHOEA

This is due to infection of the mucous membrane of the genito-urinary tract with *Neisseria gonorrhoeae*. The eyes and anal canal may also be infected. The incubation period is about 3-10 days.

Clinical Features. In the male the infection starts in the anterior part of the urethra and tends to spread to the prostate and occasionally to the bladder or the epididymes. There is dysuria, some increased frequency of urination and a white or yellow discharge from the urethra. If untreated or inadequately treated the discharge becomes less copious or intermittent, or may be observed only on waking from sleep—a condition known as gleet.

In females the infection is mainly in the urethra, the cervix uteri and the Bartholinian glands. At the onset there is dysuria, frequency of urination, vaginal discharge and some swelling of the vulva. The symptoms may be trivial and pass unnoticed. Extension up the genital tract leads to cervicitis and acute salpingitis. The anal canal may be infected in either sex. Infection of the conjunctiva of infants born of infected mothers causes a profuse purulent discharge and often damage to sight. This condition, known as ophthalmia neonatorum, is now rare in this country, but was formerly a frequent cause of blindness. In some parts of the world the disease is still frequent. Systemic spread of gonorrhoea may cause acute or chronic arthritis (p. 543) and iritis.

Diagnosis. The clinical diagnosis is confirmed by the demonstration of intracellular gram-negative kidney-shaped diplococci in stained films of pus from the infected areas. Culture of the exudate on the appropriate medium gives a much higher percentage of positive diagnoses than reliance on microscopic examinations alone and is essential for medico-legal purposes. The complement fixation test is useful in chronic cases, in complications, and as proof of cure, but is of no value in the diagnosis of acute infections.

Treatment. A single injection of 600,000 units of procaine penicillin is in most instances sufficient to cure a recent infection in a male, but it is advisable in addition to give 500,000 units of benzylpenicillin intramuscularly and this combined therapy should be repeated in 24 hours. In the female a third injection is given and if there are any complications treatment is continued daily for one week. Larger dosage will be required if the gonoccoci are relatively resistant to penicillin. Tetracycline (250 mg.) and erythromycin (250 mg.) four times daily for five days are effective alternatives for patients allergic to penicillin or infected with penicillin resistant gonococci. Gonococcal conjunctivitis responds to penicillin solution instilled into the conjunctival sac. It should also be given intramuscularly. As many cases of gonorrhoea have superadded bacterial or coccal infections of the genito-urinary tract which do not respond to penicillin, it is necessary to treat these with sulphonamides or appropriate antibiotics. In women, infection with *Trichomonas vaginalis* is also commonly present and requires treatment with metronidazole

(Flagyl) 200 mg. thrice daily by mouth for seven days. It is essential to establish that cure of gonorrhoea and any accompanying infection is complete by carrying out a series of bacteriological examinations on the secretions from the infected area. The presence of syphilis acquired at the same time as gonorrhoea may be obscured by chemotherapy. It is therefore important that serological tests for syphilis should be carried out three months after treatment.

NON-GONOCOCCAL URETHRITIS

In Britain urethritis in males is now more commonly due to organisms other than the gonococcus. In general it is a milder and more chronic infection caused by a variety of organisms, such as *Esch. coli*, staphylococci, streptococci, *Trichomonas vaginalis* or a mixture of these. Treatment is by the appropriate chemotherapy. In a considerable number of cases, however, no organism can be detected. Some of these are accompanied by conjunctivitis or arthritis, a combination known as Reiter's syndrome (p. 543); oxytetracycline is effective in about 30 per cent. of cases.

SYPHILIS

This is a chronic infection due to *Treponema pallidum*.

It is convenient to describe untreated syphilis in three stages—primary, secondary and tertiary. It must be realised, however, that the disease is generalised and continuous from the time of inoculation, and that it may be almost completely latent during its long course which may last for over 30 years.

Clinical Manifestations. Primary Stage. The primary lesion (chancre) develops at the site of inoculation. It occurs usually on the genitals, but it may be found on the lips, in the mouth, at the anus, or on a finger. The incubation period is 10 days to 10 weeks. A small painless indurated swelling forms and usually ulcerates. The regional lymph nodes are enlarged, firm, painless, and seldom suppurate.

Secondary Stage. The primary lesions tend to heal, and from about the third to sixth month evidence of generalised infection becomes apparent. The patient may have malaise, headaches, sore throat and low irregular fever.

Four cardinal signs must be remembered, though any of them may be absent.

(1) *Cutaneous Rashes.* The most common early rash is a faint macular erythema which may be perceptible only in a good light. Later the rashes are characteristically polymorphic, symmetrical, of a dull red colour and do not itch.

(2) *Condylomata.* In moist areas, such as in the perineum, the lesions become heaped up and are known as condylomata; they contain spirochaetes and are highly infective.

(3) *Mucous Patches.* The mucous membranes of the mouth are commonly affected by shallow ulcers with a narrow red edge and a surface covered by a thin white membrane. Their appearance has given rise to the descriptive term of snail track ulcers. They are highly infective.

(4) *Lymphadenopathy.* There may be generalised painless enlargement of the lymph nodes.

In over 30 per cent. of cases changes occur in the cerebrospinal fluid, indicating that there has been some involvement of the central nervous system; the clinical features of meningitis may be present, accompanied sometimes by cranial nerve palsies. Rarely there may be clinical evidence of involvement of any other part of the body. After several months the secondary changes gradually disappear to be followed by a latent period lasting from 2 to 30 years.

TERTIARY STAGE. In this stage lesions appear almost anywhere, but particularly in the skin and subcutaneous tissues, bone, tongue, testes, liver (p. 1037), aorta (p. 260) and central nervous system (p. 1163). The affected structure is infiltrated with granulation tissue containing plasma cells and lymphocytes. There is endarteritis obliterans which causes necrosis. The formation of a localised necrotic swelling, which is characteristically painless, is known as a gumma.

Congenital Syphilis. The foetus may contract syphilis from an infected mother. There is then no primary stage. The damage done may be such that the child is born dead or skin eruptions may be present at birth. More often the child appears to be normal at birth but fails to thrive, and within a few months presents rashes, and signs of syphilitic disease of bone, liver, kidneys and other organs. In yet a third group of cases the overt manifestations may be delayed until late childhood, when such findings appear as deformities of bone and teeth, iritis, keratitis, juvenile tabes or general paralysis.

Congenital syphilis is now rare, as treatment of a syphilitic woman during pregnancy will ensure the birth of a normal baby.

Diagnosis. In the primary and early secondary stages, the spirochaete may be demonstrated in serum from the chancre, condylomata or mucous patches. The serological tests for syphilis become positive from about the fourth week of the disease onwards and are invariably strongly positive by the end of the third month in untreated cases. It should be realised that in the usual serological screening tests (W.R. and V.D.R.L.) non-specific antigen is used and hence the specificity and sensitivity of such tests are variable. False positive tests may be found temporarily in glandular fever, systemic lupus erythematosus and other generalised diseases, while negative tests may be observed in many patients with late syphilis. For conclusive results additional tests are required, including those which use specific treponemal antigen (fluorescent treponemal antibody and treponemal immobilisation tests).

Treatment. *T. pallidum*, though very sensitive to penicillin, has to be exposed to it for longer periods than most micro-organisms if a spirochaeticidal effect is to be obtained. Hence the longer acting forms of penicillin are used such as procaine benzylpenicillin in oil containing 2 per cent. aluminium monostearate (P.A.M.). Patients suffering from early primary (sero-negative) syphilis require 6 mega units in 10 days. For sero-positive primary cases and for secondary syphilis 12-20 mega units should be given in 20 days. Several of these courses may be required for patients with tertiary syphilis. If the patient is allergic to penicillin, tetracycline or erythromycin can be used.

E. B. French.
J. G. Macleod.

CHEMOTHERAPY OF INFECTIONS

(*Antimicrobial agents; Sulphonamides and Antibiotics*)

THE practice of medicine entered a new era in 1935 when Domagk introduced prontosil. This was followed by the development of more effective sulphonamides and then by the antibiotics—substances which are produced by living organisms, such as moulds, and which can destroy or inhibit the growth of other organisms. The early forties saw the first clinical use of penicillin and in the ensuing decade, streptomycin, the tetracyclines and chloramphenicol became available. The world-wide stimulus to research in this field led to the isolation of a host of other antibiotics, but only a few of these have found a place in medicine. The effective therapeutic range now covers the majority of infections with the exception of those due to viruses. This situation, however, has brought with it problems of its own. Thus careful judgement must be exercised when selecting the most appropriate therapy for an individual infection as some organisms have become resistant to certain antibiotics and most antibiotics have their adverse as well as their beneficial effects.

Several principles must be kept in mind if the best results are to be obtained from the chemotherapy of infections. In the first place a bacteriological, as well as a clinical diagnosis, is necessary. In many instances, provided the nature of the infection can be inferred from the clinical findings, treatment may proceed without bacteriological investigation, e.g. the use of penicillin in acute follicular tonsillitis. In other cases it is essential to know the exact bacteriological diagnosis from the outset as in meningitis. The bacteriologist can also assist by determining not only the nature but also the sensitivity of the infecting organism to various antibiotics, and so help the clinician to choose the most effective form of treatment. This knowledge may be of vital importance in such conditions as staphylococcal infections, and in bacterial endocarditis. Some species of organisms originally sensitive to a chemotherapeutic agent may become resistant to it. The emergence of strains of staphylococci resistant to penicillin and of tubercle bacilli resistant to streptomycin are notable examples. Such resistant organisms may be present from the outset of an infection or may become predominant during treatment and so render it ineffective. Knowledge of the sensitivity of the infecting organism before commencing treatment, and during the course of chemotherapy is thus invaluable in many cases. It is obvious, therefore, that the clinician and the bacteriologist should collaborate closely if the best results are to be obtained.

Antibiotics may have a bactericidal action whereby organisms are destroyed directly, or they may have a bacteriostatic effect which renders the organism more vulnerable to the natural defence processes, by inhibiting growth and multiplication. A bactericidal antibiotic is to be preferred to the sulphonamides or to the antibiotics whose action is only bacteriostatic, as the infection will be overcome more quickly and the organisms have less time to acquire resistance.

The need for a bacteriological as well as a clinical diagnosis has been emphasised and chemotherapy must not, save in exceptional instances, be employed in the absence of a diagnosis. It is tempting, but wrong, to prescribe a potent antibiotic with a wide range of activity, such as tetracycline or cephaloridine, for a febrile patient who is suffering from a pyrexia of unknown origin, as chemotherapy is not without its dangers. The adverse effects of sulphonamides and the antibiotics are discussed on the following pages.

Some antibiotics which are too toxic to be administered systemically may be used locally, particularly those with a bactericidal action, those to which organisms are slow to develop resistance, and those which rarely provoke allergic reactions.

Combinations of antibiotics should be used only when specific indications are present. Thus it is imperative when treating tuberculosis to use more than one chemotherapeutic agent to prevent the appearance of resistant strains. Secondly, if the infection is due to several different organisms, as in peritonitis or some cases of bronchopneumonia and in the topical treatment of wounds, a combination of antibiotics with different ranges of activity may be indicated. Thirdly, it is possible that penicillin and streptomycin may have a synergistic action and advantage of this property can be taken when treating a relatively resistant organism such as the enterococcus in bacterial endocarditis. There are few other examples of synergism between antibiotics; at the most, some combinations may have an additive effect. It must be remembered that the risk of adverse effects is increased as the treatment becomes more complex and as the range of activity becomes greater.

Finally it is important to appreciate certain economic considerations in connection with chemotherapy. Some of the more recently introduced antibiotics are very costly. It is obvious that they should not be prescribed without good reason when less expensive treatment would be equally effective.

These introductory remarks may be summarised as follows. When chemotheraphy is being considered the clinician should know, or be able to infer, the nature of the infecting micro-organism; if in doubt about effective treatment, he should seek the help of the bacteriologist. A bactericidal antibiotic is to be preferred to a bacteriostatic agent. Before a decision is made consideration must be given to any potential dangers and to the relative expense involved.

THE SULPHONAMIDES

Antibiotics have largely superseded the sulphonamides which now have only a limited sphere of usefulness. Although they have the merit of being inexpensive, especially in comparison with antibiotics of recent introduction, they have the disadvantages of being much less effective in the presence of pus and of having a wide range of potential dangers.

Preparations and Principal Indications

Sulphadimidine (Sulphamezathine). This is the sulphonamide of choice for general purposes as it combines effectiveness with low toxicity. Sulphadimidine is rapidly absorbed and relatively slowly excreted in the urine in a fairly soluble form. An effective concentration in the blood can usually be maintained by administration every four to six hours. Sodium salts are available for intravenous and intramuscular administration if the patient is vomiting or comatose (Inj. sulphadimidine sodium B.P. 1 g. in 3 ml. solution). The principal indications for the use of sulphadimidine are as follows:

Meningococcal Meningitis. An initial loading dose of 3 g. should be given followed by 1 g. four-hourly. At the outset it may be necessary to administer the soluble salt intravenously; this preparation must never be given intrathecally. Sulphadiazine may be even more effective than sulphadimidine because it attains higher concentrations in the cerebrospinal fluid.

In some areas in recent years the meningococcus has been found to have acquired a relative resistance to the sulphonamides. In these circumstances benzylpenicillin (p. 71) should be prescribed.

It may be advisable to use sulphadimidine or sulphadiazine in doses of 0·5 g. twice daily, as a prophylactic measure against meningococcal meningitis, if this condition occurs in circumstances where infection may readily be disseminated, such as in a school or barracks.

Infections of the Urinary Tract. Many infections of the urinary tract are due to *Escherichia coli* and, if the organism is sensitive, may be treated with sulphadimidine. After a loading dose of 2 g., 1 g. eight-hourly is adequate as the drug is concentrated in the urine. The development of resistant organisms limits the usefulness of sulphadimidine in this sphere (p. 815).

Phthalylsulphathiazole (Sulphathalidine). This preparation, which is poorly absorbed, is converted in the large intestine to sulphathiazole in bacteriostatic concentrations. Hence it may be given before operations on the colon since it diminishes the risk of peritonitis developing from contamination with the contents of the gut. It may also be used in the treatment of bacillary dysentery (p. 958), but in Britain many of the organisms causing bacillary dysentery are now resistant to the sulphonamides.

Sodium Sulphacetamide. This preparation is used in the treatment of uncomplicated cases of mucopurulent conjunctivitis. A 10 or 30 per cent. solution is dropped into the conjunctival sac at hourly intervals. For more severe infections and for corneal ulceration antibiotics such as benzylpenicillin (p. 71) or neomycin (p. 83) will be required.

Long-acting Sulphonamides. The long-acting sulphonamides, such as sulphamethoxypyridazine (Lederkyn), are rapidly absorbed and very slowly excreted so that one daily dose may suffice. Apart from the convenience of less frequent administration these sulphonamides have no other advantages over their predecessors and, as they are more extensively bound to plasma proteins, their antibacterial action is less effective. Accordingly their use is not recommended.

Dangers of Sulphonamides

Although the sulphonamides carry a wide range of potential hazards, the incidence of these is low when a preparation such as sulphadimidine is used. Rashes, fever, agranulocytosis, haematuria and anuria are sometimes encountered. The risks of haematuria and anuria can be decreased by ensuring an ample output of urine. Serious but rare complications are haemolytic anaemia, aplastic anaemia, purpura and the Stevens-Johnson syndrome which may be induced by the long-acting sulphonamides. When any of the above complications develops, the drug must be withdrawn at once. Cyanosis due to methaemoglobinaemia, and nausea and vomiting, which were so commonly encountered with the earlier preparations, very rarely occur with sulphadimidine.

Sulphonamide preparations should not be used as local applications to the skin. Such contact may result in a reaction due to hypersensitivity to solar radiation, when exposure of any part of the skin surface to even a moderate degree of sunlight will produce eczema, and this state may persist for a number of years. This capacity to act as a photo-sensitiser is distinct from the development of hypersensitivity to the drug itself.

THE ANTIBIOTICS

The antibiotics may be divided, for practical purposes, into two main categories. Those included in the *first category* are mainly in general use and their therapeutic values are well established. This category comprises the penicillins, erythromycin, streptomycin, the tetracyclines and chloramphenicol. Although the indications for the oral use of chloramphenicol are restricted, it has a place in the treatment of topical infections and is conveniently described alongside the tetracyclines.

The *second category* consists of those antibiotics in less common use either because the indications for them are more limited or because they are deliberately kept in reserve. While the majority of infections can now be controlled by the penicillins, streptomycin, or the tetracyclines, there are special circumstances in which other antibiotics are required, either because of insensitivity of the organism or hypersensitivity of the patient. The antibiotics which may have an important part to play in these circumstances can be classified as follows:

1. Antibiotics mainly effective against gram-positive bacteria
   Fucidin
   Lincomycin
   Bacitracin.
2. Antibiotics mainly effective against gram-negative bacteria
   Kanamycin, gentamycin and neomycin
   Cycloserine
   Colistin and polymyxin.
3. Antibiotic effective against both gram-positive and gram-negative bacteria
   Cephaloridine
4. Antibiotics effective against fungi
   Nystatin
   Griseofulvin
   Amphotericin B.

CATEGORY I. ANTIBIOTICS IN COMMON USE

The Penicillins

This group of antibiotics is composed of various penicillins, some occurring naturally, and others produced by a semi-synthetic process. All have a bactericidal action and the range of the activity of the group is now wide, as both gram-positive and certain gram-negative organisms are sensitive to individual penicillins. The only adverse effect is the risk of inducing a hypersensitivity reaction in some persons, and when this occurs with one member of the group, the others have a similar, potentially dangerous effect. Even so the penicillins are the most useful antibiotics at present available.

The group can be subdivided into six sub-groups for descriptive purposes:

1. *Benzylpenicillin.* This is the original penicillin which, when given by injection, is highly effective for short periods.

2. *Procaine benzylpenicillin and benzathine penicillin.* These are long-acting penicillins which are administered parenterally.

3. *Phenoxymethylpenicillin and its synthetic analogues.* These penicillins are effective when administered by mouth.

4. *Cloxacillin and methicillin.* These penicillins are reserved for the treatment of severe staphylococcal infections resistant to benzylpenicillin.

5. *Ampicillin.* This penicillin has the additional property of being effective against gram-negative bacilli, in contrast to the other penicillins whose activity is largely limited to gram-positive organisms and gram-negative cocci.

6. *Carbenicillin.* This broad spectrum antibiotic is the first penicillin to be effective against *Ps. pyocyanea.*

1. Benzylpenicillin

The naturally occurring penicillins constitute a group of closely related acids whose sodium, potassium and other salts can be used for therapeutic purposes. Benzylpenicillin ('crystalline' or 'soluble' penicillin) is the sodium or potassium salt of one of these acids, penicillin G. It is rapidly absorbed following intramuscular injection and is excreted by the kidneys within a few hours. Half a million units (300 mg.) twice daily will suffice for most infections due to sensitive organisms. By prescribing larger doses, such as 2-6 million units of benzylpenicillin intramuscularly, very high blood levels of penicillin can be produced and therapeutic concentrations can be achieved within deep-seated or walled-off foci of infection, as occur in bacterial endocarditis or lung abscess. Quantities of this order are painful to inject and, therefore, must not be administered unnecessarily. Probenecid given concurrently with benzylpenicillin will raise the blood level of penicillin by delaying its excretion by the kidney and hence reduce the size, number and pain of the injections. The dose of probenecid is 2 g. daily by mouth.

Benzylpenicillin passes only in small quantities from the blood into the normal cerebrospinal fluid or through the normal pleural, pericardial or synovial membranes. Although in the presence of inflammation its diffusion to these sites is greater, benzylpenicillin will also have to be given by local injection when treating severe infections of the central nervous system, joints, pleura or pericardium.

2. Procaine Benzylpenicillin and Benzathine Penicillin

These are long-acting penicillins given by injection and used in the treatment of the treponemal diseases, syphilis and yaws. *Procaine benzylpenicillin* in aqueous suspension intramuscularly, in a dose of 600,000 units once daily, is relatively painless and will maintain an adequate blood level of penicillin for 24 hours. The addition of aluminium monostearate to procaine benzylpenicillin (P.A.M.) still further prolongs its action and this preparation has a limited application, e.g. in the treatment of syphilis.

Benzathine penicillin has a much longer duration of action than procaine benzylpenicillin. A single injection of 600,000 units will maintain, for about one week, blood levels suitable for the treatment of chronic diseases such as yaws, but which would be inadequate in the case of acute infections such as bronchopneumonia. Benzathine penicillin may be useful when the patient cannot be relied upon to report regularly for treatment.

3. Phenoxymethylpenicillin and its Analogues for Oral Use

Phenoxymethylpenicillin (Penicillin V) is a stable acid which, unlike benzylpenicillin, is unaffected by gastric hydrochloric acid. The oral administration of 250 mg. will produce blood levels which compare favourably with those resulting from the intramuscular injection of 200,000 units of benzylpenicillin. The usual dose of phenoxymethylpenicillin is 250 mg. every four to six hours, preferably given at least half an hour before meals to ensure maximum absorption.

The discovery in 1960 at the Beecham Research Laboratories of a process for manufacturing the penicillin 'nucleus', 6-aminopenicillanic acid, on a large scale, has made many new synthetic penicillins available by the addition of various side chains to the nucleus, e.g. phenoxyethylpenicillin or phenethicillin (Broxil) and phenoxypropylpenicillin or propicillin (Ultrapen). These compounds produce higher blood levels than phenoxymethylpenicillin but as their effectiveness *in vivo* may be less and as they are more expensive, they are not to be preferred.

Penicillin given orally has obvious advantages in ease of administration. The severe anaphylactoid reaction which occasionally follows the injection of penicillin is much less frequently encountered when the antibiotic is given by mouth. Provided the infection is due to an organism highly sensitive to penicillin and provided the patient is not seriously ill or vomiting, phenoxymethylpenicillin may be prescribed, particularly for infants and children. If the patient is seriously ill, unable to swallow, vomiting or unreliable, or if the organism is relatively inaccessible or only moderately sensitive, benzylpenicillin must be given by intramuscular injection. Provided the organism is sensitive, the antibacterial activity of benzylpenicillin is the greatest of all the penicillins.

4. **Cloxacillin and Methicillin**

Unlike benzylpenicillin, these synthetic penicillins are normally unaffected by the penicillinase produced by many staphylococci. They are, however, inactivated by the penicillinase produced by other species, e.g. *Esch. coli.* Cloxacillin and methicillin should be kept in reserve solely for the treatment of severe staphylococcal infections resistant to benzylpenicillin. *Cloxacillin* (Orbenin) is superior to methicillin in that it is ten times more active *in vitro* and is not destroyed by gastric hydrochloric acid and can, therefore, be given orally. The dose is 500 mg. six-hourly but in the case of seriously ill patients treatment should be initiated by the intramuscular injection of 250 mg. every four hours, especially if there is any doubt about the efficacy of absorption from the alimentary tract. Neither cloxacillin nor methicillin can be prescribed if the patient is sensitive to benzylpenicillin. In these circumstances erythromycin, fucidin, lincomycin or cephaloridine may be used.

5. **Ampicillin** (Penbritin)

This is a synthetic penicillin which is effective by mouth and which has a bactericidal action not only against gram-positive organisms but also against a variety of gram-negative organisms, notably Salmonella, Shigella, *H. influenzae* and certain strains of *Esch. coli* and *Proteus.* It is unaffected by acid gastric juice. Its use is limited by its destruction by penicillinase, by hypersensitivity reactions in many patients and by the development of bacterial resistance. At present its main use is in urinary tract infections due to *Esch. coli* and *Proteus* and in exacerbations of bronchitis. Ampicillin is an effective alternative to chloramphenicol in enteric fever and is preferable in the treatment of the carrier state. It is given orally in a dosage of 250 mg.-1 g. four to eight-hourly and for a period of time depending on the nature and severity of the infection. Preparations for administration by injection are now available.

6. Carbenicillin (Pyopen)

This antibiotic, introduced in 1967, has a wider range of activity than ampicillin against gram- negative organisms and, in particular, is active against *Ps. pyocyanea*. Unfortunately carbenicillin can be given only by injection and its administration by the intramuscular route is painful. The standard dose is 1 g. every six hours but larger quantities are required for *Ps. pyocyanea* infections. The usefulness of this new antibiotic remains to be determined.

Principal Indications for the Penicillins

Infections of the Respiratory System

In pneumococcal (lobar) pneumonia penicillin is preferable to sulphadimidine. Acute bronchitis or bronchopneumonia may respond to benzylpenicillin alone, but this antibiotic should be combined with streptomycin if a mixed infection is responsible, especially if *H. influenzae* is one of the invaders, as is often the case. In these circumstances ampicillin may be preferable, particularly in the elderly who tolerate streptomycin poorly. An empyema can be treated by aspiration of the pus and the injection of 500,000-1,000,000 units of benzylpenicillin into the pleural cavity, provided the organism is sensitive to penicillin.

Infections due to Streptococcus Pyogenes

In the prophylaxis and treatment of infections due to streptococcus pyogenes such as acute tonsillitis, acute otitis media, erysipelas and puerperal fever, penicillin is preferable to sulphadimidine because its bactericidal action more rapidly eliminates the organism and reduces the risk of the later development of rheumatic fever or acute nephritis. Recurrences of rheumatic fever can best be prevented by the oral administration of phenoxymethylpenicillin (Penicillin V) in a dose of 125 mg. twice daily for five years or until the child has left school, whichever is the longer.

Bacterial Endocarditis

Many cases of bacterial endocarditis are caused by *Streptococcus viridans* and can be treated successfully with benzylpenicillin in a dosage depending on the sensitivity of the organism as described on p. 216.

All patients with rheumatic or congenital valvular disease of the heart undergoing dental extractions, tonsillectomy, or any other procedures likely to result in transient bacteraemia, should be given penicillin as a prophylactic measure against bacterial endocarditis. The method recommended by the Ministry of Health is 300,000 units each of benzylpenicillin and procaine benzylpenicillin one hour before the operation followed by another 300,000 units of procaine benzylpenicillin 6 to 12 hours later. Prophylactic therapy should not be commenced earlier, as this might favour the elimination of sensitive organisms and their replacement by those that are insensitive.

Staphylococcal Infections

Unfortunately many strains of pathogenic staphylococci have emerged with a high degree of resistance to benzylpenicillin, especially in hospitals where this antibiotic is used freely. In every staphylococcal infection the possibility of the organism being resistant to benzylpenicillin must be considered and therefore its sensitivity should be determined by *in vitro* tests as soon as possible. If the staphylococcus proves to be resistant, the alternative antibiotics are cloxacillin, erythromycin, fucidin, lincomycin and cephaloridine, the last four having the additional value of being suitable if the patient is hypersensitive to the penicillins.

Meningitis

Meningococcal meningitis was formerly treated with sulphonamides alone (p. 68) but the emergence of relatively resistant organisms in some areas requires supplementary treatment with benzylpenicillin. Other forms of meningitis due to penicillin sensitive infections (pneumococcal, streptococcal) should be treated with benzylpenicillin by intrathecal and intramuscular injection for a period depending on the clinical response. Intrathecal administration may be required if penicillin given by other routes does not traverse the blood-brain barrier in adequate amounts, but the daily intrathecal dosage should not exceed 20,000 units if an irritant effect is to be avoided.

Gonorrhoea and Syphilis

Penicillin is at present the antibiotic used in the routine treatment of these diseases. There is evidence of a moderate increase in resistance of the gonococcus to penicillin and accordingly larger doses of the antibiotic are now required. In treating gonorrhoea the danger of suppressing but not curing syphilis contracted at the same time must be remembered.

Urinary Tract Infections

Ampicillin and carbenicillin are effective in disease due to sensitive strains of *Proteus* and *Esch. coli* and carbenicillin may be used in *Ps. pyocyanea* infection.

Vincent's angina, Anthrax, Actinomycosis, Tetanus and Gas Gangrene.

Benzylpenicillin is effective in these conditions and is very useful as a prophylactic measure against tetanus and gas gangrene in traumatised patients.

Dangers of Penicillin

An increasing number of patients have acquired a hypersensitivity to the systemic administration of penicillin, in the form of a skin eruption, fever or even of an acute anaphylactic reaction which has occasionally proved fatal. The patient should always be asked about any previous allergic reaction to penicillin before treatment is commenced. If such a history is given, penicillin should not be prescribed, even if a different form had previously been used. Patients who suffer from bronchial asthma or who are hypersensitive to other drugs are particularly liable to become allergic to penicillin. A mild hypersensitivity state developing during treatment may be controlled by an antihistamine drug; a more severe reaction will demand a change of antibiotic. Desensitisation is rarely practicable and even if successful may only be temporary. The treatment of anaphylactic shock is described on p. 26.

It is important to avoid accidental intravenous administration, especially when injecting procaine benzylpenicillin intramuscularly as this may result in a very severe disturbance consisting of a sensation of impending death, paraesthesiae and confusion lasting up to an hour and followed by exhaustion and anxiety for several days.

The skin may be hypersensitive to the application of an antibiotic, and this is usually the result of previous contact with the substance. Such hypersensitivity to penicillin is so frequently encountered that its routine use as an ointment is contraindicated in the common pyodermias, such as impetigo and folliculitis.

A purified form of benzylpenicillin (Purapen G) became available in 1967 from which one potent allergen had been removed. While this preparation should not be given to patients known to be hypersensitive to penicillin, its use may help to prevent the development of allergy in the future.

Erythromycin

Erythromycin has a range of activity similar to penicillin but it differs in being predominantly bacteriostatic. This antibiotic was formerly kept in reserve for the treatment of staphylococcal infections resistant to benzylpenicillin, but, with more effective antibiotics now available, erythromycin can be used for more general purposes. Its main application is in adults or children suffering from an infection which would normally be treated with an oral penicillin, but in whom this is precluded because of hypersensitivity. Erythromycin estolate gives the most satisfactory blood levels and is prescribed in a dosage of 250 mg. by mouth every six hours. It may cause liver damage if given for longer than a fortnight. Allergic reactions to erythromycin are rare unless the antibiotic is used topically.

Streptomycin

The outstanding advantage of this antibiotic is its bactericidal effect on the tubercle bacillus. Its value in controlling certain infections due to gram-negative bacilli is also of clinical importance. Its disadvantages are the serious toxic reactions which are discussed below and the fact that bacteria readily acquire resistance to the antibiotic. Kanamycin, gentamycin and neomycin which are closely related to streptomycin, are described on p. 83.

Principal Indications

Tuberculosis. Streptomycin is highly effective against the tubercle bacillus if used in conjunction with para-aminosalicylic acid (PAS) or isoniazid or both in order to prevent the emergence of resistant strains. For long term therapy the daily dose of streptomycin should not exceed 1 g. The chemotherapy of tuberculosis is discussed in detail on pages 425-429.

Bacterial Endocarditis. When this condition is due to an organism relatively resistant to penicillin, such as *Str. faecalis*, good results may be obtained by combining streptomycin with large doses of penicillin.

Certain Infections due to Gram-negative Organisms

Mixed Infections. Peritonitis, acute exacerbations of chronic bronchitis and bronchopneumonia are often due to mixed infections with gram-positive and gram-negative organisms and require antibiotics with a wide range of activity for their control. A combination of 500,000 units of benzylpenicillin and 0·5 g. of streptomycin twice daily is effective as these antibiotics are synergistic and provide the parenteral therapy which is often necessary, e.g. in a post-operative patient suffering from peritonitis.

Bacillary Dysentery. Streptomycin is not absorbed when given by mouth and hence can be used in the treatment of intestinal infections, such as dysentery due to sensitive organisms. One or two grams are given daily in divided doses for about five days.

Plague, Tularaemia and Friedländer's Pneumonia. Streptomycin is the treatment of choice in these conditions.

Urinary Tract Infections. Urinary infections due to sensitive gram-negative organisms can be treated with this antibiotic provided the urine is kept alkaline, as streptomycin, being a base, is inactive in an acid medium. It is now possible to prescribe simpler and more effective therapy with less risk of the development of resistant organisms and streptomycin has largely been superseded by other antibiotics in the treatment of urinary tract infections.

Dangers of Streptomycin

The outstanding toxic effect is on the eighth nerve. The vestibular division is affected first with resultant vertigo and incoordination. Later there may be deafness. The damage is directly proportional to the age of the patient and to the size of the dose and the duration of its administration; the smaller doses now employed have much reduced the frequency and severity of this complication. The risk is enhanced if there is any impairment of renal function and consequently streptomycin must be given with great caution to any patient with kidney disease. Sensitivity to streptomycin, usually in the form of skin eruptions and fever, may be acquired in some cases. Desensitisation may be indicated if it is essential to continue with this antibiotic. This is achieved by administering streptomycin intramuscularly in very small doses which are gradually increased daily or, in more urgent cases, by continuing with streptomycin in therapeutic doses under cover of prednisolone.

The Tetracyclines

Chlortetracycline (Aureomycin), oxytetracycline (Terramycin) and tetracycline (Achromycin) are very closely related substances which, for practical purposes, show no difference in their antibacterial actions. Their range of activity is extensive and this has led to the tetracyclines being known as 'broad-spectrum' antibiotics. This is offset to some extent by their action being bacteriostatic and not bactericidal.

An average dose for an adult is 250 mg. at six-hourly intervals, given in the form of a capsule or a tablet. This is sufficient to combat most sensitive organisms. If the patient is seriously ill, or the organism relatively resistant, larger doses may rarely be indicated but the daily total should not exceed 2 g. Oral administration is adequate unless the patient is vomiting or comatose, when parenteral therapy will be required and for this purpose rolitetracycline is the preparation of choice.

Demethylchlortetracycline (Ledermycin) and methacycline (Rondomycin) attain higher and more prolonged blood levels than other tetracyclines and hence may be given less frequently. These advantages, however, are counter-balanced by the high degree of plasma binding which occurs and which reduces the antibacterial activity of these compounds.

Principal Indications

The tetracyclines have a bacteriostatic effect against a wide variety of gram-positive and gram-negative bacteria, rickettsial infections such as typhus fever and Q fever and *Entamoeba histolytica*. They are ineffective in uncomplicated virus infections, except in those due to the psittacosis-lymphogranuloma group whose identity as viruses is disputed. The tetracyclines may limit the severity of pertussis if given in the first week of the disease and they are effective in the treatment of brucellosis. Thus this group of antibiotics is of particular value in the treatment of typhus fever, Q fever, amoebiasis, psittacosis (ornithosis), lymphogranuloma venereum, pertussis and undulant fever.

In addition to these specific indications the tetracyclines have a wide sphere of usefulness in the treatment of many other conditions more frequently encountered, such as infections of the respiratory tract. They are particularly effective in the treatment of acute exacerbations of chronic bronchitis and in pneumonia due to *Mycoplasma pneumoniae*. In other infections the tetracyclines provide a useful alternative to penicillin, for example if the response is poor or if the patient is hypersensitive to penicillin. Although the tetracyclines can be used in the treatment of bacillary dysentery and of urinary tract infection their effectiveness is limited by their bacteriostatic action and the development of resistant organisms. As in the case of penicillin, the staphylococcus, which was initially highly sensitive to the tetracyclines, is now often found to have acquired a resistance to these antibiotics, especially in hospitals. When resistance occurs it is common to all members of the tetracycline group.

Chlortetracycline is the antibiotic of choice for the local treatment of many infections of the skin as it does not cause eczematous sensitisation.

Dangers of the Tetracyclines

Many of the normal saprophytes of the alimentary tract are sensitive to the tetracyclines and may be eliminated when these antibiotics are administered. Insensitive organisms are then free to multiply and 'superinfection' may develop which can be very difficult to control. This happens particularly with fungi, such as monilia, which cause stomatitis, glossitis or an anal or vulvar pruritus which can be very distressing. Some of these lesions resemble riboflavine deficiency, but treatment with Vitamin B complex is not beneficial, whereas the antibiotic nystatin is effective. In hospital the risk of superinfection with resistant staphylococci is even more serious and the ensuing enteritis, septicaemia or pneumonia may prove fatal. The incidence of all these adverse effects is directly related to the duration of therapy; the tetracyclines should not normally be prescribed for more than one week. Should longer periods of treatment be essential, as in the management of some cases of chronic bronchitis, the patient must be kept under observation in view of the risks involved. When monilial infection threatens to interfere with the long term treatment of chronic bronchitis, tetracycline may be given in conjunction with nystatin.

The danger of 'superinfection' following the use of the tetracyclines illustrates the principle that a broad-spectrum antibiotic should not be prescribed if an antibiotic is available which is effective against the specific organism responsible for the illness. This is especially the case in hospital practice where the risk of cross-infection with resistant organisms is always present.

Severe liver damage has been reported in pregnant women with pyelonephritis treated with tetracycline administered intravenously. The tetracyclines cause staining of the deciduous teeth and interfere, temporarily, with the growth and development of bones in infants. Accordingly this group of antibiotics is contraindicated in pregnant women and young children when other effective chemotherapy is available.

Chloramphenicol

Chloramphenicol (Chloromycetin) has a range of activity similar to that of the tetracyclines but with the important difference that it is effective in typhoid and paratyphoid fever. This was the only specific therapy available for these infections until 1961 when ampicillin was synthesised. Chloramphenicol is more active than the tetracyclines against *H. influenzae* and is to be preferred to them in the treatment of meningitis due to this organism. The daily dose of chloramphenicol for an adult is 1-2 g.; 1-2 capsules, each containing 250 mg. are given at six-hourly intervals for about five days. Preparations for parenteral administration, and ointments for the local treatment of susceptible infections, are also available.

Dangers of Chloramphenicol

As in the case of the tetracyclines, chloramphenicol may cause gastrointestinal disturbances and its prolonged use may be followed by similar superinfections. Much more serious, although fortunately rare, are the blood dyscrasias which have been reported following its use. This antibiotic has in its chemical structure a benzene ring of the type known to cause bone marrow aplasia. Although the risk of the development of aplastic anaemia is remote, unless chloramphenicol is prescribed repeatedly or for prolonged periods, its use is justified only in the presence of a serious infection for which there is no alternative therapy.

Chloramphenicol should never be given to premature infants and very rarely to the newborn because of the risk of the development of the 'grey syndrome'. This is a state of peripheral circulatory failure caused by the very high blood levels of chloramphenicol found in these children in whom conjugation of the antibiotic is defective as compared with adults.

CATEGORY II. ANTIBIOTICS IN LESS COMMON USE

Antibiotics mainly effective against gram-positive bacteria

Lincomycin. This was isolated in 1961 and resembles erythromycin in its range of activity, its effectiveness against staphylococci and its low toxicity. It is particularly useful in staphylococcal osteomyelitis as it can penetrate into bone. Lincomycin is given by mouth in doses of 500 mg. six-hourly.

Fucidin. This is the sodium salt of fusidic acid and is particularly effective against staphylococci, being bactericidal in its action. It has a place in the treatment of staphylococcal infections in patients who are hypersensitive to the penicillins. Fucidin is well tolerated, rapidly absorbed and is effective by mouth in doses of 500 mg. thrice daily.

Bacitracin. This is not absorbed when given by mouth and is too toxic for parenteral administration. As in the case of certain other antibiotics with these limitations, it may be used topically for infection of the skin or for the irrigation of wounds or burns, either alone or in conjunction with an antibiotic effective against gram-negative organisms such as neomycin or polymyxin or both as in Polybactrin. Bacitracin may also be used for the treatment of superinfection of the bowel with staphylococci.

Antibiotics mainly effective against gram-negative bacteria

Kanamycin, Gentamycin and Neomycin. These are related to streptomycin but differ from it in that resistant organisms are slow to appear. *Kanamycin* is less toxic than neomycin and can be given parenterally. It should be reserved for the treatment, in hospital, of serious infections such as peritonitis or septicaemia due to *Esch. coli* or *Proteus* insensitive to safer antibiotics. As with streptomycin there is a risk of damage to the eighth nerve especially in the elderly or if renal function is impaired. The dose, which should be controlled when possible by estimating the concentration of the antibiotic in the blood, should not exceed 1 g. daily, given intramuscularly in a dose of 0·25 g. six-hourly. *Gentamycin* resembles kanamycin but has the additional advantage of being effective against *Ps. pyocyanea*. *Neomycin* is too toxic to be given parenterally but, as it rarely causes allergic reactions, ointments containing neomycin are extensively used in infections of the skin and eye. As neomycin is poorly absorbed it can be given by mouth in the treatment of intestinal infections and for the 'sterilisation' of the bowel pre-operatively or in the management of hepatic coma.

Cycloserine is a bactericidal antibiotic which is used in the treatment of urinary tract infections, particularly those due to *Esch. coli* which have not responded to other antibacterial agents. Cycloserine is administered by mouth in doses of 250 mg. twice daily for a fortnight to adults weighing more than 50 kg. (110 lb.). In patients weighing less than this the dose should be reduced to 125 mg. twice daily. At the extremes of life the dose should never exceed this level. In infants the dose is 62·5 mg. twice daily. In larger doses or if renal function is impaired it is liable to have a toxic action on the central nervous system and cause disturbances such as drowsiness or epilepsy. Recurrent infection with *Esch. coli* can be prevented by long-term treatment with 125-250 mg. cycloserine on alternate days.

Colistin and Polymyxin. Colistin is identical with polymyxin E and is also known as colimycin and the proprietary preparation Colomycin. It has a bactericidal effect against many gram-negative organisms and notably against *Pseudomonas pyocyanea*. There is evidence of an increasing incidence of infection with this organism especially in debilitated patients. Colistin is less painful to administer than polymyxin and accordingly is the antibiotic of choice and should be reserved for the treatment of infections due to *Ps. pyocyanea.* It is given by intramuscular injection in a dosage of 1-3 million units eight-hourly depending on the weight of the patient.

Polymyxin B is used in conjunction with bacitracin for the topical treatment of wounds, pressure sores, etc.

Antibiotic effective against both gram-positive and gram-negative bacteria

Cephaloridine (cephalosporin C, ceporin) became available commercially in 1964 and is the most important of a group of closely related antibiotics, which includes cephalothin, cephalosporin N (Synnematin B) and cephalosporin P. The last has a steroid structure and is closely related to fucidin.

Cephaloridine has a structure resembling penicillin and a very wide range of bactericidal activity against gram-positive and gram-negative bacteria. This antibiotic is given by injection in doses of 250-500 mg. twice daily or more frequently in very severe infections. Cephaloridine is excreted unchanged in the urine. It is resistant to penicillinase and is very well tolerated, apart from occasional renal tubular damage if very large doses are given. It is useful in severe staphylococcal infection when the penicillins are contraindicated, in pyelonephritis or in resistant bacterial endocarditis and in septicaemia due to gram-negative infections. Meantime the facts that cephaloridine is expensive and that it has to be given parenterally, detract from its value, except in severe infections not responding to standard therapy.

Antibiotics effective against fungi

Nystatin is effective against *Candida albicans*, a normal inhabitant of the mouth and intestine but which may proliferate to cause thrush in debilitated, diabetic or pregnant patients, or if the normal flora is suppressed by a broad spectrum antibiotic such as tetracycline. Lesions of the alimentary tract are treated with tablets, containing 500,000 units, thrice daily for three weeks. Pessaries are available for the treatment of vaginal infections and are inserted once or twice daily.

Griseofulvin is effective by mouth in dermatophytic infections causing ringworm of the skin, hair, and nails, where it appears to be taken up by newly formed keratin which is then resistant to further invasion by the fungus. Superficial skin lesions respond promptly but many months of treatment may be required to eradicate the infection from slowly growing tissues such as the nails. The antibiotic is given in doses of 1 g. daily and is well tolerated.

AMPHOTERICIN B is indicated only in the treatment of severe systemic mycoses such as coccidioidomycosis. It is given in increasing doses by intravenous injection and is very toxic.

SUMMARY OF PRINCIPAL INDICATIONS

The principal indications for the use of the sulphonamides and the antibiotics in the chemotherapy of the more common or important infections may be summarised as follows:

The Sulphonamides. Meningococcal meningitis; some infections of the urinary tract and colon; mucopurulent conjunctivitis.

ANTIBIOTICS IN GENERAL USE

The Penicillins

1. BENZYLPENICILLIN; PROCAINE BENZYLPENICILLIN; PHENOXYMETHYLPENICILLIN AND ITS ANALOGUES FOR ORAL USE. For infections of the respiratory system, haemolytic streptococcal infections, bacterial endocarditis, sensitive staphylococcal infections, pneumococcal or streptococcal meningitis, gonorrhoea, syphilis, Vincent's angina, etc. The choice of the penicillin depends on the sensitivity and the severity of the infection, benzylpenicillin being the preparation of choice for a seriously ill patient.

2. CLOXACILLIN. Reserved for the treatment of severe staphylococcal infections resistant to benzylpenicillin.

3. AMPICILLIN. For some urinary tract infections and exacerbations of bronchitis; an alternative to chloramphenicol in the enteric fevers.

4. CARBENICILLIN. For *Ps. pyocyanea* infections.

Erythromycin

An alternative to phenoxymethylpenicillin especially in those patients hypersensitive to the penicillins.

Streptomycin

For tuberculosis; in conjunction with benzylpenicillin in some cases of bacterial endocarditis and in mixed infections such as peritonitis.

Tetracyclines

For rickettsial infections, psittacosis-lymphogranuloma group of infections, amoebiasis, undulant fever, pertussis in its early stages, acute and chronic bronchitis and in infections due to *Mycoplasma pneumoniae*.

Chloramphenicol

For enteric fever and *H. influenzae* meningitis.

Antibiotics in Less Common Use

Antibiotics mainly effective against gram-positive bacteria

1. Lincomycin and Fucidin. For staphylococcal infections in patients hypersensitive to the penicillins.
2. Bacitracin. For topical use in conjunction with neomycin and polymyxin.

Antibiotics mainly effective against gram-negative bacteria

1. Kanamycin. Reserved for the parenteral treatment of severe infections due to gram-negative organisms.
2. Gentamycin. For *Ps. pyocyanea* infections.
3. Neomycin. For topical treatment of infections of the skin and eyes and for 'sterilisation' of the gut.
4. Cycloserine. For *Esch. coli* urinary tract infections.
5. Colistin and Polymyxin. Colistin (Polymyxin E) for infection due to *Ps. pyocyanea*. Polymyxin B for topical use in conjunction with bacitracin.

Antibiotic effective against both gram-positive and gram-negative bacteria

Cephaloridine. Should be reserved for the treatment of serious infections not responding to standard therapy.

Antibiotics effective against fungi

1. NYSTATIN. For monilial infections (thrush).
2. GRISEOFULVIN. For superficial dermatomycoses (ringworm).
3. AMPHOTERICIN B. For systemic mycoses.

J. G. MACLEOD.

ACUTE POISONING

Introduction

The great increase in the production in recent years of potent and dangerous drugs has been accompanied by a marked rise in the incidence of acute poisoning. This chapter deals with the clinical features, diagnosis and management of acute poisoning. The diagnosis and treatment of food poisoning are discussed on pp. 930-935. Only brief reference is made to industrial and agricultural poisons and none to poisoning by ionising radiation.

The incidence of acute poisoning is steadily rising and has now reached the alarming stage where one in every thousand of the adult population in Edinburgh is admitted to hospital each year suffering from intentional poisoning. Accidental poisoning in the home is also showing a steady increase, especially in children. The rate of poisoning in industry and agriculture, however, remains low despite the introduction of toxic substances for an increasing number of procedures. The deaths in Britain from all forms of poisoning amount to almost 7,000 per annum, a figure almost equal to the number of deaths from road accidents.

CLASSIFICATION OF POISONING

Persons poisoned can be classified into one of three groups: (*a*) accidental poisoning in the home, (*b*) intentional poisoning, and (*c*) industrial and agricultural poisoning.

Accidental Poisoning. Death from accidental poisoning has increased almost threefold in the past 30 years, women being more likely than men to die in this way. The frequency rate of accidental poisoning for Scotland is the highest in Europe and shows no sex difference. However, except in children it is doubtful if the official statistics reflect the true incidence of accidental poisoning. For example, many more adults are certified as dying each year from accidental poisoning by barbiturates than from suicidal poisoning by this drug. It is, however, difficult to believe that more than a few adults in a year accidentally consume a lethal dose of barbiturates. Licence in certification is most likely to account for the large numbers apparently dying from accidental poisoning.

Substances involved in Accidental Poisoning. Death from accidental poisoning is the result most commonly of (*a*) carbon monoxide inhalation from domestic gas or fumes of incomplete combustion from stoves or motor car exhaust pipes, or (*b*) ingestion by children of household substances (e.g. paraffin or bleach), medicines (e.g. aspirin or iron tablets and liniments) and, rarely, poisonous berries; the highest death rate is in the age-group 1-4 years.

Intentional Poisoning. This covers a broad spectrum of patients ranging from a minority who are determined on self-destruction, i.e. 'suicidal poisoning', to the large group who till recently have been designated 'attempted suicidal poisoning' but who are more accurately described as 'indulging in self-poisoning'. The term 'attempted suicide' is best discarded, for it purports to provide an interpretation of the motives of the act of self-poisoning, an interpretation which is frequently incorrect. The majority of people who deliberately take poison do not have any strong intentions of self-destruction in mind; in fact, they often take steps to ensure that measures to bring about their recovery will be put in train immediately following the act. Self-poisoning is usually a conscious, often impulsive act, undertaken to manipulate a situation in order to secure redress of some circumstances which have become intolerable. Frequently relatives and society rally to the help of the unfortunate victim and the situation which has caused so much distress is rectified. Accidents, however, do occur through misjudgment of dosage or of a failure to ensure that help would be to hand, and an act which was committed merely to draw attention to a particular situation may end in death. Self-poisoning often occurs in a setting of poverty and alcoholism and with a background of a broken home in childhood. The alarming increase in the incidence of acute poisoning is largely due to self-poisoning. Out of every 100 adult poisoned patients admitted to hospital, at least 90 will be suffering from self-poisoning and this proportion is greater in countries where the welfare state is more highly organised.

Under the heading of intentional poisoning, in addition to suicidal and self-poisoning, homicidal poisoning should be included for the sake of completeness.

Substances and Methods used in Intentional Poisoning. *Self-poisoning.* Almost any substance may be taken for self-poisoning, but the choice is approximately as follows, as based on the statistics of poisoned patients admitted to the Poisoning Treatment Centre of the Royal Infirmary, Edinburgh:

1. Barbiturates, 50 per cent. The frequency with which this group of drugs is taken rises with age.
2. Salicylates, 15 per cent. A marked preponderance of younger people who take poison are in this group.
3. Tranquillisers and antidepressants, 15 per cent. The proportion resorting to these drugs has steadily increased in recent years.
4. Coal-gas, 7 per cent. The older age-group show a definite preference for coal-gas. It may be difficult to determine whether coal-gas poisoning is accidental or self-poisoning, but it is not a real kindness to regard the incident as accidental when in fact it was due to a state of depression requiring investigation and treatment.
5. Non-barbiturate hypnotics, 8 per cent.
6. Other drugs, e.g. iron, quinine and digitalis, 5 per cent.

Combinations of drugs are frequently taken and alcohol, which enhances the effect of certain drugs, may also be involved.

Suicide. The methods adopted for deliberate self-destruction vary from country to country and between the sexes. In Britain domestic gas poisoning is by far the most common method employed by both sexes. In women the second choice is drugs and the third drowning. In males the second choice is by self injury, such as hanging or strangulation and the third choice poisoning with drugs. In America where firearms are more readily available this is the first choice by males but only the second by females. Poisoning by drugs is the first choice of females. Recently coal-gas in America has largely been replaced for domestic use by natural gas which is in itself not toxic; this has resulted in a steep decline in the use of gas for suicidal purposes and as a cause of accidental poisoning. Despite this decline the total incidence of poisoning has not fallen.

Industrial and Agricultural Poisoning. It is not intended to discuss the incidence or methods of acquiring poisoning in industry or agriculture. Suffice it is to record that lead (p. 1219), cyanide (p. 103), mercury, beryllium (p. 433) and cadmium are potential causes of industrial poisoning. In agriculture many highly toxic weedkillers of the dinitro-ortho-cresol group and the insecticides belonging to the organo-phosphorus compounds have been developed in recent years. They have been responsible for only a small number of cases of acute poisoning in Britain owing to adequate and effective legislation for controlling their use. In some countries, however, they have caused many deaths each spring.

DIAGNOSIS OF ACUTE POISONING

Information Service. With the increasing frequency of accidental and intentional poisoning it is important to determine whether the substance ingested is noxious. In Britain a Poisons Information Service is available to doctors telephoning one of the following numbers:

Belfast: Royal Victoria Hospital. Tel. 0232-30503.
Cardiff: Royal Infirmary. Tel. 0222-33101.
Edinburgh: Royal Infirmary. Tel. 031-229 2477.
Eire: Jervis Street Hospital. Tel. Dublin 45588.
Leeds: General Infirmary. Tel. 0532-32799.
London: Guy's Hospital. Tel. 01-HOP 7600.
Manchester: Booth Hall Children's Hospital. Tel. 061-CHE 2254.
Newcastle: Royal Victoria Infirmary. Tel. 0632-25131.

Information can be immediately obtained regarding the ingredients of a substance, the fatal dose of a poison and the best method of treatment can be discussed with a physician trained in clinical toxicology.

Differential Diagnosis. The diagnosis of acute poisoning is usually made on the history obtained from relatives or friends, from circumstantial evidence, such as finding tablets at the bedside and from a prompt physical examination with special reference to the degree of unconsciousness and circulatory and respiratory failure. It is very important to exclude other causes of coma (p. 1113). In addition, a decision should be reached as to whether the poison has been swallowed, inhaled or absorbed from the skin. Few poisons produce diagnostic clinical features, but the smell of coal-gas associated with the classical but somewhat uncommon cherry-pink colour of the lips, the hyperpnoea and initial sweating of salicylate poisoning, the markedly depressed respiration and pin-point pupils of opiate poisoning will be helpful on occasions in arriving at a precise diagnosis. It is important that the start of treatment should not be delayed by spending excessive time in attempting to identify precisely the poison involved, since there is seldom a specific antidote and the essential immediate treatment of poisoning is dependent on the application of well established basic therapeutic principles. Every hospital, nevertheless, should have some scheme for making easier the identification of capsules and tablets which are often used in poisoning. For this purpose a coloured diagram or even examples of the more common drugs can be mounted on a board. The marking of tablets with code letters and numbers has recently been introduced to a limited extent and has already proved of value in identification. Laboratory analysis of gastric aspirate, blood or urine will confirm the diagnosis. Qualitative and quantitative estimation of carboxyhaemoglobin, salicylate, barbiturate (with group identification) and of alcohol and iron should be possible within 90 minutes of the receipt of the specimen. These results will, in addition to confirming the diagnosis, be of some value in deciding on further treatment. They may also be of value for medico-legal purposes.

General Therapeutic Measures

1. Removal or Inactivation of the Poison. It cannot be emphasised too strongly that it is very important that the poison should be got rid of as quickly as possible. This first-aid treatment will often be given by the general practitioner in the patient's home while awaiting the arrival of an ambulance. The patient who is inhaling a poisonous gas must be removed to fresh air as quickly as possible. When a liquid or solid poison is in contact with the patient's clothes these must be discarded at once and any poison on the skin must be washed off to prevent absorption. When poison has been swallowed the decision as to whether emesis and gastric aspiration and lavage should be undertaken will depend on three factors: (*a*) the substance ingested, (*b*) the state of consciousness of the patient, and (*c*) the length of time since the poison was ingested.

Regarding the substance ingested, the only contraindication to inducing emesis or passing a stomach tube is the knowledge that paraffin oil (kerosene) or other petroleum distillates have been swallowed, as the entry of even a small quantity of these substances into the lungs will lead to a severe pneumonitis. Great care must be exercised in passing a stomach tube in corrosive poisoning, in alcoholics, in patients who have had gastric surgery and in the very young and elderly, but the benefits from gastric aspiration and lavage outweigh the potential dangers of perforating the oesophagus or stomach.

The second factor to be considered is the state of consciousness. Fully conscious patients should be made to vomit by putting one's finger into the throat; if initially unsuccessful this can be repeated after giving a tumblerful of tepid water containing a dessertspoonful of common salt. When this is impracticable as in a hysterical, violent patient, apomorphine hydrochloride, 5 mg. may be given intramuscularly. It is a powerful emetic but unfortunately it can produce hypotension, dangerous collapse and persistent vomiting. These effects can, however, be antagonised by administering 15 mg. of nalorphine. Syrup of Ipecac, 15 ml., recommended by certain authorities as worthy of a place in every home medicine cupboard, is in practice almost invariably too slow in action to be of any value. After successful emesis, gastric aspiration and lavage is still essential.

In a semiconscious patient emetics are to be avoided in view of the danger of aspiration pneumonitis, but gastric aspiration and lavage can be employed provided the cough reflex is still present. Gastric lavage in the deeply unconscious patient without this reflex is a highly dangerous procedure unless the lungs can be protected by the insertion of a cuffed endotracheal tube.

The third factor to be considered is the time which has elapsed since the ingestion of the poison. If four hours have elapsed since a barbiturate was taken very little or no recovery of the drug will be achieved by undertaking emesis and gastric lavage; if it is known that the barbiturate was taken less than four hours previously aspiration and lavage may be helpful. In salicylate poisoning, because of the almost inevitable pylorospasm which prevents the drug from leaving the stomach, it is virtually never too late to undertake these procedures and large amounts of salicylates may be recovered up to 24 hours after ingestion. In other forms of poisoning, provided the two factors already discussed have been considered, gastric aspiration and lavage should be undertaken if less than four hours have elapsed since the drug was taken.

Technique of Gastric Aspiration and Lavage. With the foot of the bed raised some 18 in. and the patient lying on his left side a wide-bore Jaques rubber stomach tube, English gauge 30, should be passed. A gag may be necessary to prevent biting on the tube. When the tube has been passed, its position in the stomach is verified by aspiration of stomach contents or by blowing a little air through it and auscultating over the abdomen when a bubbling sound will be heard. Aspiration may then be attempted with either a Dakin's syringe or a Senoran's evacuator, but in the writer's opinion they are of little value; it is best achieved by lowering the funnel to which the stomach tube is attached, to a level well below the patient's head. Aspiration is advisable prior to lavage as initial lavage will drive some of the stomach contents into the duodenum and promote absorption. When no further material can be aspirated repeated careful lavage with tepid water should be undertaken, using no more than 300 ml. for each single washout. Lavage should be continued until the returning fluid is clear. Except in the specific instances of opiate, cyanide or iron poisoning, little is achieved by employing lavage fluid other than water. If an opiate has been ingested, lavage should be undertaken with tepid water. Potassium permanganate (1 in 15,000-10,000) solution is recommended by some, but it is doubtful if this addition is of any real value. If cyanide has been ingested, the stomach should be washed out with 25 per cent. sodium thiosulphate. In acute iron poisoning lavage should be undertaken with 1 per cent. sodium bicarbonate.

After lavage no effort should be made to promote intestinal evacuation by leaving a laxative in the stomach, as in ill patients the ensuing diarrhoea may increase any existing electrolyte imbalance. It must be realised that on occasions, after lavage, some further impairment of consciousness may occur; hence except in iron poisoning the value of leaving fluid in the stomach may be outweighed by the dangers of subsequent aspiration pneumonitis if the patient has had no cuffed endotracheal tube inserted. However, with this possibility in mind and provided that no delay in further treatment is occasioned by the preparation of solutions, the following may be left in the stomach after lavage: 300 ml. milk on account of its demulcent properties in corrosive poisoning; the chelating agent desferrioxamine (Desferal) in acute iron poisoning (p. 102). It is frequently advised that on completion of gastric lavage for salicylate poisoning a solution of sodium bicarbonate should be left in the stomach. In the writer's opinion this is not recommended. Although the bicarbonate counteracts the irritation of the gastric mucosa and when absorbed will promote excretion of salicylate by rendering the urine alkaline, its presence in the stomach encourages absorption of further salicylate.

If considerable absorption has occurred the patient may be gravely ill, hence measures to enhance elimination of the poison may require to be undertaken. These can only be carried out in hospital because of the technical skill and special apparatus required. For this purpose the following procedures can be employed: (*a*) diuresis, (*b*) forced diuresis, (*c*) peritoneal dialysis, (*d*) haemodialysis, (*e*) exchange transfusion.

2. MAINTENANCE OF RESPIRATION. It is essential that there should be a clear airway. This can be ensured by removal of dentures, vomitus, foreign bodies and excess mucus. The patient should be turned on his side to prevent the tongue falling backwards and to avoid aspiration of vomitus and mucus. An oropharyngeal or cuffed endotracheal tube may have to be inserted to maintain a free airway. Artificial respiration is required if respiration is depressed, using preferably the method of expired air resuscitation (p. 181). Oxygen should be given through an oronasal mask (p. 321). Prophylactic antibiotics to 'protect' the lungs are not recommended. Any infection which develops should be treated energetically.

3. MANAGEMENT OF CIRCULATORY FAILURE. If the patient shows any degree of shock the foot of the bed should be raised. Warmth should be applied but excessive heat is to be avoided. Drugs should be given to counteract hypotension. For severe shock metaraminol should be given intramuscularly in a dose of 2 to 10 mg. Intravenous hydrocortisone is of value in severe shock but should only be given in hospital. Acute circulatory failure may also require treatment by infusion of whole blood, plasma or dextran (p. 179).

4. TREATMENT OF PAIN. Pain is an uncommon feature in poisoning except in corrosive poisoning in which it will require to be relieved by generous doses of morphine combined with cyclizine.

5. TREATMENT OF CONVULSIONS. Convulsions should be controlled with intramuscular injection of paraldehyde 5-10 ml. or sodium pentobarbitone, 100-200 mg.

As already noted 75 per cent. of all cases of poisoning admitted to hospital are due to the ingestion of barbiturates or salicylates, or to the inhalation of gas or fumes containing carbon monoxide. Accordingly it has been decided to limit the description of the clinical features and treatment to these three methods of poisoning. However, the treatment of poisoning by tranquilliser drugs, the non-barbiturate hypnotic drugs and antidepressants except the monoamine oxidase inhibitors, is essentially the same as that for barbiturate poisoning.

BARBITURATE POISONING

Clinical Features. In poisoning of moderate to severe degree there may be:

1. Impaired Consciousness. The degree of unconsciousness will vary and is best expressed by the following classification: Grade 1, response to vocal commands; Grade 2, maximal response to minimal painful stimulation; Grade 3, minimal response to maximal painful stimulation; Grade 4, Total unresponsiveness to maximal painful stimulation.

2. Hypotension. Hypotension is produced mainly by the toxic action of barbiturate on the heart and smooth muscles of the blood vessels. The heart rate is normal or only slightly increased.

3. Respiratory Depression. Both the rate and depth will be depressed. The clinical assessment of the degree of respiratory depression is very difficult. It can best be measured with Wright's spirometer; a minute volume of expired air of less than 3 litres per minute indicates severe depression necessitating immediate measures to improve ventilation.

4. Abnormal Reflexes. Diminution or absence of the limb reflexes varies and is not a good measure of the severity of the poisoning nor is the size of the pupils or the presence or absence of the light reflex.

5. Oliguria or Anuria. Urinary output may be severely reduced owing to a number of factors such as hypotension, anoxia, a central antidiuretic effect, and a toxic action of barbiturate on the renal tubular cells.

6. Hypothermia. For its accurate detection the use of a low temperature recording rectal thermometer will be required. Hypothermia, since it reduces the oxygen demands of the tissues,

is not a deleterious feature unless severe, e.g. below 35° C., when it may exaggerate hypotension, produce sludging of the blood and lead to other complications.

7. SKIN LESIONS. Bullous lesions occur in 8 per cent. of cases and appear mainly on the pressure bearing areas but are also found on the hands and feet. The initial lesion is a slightly raised patch of erythema with a sharp outline which may proceed to bullous formation. Bullous lesions are most helpful in differentiating the coma of barbiturate poisoning from other causes of coma.

8. RAISED BLOOD LEVEL OF BARBITURATE. The longer acting barbiturates produce higher levels than do the shorter acting preparations, e.g. in a patient severely poisoned with phenobarbitone the level may reach 15 mg. per 100 ml. whereas with a medium acting preparation such as amylobarbitone, the patient may show features of poisoning of a similar degree when the blood level is only 5 mg. per 100 ml. It should be remembered that high blood levels with few features of poisoning may be found in epileptics and others habituated to the drug. Pre-existing liver or renal disease will exaggerate and prolong the toxic effects of barbiturates.

Complications. The complications can be deduced from study of the above list of clinical features. Briefly they are: (1) acute respiratory depression; (2) hypostatic pneumonia and aspiration pneumonitis; (3) severe shock; (4) anuria; (5) fluid and electrolyte imbalance with acid-base disturbance; (6) withdrawal fits and psychoses on recovery of consciousness.

The following complications are the direct effects of treatment: (*a*) Aspiration pneumonitis from injudicious gastric lavage; (*b*) pulmonary oedema from overloading of the circulation during forced diuresis; (*c*) the hazards associated with haemodialysis and peritoneal dialysis; (*d*) Convulsions, cardiac arrhythmias and psychoses from analeptic drugs.

Treatment. As a result of effective treatment the mortality rate for patients suffering from barbiturate poisoning admitted to a well equipped and staffed hospital has fallen from 25 per cent. to 1 per cent. in the past 10 years.

Treatment is based on the adoption of basic therapeutic principles to maintain respiration (p. 320), support the circulation (p. 178), correct electrolyte imbalance (p. 863) and prevent further absorption of the drug by removal of poison from the stomach. In poisoning producing Grades 1 and 2 unconsciousness and usually in Grade 3 unconsciousness no additional medical treatment is required but under careful nursing supervision the patient should be left to sleep off the effects of the drug. In the severely poisoned patient, treatment in hospital includes assisted respiration (p. 181) measures to combat shock and dehydration (p. 845) and possibly measures for enhanced elimination of barbiturate from the body. These subjects are discussed under General Therapeutic Measures (p. 92) and in other chapters of this book. There is no specific barbiturate antagonist and bemegride (Megimide) is merely a respiratory stimulant and is no better than nikethamide for this purpose.

CARBON MONOXIDE POISONING

Poisoning by this gas carries by far the highest mortality both in and out of hospital. The mortality rate is 8 per cent. for patients admitted to the Poisoning Treatment Centre of the Edinburgh Royal Infirmary. However, it is hoped that the amount of carbon monoxide in domestic gas in Britain will be reduced to below lethal levels within the next two years.

The smell of household gas is usually evident but may be absent if the gas coming from a broken pipe has seeped through a layer of earth. It is rare to encounter a deeply comatose patient in hospital because victims who reach that stage usually die at the site of poisoning. Since the carbon monoxide in coal gas combines so strongly with haemoglobin to form carboxyhaemoglobin, which is two hundred and ten times more stable than oxyhaemoglobin, the clinical features will be those due to varying degrees of anoxia.

Clinical Features

1. Disorientation or coma.
2. Skin and Mucosae. A cherry-red colour may be present but is not as commonly seen as is supposed. There may be extensive areas of erythema in the skin which may eventually blister and slough.

3. Respiratory System. Contrary to what might be expected, breathing is usually rapid and deep.

4. Cardiovascular System. In cases of average severity the heart rate will be approximately 100 with a slightly raised blood pressure. Arrhythmias are commonly present in the form of ectopic beats or atrial fibrillation. Congestive heart failure may set in rapidly. In severe poisoning with concomitant shock the fall in blood pressure may be marked.

5. Reflexes. The limb reflexes are increased and the pupils dilated. The plantar responses may be extensor in severe poisoning.

6. Temperature. The rectal temperature is usually low and the skin cold.

7. Renal System. Output of urine is seldom reduced unless in association with shock. Albumen and glucose are often present.

8. Carboxyhaemoglobin. By itself the percentage saturation by carboxyhaemoglobin is not a reliable indication of severity nor a good prognostic index. It will be about 30 per cent. for moderate poisoning and about 50 per cent. for severe poisoning, provided there is no associated anaemia.

Complications. Carbon monoxide poisoning being so frequently encountered in the older age-groups and the features being the result of anoxia, the state of the patient's coronary and cerebral circulation prior to poisoning will be a very important factor in determining the presence or absence of the complications which most frequently occur, namely, (1) congestive heart failure, the result of myocardial ischaemia or actual infarction; (2) pulmonary oedema due to congestive heart failure and the effects of severe anoxia on the bronchi and alveoli; (3) prolonged unconsciousness which may be due either to permanent cerebral damage or to cerebral oedema. Cortical atrophy and Parkinsonism are late complications.

Treatment. The basic necessity is to remove the sufferer immediately from the source of gas and without any delay apply artificial respiration if indicated. Oxygen and 5 per cent. CO_2 should be given. Admission to hospital is essential, resuscitative measures being maintained during transportation. In hospital the dangers of anoxia, especially to the cardiac muscle, must be remembered and the patient should be kept resting quietly for several days until it is certain that the heart has escaped damage

Acute cerebral oedema may be promptly reduced by the rapid infusion of mannitol. At the present time the hyperbaric oxygen chamber is of limited value in the treatment of carbon monoxide poisoning because of the time which usually elapses before the patient reaches hospital. However in the future the provision of portable hyperbaric pressure chambers, which can be rushed to the scene of the poisoning, may prove of value.

SALICYLATE POISONING

The victim is almost always conscious, hence simple questioning regarding consumption of salicylates will usually prevent the condition from being misdiagnosed as diabetic precoma or a severe infection, especially of the respiratory tract. Salicylates are often taken in compound tablets with codeine and phenacetin but the important acute toxic ingredient is the salicylate.

A moderately to severely poisoned patient may show some or all of the following clinical features.

1. Roaring in the Ears, Deafness and Blurring of Vision.
2. Restlessness. This is the result of the stimulant effect.
3. Hyperventilation. The drug acts as a stimulant to the respiratory centre increasing depth and rate, thereby washing out CO_2 and producing a respiratory alkalosis.
4. Sweating. The increased metabolic rate leads to fluid loss by sweating.
5. Epigastric Pain and Vomiting. The combination of loss of gastric contents, hyperventilation and profuse sweating leads to severe dehydration and a reduced urinary output.
6. Biochemical Changes. The initial respiratory alkalosis may be replaced, especially in children, by a metabolic acidosis. The serum potassium, despite dehydration, will be low as a result of the initial repiratory alkalosis.
7. Urinary Changes. There may be albumen and renal tubular casts. A purple colour will appear on Phenistix testing.
8. Raised Serum Salicylate. The level will be 50 mg. or more per 100 ml.

Complications. Profound disturbances of acid-base equilibrium, especially when associated with impaired consciousness, are to be regarded as a very serious feature and may herald sudden death.

The underlying mechanism is not fully understood but it is postulated that death is the result of cellular depletion of potassium.

Despite the tendency for salicylates to cause gastric erosion and hypoprothrombinaemia, haematemesis rarely occurs and blood-stained gastric contents evacuated by lavage are seldom seen.

Although albumen and renal tubular cells are often present in the urine during the acute stage, permanent renal damage has not been recorded.

Treatment. Moderate to severe salicylate poisoning is best treated in an adult by gastric aspiration and lavage (p. 94) which should never be omitted irrespective of the time that has elapsed since the drug was taken. Salicylate can best be eliminated from the body by forced alkaline diuresis. The urine must be rendered alkaline since a rise in urinary pH from 6 to 7·7 increases the excretion of free salicylate tenfold. For this purpose consecutive infusions of 500 ml. each of 0·87 per cent. saline, 5 per cent. dextrose, and 1·26 per cent. sodium bicarbonate are given intravenously. The rate of infusion is extremely important and should be 2 litres per hour for three hours. Control of serum potassium is essential and the addition of potassium to the infusion is necessary. If forced alkaline diuresis cannot be undertaken or if a diuresis is not achieved, peritoneal dialysis or haemodialysis will be required. In view of the bleeding tendency, vitamin K_1 (Phytomenadione) 10-20 mg. should be given parenterally (p. 668).

The mortality from salicylate poisoning is 1 per cent. if effective forced diuresis is employed.

ACUTE POISONING IN CHILDREN

Accidental poisoning in children under 4 years of age is an all too common event. Two-thirds of the enquiries dealt with by the Poisons Information Service are about children who have taken a substance which may be noxious. Analysis of the enquiries has shown that whilst sugar coating and colouring of tablets is frequently attractive, an unpleasant odour or taste does not prevent toddlers from sampling a substance. Domestic bleaches and detergents are amongst the most common substances taken; fortunately they are relatively innocuous and, apart from symptomatic treatment for the irritant effects on the alimentary tract, require no particular management. Poisoning by drugs can be serious in children, especially when salicylate or iron tablets have been taken. Most of the clinical features of salicylate poisoning resemble those already described in adults but it should be remembered that children are especially susceptible to the severe acid-base disturbance which occurs in this form of poisoning and which may develop at blood levels of salicylate which are not considered dangerous in adults. Exchange transfusion is a valuable therapeutic procedure in severe salicylate poisoning in little children. Poisoning with iron salts which formerly carried a high mortality, is now effectively treated with the chelating agent, desferrioxamine (Desferal). The agent is given via the gastric tube, intramuscularly and by intravenous infusion. Speed is essential in starting treatment which may be summarised as follows:

1. An intramuscular injection of 2 g. of desferrioxamine is given immediately.

2. After gastric lavage with 1 per cent. sodium bicarbonate 5 g. of desferrioxamine in 100 ml. of water or saline is left in the stomach.

3. This is followed by an intravenous infusion of desferrioxamine in saline, dextrose or blood. The amount should not exceed 15 mg./kg. body weight/hour up to a maximum of 80 mg./kg. in 24 hours.

4. Full supporting therapy for convulsions, shock, acidosis, blood loss and electrolyte disturbance is essential.

ANTIDOTES

It is widely but erroneously believed that for each toxic substance there is a specific antidote. As will have been appreciated from reading the sections on barbiturate, salicylate and carbon monoxide poisoning there is no antidote for these substances which are responsible for 75 per cent. of poisoning in adult patients admitted to hospital. In about 2 per cent. of instances, however, certain pharmacological antagonists are of value. An example is desferrioxamine for iron poisoning which has already been discussed; others are mentioned in Table 3.

TABLE 3

Some Features and Treatment of Poisoning by less Common Agents

Poison	Signs and Symptoms	Treatment
Amphetamine Group.	Excitement. Flushing. Tremor. Fits. Insomnia. Psychoses. Tachycardia. Hypertension.	1. General Measures. 2. Chlorpromazine, 100 mg. intramuscularly. If forced diuresis is indicated the urine must be rendered acid.
Corrosives.	Stains and burns of corners of mouth and chin. Burns of fauces. Pain. Shock.	1. General Measures. 2. Gastric lavage with care. 3. Neutralize acid or alkali. 4. Relieve pain.
Cyanides and Hydrocyanic Acid.	Odour of bitter almonds. Shallow breathing. Pink colour of skin and mucosae. Shock. Widely dilated pupils.	1. General measures. 2. Inhalation of amyl nitrite. 3. Sodium nitrite 3 per cent. 10 ml. intravenously in 3 minutes. 4. Sodium thiosulphate 50 per cent. 25 ml. intravenously very slowly. 5. If ingested, gastric lavage with 25 per cent. sodium thiosulphate.
Dinitro-ortho-cresol Weedkillers.	Yellow skin. Severe sweating. Thirst. Fatigue. Tachycardia. Tachypnoea. Raised temperature.	1. Wash skin. 2. Sedatives. 3. Reduce temperature.
Domestic Bleach.	Burning sensation in mouth and fauces. Gastroenteritis.	Gastric lavage with sodium thiosulphate 0·1 per cent. if symptoms severe.
Iron Salts.	Vomiting and diarrhoea. Haematemesis. Shock. Dehydration. Convulsions.	p. (102).
Opiates.	Depressed respiration. Pin-point pupils. Pallor. Vomiting. Coma.	1. If ingested gastric lavage with very dilute pot. permanganate—1 in 10,000.— 2. Nalorphine, 15 mg. intravenously and repeat every 15 min. till consciousness regained.

TABLE 3—*continued*

Poison	Signs and Symptoms	Treatment
Organophos-phorous Compounds.	Cold. Sweating. Constricted pupils. Salivation. Twitching. Convulsions. Slow pulse. Bronchospasm. Acute pulmonary oedema. Diarrhoea.	1. Remove contaminated clothes and wash skin. 2. General measures. 3. Atropine, 2 mg. intravenously and repeat 1 mg. intravenously hourly. 4. Pralidoxime (P_2S) 1 g. in 5 ml. water intravenously. Repeat in 1 hour.
Paraffin and Petroleum Distillates.	Vomiting and diarrhoea. Pallor. Cough and dyspnoea.	1. Do NOT wash out stomach. 2. Mag. sulph. to drink. 3. Antibiotics if aspiration has occurred.

PSYCHIATRIC ASSESSMENT

As most instances of poisoning in adults are deliberate acts o self-poisoning it is very important that all patients whether suffering from accidental or intentional poisoning should be seen by a psychiatrist. Self-poisoning is often an important feature of various psychiatric disorders and even if there is no psychiatric disorder the techniques of psychiatry are well suited for unravelling the underlying situation. It is greatly to the benefit of the patient if the initial psychiatric interview takes place as soon as possible after the act and before the patient and his relatives have time to discuss the event and thereafter present the same rationalised and often false picture.

HENRY MATTHEW.

Book Recommended:

Matthew, H. & Lawson, A. A. H. (1967). *Treatment of Common Acute Poisonings*. Edinburgh: Livingstone.

GENETICS IN RELATION TO MEDICINE

During the first part of this century infection and malnutrition were the main medical problems and as a result of research great advances in their control have been achieved. In the last 15 years interest has turned increasingly to the study of genetics in relation to medicine. There are several reasons for this. Whereas congenital malformation used to be a relatively unimportant cause of infant deaths, now, because of a decline in the number of deaths from other causes, it accounts for one in four. It has been realised that many prevalent diseases can be partly determined by genetic factors. There are grounds for believing that cancer might be due to alteration of the genetic material that is contained in every dividing cell. Parents are more aware than previously of the risks of transmission of established abnormal genes to their children. The effect of accumulating ionising radiation in our environment on ourselves, and on the whole future of the human race is debated widely. It has been discovered that reactions to certain drugs and chemicals can be due to inherited sensitivity. This applies to patients with a type of porphyria (p. 1219) who develop dangerous exacerbations on receiving barbiturates and to patients possessing an abnormal variety of the enzyme cholinesterase who are unduly responsive to the muscle relaxant, suxamethonium, used in general anaesthesia. Most inherited traits are advantageous to the individual and these are as important as the traits which are harmful; there are deleterious traits that persist in a population because of a less obvious beneficial effect. Examples are the sickle cell trait (p. 632) and a disorder of the erythrocyte due to deficiency of the enzyme glucose-6 phosphate dehydrogenase (p. 632) which under certain circumstances also gives rise to haemolytic anaemia. Both of these conditions, which are common in some of the areas where malaria is endemic, confer on an affected individual a degree of protection against malarial infection. Anaemia associated with the red cell enzyme deficiency is also an example of a drug-induced disease since the episodes of haemolysis follow exposure to the antimalarial drug primaquine, other aniline compounds and the bean and pollen of the fava plant (favism).

Modern medicine, by keeping people alive who would previously have died before reaching reproductive age, may well be increasing the frequency of genetically determined diseases in the population. It is essential that students and doctors should know about developments in the field of genetics so that they are able to appreciate the implications of inherited predisposition to certain disabilities; in addition they can use this knowledge to advantage in the anticipation and early recognition of disease, and can discuss intelligently problems arising from genetic factors with patients who nowadays are often well informed about these matters through the press, radio and television.

Cell Division and Reproduction

One of the fundamental characteristics of a living organism is the ability to reproduce itself. This can be achieved in the simpler plants and animals by binary fission. However, unless there is a mechanism for conjugation with other individuals with exchange of genetic material the stock soon becomes degenerate. In higher organisms the two processes of fission and conjugation have become highly specialised. The first is represented by mitosis (Fig. 3), a mechanism for maintaining the constancy of genetic material in the cells of any one organism. In this process, granularity appears in the nucleus which resolves into fine intertwining threads. These shorten and thicken into rods, the chromosomes, which split longitudinally into two identical pairs, or chromatids (prophase). At metaphase the chromosomes become arranged in the equatorial plane of the cell. In the next stage of division, anaphase, the chromatids separate and move to opposite poles of the cell to be reconstituted as resting nuclei; then with cleavage of the cytoplasm (telophase) two new cells with the same genetic constitution as the parent cell have been formed.

The second process, termed meiosis (Fig. 3) is concerned in the formation of germ cells for reproduction of a new organism. It ensures sufficient interchange of genetic material to preserve or even improve vitality of the stock. Normal somatic cells in a particular species have a constant number of paired chromosomes

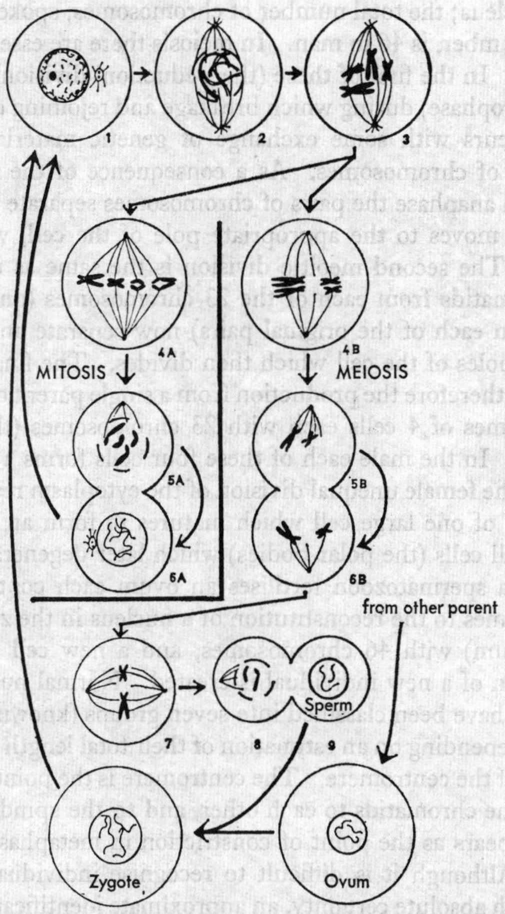

FIG. 3

A diagram to indicate the processes in cell division; for illustrative purposes only four chromosomes are shown in the nucleus. On the left is the common division, mitosis. Stages 1, 2 and 3 show the appearance of chromosomes and chromatids (prophase). Stage 4A is metaphase when the chromosomes are arranged in the equatorial plane of the cell. Stages 5A and 6A, anaphase and telophase respectively show the separation of the chromosomes and cleavage of the cytoplasm to give rise to two daughter cells identical with the parent cell. On the right is meiosis. In the first division (reduction division), Stages 1, 2, 3 and 4B to 6B, two cells are produced each containing one member of every pair of chromosomes in the parent cell. Then follows a second division, Stages 7, 8 and 9 similar to mitosis which gives rise to spermatozoa and ova. (Romanes, 1964) in the nucleus; the total number of chromosomes, spoken of as the diploid number, is 46 in man. In meiosis there are essentially two divisions. In the first of these (the 'reduction' division) there is a period (prophase) during which breakage and rejoining of chromosomes occurs with some exchange of genetic material between each pair of chromosomes. As a consequence of the first metaphase and anaphase the pairs of chromosomes separate and one of each pair moves to the appropriate pole of the cell, which then divides. The second meoitic division is the same as in mitosis; two chromatids from each of the 23 chromosomes (one chromosome from each of the original pairs) now separate and move to opposite poles of the cell which then divides. The final result of meiosis is therefore the production from a single parent cell with 46 chromosomes of 4 cells each with 23 chromosomes (the haploid number). In the male each of these four cells forms a spermatozoon; in the female unequal division of the cytoplasm results in the formation of one large cell which matures to form an ovum and three small cells (the polar bodies) which later degenerate.

When a spermatozoon fertilises an ovum each contributes 23 chromosomes to the reconstitution of a nucleus in the zygote (fertilised ovum) with 46 chromosomes, and a new cell capable of production of a new individual is created. Normal human chromosomes have been classified into seven groups (known as groups A to G) depending on an estimation of their total length and on the position of the centromere. The centromere is the point of attachment of the chromatids to each other, and to the spindle (Fig. 4) which appears as the point of constriction in metaphase chromosomes. Although it is difficult to recognise individual chromosomes with absolute certainty, an approximate identification can be achieved using these characteristics and the presence or absence of small satellites which are attached to some chromosomes.

Of the 23 pairs of normal human chromosomes, 22 are homologous; they are known as *autosomes* and when arranged in order of diminishing length they may be numbered from 1 to 22. It is by these numbers that they are known at present. The members of the remaining pair of chromosomes are known as the *sex chromosomes*. In the female, sex is determined by inheriting from each parent two sex chromosomes that are alike, the X chromosomes. In the male the members of the pair are dissimilar; his sex is determined by an X chromosome from his mother and a smaller and different one called the Y chromosome from his father. Hence in the normal somatic cell nucleus of the female there are 22 pairs of autosomes plus XX sex chromosomes, while in the male there are

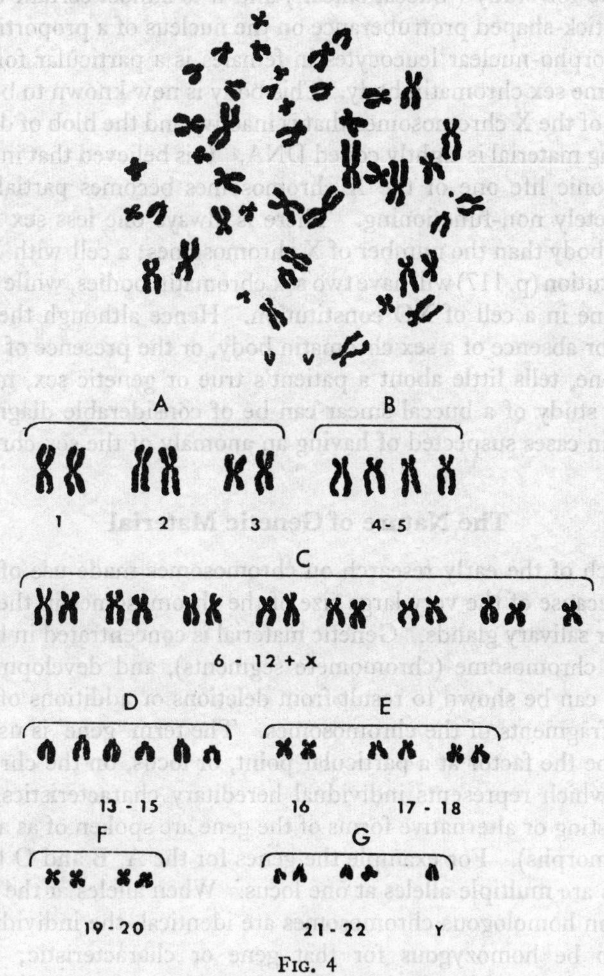

FIG. 4
Normal human male karyotype.

22 plus XY. A typical normal human male karyotype is illustrated in Figure 4.

In cells from normal females a minute condensation of nucleur chromatin can be seen lying against the nuclear membrane (Plate

III). Such female cells are sometimes spoken of as *chromatin-positive* (or Barr-positive); male cells are *chromatin-negative* (or Barr-negative). Cells from the buccal mucosa are particularly suitable for study ('buccal smear') and it is almost certain that a drumstick-shaped protruberance on the nucleus of a proportion of polymorpho-nuclear leucocytes in females is a particular form of this same sex chromatin body. This body is now known to be due to one of the X chromosomes that is inactive and the blob of deeply staining material is tightly coiled DNA. It is believed that in early embryonic life one of the X chromosomes becomes partially or completely non-functioning. There is always one less sex chromatin body than the number of X chromosomes; a cell with XXX constitution (p. 117) will have two sex chromatin bodies, while there are none in a cell of XO constitution. Hence although the presence or absence of a sex chromatin body, or the presence of more than one, tells little about a patient's true or genetic sex, microscopic study of a buccal smear can be of considerable diagnostic value in cases suspected of having an anomaly of the sex chromosomes.

The Nature of Genetic Material

Much of the early research on chromosomes made use of fruit flies because of the very large size of the chromosomes in the cells of their salivary glands. Genetic material is concentrated in bands in the chromosome (chromomere segments), and developmental effects can be shown to result from deletions or additions of very small fragments of the chromosomes. The term 'gene' is used to describe the factor at a particular point, or locus, on the chromosome which represents individual hereditary characteristics, and contrasting or alternative forms of the gene are spoken of as alleles (allelomorphs). For example the genes for the A, B and O blood groups are multiple alleles at one locus. When alleles at the same locus on homologous chromosomes are identical, the individual is said to be homozygous for that gene or characteristic; when different he is said to be heterozygous.

The first advance in the understanding of the nature of inheritance came from the finding of deoxyribonucleic acid (DNA) in the chromomeres and then the demonstration that this was the substance in extracts from pathogenic capsule-forming pneumococci which could confer pathogenicity and capsule formation on pneumoccoci without these features. DNA has now been established as the ultimate carrier of genetic information; except for certain viruses which contain only ribonucleic acid (RNA), it is present in the cells of all reproducing organisms.

The capacity of genes for identical replication is due to the unique structure of the DNA molecule, a long double strand in helical formation made up of many thousands of mononucleotides. According to the Watson-Crick DNA model, the two spirals are formed from phosphate and sugar and are united by side chains each of which contains two of the four bases, adenine, cytosine, thymine and guanine. Experimental work on a bacteriophage indicates that it is the sequence of these base pairs that determines the genetic information transmitted; a change in the sequence causes a change in genetic information or mutation.

It is now generally agreed that the primary action of genes is to specify the amino acid sequence of a particular protein or of one polypeptide component of a protein. These proteins may be either definitive proteins (e.g. collagen, haemoglobin) or enzymes and it is a useful concept that one particular gene or group of genes is concerned exclusively with the production of one protein. The genetic 'code', the specific information which controls protein synthesis and determines the structure of individual proteins, is contained in the chromosomal DNA; protein synthesis however occurs mainly in the ribosomes in the cell cytoplasm. The precise mechanism of transference of genetic instruction from the chromosomes to the ribosomes is still uncertain but it seems likely that this is a function of RNA (a smaller molecule than DNA in which ribose replaces deoxyribose and uracil replaces thymine). One hypothesis suggests that some molecules of RNA bring amino acids from the cytoplasm to the ribosomes while other molecules of RNA (messenger-RNA) are concerned with bringing instrunc tion, the genetic code, from the chromosomes regarding the specific make-up of individual proteins. Messenger-RNA then acts as a form of template on which the amino acids can be laid down in the correct sequence.

If mutation occurs in the chromosomal DNA, and there are many base pairs concerned with the synthesis of a complex protein that are vulnerable, then the mutant gene could give rise to a different protein (or enzyme) or perhaps to no protein at all. An example of the production of a different protein is sickle cell disease (p. 632) in which the main lesion is a form of haemoglobin with properties differing from normal adult haemoglobin due to the replacement of glutamic acid by valine in the β polypeptide chain of the globin moiety; sickle haemoglobin is much less soluble than normal haemoglobin and tends to precipitate in the circulation producing misshapen red cells (sickle cells) which are haemolysed abnormally easily. A typical example of loss of an enzyme is phenylketonuria which results from the deletion of a specific liver enzyme (L-phenylalanine hydroxylase) necessary for the conversion of phenylalanine to tyrosine; in consequence phenylalanine and related compounds accumulate in the body in excessive amounts, causing mental retardation.

The Pattern of Familial Disorders

One of Mendel's pioneer concepts was that the genetic information from both parents is transmitted to the next generation unchanged and new characteristics appearing are due to the combined effect of unaltered paternal and maternal genes. When hybrids in respect of a particular characteristic are produced then the result depends on the 'dominance' or 'recessiveness' of the gene for that characteristic in relation to its allele. Such simple Mendelian laws are the basis of inheritance in man but it is with mutant genes having harmful effects that this pattern of behaviour in families can be most easily discerned.

Many factors influence a pedigree pattern. There are two main ones. The first relates to the 'expression' (i.e. the production of disease which is evident clinically) of the mutant gene and the second to the type of chromosome on which it is located. If the effects of the gene are evident in a single dose, i.e. the abnormal gene has been transmitted from only one parent and the individual is heterozygous for the particular trait then the gene is said to be 'dominant'. If on the other hand, the character is only expressed when the mutant gene has been inherited in double dose, i.e. from both parents and the individual is homozygous for the trait, then the mutant gene is said to be 'recessive'. In addition to these considerations the mutant gene may be located on the autosomal chromosomes or on the sex chromosomes; the inheritance of the abnormal trait is then described as autosomal or sex-linked respectively.

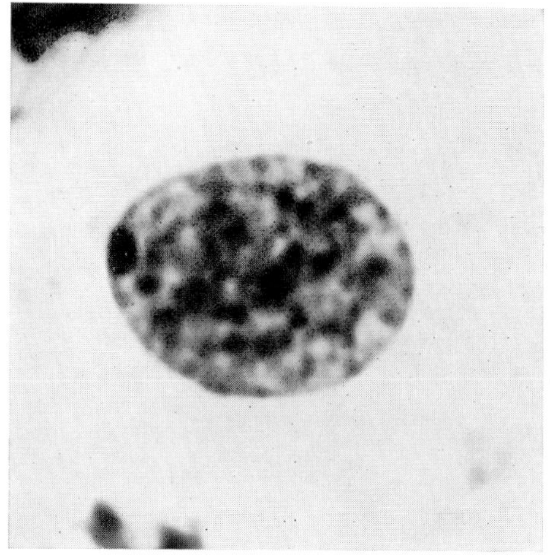

A

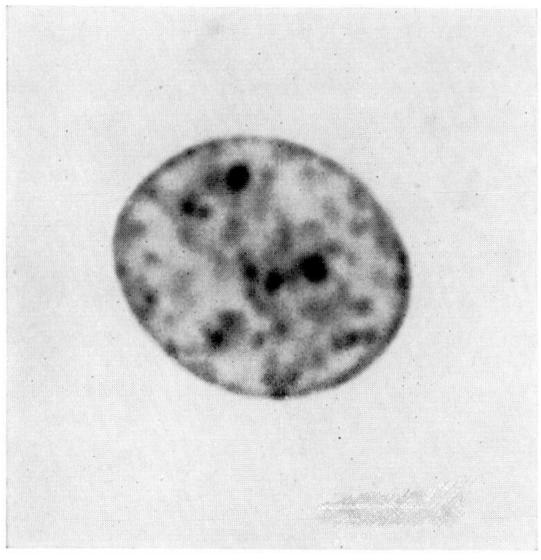

B

PLATE III

THE SEX CHROMATIN BODY.

A Chromatin-positive cell from a female patient showing the condensation of nuclear chromatin lying against the nuclear membrane.
B Chromatin-negative cell from a male patient; no sex chromatin body is present.

[*Facing page* 112

Autosomal Dominant Traits. The mutant gene is contributed by the affected parent on one of the autosomes and in the classical examples such as neurofibromatosis (p. 1206) and hereditary haemorrhagic telangiectasia (p. 672), there is a 1 in 2 chance of the children being affected, be they males or females. In general dominant traits tend to be less severe than recessive. This is probably because when a gene mutation gives rise to a serious disorder it mitigates against reproduction and hence tends to die out quickly. An exception to this is Huntington's chorea (p. 1195) which although serious does not become manifest until towards the end of reproductive life.

The inheritance of dominant traits is not always straightforward in terms of Mendelian laws. In many conditions there tends to be a wide variation in severity. The term 'penetrance' is used in connection with the expression or non-expression of abnormal genes and when detailed family studies are made it is possible to speak of 90 per cent., 50 per cent. or 10 per cent. penetrance of a particular mutant gene as the case may be. A dominant trait, frequently showing variable penetrance, is hereditary spherocytosis (p. 630); whole generations may be skipped—at least the trait is not detectable in them by present methods. Variation in expression of a dominant gene is difficult to explain; when it occurs it may be due to modification of the action of the abnormal gene by the recessive allele on the other chromosome.

Autosomal Recessive Traits. These also occur equally in the two sexes. Both parents, if outwardly normal, will be heterozygous for the recessive trait and each affected child will be homozygous, having a double dose of the mutant gene. In general there is a one in four chance of the progeny from parents who are heterozygous carriers of an abnormal recessive gene being homozygous for the trait and showing clinical stigmata; one quarter may be expected to be homozygous for the normal allele and will be normal in respect of the particular characteristic, and one-half will be heterozygous like the parents. Because related individuals will tend to be heterozygous for a particular mutant gene more frequently than the general population, recessive disorders, particularly the rarer ones, tend to arise more often in children of consanguineous matings than in random marriages.

Sometimes in recessive traits the terms 'dominance' and 'recessiveness' are relative. Biochemical disturbances can occasionally be shown in the heterozygous individual, although no clinical disease is present. Examples are phenylketonuria (p. 112) and hepatolenticular degeneration (p. 1191); in the former special studies of the carrier individual will show impaired ability to convert phenylalanine to tyrosine, while in the latter the synthesis of plasma copper oxidase is suppressed, suggesting in both instances partial (but subclinical) expression of the defect that causes disease in the homozygous state.

Intermediate inheritance and Codominance. Not all genetically determined diseases are easily classified since they may present clinically in both the heterozygous and homozygous state, the effect differing in severity and quality. Examples are thalassaemia (p. 632) and sickle cell disease (p. 632). In both, the heterozygous individual shows mild but definite and easily recognised clinical illness (thalassaemia minor and sickle cell trait respectively), whereas the homozygous has more marked haemolytic disease and shortened life expectancy. This phenomenon is described as 'intermediate' inheritance.

Another pattern in which allelomorphic genes in a heterozygous individual have equal importance is described as 'codominance'. The best example is seen in the inheritance of ABO blood groups; the heterozygote who acquires the A antigen from one parent and the B antigen from the other, produces red cells of group AB.

Sex-linked Inheritance. Some traits appear to be transmitted by mutant genes on the X chromosome; disease due to location of a mutant gene on the Y chromosome has not been described in man.

In the female who has two X chromosomes, sex-linked characteristics may be dominant or recessive and may be produced by homozygous or heterozygous inheritance. Since the male has only one X chromosome he is said to be 'hemizygous' in respect of characteristics on this chromosome; there is no allele on the Y chromosome corresponding to an abnormal gene on the X; hence sex-linked traits whether dominant or recessive in the female are always fully expressed in the male. Another feature of sex-linked inheritance is that a father cannot transmit a mutant gene (dominant or recessive) from his X chromosome to his sons because he gives his X chromosome exclusively to his daughters.

The best example of sex-linked recessive inheritance is haemophilia (p. 663). A haemophilic male must have obtained the mutant gene on the X chromosome contributed by his mother. He will transmit the characteristic to all his daughters (who will be heterozygous carriers) but to none of his sons. Sex-linked recessive traits are not exclusively male diseases but are nearly always so. A female haemophilic would require to inherit the gene from an affected father and from a heterozygous carrier mother. Such an event is, of course, very rare in haemophilia. A much more common example of a sex-linked recessive trait in females is the one for colour blindness.

Sex-linked dominant inheritance occurs but is very rare. Both males and females are affected and both may transmit the disorder to their offspring. Superficially, sex-linked and autosomal dominant inheritance may appear to be similar; the critical difference is that an affected father in the former type transmits the disease to none of his sons but to all his daughters.

In addition to these classical familial disorders that follow simple laws, albeit sometimes with incomplete penetrance, there is a whole range of conditions that cannot be so easily defined. Many common diseases, e.g. hypertension (p. 226), pernicious anaemia (p. 621), diabetes mellitus (p. 738), thyroid disorders (p. 690), rheumatoid arthritis (p. 538) and schizophrenia (p. 1266) fall into this category. In each, a familial incidence can be established but it would appear that in these the interplay of a number of mutant genes may be conferring on the individual a predisposition to the disease rather than the disease itself. In peptic ulceration (p. 900) which may be another example of multifactorial inheritance, the patient's sex, blood group status, gastric secretion, pancreatic secretion and the exercise of environmental factors such as psychological stress all combine for the full development of recognisable clinical illness. Although unsatisfactory, some such explanation is required for the irregular pedigree patterns that these diseases produce.

Visible Abnormalities of the Chromosomes

The first visible chromosomal abnormality in association with disease was reported in 1959. Since then, there have been many further discoveries involving change in the total number of chromosomes and in the appearance of individual chromosomes. Research has been facilitated by improved techniques for analysis. Cells from bone marrow, skin and peripheral blood seem to be best for study and are grown in tissue culture. Colchicine is used to arrest cell division at metaphase since this seems to be the best stage for recognition of individual chromosomes; hypotonic solutions help to swell the cell nuclei and separate the chromosomes. Suitable cells may then be photographed and enlarged so that the chromosomes may be counted accurately and examined in detail.

'Aneuploidy', the term used when the chromosome number differs from the usual diploid number, is relatively common. The cause is failure of separation (non-disjunction) of a pair of chromosomes during meiosis and when this arises two aneuploid gametes are produced, one with 24 chromosomes, and one with 22, the former containing the unseparated pair. When gametes of this type are then fertilised by a normal gamete, the resulting fertilised ova contain 47 and 45 chromosomes respectively. In the former the chromosome affected by non-disjunction will be represented three times instead of twice (the unseparated pair from the aneuploid gamete and one from the fertilising gamete) and the cell is said to be 'trisomic'; in the latter only the chromosome provided by the fertilising gamete will be present and the cell is 'monosomic'. The cause of aneuploidy is not known. Some trisomic syndromes, e.g. mongolism, are more common with advancing maternal age but this is the only association that has been found. Ionising radiation used for therapeutic purposes has been shown to produce mainly chromosome breakage and abnormal chromosomes from joining of fragments rather than aneuploid cells.

Morphological abnormalities of the chromosomes are now known to be relatively common in the population. Although they are frequently not associated with clinical abnormality in the individual showing the aberration, they are of importance because they are transmitted from one generation to the next and may give rise to an increased incidence of abortion (p. 119) or to abnormality in the offspring. The most common are 'translocation meaning transfer of a segment of a chromosome to a different site on the same chromosome or to a different chromosome and 'deletion' which means complete omission of a segment of a chromosome from a chromosome set.

Sex Chromosomes. Studies of the nuclear sex chromatin body (p. 109) and also of the chromosomes have shown clearly that in a few interesting conditions the nuclear sex does not accord with the patient's apparent or phenotypic sex. The most important or these is Klinefelter's syndrome (p. 736), a condition characterised by testicular dysgenesis (only a rudimentary gonad is present), azospermia and variable degrees of gynaecomastia, and eunuchoid conformation. The patients with this syndrome are apparent males but are usually chromatin positive. The first studies on one such chromatin positive male showed 47 chromosomes and a sex chromosome constitution of XXY pattern instead of the normal XY. Since then it has been demonstrated that this is by no means the only chromosome pattern in these abnormal males. XXXY and XXXXY patterns and even patients in whom the somatic cells may have differing chromosome make-up have been described. The last group are spoken of as sex chromosome 'mosaics'. The term Klinefelter's syndrome has come to be applied to all males with more than one X chromosome. Recent surveys of live male births suggest that as many as 2 per 1,000 infants are chromatin positive, indicating that the problem is not unimportant.

A second condition is Turner's syndrome in which the clinical features include short stature, amenorrhoea, ovarian dysgenesis, poor development of secondary sex characteristics, webbing of the neck and cubitus valgus deformity as well as various other congenital abnormalities including coarctation of the aorta. Patients with Turner's syndrome are apparent females but are chromatin negative. They have only 45 chromosomes with a sex chromosome constitution XO. The XO type is now known to be one of several abnormal sex chromosome patterns that can be found in patients with ovarian dysgenesis; it would appear that some are mosaics, one of the cell lines having an XO complement while, more rarely, others show morphological abnormality of one of the X chromosomes. The importance of such aberrations lies in the fact that they are a major cause of primary amenorrhoea in gynaecological practice.

Other sex chromosome abnormalities include XXX and XXXX constitutions, neither showing any gross deviations from the normal female phenotype. The majority of adult cases described have had normal sex development and some have borne children. A very recent study suggests that there is a significant number of patients in delinquent institutions with an extra Y chromosome

(XXYY, XYY). These patients tend to be high grade mental defectives aggressive in behaviour and tall in stature.

While some patients with sex chromosome abnormalities may be mentally retarded this is by no means the rule and many patients with Klinefelter's syndrome, for example, are highly intelligent people.

Autosomes. In contrast to the abnormalities of the sex chromosomes, relatively few abnormalities of the autosomes have been described and none have been due to monosomy. This is probably because many are lethal *in utero* or even before implantation of the ovum.

Three autosomal trisomic states are now recognised; one affecting a chromosome in the 13-15 group and another affecting a chromosome in the 17-18 group are both characterised by severe physical abnormalities and mental retardation. The third and best known is Down's syndrome, mongolism, which appears to be due to trisomy of chromosome 21. In this condition the main abnormalities are mental retardation and stunting of growth in association with a number of distinctive features which include absence or poor development of the bridge of the nose, an oriental slant to the eyes, short curved little fingers, hyperextensible joints, broad palms with a single transverse palmar crease and spots of depigmentation in the iris.

Generally speaking the likelihood of occurrence of Down's syndrome is related to maternal age, presumably because of an increased risk of non-disjunction occurring in the ageing ovary. However, if a young mother (under 35 years) produces a mongol there is a very high chance of her producing another. This is because some of the mongols born of young mothers are due to chromosome translocation. When this occurs the mother (or rarely the father) has only 45 chromosomes, one of which is abnormal, usually comprising chromosome 15 or chromosome 22 and genetic material translocated from chromosome 21. This abnormal translocation chromosome is transmitted along with a normal chromosome 21 to the mongol child who also acquires a chromosome 21 from the other parent. Such 'translocation mongols', who only show 46 chromosomes are effectively trisomic for chromosome 21, like the 'age dependent' mongols due to non-disjunction who show 47.

A well marked syndrome which includes mental retardation, microcephaly and transverse palmar creases has recently been described in association with deletion of part of the short arms of one of the 4 or 5 autosomes. It has been found to be relatively common in studies of mental defectives. Since the most characteristic feature is a plaintive cat-like noise made by affected infants the condition has been described as the *cri du chat* syndrome.

A most interesting development has been the finding that in most cases of chronic myeloid leukaemia (p. 650) one of the smallest chromosomes (of pairs 21 or 22, but probably the former) has almost half of its substance missing. The abnormal chromosome has come to be known as the 'Philadelphia chromosome'. It has not yet been decided whether the loss of substance is due to deletion or translocation; nor is it known how the aberration is caused or what it means. The Philadelphia chromosome has diagnostic usefulness in doubtful cases of myeloid leukaemia. So far, though chromosome abnormalities are seen frequently in the other types of leukaemia and other malignant diseases, no consistent pattern has emerged.

Since ionising radiation is known to cause chromosome damage it is relevant to mention here the increased incidence of leukaemia that has been described in a number of groups exposed to excessive amounts, namely, the early X-ray workers, the radium watch-dial painters, the survivors of the atomic bomb explosions in Hiroshima and Nagasaki (about four times that in a comparable population) and those receiving irradiation therapy for ankylosing spondylitis (about five to ten times that in a comparable population depending on the treatment dose).

Another new fact which has been emerging in the past few years is the relation of genetic constitution to abortion. Not only do some families with chromosome abnormalities show an increased tendency to abortion, but also about 25 per cent. of spontaneous abortions appear to be associated with visible chromosome abnormalities in the foetus. These findings indicate that many spontaneous abortions are not affecting normal foetuses; instead they are having considerable eugenic importance by reducing the total number of children born with chromosomal aberrations.

Genetic Advice

Doctors are being asked increasingly by their patients about genetic risks. Questions are raised by parents or young people contemplating marriage, who themselves have some disorder like epilepsy or some malformation like a hare-lip, about the danger of transmitting this to a child. Most enquiries come from parents who, having already produced an abnormal child, e.g. a mongol, wish to know the chances of subsequent children being affected. Cousins (there are 6 cousin marriages per 1,000 unions) will often wish to discuss the hazards of consanguinity. Adoption societies have special problems when handling children of mentally defective mothers. The doctor's responsibility for giving sensible advice on these matters is considerable because the whole subject is pervaded by emotion and superstition and much of the importance of genetic counselling lies in allaying the fears of the ill-informed.

Although it is not possible for the family doctor to be familiar with the many hundreds of conditions that are known to be due to mutant genes, he should have some knowledge of those disorders in which special genetic risks are involved. He also requires to know the principles underlying genetic counselling and where expert advice for his patients can be obtained. It is to meet this latter need that genetic counselling clinics are being established in main centres in this and other countries.

Some examples of conditions transmitted by autosomal dominant inheritance when the risk to children of an affected parent is one in two have already been given, e.g. Huntington's chorea. Another disease worthy of special mention because it illustrates the scope of the problem is multiple polyposis of the colon. This rare disorder, if inherited, carries a sufficiently high risk of malignant disease to justify prophylactic colectomy. Hence children of affected families require regular investigation of the colon until it is known which are at risk.

Recessive traits appear unexpectedly in the first affected child and the diagnosis may well not be made until it is too late for successful treatment. The risk that subsequent siblings will inherit the disease is one in four, and in the case of phenylketonuria, for example, if there is to be any value in treatment, prompt diagnosis soon after birth is essential. It is probably with recessive genes that genetic counselling before marriage will have its greatest value, particularly when further methods develop for recognising the carrier state. Already this is being applied to the problem of thalassaemia in parts of Italy where as many as 1 in 10 of the population carry the mutant gene. The object of detection of the carrier state for thalassaemia by routine examination of school children is to warn and, if possible, prevent the intermarriage of carriers, as by this means the disease could be prevented. Elsewhere in Europe recessive genes do not cause the same public health problems but means of demonstrating with certainty the carrier for fibrocystic disease of the pancreas (p. 688) and haemophilia would be valuable. As stated above, the detection of the carriers of phenylketonuria and hepatolenticular degeneration is already possible. In addition, 70 per cent. of the female carriers of the Duchenne type muscular dystrophy (a sex-linked recessive trait) can be recognised by estimation of the enzyme creatinekinase in the serum (p. 1232).

The conditions to which reference has been made are due to mutations in single genes. It is now known that mutations may affect whole chromosomes or even several chromosomes. As has been discussed, the risk of a further mongol child being born to a woman over 35 is not increased since this child has probably been produced by an accident of disjunction. However, the young mother may have produced a translocation mongol due to a fixed abnormality in her genetic make-up and the chance of her producing another mongolian imbecile is about one in five or greater. Such a problem can only be resolved by a knowledge of genetic prognosis based on chromosome examination. Hence the value of having genetic laboratories associated with genetic clinics.

Even with complex and partly genetic conditions accumulating experience will allow the geneticist to assess the risk or give a statement of the odds. For example, it has been estimated that the risk of anencephaly (absence of a large part of the brain) in a later sibling of an affected child is about 1 in 8, of epilepsy about 1 in 40, while if a parent and child both have a hare lip, the chance of a subsequent child being affected is about 1 in 10.

The risk of a normal woman with a normal husband producing a child with serious congenital malformation is about 1 in 40. This gives the geneticist some degree of perspective on which to base his assessment and his advice. It is generally agreed that a genetic risk exceeding 1 in 10 is a bad risk, while one of less than 1 in 20 is a good risk. Fortunately most genetic problems divide clearly into one or other of these categories.

JOHN RICHMOND.

Books recommended:

Clarke, C. A. (1964). *Genetics for the Clinician*, 2nd ed. Oxford: Blackwell.

Thompson, J. S. & Thompson, M. W. (1966). *Genetics in Medicine.* Philadelphia: Saunders.

Watson, J. D. (1965). *Molecular Biology of the Gene.* New York: Benjamin.

DISEASES OF THE CARDIOVASCULAR SYSTEM

INTRODUCTION

Coronary atherosclerosis and hypertension are the principal causes of heart disease in middle and old age. Rheumatic fever is by far the most common cause in childhood, adolescence and early adult life. The incidence of ischaemic heart disease appears to be increasing but that of rheumatic heart disease is falling. Hypertensive heart disease is becoming less common owing to the efficacy of drugs which lower the blood pressure. All other forms of heart disease are relatively uncommon.

The approximate incidence of each form as regards hospital practice in the British Isles is shown in the following table. In certain districts, e.g. in industrial areas, the incidence of pulmonary heart disease is much higher. In some countries the incidence of syphilitic heart disease is higher, and in others, e.g. Africa, that of hypertensive and ischaemic heart disease is lower.

	Per cent.
Ischaemic heart disease (coronary atherosclerosis) / Hypertensive heart disease	60
Rheumatic heart disease	20
Pulmonary ,, ,,	10
Congenital ,, ,,	3
Thyrotoxic ,, ,,	1
Other forms of heart disease	6

Diagnosis in heart disease can usually be made from a carefully taken history, a detailed physical examination and electrocardiography, but occasionally it is necessary to make use of highly specialised techniques such as cardiac catheterisation and angiocardiography.

In clinical diagnosis it is impossible to exaggerate the importance of the history, which frequently requires much patience and skill to elicit accurately. Time taken over this part of the examination is never wasted. Patients with heart disease usually complain either of breathlessness, pain in the chest or swelling of the ankles. Other symptoms such as dizziness, faintness or palpitation are more commonly associated with anxiety or neurotic ill-health. Apart from the analysis of specific complaints each patient should be assessed as an individual and due allowance made for powers of exaggeration or understatement. The patient should be encouraged to tell his or her own story as far as possible, but prompting with leading questions may be necessary on occasion. The patient should be asked to describe the very first symptom, and the development of this together with subsequent manifestations should then be followed. It is important to distinguish symptoms due to organic disease from those which are due to associated anxiety.

It must not be forgotten that the common manifestations of heart disease can be produced by disease elsewhere in the body. For example, breathlessness may be due to disease of the lungs, pain in the chest may be based on psychoneurosis and not on organic disease and oedema may be due to disease of the kidneys. The most frequent cause of oedema, especially in women, is incompetence of the venous valves of the lower limbs. Whenever possible, therefore, objective evidence should be sought in confirmation of the diagnosis.

Various tests of cardiac function have been devised, but of far more value is a careful appraisal of the history as regards capacity for familiar effort. If necessary, confirmation of the patient's statements may be obtained by witnessing the effects of such exercise.

Palpation of the pulse may give important information. Some disturbances of rate and rhythm are physiological and others are of serious significance.

The presence or absence of cardiac enlargement and abnormal heart sounds and murmurs must always be determined. Whilst familiarity with gross abnormalities may readily be learned, the finer details of auscultation require much experience in interpretation. Misinterpretation of these signs may give rise to serious errors of judgment.

Radiology is of great value in diagnosis and in the assessment of cardiac enlargement and its progression or regression.

Electrocardiography has become so complex that detailed analysis must be left to specialists in this field. However, it is important not only to be able to recognise the common abnormalities but to know the indications for taking an electrocardiogram and the type of information which may be expected from it.

PHYSICAL EXAMINATION

The best means of avoiding errors in diagnosis is adherence to a systematic plan of examination. The part of such an examination which applies to the cardiovascular system is outlined below.

(*a*) General Observations.
(*b*) Examination of the Pulse.
(*c*) Examination of the Neck Veins.
(*d*) Examination of the Heart.
(*e*) Examination for Signs of Cardiac Failure.
(*f*) Examination of the Lungs.
(*g*) Estimation of the Blood Pressure.
(*h*) Examination of the Retina.
(*i*) Examination of the Urine.

(*a*) GENERAL OBSERVATIONS

Whilst taking the history and before examining the cardiovascular system, certain pertinent observations may be made.

Does the patient look ill? Many patients with hypertension or angina pectoris appear to be in robust health. On the other hand, those suffering from myocardial infarction may be pale, sweating and cold, those with bacterial endocarditis may look pale and ill, and those with chronic congestive cardiac failure may appear wasted.

Cyanosis. Cyanosis depends on the absolute amount of reduced haemoglobin in the blood of the superficial vessels and is usually evident when this exceeds 5 g. per 100 ml.; thus it will be readily apparent in polycythaemia and cannot occur in severe anaemia even with extreme oxygen undersaturation.

Peripheral cyanosis is due to an excessive abstraction of oxygen from the blood when the circulation is impaired from vasoconstriction, a low cardiac output or stasis. A blue tinge is seen in the lips, in the nails and in the skin, especially of the ears, cheeks, hands and feet. When due to cold the cyanosis is peripheral in origin and disappears when the patient is warm. Central cyanosis is due to oxygen undersaturation of the arterial blood from poor gaseous exchange in the lungs in such conditions as emphysema, pulmonary oedema and pneumonia, or when there is a veno-arterial shunt in congenital heart disease. If the affected parts mentioned above and in addition particularly the tongue, are both warm and cyanosed, it may be deduced that the cyanosis is central in origin. A combination of central and peripheral cyanosis may occur and is often seen in cardiac failure. Cyanosis is not in itself a sign of cardiac failure.

In addition it must be remembered that there are disorders in which abnormal pigments such as methaemoglobin or sulphaemoglobin are present in the blood and these may cause a blue tinge similar to that produced by an excess of reduced haemoglobin.

Anaemia. Angina or cardiac failure may be aggravated or even brought about by anaemia. It is therefore imperative to examine the blood in patients with symptomatic heart disease in order to determine if anaemia is present and if so which type and to provide the appropriate treatment. Anaemia in a patient with valvular disease may be secondary to active rheumatic fever or to bacterial endocarditis.

Breathlessness at rest may be observed, especially if the patient is asked to lie flat. If of cardiac origin, it indicates pulmonary venous congestion or pulmonary oedema.

Obesity will aggravate, or may entirely account for, breathlessness on exertion and decreases exercise tolerance in patients with angina.

Loss of weight is a common sequel to chronic congestive cardiac failure. It is also a feature of thyrotoxicosis which, particularly in the elderly, may readily be overlooked as a cause of heart disease.

Skin temperature varies with skin blood flow. In an equable temperature and with normal arteries the skin temperature usually reflects the cardiac output. Thus in low output failure the nose, ears and hands are usually cold; conversely in high output failure (p. 170) they are usually warm.

Hands. Unduly moist palms suggest anxiety or thyrotoxicosis. In anxiety the hands are usually cold whereas in thyrotoxicosis they are warm. Clubbing of the fingers occurs in cyanotic congenital heart disease and in advanced bacterial endocarditis, but is more often found in other conditions, such as intrathoracic suppuration and bronchogenic carcinoma. Flattened, brittle nails (koilonychia) suggest iron deficiency anaemia (p. 612).

'Splinter' haemorrhages under the nails may be present in bacterial endocarditis but are not diagnostic of this condition. Painful subcutaneous nodules, especially in the fingers or palms may also occur (p. 219).

(*b*) EXAMINATION OF THE PULSE

The radial pulse should be examined for rate, rhythm, volume, the character of the pulse wave and the condition of the vessel wall.

Rate

Bradycardia may be physiological or due to heart block. Excessive administration of digitalis is a common cause.

Tachycardia with regular rhythm may be due to emotion, thyrotoxicosis, fever, cardiac failure or occasionally to an ectopic rhythm, e.g. paroxysmal tachycardia.

Rhythm

An irregular pulse is commonly due to sinus arrhythmia, extrasystoles or atrial fibrillation, and less frequently to dropped beats, to atrial flutter with varying block or to rarer causes.

Pulse Deficit. This term signifies a difference between the heart rate as recorded by auscultation and the pulse rate as counted at the wrist. It may be a feature of extrasystoles and of atrial fibrillation and is discussed under these headings.

Pulse Volume

By pulse volume is meant the amplitude of expansile movement of the vessel wall during the passage of the pulse wave. The pulse volume provides a useful clinical estimate of the left ventricular output per beat (stroke volume). It is modified by vasomotor tone and local conditions such as a sclerotic or anatomically small artery.

A pulse of small volume is characteristic of shock and of low output heart failure and may occur with severe stenosis of any valve or severe pulmonary hypertension. A pulse of large volume is found in fevers, aortic incompetence, atherosclerosis of the aorta, extreme bradycardia as with heart block and in diseases in which there is an increased cardiac output, e.g. severe anaemia, thyrotoxicosis and some patients with cor pulmonale. If the brachial pulses are unequal, it can be inferred that there is a vascular block of which the most common causes are embolism, thrombosis and atherosclerosis of the aorta.

Character of the Pulse Wave

Anacrotic Pulse. In aortic stenosis a notch may sometimes be felt on the upstroke of the pulse, and the wave may be prolonged and of small amplitude ('Plateau' type).

Dicrotic Pulse. Accentuation of the dicrotic wave, sometimes so marked as to give the impression of a double pulse at the wrist, may be found in any condition associated with vasodilatation, e.g. high fever.

Collapsing or 'Water-hammer' Pulse. In aortic incompetence a characteristic pulse wave may be felt at the wrist if regurgitation is free. There is a sharp impact from the rapid filling and sudden rise of pressure associated with a large systolic discharge from the left ventricle and a rapid falling away or collapse from the subsequent sudden fall of pressure due to regurgitation of blood through the incompetent aortic valve. Such a pulse is frequently accompanied by capillary pulsation due to arteriolar dilatation. The diastolic pressure will be low or even zero. A high pulse pressure and bounding pulse may occur in any condition associated with vasodilatation, e.g. anaemia, fever or thyrotoxicosis.

Pulsus Alternans. The pulse is regular but the amplitude is larger and smaller in alternate beats (Fig. 5). It is a serious sign of left ventricular failure, most commonly from hypertension, and is usually best detected with the sphygmomanometer. There will be a difference of 10-40 mm. between strong and weak beats.

Pulsus bisferiens. A pulse with a double peak is characteristic of combined aortic stenosis and incompetence (Fig. 6).

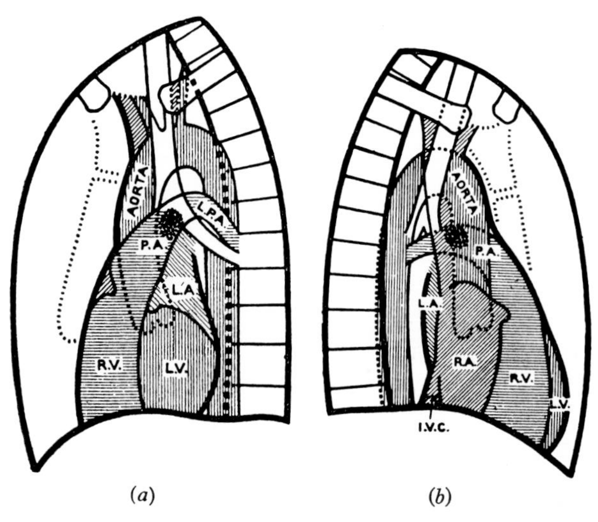

(*a*) (*b*)

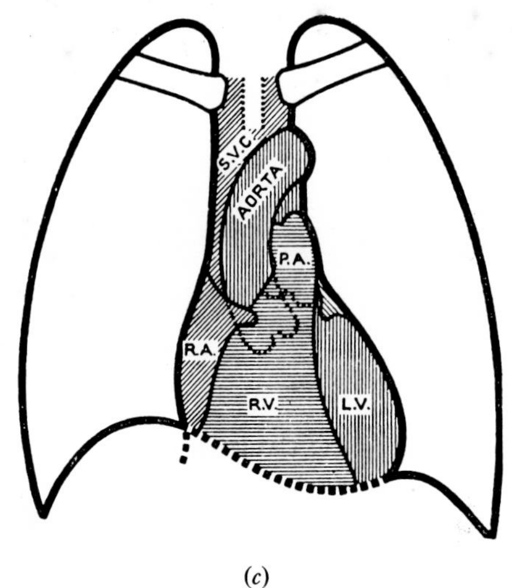

(*c*)

PLATE IV

RADIOLOGICAL ANATOMY OF THE HEART

(*a*) Left oblique view. (*b*) Right oblique view. (*c*) Anterior view.

(*By courtesy of Sir John Parkinson and 'The Lancet'*.)

[*Facing page* 128

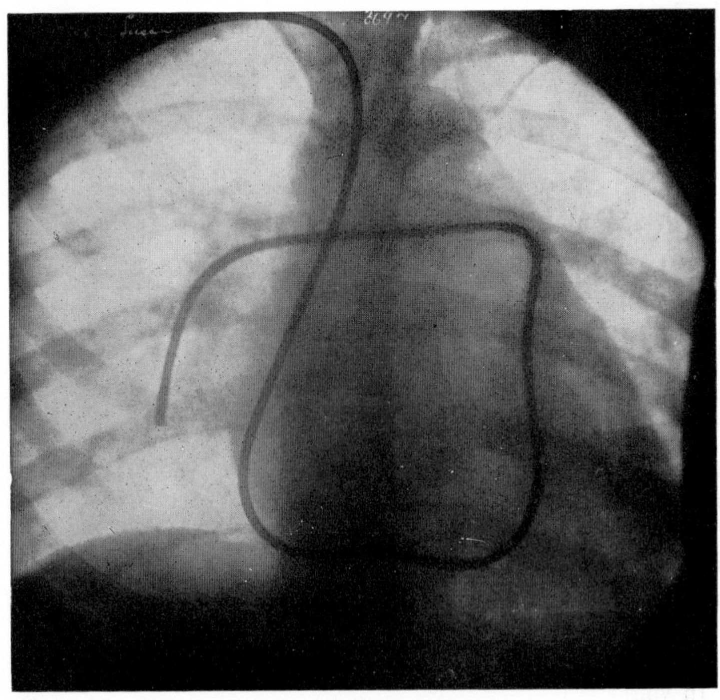

PLATE V

CARDIAC CATHETERISATION

The catheter has been passed through an antecubital vein into the right subclavian vein, superior vena cava, right atrium, right ventricle, main pulmonary artery, right pulmonary artery and its branch to the lower lobe of the lung.

Pulsus Paradoxus. In pericarditis with effusion or in constrictive pericarditis the normal increase in venous return to the right side of the heart during inspiration cannot be accommodated. The normal increase in capacity of the pulmonary vascular bed which occurs during inspiration results in a diminished return of blood to the left side of the heart. Hence the volume of the pulse is decreased by inspiration. Pulsus paradoxus is also found in asthma or stridor, where there is an increased change in intrathoracic pressure with respiration.

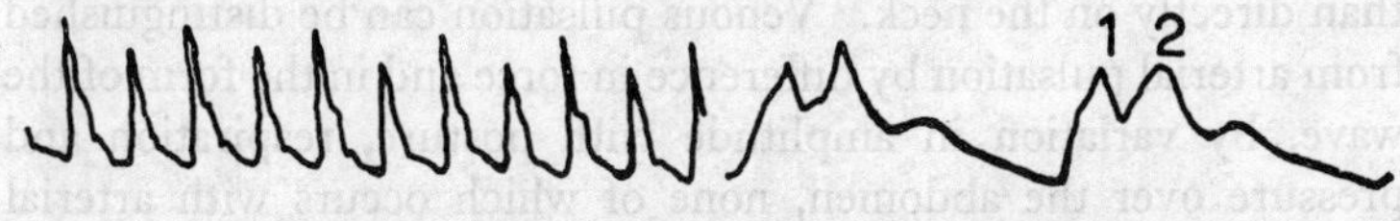

FIG. 5
PULSUS ALTERNANS

FIG. 6
PULSUS BISFERIENS

VESSEL WALL

The condition of the vessel wall should be noted for evidence of arterial thickening and undue mobility. Medial sclerosis is unrelated to hypertension or narrowing of the lumen. Obliteration of the blood column proximal to the examining finger is necessary, otherwise a full tension pulse in hypertension may be mistaken for hardening of the vessel wall.

PERIPHERAL (LOWER LIMB) PULSES

In younger hypertensives and in children suspected of having congenital heart disease the femoral pulses should always be examined. Absence, weakness or delay may be due to coarctation of the aorta, in which case the blood pressure in the lower limbs will be reduced, in contrast to the raised pressure in the upper limbs.

In peripheral vascular disease, the pulses should be felt and compared in the femoral, popliteal, posterior tibial and dorsalis pedis vessels.

ARTERIAL PULSATION IN THE NECK

Excessive arterial pulsation in the neck may be seen in aortic incompetence, coarctation of the aorta or sometimes from kinking of the carotid artery due to unfolding of an atheromatous aorta.

(*c*) EXAMINATION OF THE NECK VEINS

Examination of the jugular veins is of great value in estimating the venous pressure and in studying abnormalities of the jugular venous pulse. These veins reflect the pressure and pulsations in the right atrium and serve as convenient clinical manometers. It should be made with the patient reclining comfortably with the neck in the position in which pulsation is shown most distinctly. Each side should be inspected in turn, with the head slightly rotated. When possible the light should be shining across rather than directly on the neck. Venous pulsation can be distinguished from arterial pulsation by difference in force and in the form of the wave, by variation in amplitude with posture, respiration and pressure over the abdomen, none of which occurs with arterial pulsation. Venous pulsation can be obliterated by light pressure below the level of pulsation. The difference in vertical height between the sternal angle as reference point and the highest point of pulsation over the internal jugular vein, or highest point of pulsation or distension in the external jugular vein, provides an index of the venous pressure and is usually recorded in centimetres. It should be realised that increased venous pressure may be reflected in pulsation without obvious distension, and that this may show better in the deep than in the superficial veins. Distension of the external jugular veins may be an unreliable index because 'kinking' may give a falsely high estimate of the venous pressure, in which case there will be distension without pulsation. In obesity or with marked carotid pulsation, the pulsation in the deep jugular veins may be obscured. Venous pulsation or distension is not normally seen when the patient is reclining at 45°, but may appear in the horizontal position. Where doubt exists as to its presence pressure should be exerted over the abdomen. This produces what is sometimes referred to as the hepatojugular reflux, but it is not necessary to press over the liver itself, which may be tender, and it is important that the breath should not be held. The venous return to the heart is temporarily increased and reflected in the neck veins by increased distension and pulsation. It is very useful in bringing to light borderline cases of congestive failure.

Increased venous pressure occurs as a result of congestive cardiac failure, of pulmonary embolism or of pericardial effusion or constriction. Venous obstruction, e.g. by a mediastinal tumour compressing the superior vena cava, causes distension without pulsation.

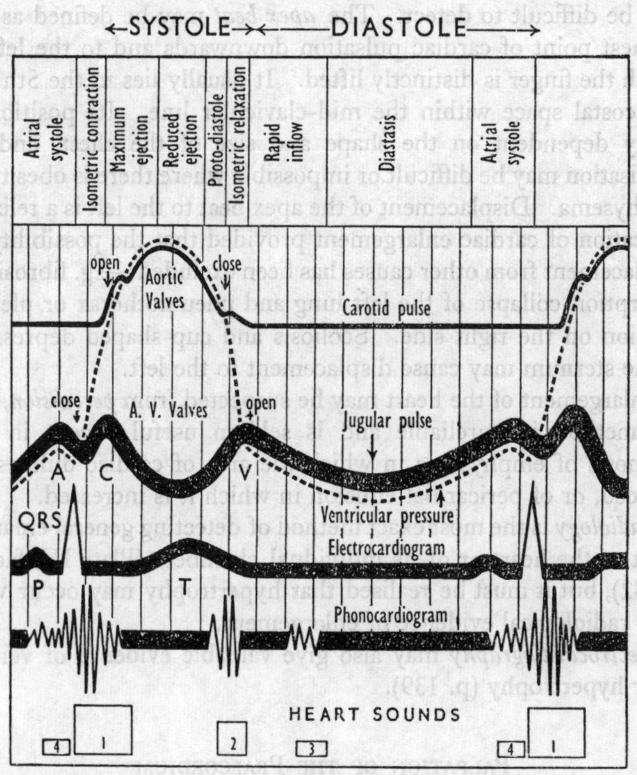

FIG. 7
TIMING OF EVENTS IN THE CARDIAC CYCLE

Examination of the jugular veins for the normal 'a' (atrial, presystolic) and 'v' (ventricular) waves may give useful information —thus in tricuspid stenosis, pulmonary stenosis or pulmonary hypertension from any cause the 'a' wave will be exaggerated, and in functional or organic tricuspid incompetence a positive, systolic wave will replace the usual dip in pressure in early systole. The 'c' wave recorded by physiologists can rarely be seen (Fig. 7).

(*d*) EXAMINATION OF THE HEART

Signs of Cardiac Enlargement

Cardiac enlargement is always significant, but minor degrees may be difficult to detect. The *apex beat* may be defined as the furthest point of cardiac pulsation downwards and to the left at which the finger is distinctly lifted. It usually lies in the 5th left intercostal space within the mid-clavicular line. Its position is partly dependent on the shape and size of the chest, and its localisation may be difficult or impossible where there is obesity or emphysema. Displacement of the apex beat to the left is a reliable indication of cardiac enlargement provided that the possibility of displacement from other causes has been excluded—e.g. fibrosis or absorption-collapse of the left lung and pneumothorax or pleural effusion on the right side. Scoliosis and cup-shaped depression of the sternum may cause displacement to the left.

Enlargement of the heart may be suspected from *percussion*, but the method is unreliable and is seldom useful except in the diagnosis of emphysema in which the area of cardiac dullness is reduced, or of pericardial effusion in which it is increased.

Radiology is the most exact method of detecting general enlargement of the heart or of its individual chambers (Plate IV, facing p. 132), but it must be realised that hypertrophy may occur with little radiological evidence of enlargement.

Electrocardiography may also give valuable evidence of ventricular hypertrophy (p. 139).

Palpation of the Praecordium

On palpation, not only should the *position of the apex beat* be located as a guide to cardiac enlargement or displacement but the *quality of the impulse* should be noted. A heaving impulse at the apex suggests hypertrophy of the left ventricle. Hypertrophy of the right ventricle may give rise to a lift in the epigastrium and of the lower sternum. A tapping impulse is due to closure of the mitral valve and corresponds in mechanism to the loud first heart sound. It should be remembered that a forceful impulse may be felt in the over-acting heart of nervous individuals, but in practice there is rarely any difficulty in differentiating this from the sustained heave which is characteristic of hypertrophy. The presence or absence of *thrills* should be noted. Thrills frequently accompany valvular or congenital heart disease. The position of maximal intensity should be determined. An apical thrill is best felt with the patient lying on the left side. During palpation for thrills in other areas the patient should lean forward and hold his breath in expiration. The most common thrills are:

Mitral Area: Systolic—mitral incompetence; diastolic—mitral stenosis.

Pulmonary Area: Systolic—pulmonary stenosis; patent ductus arteriosus.

Aortic Area: Systolic—aortic stenosis.

Lower Left Sternal Edge: Systolic—ventricular septal defect.

Heart Sounds and Murmurs

Sounds. The first heart sound is mainly produced by closure of the mitral and tricuspid valves. The second heart sound is due to closure of the aortic and pulmonary valves and marks the end of systole. In auscultation attention should be paid to each sound separately. It should be noted whether both sounds are present and if so whether they are normal. If not, then it must be decided whether the first or second sound is accentuated, diminished or absent. Both heart sounds may be diminished in the presence of obesity or emphysema. Accentuation of the first sound at the apex may be present with mitral stenosis, emotion, thyrotoxicosis or hypertension. This sound may be diminished in mitral incompetence, rheumatic carditis or in severe cardiac failure, or may largely be obscured by a loud systolic murmur. Accentuation of the aortic second sound is found in hypertension, atherosclerosis and syphilitic aortitis. It may be diminished in aortic stenosis. The pulmonary second sound may be accentuated in pulmonary hypertension, which is most often due to pulmonary congestion, e.g. from mitral stenosis or left ventricular failure. It may be diminished in some cases of pulmonary stenosis. Sometimes more than two heart sounds can be detected.

Splitting of the First Sound (Fig. 8.) The importance of splitting of the first heart sound, which is not uncommon in normal people, lies solely in its correct identification and an appreciation of the fact that the condition is usually innocent and quite unconnected with any form of heart disease. It is due to asynchronous closure of the mitral and tricuspid valves. The two components have much the same quality and are separated from one another by a very short interval. Splitting of the first sound may be

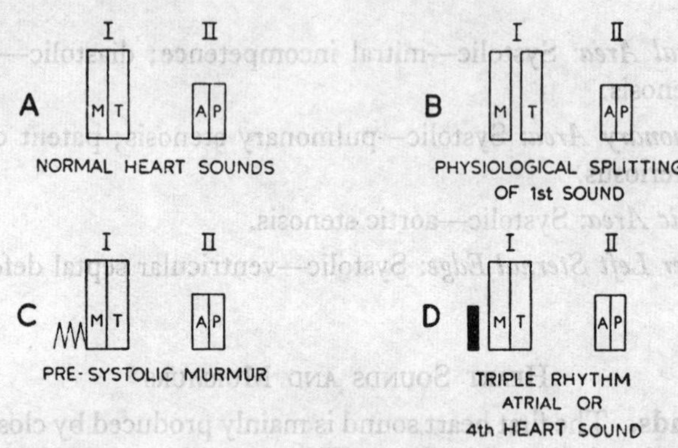

FIG. 8
DIFFERENTIAL DIAGNOSIS OF SPLIT FIRST SOUND

mistaken for the pre-systolic murmur of mitral stenosis. It must also be distinguished from the pre-systolic variety of triple rhythm in which the extra sound coincides with atrial contraction.

SPLITTING OF THE SECOND SOUND (Fig. 9.) Splitting of the second sound at the base of the heart is due to slightly asynchronous closure of the aortic and pulmonary valves and as such it is of no pathological significance. Physiological splitting increases with inspiration. Its main importance lies in distinguishing it from one of the forms of triple rhythm (referred to below). Splitting must also be distinguished from the additional sound, sometimes referred to as the '*opening snap*' of the mitral valve, which so often immediately precedes the mid-diastolic murmur of mitral stenosis and is best heard at the lower, left sternal margin. This 'opening snap' should serve as a reminder to listen carefully for such a murmur.

TRIPLE RHYTHM: Triple rhythm may be said to occur whenever three sounds can be heard instead of the normal two. It is important to recognise that there are physiological and pathological forms of triple rhythm and to differentiate between them, otherwise serious errors in diagnosis may be made and unwarranted fears engendered. It is far better to ignore all such added sounds than to misinterpret them. Nevertheless they are a common source of confusion in practice. It is not the mechanism (which is often obscure or debatable) but the significance of the sounds which

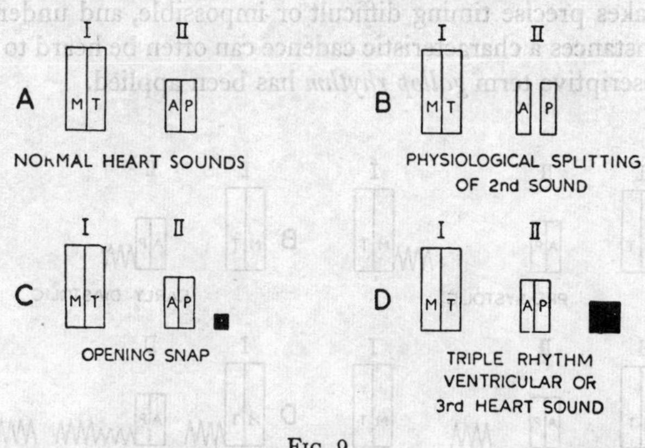

FIG. 9

DIFFERENTIAL DIAGNOSIS OF SPLIT SECOND SOUND

matters most. If the doctor has any doubt in his mind about the nature of additional heart sounds he should refer the patient to a cardiologist.

In the first place, triple rhythm should be distinguished from splitting of the first or second heart sounds and from short diastolic murmurs.

An extra heart sound, in diastole, may be *physiological*, especially in children or young persons and in pregnancy, or *pathological* in failure of the left or right ventricle. The differentiation between a physiological and pathological triple rhythm cannot be made by auscultation alone, but only by the presence or absence of other evidence of heart disease, i.e. by consideration of the symptoms and signs and by the detection of some aetiological factor which might be responsible for cardiac failure (e.g. hypertension). *One should always beware of drawing conclusions from an isolated sign.* In established heart disease triple rhythm is usually of serious prognostic significance.

The extra sound may precede the normal first heart sound (when it is referred to as an atrial or 4th heart sound, Fig. 8 D) or follow the normal second sound (when it is referred to as a ventricular filling or 3rd heart sound, Fig. 9 D). The extra sound when pathological in origin is separated from the normal sound by a readily appreciable gap and has a different quality, being dull or muffled. The tachycardia which often accompanies cardiac failure makes precise timing difficult or impossible, and under these circumstances a characteristic cadence can often be heard to which the descriptive term *gallop rhythm* has been applied.

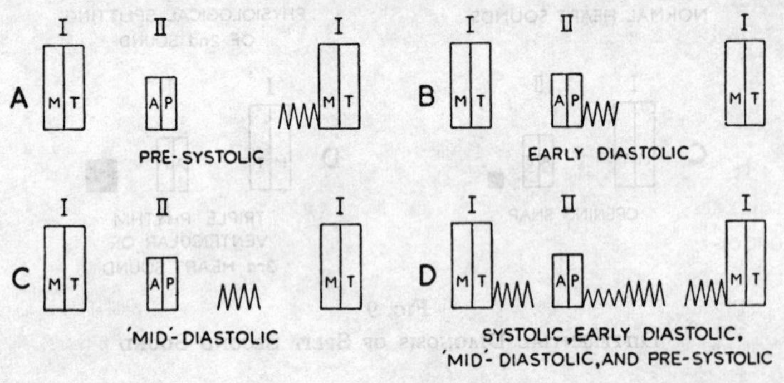

FIG. 10
HEART MURMURS

Murmurs. If a murmur is heard it is important to note the *intensity*, e.g. faint, moderate or loud; the *position of maximal intensity*; the *timing*, e.g. systolic or diastolic; the *quality*, e.g. blowing or harsh; the *pitch* and the direction in which it is *conducted*. Some murmurs are characteristic, e.g. a harsh, crescendo presystolic murmur at the apex leading up to a sudden, loud first sound in mitral stenosis or the blowing early diastolic murmur of aortic incompetence best heard down the left sternal border. It will be appreciated that in the presence of tachycardia it may be difficult to define the position of a murmur in diastole. In these circumstances interpretation of the murmur depends upon its other characteristics. Further details of heart murmurs are discussed under Valvular Heart Disease, pp. 199-206, and are summarised in graphic form in Fig. 10.

(*e*) EXAMINATION FOR SIGNS OF CARDIAC FAILURE

The signs of cardiac failure are fully described on pp. 169-176.

(*f*) EXAMINATION OF THE LUNGS

The pulmonary manifestations of heart disease are due to pulmonary hypertension or pulmonary oedema, and include dyspnoea, cough, sputum, crepitations and haemoptysis. Pulmonary infarction frequently accompanies heart failure and is described on p. 253. In addition, certain diseases of the lung, notably chronic bronchitis and emphysema, may themselves be responsible for heart failure.

(*g*) ESTIMATION OF THE BLOOD PRESSURE

It is important that the patient should be comfortable and relaxed and that the arm should be laid bare to the shoulder in order to avoid any constriction by a rolled-up sleeve and to facilitate the proper application of the armlet.

The cuff, deflated, should be applied evenly to the middle of the upper arm with the middle of the rubber bag over the inner side.

A preliminary approximate reading of the systolic pressure should be taken by palpation; the pressure in the armlet should be raised quickly in steps of 10 mm. until the radial pulse disappears and then allowed to fall rapidly.

The stethoscope should be applied *lightly* and accurately over the brachial artery.

After inflating the cuff to a pressure of about 30 mm. above the systolic pressure as found by palpation, auscultation should be conducted during slow deflation. The systolic pressure is the highest pressure at which successive sounds are heard.

With the pressure continuing to fall slowly and uniformly the sound increases to its maximum intensity and then decreases at first gradually and later suddenly and soon disappears. The point where the loud, clear sounds change abruptly to the dull and muffled sounds and the point where they disappear should be recorded. The latter probably reflects the true diastolic pressure more accurately.

The blood pressure depends principally on the cardiac output and the peripheral resistance. The range of normal varies considerably not only with age but from patient to patient and from time to time and with the circumference of the arm in relation to the width of the cuff. The blood pressure varies greatly with exercise and emotion, and to a slight extent with meals and smoking. *Casual* readings in the consulting room or out-patient department may be very different from resting readings taken in bed after a night's sleep, reassurance and repeated recordings on different occasions. The information to be gained from a single reading is limited. There is still some difference of opinion as to what level constitutes hypertension. A consistent level of 150/90 in young people is suspicious and a pressure of 160/100 should be regarded as abnormal, but not necessarily of bad prognostic significance or requiring treatment.

It is important to distinguish predominantly systolic from diastolic hypertension. Emotion chiefly affects the systolic pressure. *Systolic* hypertension is also found in elderly patients with atherosclerosis of the aorta (and hence loss of elasticity) and in aortic incompetence, heart block and thyrotoxicosis. It is of far less significance in prognosis than diastolic hypertension. *Diastolic* hypertension largely depends on constriction of the arterioles and is most commonly associated with essential hypertension, renal disease and toxaemia of pregnancy.

Pulse Pressure. The pulse pressure is the difference between the systolic and diastolic pressures. The normal range is 40-70 mm. Hg. In hypertension the pulse pressure is commonly increased (e.g. 220/120), and particularly if there is atherosclerosis of the aorta as mentioned above (e.g. 200/95). It is often raised in thyrotoxicosis, and in aortic incompetence it may be very high (e.g. 200/40). In aortic stenosis it is characteristically low (e.g. 110/90).

(*h*) EXAMINATION OF THE RETINA

Ophthalmoscopy permits direct inspection of the optic disc, the retina and the retinal vessels (see Frontispiece). In particular, very useful information as regards diagnosis and prognosis may be obtained in hypertension (p. 232).

The optic discs should first be examined, after which the four quadrants in each eye should be studied and attention paid to the vessels and the presence or absence of haemorrhages and exudates. The central retinal artery and its primary and secondary branches correspond in size to small arteries and are prone to atherosclerosis (pp. 278-283), and consequently thrombosis. Thrombosis may also occur in the veins. Beyond the second bifurcation the vessels are arteriolar in character and therefore prone to arteriolar sclerosis (p. 277). Important vascular changes may occur in essential hypertension (p. 232), nephritis (p. 797), diabetes (p. 738) and eclampsia, or as a result of degenerative arterial disease independent of such conditions. Haemorrhages and exudates result from rupture of capillary walls or from increase in their permeability. Papilloedema is due to transudation of fluid into the nerve head and occurs from a number of causes (p. 1096), including severe hypertension. Papilloedema may also accompany the transient hypertension of acute nephritis or toxaemia of pregnancy.

(*i*) EXAMINATION OF THE URINE

In congestive cardiac failure protein and a few red cells and granular casts may be found in the urine. They are the result of renal congestion and will disappear when the congestive cardiac failure has responded to treatment. Microscopic haematuria is a common finding in bacterial endocarditis. In hypertensive heart disease proteinuria may be the consequence of concomitant congestive cardiac failure or of a renal lesion, e.g. chronic nephritis or pyelonephritis, that was primarily responsible for the hypertension. It should be noted that proteinuria does not develop until the course of idiopathic hypertension is well advanced, and therefore is of serious prognostic importance (p. 228).

ELECTROCARDIOGRAPHY

Electrocardiography plays an important part in the diagnosis and investigation of all forms of heart disease. Its main value lies in the elucidation of cardiac arrhythmias (p. 155) and conduction defects (p. 152), and in the information which it provides about the state of the myocardium. Electrocardiography has achieved a high degree of accuracy in the diagnosis and location of myocardial infarction and is of particular value in cases of unexplained chest pain or collapse.

A normal electrocardiogram (ECG) will go far to refute a diagnosis of myocardial infarction, but it must be realised that in some cases the electrocardiographic changes of infarction are slow to develop, and accordingly a series of electrocardiograms is indicated in doubtful cases. In cases of minor or intramural infarction the electrocardiogram may be normal.

Electrocardiograms must always be interpreted in the light of the entire clinical picture. For instance, digitalis and quinidine, myxoedema, and certain electrolyte disturbances cause electrocardiographic changes which may easily be misinterpreted.

The electrocardiograph is a sensitive meter which amplifies and records the difference in electrical potential between any two points on the surface of the body. It is capable of detecting the electrical activity (depolarisation and repolarisation) which accompanies muscle fibre contraction, and the electrocardiogram is the graphic representation of these electrical changes. It does not represent the actual muscular contraction.

The simplest type of electrocardiograph consists of a galvanometer and two metal plates (electrodes) which are attached to two points on the body surface. The resulting tracing is termed a *lead*, and because two electrodes are used it is termed a *bipolar lead*. Three such bipolar leads are used, the electrodes being placed as follows:

Lead I	left arm—right arm
Lead II	left leg—right arm
Lead III	left leg—left arm

For many years bipolar leads alone were used in clinical electrocardiography, but they have largely been supplemented by the so-called *unipolar leads* which give more accurate information about the state of the myocardium.

The waves which are seen in unipolar leads can be understood in relation to the changes which occur during stimulation of a single muscle cell. In its resting condition, a cell is in a state of electrical balance. When the cell is stimulated at one end, the activation process spreads rapidly through the cell, and for a very short space of time a potential difference exists between that part of the cell which has been activated and the part which is still in its resting state. This transient potential difference can be detected by a galvanometer, which will show a deflection. (The P wave and QRS complex of an ECG correspond to this deflection.) As the impulse spreads through the cell, contraction occurs, and after a short interval a recovery process takes place, restoring electrical balance. (The T wave of an ECG corresponds to this recovery process.)

If the passage of an impulse along a strip of heart muscle is recorded by a unipolar lead, the deflections of the galvanometer, and hence the waves of the ECG, will vary according to the position

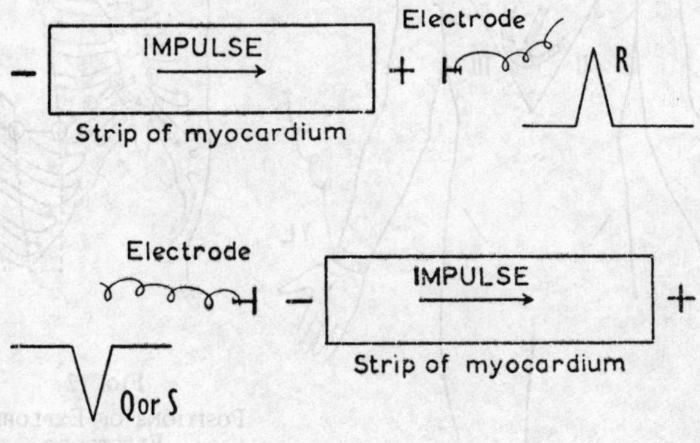

FIG. 11

of the exploring electrode in relation to the muscle strip (Fig. 11). When the impulse moves towards the electrode, a positive wave (R) is recorded. When the impulse moves away from the electrode, a negative wave (Q or S) is recorded.

The use of unipolar leads is based on Einthoven's hypothesis that the heart may be considered to lie at the centre of an equilateral triangle, the angles of which are at the right arm, the left arm and the left leg, and that the algebraic sum of the potential differences between these three points at any instant is zero. If these points are connected to a common terminal, no current will flow. This terminal is connected to one pole of the galvanometer, and the other pole is then connected to an electrode which can be placed anywhere on the body surface, and which is termed the *exploring electrode*. Such an electrode detects the electrical events of the heart as if it were situated on that part of the heart to which it lies closest. Tracings obtained in this way are termed *V leads*, and usually these are recorded from nine positions—the right arm

(VR), the left arm (VL), the left leg (VF), and six positions on the chest wall (V_1-V_6) (Fig. 12). As a rule, the amplitude of the unipolar limb leads (VR, VL and VF) is 'augmented' to make them more easily interpreted, and they are then termed aVR, aVL and aVF.

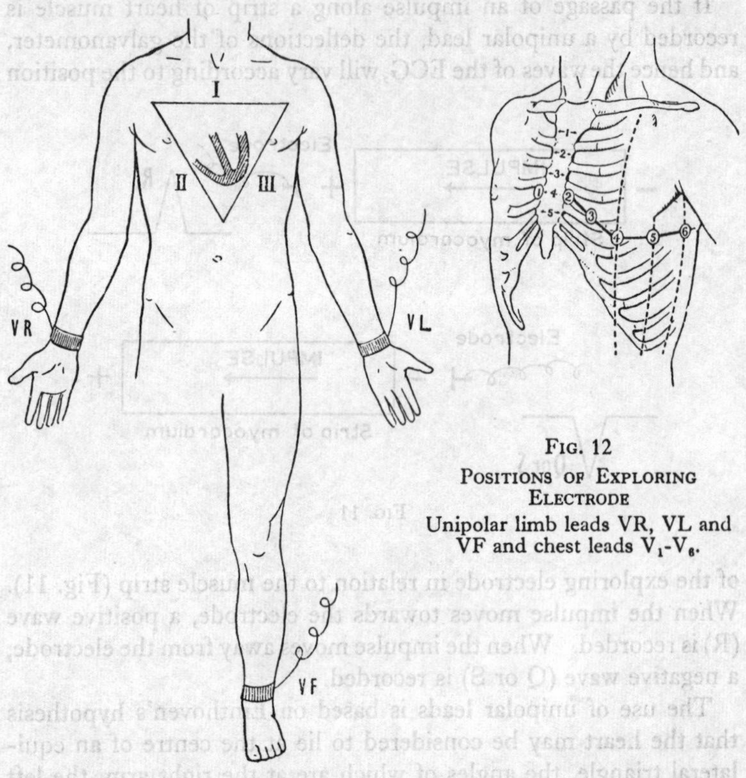

FIG. 12
POSITIONS OF EXPLORING ELECTRODE
Unipolar limb leads VR, VL and VF and chest leads V_1-V_6.

An example of a single lead of an ECG is shown in Figure 13. The letters P, Q, R, S and T were applied to the various waves many years ago by Einthoven. The P wave represents the passage of the activating impulse through the atria. The QRS complex represents the passage of the activating impulse through the ventricles, Q being applied to an initial negative deflection, R to the first positive deflection (whether preceded by a Q wave or not), and S to a negative deflection following an R wave. The PR interval is measured from the start of the P wave to the start of the ventricular complex (i.e. if a Q wave is present, it is strictly speaking the PQ interval). The T wave represents ventricular recovery. The S-T segment extends from the end of the QRS complex to the commencement of the T wave. The heavy vertical lines on the paper, on which the electrocardiogram is recorded, are one-fifth of a second apart and the fine vertical lines are 0·04 seconds apart. The approximate rate of the heart per minute can be calculated by dividing 1500 by the number

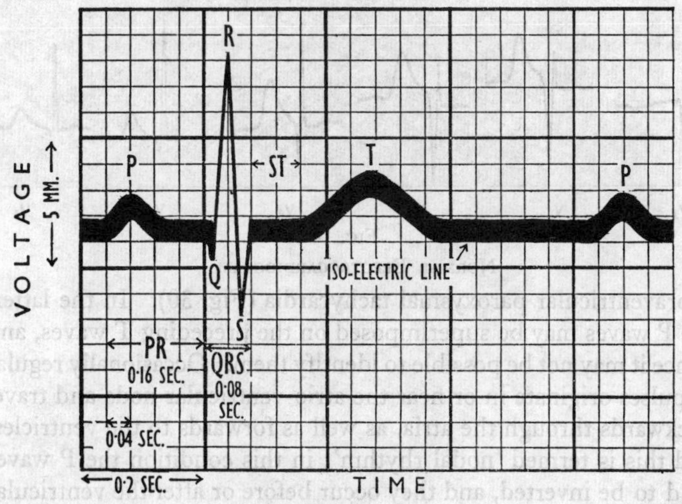

Fig. 13

An Example of an Electrocardiogram

of fine divisions between two successive corresponding points on the electrocardiogram, e.g. the peaks of the R waves.

The various waves in the ECG of a normal person (Fig. 14) will now be considered in more detail, and thereafter some of the abnormalities which may occur.

P Wave

Abnormalities of P Waves. Prominent P waves may occur in atrial hypertrophy, being broad and bifid in the left atrial hypertrophy of mitral stenosis, and tall and peaked in the right atrial hypertrophy which accompanies tricuspid stenosis or right ventricular hypertrophy from pulmonary stenosis or pulmonary hypertension from any cause.

The P wave tends to be of abnormal form if the activating impulse originates at some point in the atria other than the sino-atrial node. This occurs in supraventricular extrasystoles and in

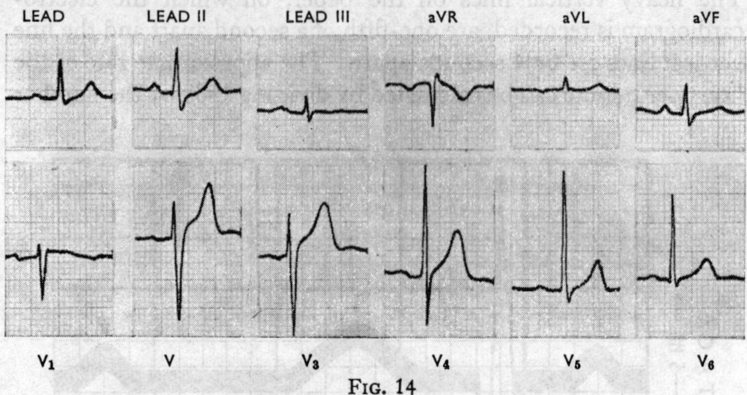

FIG. 14

NORMAL ELECTROCARDIOGRAM

supraventricular paroxysmal tachycardia (Fig. 30). In the latter, the P waves may be superimposed on the preceding T waves, and hence it may not be possible to identify them. Occasionally regular impulses originate in or near the atrio-ventricular node and travel backwards through the atria, as well as forwards to the ventricles, and this is termed 'nodal rhythm'; in this condition the P waves tend to be inverted, and they occur before or after the ventricular complexes, or coincide with them and hence be hidden. Another condition, in which the P waves and ventricular complexes may coincide, is complete heart block, where the atria and ventricles beat independently of one another.

P waves are absent in atrial fibrillation and flutter, their place being taken by fibrillary 'f' (Fig. 28), or flutter 'F' waves (Fig. 29). Disturbances of rhythm are considered on p. 155.

P-R INTERVAL

This represents the time interval from the moment when the impulse leaves the sino-atrial node until the moment when it starts to activate the ventricular muscle. The P-R interval is normally less than 0·20 of a second.

PROLONGATION OF THE P-R INTERVAL, and intermittent or complete failure of atrio-ventricular conduction (p. 165), constitute varying degrees of heart block (Figs. 33, 34 and 35).

QRS Complex

The first part of ventricular muscle to be activated is the septum, and this activation occurs from the left bundle branch (Fig. 17). Subsequently, the impulse spreads out simultaneously through both ventricles from endocardial to epicardial surfaces. The amplitude, and to some extent the duration, of the QRS complexes depend on the bulk of muscle tissue through which the impulse is passing; as the left ventricle is normally much thicker than the right, most of the QRS complex is due to activation of the left ventricle.

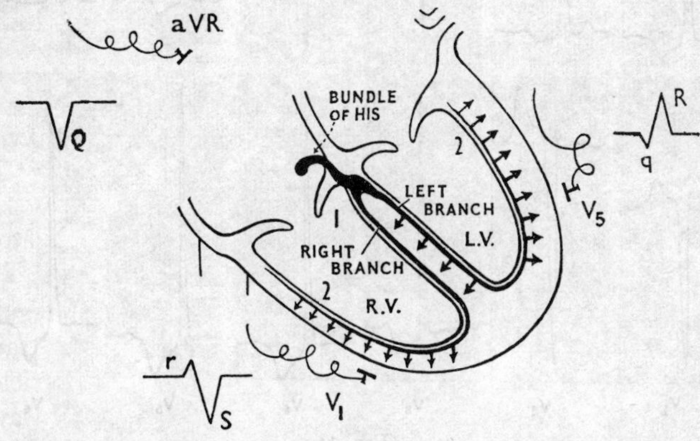

Fig. 15

This can be illustrated by consideration of two unipolar chest leads, one (e.g. V_1) lying over the surface of the right ventricle and the other (e.g. V_5) lying over the surface of the left ventricle (Fig. 15). In both these leads the initial wave (small *r* in V_1 and small *q* in V_5) is due to the same activation of the septum from left to right, and the subsequent wave (S in V_1, and R in V_5) is due to the spread of the same impulse through the left ventricle. A lead taken with an electrode which faces the cavities of the ventricles (e.g. aVR) shows a negative wave (deep Q) because the impulse is moving away from the electrode.

There is considerable individual variation in the pattern of the QRS complexes of the 12-lead ECG in normal people. This is partly related to variation in the anatomical position of the heart; for example, a long, narrow heart gives a different ECG from a broad, transverse heart.

Abnormalities of the QRS Complex

1. *Ventricular hypertrophy.* In left ventricular hypertrophy there is a greater preponderance than usual of the left ventricle over the right ventricle, with the result that the R waves in the left chest leads (V_5, V_6) and the S waves in the right chest leads (V_1, V_2) are of greater amplitude than usual (Fig. 16).

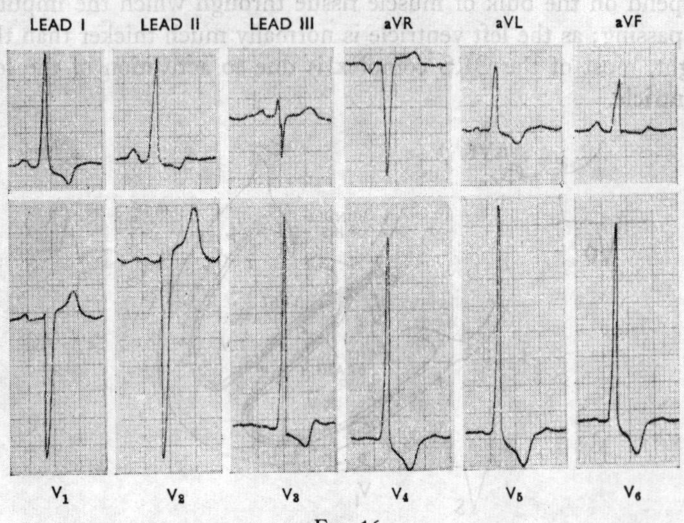

Fig. 16

Left Ventricular Hypertrophy

Note: (1) tall R waves over left ventricle;
(2) deep S waves over right ventricle;
(3) ST depression and asymmetrical inversion of T wave in leads I, aVL, and V_3-V_6.

In right ventricular hypertrophy the wall of the right ventricle is thicker than usual though still less thick than the wall of a normal left ventricle, so that activation of the right ventricle is no longer overshadowed by activation of the left ventricle; it therefore causes changes in the ECG of which a prominent R wave in V_1 is the most important (Fig. 17).

2. *Bundle branch block.* This may be partial or complete, and may involve either the right or left branch of the bundle. Conduction of the activating impulse has to occur by unusual routes, and this leads to a prolongation of the conduction time, seen as a widening of the QRS complex, and to distortion of the normal pattern (Figs. 18 and 19).

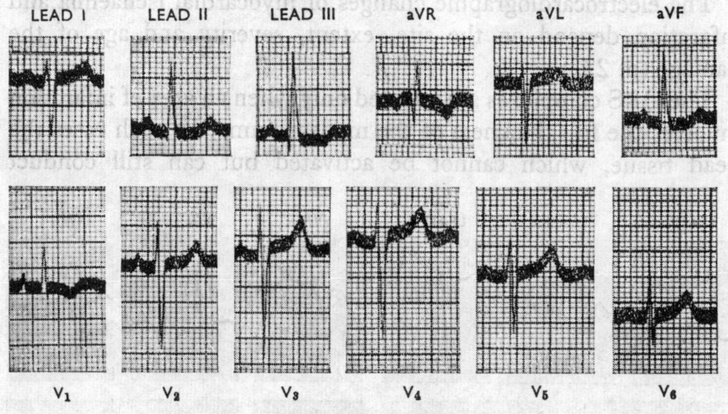

FIG. 17

RIGHT VENTRICULAR HYPERTROPHY

Note: (1) R wave exceeds the S wave in amplitude in V_1;
(2) negative T wave in V_1.

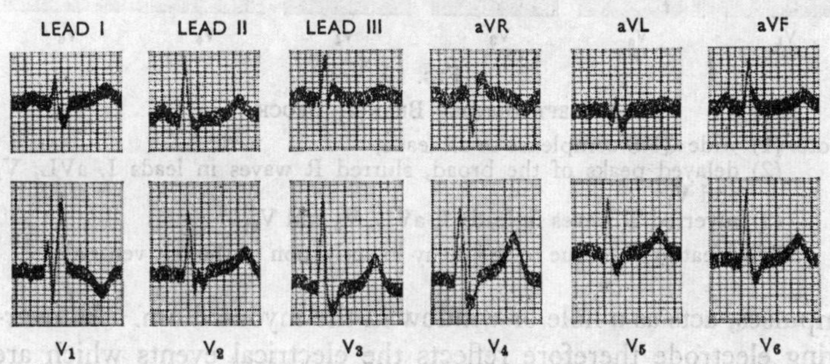

FIG. 18

RIGHT BUNDLE BRANCH BLOCK

Note: (1) wide QRS complexes in all leads;
(2) delayed peak of the main upright wave in V_1
(3) slurred S waves in leads I, aVL, V_3-V_6;
(4) inverted T wave in V_1.

These features are due to the delay in activation of the right ventricle.

3. *Myocardial infarction.* As a rule myocardial infarction occurs in the wall of the left ventricle and in the interventricular septum; the wall of the right ventricle is usually only affected in areas adjacent to a large septal infarct, and infarction of this wall can seldom be diagnosed electrocardiographically.

The electrocardiographic changes of myocardial ischaemia and infarction depend on the site, extent, severity and age of the damage (p. 221).

The QRS complexes are affected only when an area of infarction involves the full thickness of the myocardium. In such cases the dead tissue, which cannot be activated but can still conduct

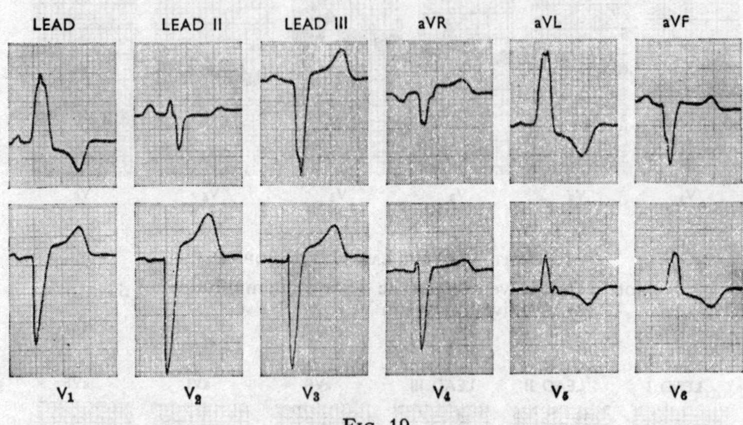

FIG. 19

LEFT BUNDLE BRANCH BLOCK

Note: (1) wide QRS complexes in all leads;
(2) delayed peaks of the broad, slurred R waves in leads I, aVL, V_5 and V_6;
(3) inverted T waves in leads I, aVL, V_5 and V_6.

These features are due to the delay in activation of the left ventricle.

impulses, acts as a hole or window in the myocardium. An overlying electrode therefore reflects the electrical events which are occurring in the septum and the opposite wall of the heart, shown in the electrocardiogram as a negative wave (deep Q) for the reasons explained above. This is the characteristic sign of an infarct which involves the entire thickness of the ventricular wall.

S-T SEGMENT AND T WAVE

The S-T segment represents the period when activation of the ventricles is complete, but before recovery has started. It should be iso-electric, i.e. it should not deviate from the base line.

The T wave represents recovery of the ventricular muscle. It should normally be upright in all leads except aVR, and sometimes leads III, and V_1.

ABNORMALITIES OF S-T SEGMENT AND T WAVE. This part of the electrocardiogram is altered by many factors. Among these are drugs (e.g. digitalis), disturbances of electrolyte balance (especially potassium), certain endocrine diseases (e.g. myxoedema) and—most important of all—myocardial ischaemia with or without subsequent infarction. The S-T segment and the T wave are also

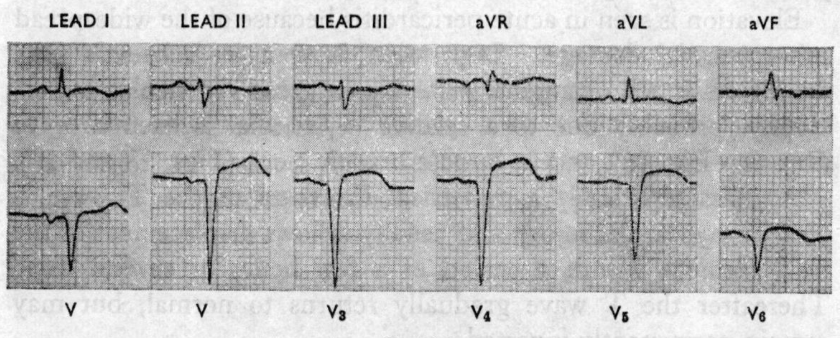

FIG. 20

ANTERIOR MYOCARDIAL INFARCTION

Note: (1) deep abnormal Q waves in V_1-V_6;
(2) S-T elevation in V_3-V_6 (elevation in V_1 and V_2 could be normal).
(3) shallow inverted T waves in I, II, aVL and V_6 (inversion in III could be normal).

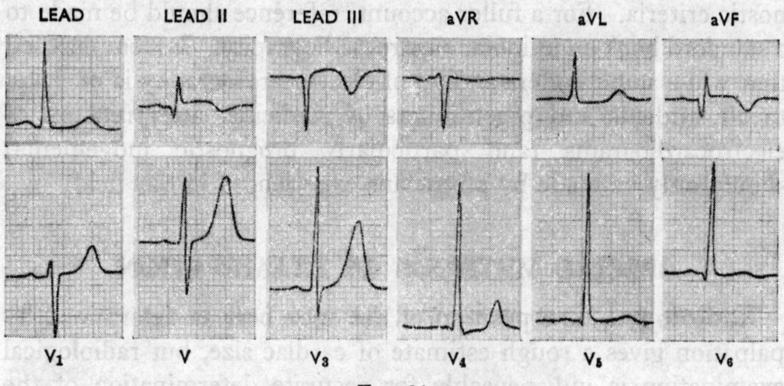

FIG. 21

POSTERIOR MYOCARDIAL INFARCTION

Note: (1) deep abnormal Q waves in leads III and aVF;
(2) S-T elevation in leads II, III and aVF.
(3) inverted T waves in leads II and III and aVF
(4) 'reciprocal' S-T depression in leads I and aVL.

affected by primary myocardial disease-myocarditis or cardiomyopathy.

Ischaemia causes a change in the electrical state of the affected area of the myocardium, and this results in elevation or depression of the S-T segment, depending on whether the sub-epicardial or sub-endocardial layer of muscle is mainly involved, and also on the position of the exploring electrode (Figs. 20 and 21).

Elevation is seen in acute pericarditis because of the widespread sub-epicardial damage. Depression is seen in ischaemia (e.g. during an attack of angina pectoris), in gross ventricular hypertrophy (probably due to a relative myocardial ischaemia or to fibrosis—Fig. 16), and in bundle branch block (Figs. 18 and 19).

A characteristically symmetrical inversion of the T wave is seen in myocardial injury and usually follows displacement of the S-T segment within a period of a few hours or several days. Thereafter the T wave gradually returns to normal, but may remain permanently inverted.

By means of these ST-T wave changes, the age of a myocardial infarct can often be assessed, and serial electrocardiograms are particularly valuable in this respect.

The preceding account of electrocardiography is greatly simplified, and details have not been given of the many normal variants which may be encountered, nor of the minutiae of diagnostic criteria. For a fuller account, reference should be made to a standard book on unipolar electrocardiography. It is emphasised that while some understanding of electrocardiography is of value to all students and practitioners of medicine, interpretation of electrocardiograms (and particularly prognostic judgements) should only be made by physicians experienced in this field.

SPECIAL METHODS OF EXAMINATION

Radiology. The position of the apex beat as determined by palpation gives a rough estimate of cardiac size, but radiological examination is indispensable for accurate determination of the size and shape of the heart (p. 132). Radiology enables not only the width but also the depth of the heart to be seen. The oesophagus can be outlined by giving the patient some barium emulsion to swallow. This will help to show backward enlargement of the left atrium in mitral stenosis in the right oblique position.

Films are useful for record purposes and for studying the details of abnormalities in the lung fields. Screening (radioscopy) is invaluable on account of its technical simplicity and for allowing the heart and great vessels to be viewed from every angle and abnormal pulsations observed. Not only can the size of the heart as a whole be determined but also the size of individual chambers and of the great vessels. The presence or absence of valvular calcification can also be determined.

Characteristic configurations are often to be seen in the various forms of valvular and congenital heart disease, in syphilitic aortitis and in aneurysm of the heart.

Congestion and oedema of the lungs and small pleural effusions can be shown radiologically before they can be detected clinically.

Angiocardiography. The individual chambers of the heart and the great vessels may be visualised by the injection of a radio-opaque material into a vein or by catheter directly into the heart before taking a series of radiographs in rapid succession. Such studies are very useful in the differentiation of various congenital cardiac lesions and of vascular from other abnormal mediastinal shadows.

Phonocardiography. The phonocardiograph records heart sounds and murmurs and may help to elucidate difficult problems of auscultation.

Cardiac Catheterisation. A radio-opaque catheter can be passed from a vein into the right atrium, right ventricle, pulmonary artery and its right or left branches (Plate V, facing p. 133) or from an artery into the aorta or left ventricle. If necessary the left atrium or left ventricle can be punctured with a needle. The pressures in these chambers can be recorded and the oxygen saturation of extracted blood samples estimated. Valuable information may be obtained in cases of congenital heart disease and in certain types of acquired heart disease. For example, in pulmonary hypertension the pressure in the pulmonary artery and right ventricle will be increased; in pulmonary stenosis the pressure will be higher in the right ventricle than in the pulmonary artery; and in aortic stenosis it will be higher in the left ventricle than in the aorta; in atrial septal defect the oxygen content of the blood in the right atrium will be higher than that in the vena cava; in ventricular septal defect the oxygen content of the blood in the right ventricle will be higher than that in the right atrium. In some cases the volume of a shunt or the area of a valve can be calculated. If the oxygen content of blood from the right atrium and brachial artery, and also the oxygen consumption, is known, then the cardiac output can be calculated from the Fick formula:

$$\text{Cardiac Output} = \frac{\text{oxygen consumption}}{\text{arterio-venous difference}}$$

Dye Dilution Curves. By the injection of a dye into a vein or directly into the heart through a catheter and estimation of its time of arrival and concentration in a peripheral artery, the presence of a shunt can be detected and the cardiac output measured.

TESTS OF CARDIAC FUNCTION

The reserve power of the heart is normally very great and it is important to elicit any evidence of impairment of this reserve. At first this will be apparent only on considerable effort, the patient becoming breathless after exertion which he could formerly carry out without distress. Thereafter the disability is usually progressive until breathlessness is present on slight exertion and finally even at rest. Sometimes it is pain rather than breathlessness which limits exertion (angina pectoris).

Various forms of '*exercise tolerance test*' have been devised to measure the reserve power of the heart. The patient may be submitted to a standard amount of effort and the reaction estimated by the degree of dyspnoea, tachycardia or pain. The value of such a test is seriously limited by the fact that other factors, such as emotion, infection, obesity and lack of physical fitness may give rise to undue tachycardia after exertion in the absence of organic heart disease. Of far more value is a careful appraisal of the history as regards capacity for familiar effort such as normal occupation and climbing stairs or hills.

DISORDERS OF CARDIAC CONDUCTION

Physiology and Anatomy

The impulse initiating cardiac contraction originates in the sino-atrial (S-A) node which lies at the junction of the superior vena cava and the right atrium. From the S-A node the impulse spreads through the atria to the atrio-ventricular (A-V) node at the base of the interatrial septum, and from there it is conducted down the A-V bundle to the ventricles. This bundle of specialised conducting tissue divides into right and left branches which pass down on either side of the interventricular septum and ramify widely beneath the endocardium in a syncytial network which then extends

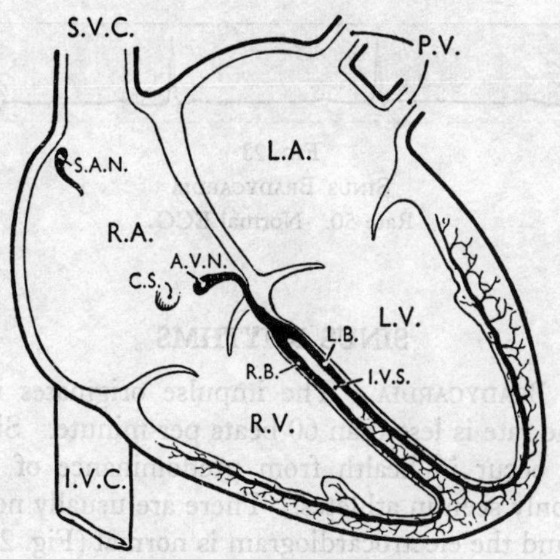

FIG. 22

CONDUCTION SYSTEM OF THE HEART

R.A., right atrium; R.V., right ventricle; L.A., left atrium; L.V., left ventricle; I.V.S., Interventricular septum; P.V., pulmonary vein; S.V.C., superior vena cava; I.V.C., inferior vena cava; C.S., coronary sinus; S.A.N., sino-atrial node: A.V.N., atrio-ventricular node; R.B., right branch; L.B., left branch.

outwards towards the pericardium (Fig. 22). The A-V node and bundle have a special blood supply from the circumflex branch of the right coronary artery, and hence localised vascular disease may cause serious impairment of its nutrition.

The inherent rhythm of cardiac contraction is under the influence of the autonomic nervous system and may be affected by emotion, various vagal and sympathetic reflexes, or by chemical substances, e.g. adrenaline. The normal pacemaker of the heart, the S-A node, has an inherent rate of 75/min. but if it is depressed for any reason, e.g. by ischaemia or nervous impulses, the A-V node (60/min.) takes over control and initiates the impulse. The ventricles may develop an inherent rhythm if stimuli from the

S-A and A-V nodes fail to reach them (as in complete heart block 30-40/min.).

The normal heart rate in adults varies between 60 and 90 beats per minute. The rate gradually slows from 120-140 in infants to about 80 at puberty.

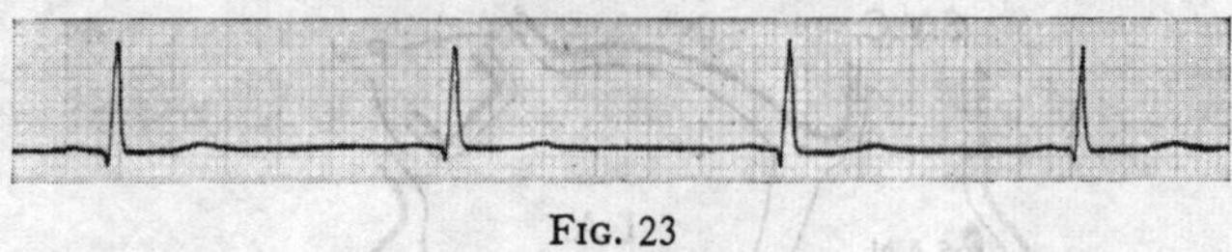

FIG. 23
SINUS BRADYCARDIA
Rate 50. Normal ECG.

SINUS RHYTHMS

1. SINUS BRADYCARDIA. The impulse originates in the S-A node but the rate is less than 60 beats per minute. Sinus bradycardia may occur in health from predominance of vagal tone. It is commonly seen in athletes. There are usually no associated symptoms and the electrocardiogram is normal (Fig. 23). It may

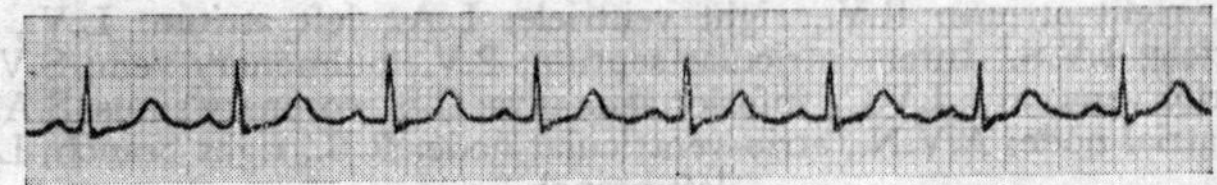

FIG. 24
SINUS TACHYCARDIA
Rate 110. Normal ECG.

occur pathologically, e.g. in convalescence from infective fevers, raised intracranial pressure, myxoedema, jaundice or excessive dosage with digitalis.

2. SINUS TACHYCARDIA. The impulse originates in the S-A node but the rate is greater than 90 (adults). Sinus tachycardia may be associated with exercise or emotion or it may accompany fever, thyrotoxicosis, shock, acute haemorrhage, constrictive pericarditis or cardiac failure. The rate rarely exceeds 160 beats per minute and the electrocardiogram is normal (Fig. 14).

3. Sinus Arrhythmia. The impulse originates in the S-A node but the rhythm is irregular. The heart rate increases in inspiration and slows in expiration. Hence deep breathing may help in its differentiation from other arrhythmias. This rhythm is of no pathological significance and is most commonly seen in the young. The electrocardiogram shows rhythmic variations in the length of the cardiac cycles but is otherwise normal (Fig. 25).

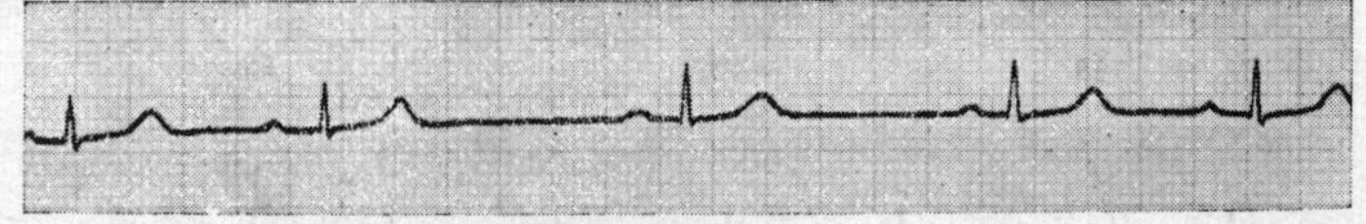

Fig. 25

Sinus Arrhythmia

Rate approx. 50-60. Note varying intervals between ventricular complexes. Normal ECG.

ECTOPIC RHYTHMS

When the impulse arises elsewhere than in the S-A node, e.g. in atria, A-V node or ventricles, it is referred to as an ectopic rhythm. The rhythm may be regular or irregular.

1. Extrasystoles

Extrasystoles arise from some abnormal focus in the heart and are really premature beats coming earlier than expected in the cardiac cycle. The term extrasystole is really a misnomer because, except in rare instances, there is in fact no 'extra' or additional beat. Very occasionally a true interpolated extra beat occurs between two normal beats. Since the heart muscle is rendered refractory by the extrasystole, the next normal impulse usually fails to cause a contraction and there is a long (compensatory) pause with increased diastolic filling so that the next normal contraction is augmented. The site of origin may be in the atria, ventricles or occasionally in the A-V node and can be recognised only by means of an electrocardiogram (Figs. 26 and 27).

Aetiology. Extrasystoles are often found in healthy people with normal hearts. They occur in males more often than in females and are particularly common in the elderly. They may be caused by over-indulgence in tea, coffee, tobacco or alcohol, or in association with dyspepsia or anxiety. Extrasystoles may also

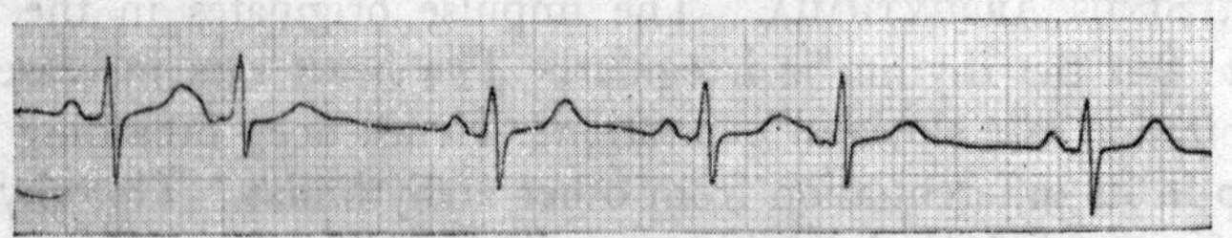

FIG. 26

SUPRAVENTRICULAR EXTRASYSTOLE

The second and fifth complexes occur earlier in the cardiac cycle than expected and are followed by compensatory pauses. Note normal PQST of extrasystole.

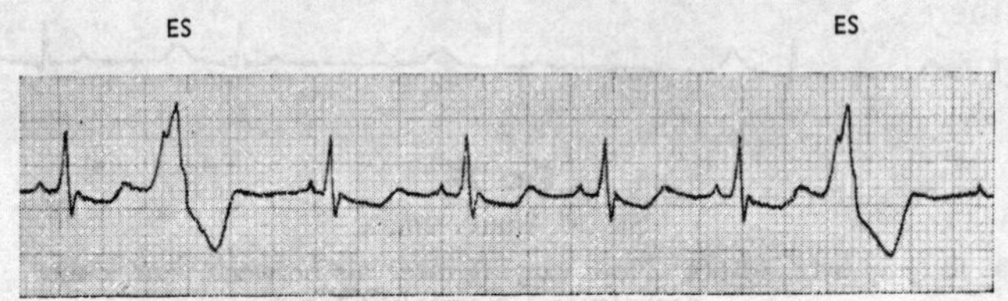

FIG. 27

VENTRICULAR EXTRASYSTOLES

Normal complexes followed by an extrasystole (large abnormal complex) and compensatory pause.

be found in association with organic heart disease, especially rheumatic carditis, ischaemic heart disease and hypertension. They may be induced by overdosage with digitalis. By themselves they have no pathological significance, and their importance is entirely due to any associated disease to which they may sometimes draw attention.

Symptoms. Usually there are no symptoms and the rhythm is discovered on routine examination. Sensitive individuals may complain of palpitation or of the heart missing a beat or of a thud from the augmented beat following the extrasystole. Unwarranted anxiety is often engendered.

Diagnosis. The small premature beat, the long pause after it or the subsequent augmented beat may be detectable at the wrist. When the extrasystole occurs too soon for adequate ventricular filling there may be no corresponding pulse beat and ventricular systole can only be detected by auscultation.

Pulsus bigeminus is the name which is applied to the rhythm produced when an extrasystole and its compensatory pause succeed each normal beat. The heart beats are 'coupled'. This is seen especially in digitalis poisoning. Sometimes the extra-systolic contraction will be too weak to be appreciated at the wrist in which case the pulse rate will be halved, but the extra ventricular beat will be heard on auscultation. Hence the importance of auscultation of the heart as well as palpation of the pulse in any patient who is receiving digitalis.

Treatment. If extrasystoles are discovered and are not giving rise to symptoms, the patient should not be told of their presence and no treatment is required. When palpitation is complained of but there is no evidence of cardiac disease the patient should be reassured. Excessive tea-drinking or smoking, should be reduced and dyspepsia investigated. A sedative such as phenobarbitone may be given as a temporary measure. If any organic disease is associated it should be treated in the ordinary way. Coupled extrasystoles due to digitalis are a warning to reduce the dose of the drug unless the ventricular rate cannot otherwise be controlled. Occasionally extrasystoles are really troublesome and may require for their control quinidine (p. 193), 0·2-0·4 g. q.d.s., potassium salts or procainamide by mouth (p. 195). In an emergency after myocardial infarction, lignocaine by injection may be required (p. 195).

2. Atrial Fibrillation

Atrial fibrillation is a common and important disorder. Rapid fibrillary waves take the place of normal atrial contractions and the ventricles respond erratically. The precise mechanism is obscure but is probably due to multiple ectopic foci discharging at variable rates. The condition may be permanent or paroxysmal. The atrial rate is about 350-600 per minute but the A-V bundle cannot conduct so many impulses and varying degrees of heart block always exist in untreated cases. The ventricular rate is usually about 100-150 per minute and the rhythm is totally irregular. Paroxysmal fibrillation is sometimes the precursor of established fibrillation.

Aetiology

1. Rheumatic heart disease; usually in young or middle-aged individuals.

2. Ischaemic heart disease and/or hypertension; usually in those past middle-age. Temporary atrial fibrillation may follow myocardial infarction.

3. Thyrotoxicosis, especially in older patients with nodular goitre.

Rarer causes include acute infections, e.g. diphtheria and pneumonia, operations (especially thoracic, e.g. for carcinoma of lung), pericarditis and idiopathic fibrillation.

It is important to realise that fibrillation may occur in the absence of any other evidence of heart disease and persist for many years. It is uncommon in congenital and pulmonary heart disease and in aortic valvular disease.

Diagnosis. The pulse is completely irregular in time and force but the diagnosis is often more easily made by auscultation, when the gross cardiac irregularity is usually unmistakable. There may be a pulse deficit, e.g. the rate may be 120 at the apex but only 100 at the wrist, due to the fact that some of the weaker beats following a short diastole are not strong enough to open the aortic valve. In cases of mitral stenosis the pre-systolic murmur, which is dependent on atrial contraction, disappears with the onset of atrial accentuation, though the mid-diastolic murmur persists.

Differential Diagnosis

(*a*) Multiple extrasystoles.

(*b*) Partial heart block with dropped beats.

(*c*) Atrial flutter with a varying degree of A-V block and hence an irregular ventricular rhythm.

When the pulse rate is normal, and provided the patient is sufficiently well, exercise usually reduces the irregularity due to extrasystoles but increases that due to atrial fibrillation. If the pulse rate is above 100, atrial fibrillation is probably the cause of the irregularity. The electrocardiogram of atrial fibrillation is diagnostic, since it shows that the P waves are absent and usually replaced by irregular fibrillary (f) waves (Fig. 28). In cases of

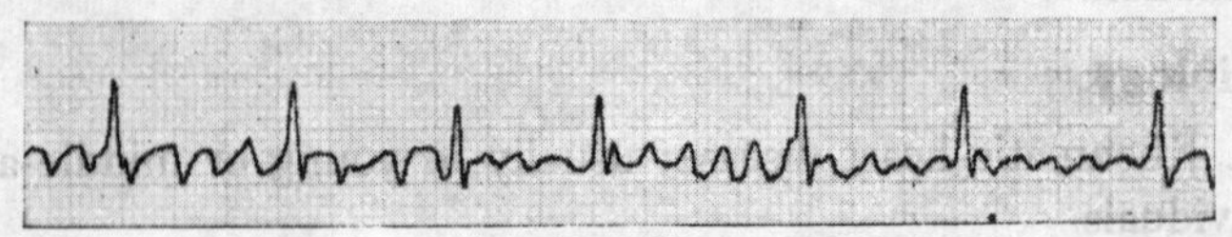

Fig. 28

Atrial Fibrillation

Ventricular rate approx. 75. Note absence of P waves and continuous rapid irregular 'f' oscillations and varying intervals between ventricular complexes.

partial heart block with dropped beats and in atrial flutter with varying block, it can often be appreciated that runs of completely regular beats are occurring. If there is any doubt, an electrocardiogram must be taken for accurate diagnosis.

Prognosis. Atrial fibrillation impairs the efficiency of the heart. The prognosis varies with the cause and is best when the underlying disease can be cured, e.g. thyrotoxicosis, or where no cause is found (idiopathic atrial fibrillation). In mitral stenosis the sudden onset of atrial fibrillation may precipitate cardiac failure or systemic or pulmonary embolism. In older subjects untreated atrial fibrillation is often associated with a normal ventricular rate and there may be little disability.

Treatment. Where, as is usually the case, atrial fibrillation occurs as a feature of heart disease, digitalis is used to reduce a rapid ventricular rate. This may result in a striking improvement and is a most valuable effect. In selected cases an attempt may be made to restore sinus rhythm, for example, in patients with fibrillation in whom there is no obvious underlying disease or if fibrillation has apparently been precipitated by an acute infection, myocardial infarction or thoracotomy. This may be achieved with quinidine or procainamide, drugs which decrease conduction and increase the refractory period or by conversion with a direct current defibrillator. Normal rhythm can usually be restored in thyrotoxicosis if this has not been achieved by thyroidectomy or antithyroid drugs. In cases of mitral stenosis there is little to be gained from the restoration of normal rhythm, since the arrhythmia is almost certain to return, except when fibrillation has followed valvotomy. Clot is liable to form in a fibrillating atrium, and with the restoration of normal rhythm there is always the risk of dislodging emboli from the left atrium into the peripheral circulation or from the right atrium into the lungs.

In most cases the object of treatment is to control the ventricular rate and this can usually be done satisfactorily with digitalis. The details of digitalis and quinidine administration are discussed on pp. 185 and 193.

3. Atrial Flutter

There is rapid, regular atrial action at a rate of 250-350 per minute and the ventricles usually respond to every other beat (i.e. 2 : 1 heart block). Sometimes the response is slower, e.g. 3 : 1 or 4 : 1 block, and occasionally the degree of heart block varies so that the rhythm is irregular.

Aetiology. The aetiology of atrial flutter is essentially the same as atrial fibrillation but the condition is far less common.

Diagnosis. When the patient has constant regular tachycardia of about 160 beats per minute which is uninfluenced by changes of posture or mild exercise, atrial flutter may be the cause. Occasionally the atrial waves may be seen in the jugular veins, but most often an electrocardiogram is needed to confirm the

A

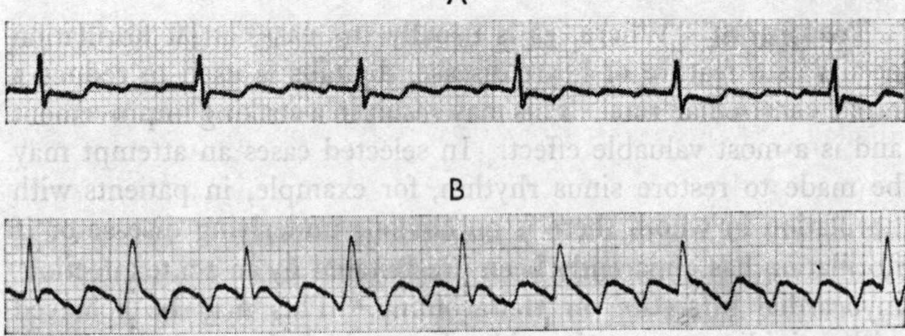

Fig. 29

Atrial Flutter

A. 4 : 1 A-V ratio. Atrial flutter rate 300. Ventricular rate 75.
B. Varying A-V ratio.

diagnosis (Fig. 29). Flutter waves have a regular saw-like appearance and are interrupted by the ventricular complexes. Sometimes the ventricular rate may suddenly double or halve itself. Vagal stimulation, e.g. pressure over the carotid sinus in the neck, may halve the rate temporarily, but sinus rhythm is not restored. By contrast, in paroxysmal supraventricular tachycardia vagal stimulation will either terminate the paroxysm or have no effect. With varying AV block the radial pulse may be indistinguishable from that in atrial fibrillation.

Treatment. Digitalis should be given in full dosage and this may produce atrial fibrillation. When the drug is stopped normal rhythm may return. If not, treatment with quinidine, procainamide or a defibrillator as for atrial fibrillation, may be tried.

4. Paroxysmal Tachycardia

Paroxysmal tachycardia is the name given to a condition characterised by attacks of tachycardia due to rapidly recurring extrasystoles lasting from a few seconds to several days. The electrocardiogram of an attack distinguishes the following types.

Supraventricular

(*a*) Atrial; originating somewhere in the atria other than in the S-A node. Paroxysmal atrial tachycardia is by far the most common type and usually occurs in young people without organic heart disease. The cause is unknown. The onset of the paroxysms may be influenced by nervousness but usually occurs for no obvious reason. Occasionally tobacco, alcohol, overeating or gastric distension is responsible.

(*b*) Atrial tachycardia with AV block. This may be a sign of digitalis toxicity, especially if hypokalaemia is present.

(*c*) Nodal: originating in the A-V node.

Ventricular

This originates in the ventricles. Paroxysmal ventricular tachycardia is much less common and more serious than atrial tachycardia. It is usually seen in people with ischaemic heart disease. It may be an immediate sequel of coronary occlusion and it is sometimes caused by over-dosage with digitalis.

Symptoms and Signs. If the paroxysm is brief, symptoms may be absent. Usually there is a sudden sensation of fluttering in the chest, often described as palpitation. Sometimes the attack is very distressing. If the paroxysm is prolonged, and especially if the heart is diseased, cardiac failure may develop secondary to the tachycardia. The heart rate is about 180 per minute (150-250) and quite regular. The rate is uninfluenced by rest, posture or

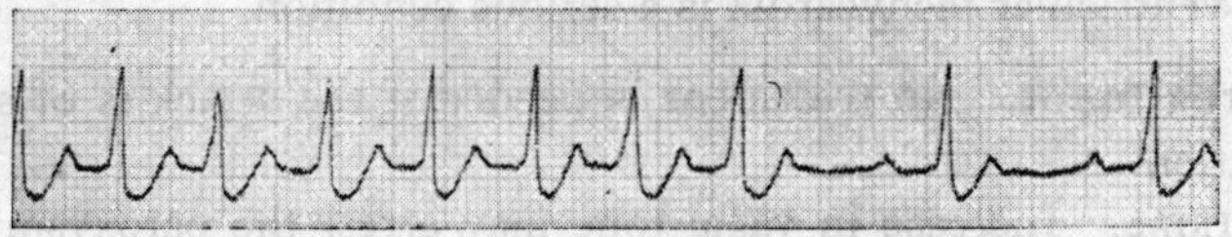

Fig. 30

Paroxysmal Supraventricular Tachycardia

Rate=180. P waves not visible. Return to sinus rhythm.

exercise. Supraventricular tachycardia may be terminated abruptly by carotid sinus massage as described on p. 163. The pulse may be scarcely palpable and sometimes there is pulsus alternans. The electrocardiogram shows a series of rapidly occurring extrasystoles of supraventricular or ventricular type. The cessation often appears to the patient to be less abrupt than the onset, and this is usually due to a period of sinus tachycardia following the paroxysm (Figs. 30, 31).

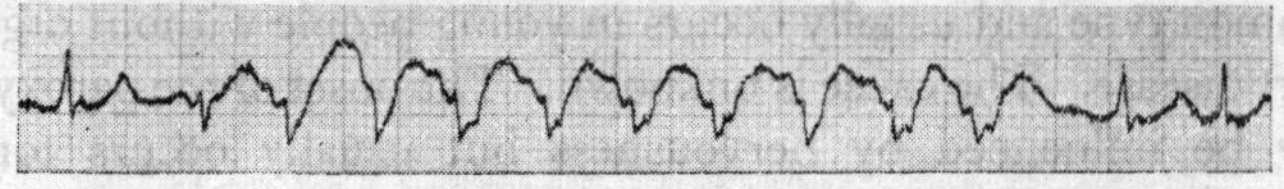

FIG. 31

PAROXYSMAL VENTRICULAR TACHYCARDIA

Rate 150. QRS 0·10 sec. Note run of large, slurred complexes each resembling a ventricular premature beat followed by return to sinus rhythm.

Differential Diagnosis

SINUS TACHYCARDIA. The rate in sinus tachycardia is rarely so fast and is influenced by emotion, exercise and posture. The onset and cessation are gradual. Palpitation caused by panic is often wrongly diagnosed as paroxysmal tachycardia.

ATRIAL FLUTTER. The rate in atrial flutter rarely exceeds 160, and although, as with paroxysmal tachycardia, the rate is uninfluenced by exercise and posture, in flutter it may be suddenly halved by change in the degree of A-V block.

Prognosis. The majority of paroxysms of supraventricular tachycardia give rise to few symptoms and cease spontaneously but they can be unpleasant. If the attack is prolonged, cardiac failure may develop, but usually improves rapidly with the return of sinus rhythm. Death is rare in a paroxysm. The prognosis depends on the underlying disease and it is largely for this reason that ventricular tachycardia is a serious condition.

Treatment. No treatment is needed if the attack is of short duration.

ATRIAL. Increase in vagal tone may arrest the paroxysm and this is most effectively achieved by carotid sinus massage. All clinicians should be adept at carotid sinus massage which should be carried out as follows. The sinus is situated close to the bifurcation of the common carotid artery opposite the angle of the jaw. With the head turned to one side, the thumb should be placed over the position of maximum pulsation and firm massage applied up and down over the vessel and against the spine for not longer than 10 seconds, first on one side and, if necessary, then on the other side, but never on both sides together. Mere pressure is rarely sufficient. The radial pulse should be felt with the other hand and the heart auscultated with the chest-piece of the stethoscope held over the apex beat by the patient or an assistant. If possible, the procedure should be monitored by a continuous ECG record. Simpler methods which can be used at home are sometimes effective, such as holding the breath for as long as possible or by performing the Valsalva (forcible expiration with glottis closed) or Muller (deep inspiration with glottis closed) manœuvre. Retching or vomiting may terminate the attack and this may be induced by putting a finger down the throat or taking an emetic such as tinct. ipecac. 8-16 ml. or salt or mustard in water. Direct current conversion is preferable to treatment by drugs if the apparatus and an anaesthetist are available.

Digitalis is often the most effective drug for arresting an attack and can be given in the form of digoxin, 1 mg. intravenously, or an initial dose of 1 mg. may be given orally followed by 0.25 mg. four-hourly until nausea or vomiting results. Should digitalis fail, drugs to stimulate the parasympathetic should be tried, e.g. neostigmine 1-2 mg. or acetylmethylcholine 10-25 mg. subcutaneously. Occasionally unpleasant side-effects result from such drugs, e.g. vomiting, abdominal colic or even collapse. Atropine is the antidote which should always be on hand, 1·0 mg. ($\frac{1}{60}$ gr.) being injected intravenously should symptoms be alarming. Quinidine 0·4 g. by mouth every two hours up to eight doses if necessary or intravenously in severe cases (p. 193), or procainamide or propranolol (p. 195), may arrest the attack when the above measures have failed.

VENTRICULAR. Measures which increase vagal tone are ineffective and should never be used in the treatment or prevention of ventricular tachycardia. Quinidine, as above, may arrest the paroxysm. If this fails, procainamide at the rate of 100 mg. a minute up to a maximum of 2·0 g. by intravenous injection may be effective. The injection should be given slowly and stopped immediately if there is a significant fall in the blood pressure.

Since digitalis may be the cause this drug should not be given unless other drugs have failed. Direct current conversion is the simplest and safest form of treatment if the apparatus is available.

Prevention of Further Attacks. This is difficult. Exciting causes should be guarded against wherever possible. Sedatives may be given as required. Digitalis by mouth usually reduces the frequency of attacks of supraventricular tachycardia. Antiarrythmic drugs are discussed on pp. 193-195.

HEART BLOCK

The term heart block denotes depression of impulse formation or conduction. It may be slight and reflected only in prolongation of the P-R interval in the electrocardiogram; or moderate so that delay in conduction of the impulse from the atria results in a 'dropped' ventricular beat; or so great that the ventricles adopt an independent rhythm of their own.

S-A Block

A complete cardiac cycle is missed so that a gap appears in the pulse. This condition is uncommon and of little clinical importance, being due to increased vagal tone. The electrocardiogram shows that both atrial and ventricular complexes are absent (Fig. 32).

A-V Block

Conduction between the atria and ventricles is impaired.

(*a*) First degree or Latent Heart Block.

P-R interval is prolonged beyond the upper limit of normal (0·2 of a second) (Fig. 33).

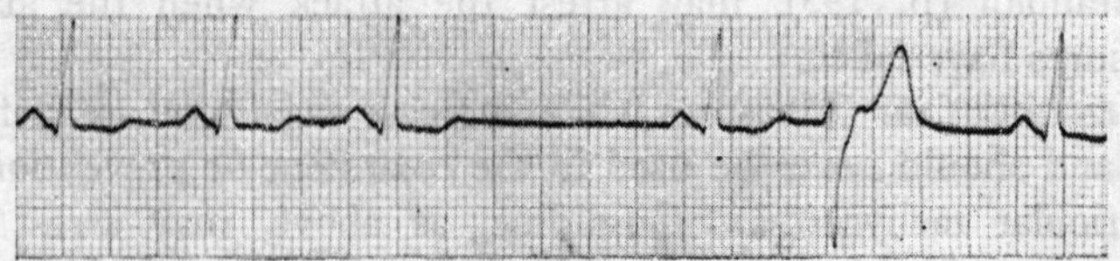

Fig. 32
Sino-Atrial Block
Rate 68. Note pause due to absence of entire PORST. A ventricular extrasystole follows the fourth complex.

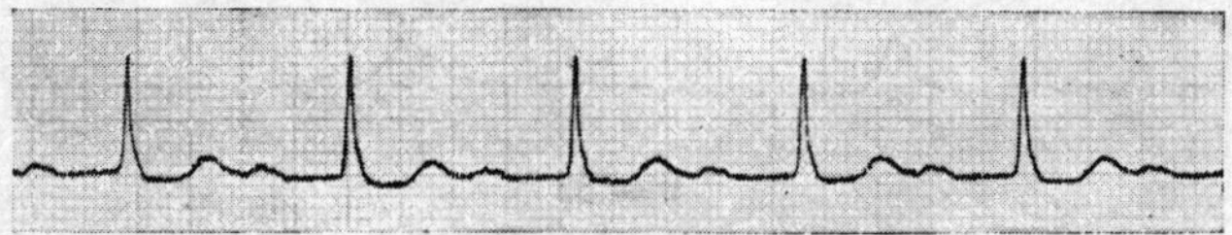

FIG. 33
LATENT A-V BLOCK
1st degree heart block. Rate 66. P-R interval 0·36 of a second.

(*b*) Second degree or Partial Heart Block
Some impulses from the atria fail to get through to the ventricles, i.e. dropped beats occur (Fig. 34). Sometimes there is progressive lengthening of successive P-R intervals followed by a dropped beat.

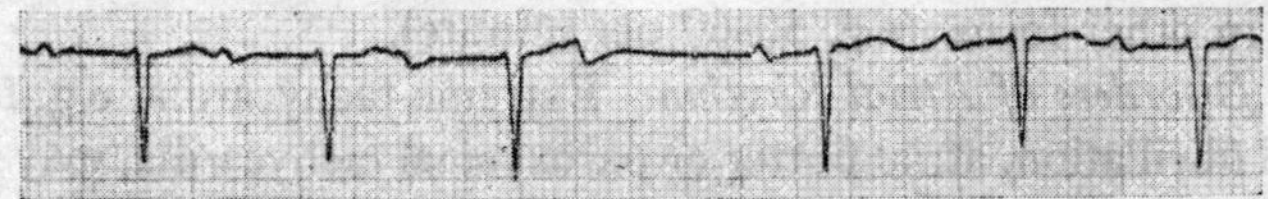

FIG. 34
PARTIAL A-V BLOCK (WENCKEBACH'S PHENOMENON)
Second degree heart block. Rate 88. Progressive lengthening of successive P-R intervals (Wenckebach periods) followed by dropped ventricular beat.

(*c*) Third degree or Complete Heart Block
No impulses from the atria reach the ventricles, which beat at their intrinsic rate (Fig. 35).

Aetiology. Depression of conductivity is most commonly due to ischaemia, fibrosis or inflammation of the bundle of His, or to vagal stimulation.

1. *Coronary Artery Disease.* This is the chief cause of permanent heart block.

2. *Aortic Stenosis.* This may result in functional coronary insufficiency (p. 204), or the degenerative process responsible for the stenosis may extend into the interventricular septum and thus interfere with the conducting tissues.

3. *Rheumatic Fever.* This is commonly responsible for latent heart block and rarely for more severe grades.

4. *Digitalis.* This drug is a frequent cause of the milder degrees of impaired conduction. This action is, of course, beneficial when it is used to reduce the rapid ventricular rate accompanying

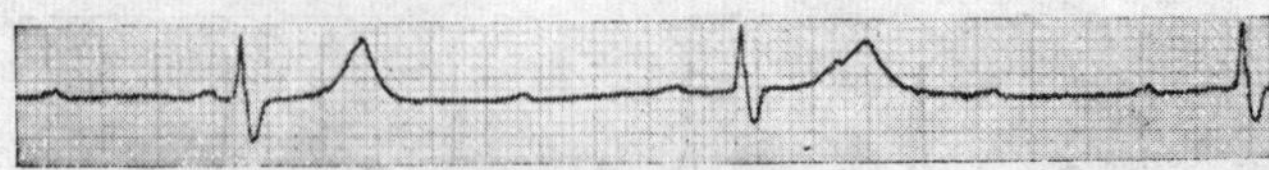

Fig. 35

Complete A-V Block

Atrial rate 100. Ventricular rate 34. Note complete dissociation of atrial and ventricular complexes.

atrial fibrillation. Complete heart block may be a late manifestation of digitalis poisoning.

5. *Diphtheria* and *Syphilis* are now rare causes of heart block.

6. *Cardiomyopathies.*

7. *Congenital Heart Disease.* Complete heart block occasionally results from a congenital maldevelopment of the bundle. The condition is benign and the degree of bradycardia often less marked than in other forms (e.g. 50-60 per minute).

8. *Disorders of Atrial Rhythm.* Extreme tachycardia, e.g. from atrial fibrillation, atrial flutter or paroxysmal tachycardia, may lead to fatigue and refractoriness of the A-V node and bundle.

Diagnosis. Heart block is readily diagnosed electrocardiographically. With patience and practice, however, it is possible to recognise many cases of heart block by inspection of the jugular venous pulse and simultaneous palpation of the opposite carotid artery.

Latent Heart Block cannot be diagnosed clinically but only on the electrocardiogram. Its recognition is sometimes of help as an indication of active rheumatic carditis.

Partial Heart Block. When the atrial and ventricular contractions bear a simple ratio to one another such as in 2 : 1 and 3 : 1 block, the pulse is slow and regular. Change in the degree of partial heart block may give rise to sudden changes in pulse rate. The degree of block may be diagnosed by comparing the number of atrial contractions ('a' waves in the jugular pulse) with the carotid pulse. More complex ratios between atrial and ventricular contractions such as 3 : 2 or 4 : 3 block give rise to 'dropped beats'. On auscultation it can be appreciated that there has been no ventricular beat, thus distinguishing the condition from dropped beats at the wrist due to extrasystoles. The first heart sound may vary in intensity. Sometimes the electrocardiogram shows repetitive cycles in which the P-R interval increases progressively until a ventricular complex is 'dropped'. This is termed the Wenckebach phenomenon and is due to progressive fatigue of the A-V bundle with recovery following the rest period when the dropped beat occurs (Fig. 34). Partial heart block is usually transient and occurs during an acute infection or from digitalis overdose. If due to coronary disease, the degree of block may increase as time goes on.

COMPLETE HEART BLOCK should be suspected when the pulse rate is slow (30-40) and regular, and does not vary with exercise. There is complete dissociation between the 'a' waves in the jugular and carotid pulses. There may be noted varying intensity of the first heart sound and audible atrial sounds. Venous 'cannon' waves in the neck may be seen when the right atrium contracts against a closed tricuspid valve.

Treatment. When practicable, treatment should be directed to the underlying cause. Digitalis should not be given unless cardiac failure is present because it may aggravate the degree of block. The treatment of Adams-Stokes attacks is discussed below.

ADAMS-STOKES SYNDROME

When cerebral blood flow ceases as a result of ventricular asystole, tachycardia or fibrillation, syncope occurs rapidly. Convulsions will occur if the heart does not begin to beat again within about 10 seconds, and death will result if asystole is prolonged for 2-3 minutes. The skin blanches and later cyanosis occurs. When the heart starts beating again there is a characteristic flush as the emptied vessels are filled with blood. Such attacks take their name from the two Irish physicians who first described them. The syndrome is a complication of complete heart block or less commonly partial heart block. Patients who have repeated attacks may be aware of the imminence of unconsciousness, but frequently syncope occurs without warning. Breathing continues after the heart has stopped.

Treatment

Adrenaline hydrochloride, 0·3-0·6 ml. 1 : 1,000 solution should be given by intramuscular or intravenous injection as quickly as possible. An alternative drug is methylamphetamine (Methedrine) 30 mg. If attacks are recurring at short intervals an injection of

0·5-1·0 ml. of adrenaline in oil for slow absorption should be administered. Each ml. contains the equivalent of 2 ml. of adrenaline hydrochloride 1 : 1,000 solution. If the attack is prolonged for more than a minute, so that life is in danger, closed-chest cardiac resuscitation, as described on page 180 should be begun immediately. An injection of adrenaline may be given into the heart. Whenever possible an ECG should be recorded in an attack because apparent cardiac standstill may occasionally be due to other causes, e.g. ventricular tachycardia or fibrillation. Digitalis is contraindicated unless cardiac failure is present. Recovery from the seizure usually takes place spontaneously so that the necessity for treating individual attacks seldom arises and it is also difficult to assess the value of any particular treatment.

Prevention of Attacks. Ephedrine, 60-120 mg. three times daily should first be tried as a sympathetic stimulant. Sustained action isoprenaline tablets (30 mg.) for oral administration have now replaced the short action sublingual tablets and may be given every four to six hours. Thyroxine, 0·5-1·0 mg. three times daily, may also be tried with a view to sensitising the sympathetic nervous system to the action of ephedrine or adrenaline. Cortisone has been used with some success. Unfortunately all these drugs are apt to be disappointing.

Should these measures fail a battery powered pacemaker can now be inserted subcutaneously with wires leading to electrodes implanted into the myocardium. As a temporary measure the heart can be stimulated by an electrode catheter passed through a vein to the apex of the right ventricle.

Prognosis

The outlook is usually serious since the most common cause is severe coronary disease.

Bundle Branch Block

This term is applied to the electrocardiographic finding of delay in conduction in either the right or left branch of the A-V bundle. Most cases are due to coronary artery disease. Rheumatic heart disease accounts for a few. Congenital heart disease, syphilis and diphtheria are occasional causes.

The diagnosis can only be made by means of an electrocardiogram. The QRS interval is increased above the upper limit of normal, 0·1 of a second. Examples of right and left bundle branch block are shown in Figures 18 and 19. The clinical manifestations, treatment and prognosis are those of the underlying disease.

* * * * * *

CARDIAC FAILURE

Cardiac failure may be said to exist when the output of the heart is insufficient for the needs of the tissues. It may be acute or chronic. The clinical picture of acute failure is very similar to that which occurs in peripheral circulatory failure or shock (p. 176). The term 'congestive cardiac failure' is used to describe the clinical syndrome which usually results from chronic failure. The term 'congestive cardiac failure' has sometimes been confined to patients in whom evidence of congestion has appeared in the peripheral circulation, i.e. distended neck veins, engorgement of the liver, and oedema. However, in patients with primary left-sided failure (as defined below), congestion may sometimes be confined to the lungs, at least for a considerable time. Ultimately it is often followed by evidence of congestion in the peripheral circulation. In other instances, congestion in the lungs and in the peripheral circulation appears simultaneously.

In the discussion that follows, an attempt is made to present a unified conception of congestive failure and to explain the underlying mechanisms of failure and its clinical manifestations. The term 'congestive failure' is in fact applicable whenever and wherever congestion appears as the result of heart failure. In most cases there is a general cause for congestion, namely an increased blood volume, which results from the retention of sodium and water by the kidneys, and a localising factor which determines whether congestion is solely or principally confined to the lesser (i.e. pulmonary) or greater (i.e. systemic) circulations.

The heart may apparently fail as a whole, but it is helpful to consider failure of the left and right sides of the heart separately. In the early stages, and sometimes throughout the whole course, failure of the left or of the right side of the heart may be recognised as an isolated clinical condition. Left ventricular failure is usually due to hypertension, coronary atherosclerosis or aortic valvular disease. Left-sided failure may be said to occur when the left atrium cannot empty its blood satisfactorily into the left ventricle, as occurs in mitral stenosis. Right ventricular failure is most often secondary to preceding left-sided failure. It may, however, result from certain diseases of the lungs, notably emphysema; congenital heart disease, e.g. pulmonary stenosis or septal defects; or conditions which impede the inflow of blood into the right side of the heart, e.g. tricuspid stenosis or some cases of constrictive pericarditis. In such instances the left side of the heart is unaffected.

Left-sided failure leads to manifestations of 'forward failure' such as weakness and lethargy from a decreased blood supply to the tissues and to dyspnoea from 'backward failure' causing pulmonary congestion. These two terms, 'forward failure' and 'backward failure', though hallowed by long usage, are confusing because the two conditions are not really distinct but interdependent.

The principal manifestations of right-sided failure are engorgement of the systemic and portal venous systems, the appearance of peripheral oedema, and enlargement of the liver.

Cardiac failure is usually accompanied by a reduction in cardiac output, and as a result various compensatory mechanisms are brought into play. The chief of these is an increase in the circulating blood volume. Although this serves for a time to increase the failing output, it is also largely responsible for many of the clinical features of cardiac failure. Most cases of cardiac failure are in fact accompanied by a low cardiac output, but certain conditions in which the circulatory needs of the tissues are above normal, e.g. thyrotoxicosis (increased metabolic rate), anaemia (decreased oxygen-carrying power) and emphysema (decreased oxygen saturation), may result in cardiac failure while the cardiac output is still above normal though lower than before the onset of failure. Cardiac failure may be very gradual in onset or precipitated by tachycardia from any cause or by a respiratory infection, anaemia or pregnancy.

LEFT-SIDED HEART FAILURE

Although pulmonary congestion and oedema are the cardinal features of all forms of left-sided failure, the clinical course of primary failure of the left ventricle is not the same as when failure is secondary to mitral stenosis (in which case the left ventricle is unaffected).

In rheumatic heart disease when the mitral valvular defect is the predominant factor and the myocardium is relatively little affected, dyspnoea is usually present for many years. The long-standing increase in pressure in the pulmonary circulation gradually leads to right-sided failure with its peripheral signs of venous congestion and oedema. With adequate care this often responds to treatment and it is common for episodes of congestive failure to recur again and again, though at ever-decreasing intervals and with ever-increasing severity. With severe mitral stenosis attacks of pulmonary oedema may occur and be precipitated by exercise, emotion, tachycardia from any cause, e.g. paroxysmal atrial fibrillation, or by pregnancy.

Left ventricular failure from coronary occlusion may be of acute onset but when the underlying disease is of long standing, as is usually the case in hypertension or aortic valvular disease, the powerful left ventricle has time to compensate for the mechanical burden by gradual hypertrophy. In such cases dyspnoea is not usually evident for many years. When failure does occur it tends to be steadily progressive and life is rarely prolonged for more than one to three years.

Left Ventricular Failure

Symptoms and Signs. The principal manifestations of left ventricular failure are dyspnoea, cough, crepitations at the bases of the lungs, enlargement of the heart due to hypertrophy and dilatation of the left ventricle, triple rhythm and pulsus alternans.

Dyspnoea. Dyspnoea is usually the earliest manifestation of heart failure. It may occur on exertion or at rest.

Dyspnoea at rest is always pathological. Dyspnoea on exertion occurs in normal people and hence must be assessed in relation to age, obesity and physical fitness. Progression or regression of dyspnoea on exertion is a valuable guide to the course of the underlying heart disease.

Cardiac dyspnoea is nearly always due to pulmonary venous congestion from failure of the left side of the heart. This renders the lungs inelastic, increases the work of breathing, stimulates the Hering-Breuer reflex and results in rapid shallow respiration. The vital capacity is correspondingly reduced. Subsequent right-sided failure may partially and temporarily relieve the dyspnoea by reducing the amount of blood pumped into the lungs. In such circumstances the patient may be agreeably but mistakenly encouraged as to his progress.

Dyspnoea on Exertion. Dyspnoea may be judged by the normal activities of the patient. The first evidence is usually breathlessness on hills, or the necessity to pause for breath after one or two flights of stairs. The housewife finds the heavier household tasks such as scrubbing and polishing too difficult. Eventually there is dyspnoea when walking on level ground which at first makes conversation impossible and then imposes a slower pace.

Dyspnoea at Rest. Later dyspnoea will be present at rest and finally the patient cannot lie flat without distress (orthopnoea). In the recumbent posture the venous return to the heart is increased. Pulmonary congestion is aggravated and this together with the elevation of the diaphragm which results from lying down reduces still further the vital capacity of the lungs.

Paroxysmal Dyspnoea. Paroxysmal dyspnoea may occur from acute pulmonary congestion and oedema in patients with left ventricular failure or less commonly with mitral stenosis. Attacks due to left ventricular failure are most often seen in patients with hypertension but may accompany aortic valvular disease or severe coronary disease. They usually occur at night, often wakening the patient. The factors mentioned above concerning orthopnoea are operative if the patient slips down in bed. During the night peripheral oedema, which has accumulated by day, with the patient up and about or sitting in a chair, tends to be reabsorbed. During sleep when the respiratory centre is not stimulated so readily, pulmonary congestion 'builds up' and on wakening fear and the struggle for breath aggravate the position further.

The patient sits up or even gets out of bed and walks to an open window gasping or choking. There is often a dry repetitive cough, but with the most severe and prolonged attacks there may be watery, frothy sputum which is often blood-stained. The patient is anxious, pale, sweaty and cyanosed. The pulse is rapid and the blood pressure often raised. The diagnosis is confirmed during the attack by the presence of pulmonary crepitations and by the discovery of some cause for left-sided heart failure. In some cases wheezing accompanies the dyspnoea (cardiac asthma).

In mitral stenosis, paroxysmal dyspnoea may be precipitated by tachycardia secondary to emotion or exertion and is particularly liable to occur during pregnancy.

The distinction between bronchial and cardiac asthma may occasionally be difficult. A long history of similar attacks, a personal or family history of allergic disorders, extreme expiratory difficulty, the tendency to occur in younger people and the absence of signs of heart disease are features of the former.

CHEYNE-STOKES RESPIRATION. Cheyne-Stokes respiration refers to a periodic form of breathing characterised by alternate phases of waxing and waning. It is particularly liable to occur in elderly patients with left ventricular failure and decreased cerebral blood flow and is also seen in patients with intracranial disease, e.g. tumour or vascular accidents, and uraemia. It is a sign of serious prognostic importance. It is aggravated by anything which further depresses the respiratory centre, e.g. sleep and the administration of sedative drugs. The principal factor in its production is depression of the medullary centres from decreased blood flow. Oxygen lack, accentuated during apnoea, sensitises the centre to the stimulus of carbon dioxide. The force and depth of respiration then increase and the resulting reduction of carbon dioxide in the blood leads to apnoea, carbon dioxide accumulates and the cycle begins again. Each phase lasts from about ½ to 1 minute. In cardiac cases with pulmonary congestion the hyperpnoeic phase may be very distressing and waken the patient from sleep. Aminophylline (0·25-0·5 g. intravenously) will usually abolish Cheyne-Stokes breathing by stimulating the respiratory centre.

COUGH. Cough may result from pulmonary congestion or oedema, from superimposed infection or occasionally from pulmonary infarction. It is frequently troublesome at night and may be responsible for insomnia. Pulmonary congestion from cardiac failure may mimic chronic bronchitis in elderly persons.

PULSUS ALTERNANS. Pulsus alternans is another serious sign in left ventricular failure (p. 128).

ENLARGEMENT OF THE HEART. Enlargement of the heart from left ventricular hypertrophy is always present when failure is due to hypertension or aortic valvular disease and the heaving impulse can be felt at the apex. Enlargement is also frequently present in long-standing coronary disease. Enlargement of the left atrium is constantly found in patients with severe mitral disease and is followed by enlargement of the right ventricle and later of the right atrium.

TRIPLE RHYTHM. An extra, atrial heart sound may be heard in

late diastole and is a serious sign in left ventricular failure. It is usually maximal at the apex and is sometimes palpable as well as audible. When tachycardia is present a characteristic cadence is heard which has been called 'gallop rhythm' (p. 136).

ACCENTUATION OF THE PULMONARY SECOND SOUND is a feature of pulmonary hypertension. It tends to be more marked in cases of mitral stenosis than of systemic hypertension owing to the longer duration of the underlying cause with consequent secondary changes in the pulmonary arterioles. In mitral stenosis the 'opening snap' of the mitral valve may simulate wide splitting of the second sound as explained on p. 134.

CREPITATIONS AT THE BASES OF THE LUNGS which persist after coughing are the most important sign of pulmonary oedema. Rhonchi may also be present from the same cause.

HYDROTHORAX on one or both sides may occur (p. 258).

RADIOLOGICAL EXAMINATION may reveal evidence of enlargement of the heart and its individual chambers, of congestion of the lungs (i.e. increased vascular markings and/or pulmonary oedema), and possibly hydrothorax.

ELECTROCARDIOGRAPHY may show evidence of ventricular hypertrophy or of ischaemic heart disease.

RIGHT-SIDED HEART FAILURE

It must be emphasised again that right-sided failure is usually secondary to left-sided failure and is therefore associated with pulmonary congestion and dyspnoea. Increasing pressure in the lesser circulation is followed by dilatation and hypertrophy of the right ventricle. Sometimes the heart will fail as a whole and in such cases the clinical manifestations are principally those of right-sided failure. Isolated right-sided failure may occur as a result of pulmonary disease, e.g. chronic bronchitis, emphysema, and in certain forms of congenital heart disease, e.g. pulmonary stenosis. When the right ventricle begins to fail, oedema and systemic venous congestion occur.

Symptoms and Signs. OEDEMA. The principal factors in the pathogenesis of cardiac oedema are:

1. Retention of water in the body due to increased reabsorption of sodium from the proximal tubules. The precise mechanism

by which sodium is retained by the kidney is uncertain but both haemodynamic and endocrine factors may be involved.

2. Passive engorgement of the vessels behind the failing heart so that the hydrostatic pressure in the capillaries exceeds the colloid osmotic pressure of the plasma proteins.

It used to be thought that the occurrence of oedema could be explained on the simple basis of back pressure from a failing right ventricle. Emphasis has now been shifted to the retention of sodium and water by the kidneys. As a result the extracellular fluid, including the circulating blood volume, is increased and hence also the venous pressure. This determines the occurrence of peripheral oedema. In the same way a rise of pressure in the pulmonary circulation determines the occurrence of pulmonary oedema in left-sided failure. From what has been said it is apparent that an increase in blood volume is an important factor in the causation of oedema while its localisation is largely determined by which chamber is failing.

Minor factors which may play a secondary part in the production of oedema include increased capillary permeability secondary to anoxaemia and reduction in colloid osmotic pressure. The latter may be due to hypoproteinaemia resulting from anorexia, malabsorption from venous congestion in the intestine, defective metabolism from congestion of the liver and perhaps to loss of protein in the urine or in transudates.

Cardiac oedema usually occurs in the dependent parts of the body in the first place, i.e. it is found in the loose tissues round the ankles if the patient is up and about or in the sacral region if confined to bed.

Hydrothorax is usually bilateral, but may be confined to one side (p. 258).

Ascites is usually a later manifestation of failure than peripheral oedema but tends to be especially prominent in constrictive pericarditis and whenever prolonged cardiac failure has led to cirrhosis of the liver with portal hypertension.

Distension and Pulsation of the Neck Veins. The importance of distension of the neck veins as evidence of increased venous pressure from cardiac failure is discussed on p. 130. An expansile wave in systole is frequently present from functional tricuspid incompetence.

Enlargement of the Liver. The inability of the right ventricle to deal with the increased venous return to the heart is also reflected in engorgement of the liver which becomes enlarged, tender and often pulsating. In the early stages there may be abdominal pain from stretching of the capsule.

GASTROINTESTINAL SYMPTOMS. Anorexia and abdominal distension may be troublesome features of portal venous engorgement.

OLIGURIA. A reduction in the secretion of urine commonly accompanies severe congestive failure and the onset of diuresis is a favourable prognostic sign.

NOCTURIA. The reabsorption into the blood of tissue oedema which has accumulated during the day and the excretion of this fluid by the kidneys is facilitated by the recumbent posture. Nocturia is therefore a common complaint in cardiac failure, particularly in ambulant patients.

PROTEINURIA. Proteinuria is a frequent manifestation of renal congestion and disappears when improvement in the circulation occurs.

ACUTE CIRCULATORY FAILURE

Acute cardiac failure and cardiac arrest

Acute cardiac failure may result from:

1. Ventricular asystole or extreme bradycardia in ischaemic heart disease, e.g. angina pectoris, myocardial infarction or heart block; or in acute myocarditis, e.g. in diphtheria.

2. A great reduction in the cardiac output may also occur with massive myocardial infarction, an attack of paroxysmal tachycardia, fibrillation or flutter, a large pulmonary embolism or a rapidly developing pericardial effusion (e.g. from haemorrhage).

The clinical picture of acute cardiac failure is very similar to that which occurs in peripheral circulatory failure, i.e. it is that of shock. Syncope or sudden death may occur.

Peripheral Circulatory Failure

The fundamental basis of peripheral circulatory failure (shock) is a decrease in the circulating blood volume. This is associated with a reduction in the venous return to the heart and therefore of the cardiac output, and hence with a generalised tissue anoxia. As a result compensatory mechanisms are brought into play to try and maintain an adequate circulation to the more vital parts of the body.

This conception is fundamental to an understanding of the great variety of clinical conditions in which shock may occur. Shock is usually divided for convenience into surgical, medical and neurogenic shock although the underlying mechanism is similar in all three. More than one such factor may be involved in any particular case.

It must be emphasised that a similar clinical picture to that of acute peripheral failure may be seen in circulatory failure of central origin.

Aetiology

SHOCK. Shock arises from a reduction in circulating blood volume due to loss of blood or plasma.

1. *Haemorrhage.* This may result from accidents, operations, diseases, ruptured ectopic pregnancy and ante- or post-partum haemorrhage.

2. *Shock following trauma and burns.*

These conditions are due to the very considerable loss of fluid into the tissues, with consequent reduction of circulating blood volume. Post-operative shock may be due to a combination of loss of blood and excessive handling of the tissues, which result in loss of fluid and dehydration.

In some forms of shock there is no loss of blood or plasma, but reduction in circulating blood volume is due to loss of fluid and electrolytes. Reference has already been made to the close association of sodium to water retention and fluid balance. Loss of fluid and electrolytes may occur in diarrhoea, vomiting, excessive sweating, diabetes (p. 738) and Addison's disease (p. 724).

Shock may also result from severe bacterial infections, particularly with gram-negative organisms, but the mechanism is not clear.

NEUROGENIC SHOCK. Neurogenic shock occurs suddenly without loss of blood, plasma or fluids from reflex vasodilatation with consequent pooling of blood in the small vessels, particularly in the splanchnic area, deficient venous return to the heart and hence reduced cardiac output. The precise mechanism is obscure but this form of shock may be seen in various clinical conditions, which are usually accompanied by pain, e.g. perforation of a peptic ulcer, a blow on the 'solar plexus' or testicles, acute pancreatitis or severe pain from any other cause. In some of these conditions there may also be a loss of fluid, e.g. into the peritoneal cavity.

Other Forms of Shock. In some cases the aetiology of shock is obscure even though the fundamental mechanism is the same, i.e. reduction of circulating blood volume. In this group must be included anaphylactic shock and histamine shock, which are believed to result from direct impairment of vascular tone and permeability.

Symptoms and Signs of Peripheral Circulatory Failure

1. Apathy or sometimes restlessness.
2. Extreme weakness.
3. Pale, cold, clammy skin.
4. Rapid, thready pulse.
5. Hypotension.
6. Oliguria.

These clinical features are explained on a basis of diminished cardiac output and the various compensatory mechanisms which are brought into play in an attempt to restore the situation. The reduction in blood volume necessitates the redistribution of blood to such vital organs as the brain and heart and the maintenance of an adequate blood pressure. This is achieved by vasoconstriction in relatively non-essential parts of the body, e.g. the skin and splanchnic area. If severe shock is prolonged it becomes irreversible and the cardiac output and blood pressure continue to fall despite all methods of treatment.

Prophylaxis. Much can be done to prevent the onset of shock by gentle handling of injured parts and by protection from cold; by prompt attention to the control of haemorrhage and pain; by minimising the loss of fluid from the body and the early correction of dehydration and electrolyte loss. Early diagnosis is all-important.

Treatment. Treatment should be directed towards the cause of the circulatory failure whenever possible, e.g. a bleeding vessel, perforated ulcer or diabetes. Pain must be relieved, e.g. by morphine. Warmth, e.g. by blankets, hot water bottle or an electric pad, should be applied to conserve body heat but sweating should be avoided, since this will result in further fluid loss. Raising the foot end of the bed will facilitate the venous return to the heart and help to maintain the cerebral circulation. For severe cases of shock with marked hypotension the intravenous infusion of hydrocortisone, metaraminal (Aramine) or noradrenaline may be of value but caution is required in the treatment of shock following myocardial infarction (p. 221). Metaraminol and noradrenaline are of no value if vasoconstriction is maximal.

Replacement of Fluid. Transfusion of blood is a most important measure in the treatment of shock due to loss of blood. Transfusion of plasma may be given when blood is not available and in the treatment of burns. Transfusion of plasma substitutes, e.g. dextran or rheomacradex, should be particularly valuable in time of war and whenever blood or plasma is not available.

Disturbances of water and electrolyte balance and their treatment are discussed on p. 839.

CARDIAC ARREST

Cardiac arrest in an emergency which will often respond to appropriate treatment if this is given within approximately five minutes, after which irreversible cerebral damage occurs. The development of the technique of closed-chest cardiac massage (sometimes described as external cardiac massage) together with mouth to mouth artificial respiration has greatly improved the prognosis of cardiac arrest. Hence doctors, nurses, ambulance drivers and attendants should all receive instruction in this vitally important form of first aid.

The most frequent causes are anaesthesia, surgical operations, special diagnostic procedures, drug sensitivity or toxicity, myocardial infarction, heart block and electrocution.

Cardiac arrest may be due to ventricular asystole or ventricular fibrillation, but these two conditions can only be distinguished by electrocardiography or by direct inspection of the heart.

The diagnosis is based on the absence of the pulse in the carotid or femoral artery, and of the heart sounds on auscultation.

The immediate objective of the treatment is to restore an oxygenated blood supply to the brain and to the heart muscle, and for this purpose the following actions should be taken immediately.

Give a smart blow to the chest with the fist and elevate both legs to 90° for 15 seconds. If the heart does not start beating immediately, as indicated by the return of the carotid or femoral pulse, cardiopulmonary resuscitation must be started.

Technique of cardiopulmonary resuscitation

The object of closed chest cardiac massage is to empty the blood from the ventricles by compressing the heart between the sternum and the spinal column (Fig. 37D). This is accomplished by laying the patient on his back on a hard surface, e.g. the floor. The operator places his hands, one on top of the other, on the lower end of the patient's sternum immediately above the xiphisternum and commences forcible rhythmic compressions at the rate of 60 to 80 per minute. The force of the compression must be sufficiently great to produce pulsation in the carotid and femoral arteries.

When cardiac arrest occurs, respiration usually stops or respiration may have ceased prior to cardiac arrest. Hence measures for the relief of this emergency are essential and must be taken immediately. Direct mouth-to-mouth breathing or breathing through a specially designed tube if this is available must be started at once (Figs. 36 and 37).

Closed-chest cardiac massage and artificial respiration must be continued so long as there seems any chance of the heart beating again. This may occur spontaneously if the cause of the cardiac arrest is ventricular asystole, but it is very unlikely if the arrest is due to ventricular fibrillation. Hence it is essential that an electrocardiogram should be taken to establish the cause of the arrest. If ventricular fibrillation is present it must be corrected by means of an electric defibrillating machine which is effective when applied externally to the chest wall. As a result ventricular fibrillation is changed to ventricular asystole and in a proportion of cases the heart will start beating again either spontaneously or after a short period of continued closed-chest cardiac massage. If cardiac contractions are restored but the blood pressure remains low adrenaline hydrochloride (1 : 10,000) 0·5 ml. should be given intravenously and repeated as required. If electrical defibrillation fails it may be successful after an injection of procainamide 1 g. If the contractions do not start, the heart can be stimulated by an electrical pacemaker. The acidosis which immediately follows even temporary arrest must be corrected by the intravenous administration of 150 m.Eq of bicarbonate in the first 10 minutes and repeated as long as the circulation remains inadequate. Persistence of fixed dilatation of the pupils indicates that cerebral damage is irreversible.

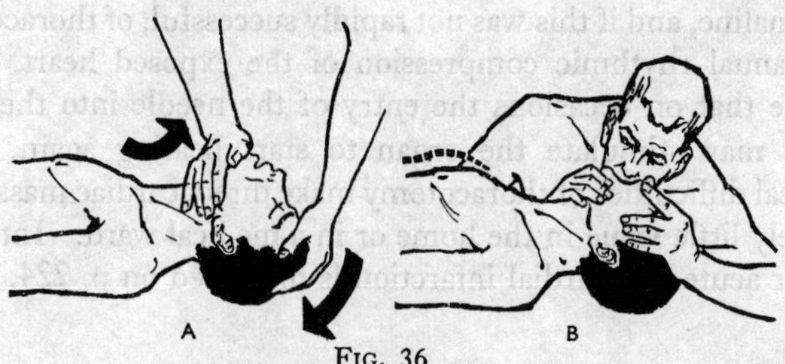

FIG. 36

INTERMITTENT POSITIVE-PRESSURE BREATHING

(A) Head hyperextended and chin raised. (B) Mouth-to-mouth resuscitation. Look for chest rise with each inflation.

(*By courtesy of the British Medical Journal*)

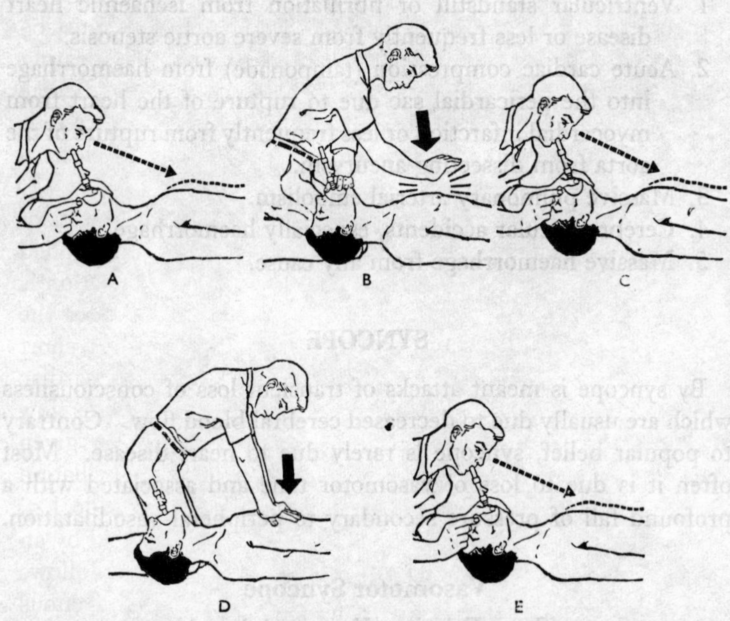

FIG. 37

EMERGENCY RESUSCITATION

(*By courtesy of the British Medical Journal*)

Prior to the development of closed-chest cardiac massage, the treatment of cardiac arrest consisted of the intracardiac injection of adrenaline, and if this was not rapidly successful, of thoracotomy and manual rhythmic compression of the exposed heart. It is possible that on occasions the entry of the needle into the heart muscle may stimulate the organ to start beating again. The technical difficulties of thoracotomy make direct cardiac massage of relatively little value in the home or in a medical ward. Intensive care for acute myocardial infarction is discussed on p. 224.

SUDDEN DEATH

Failure of the cerebral circulation leads to unconsciousness within 10 seconds and death within a few minutes.

The most common cardiovascular causes of sudden death are:

1. Ventricular standstill or fibrillation from ischaemic heart disease or less frequently from severe aortic stenosis.
2. Acute cardiac compression (tamponade) from haemorrhage into the pericardial sac due to rupture of the heart from myocardial infarction or less frequently from rupture of the aorta from dissecting aneurysm.
3. Massive pulmonary arterial embolism.
4. Cerebrovascular accidents, especially haemorrhage.
5. Massive haemorrhage from any cause.

SYNCOPE

By syncope is meant attacks of transient loss of consciousness which are usually due to decreased cerebral blood flow. Contrary to popular belief, syncope is rarely due to heart disease. Most often it is due to loss of vasomotor tone and associated with a profound fall of pressure secondary to peripheral vasodilatation.

Vasomotor Syncope

(Syn.: Fainting, Vasovagal Attack)

This type of syncope is responsible for ordinary fainting. The usual cause of fainting is psychogenic and due to strong emotional stimuli such as fear, disgust or surprise, e.g. at the sight of blood or witnessing an accident. Occasionally it may be due to pain. Lack of food and hot stuffy atmospheres are sometimes predisposing factors. Postural hypotension is a cause of fainting which may occur on standing up suddenly or standing still on the parade ground. It is especially liable to occur in patients who are convalescing from some debilitating illness. It may occur after sympathectomy for hypertension or following the administration of ganglion or sympathetic blocking drugs which paralyse the transmission of nerve impulses. Both these procedures reduce vasomotor tone.

Some individuals have hypersensitive carotid sinuses, and loss of consciousness may follow pressure on the sinus such as occurs with abrupt movements of the neck.

Syncope may occasionally result from the strain of coughing or micturition, each being the equivalent of performing a valsalva manoeuvre which raises the intrathoracic pressure and causes peripheral vasodilatation.

Clinical Features. The attack comes on rapidly and usually unexpectedly, although the cause may be apparent. Weakness, light-headedness, nausea and a sinking feeling in the epigastrium are followed by a period of unconsciousness which usually lasts for a few seconds or minutes, but may be longer, The subject is pale and clammy, the blood pressure low and the pulse rate usually slow but sometimes rapid. Recovery follows because fainting often removes the precipitating factor and the inevitable assumption of the recumbent posture facilitates the venous return to the heart and hence cerebral flow.

Differential Diagnosis. It is important to distinguish vasomotor syncope from other causes of loss of consciousness such as epilepsy. An accurate history and if possible an eye-witness account of an attack are all-important. In syncope there are usually warning sensations of an impending attack and often some obvious precipitating factor. In epilepsy, apart from the occasional occurrence of an aura, loss of consciousness is instantaneous and occurs for no obvious reason. In vasovagal syncope the patient is usually pale and flaccid, and in epilepsy cyanosed and rigid. When syncope develops the patient is usually standing, but an epileptic attack may occur in any position, and even during sleep.

Treatment. The recumbent posture with the head low, fresh air, smelling-salts and a cold drink will facilitate recovery. When possible, predisposing and precipitating factors should be avoided.

Cardiac Syncope

Syncope may be due to cardiac standstill as occurs in Adams-Stokes attacks from heart block (p. 167). It may also result from extreme degrees of tachycardia or from temporary ventricular standstill at the onset or end of any paroxysmal arrhythmia. It may occur in severe valvular stenosis when the cardiac output cannot increase with exertion and there is vasodilation in the muscles, and in cyanotic congenital heart disease from cerebral anoxia.

TREATMENT OF CARDIAC FAILURE

General Principles. Whenever heart disease is diagnosed its nature and degree must be assessed with meticulous accuracy in order to decide whether any treatment is necessary. There are many structural defects of such slight degree that no treatment is indicated other than reassurance. Much unwarranted anxiety is engendered by failure to take sufficient care to explain the position in detail both to the patient and relatives. Restrictions and drugs are rarely required unless exertion results in dyspnoea or pain. However, certain disorders, such as valvular disease and hypertension, are in time potential causes of heart failure. This eventuality may be prevented or at least postponed by suitable advice with regard to occupation, the limitation of physical activities and the reduction of obesity. The development of a serious degree of cardiac failure may be avoided or minimised by early recognition of its clinical manifestations and prompt treatment.

Whenever possible, treatment should be directed towards the underlying cause or precipitating factor, e.g. thyrotoxicosis, syphilis, anaemia, pregnancy, acute respiratory infections or extreme tachycardia. In addition certain conditions such as congenital defects, acquired valvular disease and constrictive pericarditis are often amenable to surgical treatment.

REST AND SLEEP

Rest and sleep are of fundamental importance in the management of every patient with cardiac failure. However, in the past rest has often been abused. Unnecessarily prolonged confinement to bed is harmful as will be explained below. When signs of heart failure are first manifest complete rest in bed should be enforced until treatment has resulted in the maximal benefit which can be obtained. Thereafter the return to activity must be graduated and it will become apparent how much rest during the day and how much general restriction of exertion are required to prevent further failure. There should be no fixed rules such as the 'six weeks in bed' formerly advised following myocardial infarction. Each case must be assessed on its merits. The use of sedatives and hypnotic drugs for allaying restlessness and anxiety and for inducing sleep is discussed on p. 195.

Disadvantages of Bed Rest. When breathlessness is extreme the patient is compelled to sit up (orthopnoea). The vital capacity is increased in this position and on occasion it will be found that sitting in a chair is more comfortable than sitting up in bed. Moreover, the central venous pressure is increased in the recumbent posture and this adds to the work of the heart. Oedema will tend to collect in the legs rather than in the lungs when the patient is sitting and this may be an advantage when fluid retention is difficult to combat. Confinement to bed necessitates the use of the bed pan, but this may be a considerably greater strain than a bedside commode or sani-chair which should be used whenever possible. In bed the circulation rate is slowed and the risk of venous thrombosis and its attendant dangers is increased. Finally hypostasis in the lungs predisposes to pneumonia.

DIGITALIS

Digitalis is still the most useful drug available for the treatment of cardiac failure whatever its cause. Apart from a few conditions which are amenable to cure, once given it should usually be taken permanently. It is most effective in patients with atrial fibrillation accompanied by tachycardia, but it is also of value when sinus tachycardia is accompanied by failure. It is of value for the treatment of paroxysmal atrial tachycardia or flutter and also for the prevention of these conditions. Digitalis will be most effective when the left ventricle is failing from hypertension or ischaemic heart disease. It is of less value in aortic stenosis or incompetence. In right ventricular failure due to disorders of the pulmonary circulation its clinical benefits are more difficult to assess, but it should not be withheld on this account. It is contraindicated in the treatment of uncomplicated sinus tachycardia, constrictive pericarditis, ventricular tachycardia or fibrillation, peripheral circulatory failure, and of heart block unless associated with cardiac failure.

Action

1. **Improvement of Myocardial Efficiency.** The strength of systolic contraction is increased from direct stimulation of the failing myocardium. The ventricles empty more completely, the cardiac output is increased and the venous pressure is lowered. The work of the heart is more efficient in that relatively less oxygen is used by the myocardium for a given amount of work.

2. **Slowing of the Heart Rate.** In cardiac failure the heart rate is usually increased, especially if there is atrial fibrillation. Digitalis slows the heart by direct depression of the conducting tissues and by vagal stimulation. Improvement of function and slowing of rate are closely related.

3. **Diuretic Action.** Digitalis acts as a diuretic in patients with oedema due to cardiac failure, consequent on the improved blood supply to the kidneys which results from its action on the myocardium.

Preparations

The preparations in most common use (with equivalent strengths for maintenance) are:

Digitalis Leaf	100 mg.
Digoxin (Lanoxin)	0·25 mg.
Digitoxin (Digitaline, Nativelle)	0·1 mg.

There are many different preparations on the market. Proprietary preparations are usually relatively expensive. It is better for the practitioner to become thoroughly familiar with one or two preparations than to experiment with many different products. Digoxin is probably the best drug to be used for all purposes because it is chemically pure, well and quickly absorbed and can be given by mouth or injection.

Rapid absorption of preparations such as digoxin is an advantage when speed of action is important and it is desired to avoid parenteral administration.

Administration

The aim of digitalisation is to achieve initial saturation and thereafter to give a maintenance dose for as long as is necessary. This will often be for life. Patients vary in their requirements but the average dose will mainly depend on body weight. Urgent digitalisation by parenteral administration is rarely required because some preparations act so quickly when given by mouth that the situation can be brought under control within a few hours. Whenever possible digitalisation over a few days or a week is much to be preferred, and toxic symptoms will thereby be minimised. During this time a patient who has been ambulant will also have had the opportunity to experience the benefits of rest in bed, which is often remarkably effective in reducing dyspnoea and inducing a diuresis. However, on occasion, e.g. for paroxysmal fibrillation or tachycardia or for urgent congestive cardiac failure, the danger may be such that full digitalisation by the intravenous injection of a suitable preparation is warranted.

Full digitalisation can be achieved by oral dosage within a few hours, a day, three days or a week according to the degree of urgency. In cases of real urgency digoxin, 1 mg. for a 63 kg. (10 st.) patient, may be given by intravenous injection. The effect will be noticeable within 10 minutes. The effect of a large single dose of digoxin by mouth begins within an hour. If 1·5 mg. (for a 63 kg. patient) is given by mouth a very beneficial effect will be noticeable within the following six hours, that is before the next dose is due. Digitalisation within 24 hours can be achieved if necessary by giving digoxin, 1·5, 0·5, 0·5 and 0·5 mg. at intervals of six hours.

When there is no urgency (as is usually the case) a suitable regime is to give digoxin, 0·5 mg. t.d.s. the first day, 0·25 mg. q.d.s. the next day, and thereafter 0·25 mg. t.d.s. until the heart rate is controlled and symptoms and signs of failure are relieved, or mild toxic symptoms ensue.

Individuals vary in their requirements and the most suitable dose must be discovered by trial in each case. In practice this means that each patient must learn to recognise his early toxic symptoms. If necessary the drug can then be omitted for a day and thereafter continued at a slightly lower dosage. It is not advisable to omit the drug as a routine during the weekends as sometimes recommended. Very occasionally vomiting is of local and not central origin, in which case the preparation can be changed for another.

Toxic Effects. Individuals vary considerably in their tolerance to digitalis. Toxic effects are always a sign of overdosage and, if ignored, may prove serious. The toxic and therapeutic doses may be close together. Toxicity is readily induced in the elderly who require relatively small dosage, and likewise in those with renal failure.

The earlier clinical features of overdosage are anorexia, nausea and headache, followed by vomiting, occasionally diarrhoea and blurring of vision. The pulse rate may become unduly slow (under 60 beats per minute). Ventricular extrasystoles are a common occurrence and a warning to stop treatment for 24 hours (Fig. 27, p. 156). Coupled beats, i.e. alternate extrasystoles (pulsus bigeminus) are characteristic of digitalis poisoning. It is important to listen to the apex beat because the presence of extrasystoles may be missed at the wrist. Before giving digitalis by injection or in large doses by mouth it is important to ensure that the patient has not been taking the drug within the previous few days, or serious toxicity may result. Hypokalaemia may be responsible for hypersensitivity to digitalis and predisposes to the dangerous arrythmia of atrial tachycardia, usually with AV block (p. 161).

If administration of the drug is continued after toxic effects have developed, any degree of heart block may follow, and there is a risk of ventricular tachycardia. Occasionally ventricular fibrillation occurs and is one cause of sudden death.

Once experienced, early toxic symptoms are readily recognised by the patient, who is often the best judge of his optimal maintenance dosage.

Symptoms of cardiac failure, e.g. anorexia, nausea and vomiting, may sometimes be confused with those of digitalis intoxication. Differentiation can usually be made by considering the amount of digitalis administered and other evidence of overdosage, e.g. bradycardia and extrasystoles.

Strophanthus

Ouabain (strophanthin) is a rapidly acting cardiac glycoside for intravenous use only. It has no advantage over intravenous digoxin. The dose is 0·5 mg.

DIURETICS

The applied pharmacology of the various diuretics in use at the present time is discussed on pp. 853-857.

Diuretics are as effective in left ventricular failure as in right-sided congestive failure with peripheral oedema, and indeed in the former group they are often of more value than digitalis and may protect the patient from attacks of nocturnal dyspnoea (cardiac asthma). This is because left ventricular failure commonly occurs with normal rhythm and in such circumstances digitalis is less beneficial than when cardiac failure is accompanied by atrial fibrillation. Digitalis should nevertheless also be given.

Regular weighing of the patient is a good guide to the early recognition of fluid retention or fluid loss. Apart from obvious oedema, patients can often tell when they are in need of a diuretic by a feeling of increasing tightness in the chest or abdomen and by dyspnoea.

Oral Diuretics. Oral diuretics are the first choice in the treatment of the oedema of cardiac failure, provided nausea or vomiting does not prevent their administration. In acute left ventricular failure (cardiac asthma, p. 172) parenteral administration is indicated. During the last few years the thiazide group of drugs, which includes chlorothiazide, bendrofluazide, hydroflumethiazide, hydrochlorothiazide and polythiazide, has become established as the first choice, but the recently introduced drugs frusemide and ethacrynic acid have proved superior in some cases. In terms of diuretic effect and toxicity there is little to choose between the thiazide drugs and usually the choice should be determined by price. If given over a prolonged period in doses approaching the maximum, depletion of body potassium with all its possible consequences (p. 845,) is liable to be produced. Hence it is essential to prescribe a supplement of potassium when oral diuretics are given more than twice a week (p. 846). The prophylactic dose is 3 g. of potassium chloride daily or other equivalent of potassium salt.

The dosage of chlorothiazide and its related compounds varies according to the preparation used. The maximum recommended dose of chlorothiazide in one day is 2 g. It may be given in a single dose at 8 a.m. or in divided doses at 8 a.m. and 2 p.m. The thiazide drugs are rapidly absorbed from the gastrointestinal tract and diuresis usually begins within two hours, reaching its maximum in four to six hours; it is largely completed in 12 hours. Oral diuretics should rarely be given on more than three days a week. Some patients who are resistant to them respond to mersalyl, and vice versa. In resistant cases a combination of the two diuretics given on the same day or on alternate days may be successful. Should this fail aminophylline or spironolactone should be given in addition.

Chlorthalidone (Hygroton, p. 855) has a gentler but much longer duration of action than chlorothiazide and its derivatives, and when there is no urgency for a prompt diuresis it may be the drug of choice. The average dose is 100-200 mg. by mouth once or twice weekly. It may also be used as adjuvant therapy in hypertension (p. 241). Potassium supplements may be required. Polythiazide (Nephril) is a similar preparation.

Frusemide (Lasix) is a more recently introduced diuretic. It may be given orally (40-80 mg.) or intravenously (10-20 mg.) as an alternative to mersalyl. The onset of the diuresis is extremely rapid and is generally completed within six hours. It will be appreciated that this is a great advantage for cases urgently requiring treatment, e.g. severe congestive failure and pulmonary oedema, but a disadvantage in chronic congestive failure in which a more gentle action may be desirable. Frusemide given intravenously has superseded intravenous mersalyl as the first choice in acute emergencies. It should be noted that it is more expensive than the thiazide drugs.

Ethacrynic acid (Edecrin) is another potent oral diuretic (p. 855) which may be effective in promoting a diuresis when other drugs have failed. It may be given orally in a dose of 50-200 mg. per day. An intravenous preparation is also available.

Contrary to original claims both frusemide and ethacrynic acid may cause an excessive loss of potassium so that dosage must be carefully regulated and supplements of potassium given (p. 847).

Triamterene (Dytac) is a less potent diuretic but has the advantage of producing a relatively small excretion of potassium. It is best given in combination with a small dose of another oral diuretic.

SPIRONOLACTONE. Spironolactone (p. 855) inhibits the action of aldosterone and thus promotes diuresis. The dose is 25 mg. four times a day. It is only of limited value in the treatment of the oedema of cardiac failure but is sometimes of use when intractable oedema is present. This drug is ineffective alone and should only be given in combination with another diuretic.

MERCURIAL DIURETICS. The introduction of the newer diuretics discussed above given by mouth or intravenously in emergency has resulted in the mercurial diuretics being very rarely used at the present time. The official preparation in Britain is inj. Mersalyl B.P., 1 ml. of which should be given intramuscularly in the first instance, followed by 2 ml. two days later. The latter dose is therapeutically equivalent to 2 g. of chlorothiazide.

Intravenous injection is the most effective method of giving mersalyl. However, the solution is irritating if it gets outside the vein. Intramuscular injections are more convenient and the risk of an occasional serious or even fatal general reaction is certainly less. The effect of a 1 ml. dose should always be determined before a 2 ml. dose is given, and the effect of an intramuscular injection before an intravenous one.

Diuresis begins within half an hour of an injection and lasts for 12 or more hours. The effect is enhanced by giving 4 tablets, each of 0·5 g., containing ammonium chloride or better still equal parts of ammonium and potassium chloride before each injection.

Toxic effects rarely occur, e.g. stomatitis, colitis or dermatitis. The only absolute contraindications are active nephritis or severely impaired renal function from any cause other than cardiac failure.

SALT AND WATER RESTRICTION

The accumulation of sodium in the body is mainly responsible for the retention of water in oedema. The average daily intake of salt is normally about 10 g.; if no salt is added at table it is about 5 g. and if salt is withheld from cooking about 3 g. Special diets can be devised which contain less than 1 g. of sodium (Diet 8, p. 1293), but to achieve this it is necessary to take salt-free butter or margarine, salt-free bread, little milk or cheese, no bacon, salty fish, sauces, meat extracts or tinned foods (except fruit). Care must be taken not to prescribe medicine containing sodium, e.g. stomach powders, and to avoid baking powder in cooking. Sodium-free 'salt' is available for table use. Such severe restrictions are only necessary if oedema cannot otherwise be controlled and this is rarely the case since the introduction of the oral diuretics and mersalyl. For practical purposes if no salt is added at table and a thiazide or other effective diuretic is given as required there need be little or no limitation of the amount of fluid taken by mouth.

OTHER MEASURES

Diet

Weight reduction is advisable in obese patients. Small, dry meals at relatively frequent intervals, with fluid in between, will help to minimise abdominal distension. An adequate vitamin content should be ensured, particularly as regards the B group and vitamin C. Diet No. 4 (p. 1288) will be suitable for a case of severe congestive cardiac failure.

Oxygen

The only real indication for oxygen therapy in cardiac disease is when the arterial oxygen saturation is reduced, e.g. in cardiac failure with pulmonary congestion or with associated disease of the lungs, or in severe myocardial infarction. The need for oxygen is usually indicated by the presence of central cyanosis (p. 125) which however may be masked by shock or anaemia. For details of administration see p. 318.

Venesection

Venesection (phlebotomy) is rarely indicated and only if pulmonary congestion or venous engorgement is extreme and other measures are not rapidly effective. It acts by reducing the circulating blood volume and the viscosity of the blood.

Paracentesis

Pleural effusions and ascitic fluid should be removed whenever large enough in volume to contribute towards dyspnoea or to cause marked discomfort.

Mechanical removal of subcutaneous fluid is sometimes required and is still a very useful measure in cases of gross, intractable oedema.

The subject sits in a chair or cardiac bed until distension of the legs is extreme, and Southey's tubes are then inserted or multiple incisions made with a scalpel. Little discomfort is caused by the procedure and large volumes of fluid may be drained away with great relief. Penicillin should be given to minimise the risk of infection.

OTHER DRUGS OF VALUE IN THE TREATMENT OF HEART DISEASE

Quinidine

If facilities for electric conversion are not available quinidine is a useful drug for restoring normal rhythm in selected cases of cardiac arrhythmia, particularly atrial fibrillation, and for the prevention of recurrent attacks. Its administration is not without risk but this is slight in experienced hands when the patient is under close observation, preferably with facilities for electrocardiographic control. For this reason treatment should rarely be undertaken in general practice.

Actions. The principal action of quinidine is to prolong the refractory period of atrial muscle. It also depresses conduction. It is a vasodilator.

Indications

Atrial Fibrillation. Quinidine is rarely indicated if fibrillation has been present for more than a few months or if congestive cardiac failure, gross enlargement of the heart or other evidence of severe underlying disease is present. On occasion, however, it may be useful if digitalis fails to control the ventricular rate. It is most likely to be effective in cases of recent origin and without evidence of serious underlying disease (p. 157).

ATRIAL FLUTTER. Quinidine may be used to try and restore normal rhythm where digitalis, the drug of choice, has not been effective.

PAROXYSMAL TACHYCARDIA. Quinidine should be used for the treatment of paroxysmal supraventricular tachycardia if other measures fail. It is effective in the treatment and prevention of attacks of paroxysmal ventricular tachycardia or ventricular fibrillation.

PROPHYLAXIS. Quinidine is useful for the prevention of recurrent attacks of most forms of paroxysmal cardiac arrhythmia, but is most often used in cases of atrial fibrillation. It may even be useful for preventing extrasystoles in the occasional instances where they give rise to unpleasant symptoms which cannot otherwise be controlled.

Administration. Quinidine is normally given by mouth, but for urgent cases a preparation suitable for intravenous injection is available. It is desirable to digitalise the patient first in order to prevent the speeding up of the ventricular response which quinidine may produce.

DOSAGE. Very occasionally idiosyncrasy is present. If no toxic effects (see below) develop after the first dose, treatment should be continued. Some physicians advise giving 0·4 g. every two hours for 6-8 doses but since many patients revert to sinus rhythm on a small dose it is better to begin with 0·2 g. t.d.s. and gradually increase the daily dose until the desired effect is obtained. Should normal rhythm be restored a maintenance dose of 0·2-0·4 g. t.d.s. should be given until normal activities have been resumed. For intravenous administration 3 g. of quinidine sulphate are dissolved in 500 ml. of 5 per cent. glucose solution and given at the rate of 100 ml. per hour until the desired effect is obtained or toxic symptoms develop.

Toxic Effects. Toxic symptoms are not common. The symptoms are similar to those of quinine or salicylate poisoning, i.e. headache, tinnitus, blurring of vision, nausea, vomiting, diarrhoea and occasionally mental disturbances. Purpura may occur. Rarely, sudden death has been reported from cardiac standstill or ventricular fibrillation. Warning signs may be disclosed by serial electrocardiograms, notably widening of the QRS interval.

Procainamide

Procainamide has similar properties to those of quinidine, and in particular it depresses the irritability of ventricular muscle. It may be used for the treatment of ventricular tachycardia. Toxic effects include hypotension and gastrointestinal disturbances, and the drug must be used with caution.

Propranolol

This drug blocks the adrenergic beta receptors and thus counteracts the stimulating action of sympathomimetic amines on the rate and force of myocardial contraction. It is often effective in reducing the ventricular rate or restoring sinus rhythm in attacks of paroxysmal tachycardia especially if induced by digitalis. By modifying the circulatory response to exercise it reduces relative myocardial ischaemia in patients with coronary disease and is of value in the treatment of intractable angina.

Propranolol (Inderal) should be given cautiously to patients with heart failure because this may be exacerbated and a fall of blood pressure induced. Oral administration is preferable (5-30 mg. every six hours for an arrythmia and up to 300 mg. for angina) but in an emergency up to 5 mg. may be given by slow intravenous injection.

Phenytoin

This anticonvulsant drug has recently been used with some success in the treatment of paroxysmal supraventricular and ventricular tachycardias. It can be given either as a slow intravenous injection of 250 mg. or orally in a dose of up to 4 g. per day. As with other cardiac depressants hypotension may be induced by excessive administration.

Lignocaine

For the treatment of extrasystoles after myocardial infarction 50-100 mg. of lignocaine (Xylocaine) may be given or 250 mg. in 500 ml. glucose as a slow intravenous drip.

Sedatives

Sedatives are useful for allaying restlessness and anxiety and for inducing sleep. Oversedation must be avoided owing to the dangers of undue depression of respiration, and of excessive lethargy which increases the risk of venous thrombosis.

When severe pain, dyspnoea or unproductive cough prevent sleep an opiate is usually required and may be the most important measure in treatment. It may be given either in the form of morphine by injection or tincture of opium by mouth. Opiates have sedative as well as analgesic properties and an injection of morphine is usually sufficient by itself to procure sleep. The sedative action of tincture of opium may however have to be supplemented with a hypnotic such as chloral or one of the barbiturates.

TABLE 4

DURATION OF ACTION	OFFICIAL NAMES	OTHER NAMES	DOSAGE BY MOUTH mg.
>8 hrs.	Phenobarbitone	Luminal	30-120
<8 hrs.	Amylobarbitone Sodium	Sodium Amytal	100-200
	Butobarbitone	Soneryl	100-200
	Cyclobarbitone	Phanodorm	200-400
	Pentobarbitone Sodium	Nembutal	100-200
	Quinalbarbitone Sodium	Seconal	100-200

A wide range of barbiturates is available for the treatment of insomnia *per se*, and the choice is largely an individual one depending on the duration of action required. Table 4 summarises some of the preparations in common use which have received official sanction. All these drugs may be taken by mouth and their hypnotic effect will usually be evident in about half an hour. Phenobarbitone is widely prescribed for anxiety and nervousness but has relatively little hypnotic effect.

ANALGESICS

Morphine. After more than 100 years morphine remains supreme as the most effective drug for severe pain such as that experienced by patients with myocardial infarction. The dose must be sufficient to secure complete relief, 15 mg. being administered intramuscularly or even intravenously, as absorption from subcutaneous injection is relatively slow. This dose may have to be repeated once or even twice, but not more than 60 mg. should be given in all during the first 12 hours for fear of producing undue depression of the respiratory centre.

Apart from its use in the treatment of pain, morphine is an invaluable drug in the management of left-sided heart failure, especially for the relief of orthopnoea, paroxysmal dyspnoea and acute pulmonary oedema. This action is presumably due to depression of the respiratory centre and of the Hering-Breuer reflex and to the relief of restlessness and anxiety. For a few days after the onset of nocturnal dyspnoea it is reasonable to give a prophylactic injection at bedtime or an opiate by mouth.

Unfortunately morphine is apt to produce vomiting which is particularly undesirable in a patient who is seriously ill. Vomiting can usually be prevented by giving an antihistamine tablet, e.g. cyclizine (Marzine) or chlorpromazine at the same time.

Pethidine. Undesirable side-effects, tolerance and addiction are less likely to develop with pethidine than with morphine. Its analgesic effects are less powerful and more transient but this can be overcome by giving the drug in appropriate doses every few hours. It may be taken by mouth or given intramuscularly (100 mg.) and repeated once or twice within the hour if necessary.

Methadone (Physeptone). Methadone, 15-30 mg. is roughly equivalent to a similar dose of morphine. Side-effects and addiction are less common. The drug can be given by mouth or by subcutaneous or intramuscular injection. It is particularly useful for allaying cough, for which purpose linctus methadone should be used.

Codeine. By itself codeine is an unsatisfactory analgesic. Combined with aspirin and phenacetin in a tablet (Tab. codein. Co. B.P.C.) it is widely prescribed for the relief of pain of mild to moderate intensity. Each tablet contains aspirin 0·25 g., phenacetin 0·25 g. and codeine 8 mg., and 2-3 tablets may be taken at a time.

Paracetamol (Panadol). Many analgesic drugs have been synthesised in recent years, the potency of which is approximately equal to that of aspirin. One of the most widely used of these drugs is paracetamol which is indicated instead of aspirin if there is evidence that the patient has a tendency to gastric haemorrhage.

The dose is 2 tablets, each containing 500 mg., every three or four hours.

TREATMENT OF PAROXYSMAL DYSPNOEA AND ACUTE PULMONARY OEDEMA (CARDIAC ASTHMA)

The first essential is to place the patient in the upright sitting posture in order to drain as much blood as possible into the dependent parts of the body and increase the vital capacity. Morphine 15 mg. should be injected, preferably intravenously. The response is usually dramatic. Oxygen should be administered if central cyanosis is present. In patients with left ventricular failure (who have not been taking digitalis for 14 days) digoxin 1 mg. should be given intravenously. A potent diuretic such as frusemide or ethacrynic acid should be given when the acute phase is over. For the prevention of further attacks they are also of value. The intravenous injection of aminophylline 0·5 g. is useful if bronchospasm is present.

If these measures are not sufficient, pressure cuffs should then be applied to the thighs as far proximally as possible and inflated to just above diastolic pressure, and preparation made for venesection. Artificial ventilation by intermittent positive pressure may be necessary in a prolonged attack.

THE SURGICAL TREATMENT OF HEART DISEASE

Progress is being made in the field of cardiac surgery and it is now possible to correct or alleviate a considerable number of congenital or acquired defects. Some operations can be performed under normal circulatory conditions. Others require opening the heart with temporary occlusion of the circulation. In such cases increased time for intracardiac surgery can be obtained either by cooling the blood or the whole body (hypothermia) which decreases the oxygen requirements of the tissues or by the use of an extracorporeal circulation (pump-oxygenator) so that the heart can be temporarily excluded from the circulation. It is important, therefore, for the practitioner to know which defects can be so treated, the criteria for diagnosis, the natural history of the condition without surgical treatment, the operative risk, the degree of improvement in symptoms and altered prognosis for life which is likely to be obtained by operation and therefore the indications for advising surgical treatment. In suitable cases the following conditions can be treated by operation:

(1) Patent ductus arteriosus (p. 245).
(2) Coarctation of the aorta (p. 247).
(3) Atrial septal defect (p. 248).
(4) Ventricular septal defect (p. 249).
(5) Pulmonary stenosis (p. 250).
(6) Fallot's tetralogy (p. 251).
(7) Mitral stenosis and incompetence (pp. 200, 201).
(8) Aortic stenosis and incompetence (pp. 203, 204).
(9) Tricuspid stenosis and incompetence (p. 206).
(10) Constrictive pericarditis (p. 269).
(11) Intractable angina pectoris (p. 220).

* * * * * *

VALVULAR DISEASE OF THE HEART

It has been decided to group together the descriptions of all forms of valvular disease because the manifestations are largely independent of the aetiology.

Since the medical treatment of the sequelae of valvular disease has been described under Cardiac Failure, reference to treatment in this section will be confined to the value of surgical procedures.

Aetiology. The principal cause of valvular disease is rheumatic endocarditis. This most commonly affects the mitral valve, next the aortic valve, and comparatively rarely the triscupid valve. Syphilis may affect the aortic valve but not the others. Congenital lesions are frequently responsible for most cases of pulmonary valvular disease, some cases of aortic disease and occasionally for tricuspid disease. Sub-acute bacterial endocarditis may be superimposed on rheumatic or congenital lesions and cause further damage. Trauma is a very occasional cause of a ruptured cusp. Functional incompetence of a valve may be present without structural changes in the cusps, e.g. from dilatation of the mitral valve ring in left ventricular failure, the tricuspid valve ring in right ventricular failure or the pulmonary valve ring in pulmonary hypertension.

MITRAL VALVULAR DISEASE

Rheumatic fever is responsible for almost all cases of mitral valvular disease. All degrees of disability may be present, from mild cases without relevant symptoms to severe ones with marked dyspnoea and subsequent cardiac failure. In the early stages incompetence is frequently present, but later stenosis usually develops and becomes the predominant lesion. Pure mitral incompetence does occur but is relatively uncommon.

Pathology. Rheumatic endocarditis leads to inflammation, thickening, fibrosis and deformity of the valve cusps, the chordae tendineae and the valve ring. This leads to varying degrees of imperfect closure and of narrowing of the valve. Adhesions of the cusps, rigidity and sometimes calcification lead to narrowing of the orifice and sometimes to a slit-like 'buttonhole' aperture. Shortening of the chordae may produce a 'funnel-shape' which further accentuates the narrowing.

Mitral Incompetence

In mitral insufficiency the left atrial volume increases with ventricular systole and the left ventricle is over-filled during diastole, but its output per beat into the aorta is unchanged until left ventricular failure develops.

Symptoms. In mild cases the left ventricle can compensate for this increase in diastolic volume and there will be no symptoms. Severe cases of pure or predominant mitral incompetence are relatively uncommon. Symptoms and eventual signs of cardiac failure are similar to those of mitral stenosis.

Signs

1. A pan-systolic murmur maximal at the apex and often conducted towards the left axilla. The murmur may be accompanied by a thrill.

2. The first heart sound and the opening snap are weak or absent in contrast to mitral stenosis, and a third sound may be present.

3. Enlargement of the left atrium. This can only be detected radiologically.

4. Enlargement of the left ventricle, which may be felt as a distinct thrust at the apex of the heart or seen radiologically.

5. Left ventricular hypertrophy may be demonstrated by electrocardiography.

Differential Diagnosis. The differentiation of the organic murmur of mitral incompetence from physiological or functional systolic apical murmurs is often impossible.

Physiological murmurs are common in children and adolescents and in the presence of fever, anaemia or thyrotoxicosis when the circulation rate is increased. The discovery of any murmur should invariably be followed by a thorough examination. If the individual is otherwise well, there is no history of rheumatic fever, no enlargement of the heart, a normal blood pressure and no other signs of valvular disease, the murmur can be ignored from a practical point of view. It is most important that unwarranted restrictions should not be imposed or an anxiety neurosis engendered.

The problem is rather more difficult from a life insurance point of view because there is no doubt that the differentiation of apparently innocent murmurs from mild organic heart disease may be important and yet impossible. It cannot be told from a single examination whether or not the condition is progressive. Also, a patient with rheumatic heart disease is liable to further attacks of rheumatic fever and even a mild mitral valvular lesion is prone to become the seat of subacute bacterial endocarditis.

Surgical Treatment. Satisfactory surgical treatment using the pump-oxygenator has recently been introduced. The valve may be repaired or replaced according to circumstances.

Mitral Stenosis

In moderate or severe cases the left atrium tends to dilate and hypertrophy. However, the atrial muscle is thin and may be affected by rheumatic myocarditis, so that back pressure soon leads to pulmonary congestion and pulmonary hypertension and in time to dilatation, hypertrophy and eventually failure of the right side of the heart. Atrial fibrillation is very common and adds to the disability.

Symptoms. Long-standing pulmonary congestion is responsible for the dyspnoea so characteristic of mitral stenosis. Attacks of acute pulmonary oedema may occur but are less common than in left ventricular failure. Palpitation is often a distressing complaint and cough may be very troublesome. Haemoptysis may occur, especially in those with severe pulmonary venous hypertension and sometimes from pulmonary infarction.

Signs

1. Peripheral cyanosis and a small volume pulse may be present and are due to vasoconstriction.

2. The apical impulse is often 'tapping' in quality, and a right ventricular thrust may be felt behind and to the left of the lower sternum and in the epigastrium.

3. A diastolic thrill is often palpable at the apex.

4. A diastolic murmur maximal at, or confined to, the region of the apex beat is the hallmark of mitral stenosis. The murmur may be pre-systolic in time or fill most of diastole with apparent pre-systolic accentuation. It is usually low-pitched and rumbling in quality and best heard with a bell stethoscope and the patient lying on the left side.

In early cases it may only be heard if the heart rate is increased, e.g. by exercise. The pre-systolic part of the murmur is dependent on atrial systole, and hence disappears with the onset of atrial fibrillation.

5. The first heart sound at the apex is characteristically loud and sudden. The second heart sound at the base may be accentuated from pulmonary hypertension. An added sound may frequently be heard immediately preceding the mid-diastolic murmur. It coincides in time with the opening of the mitral valve and is referred to as the 'opening snap' of the mitral valve (p. 134).

6. Enlargement of the left atrium can readily be seen on radiological examination, especially in the right oblique position, in which it will be seen projecting backwards and indenting the barium-filled oesophagus (Plate IV, facing p. 132). Calcification of the mitral valve may be observed. Later enlargement of the pulmonary artery and of the right ventricle occurs.

7. Right ventricular hypertrophy may be detected by electrocardiography.

Surgical Treatment. Mitral valvotomy not only reduces the back pressure on the lungs and hence by relieving pulmonary congestion alleviates dyspnoea but also permits of a greater increase in cardiac output especially on exertion. It must be appreciated that the degree of mechanical obstruction at the mitral valve is rarely the only factor of importance in mitral stenosis. What matters too is the amount of myocardial damage, the presence or absence of other valvular defects, the occurrence of narrowing in the pulmonary arterioles and the changes in the lungs which result from prolonged congestion. However, the mechanical factor is frequently predominant.

The most suitable patients for operation are those with uncomplicated mitral stenosis, with sinus rhythm and no great enlarge- of the heart. The possibility of surgical treatment should be considered whenever there is a considerable disability or evidence of progression of symptoms and signs and the patient should be referred to a special unit. Pulmonary oedema and recurrent haemoptysis are strong indications for operation, while atrial fibrillation is a disadvantage but not an absolute contraindication. Not only does atrial fibrillation mean that the myocardium has been involved by the rheumatic process but also that clot is more likely to be formed in the atrium than if normal rhythm is present and consequently there is an increased risk of systemic embolism. Some cases are complicated by mitral incompetence and others by aortic valvular disease and it is important to decide that these defects are not predominant. Remarkable clinical improvement can be achieved by this operation in suitably selected cases and this usually persists for some years. However, many patients require a second valvotomy for re-stenosis. If the valve is severely damaged it can be replaced by a prosthesis. It must be remembered that surgical treatment is but an incident in the relentless progress of rheumatic heart disease whether from activity of the rheumatic process or from the progressive fibrosis which follows activity.

AORTIC VALVULAR DISEASE

Aortic Incompetence

Aetiology. Most cases are due to rheumatic fever and some to syphilitic aortitis. Occasional cases may be due to bacterial endocarditis or trauma. Functional incompetence may be secondary to hypertension or atheroma of the aorta.

Pathology. The pathology of rheumatic endocarditis is described on p. 207 and of syphilitic aortic incompetence on p. 260.

Symptoms. Owing to the ability of the powerful left ventricle to deal with the reflux of blood which occurs in diastole, compensation may be excellent for many years. In time left ventricular failure occurs and progressive dyspnoea on exertion is soon followed by paroxysmal dyspnoea at rest, orthopnoea and finally congestive cardiac failure (p. 169).

Signs

1. The characteristic and most important sign of aortic incompetence is a high-pitched, blowing, early diastolic murmur commencing immediately after the second heart sound and best heard down the left sternal edge with the patient standing or sitting and the breath held in expiration. A blowing systolic murmur is a common accompaniment.
2. Enlargement of the left ventricle leads to displacement of the apex beat downwards and to the left and to a heaving impulse.
3. Low diastolic blood pressure with high pulse pressure.
4. Peripheral signs of aortic incompetence (free regurgitation).
(*a*) Collapsing or 'water-hammer' radial pulse. There is an abrupt upstroke with sudden impact against the examining finger and a rapid falling away or 'collapse'.
(*b*) Visible arterial pulsation, e.g. in the carotids.
5. Associated peripheral vasodilatation gives rise to pink and warm extremities and to capillary pulsation, e.g. in the nail beds.
6. Radiography will show the degree of left ventricular enlargement and the electrocardiogram may show the pattern of left ventricular hypertrophy.

Surgical Treatment. Occasionally it is possible to repair the valve. Usually it must be replaced by a prosthesis.

Aortic Stenosis

Aetiology. Some cases are due to rheumatic fever, usually in association with other valvular lesions. Aortic stenosis with calcification of the valve often occurs as an isolated lesion commonly in association with a congenital bicuspid valve.

Symptoms. The clinical features will depend on the degree of narrowing and the presence or absence of other valvular lesions.

In recent years it has been realised that mild cases of stenosis are relatively frequent but often unrecognised. In the compensated phase symptoms may be entirely absent. When left ventricular failure occurs its symptoms and signs are similar to those occurring in aortic incompetence. The degree of ventricular hypertrophy is usually greater.

In addition, faintness and dizziness, syncope, anginal pain, heart block and sudden death all tend to be associated. Such symptoms are probably due to myocardial or cerebral ischaemia.

In established cases some or all of the following signs are usually present.

Signs

1. The apical impulse is thrusting in quality as a result of ventricular hypertrophy.
2. A systolic thrill maximal in the same areas as the murmur and likewise transmitted into the neck is a common, but not invariable accompaniment. As with the diastolic murmur it is best appreciated with the patient leaning forward and the breath held in expiration.
3. A harsh murmur maximal in mid-systole to the right of the upper sternum and transmitted into the carotid arteries.
4. Faint or absent component of the aortic second sound.
5. An aortic diastolic murmur is often present but without peripheral signs of free aortic incompetence, i.e. undue arterial pulsations.
6. Pulse of small amplitude and rising slowly to a delayed peak.
7. Lowered systolic blood pressure and decreased pulse pressure.
8. Left ventricular enlargement or hypertrophy may be confirmed by radiography and electrocardiography.
9. Calcification of the aortic valves may be seen on the radiological screen, particularly with an image intensifier.

The severity of aortic stenosis must be judged by symptoms and the degree of left ventricular hypertrophy. Auscultatory findings and blood pressure readings may be misleading.

Surgical Treatment. Aortic valvotomy is best done under direct vision. If calcification is present the valve will have to be replaced by a prosthesis or homograft.

PULMONARY VALVULAR DISEASE

Pulmonary Incompetence

This is usually functional in origin from pulmonary hypertension, e.g. in mitral stenosis. An early diastolic murmur can be heard to the left of the upper sternum (Graham Steell murmur). Dilatation of the pulmonary artery and hypertrophy of the right ventricle are associated. Most diastolic murmurs heard in this area originate at the aortic valve and can often be distinguished by the presence of other signs of aortic incompetence (p. 203).

Pulmonary Stenosis

This is almost always congenital in origin and may occur as an isolated lesion but is more commonly associated with a ventricular septal defect particularly as part of the tetralogy of Fallot (p. 251).

TRICUSPID VALVULAR DISEASE

Aetiology. Occasional cases are congenital in origin. Most cases are due to rheumatic fever and are associated with severe mitral stenosis and often aortic valvular disease as well. These valvular defects tend to obscure the characteristic clinical features of triscupid disease. Functional tricuspid incompetence often occurs in right ventricular failure from dilatation of the heart.

Diagnosis. This may be difficult for the reasons mentioned above but may be suggested by:

1. A systolic or diastolic murmur maximal near the lower sternum and becoming louder in inspiration.
2. Exaggerated pulsation (p. 130) of the jugular veins.
3. Expansile pulsation of the enlarged liver.
4. Relatively little dyspnoea or orthopnoea in cases of mitral stenosis owing to 'protection' of the pulmonary circulation by the diminished output of the right ventricle into the lungs.
5. Electrocardiographic evidence of right atrial hypertrophy.
6. Radiographic evidence of right atrial dilatation.

Treatment. Repair, valvotomy or replacement can be carried out according to circumstances.

* * * * * *

RHEUMATIC FEVER AND RHEUMATIC HEART DISEASE

Heart disease is the most serious manifestation of rheumatic fever and indeed its only important consequence. Rheumatic fever is therefore best considered under Diseases of the Cardiovascular System. The nomenclature is unsatisfactory because the term 'rheumatic' is applied to a large number of diseases characterised by aches and pains, and fever is often absent or too slight to be recognised. Rheumatic fever, nevertheless, is a well-recognised, specific entity.

RHEUMATIC FEVER

The incidence of rheumatic fever is greatest in childhood and adolescence, 90 per cent. of cases commencing between the ages of 5 and 15. It tends to develop into a chronic stage and recurrences are frequent. Mild and subclinical forms occur and about half the patients who are found to have valvular disease of the heart of rheumatic origin give no history of any such preceding infection.

Aetiology. The precise cause of rheumatic fever is unknown. However, there is much evidence that rheumatic fever is related to infection with group A haemolytic streptococci, probably on the basis of tissue allergy. There is no diagnostic laboratory test which is specific for the disease. Rheumatic fever is mainly a disease of temperate climates and is less common in the tropics. It tends to occur in families, but this may be due to environment rather than heredity. Most cases in Britain occur in autumn and spring.

Rheumatic fever commonly affects the lower income groups and town dwellers. Poor housing and overcrowding are important factors. The disease is often preceded by tonsillitis or pharyngitis one to three weeks before.

Pathology. The fibrous tissues of the body are involved. Joints, muscles, tendons, heart valves, subcutaneous tissues and blood vessels are all affected. In the exudative stage there is hyperaemia, oedema of the collagen tissue and infiltration with leucocytes. The hallmark of rheumatic fever is the Aschoff nodule, which may be found in the interstitial tissues of any part of the heart, most frequently under the endocardium and in close relation to small blood vessels. Its microscopic appearance is that of a central area of necrosis surrounded by small round cells, histiocytes and giant cells. The lesions of rheumatic fever never suppurate.

Clinical Manifestations

ONSET. There may be a sudden onset of pain, swelling and stiffness in one or more joints, with fever, sweating and tachycardia, or the onset may be insidious with fatigue, malaise and loss of weight.

FEVER. Fever is usual in acute attacks but variable in degree and duration and much influenced by the administration of salicylates which have a marked antipyretic effect. Sweating may be profuse and tends to be accentuated by salicylates. Other accompaniments of fever, such as anorexia, furred tongue, constipation and albuminuria, are often present.

TACHYCARDIA. Tachycardia tends to be out of proportion to the degree of fever and may persist after the latter has settled. The sleeping pulse rate will differentiate tachycardia due to anxiety or excitement, and this observation is exceedingly useful in deciding when more physical activity can be permitted.

POLYARTHRITIS. This manifestation is more marked in adults than in children. The big joints are principally affected, e.g. knees, ankles, shoulders and wrists, but almost any joint may be involved. Characteristically there is a migrating polyarthritis, that is to say the pain tends to move from one joint to another, one getting better as another becomes worse. In severe cases the joints become hot, swollen, red and exquisitely tender. The peri-articular tissues are principally involved. Sterile effusions may develop. However, there are no residual effects in the joints once the acute attack is over.

RHEUMATIC NODULES. These are seen most often in childhood and their principal importance lies in the almost invariable association with active carditis. They are situated subcutaneously, are painless, not attached to the skin and tend to occur over bony prominences or be attached to tendons. Elbows, backs of hands, knees, malleoli, skull, scapulae and vertebrae are the most common sites. Rheumatic nodules are seen far less frequently than 20 years ago.

ERYTHEMA MARGINATUM (ERYTHEMA ANNULARE). Reddish patches appear mainly on the trunk and rapidly enlarge to form irregular crescent shapes which join together to form larger areas. The margins are slightly elevated. The lesions tend to disappear and reappear over a short period of time.

ERYTHEMA NODOSUM. Erythema nodosum is an occasional manifestation of rheumatic fever or streptococcal infection. It is always important to exclude tuberculosis and sarcoidosis as the cause (pp. 416 and 433).

CARDITIS. This is considered under the heading of Rheumatic Heart Disease (p. 207).

BLOOD. A polymorph *leucocytosis* of 10,000 to 15,000 cells per c. mm. is common in the acute stage and hypochromic *anaemia* often accompanies active rheumatic infection. A raised *erythrocyte sedimentation rate* is usually present in the active stages and may persist as evidence of activity of the rheumatic process when all other manifestations have subsided.

CHOREA (SYDENHAM'S CHOREA). There is no doubt about the close relationship of chorea to rheumatic fever in many cases. The majority of children with chorea either show evidence of rheumatic valvular disease or develop such evidence subsequently. The clinical features suggest involvement of the basal ganglia, and when the opportunity for study has occurred changes suggesting an encephalitis in this region of the brain have been found, although they are surprisingly mild. For this reason the clinical features of chorea are described under the Diseases of the Nervous System (p. 1212).

Differential Diagnosis. The differential diagnosis of rheumatic fever in the absence of any cardiac abnormality must sometimes be considered when fever and joint pains are the principal manifestations of illness. A raised antistreptolysin titre may be present in the blood. It is a fallacy to assume that rheumatic fever may be excluded because only one joint is involved. It is, however, true that rheumatic fever is unlikely to be responsible for joint symptoms which are not markedly alleviated by salicylates within 48 hours. Diagnosis may be difficult and must include the consideration of acute rheumatoid arthritis, osteomyelitis, tuberculosis, allergic conditions, undulant fever, gonococcal and meningococcal arthritis, disseminated lupus erythematosus, bacterial endocarditis and septicaemia. In rheumatoid arthritis the onset is rarely so acute, the small joints are principally affected and often assume a characteristic abnormality, morning stiffness in the affected parts is usual and flitting pains are uncommon.

In cases of osteomyelitis careful examination will reveal that pain and tenderness are maximal over the neighbouring bone rather than joint. The diagnosis will subsequently be confirmed by radiological examination. In gonococcal arthritis the condition is usually monarticular and there is either a history of a discharge or positive smears will be obtained from the urethra or cervix. Brucellosis (p. 59) may be suggested by the temperature chart, a history of a possible source of infection and a positive blood culture or agglutination reaction.

Prophylaxis. The problem of prevention, which is largely a social and economic one, is discussed on p. 274. This is a very important aspect because there is no specific treatment for rheumatic fever, and very little can be done to mitigate the damage done to the heart. The heart is liable to be further affected in subsequent attacks. Relapses may be largely prevented by giving a small daily dose of oral penicillin, phenoxymethylpenicillin V 125 mg. b.i.d. for five years after the first attack. Relapses occur most frequently during this period, but their incidence diminishes with age. Fortunately streptococci do not develop resistance to penicillin. Reactions, e.g. urticaria or joint pains, occasionally occur, in which case sulphadimidine, 0·5 g. daily may be given instead.

Treatment. There is no specific treatment.

Rest in Bed is essential throughout the active stage of the disease, i.e. until symptoms and fever have subsided, the sleeping pulse rate, white count and haemoglobin level and blood sedimentation rate have returned to normal, and weight is being gained. This may entail rest in bed for six weeks to six months or even longer. Thereafter, the return to activity should be gradual.

The blood sedimentation rate is a very useful guide to progress. Relapse may follow if the patient is allowed up before the rate is normal, but on occasion this rule may have to be ignored when a slightly raised rate persists for an undue length of time.

Nursing Care is important for ensuring proper rest and sleep. for encouraging appetite and for maintaining adequate nutrition,

There may be much sweating in the active stages necessitating sponging and frequent changes of clothing. For the same reason, extra fluids must be given. Posture in bed should be determined solely by the position of maximum comfort. Affected joints should also be supported in the most comfortable position. Cottonwool and bandages are usually sufficient for this purpose, but light splints may be required. In the acute stage a lead and opium lotion applied to the painful joints is soothing.

DRUGS. *Penicillin* should be given for 7 to 10 days routinely at the start of treatment with the object of killing haemolytic streptococci in the nose and throat There is no evidence that antibiotics and chemotherapy are of the slightest value in treatment except for this purpose. If tonsillectomy is deemed to be necessary it should be carried out after the acute stage of the disease has subsided.

Salicylates have long been used to combat fever and pain, and there is no doubt about their efficacy in this respect. Acetylsalicylic acid (aspirin) is preferable to sodium salicylate because it is better tolerated and has a greater analgesic effect. Calcium aspirin has the advantage over aspirin in that it is more soluble and hence is less liable to cause gastric irritation. It may be given every two hours for the first day or two and thereafter four-hourly with a double dose at night to save waking the patient. The total daily dose of aspirin is from 4-8 g. depending on age and body weight. If sodium salicylate is prescribed the total daily dose for an adult varies from 6-10 g. This dosage should be continued until fever and symptoms have been controlled for at least 10 days and then gradually reduced. Should rheumatic manifestations return, treatment will have to be resumed. If toxic symptoms develop, the dose must be reduced and then maintained at the highest level which can be tolerated. Nausea, headache, dizziness, tinnitus and deafness are the early toxic symptoms, followed by vomiting, hyperventilation and mental symptoms. Occasionally haemorrhage may occur from hypoprothrombinaemia (p. 667).

Clinical trials have shown that the combination of prednisolone with salicylates in high dosage is the most effective treatment for *severe* cases but has no effect on long term results.

There is little convincing evidence that salicylates influence the important cardiac complications, or materially shorten the course of the disease. Nevertheless they add to the patient's comfort and well-being and it is difficult to believe that they can benefit the joints so markedly without influencing to some extent the other structures involved. In addition, they are of some value in the differential diagnosis of polyarthritis. Should symptoms not rapidly subside it is improbable that they are due to rheumatic fever and some other cause should be sought. However, other somewhat similar illnesses may be benefited to some degree and occasionally rheumatic fever is slow to respond so that too much reliance should not be placed on this test.

Other drugs may be needed for complications, e.g. cardiac failure.

CONVALESCENCE in a suitable environment will be required when the active stage is over and before return to school or work. Its duration will depend on the length of the preceding illness and the presence or absence of cardiac complications.

RHEUMATIC HEART DISEASE

The heart is affected in most cases of rheumatic fever and this occurs too commonly to be referred to merely as a complication. There are about 25,000 deaths from rheumatic heart disease in Britain each year, and these form about 20 per cent. of all cardiac deaths. Rheumatic fever is in fact the most common cause of heart disease under the age of 50.

(*a*) ENDOCARDITIS. In the early stages this may be suspected from diminished intensity of the first heart sound or from the development of a blowing systolic murmur. A transient diastolic murmur may be heard. There may, of course, be evidence of previous rheumatic infection, e.g. mitral stenosis or aortic incompetence.

(*b*) PERICARDITIS (p. 265). Pericarditis may be suspected as a complication when there is a recrudescence of fever with the development of malaise, restlessness and pallor. Retrosternal or praecordial pain is common and pericardial friction may be heard. Characteristic changes may occur in the electrocardiogram (p. 266). An effusion may develop. Pericarditis itself is not a serious manifestation of rheumatic fever, but its association with myocarditis is almost invariable.

(*c*) MYOCARDITIS. Myocarditis may be assumed in the presence of endo- or pericarditis, but its clinical manifestations may be difficult to recognise. Active myocarditis is suggested by undue tachycardia, decreased intensity of the first heart sound, increasing enlargement of the heart, evidence of cardiac failure and abnormalities in the electrocardiogram (prolongation of the P-R and Q-T intervals).

It is important to emphasise that rheumatic carditis may occur without other evidence of rheumatic fever.

The active and inactive forms of rheumatic heart disease must be distinguished. Persistent activity is suggested by the presence of fever, tachycardia, anaemia, changing cardiac signs, failure to gain weight, a raised blood sedimentation rate and abnormalities in the electrocardiogram. Activity implies progressive damage to the heart by the rheumatic process. It may be followed by a period, probably for as long as two years, when the contraction of fibrous tissue leads to increasing deformity of the involved valves. Thereafter, unless further attacks of rheumatic infection occur, deterioration is due to the mechanical effects of valvular disease, which in time may lead to failure of the heart muscle.

The effects of chronic valvular disease of the heart resulting from rheumatic fever are described on p. 199.

* * * * * *

BACTERIAL ENDOCARDITIS

Bacterial endocarditis should logically be classified on an aetiological basis depending on the bacterial cause. In practice, however, it is divided into acute and subacute forms (of which the latter is the more frequent) largely because the clinical and pathological courses are usually distinctive and the responsible organisms are also different. Overlapping between the two groups, however, may occur.

As a result of modern treatment of acute infections by antibacterial drugs, acute bacterial endocarditis has become much rarer. It is a complication which results from an infection of the blood stream with virulent organisms, e.g. staphylococci, streptococci or pneumococci, and may attack healthy valves. High fever, sweats, rigors, wasting and septic emboli in various parts of the body are characteristic. Treatment with the appropriate antibiotic will be required, and in view of the seriousness of the condition the drug should be given in high dosage. The source of infection is usually apparent and often of a surgical nature, e.g. osteomyelitis or a septic abortion, and will itself require appropriate treatment.

The subacute form mainly affects hearts previously rendered abnormal from rheumatic valvular or congenital heart disease. It is usually due to infection with non-haemolytic streptococci, though occasionally other organisms, e.g. streptococci, gonococci, meningococci, brucellae or influenza bacilli are responsible. It nearly always affects those with well compensated heart disease and is a rare complication when congestive cardiac failure or atrial fibrillation is present. It was almost invariably fatal but since the introduction of antibiotics it can now generally be arrested. This renders early diagnosis very important before further cardiac damage or serious complications ensue.

Predisposing Factors

1. *Rheumatic valvular disease.* The mitral and aortic valves are those most commonly affected by rheumatic endocarditis and hence the most usual sites for subacute bacterial endocarditis.

2. *Congenital heart disease.* Patent ductus arteriosus, ventricular septal defect, a bicuspid aortic valve and pulmonary stenosis are the most common congenital lesions associated with this condition.

3. *Focal infection.* Non-haemolytic streptococci are the most common organisms to be found in infected gums, teeth and tonsils. It is known that transient bacteraemia frequently follows even minor surgical procedures in such infected regions. Although this is quite harmless in normal individuals the organisms may settle in the endocardium of abnormal hearts. A preceding history of recent tonsillectomy, dental extractions or even scaling of tartar from the teeth, or more rarely urethral catheterisation is frequently obtained in cases of subacute bacterial endocarditis.

4. *Upper respiratory infections.* A history of a cold in the head or influenza may be obtained prior to the onset of subacute bacterial endocarditis, though the symptoms may be difficult to differentiate from the onset of the disease itself. Since non-haemolytic streptococci are normal inhabitants of the upper respiratory tract it may well be that an acute infection facilitates their entry into the blood stream.

Clinical Features

1. Malaise, fatigue, anorexia, and pain in the joints.

2. *Persistent fever.* Bacterial endocarditis should always be con-

sidered in the differential diagnosis of a case of obscure fever, especially in a patient known to be suffering from heart disease.

3. *General appearance.* Apart from pallor due to anaemia a curious earthy 'café-au-lait' complexion was not uncommonly seen in the late stages of the disease prior to the antibiotic era.

4. *Skin.* Petechial haemorrhages into the skin and conjunctivae are frequent. Splinter haemorrhages may be seen under the nails. Osler's nodes are small, raised, pink, painful, tender areas on fingers or toes, palms or soles, which come and go, persisting for a few days.

5. *Clubbing of the fingers.* This is a common finding in long-standing cases but the changes are rarely gross.

6. *Examination of the heart* will almost always show evidence of previous rheumatic valvular disease or some congenital defect. Active rheumatic carditis is known to be frequently associated and may account for some of the instances of cardiac failure which occur even though the bacterial infection is apparently controlled.

7. *Spleen.* Moderate enlargement is usual.

8. *Kidney.* Microscopical haematuria is commonly found at some stage. This may arise from local vascular changes, nephritis or embolisation. Renal failure is frequent in fatal cases as a result of multiple renal infarction or from nephritis.

9. *Peripheral embolism.* Emboli from the vegetations on the endocardium may lodge in spleen, kidneys, retinae, brain, limb or mesenteric vessels. The effects will depend on the number and size of the emboli and may consist, for example, of sudden pain in the affected organs, blindness or segmental loss of vision, hemiplegia or possibly a subarachnoid haemorrhage. Suppuration does not occur in such infarcts.

10. *Blood.* A progressive hypochromic anaemia occurs. There may be a moderate leucocytosis. The ESR is raised.

11. *Blood culture.* A positive blood culture may be obtained in most cases, especially if repeated specimens are taken and meticulous care is taken over the technique. However, treatment should not be delayed for more than a day or two on this account if the diagnosis is reasonably certain on clinical grounds.

12. There may be evidence of active rheumatic fever.

Prophylaxis. Penicillin cover (p. 75) should be given to any individual with congenital or rheumatic heart disease, who has to have tonsillectomy or extraction of teeth, because these surgical procedures may well precipitate endocarditis. Prompt treatment of all upper respiratory infections is also important.

Early Diagnosis. Every patient with valvular or congenital heart disease who develops an obscure fever which persists for more than a few days should be suspect, and steps should be taken to confirm or exclude the diagnosis of bacterial endocarditis.

Prognosis. If the diagnosis is made early the infection can probably be eliminated in more than 90 per cent. of cases by giving adequate doses of the appropriate antibiotic for a sufficient length of time. If, however, the diagnosis is delayed, which is not infrequently the case, the underlying cardiac disease may progress and the prognosis is much more serious.

Treatment. Whenever possible the organism should be isolated by blood culture and its sensitivity to antibiotics assessed in the laboratory. The selection of the antibiotic, the assessment of dosage and the duration of treatment will depend on the results of the sensitivity tests and on the clinical response to treatment. If the organism is very sensitive, benzylpenicillin should be injected twice daily, usually for four to six weeks. If the organism is sensitive to penicillin and the temperature returns to normal within a few days benzylpenicillin may be replaced by phenoxymethylpenicillin given orally in a dose of 250 mg. four-six hourly, in combination with probenicid, to ensure high blood levels. Larger doses of benzylpenicillin or the concurrent administration of streptomycin might be required for more resistant organisms. Depending on the bacteriologist's findings as regards sensitivity, other antibiotics may be necessary. With very resistant organisms the dose of streptomycin may have to be increased to 2 g. per day for a short time. Unfortunately toxicity is a serious problem with some drugs.

* * * * * *

ISCHAEMIC HEART DISEASE

Ischaemic heart disease or coronary insufficiency implies an inadequate blood supply for the needs of the heart. This may be manifest clinically as:

I. Cardiac pain (angina pectoris or myocardial infarction).
II. Cardiac failure.
III. Various arrhythmias, e.g. atrial fibrillation or heart block.
IV. Heart block.

In addition ischaemic fibrosis of heart muscle may be found histologically in cases where there have been no relevant symptoms during life.

Most cases of ischaemic heart disease are due to narrowing of the coronary arteries from atherosclerosis, the cause of which is discussed on p. 278.

I. CARDIAC PAIN

Angina pectoris is the term commonly used to denote attacks of cardiac pain of short duration and without evidence of lasting damage to the myocardium. The term 'coronary thrombosis' is used to denote attacks of cardiac pain of longer duration and which are accompanied by evidence of cardiac infarction. Both the conditions referred to are based on myocardial ischaemia, and their characteristic features are described in detail below. They are not altogether satisfactory terms. There are causes of coronary occlusion other than thrombosis, e.g. haemorrhage into an atheromatous plaque. Coronary occlusion does not always result in myocardial infarction and myocardial infarction may occur without coronary occlusion, e.g. from transient coronary insufficiency when there is imbalance between the needs of the heart and the available blood supply. Such an imbalance may be precipitated by exertion, emotion, haemorrhage or shock from any cause. When a patient is first seen following the onset of angina of effort electrocardiographic evidence of previously unsuspected myocardial infarction is often found. On the other hand, prolonged attacks of anginal pain may occur without evidence of myocardial infarction. Temporary ischaemic changes may be recorded in the electrocardiogram during attacks of angina, while more lasting but reversible changes are shown if the period of coronary insufficiency is prolonged. If muscle necrosis has taken place the characteristic picture is recorded.

Whether or not myocardial infarction takes place following coronary occlusion depends on the size of the obstructed vessel and the presence or absence of an adequate collateral circulation. In normal hearts, small but functionally inadequate inter-coronary collateral channels can be demonstrated. In patients with coronary artery disease these channels are much wider, and it is believed that pathological narrowing of the coronary vessels is the stimulus for their enlargement.

In the past it has been customary to draw a sharp distinction between angina pectoris and myocardial infarction. Tables have been constructed to emphasise the different features and up to a point such a distinction serves a useful purpose. It will be appreciated, however, from what has been said above that from the clinical and electrocardiographic point of view differences between the various forms of ischaemic pain are really matters of degree and stages can be recognised between angina pectoris and myocardial infarction.

Pathogenesis. Cardiac pain is almost invariably based on myocardial ischaemia and is similar in nature to pain in the legs in intermittent claudication (p. 284). It is probably due to local accumulation of the products of metabolism.

Aetiology. Most cases of cardiac pain are associated with coronary disease, but, before concluding that this is the basis, certain other causes of relative myocardial ischaemia should be remembered and excluded:

(*a*) *Aortic valvular disease*—in which the work of the left ventricle is increased and coronary blood flow decreased.

In aortic stenosis the intraventricular pressure is raised and during ventricular systole the coronary vessels are unduly compressed. In aortic incompetence the diastolic pressure in the aorta is decreased and coronary blood flow is diminished.

(*b*) *Syphilitic aortitis*—in which the orifices of the coronary arteries may be obstructed although the vessels themselves are unaffected.

(*c*) *Severe anaemia*—in which the oxygen-carrying power of the blood is diminished.

(*d*) *Paroxysmal tachycardia*—in which the work of the heart is increased and coronary blood flow is decreased owing to the shortened duration of diastole.

Clinical Features

SITE The pain is characteristically felt behind the sternum or across the chest.

Quality. It is usually described as being constrictive or crushing in character and may be very severe. Sometimes there is no actual pain but rather a feeling of discomfort or an unpleasant sensation of pressure or weight. It may be described as 'only indigestion', but indigestion felt in the chest should always be suspect. The pain is rarely sharp, stabbing or knife-like, but individuals vary in their use of adjectives.

Radiation. There may be no radiation or the pain may be referred down one or both arms, more commonly the left, sometimes to the fingers. The hand may turn pale from vasoconstriction or be drawn up from muscular contraction. The pain may extend into the throat, jaws or neck or pass into the shoulders, to the upper abdomen or through to the back.

Angina Pectoris

Diagnosis. In angina pectoris the pain usually bears a quantitative relationship to exertion and forces the patient to stop; whereupon it passes away within a few minutes. Pain is more readily induced after meals and in cold weather. It may be precipitated by emotion. It is rapidly relieved by glyceryl trinitrate (trinitrin) which dilates the coronary vessels. As the diagnosis often depends solely on the interpretation of subjective symptoms the doctor's responsibility is great. Frequently there will be no additional assistance from clinical or radiological examination, although sometimes coronary artery calcification may be seen. Standard electrocardiograms are often negative, but abnormalities are more likely to be found if multiple leads are recorded or if the electrocardiograms are repeated after exercise.

Treatment. The patient must always be reassured, but some relative must be told that the future is unpredictable. It is sensible to avoid excessive exertion and, as far as humanly possible, emotional conflicts but moderate exercise is beneficial. Encouragement can be given to adopt a more philosophical attitude, to be more tolerant of the weaknesses of others and to make allowance for differences in temperament, outlook and ambition. There is often a price to be paid for health and this may lie in the direction of delegated responsibility, change of work, early retirement, refusal of invitations and the acceptance of the fact that few are indispensable. Some occupations such as train driving are unsuitable because they involve responsibility for the lives of others. Treatment should be directed to limiting the work of the heart while the all-important inter-coronary collateral circulation develops. Slight ischaemia is the stimulus to its development but severe ischaemia results in muscle necrosis. Hence it is important to avoid any unnecessary work by the heart which calls for a sudden and marked increase in coronary blood flow. In time the collateral circulation may become such that even the occlusion of a major vessel may be survived. Attacks of pain must be prevented as far as possible by avoiding the precipitating factors discussed above. Tablets of trinitrin B.P., 0·5 mg should always be carried by the patient so that one may be allowed to dissolve in the mouth should pain develop. A tablet may also be taken before doing anything likely to bring on pain. Trinitrin can be taken very freely. There are no harmful side-effects, though headache and flushing may be experienced, nor does tolerance develop. Amyl nitrite acts more quickly but is more violent in its side-effects, less convenient and rarely necessary. Longer acting nitrites, e.g. pentaerythritol tetranitrate, have proved disappointing. Propranolol (p. 195) is sometimes effective. Sedatives, such as phenobarbitone, are useful to reduce anxiety and emotional disturbances. Constipation should be avoided because straining at stool may be dangerous. Obesity is an added burden on the heart and should be reduced whenever possible (p. 444). Anaemia must be corrected. Meals should be small, eaten slowly and followed by a period of rest. Cigarette smoking should be given up. The relation of ischaemic heart disease to atherosclerosis is discussed on p. 278. Operation may be considered for intractable cardiac pain. Sensory impulses from the heart are conducted by the sympathetic nervous system, and these pathways may be interrupted by the injection of alcohol or by surgical section. It is important to realise that sympathectomy is only a palliative procedure to reduce pain, and there is no evidence that the blood supply to the heart is thereby increased. As an alternative hypothyroidism may be induced with antithyroid drugs or with radio-iodine and although sometimes remarkably effective in relieving pain the result is often rather shortlived. Re-vascularisation of the myocardium, using the internal mammary or splenic artery, is under trial.

Myocardial Infarction

Diagnosis. In myocardial infarction the pain is similar in situation, distribution and quality to that of angina pectoris, but is generally more severe and prolonged and is not relieved by rest or glyceryl trinitrate. In addition there is usually evidence of muscle necrosis (infarction) such as fever, leucocytosis and an increased blood sedimentation rate. The blood pressure usually falls and may never recover its former level. There may be evidence of central or peripheral circulatory failure. A pericardial rub may be heard if the infarct extends to the epicardial surface. Characteristic changes occur in the electrocardiogram. The S-T segment is elevated above the iso-electric line and bowed convexly upwards, the T waves become inverted, and if the infarct extends right through the ventricular wall Q waves also appear. These changes occur in chest leads recorded over the affected area of muscle and may be reflected in the limb leads (Figs. 20 and 21). The finding of a raised concentration of the enzymes glutamic oxalacetic transaminase (SGOT) and lactose dehydrogenase (LDH) in the serum may be of diagnostic value in difficult cases.

The diagnosis is by no means always easy. Pain may be absent or atypical in situation, radiation or quality. The presenting feature may be a cerebrovascular disturbance from the fall in cardiac output, an acute arrythmia or heart block.

Complications

1. *Cardiac failure.* Since it is the left ventricle which is predominantly affected by coronary disease the principal manifestation of failure will be dyspnoea and crepitations in the lungs. Venous congestion and peripheral oedema may follow.

2. *Shock.* The aetiology of shock following myocardial infarction is complex. Central and peripheral factors are involved (p. 176). If a major degree of infarction has occurred, the patient is pale, cold, sweating and mentally retarded, with hypotension and oliguria, and usually fails to respond to the customary measures for combating shock. When a severe state of shock is present the prognosis is bad (80 per cent. mortality).

3. *Arrythmias*

4. *Defects of conduction*

5. *Pulmonary or systemic embolism.* Pulmonary embolism may

follow thrombosis in the right side of the heart, e.g. in the right atrium, from atrial fibrillation or in the right ventricle from extension of the infarct to the endocardial surface. Pulmonary embolism may also result from peripheral venous thrombosis, usually in the legs. Systemic embolism may occur if the infarct extends to the endocardial surface of the left side of the heart.

6. *Rupture of the heart.*

Treatment

Since the cause of myocardial infarction is usually atherosclerosis of the coronary arteries, no specific measures for prevention and treatment will be available until the pathogenesis of atherosclerosis is understood. This problem is discussed in detail on p. 278.

Relief of Pain. The first step must always to be relieve pain. Morphine 15 mg. can be given intravenously in severe cases or by intramuscular or subcutaneous injection and repeated as required. Not more than 60 mg. should be given in 12 hours. Some patients are sensitive to morphine, with resultant vomiting (p. 196). Recently it has been suggested that heroin may be superior. If less severe, pethidine (100 to 200 mg. subcutaneously or by mouth), tab. codein. co. (2-4 tablets) or one of the newer analgesic drugs may suffice.

Measures to Combat Shock. The customary first aid measures are warmth, oxygen, raising the foot of the bed and the relief of pain. For the treatment of severe shock, hydrocortisone, 200 mg. by intravenous injection should be tried first. Vasoconstrictor drugs have been shown to be ineffective in most cases because vasoconstriction is often already maximal, in which case they may be actually harmful. Digoxin (1 mg. by intravenous injection) is sometimes given to stimulate the myocardium. Cardiac failure should be treated in the usual way. If treatment is to have any chance of success it must be started as soon as possible. There is far from universal agreement about the value of these methods of treatment. As already indicated, the prognosis of severely shocked patients is bad.

Cardiac Arrest. Should cardiac arrest occur, treatment by closed-chest cardiac massage, as described on p. 180, must be instituted immediately.

Rest. Physical and mental rest is of primary importance. The duration of rest in bed will naturally depend on the severity of the infarction. Three weeks should be the average period, but after a small infarct sitting in a chair should be allowed after about 10 days, and six weeks or more in bed may be necessary after a large infarction or if cardiac failure has developed. The return to physical activity should thereafter be gradual. Nowadays severe restrictions are no longer imposed and those who feel well should be allowed to sit up in bed and to feed and wash themselves after the first day or two. A 'sani-chair' which can be wheeled over an ordinary lavatory outside the ward is usually preferable to the bed-pan. In severe cases with restriction to bed for longer periods physiotherapy is advisable.

OXYGEN. Oxygen should be given if there is dyspnoea or shock; it may help to relieve pain.

TREATMENT OF ARRYTHMIAS. Multiple extrasystoles, especially if superimposed on the preceding T waves, which may precede ventricular fibrillation, should be treated with lignocaine and other arrythmias by the drugs described on page 195. Ventricular fibrillation should be treated by immediate electrical countershock and asystole by electrical pacing. Bradycardia should be treated by atropine.

ANTICOAGULANTS. There is a considerable difference of opinion as to the value of anticoagulant drugs in the treatment of myocardial infarction. Some physicians are convinced that the mortality rate has been materially reduced by their use, whereas others in apparently well controlled series have shown no material benefit except in regard to thrombo-embolic complications. In view of the prevailing uncertainty after 15 years of use, it must at least be concluded that the benefit derived is relatively small and less than used to be claimed. Certainly there is a general trend to reserve their use for relatively severe cases and to give these drugs for a shorter period of time. It will be appreciated that selection of the latter group may be very difficult in the early stages, but intractable pain, shock, gallop rhythm, cardiac failure or the development of an arrhythmia are all serious signs. The precise mode of action of these drugs is undecided. Heparin has a rapid and transitory action. It is expensive and must be given by injection. The coumarin anticoagulant drugs such as dicoumarol, phenindione and warfarin prolong the 'prothrombin time' by interfering with the generation of thromboplastin. They have the disadvantage of not being effective for 24 hours and of requiring facilities for estimation of the prothrombin time if dosage is to be adequately controlled. The object of anticoagulant therapy is to limit extension of the coronary thrombosis and to reduce the risk of thrombosis occurring on the endocardium or in another coronary vessel, or in a peripheral vein, e.g. in the legs, with subsequent risk of pulmonary embolism. Anticoagulants are usually continued for three to four weeks after which the immediate danger period is over. Large numbers of patients have been placed on long-term anticoagulant therapy, especially for recurrent angina or infarction, particularly in the relatively young, but it is doubtful if benefit lasts for more than 12 months.

Heparin. Initial dose 15,000 units intravenously followed by 10,000 units every six hours for 24-36 hours or as indicated by the coagulation time.

Phenindione. The initial dose is 200-300 mg. by mouth and the average daily dose is usually 25-50 mg. twice daily. The prothrombin activity of the patient should be kept as near as possible to 20-30 per cent. that of a normal individual tested each day by the same method.

Warfarin. This is an alternative preparation which is being increasingly used because of the frequency with which sensitivity reactions to phenindione have occurred. The initial dose is 30-50 mg. and the average daily dose is 5-10 mg.

HAEMORRHAGE FROM OVERDOSAGE. An antidote to heparin exists in the form of protamine sulphate which should be given intravenously in the proportion of 1 ml. of a 1 per cent. solution to each 1,000 International Units of heparin given in the last dose. Fresh blood may also be required. Following overdosage of phenindione vitamin K_1 (phytomenadione) by mouth in a dose of 10-20 mg. will usually restore the prothrombin time to normal within eight hours. Fresh or stored blood may also be required.

CORONARY CARE UNITS. In many hospitals Coronary Care Units have recently been established to which all patients with suspected acute myocardial infarction are admitted. This followed appreciation of the fact that most deaths occur within the first 48 hours and that some patients with relatively mild coronary disease can have their lives saved if trained staff and appropriate equipment are available because death is due to a reversible arrhythmia or cardiac arrest. Emphasis has shifted from resuscitation to anticipation of serious arrhythmias and their prevention or prompt treatment and heart block can be treated by electrical pacing. Each patient is monitored so that an electrocardiogram can be seen on the oscilloscope and an alarm bell rings if the heart rate increases or falls beyond a set level.

Differential Diagnosis of Cardiac Pain. The pain of myocardial infarction may be mistaken for acute pericarditis (p. 265), pulmonary embolism (p. 253), dissecting aneurysm of the aorta (p. 283) or acute abdominal disease, e.g. perforation of a peptic ulcer. In addition difficulty may less commonly be experienced with a variety of other pains. Pain may be referred to the neck, arms or chest wall as a result of disease in the spine, ribs, joints, muscles, or fascia or from the involvement of nerves, e.g. in tabes dorsalis or herpes zoster. Pain may arise in the *oesophagus*, e.g. from hiatus hernia, peptic ulceration or carcinoma. Pain may be referred to the *abdomen*, e.g. in cases of pancreatitis, pylorospasm or biliary disease. Accuracy in diagnosis is most desirable in view of the seriousness of many of the underlying conditions, the importance of appropriate treatment, the apprehension so often experienced by the patient and the unwarranted restrictions which are sometimes imposed.

Prognosis in Coronary Artery Disease. There is no condition in which it is more difficult to foretell the future than coronary artery disease. Analyses of large series do not help in the individual case but statistics do, of course, give some guidance, particularly as regards complicating factors. Angina from syphilitic aortitis or aortic stenosis has a more serious prognosis.

Some 25 per cent. of individuals die within four weeks of myocardial infarction, mostly within 48 hours. A study of various statistical surveys on the mortality of myocardial infarction suggests that following recovery from an acute attack 20 per cent. will die within a year, 30 per cent. within five years and 70 per cent. within 10 years. Thus the prognosis is not so gloomy as sometimes thought. Mortality increases with age, a past history of myocardial infarction, prolonged pain, cardiac failure, shock, arrhythmias or embolism. The prognosis of patients with angina pectoris from coronary atherosclerosis has been shown to be very similar to that of patients who survive a first attack of myocardial infarction. The prognosis is likely to be better if the patient accepts advice in regard to giving up smoking and takes regular moderate exercise, reduces excessive weight and, if hypertension is found, receives the appropriate treatment.

II. CARDIAC FAILURE

Cardiac failure in the older age groups frequently results from an impaired blood supply to the myocardium secondary to coronary artery disease. Such failure may occur in the absence of pain. Progressive dyspnoea on exertion precedes signs of manifest failure. Hypertension is commonly associated with coronary atheroma and increases the cardiac burden.

III. ATRIAL FIBRILLATION AND HEART BLOCK

Coronary disease is the most common cause of atrial fibrillation in persons over the age of 50 and also of the more severe grades of heart block. It is noteworthy that patients with atrial fibrillation rarely develop cardiac pain.

HYPERTENSION

The normal range of blood pressure, the importance of casual and resting readings and the significance of systolic and diastolic hypertension have already been discussed (p. 137). Although in most cases of hypertension the cause is obscure some cases are *secondary* to recognisable disease. For this reason each patient is worthy of thorough investigation in the hope that some remediable underlying condition may be found.

CAUSES OF SECONDARY HYPERTENSION

RENAL DISORDERS (p. 781 *et seq.*).

(*a*) Acute glomerulonephritis.
(*b*) Chronic glomerulonephritis.
(*c*) Chronic pyelonephritis.
(*d*) Polycystic disease.
(*e*) Unilateral renal disease associated with renal ischaemia.
(*f*) Prostatic obstruction.

ENDOCRINE DISORDERS

(*a*) Phaeochromocytoma (p. 733).

(*b*) Cushing's syndrome (p. 731).
(*c*) Primary aldosteronism (Conn's syndrome) (p. 733).

Coarctation of the Aorta (p. 247)

Toxaemia of Pregnancy. Hypertension in pregnancy may be due to coincidental essential hypertension, to pre-existing renal disease or may be directly related to the pregnancy.

In the latter instance the conditions are referred to as pre-eclamptic or eclamptic toxaemia of pregnancy.

The conditions mentioned above may usually be excluded by a careful history, physical examination, testing of the urine and in selected cases pyelography or occasionally aortography.

ESSENTIAL (IDIOPATHIC) HYPERTENSION

Essential hypertension is the name given to the type of hypertension for which no cause can be found. The diagnosis is accordingly made by a process of exclusion. It is by far the most common form of hypertension and affects the sexes about equally. The main incidence falls between the ages of 40 and 60. Essential hypertension is often a serious condition and accounts for about 20 per cent. of all deaths over the age of 50.

Heredity is important and the disease certainly tends to run in families. It has been estimated that if both parents have hypertension the incidence of the disease in the children is about 45 per cent. and if one parent has hypertension about 30 per cent. If the patient is under 35 years and there is no family history of hypertension, an underlying cause is likely to be present.

The part played by temperament and emotional factors is difficult to assess. Many authorities consider that hypertensives have exceptionally labile vascular systems and react to nervous stimuli by rises in blood pressure, but the evidence for a specific personality type is not convincing.

Although hypertension occurs more frequently in thickset 'broad' individuals than in linear 'narrow' persons it may occur in individuals of any build. Obesity is associated with an increased tendency to hypertension. When obesity and hypertension co-exist the chance of developing cardiovascular disease is greatly increased.

Insurance statistics show that those in whom the blood pressure lies above the average level, though within the normal range, are more prone to develop subsequent hypertensive cardiovascular disease than those whose pressure is below the average level. Also those liable to exaggerated transient rises of blood pressure are predisposed to the development of essential hypertension in later life.

Pathogenesis. In most cases of hypertension the high blood pressure must be secondary to increased peripheral resistance because the other two factors which determine the height of the blood pressure, i.e. cardiac output, and the viscosity of the blood, are unchanged.

It has been shown that this increased resistance occurs chiefly in the arterioles and is more severe in the renal vessels than elsewhere. Except in advanced cases the blood pressure is labile, and any measure which reduces sympathetic tone and causes vasodilatation will result in a substantial fall of blood pressure. It follows that the hypertension must at first be due to vasoconstriction rather than to narrowing of the vessels from organic disease. Such organic narrowing does occur in time and is common as age advances (even in those without hypertension) but is patchy in distribution and variable in extent.

Vasoconstriction might be due to neurogenic stimuli, i.e. increased sympathetic tone, or to humoral stimuli, i.e. a circulating pressor substance acting directly on the arterioles.

In animals it has been shown that the experimental production of renal ischaemia by partial occlusion of one renal artery results in hypertension which is independent of the nerve supply to the kidneys and is due to the liberation into the circulation of a pressor substance formed in the damaged kidney (renin).

Renin is an enzyme which enters the blood stream by the renal vein and acts on its alpha or globulin precursor in the plasma (hypertensinogen) to produce the active vasoconstrictor agent angiotensin. However, no humoral hypertensive substance has been isolated in patients with essential hypertension.

Chronic renal disease of all types is often associated with hypertension, and it may be that in this group the mechanism is similar to that of experimental renal hypertension, i.e. reduced renal blood flow. Moreover, in cases of unilateral renal disease removal of the affected kidney or restoration of the lumen of an occluded artery will sometimes lead to cure of the hypertension. In human essential hypertension the haemodynamic effects and the pathological changes are essentially the same as in experimental renal hypertension, but it is still undecided whether the kidney is primarily or secondarily involved. It has been shown that, while in young people hypertension may be manifest before any structural changes can be demonstrated in the arterioles, in older subjects it is almost invariably accompanied by arteriolosclerosis. This progression suggests that the changes are secondary to the hypertension rather than the reverse. A vicious circle may be set up whereby vascular narrowing leads to hypertension and hypertension to further vascular narrowing.

It has been suggested that primary renal ischaemia occurs in the first place as a result of neurogenic stimuli from the hypothalamus, and that this sets the humoral mechanism in motion and produces hypertension which is later aggravated further by vascular changes. This process, if rapidly progressive, may produce hypertension of the malignant type. In conclusion it may be said that in spite of much experimental and clinical work all over the world, the pathogenesis of essential hypertension remains obscure.

Clinical Features and Course. High blood pressure is often found on routine examination, e.g. for Life Insurance. Usually there are no relevant symptoms for many years although symptoms due to anxiety (about having high blood pressure) may be present. Unfortunately the doctor is often responsible for sowing the seeds of anxiety.

The clinical features are very variable. Early symptoms which are frequently attributed to hypertension are difficult to differentiate from those associated with psychological factors, e.g. nervousness, irritability, loss of energy, easy fatigue and insomnia. Headaches, dizziness and impairment of memory and concentration are later features which may be troublesome. Contrary to popular belief, many patients with severe hypertension do not suffer from headache. In the early stage there are usually no abnormal physical signs other than the hypertension.

The precise level of the blood pressure is not necessarily the most important criterion of severity of the disease. More valuable information will be obtained by examining the optic fundi, the heart and renal function. In cases of similar severity as judged by the height of the blood pressure the disease may run very different courses. In some the condition is remarkably benign.

In the early stages, hypertension is intermittent. The blood pressure is unusually labile, rising to an abnormal degree under the influence of such stimuli as emotion, exercise and cold. Later the resting blood pressure becomes permanently elevated. Only in the late stages is there evidence of impaired renal function, and most patients nowadays die from the effects of atherosclerosis in heart or brain while still maintaining adequate renal function.

The approximate incidence of the three major causes of death in hypertensive disease used to be given as cardiac failure 60 per cent., cerebrovascular accidents 35 per cent. and renal failure 5 per cent., but there is no doubt that with the advent of modern treatment for hypertension few patients die from congestive failure.

Complications. HYPERTENSIVE HEART DISEASE. Involvement of the heart is the complication of outstanding importance. At first the left ventricle overcomes the increased peripheral resistance and maintains a normal blood flow to the tissues by increasing its force of contraction. This is achieved by dilatation of the heart and subsequent hypertrophy of the muscle fibres. This is the compensated phase of hypertensive heart disease. In due course the burden proves too great. Left ventricular output can no longer be maintained and signs of cardiac failure become manifest (p. 170). Coronary artery disease is frequently associated with hypertension and aggravates the position further.

1. *Compensated Phase.* Breathlessness may occur on exertion because of the diminished cardiac reserve which results in pulmonary congestion. Enlargement of the heart may be recognised by outward displacement of the apex beat with a heaving impulse. The first heart sound in the mitral area and the second heart sound in the aortic area are accentuated. Radiological examination will confirm the enlargement of the heart and electrocardiography will show evidence of left ventricular hypertrophy. (Fig. 16, p. 146).

2. *Decompensated Phase.* Breathlessness is present at rest and attacks of paroxysmal dyspnoea may occur. Regular sinus rhythm is usually maintained, but there may be a triple heart rhythm and pulsus alternans, both of which are serious signs. The blood pressure may become 'decapitated', i.e. there is a disproportionate fall in the systolic pressure as compared to diastolic pressure, e.g.

from 210/120 to 150/110, but in some cases there is no fall in the blood pressure. Crepitations are audible at the bases of the lungs and there are radiological signs of congestion. Finally all the peripheral signs of congestive cardiac failure will appear.

Cerebral Manifestations of Hypertensive Disease. Minor manifestations include headache, dizziness and vertigo. These are difficult to differentiate from primary vascular disease. Major disturbances are hypertensive encephalopathy, cerebral haemorrhage and cerebral thrombosis. Gradual cerebral deterioration with changes in temperament and mental powers may develop and are probably the result of a defective blood supply due to concomitant cerebral atheroma. Less frequently transient impairment of function may arise from partial or complete obstruction of the carotid or basilar artery.

Headache in hypertension is probably based on vasodilatation principally in branches of the external carotid artery with stimulation of the pain sensitive nerve endings in their walls. It is thus similar in origin to headache in migraine (p. 1133). It is not related to raised intracranial pressure in most cases. Headache in hypertension is often situated in the occipital region and is noticed on waking in the morning and improves as the day advances. Vertigo may be a symptom of hypertension and it should be distinguished from dizziness, which is a mere feeling of unsteadiness. In vertigo there is a definite sensation of rotation, either of the individual or of his environment, from stimulation of the labyrinth or of its central connections. Patients suffering from hypertension, whether essential or due to nephritis or eclampsia, may develop transitory disturbances of cerebral function. Such episodes are referred to as hypertensive encephalopathy.

Hypertensive Encephalopathy. This condition is due to acute focal cerebral ischaemia in which hypertensive spasm, oedema or minor degrees of haemorrhage or thrombosis plays a part. It is not due to uraemia. Attacks may be heralded by severe headaches, nausea, vomiting or somnolence. Transient disturbance of vision or speech, transient pareses, paraesthesiae, disorientation and fits or loss of consciousness may occur. The blood pressure and often the cerebrospinal fluid pressure rise considerably during the attack. Cardiac failure may be precipitated. Recovery usually takes place and there is no permanent loss of function.

Hypertensive encephalopathy has to be distinguished from cerebrovascular accidents, from other causes of convulsions, e.g. epilepsy and Adams-Stokes attacks, and from cerebral tumours, in which symptoms and signs tend to be more constant and not paroxysmal, and the blood pressure may be normal.

If it is reasonably certain that the attack is not due to a small cerebral thrombosis the blood pressure may be reduced by the intravenous injection of small doses of a ganglion blocking drug. Venesection, the intravenous injection of 100 ml. 50 per cent. sucrose, or lumbar puncture with removal of cerebrospinal fluid are alternative methods of proved value. When convulsions are occurring paraldehyde or sodium phenobarbitone should be given as for status epilepticus (p. 1121). In all cases the underlying hypertension should be investigated (p. 235) and if a cause is found it should receive appropriate treatment.

Cerebral Haemorrhage and Cerebral Thrombosis commonly occur and are described under Diseases of the Nervous System (p. 1138).

The Eye in Hypertension. The patient may complain of a bloodshot eye (subconjunctival haemorrhage), and though alarming to the individual concerned this is not a serious condition and does not require local treatment. It may, however, call attention to the presence of hypertension. Vascular lesions secondary to hypertension may be responsible for haziness of vision, progressive deterioration of vision or sudden loss of vision, visual field defects or diplopia (from defective ocular movements).

Retinal Changes. Very useful information regarding the severity of the condition and the prognosis may be obtained with the ophthalmoscope (p. 138 and Plates I & II). In fact, the state of the fundi is a better guide to prognosis than the height of the blood pressure.

The earliest changes consist of straightening and narrowing of the peripheral arterioles with increase in the light reflex but these changes are difficult to detect. Variations in calibre follow as a result of changes in the vessel wall. Later the outer walls become thickened and thereby visible (increased light reflex, 'copper or silver wiring'). As a result of this sclerosis the veins are deflected and compressed where crossed by the arteries and a clear area can be seen in the line of the vein corresponding to the width of the thickened arterial wall.

Haemorrhages may be linear, striate, flame-shaped or rounded according to their position in the different layers of the retina. Exudates appear as white areas which may be ill-defined, 'soft' and fluffy (cottonwool patches) if due to transudation of serum and fibrin, or smaller, well-defined and 'hard' when due to fatty degeneration and hyaline changes in areas from which exudate has been absorbed. The macular 'star' consists of a collection of small, white dots. Exudates in particular are usually evidence of serious hypertensive or degenerative arterial disease, and vision may be grossly affected if they develop in the region of the macula.

The most advanced stage in the evolution of the fundal changes in hypertension is the development of papilloedema. This usually denotes a serious prognosis, most patients dying within 12 months of its appearance unless modern treatment is given. (See Malignant Hypertension, p. 234). Similar changes in the fundi of equally serious significance may be seen in chronic renal disease (p. 807).

It has become customary to grade the various retinal changes according to severity.

Grade 1. General narrowing of the arterioles with varying calibre and increased light reflex.

Grade 2. Further reduction in the arterio-venous ratio and constriction of the veins where crossed by the arterioles.

Grade 3. Exudates and/or haemorrhages *in addition* to 1 and 2.

Grade 4. Papilloedema with or without grade 3 changes.

There are disadvantages in using such a classification because there is a tendency to state the grade and ignore important variations in detail. It is essential to describe precisely the changes which are observed in addition to stating the grade.

These changes are discussed also on p. 138.

Renal Manifestations of Hypertension. The possible rôle of the kidney in the pathogenesis of hypertension has already been discussed. Renal arteriolosclerosis is progressive as hypertension advances but impairment of renal excretory function occurs late or not at all in benign essential hypertension. In malignant hypertension arteriolar necrosis usually occurs in the renal vessels and consequently impairment of renal function is usually rapid and progressive and death frequently occurs from uraemia. Large amounts of protein are not passed until the late stages of benign essential hypertension and the quantity rarely exceeds 2 g./day. Larger amounts would suggest the presence of chronic nephritis or malignant hypertension. Similarly the presence of hyaline and granular casts and less frequently of red cells has the same significance.

Polyuria by day is usually a sign of tubular dysfunction, but nocturia may be secondary to the reabsorption of oedema fluid which tends to occur in the recumbent posture. Renal function is rarely improved by treatment of hypertension.

MALIGNANT HYPERTENSION. Essential hypertension is sometimes divided into benign and malignant groups, the diagnostic criterion of the second group being the presence of papilloedema. Papilloedema may occur after long years of known benign essential hypertension or develop rapidly in one whose blood pressure was known previously to have been normal, the whole course of the disease taking less than two years. Papilloedema may complicate chronic nephritis or develop during an attack of hypertensive encephalopathy or occur in cases of transient hypertension such as acute nephritis or toxaemia of pregnancy. It is not therefore a satisfactory criterion by itself on which to differentiate the various forms of hypertension.

It has been disputed whether malignant hypertension is a separate condition or merely a terminal phase of benign hypertension. From the pathological point of view it has been suggested that its development can be explained on the severity and rapidity of onset of the arteriolar lesions, and the essential difference is that between arteriolosclerosis and arteriolonecrosis (p. 277). It has been postulated that a vicious circle develops.

If the term malignant hypertension is to be used it should be confined to the clinical syndrome of severe diastolic hypertension with papilloedema and renal failure which occurs mainly in males in the third and fourth decades and which pursues a rapidly downhill course to death from uraemia within a year unless suitable treatment is instituted. Most cases of malignant hypertension before the age of 30 are caused by chronic pyelonephritis or nephritis. When papilloedema and renal failure develop in a person known to have essential hypertension this disease is sometimes described as having entered the 'malignant phase'.

Assessment of a Patient with Hypertension. Treatment and prognosis depend on the assessment of the severity of hypertension and its complications.

A distinction should be drawn between patients who only have high blood pressure and those who also have evidence of hypertensive disease, i.e. of pathological change in heart, kidneys or retinal vessels, because there is no doubt that the prognosis is quite different in the two groups.

When hypertension is first discovered, whether on account of relevant symptoms or on a routine examination, the problem should be carefully assessed according to a systematic plan.

HISTORY. A family history of hypertension or a past history of renal disease should be noted. Symptoms such as headaches and dizziness may be due to the high blood pressure or to an anxiety state. If undue breathlessness accompanies the hypertension, it must be decided whether it is of cardiac or pulmonary origin or due to some general condition such as anaemia, obesity or anxiety. If of cardiac origin there will be other evidence of left ventricular failure. Certain clinical features may suggest a phaeochromocytoma or Conn's Syndrome (p. 733).

ASSESSMENT OF BLOOD PRESSURE. *Casual* readings should be recorded on a number of occasions and *resting* readings taken in bed after a night's sleep. A pressure taken during sleep after sedation is sometimes useful.

EXAMINATION OF THE CARDIOVASCULAR SYSTEM. The chief points to be noted concern the heart—evidence of left ventricular hypertrophy and signs of cardiac failure. It is important to examine for evidence of ischaemic heart disease and cerebrovascular disease because lowering the blood pressure may aggravate the effects of these conditions. Examination of the optic fundi is of particular importance with reference to the vessels and the presence or absence of haemorrhages, exudates and papilloedema. The femoral pulses must be palpated as a routine if cases of coarctation of the aorta are not to be overlooked.

EXAMINATION OF RENAL FUNCTION

(a) *Assessment of Renal Function.* The urine should be examined for protein, cells and casts. Glomerular function can be assessed by a urea or creainine clearance test and tubular function by the specific gravity test or by phenolsulphonephthalein excretion test.

In patients with hypertensive disease renal failure is present if the blood urea is raised.

(b) *Exclusion of Primary Renal Disease.* In the younger age groups, an intravenous pyelogram and preferably an isotope renogram should be made to exclude the presence of unilateral renal disease that might be amenable to treatment by nephrectomy. If unilateral shrinkage is demonstrated aortography may be indicated. The urine should be cultured for evidence of infection. The differential diagnosis between the late stages of hypertension and chronic renal disease may be impossible and is immaterial with regard to treatment and prognosis.

RADIOLOGY. Radiological examination of the heart (for enlargement) and of the lungs (for congestion) should always be carried out.

ELECTROCARDIOGRAPHY. Evidence of left ventricular hypertrophy and of myocardial (coronary) disease may be found.

EXAMINATION OF OTHER SYSTEMS may be of special value in particular cases, e.g. the central nervous system when there are cerebral symptoms. A careful routine examination of the abdomen may disclose the presence of one large kidney (in hydronephrosis) or of two large kidneys (as in polycystic disease). Auscultation may reveal a bruit from renal artery stenosis.

If a phaeochromocytoma is suspected estimation of catecholamine excretion in the urine is indicated (p. 733).

Prognosis. It will be appreciated that a consideration of the family history, the age of the patient, the information obtained by the plan of assessment suggested above and an estimation of the rate of progression of the various manifestations will give the necessary data on which to judge the probable course of the disease. The condition is mild, the heart is not enlarged, the fundi show no abnormalities and there is no albuminuria or evidence of impaired renal function. Sometimes the examination must be repeated every few months before an opinion can be reached. Patients with untreated malignant hypertension rarely live for more than a year. Cases of 'benign' essential hypertension vary considerably in degree of severity and the condition may be compatible with a life of normal span or nearly so. On the other hand, without treatment once signs of left ventricular failure appear the patient rarely lives for more than two or three years, although there are exceptions. On the whole, women appear to withstand hypertension better than men.

Insurance statistics show that, in general, expectation of life is considerably reduced in those who have high blood pressure compared with those in whom the pressure is within the normal range. However, it does not follow that *all* who have high blood pressure necessarily have a bad prognosis. Many live a life of normal span free from relevant illness. Included in this category are individuals who have labile blood pressures with hypertension due to emotional causes and others in whom casual readings are raised but who have normal pressures at rest. Many middle-aged women in whom pressures whenever recorded are of the order of 220/120 but who have no relevant symptoms and no changes in fundi or heart, remain in good health for many years.

Other individuals, particularly relatively young men, who when first seen have high diastolic pressures together with secondary manifestations in the fundi or heart, undoubtedly require optimal control of the blood pressure without delay.

When properly administered to a suitable patient modern treatment is effective in relieving symptoms, preventing or postponing complications and in prolonging life, but treatment of hypertension continues to be difficult and necessitates much attention to detail and considerable patience on the part of both patient and doctor. There is, as yet, no entirely satisfactory preparation for lowering the blood pressure; that is to say one which does not produce in many patients tolerance, undesirable side-effects or occasional unpredictable hypotension. In addition, it should be remembered that, once begun, treatment will probably have to be continued for life. It is therefore evident that most careful consideration should be given to the issues discussed above before making the decision to administer antihypertensive drugs.

Treatment. There is as yet no specific treatment because the cause of essential hypertension is not known. The aim of treatment is merely to lower the blood pressure. Some physicians, though relatively few in Britain, consider that treatment should be given prophylactically whenever high blood pressure is found in order to prevent trouble in the future. Most consider that if symptoms are indefinite and no abnormality is discovered apart from the high blood pressure, treatment should not be prescribed and the patient should be firmly reassured. In most cases, however, it is wise to recommend a yearly review.

Strong indications for treatment include left ventricular failure or progressive left ventricular hypertrophy, and hypertensive encephalopathy or retinopathy. Moderately strong indications include a cerebrovascular accident or angina pectoris, but caution is required as discussed below. Treatment is also indicated in young adults (particularly men) even without these complications if there is severe diastolic hypertension and if there is a family history of hypertension.

Contraindications include considerable renal failure (blood urea 100 mg./ml.) and, with certain exceptions noted above, absence of objective evidence of secondary hypertensive disease. Caution is required in the treatment of patients with evidence of associated atherosclerosis, particularly in the heart, brain or kidneys. In such cases the blood pressure should be lowered gradually and only to a moderate degree, and postural hypotension avoided; otherwise cardiac pain or myocardial infarction, aggravation of mental changes or cerebral infarction and a rise in blood urea or fluid retention may occur.

Coronary artery disease will be indicated by a history of cardiac pain, atrial fibrillation, or by ECG evidence of ischaemia or defects of conduction.

Cerebral atherosclerosis will be indicated by a history of cerebral thrombosis or infarction, or minor cerebral vascular accidents or by mental changes such as emotional lability, defective memory, alterations in the intellect, personality or habits, or by difficulty with speech.

Atherosclerosis in the carotid artery and in the basilar-vertebral system is also an important cause of cerebral symptoms.

Renal atherosclerosis is suspected if there is a sudden onset or worsening of hypertension at any age, a history of pain in the loin, or the detection of a murmur over the abdomen and should, in particular, be excluded in young patients with severe hypertension.

The management of the patient rather than the disease must be stressed. Moderation in all things should be the guiding principle. Psychological factors are all-important and the family doctor can do much to help his patient to deal with the stresses and anxieties to which nearly everyone is submitted to a greater or lesser degree.

Concern over the height of the blood pressure is often a potent source of such anxiety.

Rest. In the early stages of established hypertensive disease, rest in bed is not important but it may be best to advise slight restrictions, e.g. going to bed early, resting after meals whenever possible and perhaps also at the week-ends. It is important to cultivate the art of relaxation. As the condition develops longer periods of rest are required and when cardiac failure is manifest, rest in bed is essential, at least until it is clear that the failure will no longer respond to treatment.

Restriction of Activities. There is no evidence that moderate exertion is harmful, and walking or playing golf, within the limits of dyspnoea or undue tiredness, is to be encouraged. Strenuous occupations, sudden stress and prolonged exertion are to be avoided. Overwork, worry and emotional stress are just as harmful as over-exertion.

Diet. Overeating is harmful and reduction of weight in obese persons beneficial. There is no scientific evidence to support the restriction of protein which used to be recommended. A low salt diet, i.e. less than 1·0 g. sodium per day (Diet No. 8, p. 1293) will often result in a significant reduction of blood pressure, but such a strict diet is so irksome that few can be persuaded to take it for more than a few weeks. Hence it is not recommended for the treatment of hypertension unless all other methods have failed. It is doubtful if a moderate restriction of salt is of any therapeutic value for hypertension.

Sedatives. Barbiturates and other sedatives are very useful for the relief of anxiety, emotional tension and insomnia but care must be taken to avoid excessive consumption.

Hypotensive Drugs. In recent years, as more effective hypotensive agents have been introduced, the trend in treatment has been away from surgical sympathectomy and strict sodium restriction in the diet, to the use of drugs. It is important that the physician should be thoroughly familiar with details of administration and possible side-effects or toxic reactions. It is advisable in the first place for the dosage to be stabilised in a hospital where there are adequate facilities for close observation and control and where the intelligence of the patient and his ability to cooperate can be assessed.

A number of hypotensive drugs are now available which have the effect of lowering the blood pressure by producing vasodilatation through a central or peripheral action.

There can be no fixed standards of optimal dosage for hypotensive drugs because individual requirements vary widely. In general the important principle is to start with a small dose and gradually increase it until the maximum control of blood pressure is obtained without undue side-effects. Some drugs are best used in combination.

Rauwolfia. Rauwolfia and its derivatives (e.g. reserpine) are taken by mouth and have a mildly hypotensive action and are also sedative. They are, therefore, useful for patients with anxiety and other emotional disturbances. The effects develop slowly over several days and not all patients respond. There are many side-effects, e.g. nasal congestion, fatigue, lethargy, drowsiness, dizziness, unpleasant dreams and diarrhoea. The only serious one which is at all common is depression, often with agitation and occasionally with suicidal tendencies. *It is most important to be on the alert for this complication and stop the drug.* Parkinsonism has also occurred. The recommended dose of reserpine is 0·5 mg. b.d. for a week and thereafter 0·25 mg. b.d. It is frequently used in combination with other agents.

Veratrum Viride (*Veriloid*) and hydrallazine (Apresoline) are so little used in Britain that it is not proposed to describe them.

Ganglion blocking drugs. The treatment of hypertension was greatly improved by the introduction of ganglion blocking drugs which act by interfering with the transmission of sympathetic and parasympathetic impulses through autonomic ganglia. The sympathetic effect results in reduction of neurogenic vasoconstricter tone. As a result the 'standing' blood pressure can be reduced to normal or near normal levels in most cases but the recumbent pressure is little affected. The accompanying parasympathetic blockade may be sufficiently marked to produce unpleasant and even dangerous side-effects such as paralysis of accommodation, dry mouth, constipation or paralytic ileus.

The earlier compounds methonium and pentolinium were superseded by mecamylamine and pempidine. These have in turn been replaced by drugs which have a selective post-ganglion action on the sympathetic nerve impulses and hence are free from the unpleasant side-effects of parasympathetic blockade. Since ganglion blocking drugs are very little used nowadays no further information about them will be given.

Sympathetic blocking drugs. Probably the two drugs in most frequent use today in the treatment of hypertension are guanethidine and methyldopa given alone or in combination with an oral diuretic but more promising preparations are under trial.

Guanethidine should be administered initially in a small dose (10 mg.) which should be increased gradually by 10 mg. every three to seven days until the standing pressure is controlled. This is achieved in most patients by a daily dose of approximately 50 mg. but the range may be as wide as 25-150 mg. By these means satisfactory results can be achieved in about 75 per cent. of cases. Side-effects include diarrhoea, muscular weakness, nasal stuffiness, frequency of micturition and sexual difficulties in the male, but these can usually be reduced in frequency and severity if dosage is carefully adjusted to each patient's requirements.

Methyldopa has a somewhat different mode of action in that it antagonises the synthesis of pressor amines and thereby interferes with the transmission of sympathetic impulses. It is relatively free from side-effects which are usually mild. They include drowsiness, fatigue, malaise and dryness of the mouth. More serious toxic effects are haemolytic anaemia, fever and jaundice. Treatment should be commenced with 250 mg. thrice daily and the dose increased by 250 mg. each day until the desired hypotensive effect is achieved.

Mention must be made of two promising new drugs.

Bethanidine (Esbatal) has a somewhat similar action to guanethidine but is more quickly absorbed and excreted, and side-effects are milder. It is being increasingly used in practice.

Debrisoquine is a more recent preparation which is remarkably free from side-effects, but the incidence of tolerance may be somewhat higher.

Oral diuretics. Oral diuretics such as chlorothiazide or chlorthalidone and their derivatives have themselves a mild anti-hypertensive effect but their principal use in the management of hypertension is as an adjuvant when the blood pressure is difficult to control with ganglion or sympathetic blocking drugs, either because of resistance or the incidence of side-effects. A small dose of chlorthalidone (50 mg.) daily is often sufficient.

As already mentioned the combined effect of two drugs may be unexpectedly potent.

SURGICAL TREATMENT. Various forms of sympathectomy, splanchnicectomy and adrenalectomy have been practised for many years with a view to lowering the blood pressure by reducing vasomotor tone. Even when the blood pressure is not appreciably or permanently lowered by these procedures prolonged symptomatic relief is sometimes achieved. The operations vary greatly in extent and therefore severity, but since they do not strike at the root of the trouble and hold no hope of cure, they are unlikely to have a permanent place in treatment. They are rarely used today.

THE CARDIOMYOPATHIES

Definition. The cardiomyopathies are acute, subacute or chronic disorders of heart muscle of unknown, unusual or obscure aetiology, and sometimes associated with pericardial and endocardial involvement.

They may be divided into (a) *primary*, in which the heart is initially or solely involved, and (b) *secondary*, in which disease elsewhere in the body has involved the heart secondarily.

The cardiomyopathies occur more frequently than was formerly believed to be the case. This is due partly to the fact that the disorder is frequently overlooked or mistaken for other types of cardiac disease, and partly because the diagnosis may have to be a presumptive one based on the absence of evidence for the nature of any underlying disease.

Aetiology. The cardiomyopathies may occur as an isolated myocardial disorder in which the aetiology is obscure (primary cardiomyopathy), or in association with certain infections, infiltrative diseases or deficiency states (secondary cardiomyopathy).

Acute cardiomyopathies usually occur secondarily as a complication of infections, the majority beingdue to the toxic effects of disorders such as diphtheria, pneumonia, typhoid fever, scrub typhus fever and meningitis. They may also occur in protozoal infections such as Chagas' disease (American trypanosomiasis, p. 576), and may follow virus diseases such as influenza, poliomyelitis, infectious mononucleosis and coxsackie infectious.

In infancy and early childhood cardiomyopathy may be associated with endocardial fibro-elastosis or with glycogen storage disease. In later life it may be due to involvement of the myocardium in sarcoidosis, amyloidosis, haemochromatosis and the collagen disorders. It may also be associated with pregnancy and, not infrequently, with chronic alcoholism. Cardiomyopathy may occur as a familial disease in which several members are affected.

In underdeveloped countries in which dietary deficiency of calories, proteins and vitamins is common, nutritional factors have long been believed to be a cause of cardiomyopathy. The cardiac failure of beriberi is due to thiamine deficiency. More recently, clinical and pathological investigations carried out in various tropical and subtropical countries have clearly shown that an obscure cardiomyopathy is a common cause of unexplained cardiac failure. This disorder is possibly nutritional in origin, and if diagnosed early it may respond well to orthodox treatment, supplemented by a good mixed diet with adequate supplies of protein and the whole vitamin B complex, but not to thiamine. In some parts of Africa a type of cardiomyopathy frequently seen is endomyocardial fibrosis. This is a disorder in which extensive fibrosis of the endocardium develops and later involves the myocardium of one or both ventricles. Endomyocardial fibrosis is rarely, if ever, encountered in Britain except in immigrants. It is possible that some infective cause, perhaps a virus, acting alone or in combination with malnutrition, may be responsible.

Clinical Features. The clinical presentation of the cardiomyopathies is usually insidious but the disease may be suspected by the detection of cardiomegaly, gallop rhythm, embolism or congestive cardiac failure for which the usual cardiac causes have been excluded. These patients fall into three main types according to the effect of the myocardial disorder on the function of the heart. (1) The most common is progressive congestive heart failure, often with functional incompetence of the atrioventricular valves. (2) Hypertrophy of the interventricular septum may be present and lead to obstruction of the ventricular outflow tracts and the condition may simulate aortic or pulmonary stenosis. (3) Rigidity of the myocardium may prevent relaxation in diastole and simulate constrictive pericarditis (p. 269). Cardiomegaly is most marked in the first type in which atrial fibrillation, triple rhythm, pansystolic murmurs and conduction defects are most likely to occur. The course of the cardiomyopathies is very variable. In a few cases complete recovery occurs, more often the course is chronic, while occasionally there may be sudden death without premonitory symptoms.

Diagnosis. The diagnosis of cardiomyopathy should only be considered after other forms of heart disease have been excluded, e.g. rheumatic, hypertensive, ischaemic, thyroid or congenital.

Treatment. Treatment remains unsatisfactory for a heterogeneous group of disorders in which the cause may be unknown, cannot be removed, or for which no specific treatment is available. A well balanced diet, supplemented by natural sources of the vitamin B complex (yeast, wheat germ), is obviously indicated in those cases in which nutritional deficiency is of aetiological importance. Corticosteroid therapy is sometimes of value for the treatment of cardiomyopathy due to sarcoidosis or associated with collagen diseases. In all cases rest in bed is of importance, supplemented when necessary by digitalis, diuretics and restriction of the intake of sodium.

Surgical resection of the hypertrophied myocardium is sometimes beneficial in the obstructive type, and thoracotomy may be necessary when the clinical features resemble those of constrictive pericarditis.

CONGENITAL HEART DISEASE

The incidence of congenital abnormalities is about 6 per 1,000 births. All degrees of severity occur. Many defects are not compatible with extra-uterine life, or only for a short time. Most cases are diagnosed in childhood, usually on account of cyanosis or the discovery of a murmur. Inevitably these conditions become less common in practice as age advances. Some are particularly important to recognise because they may be amenable to surgical treatment. Bacterial endocarditis is an important potential complication.

A precise diagnosis may be impossible in infancy but with

modern methods of investigation can usually be made in childhood. Symptoms may be absent altogether or consist principally of breathlessness and failure of development. Local signs vary with the anatomical lesion. Central cyanosis occurs only when venous blood enters the systemic circulation. The most common cause of this is a septal defect combined with a severe grade of pulmonary stenosis or pulmonary hypertension. Often the signs are characteristic, e.g. in patent ductus arteriosus or in ventricular septal defect, but sometimes diagnosis is very difficult and special investigations are required. Additional help can be obtained from:

(*a*) Radiology—to determine the size of the various chambers of the heart, the size and position of the great vessels and the presence of plethora or of relative avascularity of the lungs.

(*b*) Electrocardiography—principally to determine the presence and type of ventricular hypertrophy.

(*c*) Angiocardiography—to outline the individual cardiac chambers and to assist in the detection of abnormal shunts.

(*d*) Cardiac Catheterisation—to record the pressures and also the oxygen content of the blood in the cardiac chambers and great vessels and to estimate pulmonary blood flow.

(*e*) Dye Dilution Curves (p. 152).

Only the relatively common disorders likely to be met with in practice and those which are of practical importance will be described.

In most cases the underlying cause of the abnormality is unknown, but there is evidence that some foetal defects are due to maternal infections in the early weeks of pregnancy, e.g. German measles.

PATENT DUCTUS ARTERIOSUS

During foetal life, before the lungs begin to function, most of the blood from the pulmonary artery passes through the ductus arteriosus which joins the aorta just below the origin of the left subclavian artery (Fig. 38).

Normally the ductus closes soon after birth but, for reasons which are obscure, this sometimes fails to take place. Since the pressure in the aorta is normally higher than that in the pulmonary artery there will be a continuous arterio-venous shunt, the volume of which will depend on the size of the ductus. As much as 50 per cent. of the left ventricular output may be passed through the lungs again with a consequent increase in the work of the heart.

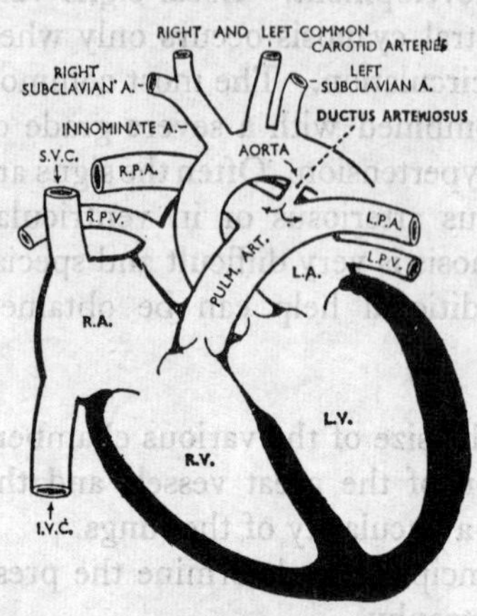

Fig. 38
Patent Ductus Arteriosus

The condition is much more common in females. Other congenital abnormalities may be associated.

Clinical Features. There may be no relevant symptoms for many years, but growth and development will be retarded if the defect is a severe one. In mild cases there will be no disability, but in cases of moderate severity undue dyspnoea on exertion and later the usual features of cardiac failure gradually develop.

A continuous 'machinery' murmur is heard (first described by Gibson of Edinburgh) with late systolic accentuation and maximal in the second left intercostal space near the sternum. It is frequently, but not always, accompanied by a thrill.

Enlargement of the pulmonary artery, but little enlargement of the heart, may be detected radiologically. Abnormal pulsation of the main pulmonary arteries sometimes occurs, but not to the extent observed with an atrial septal defect.

The electrocardiogram is usually normal. Any abnormality should suggest the possibility that some other congenital defect may be associated.

Treatment. In uncomplicated cases, the patent ductus can be divided with very little risk, especially in children, and there is general agreement that this should be carried out in all cases, preferably between 6 and 10 years of age.

Prognosis. In untreated cases few live beyond the age of 40. Death is usually from cardiac failure or subacute bacterial endocarditis. Following successful surgical treatment expectation of life is normal.

COARCTATION OF THE AORTA

Narrowing of the aorta occurs in the region where the ductus arteriosus joins the aorta, i.e. just below the origin of the left subclavian artery (Fig. 39). The condition is more common in males.

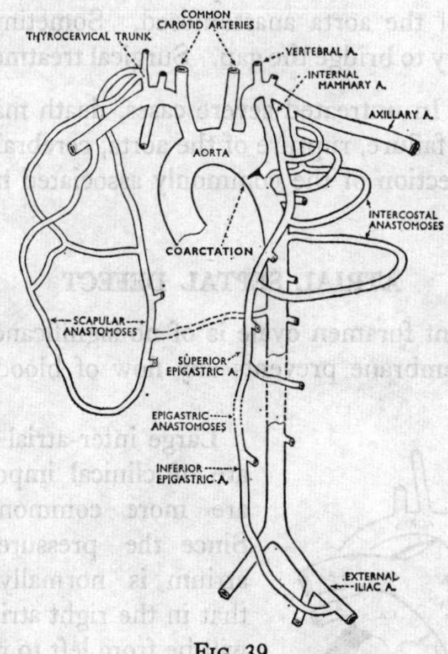

FIG. 39

COARCTATION OF THE AORTA

Clinical Features. The clinical manifestations depend on the degree of coarctation. Symptoms are often absent altogether. Headaches and dizziness may occur from hypertension in the upper part of the body and weakness or cramps in the legs from decreased circulation in the lower part of the body.

The blood pressure is raised in the arms but is normal or low in the legs. Unduly large arterial pulsations may be visible in the neck. The femoral pulses are weak and delayed after the radial. A systolic murmur is often present over the sternum but is usually loudest posteriorly.

Evidence of collateral circulation is present. Dilated, tortuous vessels exhibiting arterial pulsation may be visible or palpable around the scapulae or in the axillae, especially if the patient bends down. A systolic murmur may be heard over the collateral vessels.

Radiological examination may show changes in the contour of the aorta and notching of the under surface of the ribs from tortuous loops of enlarged intercostal arteries.

The electrocardiogram may show left ventricular hypertrophy.

Treatment. The constricted portion can be resected and the divided ends of the aorta anastomosed. Sometimes an arterial graft is necessary to bridge the gap. Surgical treatment is curative.

Prognosis. In untreated severe cases, death may occur from left ventricular failure, rupture of the aorta, cerebral haemorrhage or bacterial infection of the commonly associated bicuspid aortic valve.

ATRIAL SEPTAL DEFECT

A small patent foramen ovale is of no significance. Normally a valve-like membrane prevents any flow of blood between the two chambers.

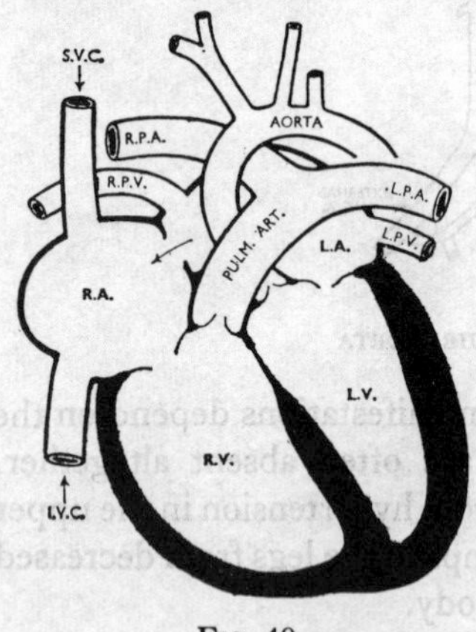

Fig. 40
Atrial Septal Defect

Large inter-atrial septal defects are of clinical importance. They are more common in females. Since the pressure in the left atrium is normally higher than that in the right atrium, the shunt will be from left to right (Fig. 40). As a result there is gradual enlargement of the right side of the heart and of the pulmonary artery and its main branches. In time the pressure in the right side of the heart will increase until the shunt is reversed and it is at this time that the diagnosis is often first made.

Clinical Features. There may be no symptoms for many years until the shunt is reversed. Dyspnoea, cyanosis and later cardiac failure then develop. There are no characteristic physical signs but a systolic or diastolic murmur may be heard to the left of the sternum, with wide splitting of the pulmonary second sound. Enlargement of the pulmonary artery and its main branches is seen radiologically and a dynamic pulsation observed on the screen ('hilar dance'). The right ventricular enlargement can also be seen and may be reflected in the electrocardiogram. Incomplete right bundle branch block is common. Mitral stenosis is sometimes associated (Lutembacher's syndrome).

Treatment. Surgical closure of the defect should be carried out, preferably before the age of 10.

Prognosis. When the shunt reverses, cardiac failure soon follows. Most patients used to live to middle age but now, following surgical treatment, the expectation of life is probably normal.

VENTRICULAR SEPTAL DEFECT

Since the pressure in the left ventricle is higher than that in the right ventricle, the shunt is normally from left to right (Fig. 41).

Clinical Features. Usually there are no relevant symptoms. The characteristic signs are a harsh systolic murmur and thrill maximal in the 4th intercostal space to the left of the sternum. In time pulmonary hypertension develops, the right ventricle hypertrophies, the shunt reverses and congestive cardiac failure may ensue.

Radiological and electrocardiographic examinations are normal except in the more severe cases when the heart is enlarged.

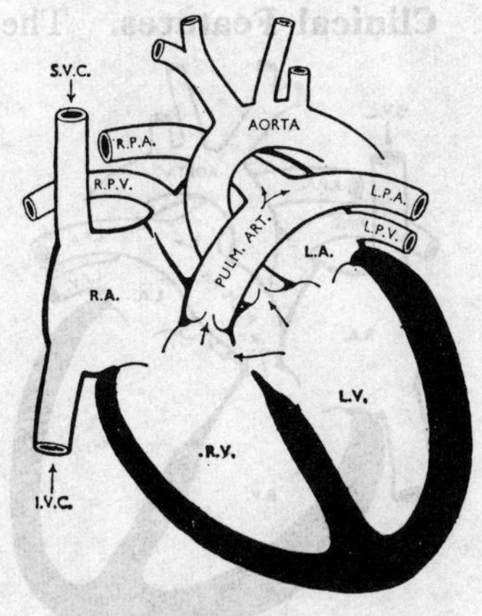

FIG. 41
VENTRICULAR SEPTAL DEFECT

Treatment. The defect can be repaired by 'open heart' surgery. Surgical treatment has recently been introduced using the by-pass technique.

Prognosis. This depends on the size of the defect. Duration of life may be unaffected, but in severe cases congestive failure may develop at any age. Bacterial endocarditis is an occasional complication. Surgical treatment is curative if carried out before the heart is much enlarged.

PULMONARY STENOSIS

Pulmonary stenosis may occur as an isolated anomaly in which case cyanosis may be absent, or in association with an atrial or ventricular septal defect in which case there may or may not be cyanosis depending on the relative pressures on the two sides of the shunt.

Surgical treatment is required if the stenosis is of sufficient severity to cause an important limitation in pulmonary blood flow and an increase in right ventricular pressure (as indicated by hypertrophy). Stenosis may occur at the level of the pulmonary valve or in the infundibular region of the right ventricle.

Pulmonary Stenosis with Closed Interventricular Septum

Clinical Features. The principal symptoms are dyspnoea, fatigue and occasionally syncope. The characteristic signs are a harsh systolic murmur and thrill, maximal in the second intercostal space to the left of the sternum. The pulmonary second sound is diminished. The pulmonary artery is usually dilated beyond the stenotic valve. The right ventricle is hypertrophied (Fig. 42). There may be an associated atrial septal defect.

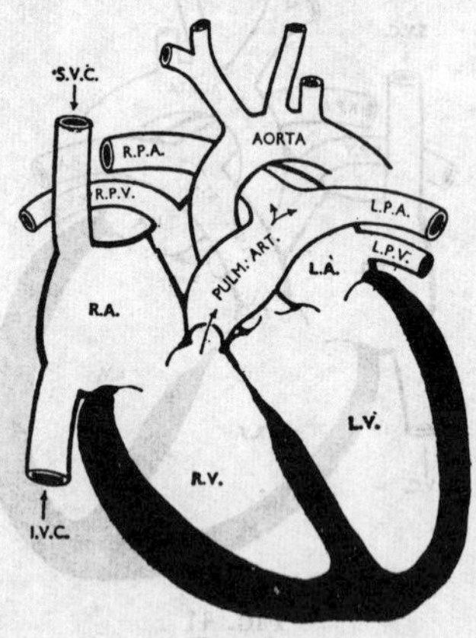

Fig. 42
Pulmonary Stenosis

Treatment. In selected cases pulmonary valvotomy can be carried out.

Prognosis. Sudden death is liable to occur. Where symptoms are progressive cardiac failure is inevitable unless surgical relief is possible.

PULMONARY STENOSIS WITH PATENT INTERVENTRICULAR SEPTUM (FALLOT'S TETRALOGY)

This is the most common form of cyanotic congenital heart disease in children or adults (Fig. 43). The usual combination of lesions is:

(*a*) Pulmonary stenosis.
(*b*) Interventricular septal defect.
(*c*) Dextro-position of aorta overriding the septal defect.
(*d*) Right ventricular hypertrophy.

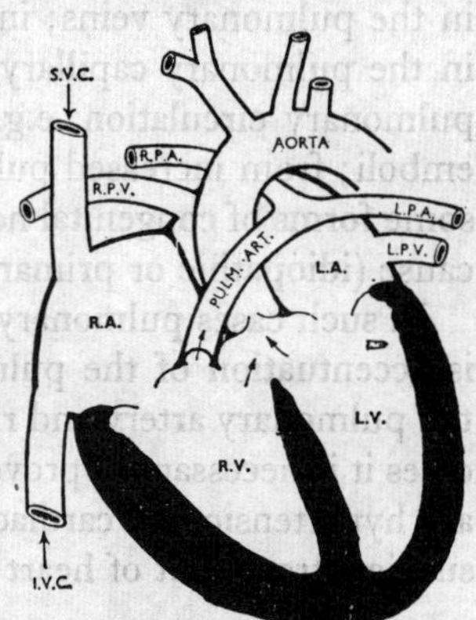

FIG. 43
FALLOT'S TETRALOGY

Clinical Features. Dyspnoea and fatigue are the principal symptoms and when present the child characteristically assumes the squatting position. The principal signs are cyanosis, polycythaemia and clubbing of the fingers; a loud systolic murmur, and often a thrill, maximal to the left of the upper sternum; soft pulmonary second sound; enlargement of the right side of the heart; absence of the normal pulmonary artery curve on radiological examination.

Treatment. In suitable cases a palliative operation in the form of an anastomosis can sometimes be made either between the left or right pulmonary artery and the corresponding subclavian artery (Blalock's operation) or between the left pulmonary artery and the aorta (Potts' operation) thereby increasing the blood supply to the lungs. More recently direct pulmonary valvotomy has been carried out, and the ventricular septal defect repaired.

Prognosis. It is difficult to generalise about prognosis because the outlook depends on the degree of severity of the defect and the possibility of surgical treatment. Experience is still limited but the risks of operation are steadily decreasing. There is no doubt that the outlook has improved for those who survive operation, but there has been insufficient time to judge the ultimate prognosis.

PULMONARY HYPERTENSION

An increase of pressure in the pulmonary arterial circulation may occur in mitral stenosis or in left ventricular failure and is secondary to a passive rise of pressure in the left atrium and hence in the pulmonary veins; in emphysema as a result of diminution in the pulmonary capillary bed; as a result of obstruction to the pulmonary circulation, e.g. from arterial narrowing or recurrent emboli; from increased pulmonary blood flow in association with some forms of congenital heart disease; or, rarely, without obvious cause (idiopathic or primary pulmonary hypertension).

In such cases pulmonary hypertension may be inferred if there is accentuation of the pulmonary second sound, enlargement of the pulmonary artery and right ventricular hypertrophy. In some cases it is necessary to prove the existence or otherwise of pulmonary hypertension by cardiac catheterisation before deciding on the surgical treatment of heart disease.

THYROTOXIC HEART DISEASE

This is an important condition to recognise because it is potentially curable. Thyrotoxic heart disease is most often seen in older patients with nodular goitre and is rare under the age of 40. The physiological disturbances as regards the circulation are tachycardia, increased cardiac output and vasodilatation. Thyrotoxicosis is an important cause of atrial fibrillation and should be always kept in mind when no other cause can be found, especially if the extremities are warm. Paroxysmal attacks often precede established fibrillation. The mechanism responsible is unknown.

Pathology. No specific morphological changes have been found in the hearts of patients who have died with thyrotoxicosis. There may, however, be metabolic or biochemical changes which affect function and yet leave no distinctive histological changes. It is possible that thyrotoxicosis may be a primary cause of heart disease but it is more commonly a contributory or precipitating factor in heart failure from other causes.

Symptoms and Signs. Palpitation, dyspnoea and tachycardia are more often related to the circulatory disturbances than to heart disease. Owing to the increased rate of blood flow there is a full bounding pulse and the hands are warm. The first heart sound is often accentuated and simulates that found in mitral stenosis. A systolic murmur, usually maximal in the pulmonary area, is common. The systolic blood pressure is often raised, and since the diastolic pressure is usually normal or somewhat reduced, the pulse pressure is raised (e.g. 170/60).

Treatment. Thyrotoxic heart disease can be prevented by early recognition and treatment of the underlying condition. Treatment is primarily directed towards the hyperthyroidism (p. 702). The customary measures for the treatment of congestive cardiac failure are all appropriate (p. 184). Should normal rhythm not be restored by antithyroid drugs, radio-iodine or thyroidectomy, quinidine or procainamide should be given (p. 195) or direct current conversion attempted.

PULMONARY COMPLICATIONS IN HEART DISEASE

PULMONARY EMBOLISM AND INFARCTION

Pulmonary embolism occurs when a portion of blood clot in a systemic vein or in the right side of the heart is discharged into the circulation and lodges in the main pulmonary artery or its branches. Pulmonary infarction is the pathological lesion which usually develops in the lung when a pulmonary artery is obstructed either by embolism or by local thrombosis. Emboli may be of any size, single or multiple and may occur in patients with heart disease or in those with normal hearts. The clinical features are largely dependent on these factors. Massive embolism may result in sudden death.

Aetiology. The most common cause of pulmonary embolism is thrombosis in the deep veins of the legs (p. 291).

Thrombi responsible for pulmonary embolism may form in the right atrium in patients with atrial fibrillation from any cause, especially if cardiac failure is present, and in the right ventricle after myocardial infarction involving the interventricular septum. However, even in those with cardiac failure the most common source of pulmonary embolism is venous thrombosis in the veins of the lower limbs. After pregnancy or a pelvic operation embolism may result from thrombosis in a pelvic vein.

Pathology. A long thrombus tends to coil up and may be found obstructing the main pulmonary artery or astride its bifurcation. Multiple emboli may be found in the smaller branches. If the patient survives for a sufficient length of time pulmonary infarction is a common sequel to pulmonary embolism, the infarct heals by absorption of the blood followed by fibrosis and contraction, the end result being a linear scar.

Infarction is most likely to develop after pulmonary embolism if pulmonary congestion is present from cardiac failure. Occasionally local thrombosis in the pulmonary arterial tree is responsible for pulmonary infarction.

In massive embolism, dilatation of the right side of the heart will result, and in long-standing cases of lesser severity, right ventricular hypertrophy may occur and constitutes one form of chronic cor pulmonale.

Clinical Features

PULMONARY EMBOLISM. With massive pulmonary embolism the patient may be suddenly seized with a sensation of great oppression in the chest and intense dyspnoea followed by peripheral cyanosis and shock. Sudden death may occur within a few minutes, an hour or two or a day or two. However, many recover. Examination of the heart and lungs is often negative but the blood pressure falls, the neck veins become engorged and cardiac failure may follow in severe cases (acute cor pulmonale). The pulmonary second sound may be accentuated and triple rhythm may develop. These signs are due to a combination of right ventricular failure and a low cardiac output.

In cases of lesser severity symptoms may be absent altogether or there may be transient dyspnoea, tachycardia or syncope.

Pain indistinguishable from that of myocardial infarction may occur and make the differential diagnosis exceedingly difficult. In some cases pulmonary embolism may actually lead to myocardial ischaemia or even infarction. This is probably due to a combination of decreased coronary blood flow and anoxaemia.

PULMONARY INFARCTION. As this is usually the result of an embolus arising in a vein of a lower limb and as phlebothrombosis in that situation is generally the result of stasis, pulmonary infarction in the vast majority of cases affects people who are confined to bed or who have just begun to get up. It is particularly liable to occur about 10 days after a surgical operation or childbirth. The existence of phlebothrombosis (p. 291) may be discovered prior to the occurrence of embolism, but often it is not recognised until afterwards. The symptoms of pulmonary infarction may be preceded by those of a fairly large pulmonary embolism (central chest pain, dyspnoea, cyanosis and circulatory collapse), but usually this is not so and the only symptoms are those due to infarction. The onset is sudden with either pleuritic pain or haemoptysis as the initial symptom. These two symptoms are not always present and the absence of one or even both of them does not necessarily exclude pulmonary infarction. The pain is often severe and the haemoptysis may be repeated. Other clinical features include tachycardia, dyspnoea and cyanosis. Pyrexia is usually present, but sometimes the temperature is subnormal. When present in the early stages it is probably due to absorption of blood from the infarct, but later it may be due to secondary infection. A polymorphonuclear leucocytosis may be present, even in the absence of infection.

Radiological Examination

(*a*) In massive pulmonary embolism the lung fields usually appear normal but in a few cases ischaemia distal to the embolus causes a reduction in the normal vascular markings of a lung or lobe.

(*b*) In pulmonary infarction there may be a pulmonary opacity, representing the infarct itself, or a linear scar caused by related pleurisy or a contracted infarct. One hemidiaphragm may be raised or paralysed. The radiological abnormalities are often multiple and bilateral. A pleural effusion may be seen.

Electrocardiography. The electrocardiogram may show a diagnostic pattern of acute cor pulmonale in cases of massive embolism but is usually normal in cases of lesser severity.

Differential Diagnosis

(*a*) Massive pulmonary embolism must be distinguished from myocardial infarction (p. 221) and spontaneous pneumothorax (p. 407).

(*b*) Pulmonary infarction must be distinguished from:

(i) Dry pleurisy of infective origin. The distinction may be impossible unless other features of pulmonary infarction, such as haemoptysis are also present, but the existence of a possible source for an embolism, e.g. phlebothrombosis in a lower limb, favours the diagnosis of infarction.

(ii) Pneumonia, by the history, the character of the sputum and the response to treatment.

(iii) Spontaneous pneumothorax, by the characteristic physical and radiological signs (p. 405).

(iv) Other causes of haemoptysis, e.g. tuberculosis, mitral stenosis, neoplasm, bronchiectasis.

Course and Prognosis. The outcome is difficult to predict. Massive pulmonary embolism is frequently fatal. Minor and medium sized emboli are much less dangerous unless they are followed by further embolisation which may itself be fatal. In retrospect it is often apparent that small 'warning' emboli have, in fact, been missed or misinterpreted. Statistical data are still inadequate but probably about 20 per cent. of patients die in their first attack, and about 30 per cent. have further attacks. Sometimes even large emboli become organised and recanalised and occasionally chronic pulmonary hypertension leads to progressive cardiac failure. An infarct may become secondarily infected and result in lung abscess or empyema.

Prophylaxis. The prevention or at least the early recognition of venous thrombosis is very important and is discussed on p. 291. An appreciation of the potential dangers of bed rest and the correct management of atrial fibrillation and of cardiac failure, together with the use of anticoagulants and occasionally of venous ligation once venous thrombosis has occurred, are the principal factors in the prevention of pulmonary embolism and infarction.

Treatment. Unfortunately little can be done to affect the course once pulmonary embolism has occurred. Morphine should be given to allay pain and apprehension. Oxygen should be given if cyanosis is present. Atropine is usually advised to reduce any vagal reflexes which may lead to constriction of the pulmonary or coronary vessels. Anticoagulants should be given in order to prevent further venous thrombosis in the legs and the occurrence of thrombosis behind the occluded vessel in the lungs (p. 223). The risk of causing haemorrhage is not great. If infection follows penicillin should be given.

Occasionally, when facilities are present, and the patient survives massive embolism for an hour or so, a large embolus has been successfully removed from the main pulmonary artery. When facilities are available open heart surgery is best for this purpose.

PULMONARY CONGESTION AND OEDEMA

Pulmonary congestion occurs whenever there is relative failure of the chambers on the left side of the heart, i.e. in mitral valvular disease and in failure of the left ventricle from aortic valvular disease, hypertension or ischaemic heart disease. Pulmonary congestion may also result from:

1. Acute pulmonary infections, such as pneumonia, in which the congestion is merely part of the acute inflammatory reaction.
2. Gravitational redistribution of blood within the lungs (hypostatic congestion), which occurs in old or debilitated persons who are confined to bed. A low-grade non-specific pneumonia (hypostatic pneumonia) may develop in the congested lungs (p. 358).

Pulmonary oedema may occur as a later stage of long-standing pulmonary congestion or with dramatic suddenness in patients with mitral stenosis or conditions prone to left ventricular failure (p. 171). It may also result from:

1. Overloading of the circulation by intravenous infusion.
2. A virulent acute respiratory infection, e.g. influenza.
3. The inhalation of an irritant gas such as chlorine or phosgene, or of an irritant liquid such as vomitus.
4. Acute nephritis (p. 797).
5. Thoracic surgical operations, particularly pneumonectomy.

Intense dyspnoea, which is usually the first symptom, is rapidly followed by cyanosis, which may become extreme, and cough with the production of large amounts of frothy sputum which is usually white, but may be pink or even frankly blood-stained. The physical signs consist of coarse, bubbling crepitations audible all over both sides of the chest. The presence of secretions in the larynx, trachea and main bronchi produces a characteristic rattling sound audible without the aid of a stethoscope.

Chronic pulmonary oedema is almost invariably of cardiac origin. Its importance from the point of view of respiratory disease is that it is readily confused with chronic bronchitis. A diagnosis of chronic bronchitis should never be accepted without a careful evaluation of the state of the cardiovascular system.

Treatment is that of the primary disease.

HYDROTHORAX

Fluid in the pleural cavity is a common occurrence in congestive heart failure and occurs without any pleural reaction such as is present in effusion secondary to pleurisy. No pain is associated with its development. The fluid is a transudate, pale yellow in colour and of low specific gravity. Hydrothorax is more common on the right side than on the left. A pleural exudate may be secondary to pulmonary infarction.

HAEMOPTYSIS

Haemoptysis in heart disease is particularly common in patients with mitral stenosis and in such cases may be due to pulmonary hypertension, pulmonary infarction or accompany attacks of acute pulmonary oedema. Pulmonary infarction associated with atrial fibrillation, peripheral venous thrombosis or local pulmonary arterial thrombosis is common in all forms of cardiac failure. In systemic hypertension haemoptysis may occur without a discoverable cause. Haemoptysis always calls for thorough investigation until either the cause is discovered or serious disease has been excluded as far as possible.

HYPOSTATIC PNEUMONIA AND ATELECTASIS

Hypostatic congestion, patchy atelectasis and infection are prone to occur in debilitated patients who are unable to move about freely in bed, to breathe deeply because of pain or to cough up secretions because of weakness, or who are given large doses of sedative drugs. For further details see p. 358.

Frequent changes of posture, encouragement to breathe deeply and to cough should be instituted together with oxygen, antibiotics and if necessary drugs such as nikethamide, to stimulate respiration.

CHRONIC PULMONARY HEART DISEASE

(Cor Pulmonale)

The term 'pulmonary heart disease' may be defined as right-sided heart disease secondary to disease of the lungs or pulmonary vessels. The principal causes of chronic cor pulmonale are emphysema and diffuse fibrosis (including pneumoconiosis). Less frequently the condition results from obstruction in the pulmonary artery or arterioles from thrombo-embolism. In certain industrial regions of England cor pulmonale from chronic respiratory disease is the most common form of cardiac failure. Acute cor pulmonale from massive pulmonary embolism is described on p. 253.

Cor pulmonale may be manifested by right ventricular failure, hypertrophy or dilatation. It should be noted that pulmonary hypertension itself does not necessarily signify heart disease any more than does systemic hypertension.

COR PULMONALE SECONDARY TO EMPHYSEMA

Pathogenesis. There is no evidence that cor pulmonale is due to primary myocardial disease. The factors involved in its pathogenesis are pulmonary hypertension, hypoxia, hypercapnia, polycythaemia, increased blood volume and increased cardiac output.

Impaired alveolar ventilation, structural abnormalities of the pulmonary vasculature and defective aeration of the blood leads to hypoxia and this is probably responsible for the polycythaemia and hypervolaemia which result in an increased cardiac output. In addition there may be carbon dioxide retention (hypercapnia). There is evidence that hypoxia itself leads to reflex hypertension.

When cardiac failure occurs it is frequently precipitated by an acute respiratory infection.

Clinical Features. The symptoms and signs of cor pulmonale are those attributed to the underlying pulmonary disease together with those of congestive cardiac failure.

The onset is usually insidious but may apparently come on suddenly following an acute respiratory infection.

Cyanosis of a moderate degree is common in emphysema but if it is severe cardiac failure is usually present.

Sinus rhythm is the rule and if there is co-existing atrial fibrillation coronary disease should be suspected.

The earliest radiographic sign is enlargement of the pulmonary artery and its two main branches followed by enlargement of the right ventricle. ECG changes with emphysema are often not diagnostic unless severe pulmonary hypertension is present.

Treatment

(*a*) Prompt and thorough treatment of any pulmonary infection is very important and is frequently the most efficacious factor in treating the cardiac failure.

(*b*) Bronchodilators should be given when airway obstruction is present (p. 345). Aerosols may be useful (p. 344). Expectoration of secretions may be assisted by the physiotherapist, or if necessary bronchoscopy or tracheostomy may be carried out to maintain an airway.

(*c*) Oxygen is indicated if central cyanosis is present with congestive failure but caution is necessary because cerebral symptoms and even coma can result from carbon dioxide retention.

(*d*) Diuretics should be given as with all forms of cardiac failure but digitalis is relatively ineffective.

(*e*) Venesection may help if polycythaemia is present.

(*f*) Morphine in particular and other sedatives must be used with great caution owing to their action in depressing the respiratory centre.

The results of treatment are often very disappointing and a recurrence of congestive failure is seldom long delayed.

* * * * * *

SYPHILITIC CARDIOVASCULAR DISEASE

Syphilitic cardiovascular disease which is much rarer today in Britain than it was 30 years ago is still an important cause of ill-health in many parts of the world. The heart itself is not primarily affected but damage results from aortitis and its complications. It occurs more frequently in men than in women. There is often a latent period of 15-20 years following infection before clinical manifestations are evident in the cardiovascular system.

Pathology. The disease begins just above the aortic valve cusps. In the adventitia there is perivascular infiltration of lymphocytes and plasma cells round the vasa vasorum, which are obliterated by intimal proliferation. Elastic tissue is gradually replaced by fibrous tissue and this leads to dilatation of the aorta. Proliferation of the intima occurs and may involve the mouths of the coronary arteries leading to myocardial ischaemia or spread along the valve cusps which become thickened, everted and incompetent.

The macroscopic changes are characteristic and consist of bluish-grey raised intimal plaques and longitudinal wrinkling of the inner surface of the aorta. Atheromatous changes with calcification are frequently associated.

Symptoms and Signs. Syphilitic heart disease occurs most frequently between the ages of 40 and 55.

1. Aortic Incompetence. The clinical manifestations are similar to those resulting from rheumatic aortic incompetence (p. 203). In the absence of other evidence of rheumatic heart disease, e.g. mitral stenosis, and especially in men between the ages of 30 and 60, syphilis should always be excluded as a possible cause of aortic incompetence by taking blood for a Wassermann reaction.

2. Angina Pectoris from coronary ostial stenosis. Sudden death is particularly liable to occur. It must be remembered that there are causes of angina pectoris other than coronary atheroma (p. 218), and it is a wise precaution to do a Wassermann reaction in all patients developing angina before the age of 45.

3. Aortitis. This diagnosis is difficult in the early uncomplicated stages. An aortic systolic murmur may be present, together with accentuation of the second sound. Dilatation and calcification of the ascending aorta may be demonstrated by radiological examination.

4. Aortic Aneurysm. An aneurysm is a localised dilatation of the vessel wall. When due to syphilis, aneurysms are most common in the proximal parts of the thoracic aorta. In contradistinction, atheromatous aneurysms are most common in the distal portions. The clinical features depend on the precise situation. Symptoms may arise from pressure on neighbouring structures and signs are similar to those of an expanding mediastinal tumour. There may be considerable difficulty in differential diagnosis especially as pulsation may be transmitted by a tumour, and an aneurysm may not pulsate owing to obliteration of the cavity by blood clot.

5. NEUROSYPHILIS. The co-existence of the clinical features of neurosyphilis with those of cardiovascular syphilis is not usual.

Treatment. If antisyphilitic drugs are given in the early stages of the infection cardiovascular manifestations in later life are prevented. In the later stages penicillin can destroy spirochaetes and relieve active inflammation but cannot restore elastic tissue which has been lost, reduce the degree of aortic incompetence or the size of an aneurysm. Treatment has been much simplified in recent years and all that is necessary in most cases is a single course of procaine penicillin, i.e. 600,000 units daily for 10 days. Some physicians recommend preceding this with potassium iodide, 0·3 g. t.d.s. for 10 days. If cardiac failure is present this should first be treated on the usual lines.

* * * * * *

DIPHTHERITIC HEART DISEASE

Owing to effective prophylaxis diphtheria has become of little importance in the Western hemisphere and hence diphtheritic heart disease is rare. Myocarditis is one of the dangerous complications of diphtheria. The toxin produced by the diphtheria bacillus causes degeneration of the muscle fibres but does not affect the valves or pericardium. Clinical features and treatment are described on pp. 33-38.

Prognosis. This is serious because sudden death is liable to occur at any time. However, should the patient survive, the heart will recover completely.

* * * * * *

HEART DISEASE IN PREGNANCY

The management of heart disease in pregnancy is a more complicated problem than in the non-pregnant state and diagnosis may be difficult owing to the altered haemodynamics.

During the second half of pregnancy the blood volume increases by about 25 per cent. due to retention of sodium by the body.

The precise mechanism is unknown but may be endocrine in origin. The cardiac output also increases by about 25 per cent., but for reasons which are obscure falls again during the last few weeks of pregnancy. Since the mean blood pressure does not alter, the work of the heart must be correspondingly increased.

Slight enlargement of the heart may be present from the increased blood volume. Breathlessness and peripheral oedema may occur even in the absence of organic heart disease. Innocent murmurs are also commonly present. Mild degrees of cardiac failure are not always easy to diagnose in pregnancy.

Pregnancy exerts an increased load on the heart and circulation, but if the heart is healthy there will be no untoward effects. Pregnancy does not cause heart disease but may inflict too great a burden on a diseased heart. The effect depends on the previous state of compensation.

About 90 per cent. of all cases of heart disease in pregnancy are due to previous rheumatic fever, and most of these have mitral stenosis. Congenital heart disease and hypertension account for most of the remainder.

It is important to emphasise that any functional classification based on the severity of symptoms is unreliable and potentially dangerous. A woman with mitral stenosis may be placed in Grade I or II early in pregnancy but die from a first attack of pulmonary oedema in the later months. Severity should be assessed on objective grounds.

In these days of planned families, the opportunity may be provided of giving advice before the patient becomes pregnant.

If signs of congestive cardiac failure are present, or have been present at any time in the past, pregnancy is not advisable. This rule applies even if the failure can be readily controlled, for the risk will be considerable to both mother and child. An exception may occasionally be allowed if the mother is extremely anxious to have a child and she and her husband are willing to take the risk; but there must be reasonably good cardiac compensation. Active rheumatic fever and bacterial endocarditis are definite contraindications. If there is no evidence of failure, the rhythm is normal, there is little or no dyspnoea and no great enlargement of the heart and the patient can be kept under close observation, then there is little added danger from pregnancy to a patient with mitral stenosis. However three children are enough for any woman with rheumatic heart disease and two if there is moderate disability. Age is important and the younger she can have her children the better from every point of view. The strain of having another child to look after may well prove greater than that of the pregnancy itself. Also most people with rheumatic mitral disease tend to develop atrial fibrillation by the age of 35-40, and the combination of fibrillation and the extra work entailed in looking after a toddler may be serious. It will be readily appreciated that economic factors are most important in that domestic help will allow the mother more adequate rest.

Although termination of pregnancy is a relatively minor matter in the early months the problem is very different later because an abdominal operation is necessary. Under medical supervision and treatment, continuation to term or until the child is viable and labour can be induced, is usually preferable. Natural delivery is probably safer than Caesarean section.

The best safeguard is repeated observation. By this means the progression of doubtful or manifest signs of cardiac failure may be detected at an early stage and appropriate treatment instituted. In such cases a period of rest in bed is important. Domestic help should be arranged if possible and extra rest is advisable during the day. Digitalis, diuretics and salt restriction will be indicated if failure is present. The therapeutic response to digitalis may assist diagnosis in the occasional difficult case. A restriction in salt intake is important. If these measures do not suffice complete bed rest will be needed and diuretics to decrease fluid retention. It is important that acute respiratory infections should be promptly treated as they may precipitate cardiac failure. Mitral valvotomy can be carried out if necessary during pregnancy but operative interference is rarely required if adequate medical treatment is given.

The periods of greatest danger are the seventh and eighth months and the first day or two after delivery. At these times congestive cardiac failure is particularly liable to occur. With due care and attention the great majority of cardiac patients can be safely shepherded through pregnancy. It is important to remember that a post-partum injection of ergometrine may be dangerous if heart failure has been present. Pulmonary oedema may result from the consequent increase in circulating blood volume.

PERICARDITIS

Pericarditis cannot be considered as a disease entity because there are many different causes and the clinical manifestations and prognosis largely depend on the underlying disease. Nevertheless certain symptoms and signs may occur whatever the aetiology and merit independent description. Adhesive pericarditis and chronic constrictive pericarditis will be discussed separately.

ACUTE PERICARDITIS

Aetiology

1. Rheumatic fever.
2. Tuberculosis.
3. Myocardial infarction.
4. Pyogenic infection.
5. Uraemia.
6. Malignant disease.
7. Trauma.
8. Idiopathic serous pericarditis.
9. Connective tissue (collagen) diseases.
10. Accidental trauma or thoracotomy.

Pathology. Pericarditis may be fibrinous, serous, haemorrhagic or purulent. In fibrinous pericarditis there is a fibrinous exudate on the surface which leads to varying degrees of adhesion formation and hence of obliteration of the pericardial cavity. In serous pericarditis there is in addition a serous exudate of anything from 100 ml. to 2 litres. The effusion is straw-coloured and often slightly turbid with a high protein content. A haemorrhagic effusion suggests a malignant origin. Purulent pericarditis is due to a pyogenic infection and the effusion is rarely large.

Clinical Features. Symptoms and signs of the underlying causative disease will be present. The clinical features will largely depend on whether or not a pericardial effusion is present.

PAIN. Pain is by no means always present and is probably dependent on involvement of the neighbouring pleura. It may occur in pericarditis of infective origin but rarely in other cases, e.g. in pericarditis secondary to uraemia, myocardial infarction or malignant disease.

A sensation of precordial oppression may be produced by a large pericardial effusion.

FRICTION RUB. Pericardial friction is the characteristic and diagnostic sign of pericarditis. It consists of a superficial scraping, scratching sound, usually best heard to the left of the sternum, often localised to a small area of the precordium and synchronous with the heart's action. It varies from time to time and may be quite transient. It may be aggravated by inspiration presumably because the adjacent pleural surface is involved.

EFFUSION. Signs of pericardial effusion are difficult to detect until about 500 ml. of fluid have accumulated. The area of cardiac dullness is increased especially to the left of the sternum and when the patient is lying down may extend beyond the apex beat when the latter can be located. The heart sounds may become muffled. An area of bronchial breathing may be found below the angle of the left scapula from compression of the lung. Many other signs of pericardial effusion have been described in the past, but they are variable and non-specific and have caused more confusion than clarification.

CARDIAC TAMPONADE. This term refers to compression of the heart by a large or rapidly increasing effusion or by constrictive pericarditis which interferes with diastolic filling of the heart. As a result the stroke output of the heart is diminished, tachycardia occurs, the blood pressure falls, the venous pressure is increased, and the clinical picture of shock may develop. Pulsus paradoxus may occur and has been described on p. 129.

RADIOLOGY. With a large effusion obliteration of the normal contours of the heart, widening of the base and diminished pulsation of the borders may be seen. Serial films may show significant changes of size over a short period of time.

ELECTROCARDIOGRAPHY. Serial electrocardiograms may reveal a diagnostic pattern in the S-T segment and the T waves.

Treatment, Course and Prognosis. This is essentially that of the underlying disease.

PARACENTESIS. Paracentesis of a pericardial effusion is rarely required but may have to be carried out for diagnostic purposes or to relieve severe symptoms from cardiac compression. The procedure is not without danger from puncture of the heart or of a coronary vessel and should only be carried out when strictly necessary. The needle may be inserted into the pericardial sac at any of the following places:

1. In the subcostal angle through the costoxiphoid notch. This is usually the best approach, the needle being directed upwards, backwards, and to the left.

2. In the 4th or 5th intercostal space just outside the cardiac impulse or just within the outer border of dullness on percussion.

3. In the 4th intercostal space 3 cm. to the right or left of the sternum.

Surgical drainage will usually be necessary if pus is found.

Aetiological Types of Acute Pericarditis

Rheumatic Pericarditis. This is the most common type of pericarditis in young people but has become much less frequent in recent years. It is invariably associated with rheumatic endocarditis and myocarditis (p. 212).

Tuberculous Pericarditis. Tuberculous pericarditis may be secondary to manifest pulmonary or mediastinal tuberculosis. The primary source may or may not be detectable. The disease sometimes begins with an acute febrile illness but is more commonly insidious in onset with vague malaise and low-grade fever. The subsequent course is chronic. An effusion usually develops and the pericardium may become thick and unyielding so that the heart is compressed (p. 269). Pleural effusions are often associated.

The diagnosis may be confirmed by aspiration of the fluid and direct examination or culture for tubercle bacilli. Injection of some of the fluid into a guinea-pig may be necessary for the isolation of the organisms. Treatment in the acute stage is by rest in bed with general nursing care and supportive measures, i.e. fresh air, good food and vitamin supplements. Streptomycin should be given together with PAS or isoniazid (p. 425). Aspiration must be carried out as required to relieve symptoms. In the inactive stage surgical relief may be necessary (p. 270).

Myocardial Infarction. Myocardial infarction may be complicated by fibrinous pericarditis if the infarct extends to the epicardial surface. The prognosis is not affected and no special treatment is required.

Pyogenic Pericarditis. Purulent pericarditis may be due to direct spread from an intrathoracic infection such as an empyema, to blood stream infection, e.g. from osteomyelitis, to extension of a subphrenic abscess through the diaphragm or to trauma through the chest wall. Treatment is by surgical drainage and chemotherapy.

Uraemic Pericarditis. This is a sign of impending death in renal failure and the diagnosis is made on discovering a pericardial rub, pain being unusual.

Malignant Pericarditis. This most commonly arises from direct extension of a bronchial carcinoma. The effusion when present may be haemorrhagic.

Traumatic Pericarditis. This may result from wounds through the chest wall and is then usually infected with pyogenic organisms (see above). It may follow injury by the steering wheel in car crashes.

Benign Serous Pericarditis. This condition has become increasingly recognised in recent years and occurs particularly in young adults. The aetiology is often obscure but a preceding upper respiratory infection is common and in some cases the Coxsackie virus has been isolated. Recovery occurs within a few weeks and there are no after effects, apart from occasional recurrences. There is no specific treatment.

Connective Tissue (Collagen) Diseases. Pericarditis may occur occasionally in this group of diseases (p. 556).

CHRONIC ADHESIVE (NON-CONSTRICTIVE) PERICARDITIS

This condition is not the same as chronic constrictive pericarditis (see below). It may be found at post-mortem examination in patients who had shown no symptoms or signs related to the heart during life and may result from any of the forms of pericarditis already mentioned. Adhesions exist between the two layers of the pericardium and apparently cause no embarrassment to the heart.

CHRONIC CONSTRICTIVE PERICARDITIS

A slowly progressive fibrosis of the pericardium develops as the result of previous infection and constricts the movement of the heart, so that it cannot expand in diastole. The fibrous tissue is far more thick, dense and inelastic than in adhesive pericarditis and calcification is common. The inflow of blood to the heart is impeded so that the cardiac output is diminished and the systemic venous pressure increased with resultant peripheral congestion. The heart is otherwise normal, though secondary atrophy of muscle fibres may occur.

The recognition of this condition is important because it is amenable to surgical treatment.

Aetiology. Most cases are probably due to tuberculosis, some to a pyogenic infection and in others the cause is obscure. Often there is no definite history of previous acute pericarditis.

Rheumatic fever may cause adhesive pericarditis as described previously but not constrictive pericarditis.

Clinical Features. Symptoms will depend on the degree of constriction around the heart.

Unlike other types of heart disease, breathlessness is relatively late in appearing and is not present at rest because the lungs are not congested, though some breathlessness on effort will occur as a result of the diminished cardiac output. Distension of the veins in the neck due to raised venous pressure is a notable feature. Enlargement of the liver and ascites occur relatively early compared with peripheral oedema. Concomitant pleural effusions are common in the tuberculous cases.

Examination of the heart is essentially normal, except that the apex beat is difficult to feel and a triple rhythm may be heard from the addition of a sound in early diastole, the pulse is rapid and of small volume, and there may be pulsus paradoxus (p. 129). An important feature in most cases is the absence of much enlargement of the heart. This would be unusual in almost all forms of congestive cardiac failure (with which this condition is often confused). Atrial fibrillation occurs in about 30 per cent. of cases.

Radiology. Calcification of the pericardium is frequently seen. Screening may show a small 'quiet' heart with diminished pulsation. Sometimes there is apparent enlargement because the pericardium is so thick. Pleural effusions may obscure the cardiac outlines.

Prognosis. The condition is serious unless pericardiectomy is performed. The operation may produce dramatic relief and considerable improvement is usual, but it may take several months for maximum benefit to be obtained. The operative mortality is 10-15 per cent., but operation has frequently been carried out too late owing to delay in diagnosis.

Treatment. Medical treatment can only produce slight or temporary improvement. The problem is a mechanical one and surgical resection of as much as possible of the pericardium is indicated. Pre-operative rest, restriction of sodium intake and administration of diuretics for a few weeks are usually advisable. Digitalis is not indicated.

SIMULATION OF HEART DISEASE

Functional Heart Disease

'Functional heart disease' is not a good term because it implies that some form of heart disease is present whereas in fact certain symptoms and signs have been misinterpreted and the heart itself is healthy. This is a common error in practice. Difficulties may arise in regard to symptoms, e.g. pain in the chest, palpitation, and the symptom complex commonly referred to as effort syndrome or in regard to signs, e.g. systolic murmurs and triple heart rhythm. The factors deemed to be of importance in the causation of functional disease are discussed on page 1248.

LEFT MAMMARY PAIN

This common symptom is apt to be mistaken for angina pectoris, an error which may be responsible for unnecessary invalidism. The pain is not felt across the middle of the chest, as in ischaemic heart disease, but usually in the neighbourhood of the left breast. It is described as a dull ache which persists for hours or even days and is often accompanied by sharp, shooting or stabbing pains. It may be referred down the left arm. The relationship to exertion is indefinite and inconstant. The pain is more likely to follow than accompany effort but may occur at any time, even in bed. There is no doubt about the reality of the pain which arises in the tissues of the chest wall but its precise cause is difficult to determine. It is rarely a single symptom but is usually accompanied by a number of other complaints as in the condition known as effort syndrome (below). Patients with left mammary pain tend to be hypersensitive individuals with unstable vasomotor systems and obvious anxiety or occasionally some more definite psychological disease. Anxiety (and left mammary pain) may, of course, be superimposed upon organic heart disease. A similar pain may be produced by muscular or ligamentous strain and it too is sometimes mistaken for angina.

Treatment. General management is discussed below under Effort Syndrome. If the pain is troublesome a local injection of 1 per cent. procaine into the painful area is worth trying.

PALPITATION

The term palpitation implies consciousness of the heart's action. It is usually due to anxiety and results from overactivity of the sympathetic nervous system. More often than not it occurs in the absence of heart disease but it may be a prominent feature of an anxiety neurosis, paroxysmal arrhythmia, thyrotoxicosis or sometimes of hypertension.

Extrasystoles may be responsible for an unpleasant sensation in the chest, sometimes referred to as a 'missed beat' or a 'thud' (corresponding to the augmented post-extrasystolic beat) or 'as though the heart turned over'. Extrasystoles are not, in themselves, indicative of heart disease (p. 155).

EFFORT SYNDROME

Effort syndrome is the term generally applied in this country to a condition formerly known as disorderly action of the heart (DAH) and referred to in the United States as neuro-circulatory asthenia.

The condition is difficult to define, but may be recognised by a characteristic series of symptoms and signs suggesting functional disorder of the autonomic nervous system. There is no evidence of organic disease. The diagnosis should not be made on the negative basis of excluding disease but on the positive evidence of recognising the syndrome. The symptoms are perfectly genuine and the pattern is far too uniform to be affected. It is a constitutional disorder usually determined by emotion. The subjects tend to be diffident, solitary, introspective and anxious. They are particularly averse to military service and fear is frequently responsible for this. The problem is also present in civilian life but these individuals have the opportunity of selecting suitable occupations, avoiding unpleasant situations and adapting themselves to their environment. War brings the condition into prominence and the various manifestations become exaggerated.

Though in common use, the term 'effort syndrome' is not a good one since the symptoms are not really similar to those produced by exertion in normal persons, although they may be unmasked by effort and limit strenuous activity. They may equally be precipitated by emotional stress. In most cases the appropriate psychological label can be attached to the individual.

Predisposing and Precipitating Factors. These are similar to any anxiety neurosis and are discussed on p. 1248.

Clinical Features

SYMPTOMS. These include breathlessness, nervousness, fatigue, palpitation, left mammary pain, dizziness, headache and sweating. Less common complaints include flushes, paraesthesiae, fainting and a variety of gastrointestinal symptoms. Left mammary pain and palpitation have already been discussed. A word may be said about breathlessness. Not only is this out of proportion to the amount of exertion undertaken but it is often present at rest. There is a sensation of inability to take a full or satisfactory breath and a deep sighing type of respiration is a characteristic feature. By contrast breathlessness at rest of cardiac origin would indicate serious disease for which an obvious cause would be present.

SIGNS. These include tachycardia, sweating, flushing, tremor and an obviously nervous manner. The hands are often cold and blue despite moist palms. Axillary sweating is also characteristic. There is no evidence of organic disease in the heart or any other system. The breath-holding test is usually positive, that is to say the breath cannot be held for more than about half the normal time of 60 seconds.

Differential Diagnosis. A thorough clinical examination supplemented by radiological examination of the heart and lungs will exclude most conditions liable to be mistaken for effort syndrome, e.g. valvular disease, hypertension and pulmonary tuberculosis. Thyrotoxicosis and anemia should be kept in mind.

Prognosis. The prognosis is excellent as regards life but very uncertain as regards the relief of symptoms.

Treatment. An initial thorough physical examination is essential but must not be repeated. Reassurance that the heart is healthy is most important. Sympathy and understanding, explanation and encouragement should be given in due proportion. Expert psychological help may be necessary (p. 1270).

Graduated physical training may be necessary in some cases. An appropriate occupation should be arranged whenever possible whether in time of peace or of war.

BENIGN SYSTOLIC MURMURS

A systolic murmur may be heard in many people in the absence of organic heart disease. Such murmurs are particularly common in the pulmonary area but may be heard at the apex or to the left of the lower sternum. Systolic murmurs not based on structural abnormalities in the heart may also frequently be heard in hyperkinetic states, e.g. anaemia, fever, thyrotoxicosis, pregnancy or tachycardia from any cause such as exercise or emotion.

Unwarranted restrictions have been imposed on the playing of games in young people and on childbearing, when in fact no heart disease is present. In the First World War innocent murmurs were often misinterpreted, down-grading was imposed and pensions subsequently granted. Once the existence of benign systolic murmurs was appreciated the pendulum began to swing too far in the other direction and between the wars there was often a tendency to ignore systolic murmurs. At the present time emphasis is placed on the careful assessment of each case in the light of all the available evidence.

The intensity of the murmur should be arbitrarily graded. The louder or harsher the murmur, the more likely it is to be of pathological significance. The presence or absence of enlargement of the heart and great vessels must be determined clinically and radiologically. Particular attention should be paid to the size of the left atrium in the right oblique position (with barium in the oesophagus) because enlargement usually accompanies mitral valvular disease. If a diastolic murmur can also be heard the systolic murmur is almost certainly due to organic disease.

The common causes of organic systolic murmurs should be considered i.e. rheumatic valvular disease and congenital defects. For practical purposes in the absence of any other evidence of relevant disease the murmur can be ignored, the patient reassured and no restrictions on activity should be enforced or suggested.

It is of course impossible to deny that slight rheumatic thickening of the valve leaflets may be responsible for a soft apical murmur.

* * * * * *

PREVENTION OF CARDIAC DISEASE

This is a most important aspect of heart disease, but is difficult to put into practice owing to ignorance of the aetiology of the principal causes, e.g. rheumatic fever, hypertension and coronary atherosclerosis.

Rheumatic Heart Disease

In Britain the incidence of rheumatic fever is falling due to improvement in the social conditions of the lower income groups and perhaps to the therapeutic effects of penicillin on streptococcal pharyngitis and tonsillitis. Rheumatic fever remains the principal cause of death from heart disease in middle-age. This is a serious economic problem from the point of view of manpower, and the cost of special facilities for treatment and convalescence. It is responsible for many children being deprived of their mother's care and upbringing at an early age.

Predisposing factors have already been mentioned (p. 207). Prolonged observation and care are necessary in the treatment of children or adults already suffering from rheumatic fever. It has been shown in epidemics that adequate treatment of a haemolytic streptococcal infection will prevent rheumatic fever.

Supervision is required to ensure that return to activity is carefully graduated. Children from poor homes undoubtedly benefit from prolonged convalescence, possibly in a special institution. Thereafter, supervision by the practitioner or in a special clinic is important to ensure early recognition of any recurrence of the rheumatic process or impairment of the general health.

Since recurrences are common following a first attack of rheumatic fever in young people prophylactic chemotherapy (p. 75) is indicated. The prompt treatment of acute upper respiratory infections, especially tonsillitis or pharyngitis, with antibiotics or chemotherapy is of paramount importance in reducing the risk of recurrences of rheumatic fever.

The general standard of nutrition in this country has greatly improved in recent years, but bad housing with the associated overcrowding and consequent increased risk of spreading infection is still a major problem in certain regions.

Bacterial Endocarditis

Subacute bacterial endocarditis occurs especially in persons who suffer from congenital heart disease or from rheumatic valvular disease. In both cases patients with mild lesions and little disability are as susceptible as those with gross lesions. Damaged valves and the site of non-valvular congenital deformities are liable to become infected even during transient low-grade bacteraemia such as so often occurs during upper respiratory tract infections or following removal of teeth or tonsils or operations on the urinary tract. Penicillin should be used for the treatment of such infections and to provide 'cover' for even minor operations which may result in transient bacteraemia (p. 75).

Hypertensive and Atherosclerotic Heart Disease

Heart disease due to hypertension or coronary atherosclerosis mainly occurs in middle and late adult life, i.e. the degenerative period. The immediate causes of these conditions are not known (pp. 227 and 216). The influence of heredity is undoubted, and obesity, insufficient physical exercise, anxiety, smoking, overwork and emotional strain are aggravating factors. Weight reduction in the obese is always advisable. The dietetic restriction of fat for the *prevention* of atherosclerosis is not warranted at the present time as its value is still debatable but it may be indicated in patients under 50 years of age who have already had cardiac infarction (p. 280).

In combating the diseases in this group, the aim must be to modify the whole life of susceptible persons in an attempt to reduce the influence of these adverse factors. This means that the early stages of the disease must be recognised. A yearly examination by a physician, though having the disadvantage of provoking introspection, has the advantage that the early stages of hypertension may be recognised and the life of the patient so ordered that the possible consequences may be delayed or averted.

Thyrotoxic Heart Disease

Cardiac complications can be avoided by early and adequate treatment of thyrotoxicosis.

Syphilitic Heart Disease

Syphilitic infection may be masked by prompt treatment for gonorrhoea without subsequent attendance for observation. Thorough treatment of all cases, education of the public to recognise the risk of neglecting the facilities for treatment which are available in all large centres, and social efforts to combat the causes which result in the spread of venereal disease are the means which will prevent cardiovascular syphilis.

Congenital Heart Disease

The factors in the germ cells or environment which determine defective development are obscure. In severe cases multiple congenital anomalies may occur, but congenital heart disease does not often run in families, and so heredity cannot be a significant factor.

It has been noted that German measles (rubella) contracted by the mother during the second or third month of pregnancy is frequently followed by the development of congenital cardiac lesions in her child. Hence women in the early stages of pregnancy must not come in contact with cases of German measles, or if they do they should be given γ globulin. In contrast no active measures should be taken to prevent children, especially girls, from coming in contact with a case of rubella.

Diphtheritic Heart Disease

Diphtheria can be prevented by immunisation in childhood and its dangers greatly reduced by early diagnosis and treatment.

* * * * * *

DISEASES OF ARTERIES

Although it must be admitted that little is known about the fundamental causes of the diseases of arteries, for clinical purposes it is convenient to classify arterial disease under the general headings of degenerative and inflammatory or allergic causes. It is important to emphasise that most of these conditions are recognised during life only when symptoms arise and that the latter are usually due to ischaemia of the tissues supplied by the affected vessels.

DEGENERATIVE ARTERIAL DISEASE

There are three main types of degenerative arterial disease:

1. Arteriosclerosis, arteriolar sclerosis and arteriolar necrosis.
2. Atherosclerosis (atheroma).
3. Medial sclerosis.

It is not at all uncommon to find at autopsy in elderly patients that all three types of arterial degenerative disease are present to a greater or lesser extent. Such changes as thickening of the intima, medial fibrosis and loss of elasticity which appear to constitute part of the normal ageing process can undoubtedly occur in the absence of hypertension. It must also be appreciated that pathological changes are largely dependent on the type of vessel involved.

ARTERIOSCLEROSIS

Arteriosclerosis is a term which in the past has been applied rather indiscriminately to various unrelated forms of arterial disease. Its retention is justified only if it is confined to the degenerative changes which are part of the normal ageing process and which affect the whole arterial tree. These changes involve the middle coat and later the intima of the vessel and are the result of a compensatory mechanism by which the vessels react to the normal intra-arterial pressure. This explains why the condition is found at its maximum in middle-aged and elderly people. Since the medium and large vessels are mainly affected and their lumina are not greatly reduced in size, clinical features are usually absent. If, however, hypertension develops these arteriosclerotic changes are accelerated and exaggerated so that the process may be said to have progressed from a physiological to a pathological state. The small arteries and arterioles are then particularly affected. In the initial stage hypertrophy of the media, splitting of the internal elastic lamina and collagenous thickening of the intima occur. Later degenerative changes develop with atrophy of muscle fibres and overgrowth of connective tissue with subsequent hyalinisation. Swelling of the intima leads to progressive narrowing of the lumen. These changes are often referred to as 'arteriolar sclerosis', and are particularly well seen in the kidneys of patients with essential hypertension. They are also found in the vessels of the pancreas, spleen and liver. Since the pathological changes in the kidney are patchy in distribution patients with arteriolar sclerosis seldom die from renal failure but succumb to cardiac failure or a cerebral vascular accident.

If hypertension develops rapidly in a severe form, as occurs in patients with malignant hypertension, still more extensive damage to the arterioles may result. These changes include necrosis of the vessel wall, which is infiltrated with a fibrin-like material, and the intima may be markedly thickened. Hence the term '*arteriolar necrosis*'.

ATHEROSCLEROSIS

Introduction. The great increase in the incidence of ischaemic heart disease in recent years is a matter of concern to doctors, research workers and laymen. There must be few persons who have reached middle age who have not lost a friend or relative at the height of his career and with his family responsibilities at a maximum as a result of disease of the coronary arteries. It is therefore important that the family doctor should be able to give his patients sound information and sensible advice on the pathogenesis, prevention and treatment of atherosclerosis and its sequelae. The fundamental causes of both atherosclerosis and intravascular thrombosis are complex.

Pathology. Atherosclerosis principally affects the aorta, large arteries and certain medium-sized vessels, particularly the coronary and cerebral arteries. It becomes increasingly common as age advances, but it is not an inevitable concomitant of ageing, and there is a great variation in its extent and severity. Although often associated with and accelerated by hypertension, atherosclerosis may be advanced even in the presence of a normal blood pressure. It may also occur in response to a local rise of pressure in the pulmonary arteries of patients with pulmonary hypertension. The pulmonary artery is not otherwise subject to atherosclerosis.

The essential lesion of atherosclerosis is the intimal thickening or plaque, the most important constituents of which are cholesterol and other lipids which may be free in the intimal tissues or inside cells. At a later stage the vessel becomes narrowed and its lining membrane roughened. During life atherosclerosis is recognised by its effects on the body, but it should be remembered that the absence of clinical features does not exclude its presence since it develops in many persons of all ages who are apparently in good health. When narrowing of a vessel occurs, serious impairment of the blood supply to important structures may result. Coronary atherosclerosis, for example, is responsible for angina pectoris, cerebral atherosclerosis for many mental changes in old age, and atherosclerosis in the vessels of the legs may be responsible for intermittent claudication. The affected vessels are liable to thrombosis and this may result for example in cardiac infarction, hemiplegia or senile gangrene. Atherosclerosis may exist for a long time without giving rise to intravascular thrombosis. A damaged arterial intima certainly predisposes to thrombus formation, but the factors actually responsible cannot be accurately stated.

In the aorta and its main branches there is widening due to replacement of elastic by fibrous tissue.

Pathogenesis. In recent years there has been a notable increase in the sequelae of atherosclerosis, and in particular of ischaemic heart disease, and also a change in the occupational and class incidences. Forty years ago ischaemic heart disease was essentially a disease of business men and members of the professions and was uncommon in a woman. Since then there has been a significant and steady increase in all classes, but especially in the working class, in men under 45, and in women over the age of 50 years.

In underdeveloped countries where the standard of living is low, the incidence of ischaemic heart disease is less than in countries where material prosperity is high. The incidence is much less in Africans and Asians living under their primitive natural conditions than in Europeans or Americans living in the same regions or in their homelands. Investigations into the incidence of ischaemic heart disease, the dietary intake of fat and the level of the cholesterol in the plasma have been carried out in many countries and in most of them a significant correlation was demonstrated between these three factors. However, a correlation can also be established between the increased incidence of coronary thrombosis and an increase in many other factors associated with the improved standard of living, e.g. increased sales of motor cars, radio and television sets, tobacco, etc. Hence the need for caution in interpreting the aetiological significance of such correlations. It has been clearly established that when Africans or Asians become prosperous and live under similar conditions to Europeans and North Americans both the plasma cholesterol and the incidence of ischaemic heart disease increase. It would appear therefore that environmental factors are of more importance than race. During the past 40 years a great increase in material prosperity has occurred, especially among the working classes, in countries which are the seat of industrial development and mechanisation. This has led to alterations in the way of living which may contribute to the pathogenesis of atherosclerosis including quantitative and qualitative changes in the diet, decrease in the amount of physical exercise and increased cigarette smoking. Perhaps of equal importance are constitutional genetically determined factors which control lipid and carbohydrate metabolism. The majority of young subjects with coronary disease have abnormally elevated plasma lipids and, within a highly developed country such as Britain, individual variations in diet are insufficient to account for this finding.

Relation of atherosclerosis and its sequelae to diet Since the lipids contained in atherosclerotic plaques are qualitatively similar to those circulating in the blood, the fat content of diet has received particular attention. However there is also evidence to suggest that the sugar content and to a less extent the protein content may be important. It has been demonstrated by clinical trials that it is possible by dietary measures to produce a coincidental decrease in the level of plasma cholesterol and β-lipoproteins. This can be achieved either by using a diet low in animal fat in which saturated fats, e.g. animal fats and dairy produce, are restricted to 30 g. or less daily, or by a diet in which unsaturated fats, e.g. vegetable oils from soya bean, maize or sunflower seed are substituted for saturated fats. Unfortunately the process of hydrogenation, which is widely used in the making of margarine and other artificial butters from vegetable oils, converts most of the unsaturated fatty acids into saturated fatty acids. The *unsaturated fat diet* is more effective in lowering the level of serum lipids than the *low fat diet*. Another advantage is that its ingestion may lead to a decrease in blood coagulability in contrast to a saturated fat diet which leads to increased coagulation. Blood coagulation is obviously a matter of great importance to persons with atherosclerosis.

Despite the clearly established fact that these diets can effectively reduce the plasma lipids, satisfactory evidence is still not available to prove that they can prevent the development of atherosclerosis or improve the prognosis of its sequelae, namely ischaemic heart disease, cerebral vascular diseases and peripheral vascular disease. Until the results of further trials have been published it is not justifiable for the prevention and treatment of atherosclerosis or its sequelae to insist on a *rigid exclusion* of animal fat from the diet and its replacement by unsaturated fats in the form of vegetable and marine oils. Nevertheless, *some restrictions of dietary fat* are indicated for patients who already have clinical evidence of atherosclerosis and for persons who are potential candidates for this disorder, namely individuals in prosperous communities who lead sedentary lives and have reached middle age, especially if they are obese and have high blood pressure. This does not mean they must partake of irrational diets or make any material change in traditional food habits. In simple language such people should restrict their intake of butter, cream and pastries; they should choose lean portions of bacon, ham, beef or mutton. Fried foods should be avoided. There is no reason for them to restrict rigidly the cholesterol content of the diet which would in fact mean the exclusion of eggs, since the level of cholesterol in the plasma is not affected by the dietary intake unless eaten in very large amounts. These dietary restrictions also have the beneficial effect of reducing obesity.

Stricter dietary measures are advisable after an attack of coronary thrombosis occurring in a patient *under the age of* 50 who is of the *male sex* and who has a *family history* of ischaemic heart disease and a *raised plasma lipid level.*

A new method of lowering raised plasma lipid levels is to use Atromid-S (ethylchlorophenoxyisobutyrate) which increases the hepatic turnover of lipid and promotes the excretion of fat from the body. No dietary changes are necessary and a daily dose of 2 g. is effective. Insufficient time has elapsed to establish its therapeutic value.

Exercise. With the mechanisation of industry and the development and widespread use of motor vehicles, the proportion of people who take hard exercise has declined and the proportion of sedentary workers, including office workers and business executives, has increased (p. 444).

Under natural conditions appetite plays an important part in the control of caloric intake and there is experimental evidence to suggest that for the accurate regulation of appetite a certain minimum amount of physical exercise is necessary. Inactivity may be an important factor in the causation of 'creeping' overweight in Western societies and in the development of atherosclerosis.

For the above reasons and because there is evidence that physical exercise *per se* lowers the plasma cholesterol, patients should be advised to be as active as possible, and to take regular exercise. Walking is especially to be recommended, as are recreations such as golf and gardening. Strenuous exercise is contraindicated in middle-aged or elderly persons, especially if they have had any clinical manifestations of atherosclerosis, since this may lead to rupture of diseased vessels or to subintimal haemorrhage in the coronary arteries.

Endocrine Glands. The observation that ischaemic heart disease is rare in women before the menopause and that after the age of 55 the difference in the incidence between the sexes becomes less, suggests the possibility that oestrogens have some protective influence. Likewise the increased incidence of coronary thrombosis which occurs in patients with myxoedema and diabetes, diseases in which the level of plasma cholesterol is raised, suggests that the secretion of the thyroid gland may also be of importance. Although the administration of oestrogens and thyroid hormones can lower the level of cholesterol in the plasma of both man and experimental animals, there is no evidence to show that the prognosis of ischaemic heart disease can be improved by their use.

SMOKING. Statistical data show that peripheral vascular disease and ischaemic heart disease, particularly myocardial infarction, occur more frequently in heavy cigarette smokers than in those who do not smoke. The mechanism by which nicotine or some other constituent of tobacco causes this adverse effect is not clear. It may be due to the vasoconstrictor action or to some undesirable effect on the level of plasma lipids or on the coagulability of the blood and the survival of platelets. Patients with ischaemic heart disease should be advised to give up smoking.

MEDIAL SCLEROSIS

This condition, sometimes referred to as Mönckeberg's sclerosis, affects the muscular coats of medium-sized peripheral and superficial arteries and is responsible for the 'pipe-stem' arteries commonly found in old age, e.g. in the radial arteries and the vessels to the lower limbs. Calcification of the media is the characteristic change. Since there is little or no narrowing of the lumen (unless there is associated atherosclerosis) the condition is of little clinical significance. It plays no part in the aetiology of hypertension.

DISSECTING ANEURYSM OF THE AORTA

In this condition a tear occurs through the intima secondary to necrosis of the media. As a result blood makes its way between the layers of the vessel wall and strips them apart to form a new channel. Death usually occurs from rupture through the adventitia into the pericardium or elsewhere. Some patients are hypertensive. In women it may occur with pregnancy. The onset is very sudden with severe, tearing, retrosternal pain which often radiates into the neck, back, abdomen or into the legs. It may be precipitated by exertion. In some cases the condition may simulate myocardial infarction. The heart sounds, however, are unchanged and the blood pressure is maintained, unless shock is present. Neurological features may result from occlusion of branches of the aorta supplying the spinal cord.

PERIPHERAL VASCULAR DISEASE

The term peripheral vascular disease is used to describe the characteristic clinical picture which develops when the blood supply to the limbs is impaired.

Peripheral vascular disease may be suggested by pain and swelling or by changes in colour, temperature or arterial pulsation in the extremities or by obvious trophic changes with ulceration or gangrene. These disturbances may result from organic obstruction of the vessels secondary to obliterative disease or from changes in vasomotor tone leading to vasoconstriction or vasodilatation. Obliterative disease and vasoconstriction are often associated.

The principal cause of obliterative disease is atherosclerosis which will therefore be discussed first. Thromboangiitis obliterans is a far less common cause and is referred to later.

Obliterative Vascular Disease secondary to Atherosclerosis

Males are more commonly affected than females and most cases occur after the age of 50. Atherosclerosis is rarely seen in the upper limbs. It is particularly common in diabetes.

Pathology. This is discussed on p. 279.

Symptoms. The principal symptoms which follow impairment of blood supply to the extremities are (1) pain, which may occur on exercise (intermittent claudication) or at rest, especially when the limb is warm at night and (2) cold extremities.

Although the pathological changes are usually present in both lower limbs, symptoms commonly present only on one side.

By intermittent claudication is meant pain which develops on exercising a limb and which disappears with rest. It most commonly occurs in the calf or foot on walking. The pain is due to relative ischaemia of the muscles and its mode of production is similar to that of cardiac pain in coronary disease. When the pain occurs at rest it signifies severe ischaemia. Pain which is relieved by elevation of the part suggests venous obstruction, and pain which is relieved by dependency suggests gross arterial obstruction. Patients seldom die from peripheral vascular disease but frequently succumb to coronary thrombosis.

Physical Examination. It is very important not only to assess the degree of impairment of the blood supply to the limbs but also to determine the relative importance of organic obstruction and of vasoconstriction in its production.

SKIN. The skin should be inspected for trophic changes, i.e. dryness and scaling, inelasticity, loss of hair, brittle nails, change of colour, delay in the return of colour after blanching with light finger pressure, ulceration or gangrene. The new technique of thermography is proving useful in the mapping out of skin temperatures.

TEMPERATURE. After exposure to room temperature for at least 20 minutes, the temperature of the two sides is compared. Where gross lesions are present in one limb the lowered temperature can be recognised by simple palpation. For the detection of temperature changes due to less marked obliterative disease, a skin thermometer or thermocouple is necessary.

ARTERIAL PULSATIONS. The examination must be made when the limbs are warm. All accessible arteries should be palpated.

Lower Limbs. Femoral, below the inguinal ligament; popliteal, behind the knee; posterior tibial, behind the internal malleolus; dorsalis pedis, between the bases of the first and second metatarsals.

The possibility of normal variations must be remembered, e.g. in 10 per cent. of healthy people one dorsalis pedis pulse and in 5 per cent. neither pulse, can be felt, even when the limbs are warm.

Upper Limbs. Axillary, brachial, radial and ulnar arteries are all readily accessible.

In addition to pulsation the condition of the vessel wall should be noted for thickness, irregularity, tortuosity or calcification.

POSTURAL CHANGES. If an ischaemic limb is first raised 45 degrees above the horizontal it will blanch more quickly than normal. If then placed in the dependent position there will be delay in venous filling and in flushing. These changes are due to arterial insufficiency.

NERVOUS SYSTEM. Peripheral neuritis may occur from impairment of the blood supply to the nerves.

Reactive Hyperaemia. The limb is warmed and raised to 45 degrees above the horizontal until the blood is drained out. A sphygmomanometer cuff is placed around the proximal end of the limb and inflated in order to obliterate the arterial pulsation for four minutes. When the pressure is released the limb should flush down to the extremity within about 10 seconds. In obliterative vascular disease there may be a delay of several minutes.

Tests for Vasomotor Tone. Temporary inhibition of sympathetic vasoconstrictor tone may be achieved in a number of ways and serves as a useful guide to the degree of improvement likely to follow operative treatment and hence for selecting cases for sympathectomy.

1. *Reflex Vasodilatation.* After exposing the affected limb to room temperature until the skin temperature is constant, the trunk, or an unaffected limb, is heated to 42° C. Normally, reflex vasodilatation occurs due to the release of vasomotor tone by the direct action of the warmed blood on the heat-regulating centre in the brain. In disease, response will be diminished.

2. *Diagnostic Procaine Block.* The sympathetic vasomotor fibres can be temporarily blocked with procaine, in the anterior spinal roots by spinal anaesthesia, in the sympathetic ganglia by paravertebral block or more peripherally by nerve block. In tests 1 and 2 the subsequent rise of temperature in the affected limb is measured and compared with that on the normal side.

Oscillometry. The approximate level of arterial occlusion may be ascertained by means of an apparatus which measures arterial pulsations. However, weak pulsation does not necessarily mean that the circulation is seriously impeded.

Radiology

1. *Radiography.* Calcification will be shown if present. Calcification is especially common in Mönckeberg's sclerosis but does not necessarily indicate that the arterial lumen is significantly narrowed.

2. *Arteriography.* Intra-arterial injection of a radio-opaque solution (Urographin) will show the site of vascular occlusion and the presence (or absence) and extent of the collateral circulation.

Treatment. Until the pathogenesis of atherosclerosis has been clearly established and until specific measures are discovered which are accepted as being effective for its prevention and cure, the treatment of peripheral vascular disease must continue to be unsatisfactory. If diabetes is present it should be treated on the usual lines (p. 750), and this also applies to obesity (p. 449). The relation of saturated and unsaturated fats to lipid metabolism and to atherosclerosis is discussed on p. 279.

COLD should be avoided and suitable woollen clothing worn especially on the limbs. Bed socks should be worn at night and sheets may with advantage be replaced by blankets. In cold weather woollen underclothes, extending to the ankles in men and to the knees in women and young girls, should be worn. Central heating in cold weather is very helpful. The application of heat to the affected limb is harmful because the local metabolism is raised but the blood flow cannot be correspondingly increased.

PROTECTION AGAINST TRAUMA and the early treatment of sepsis is most important. Detailed instructions on the care of the feet and nails must be given. The feet should be kept scrupulously clean, carefully dried after washing, especially between the toes, and dusting powder containing zinc oxide and salicylic acid applied. Nails should be cut carefully and corns pared with caution. It is wise to employ the services of a chiropodist. Socks and shoes should be well fitting. Exposure to cold must be avoided. Even the slightest abrasion should be taken seriously and medical advice sought. Rest in bed and dressings to keep the part dry are required for any breach of surface.

Fungal infection between the toes should always be treated.

The measures discussed above are of great value in the prevention of gangrene.

DRUGS are usually of little value even when an element of spasm is present, but vasodilators, such as tolazoline (Priscol) 25-50 mg. t.d.s. or the nicotinic acid derivatives, Ronicol, 25 mg. t.d.s. or Hexopal, 200 mg. t.d.s. are worthy of trial in patients with ischaemic changes involving the lower limbs.

MEASURES TO IMPROVE THE BLOOD SUPPLY

(*a*) *Reflex Dilatation.* The trunk or an upper limb is placed under a heat cage or electric blanket. The warm blood stimulates the vasomotor centre with consequent relaxation of vasomotor tone in the vessels of the affected limb.

(*b*) *Buerger-Allen Exercises.* The legs are raised and supported

45 degrees above the horizontal for one minute (or until blanched), then lowered over the side of the bed or couch for a minute until thoroughly pink. While still dependent the feet are dorsiflexed and plantarflexed alternately and the toes are moved repeatedly for two minutes. This cycle is repeated four to six times, three or four times a day. There is little evidence that this treatment is of more than psychological value.

OPERATION. Sympathectomy may be advised before an advanced stage is reached provided preliminary tests show that some improvement of the collateral circulation is possible from the release of vasomotor tone. In many cases the results are disappointing. In selected patients with localised disease arteriectomy, removal of the atherosclerotic lining or the insertion of a graft can be undertaken. Long-term anticoagulant therapy is advisable in selected cases.

SYMPTOMATIC TREATMENT. Pain and insomnia should be relieved by suitable analgesics and hypnotics (p. 196). Pain at rest may be reduced by raising the head of the bed or by lowering the limb below the horizontal and keeping it cool. *Smoking* should be forbidden because it causes vasoconstriction.

TREATMENT OF GANGRENE. Areas of gangrene should be kept clean and dry until a clear line of demarcation appears. Thereafter surgical treatment will have to be undertaken.

TREATMENT OF ASSOCIATED CONDITIONS

(*a*) Diabetes. (*b*) Obesity. (*c*) Insomnia.

SUDDEN OCCLUSION OF A MAJOR ARTERY

This may result from thrombosis or embolism. The limb becomes painful, cold, numb and pale, and pulses distal to the block are absent. The outcome depends on the collateral circulation and on subsequent treatment. Pain should be relieved and the limb kept at rest and exposed to room temperature. The other limbs and body should be kept warm and reflex vasodilatation encouraged by an electric blanket or hot-water bottles to the trunk. Smoking is forbidden. Heparin 15,000 units intravenously is given at once followed by 10,000 units six-hourly for 24 hours. At the same time an anticoagulant is commenced by mouth (p. 223). Embolectomy may have to be considered if there is not rapid improvement. Sympathectomy may be of value after the acute stage is over. Amputation may be necessary for gangrene.

INFLAMMATORY OR ALLERGIC ARTERIAL DISEASE

The principal types of inflammatory or allergic arterial disease are:

1. Syphilis (p. 260).
2. Thrombo-angiitis obliterans.
3. Polyarteritis nodosa.
4. Cranial arteritis.
5. Non-specific aortitis.

Other conditions such as rheumatic arteritis and endarteritis obliterans do not in themselves give rise to clinical manifestations and hence will not be discussed further.

Thrombo-Angiitis Obliterans

(Buerger's Disease)

This condition is a relatively uncommon cause of obliterative vascular disease.

Aetiology. This is obscure. The condition usually begins before the age of 40 and is almost confined to males. Cigarette smoking is probably an important aetiological factor. The lower limbs are principally affected, but vessels in the arms or elsewhere may be involved.

Pathology. The condition is probably inflammatory. All three coats of the arteries are infiltrated with polymorphs and the lumen is obstructed by clot. The adjacent vein and nerve are often involved and the three structures may become matted together by fibrous tissue. Recanalisation may occur in time.

Clinical Features. The symptoms and signs are essentially those of diminished blood supply to the limb (p. 284) but the severity of the pain often seems to be out of proportion to the degree of ischaemia. This may be due to associated neuritis. The method of examination and tests of function used in thrombo-angiitis obliterans are the same as those employed in peripheral vascular disease due to atherosclerosis.

In the early stages vasomotor symptoms occur as in Raynaud's disease (p. 295) and are followed by intermittent claudication and rest pain. In the leg trophic changes develop and finally gangrene so that amputation may become necessary. Superficial thrombophlebitis is seen in a proportion of cases and its occurrence should always raise the suspicion of Buerger's disease especially if migratory.

The disease is a serious one and the course is usually slowly progressive though often with prolonged remissions. Vascular accidents, e.g. coronary or cerebral thrombosis, are prone to occur.

Treatment. There is no specific treatment and the measures described on p. 286 should be applied. Sympathectomy should always be considered because the condition is often localised. It is essential that smoking should be given up completely. Any drug given intravenously which may irritate the intima, e.g. thiopentone, should never be given to patients with thromboangiitis obliterans because a severe attack of thrombophlebitis may follow.

Polyarteritis Nodosa

This is an uncommon condition of unknown aetiology, most often seen in young men. The condition may be allergic in origin. The characteristic lesions consist of multiple nodules on the smaller arteries. The vessel wall is infiltrated by polymorphs and necrosis follows with resultant aneurysmal dilatations. Thrombosis may occur in the lumen. Clinical features such as fever, tachycardia, wasting, sweating and generalised pains, are accompanied by local manifestations of ischaemia in various parts of the body. The vessels of the kidney, gastrointestinal tract, heart, peripheral nerves and skin are particularly affected giving rise to such varied manifestations as haematuria, abdominal pain, angina, pericarditis, peripheral neuritis, subcutaneous nodules or localised oedema. There may be leucocytosis or eosinophilia. Hypertension is usual at some stage. The course is usually progressive but mild cases may recover, particularly those which only involve the skin. There is no curative treatment, but steroids are worthy of trial (p. 722). Administered before vascular damage is too extensive, they have produced remarkable remissions in some patients. The outlook in more advanced cases is less hopeful. The fibrosis which follows healing of the vascular lesions may be sufficiently extensive to lead to myocardial infarction or renal failure. In view of the serious outlook, however, the administration of steroids is justified however advanced the disease.

Cranial Arteritis

Cranial arteritis may be related to polyarteritis nodosa (p. 290) or to polymyalgia rheumatica (p. 567) but it is a distinct clinical entity which is so named because the striking clinical finding is tender, thickened cranial arteries.

The vessel wall is infiltrated by mononuclear cells, plasma cells and giant cells. Focal necrosis occurs in the media. The formation of granulation tissue is followed by scarring. Thrombosis may occur in the lumen.

The vessels of the scalp, particularly the temporal arteries, are usually affected but other vessels may also be involved, for example those of the retinae and brain, and the condition may be widespread throughout the body. Intense headache, photophobia, dimness of vision and sometimes blindness are prominent features. General systemic manifestations include fever, malaise, arthralgia, anorexia, weakness and loss of weight. The cause of the disease is unknown. It affects elderly persons, and usually ends in recovery after several months. There is no specific treatment, but steroid therapy is of great symptomatic value.

DISEASES OF VEINS

THROMBOPHLEBITIS

Thrombophlebitis is the term commonly applied to all forms of intravenous thrombosis.

A distinction is sometimes made between thrombophlebitis, when the endothelium is injured by inflammation, and phlebothrombosis when simple clotting occurs. Such differentiation is not always possible.

Aetiology. Although thrombosis may occur for no apparent reason one or more of the following factors may be of importance.

1. *Injury to the endothelium of the vessel wall.* Injury may be due to inflammation or trauma and may follow accidents, operations, labour, intravenous infusions or injections. The vessel wall may be invaded by cancer cells or become involved in neighbouring inflammatory processes.

2. *Increased coagulability of the blood.* This may result from any form of tissue damage. The precise cause of the decrease in clotting time is obscure but is probably related to metabolic changes affecting clotting factors and the platelet concentration. This may occur after surgical operations, myocardial infarction, accidental injury or injury to the pelvic tissues in labour.

Increased liability to clotting also occurs in dehydration and polycythaemia due to an increase in blood viscosity.

3. *Slowing or obstruction of the blood stream.* This may result from rest in bed, especially in the elderly or when a faulty position is assumed, e.g. Fowler's position, particularly when a pillow is placed under the knees and the calves are compressed or from tight bandaging and binders. Congestive cardiac failure also leads to slowing of the circulation. Circulatory stasis is probably the most important factor in the aetiology of venous thrombosis.

Clinical Features. Venous thrombosis is most common in the lower extremities. It is usually of little local significance as regards the legs apart from pain and oedema, but the potential sequelae of embolism may be dangerous (see below).

In thrombophlebitis, local pain, tenderness and swelling are often accompanied by constitutional disturbances such as fever, malaise and leucocytosis. The clot is usually firmly attached to the wall of the vein and hence there is relatively little risk of embolism; but there is always a risk of embolism from associated phlebothrombosis in deeper veins. If the phlebitis is superficial there will be local redness of the overlying skin and the tender thrombosed vein can be felt.

In phlebothrombosis the process is relatively silent and the diagnosis is easily missed. The clot is usually not firmly attached to the wall and embolism is frequent. Dilatation of the veins and increased warmth of the affected limbs may be noted. Sometimes there is associated arterial spasm, in which case the swollen leg is pale and cold ('white leg').

Sequelae

Local. If a vessel of considerable size is occluded and the collateral venous drainage is inadequate, marked oedema of the limb will develop. If treatment is inadequate or delayed, swelling may persist and become a serious disability.

General. If the clot or a portion of it becomes detached it will pass into the right side of the heart and hence into the pulmonary circulation resulting in pulmonary embolism or pulmonary infarction. If the embolus is large, sudden death may occur (p. 253).

Early Diagnosis. In surgical wards it is now customary for the legs of all patients who have been operated upon to be examined daily. Attention should be paid to the presence of oedema and the feet and calves carefully palpated for local tenderness. Dorsiflexion of the foot may cause pain in the calves (Homans' sign). Unexplained fever or tachycardia should arouse suspicions of early thrombosis, and any complaint of pain or even discomfort anywhere in the lower extremities calls for detailed examination.

It should be remembered that venous thrombosis is also common in medical wards especially in patients with congestive cardiac failure and in elderly patients who are confined to bed.

Prophylaxis. This aspect is of the greatest importance. Obviously it is desirable to minimise operative trauma but efforts must chiefly be directed to the prevention of venous stasis. If confinement to bed is unavoidable patients should be encouraged to move about in bed as soon as possible. In hospitals exercises can be organised under the supervision of a physiotherapist. Breathing exercises are also of value. Faulty posture, tight bandages, cardiac failure and dehydration must receive attention.

Treatment. Obvious superficial thrombophlebitis and thrombosis in varicose veins are rarely dangerous to life. On the other hand thrombosis in deep veins, with or without pain or a general reaction, may be exceedingly dangerous and calls for immediate anticoagulant treatment. The occurrence of pulmonary embolism, however small, must be taken as a warning sign that further serious embolism may follow.

The treatment of phlebitis occurring in superficial veins or varicose veins is different from that in deep veins unless occurring in patients being treated in bed or for cardiac failure.

A strip of felt should be laid over the thrombosed portion of the superficial vein and covered by a supporting elastic bandage. The patient is encouraged to move about as soon as possible. Analgesics should be given when pain is present. Phenylbutazone is of value for superficial phlebitis, not only for the relief of pain but because of its anti-inflammatory action. It should rarely be given for longer than one week.

In cases of deep vein thrombosis, the patient should always be treated initially in bed. Ten days is usually sufficient. The limb should be elevated by raising the end of the bed. In severe cases it may be necessary to elevate the limb still further by suspending it in a Hodgen splint for a period of up to three weeks. The patient is then allowed up whether or not the swelling has completely disappeared. A bandage or elastic stocking is applied first thing in the morning before the patient gets out of bed. Elevation of the foot of the bed and the wearing of an elastic support may have to be continued permanently for patients who have had thrombosis of the iliac or femoral vein.

Anticoagulant therapy should be given to all patients with deep vein thrombosis, but is seldom necessary for superficial vein thrombosis. Treatment with anticoagulants should be given in the manner described on p. 223 and continued for 7-10 days at least.

General Treatment. Deep breathing exercises and straining at stool are dangerous in the early days following venous thrombosis because they tend to encourage pulmonary embolism.

Ligature of the Vein. Should the thrombosis extend proximally despite anticoagulants, surgical interruption of the vein above the involved segment is sometimes carried out.

Thrombosis in Special Sites

As already indicated, thrombosis occurs most commonly in the veins of the lower limbs, particularly in the saphenous vein and in the deep femoral vein. It occurs much less frequently in the axillary vein, in the pelvic veins following labour or after pelvic operations, or in the splenic vein as a concomitant of cirrhosis of the liver, or as a sequel to infection or trauma.

Suppurative Thrombophlebitis. This is a rare but very serious condition usually occurring in the veins of the abdomen or pelvis following sepsis or surgical operations. Extension into the portal vein and to the liver is a particular danger. Lateral sinus thrombosis may follow suppuration in the ear or nasal sinuses.

Thrombophlebitis Migrans. This is a troublesome, prolonged but usually self-limiting condition involving the superficial veins. The possibility of an association with thrombo-angiitis obliterans and with visceral cancer, particularly of the pancreas should be remembered. Thrombosis is recurrent, may occur in crops and tends to appear in different sites. Sometimes pulmonary infarction occurs, but it is usually impossible to determine whether this is from local thrombosis or from embolism from the periphery and in this disease it is not often fatal.

Recurrent phlebitis should always raise the possibility of cancer, particularly of the pancreas.

VASOMOTOR DISORDERS

Raynaud's Phenomenon

Raynaud's phenomenon is the name given to a peripheral vascular disturbance consisting of intermittent tonic contraction of the digital arteries, which is precipitated by cold, emotion and by other causative factors mentioned below. Primary Raynaud's phenomenon usually starts in childhood and may occur in either sex, being no more than an exaggerated physiological response to cold. The term 'secondary Raynaud's phenomenon' is used to describe the disorder which occurs secondary to pressure of a cervical rib, to obliterative arterial disease, or to certain occupations in which the arms and hands are exposed to high frequency vibrations from pneumatic drills, polishing tools, etc. or occasionally to cold agglutinins and cryoglobulins. The changes are virtually confined to the digits. Severe forms may lead to secondary changes in the arterioles and ultimately to gangrene.

Pathogenesis. Lewis considered that the peripheral spasm was due to increased susceptibility to cold producing a local effect on the smooth muscle of digital arterioles and that vasomotor tone was normal. More recently Raynaud's original view that the recurrent attacks of symmetrical vasospasm were due to abnormal activity of the vasoconstrictor nerves has been upheld.

Pathology. In the early, uncomplicated stages, there are no pathological changes. Later obliterating endarteritis occurs, often with thrombosis in the lumen. Prolonged asphyxia will lead to ischaemic changes in the skin of the digits and nails, superficial necrosis and finally gangrene (sclerodactyly). Sometimes sclerosis occurs in the subcutaneous tissues and is followed by diffuse contraction (scleroderma).

Clinical Manifestations. Mild forms are common in both sexes as the familiar 'dead fingers'. Severe forms are usually seen in emotional women of nervous temperament between puberty and the menopause. Symptoms are bilateral and fingers are more affected than toes, beginning at the extremities. Parasthesiae, e.g. numbness, tingling and burning, are more prominent than pain. Sensitivity to cold may be extreme and disabling.

Colour changes usually consist of three phases: pallor, cyanosis and redness. If the limb is bloodless it will be pale. If blood flow is sluggish excessive deoxygenation results in cyanosis. Redness is a rebound phenomenon due to excessive vasodilatation (reactive hyperaemia) which may follow spasm.

Diagnosis. It is important to exclude the presence of any underlying disease, as discussed above.

Treatment. Vasodilator drugs as discussed in the section on peripheral vascular disease (p. 287) may be tried, but the results are very disappointing. Protection from cold, as described on page 287, is all-important. In severe cases, sympathectomy, to remove vasomotor tone, should always be considered, but the long-term results are often disappointing. Smoking should be given up.

Acrocyanosis

This is a functional vascular disorder precipitated by cold and characterised by striking cyanosis particularly of the fingers, hands, ears and nose which disappears on warming. Arterial pulsations are normal and trophic changes do not occur. There is no pain. Chilblains are common. Warm clothing should be worn and vasodilator drugs tried. Sympathectomy should be advised for severe cases which fail to improve on the above measures.

Chilblains

Chilblains are due to local areas of vasoconstriction with vasodilatation beyond, and are usually most marked in the digits. Treatment is mainly preventive by warm surroundings, warm clothing, plenty of exercise and good food. Central heating has almost abolished chilblains in North America. Calcium, vitamin D and nicotinic acid are widely used but are of doubtful value.

Erythrocyanosis

In this condition a bluish-red discoloration of the legs occurs and is accompanied by burning and itching, which may be very troublesome. The feet feel cold. It is confined to young women with fat legs. In severe cases, there is thickening of the subcutaneous tissues, sometimes with the formation of nodules. The skin becomes atrophic. The condition develops in cold weather and clears up in the summer. Long skirts and woollen stockings alleviate the condition but such advice is often unwelcome. Sympathectomy is usually undertaken for severe cases.

Erythromelalgia

This is a rare condition and the very antithesis of Raynaud's disease. The vessels of the legs are dilated with full bounding pulses. As a result the feet become red and burning and sometimes painful to such a degree that the condition is intolerable and incapacitating. Symptoms are precipitated by exercise, heat and the dependent position. Raising the legs gives relief. Since sympathectomy may also prevent active vasodilatation as well as vasoconstriction, this operation is indicated for severe cases.

R. W. D. TURNER.

Books recommended:

Friedberg, C. K. (1966). *Diseases of the Heart*, 3rd ed. Philadelphia: Saunders.

Turner, R. W. D. (1964). *Electrocardiography*, 2nd ed. Reprint. Edinburgh: Livingstone.

Wood, P. (1965). *Diseases of the Heart and Circulation*, 2nd ed. Reprint. London: Eyre & Spottiswoode.

DISEASES OF THE RESPIRATORY SYSTEM

INTRODUCTION

ANATOMY

THE respiratory system is divided for descriptive purposes into the upper and lower respiratory tracts, the dividing line being the lower border of the cricoid cartilage. This division is an arbitrary one and must not be allowed to obscure the intimate relationship of upper respiratory disease to disease of the bronchi and lungs. For example, an upper respiratory infection such as sinusitis may under certain conditions give rise to bronchitis or even to pneumonia. Conversely, lung disease may be responsible for disease in the upper respiratory tract, as in the case of tuberculous laryngitis complicating pulmonary tuberculosis.

THE UPPER RESPIRATORY TRACT

The upper respiratory tract, which includes the nose, nasopharynx and larynx, is lined by vascular mucous membrane covered by ciliated columnar epithelium. The rich blood supply ensures that the inspired air enters the lungs at body temperature

KEY TO Fig. 44

Major Bronchi

R.M.	Right main bronchus.	L.M.	Left main bronchus.
R.U.L.	Right upper lobe bronchus.	L.U.L.	Left upper lobe bronchus.
R.M.L.	Right middle lobe bronchus.	LING.	Lingular bronchus.
R.L.L.	Right lower lobe bronchus.	L.L.L.	Left lower lobe bronchus.

Segmental Bronchi[1]

Right upper lobe.	1. Apical. 2. Posterior. 3. Anterior.
Right middle lobe.	4. Lateral. 5. Medial.
Right lower lobe.	6. Apical. 7. Medial basal (cardiac). 8. Anterior basal. 9. Lateral basal. 10. Posterior basal.
Left upper lobe.	1. Apical. 2. Posterior. 3. Anterior.
Lingula.	4. Superior. 5. Inferior.
Left lower lobe.[2]	6. Apical. 8. Anterior basal. 9. Lateral basal. 10. Posterior basal.

[1] The names of the segmental bronchi are not included in the text but are given here for future reference, numbered according to international agreement.
[2] There is no medial basal bronchus on the left side.

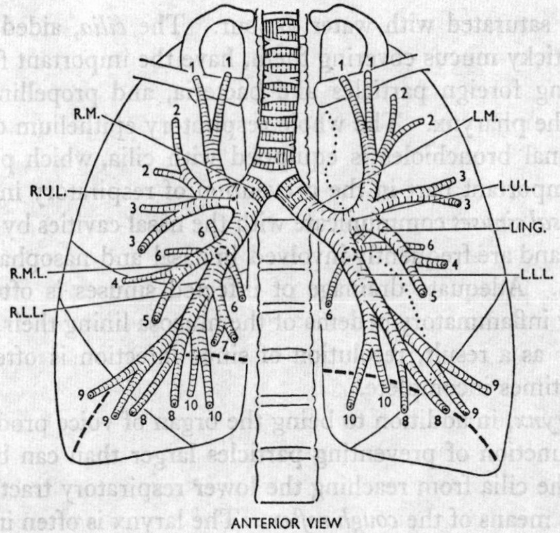

A

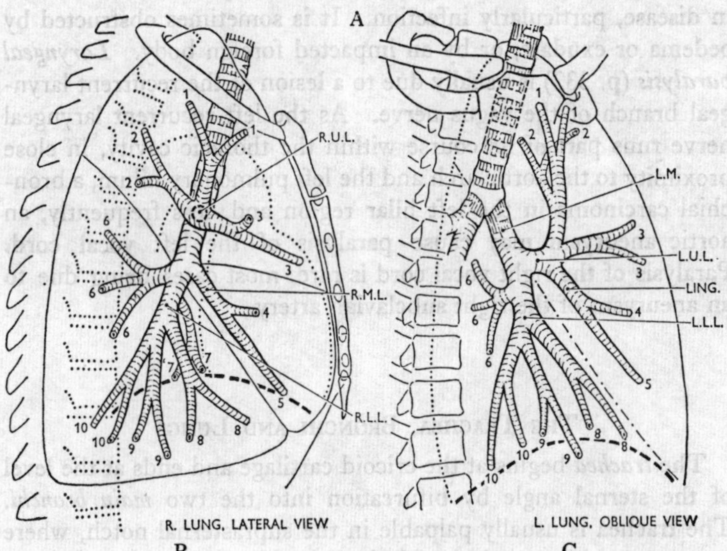

B C

FIG. 44

THE ANATOMY OF THE BRONCHI

A Right and Left Bronchi. B Right Bronchi. C Left Bronchi.

The oblique view of the left bronchi is shown in preference to the lateral view because at bronchography (p. 317) the right bronchi are normally outlined first and a lateral view of the left bronchi cannot then be obtained. The oblique view, which must be taken instead, has the additional advantage of showing the disposition of the left bronchi more clearly.

and fully saturated with water vapour. The *cilia*, aided by the layer of sticky mucus covering them, have the important function of trapping foreign particles and bacteria, and propelling them towards the pharynx. The whole respiratory epithelium down to the terminal bronchioles is equipped with cilia, which probably play an important part in the prevention of respiratory infection.

The *nasal sinuses* communicate with the nasal cavities by narrow openings and are frequently involved in nasal and nasopharyngeal infections. Adequate drainage of infected sinuses is often prevented by inflammatory oedema of the mucosa lining their narrow openings: as a result, resolution of sinus infection is often slow and sometimes incomplete.

The *larynx*, in addition to being the organ of voice production, has the function of preventing particles larger than can be dealt with by the cilia from reaching the lower respiratory tract. This it does by means of the *cough reflex*. The larynx is often involved in disease, particularly infection. It is sometimes obstructed by oedema or exudate, or by an impacted foreign body. *Laryngeal paralysis* (p. 332) is usually due to a lesion of the recurrent laryngeal branch of the vagus nerve. As the left recurrent laryngeal nerve runs part of its course within the thoracic cavity, in close proximity to the aortic arch and the left pulmonary hilum, a bronchial carcinoma in the left hilar region and, less frequently, an aortic aneurysm may cause paralysis of the left vocal cord. Paralysis of the right vocal cord is rare, most cases being due to an aneurysm of the right subclavian artery.

The Trachea, Bronchi and Lungs

The *trachea* begins at the cricoid cartilage and ends at the level of the sternal angle by bifurcation into the two *main bronchi*. The trachea is usually palpable in the suprasternal notch, where in normal subjects it is exactly in the midline. Deviation of the trachea to either side, in the absence of a local lesion in the neck, is a valuable indication of displacement of the upper mediastinum.

The *right main bronchus* is more vertical than the left, with the result that a foreign body entering the trachea in a subject standing erect is more likely to lodge in that bronchus or one of its divisions than the left. The right main bronchus first gives off from its lateral wall the *upper lobe bronchus* and then from its anterior wall the *middle lobe bronchus*, after which it continues as the *lower lobe bronchus*. The *left main bronchus* gives off the *upper lobe bronchus* from its lateral wall and continues as the *lower lobe bronchus*. The tongue-shaped part of the left upper lobe corresponding to the middle lobe on the right side is supplied by a large branch of the left upper lobe bronchus, named the *lingular bronchus* by reason of the shape of the part of lung which it supplies. The anatomical position of these bronchi is shown diagrammatically in Figure 44.

The three lobar bronchi on the right side and the two on the left divide and subdivide like the branches of a tree (the term 'bronchial tree' is in common use) until the terminal bronchi ('respiratory bronchioles') are reached. Each respiratory bronchiole communicates with a cluster of alveoli, and the 'bronchopulmonary lobule' so constituted is the basic structure of all lung tissue. The alveoli are tiny air vesicles bounded by a single layer of flattened epithelial cells which are in direct contact with the pulmonary capillaries. Exchange of the respiratory gases, oxygen and carbon dioxide, takes place between the air in the alveoli and the blood in the pulmonary capillaries.

The *right lung* differs from the left in having three lobes instead of two. The *left lung* is divided into *upper* and *lower lobes* by the *oblique fissure* which extends from the junction of the fourth or fifth rib with the vertebral column behind to the sixth costochondral junction in front, crossing the mid-axillary line at the level of the fifth rib. As the posterior end of the fissure is at a much higher level than its anterior end, the upper lobe, as well as being *above* the lower lobe, is also largely *in front of it*. It therefore follows that upper lobe lesions produce physical signs mainly on the front of the chest and lower lobe lesions on the back.

On the *right* side the oblique fissure corresponds in position to that on the left, but the lung above it is divided into *upper* and *middle lobes* by the *transverse fissure*, which runs laterally in a horizontal direction from the junction of the fourth costal cartilage with the sternum to join the oblique fissure at the level of the fifth rib in the mid-axillary line. The middle lobe is thus situated behind the lower part of the anterior chest wall.

Each lobe is composed of two or more *bronchopulmonary segments*, which represent the portions of lung tissue supplied by the main branches of each lobar bronchus.

In many diseases, e.g. pneumococcal pneumonia, atelectasis and lung abscess, the lesion is typically confined to a single lobe or segment. A knowledge of pulmonary anatomy, when applied to the interpretation of radiographs, may thus be of value in determining the nature of the lesion as well as its situation.

Pleura

Each lung is closely invested with *visceral pleura. Parietal pleura* lines the chest wall, mediastinum and diaphragm, and is continuous with the visceral pleura at the pulmonary hilum. In health the two pleural layers are separated only by a thin film of lymph, but between them there is a negative (subatmospheric) tension. This results from the natural tendency of the lung to recoil towards the hilum, a property given to it by the rich supply of elastic fibres in the bronchi and blood vessels.

If a communication develops with the atmosphere as, for example, with a penetrating wound of the chest wall or from the rupture of an emphysematous bulla, the negative intrapleural tension draws air between the pleural layers and the potential intrapleural space becomes a real one. There is then said to be a *pneumothorax*. When the space is created by the presence of clear fluid there is said to be a *pleural effusion* or a *hydrothorax*; by pus, an *empyema*; by blood, a *haemothorax;* by both clear fluid and air, a *hydropneumothorax*; by both pus and air, a *pyopneumothorax*; and by both blood and air, a *haemopneumothorax*.

When the pleural space contains air or fluid the elastic recoil of the underlying lung is to some extent released and the lung shrinks towards the hilum, this shrinkage being referred to as *pulmonary collapse*. The larger the amount of air or fluid between the pleural layers the more marked is the degree of pulmonary collapse and the greater the impairment of function of the collapsed lung. If the quantity of air or fluid is very large it causes displacement of the mediastinum towards the opposite side, with the result that function of the opposite lung is also impaired. A gross degree of mediastinal displacement may, in addition, embarrass the action of the heart. Mediastinal displacement is recognised clinically by alteration in position of the trachea and of the cardiac apex beat.

Collapse of the lung may also occur without air or fluid in the pleural space. This type of collapse, usually described as *atelectasis*, is due to bronchial obstruction (p. 366).

Mediastinum

The anatomy of the mediastinum has an important bearing on the diagnosis of intrathoracic disease, particularly tumours and aneurysms. These lesions are liable to involve mediastinal structures and, as a result, certain readily recognisable symptoms, physical signs and radiological abnormalities may be produced. The structures involved and the abnormality produced in each case are discussed in the section on mediastinal tumours (p. 380).

PHYSIOLOGY

The following is an attempt to condense and simplify the complex subject of respiratory physiology, and to select clinically important aspects.

The Control of Respiration

Rhythmic discharges originating in the reticular substance of the brain stem (the 'respiratory centre') provide the basis for co-ordinated respiratory movements. Lesions of the brain stem may thus distort the respiratory pattern and produce abnormalities such as periodic breathing. The basic rhythm of the respiratory centre is modified by centripetal impulses from many sources:

1. Those from the cerebral cortex allow conscious control of the rate and depth of breathing for a limited time.
2. An increase in the hydrogen-ion concentration in the blood or cerebrospinal fluid excites intracranial receptors which relay stimulatory impulses to the respiratory centre, thus increasing ventilation.
3. An increase in the partial pressure of CO_2 (P_{CO_2}) in the arterial blood (and therefore inside all cells) results in central stimulation of respiration by a similar mechanism.
4. A fall in the partial pressure of O_2 (P_{O_2}) in arterial blood causes hypoxia, which excites receptor cells in the carotid bodies; these send stimulatory impulses to the respiratory centre via the glossopharyngeal nerves.

CO_2 and hydrogen-ions are effective only above certain concentrations in the blood (thresholds). The hypoxic stimulus is not strong unless arterial P_{O_2} is below 60 mm. Hg. but becomes very powerful at about 30 mm. Hg. Hypoxia seems to act by increasing the sensitivity of the respiratory centre to CO_2; complete anoxia (asphyxia) depresses it. Pyrexia also increases the sensitivity of the centre, and movement of the limbs may reflexly increase ventilation. Pulmonary inflation-deflation (Hering-Breuer) reflexes are weak in man but may become important in pulmonary disease. Physiologically, respiration is stimulated most conspicuously during exercise, and depressed by sleep. Any drug which causes sleep depresses breathing; some, such as opiates, may depress it specifically.

Ventilation of the Lungs

The pulmonary ventilation-rate (minute-volume) is normally about 6 litres per minute at rest and may exceed 100 *l.*/min. during the heaviest exercise. One fifth to one third of the minute-volume ventilates the conducting airway (respiratory 'dead space'). The rest constitutes the *alveolar ventilation*, which is normally about 4 *l.*/min. at rest. Ventilation of the dead space increases when the respiration rate is raised. It follows that with a rapid rate of breathing a greater total ventilation is needed to yield a normal alveolar ventilation. Generalised hypoventilation of the alveoli occurs when respiration is depressed by sleep, narcotics, anaesthetics or intracranial disease; it may ensue when paralysisaffects the respiratory muscles, and it may be associated with gross obesity in which it is primarily due to mechanical limitation of thoracic and diaphragmatic movements. Generalised alveolar hypoventilation always produces hypoxia and hypercapnia (an increase in blood P_{CO_2}) when air is breathed. Breathing oxygen corrects the hypoxia but not the hypercapnia, as the partial pressure of CO_2 in the blood is governed solely by the level of alveolar ventilation and by the amount of CO_2 produced in the tissues. Arterial P_{CO_2} indeed reflects alveolar ventilation and CO_2-production just as the blood urea concentration reflects renal urea clearance and the metabolic production of urea.

Distribution of Gas and Blood to the Lungs

A normal alveolar ventilation is not fully effective unless it is distributed uniformly to different parts of the lungs and is matched by uniform distribution of blood. The composition of blood leaving an alveolus depends upon its composition on entering the alveolar capillaries (mixed venous blood) and upon the ratio between the ventilation of, and blood flow around, the alveolus. This *ventilation/perfusion ratio* may vary from zero (perfusion but no ventilation) to infinity (ventilation but no perfusion). Mismatching of ventilation and blood flow to the alveoli is far the commonest cause of hypoxia and hypercapnia. A minor degree of mismatching is normal, especially in the erect position. In disease, ventilation may be locally impaired by (*a*) bronchial or bronchiolar obstruction (tumour, secretions, asthma), (*b*) local destruction of elastic tissue, (*c*) pulmonary infiltration and consolidation, and (*d*) chest wall deformities. If, in response to local underventilation, total ventilation is increased, other alveoli will be overventilated. Alveolar perfusion is reduced or stopped by pulmonary embolism and thrombosis, by destruction of areas of the pulmonary capillary bed and sometimes when alveoli are densely consolidated. Increased perfusion occurs normally in the lower lobes in the erect posture.

When a substantial number of normally perfused alveoli are not being adequately ventilated, this tends to reduce P_{O_2} and O_2-saturation, and to increase P_{CO_2}, in the arterial blood. Whether it does so or not depends upon the number of perfused alveoli which are over-ventilated, and thus able to compensate to some extent for those which are under-ventilated. Three situations may exist:

1. *Arterial* P_{O_2} *and* O_2*-saturation low*: P_{CO_2} *high*. Here the overventilation of normal alveoli is insufficient to compensate for the failure of underventilated alveoli to oxygenate the blood and to eliminate CO_2.

2. *Arterial* P_{O_2} *and* O_2*-saturation low*: P_{CO_2} *normal*. The high P_{CO_2} in blood leaving underventilated alveoli has been exactly balanced by the low P_{CO_2} in blood leaving overventilated alveoli. The O_2-deficiency in blood from the underventilated alveoli is, however, greater than the extra amount of oxygen which can be added in the overventilated alveoli, because blood leaving normal alveoli is already 98 per cent. saturated with O_2.

3. *Arterial* P_{O_2} *and* O_2*-saturation low, or (rarely) normal*: P_{CO_2} *low*. Overventilation of normal alveoli has more than compensated for the failure of underventilated alveoli to eliminate CO_2. The stimulus for this overventilation is arterial hypoxia, which cannot, however, be corrected by overventilation unless the proportion of underventilated alveoli is very small.

It can be seen that when there is mismatching of the ventilation and perfusion of substantial numbers of alveoli, normal values for *both* arterial P_{O_2} and arterial P_{CO_2} cannot possibly coexist while the subject is breathing air. The effect of breathing pure O_2 will be discussed in the section on oxygen therapy (p. 318).

Diffusion of Gases in the Lungs

O_2 and CO_2 are exchanged across the alveolar membrane by diffusion from a site of higher to one of lower partial pressure. Diffusion may be hampered if the total area of the membrane is reduced (e.g. in emphysema) or if the membrane is thickened (e.g. in diffuse pulmonary fibrosis). Since CO_2 is 20 times as soluble as O_2, it diffuses much more rapidly. A pure diffusion defect thus causes hypoxia before it impairs the transfer of CO_2. Since the hypoxia causes hyperventilation, arterial P_{CO_2} is subnormal. Hypoxia and hypocapnia (a decrease in blood P_{CO_2}) may also result from distribution defects (see above). Most conditions which impair diffusion also disturb distribution; in many the distribution effect is the more important cause of the blood-gas changes.

The Work of Breathing

The respiratory muscles, in ventilating the lungs, do mechanical work of two kinds. The first kind of work is done against elastic forces in the lungs and chest wall, which together tend always to bring the chest to the position it occupies at the end of a normal expiration. Expiration or inspiration from this position of equilibrium involves the performance of 'elastic' work and the storing of potential energy which is then available to do 'viscous' work (see below) during the return to the position of rest. Thus, during quiet breathing, inspiration is 'active' and expiration 'passive'. The other kind of work is frictional or 'viscous' work and is expended in forcing air through the air-passages and in displacing soft and inelastic tissues. Work of this kind is not stored as mechanical energy but is converted into heat and motion, and it must be done during both inspiration and expiration.

Elastic work is increased when the lungs or chest wall are made more rigid by pulmonary congestion, infiltration or fibrosis, or by ankylosing spondylitis or scleroderma. Viscous work is increased by rapid breathing (with or without change in depth), by obstruction of the airway, as in tumour, asthma or emphysema, and by obesity and deformity of the chest. The work done by the respiratory muscles may be expressed in terms of their oxygen consumption; each rise of 1 *l.*/min. in ventilation normally requires an extra O_2 consumption of 0·5 to 1 ml./min. whereas patients with emphysema may need an extra 10 ml./min. or more. A person's ability to increase ventilation is reduced by old age, general unfitness (an important but neglected factor in patients who get little exercise) and by various kinds of paralysis of the respiratory muscles, as well as by the factors which increase the work of breathing.

Tests of Pulmonary Function

Disturbances of control, ventilation, distribution, diffusion and respiratory work can all be measured. Most of the tests require special skill and apparatus, but two of them are easily performed, and yield results sufficiently accurate for clinical purposes.

1. *Estimation of arterial* P_{CO_2} *(rebreathing method*[1]*)*. This test does not require arterial puncture and takes only 10 minutes to complete. Arterial P_{CO_2} is normally 36 to 44 mm. Hg., and is always increased when there is inadequate alveolar ventilation, sometimes to 80 mm. Hg. or more.

2. *Estimation of forced expiratory volume (FEV) and vital capacity (VC)*. This test requires a special recording spirometer, preferably incorporating an electronic timing device. The $FEV_{1·0}$ is the biggest volume which can be expired, from full inspiration, in one second. It provides information about ventilatory capacity (p. 311) and can be used to assess improvement or deterioration. In health the $FEV_{1·0}$ may be 3,500 ml. or more, and amounts to at least 80 per cent. of the VC. In diseases such as bronchial asthma and emphysema, which produce narrowing of the air passages during expiration, both $FEV_{1·0}$ and VC are reduced but the reduction in $FEV_{1·0}$ is proportionately greater, i.e. the FEV/VC ratio is reduced, perhaps to 40 per cent. or less. In diseases such as diffuse pulmonary fibrosis and ankylosing spondylitis, which render the lungs or chest wall more rigid, the FEV and VC are reduced proportionately and the normal FEV/VC ratio of 80 per cent. is preserved. These simple measurements are

[1] Campbell, E. J. M. & Howell, J. B. L. (1959). In *A Symposium on pH and Blood Gas Measurement*, ed. Woolmer, R. F. London: Churchill.

thus of value in distinguishing between one type of respiratory disorder and another, as well as in providing an index of its severity. Serial measurements can also be used to observe changes in functional status, whether occurring spontaneously or in response to treatment.

Estimations of pH, P_{O_2} and O_2-saturation of arterial blood are specialised laboratory procedures, but may be of considerable value in the management of severe ventilatory failure.

VENTILATORY FAILURE

The lungs exchange CO_2 for O_2 at a rate equal to the metabolic turnover of these gases; any discrepancy between tissue metabolism and external (pulmonary) respiration can only be temporary if life is to continue. The balance is achieved in such a way that blood and tissue concentrations of CO_2 and O_2 remain within limits which we recognise as 'normal'. In ventilatory failure there is a reduction in alveolar ventilation, either absolute or relative to the increased requirements imposed by pulmonary disease, and external respiration can then be maintained only at the cost of a change in the internal chemical environment. For example, a normal CO_2 output of 200 ml./min. can be achieved with a normal alveolar ventilation of 4 *l.*/min. and an arterial P_{CO_2} of 40 mm. Hg, or with an alveolar ventilation of 2 *l.*/min. and an arterial P_{CO_2} of 80 mm. Hg. Such a rise in P_{CO_2} implies, of course, a considerable increase in the body-store of CO_2; but, once achieved, this store remains constant until the alveolar ventilation changes again. Similar adjustments occur in the case of oxygen.

Ventilatory failure is thus recognised, and its degree measured, by estimation of the arterial P_{CO_2}. It may occur in the absence of pulmonary disease in conditions such as narcotic poisoning (p. 103), paralysis of the respiratory muscles and severe thoracic kyphoscoliosis. The commonest pulmonary cause is acute infection complicating chronic bronchitis and emphysema. The most severe type of ventilatory failure is that which produces both hypoxia and hypercapnia as a result of generalised alveolar hypoventilation p. 304). 'Compensated' distribution defects form a transitional type of ventilatory failure, for although there is hypoxia the arterial P^{CO_2} is normal or low (p. 305). Pure diffusion defects, if they exist, can hardly be classified as ventilatory failure, as in patients with hypoxia attributed to this cause alveolar ventilation is invariably increased.

When ventilatory failure is present and the arterial P_{CO_2} is high, a small reduction in ventilation results in a greater rise in P_{CO_2} than when the P_{CO_2} is normal. The administration of pure O_2, by removing the hypoxic stimulus, may have this effect, and the P_{CO_2} may increase to narcotic levels (120 mm. Hg. or more), with consequent further depression of breathing. The hypoxic stimulus depends on arterial P_{O_2}, not on O_2-saturation, and it is usually possible to improve saturation considerably without greatly depressing respiration, provided that the arterial P_{O_2} is not unduly raised. This can be achieved by making the patient breathe air slightly enriched with O_2, rather than pure O_2. The treatment of ventilatory failure is described on p. 320.

COMMON CLINICAL MANIFESTATIONS OF RESPIRATORY DISEASE

1. **Cough.** Cough is the most frequent of all respiratory symptoms. It may be short, painful and half-suppressed, as when dry pleurisy accompanies pneumonia. It may be loose and readily productive of sputum as in bronchiectasis, or paroxysmal, ineffectual and exhausting, as in some cases of chronic bronchitis and asthma. It may be an early symptom in bronchial carcinoma but is often relatively late to develop in pulmonary tuberculosis. Generally it is worse at night or on waking. Often it is aggravated by changes in temperature or weather. The explosive character of a normal cough is lost when laryngeal paralysis is present ('bovine cough'). Cough is accompanied by stridor in whooping-cough and in the presence of laryngeal or tracheal obstruction.

2. **Sputum.** Purulent sputum is due to infection in the respiratory tract and is typically seen in acute bronchitis, infective exacerbations of chronic bronchitis, bacterial pneumonia, bronchiectasis and lung abscess. In the last two conditions the sputum may be copious and is sometimes foetid. Mucoid sputum is due to oversecretion of bronchial mucus. It is frequently present in chronic bronchitis and bronchial asthma. In early cases of pulmonary tuberculosis the sputum is mucoid but in advanced cases it is usually purulent.

3. Haemoptysis. Haemoptysis of all grades of severity may occur, from slight streaking of the sputum with blood, which is a common symptom in acute and chronic bronchitis, to a massive haemorrhage. Frank haemoptysis, however small, must always be regarded as of potentially serious significance and demands the fullest investigation. Bronchial carcinoma, pulmonary infarction, bronchiectasis, pulmonary tuberculosis and mitral stenosis are the most common causes.

4. Chest Pain. Broadly speaking there are only two types of chest pain associated with respiratory disease:

(*a*) Central retrosternal pain of a sore, 'scratchy' character made worse by coughing, but not by deep breathing, and usually caused by inflammation of the trachea (tracheitis).

(*b*) Lateral chest pain, usually in the pectoral or axillary regions but sometimes in the back, of a sharp, stabbing character, made worse by deep breathing and coughing, and caused by inflammation of the pleura.

The second type of pain, which is referred to as *pleural* or *pleuritic* pain, is of greater clinical importance than the first and is a common symptom in respiratory disease. The pain is thought to be due to stretching of the inflamed parietal pleura (the visceral pleura is insensitive to painful stimuli) and, as would be expected, it is maximal at the end of inspiration. Patients with pleuritic pain try to minimise it by taking shallow breaths and by suppressing cough as much as possible. The pain is referred to the area of skin supplied by the same spinal nerves as those supplying the inflamed area of pleura. Usually it is referred to the chest wall, but when the pleura lining the diaphragm is inflamed it may be referred to the cutaneous distribution of the supraclavicular nerves which have the same spinal roots (third and fourth cervical) as the phrenic nerve. Pain in the front and top of the shoulder is thus characteristic of *diaphragmatic pleurisy*. Pleuritic pain may also be referred to the anterior abdominal wall, where it may be difficult to distinguish from the pain of an acute abdominal emergency.

The *pleural rub*, which is a common physical sign in dry pleurisy, is due to the rubbing together of pleural surfaces roughened by fibrinous exudate.

The effusion of fluid between the layers of the pleura diminishes pain by reducing the movement of the chest wall and abolishes the pleural rub by separating the pleural surfaces.

5. **Dyspnoea** is a subjective state in which breathing is a conscious effort. Though a symptom, it may be apparent to an observer. It is conventional to ascribe dyspnoea to the interplay of two factors. One, the maximum ventilatory capacity, is a reasonably precise concept and a rough estimate of it can be made by measuring the FEV (p. 307). The other factor is the ventilatory demand, which may have a variety of meanings; in the case of a healthy person doing submaximal exercise the ventilatory demand is simply the actual ventilation. When actual ventilation amounts to more than a certain fraction of the maximum available ventilation, such a person feels breathless—his 'ventilatory reserve' is encroached upon. The precise point at which breathlessness appears will, however, depend upon other factors, notably psychological ones—tedious activity allows more introspection than does pleasurable exercise or flight from danger. This concept of dyspnoea is useful if it is not pressed too far. It may partly account for the dyspnoea of neurosis. It provides an explanation in patients who overventilate because of abnormalities of distribution or diffusion (p. 305) or because, owing to 'stiff' lungs, they waste much of their ventilation in the respiratory dead space (p. 304). It embraces those patients whose ventilatory capacity is reduced, many of whom must also overventilate because of pulmonary disease.

Several common observations, however, do not accord with this simple formula. Why do we feel 'breathless' if we hold our breath to breaking point? This has nothing to do with actual ventilation (there is none) nor with reduced ventilatory capacity. Why do paralysed patients often feel intensely breathless while being adequately ventilated by a mechanical respirator? They are doing no respiratory work and their blood gas tensions are normal. Moreover, their 'breathlessness' may disappear as the days go by, under exactly the same mechanical and biochemical conditions. These questions illustrate the complexity of this common symptom.

Dyspnoea is a feature of some conditions other than disease of the heart or lungs. Notable among these are metabolic acidosis (ketosis, renal failure), in which the acidotic stimulus to breathing is an adequate explanation, and anaemia and hyperthyroidism, in which the cause of the dyspnoea is not properly understood.

6. **Cyanosis** (p. 125). Central cyanosis in respiratory disease may result from alveolar hypoventilation (p. 308), or from defects of distribution or diffusion (p. 304), or from combinations of these. Arterial O_2 saturation is normally above 95 per cent. Central cyanosis may not be clinically obvious unless the arterial saturation is below 80 per cent., or lower if anaemia is present. Clinical recognition of cyanosis is greatly helped by comparing the patient's tongue, buccal mucosa or nailbeds with a normal person's, side by side in daylight.

The term *hypoxaemia* denotes a reduced O_2 content of arterial blood. This may be due to undersaturation, to a reduction in O_2 capacity (as in anaemia or carbon monoxide poisoning) or to a combination of both factors. See section on O_2 therapy (p. 318).

7. **Hypercapnia.** Alveolar hypoventilation always results in a rise in arterial P_{CO_2} (normally 36-44 mm. Hg. at rest) unless metabolic production of CO_2 falls at the same time. Hypercapnia commonly arises also from mismatching of ventilation and perfusion of alveoli (p. 304). Hypercapnia at rest is therefore found (*a*) when there is diminished responsiveness of the respiratory centre to CO_2 or (*b*) when mechanical limitation prevents a normally responsive centre from producing an *adequate* alveolar ventilation. When the work of breathing is greatly increased, any extra activity of the respiratory muscles may produce CO_2 faster than it can be eliminated, and in these patients arterial P_{CO_2} *rises* when ventilation increases.

Clinical features by which hypercapnia may be recognised include warm extremities, headache, drowsiness, sweating, coma and, rarely, papilloedema. Acute hypercapnia reduces arterial pH (respiratory acidosis). If maintained for hours or days this acidosis tends to be compensated by renal retention of bicarbonate, and pH returns towards normal (p. 868).

8. **Clubbing of the Fingers and Toes.** The cause of clubbing, which is most readily recognised in the fingers, is not known but it is frequently found in patients with certain types of respiratory

disease, notably lung cancer and chronic intrathoracic suppuration such as bronchiectasis, lung abscess and empyema. It does not occur in chronic bronchitis or emphysema unless there is accompanying pulmonary suppuration, nor in pulmonary tuberculosis except in advanced cases.

Clubbing also occurs in certain other conditions. It is usually present in subacute bacterial endocarditis and cyanotic congenital heart disease; it is found occasionally in Crohn's disease, malabsorption syndrome and cirrhosis of the liver, and rarely in healthy subjects as a familial trait. The earliest indication of finger clubbing is an abnormal degree of fluctuation at the bases of the nails. With more advanced clubbing there is, in addition, an increase of the curvature of the nails and bulbous swelling of the finger tips.

THE INVESTIGATION OF RESPIRATORY DISEASE

In most respiratory diseases a reasonably accurate diagnosis can be made from the history and physical examination alone, but in several important conditions, notably pulmonary tuberculosis and bronchial carcinoma, these methods are inadequate and the diagnosis can be confirmed or excluded only by more specialised procedures such as radiological, bacteriological or endoscopic examination. In taking the history, particular enquiry must always be made about symptoms such as cough, sputum, haemoptysis, pain, breathlessness, wheeze and nasal discharge. The patient must also be asked about any previous respiratory illness, about any family history of tuberculosis and about a history of occupational exposure to dust.

Physical Examination

Before the chest itself is examined the temperature should be taken, and a note made of the rate and character of the respiration, the type and severity of any cough and the amount and character of the sputum. In addition, particular care must be taken to determine whether or not there is cyanosis, clubbing of the fingers or enlargement of the supraclavicular lymph nodes, these features being of special significance in respiratory disease.

The upper respiratory tract should be examined next, with

particular regard to nasal discharge or obstruction, oral sepsis, and infection or enlargement of the tonsils. The presence of hoarseness or a 'bovine' cough would draw attention to the need for laryngoscopic examination (p. 316). The chest wall should then be carefully inspected for soft tissue abnormalities such as cutaneous lesions, subcutaneous swellings and bulging or indrawing of intercostal spaces, and for skeletal abnormalities such as an increase of the antero-posterior diameter of the chest relative to its lateral diameter. The position of the trachea and of the apex beat should be noted and the chest expansion measured. Rib movement, vocal fremitus and the percussion note should always be compared in equivalent positions on the two sides of the chest. The terms used to describe the various types of percussion note are: hyperresonant, normal, impaired, dull and stony dull. At auscultation, attention should be directed in turn to the breath sounds, accompaniments and vocal resonance.

Breath Sounds

The following terms are used: vesicular, vesicular with prolonged expiration, diminished vesicular, absent breath sounds, high-pitched bronchial ('tubular'), low-pitched bronchial ('cavernous' or 'amphoric') breath sounds.

Accompaniments

(i) *Rhonchi* are produced by narrowing of the lumen of the bronchi by spasm of bronchial muscle, swelling of bronchial mucosa or tenacious exudate adherent to bronchial walls. Rhonchi may be high-pitched, medium-pitched or low-pitched, according to the diameter of the bronchi in which the sounds are produced.

(ii) *Crepitations* are usually produced by secretion lying within alveoli, bronchi or pulmonary cavities. They may be fine, medium or coarse in quality and often become more numerous after coughing. Crepitations of a different kind ('tinkling' crepitations) may be heard on auscultation when there is a small amount of fluid in a pneumothorax space.

(iii) *Pleural rub* (p. 393) is a diagnostic sign of pleural inflammation. It must be distinguished from a low-pitched rhonchus, fine crepitations and a 'scapular creak', which is the sound sometimes produced by movement of the scapula.

Vocal Resonance

The following terms are used: normal, increased, diminished or absent vocal resonance, aegophony, whispering pectoriloquy.

The Interpretation of Physical Signs

Certain groups of physical signs are typically associated with certain pathological changes in the lungs and pleura. Such changes are not necessarily specific for one particular disease. For example, consolidation may occur in pneumonia or tuberculosis, and fluid may be present in the pleural space in tuberculous pleurisy, empyema or congestive cardiac failure. Each group of physical signs should therefore be correlated with the gross pathological lesion by which the signs are produced rather than with any specific disease, the diagnosis of which depends on an analysis of all the clinical and other evidence.

The characteristic physical signs of the more common lesions are shown on Table 5.

Special Methods of Investigation

1. Radiological Examination of the Chest. Although radiological examination of the chest is now widely employed as a primary diagnostic measure ('mass miniature radiography') it should not be regarded as a short cut to diagnosis. In many respiratory diseases, however, clinical examination must be supplemented by radiological examination, which may provide:

(*a*) Evidence of a lesion within the thorax too small to be detected by physical examination or which because of its nature or situation does not give rise to abnormal physical signs.

(*b*) A more accurate assessment of the size and position of pulmonary, pleural and mediastinal lesions than can be obtained from physical examination. Lateral as well as postero-anterior radiographs are necessary for this purpose.

(*c*) More accurate information about the nature of the lesions than can be obtained from physical examination. For example, cavitation, which is difficult to recognise from physical signs, can in most cases be clearly demonstrated by radiological examination, using if necessary the special technique of *tomography*.

Accurate information regarding the size, shape and position of the heart.

(*e*) Information regarding the position and function of the diaphragm, which can be observed radiologically by the technique of *fluoroscopy* (p. 377).

(*f*) Evidence of disease or injury in the bony structures of the thorax.

2. Bacteriological and Cytological Examination

(*a*) SPUTUM. Bacteriological examination of the sputum seldom provides conclusive diagnostic information except when tubercle bacilli are isolated. The findings in other circumstances must be interpreted in conjunction with the results of clinical and, if necessary, radiological examination.

Cytological examination, by demonstrating cancer cells in the sputum, may enable a diagnosis of bronchial carcinoma to be made, but this examination has not yet been sufficiently developed to make it entirely reliable.

(*b*) PLEURAL FLUID. This should always be examined cytologically and bacteriologically. A special search should be made for tubercle bacilli if the fluid is serous and for pyogenic organisms and tubercle bacilli if it is purulent. When malignant disease is suspected, especially if the fluid is blood-stained, it should also be examined histologically for cancer cells.

3. **Haematological Examination.** Estimation of the total and differential leucocyte count may be of great value in distinguishing between pyogenic infection and tuberculous or virus infection.

4. **Tuberculin Tests.** (p. 417).

5. **Laryngoscopy.** (p. 332). Inspection of the larynx either by means of a mirror placed at the back of the mouth (*indirect* laryngoscopy) or through an illuminated metal tube (*direct* laryngoscopy).

6. **Bronchoscopy.** (p. 378.) Inspection of the trachea and large bronchi through an illuminated metal tube which also permits the removal of tissue for histological examination (bronchial biopsy).

7. **Bronchography.** (p. 372.) Radiological examination of the bronchi after the instillation of iodised oil, opaque to X-rays.

8. **Thoracoscopy.** (p. 399.) Inspection of the pleural surfaces by means of a telescope inserted through an intercostal space after the introduction of air into the pleural space.

9. **Pleural Biopsy.** In patients with pleural effusion it is possible to obtain a specimen of parietal pleura suitable for histological examination by means of Abrams' pleural biopsy 'punch'. The technique is simple and safe, and the procedure may be of considerable value in determining the cause of pleural effusions.

THE TREATMENT OF RESPIRATORY DISEASE

Infection

1. **Bacterial Infection.** The chemotherapy of bacterial infection of the bronchi, lungs and pleura will be described in the sections on individual diseases. Certain general principles are, however, applicable to all cases.

Before any treatment is started a specimen of sputum, a laryngeal swab (if there is no sputum) or a specimen of pleural fluid should be sent for bacteriological examination.

In acute bacterial infections it is usually necessary to begin chemotherapy before the results of bacteriological examination are available. The choice of antibiotic in these circumstances is based on clinical impressions of the nature and severity of the illness.

If a clinical diagnosis of bronchitis, pneumonia or empyema is made and the patient is not seriously ill, treatment should be started with penicillin, to which most infections of this type respond. When the acute infection is a complication of chronic bronchitis or bronchiectasis, one of the broad-spectrum antibiotics should be preferred. If the patient is gravely ill and there is any reason to suspect infection with *Staph. pyogenes*, an antibiotic to which that organism is unlikely to be resistant, e.g. cloxacillin or erythromycin, must be given.

As soon as the results of bacteriological examination and sensitivity tests are received, appropriate modifications in antibiotic therapy can be made, if necessary.

Factors which interfere with the response to antibiotics must be corrected, e.g. an empyema must be aspirated or drained and bronchiectatic cavities and lung abscesses must be kept dry by postural drainage.

2. **Viral Infection.** The viruses which infect the respiratory tract are uninfluenced by chemotherapy, but secondary bacterial infection, which occurs in many cases, often requires treatment with an appropriate antibiotic. Infection caused by organisms intermediate in size between bacteria and viruses, such as *Rickettsia burneti* and *Mycoplasma pneumoniae* (p. 353), may respond to tetracycline.

3. **Fungal Infection.** The treatment of these diseases, apart from actinomycosis which usually responds well to penicillin, is unsatisfactory. It is described on p. 365.

Oxygen Therapy

The inhalation of pure O_2 at atmospheric pressure washes nitrogen out of all ventilated alveoli, whatever their ventilation/perfusion ratio. They then contain CO_2 ($P_{CO_2} \simeq 40$ mm. Hg.), water vapour ($P_{HO_2} \simeq 47$ mm. Hg., saturated at 37° C.) and O_2. Alveolar P_{O_2} thus reaches 600-650 mm. Hg., which is more than enough to saturate all the blood perfusing these alveoli, and imparts to it a similar P_{O_2}. Dissolved O_2 in blood is proportional to P_{O_2}, and at 650 mm. Hg. amounts to 2·0 ml. per 100 ml. of blood, compared with 0·3 ml. per 100 ml. at the normal arterial P_{O_2} of 100 mm. Hg. The extra 1·7 ml. of O_2 per 100 ml. of blood is available to oxygenate blood coming from alveoli which are completely unventilated, or blood which passes through an anatomical 'right to left' shunt. In the presence of such a functional or anatomical shunt of up to 20 per cent. of the cardiac output, inhalation of pure O_2 may thus completely abolish arterial undersaturation. The P_{O_2} of arterial blood will not, however, rise nearly as much as when there is no shunt, since dissolved O_2 has been used up in oxygenating shunted blood. Blood P_{O_2} is thus a much more sensitive index of shunting than is O_2 saturation. It should be remembered that blood perfusing alveoli with some ventilation, however small, will be fully saturated by these alveoli during prolonged inhalation of pure O_2.

Pulmonary disease. The hypoxaemia of generalised alveolar

hypoventilation (p. 308) is completely corrected by breathing pure O_2; so is that of uneven distribution (p. 304) unless large regions of lung, though perfused, are completely unventilated. Such regions act as large venous-arterial shunts. Hypoxaemia due to impaired diffusion (p. 306) is completely corrected.

Anaemia; cardiac failure with low output, shock. In these conditions the arterial blood may be fully saturated with O_2 when air is breathed, but the rate of delivery of O_2 to the tissues is reduced. The increase in dissolved O_2 during O_2-breathing may, however, be valuable to seriously ill patients.

Peripheral vascular disease; carbon monoxide poisoning. Some success has been reported from the treatment of these conditions in pressure chambers by means of which O_2 can be administered at 2 to 3 atmospheres pressure. This greatly increases arterial P_{O_2} and dissolved O_2. The extra O_2 carried in the blood may tide over a patient with threatened gangrene or serious 'de-gloving' injuries. A high blood P_{O_2} rapidly dissociates carboxyhaemoglobin; for coal-gas poisoning high-pressure ('hyperbaric') oxygen is probably the best treatment, but 100 per cent. O_2 at atmospheric pressure is well worth giving when a pressure chamber is not accessible.

Technique of Oxygen Administration

Oxygen masks are of two types:

1. Those which are designed to produce a high concentration of O_2 in the inspired air but which permit the rebreathing of small amounts of expired CO_2. Examples of this type of mask are the Polymask (British Oxygen Co. Ltd.) and the Pneumask (Oxygenaire, Ltd.), both of which deliver about 60 per cent O_2 when the flow rate is 6 *l.* per min.

2. Those which are designed to produce a slight O_2 enrichment of the inspired air and do not permit the rebreathing of expired CO_2. Examples of this type of mask are the Edinburgh mask (British Oxygen Co. Ltd.) and the Ventimask (Oxygenaire, Ltd.). With the Edinburgh mask adjustments of the O_2 flow rate can provide inspired O_2 concentrations at any levels between 23 and 35 per cent. The Ventimask is available in two models, one of which delivers about 24 per cent. O_2 and the other 28 per cent. O_2 when the flow rate is 4 *l.* per min.

Nasal catheters. The single nasal catheter has now given place to the Addis double nasal catheter. This consists of a long polyethylene tube, which is slung under the nose and held loosely in place by elastic behind the head. One end is sealed off, and oxygen which is delivered into the other end flows out through two smaller side tubes placed inside the nares. The main advantages of nasal catheters such as this are that they do not permit rebreathing of CO_2 and do not interfere with eating, drinking and speaking. The inspired O_2-concentration provided by nasal catheters is somewhat unpredictable, but an O_2 flow rate of 2 *l.*/min. will usually raise it to about 30 per cent.

Oxygen tent. This is cumbersome, hampers nursing and physiotherapy and provides an extremely variable O_2 concentration because of leaks and repeated access by attendants. It has a place for patients who will not tolerate a mask (unless their confusion is due to hypercapnia) and for children.

Humidification. When a Polymask, a Pneumask or a nasal catheter is used, the oxygen must be humidified, either by passing it through a canister of warmed water or through a nebuliser. This is not necessary with the Edinburgh mask or the Ventimask, as these masks entrain a high proportion of atmospheric air.

Ventilatory Failure

1. Acute.

A clear airway is essential. In conscious patients this can often be secured and maintained by determined efforts to expectorate, every 15 minutes or so at first, strictly supervised by a doctor or nurse. If this policy fails, and particularly if the patient has become confused or unconscious, a cuffed endotracheal tube should be inserted. This is tolerated surprisingly well, without local anaesthesia, even before consciousness is completely lost, but restless patients may have to be anaesthetised before the tube can be passed. Once it is *in situ*, brisk pulmonary inflation by 'Ambu' bag or mechanical ventilator, vigorous physiotherapy for each side in turn and repeated tracheobronchial aspiration can then be carried out. These measures may quickly restore consciousness; if not, the tube can be left in place for up to 48 hours while treatment is continued. Meanwhile, a decision can be made for or against tracheostomy, which will allow tracheobronchial aspiration and mechanical ventilation to be maintained for a longer period. Tracheostomy should usually be avoided in patients who have had severe respiratory disability for several months before the onset of ventilatory failure. Bronchoscopic aspiration may be of value as an initial measure to remove tenacious secretions from the bronchi, but should seldom have to be repeated.

During manual or mechanical ventilation through an endotracheal tube the depressant effect of a high arterial P_{O_2} on respiration can be ignored, and there is no objection to ventilating the patient with a high concentration (60 per cent. or more) of O_2. When artificial ventilation is stopped, however, or in cases where it has not been employed, increasing hypercapnia is a potential hazard of O_2 administration, and the concentration of O_2 in the inspired air should initially be kept below 30 per cent. by using either a Ventimask (p. 319) or an Edinburgh mask (p. 319). It is indeed seldom necessary to increase the inspired O_2 concentration above this level. There is certainly no justification for the use of the Polymask (p. 319) or a similar type of mask to achieve high inspired O_2 concentrations, as with masks of this type gas containing 1-2 per cent. of CO_2 is inhaled from the reservoir bag and this may increase hypercapnia. When O_2, even in a concentration of 30 per cent. or less, is being administered to patients with acute ventilatory failure, the arterial P_{CO_2} (p. 307) should be estimated at regular intervals. Patients who are critically ill require a more elaborate monitoring procedure, which should include frequent measurements of arterial blood gas tensions and pH. An indwelling arterial catheter can conveniently and safely be used for obtaining blood samples. If a steady increase in P_{CO_2} is accompanied by clinical deterioration and/or by a fall in pH to below 7·25 units, artificial ventilation, either short-term via an endotracheal tube or long-term via a tracheostomy tube, should be started without delay. The disturbances in blood gas tensions and acid-base balance can usually be corrected within 24 hours, but it may be several days before the patient is capable of maintaining a sufficiently high level of alveolar ventilation to allow him to dispense with mechanical assistance.

Ventilatory failure due to potentially reversible respiratory paralysis demands early tracheostomy and mechanical ventilation.

In all cases respiratory infection should be treated (p. 317). Water and electrolyte balance should be maintained, by intravenous infusion if necessary, as dehydration increases the viscosity of bronchial mucus and makes it difficult to aspirate.

Analeptic drugs have only a minor place in treatment. Nikethamide (2-4 ml. of a 25 per cent. solution one to two-hourly) or ethamivan (infusions of up to 12 mg./min.) given intravenously for 24 hours, may successfully tide the patient over a period of hypoventilation and obviate the need for tracheostomy, particularly if bronchial secretions are not present in large amounts. Although analeptic drugs seldom produce a sustained stimulation of respiration, they may improve the level of consciousness and thus restore effective expectoration. Should sedation be necessary, paraldehyde and chlorpromazine are probably the drugs least liable to depress respiration.

2. **Chronic.**

Many patients with progressive respiratory disease eventually enter a state in which blood gas tensions never return to normal. In such patients, attempts to increase ventilation by orally administered drugs (such as the carbonic anhydrase inhibitor, dichlorphenamide) are sometimes advocated. However, there is no clear evidence that such treatment is beneficial and there is a possibility of doing harm. At present, therefore, treatment should be directed to the prevention of acute respiratory infections, the relief of asthma and the management of coincident cardiac failure. In chronic ventilatory failure a worthwhile increase in exercise tolerance has been shown to result from the use of light, portable oxygen equipment. The provision of such equipment for all patients who could derive benefit from it presents a formidable problem. However, patients confined to their homes may be helped by the intermittent use of oxygen obtained from a non-portable supply; it must be admitted that such benefit may often be psychological rather than physical.

Symptomatic Treatment

Cough, when productive of sputum, should be encouraged and not suppressed. Those who are physically weak should be exhorted at regular intervals to clear their bronchi of secretion. Those with bronchiectasis or lung abscess should practise postural drainage, and those with tenacious sputum should be given hot drinks and inhalations of either steam or nebulised water to help them to bring it up more easily.

Unproductive, distressing cough should be suppressed. Demulcent lozenges are occasionally effective, but many patients require antitussive drugs, especially if sleep is disturbed by coughing. The two most effective preparations, suitable for general use in bronchitis, pneumonia, bronchial carcinoma and pulmonary tuberculosis, are:

Pholcodine linctus (B.P.C.), 4-8 ml. (60-120 min.) and
Methadone linctus (B.P.C.), 4-8 ml. (60-120 min.).

Airways obstruction in bronchitis and asthma is treated by bronchodilator drugs (p. 345) and in certain carefully selected cases by corticosteroids (p. 345).

Chest pain. Pleural pain can usually be relieved by the application of a rubber hot-water bottle or by an electric heating pad to the chest wall, supplemented by an analgesic and, if necessary, by an antitussive drug. Kaolin poultices are messy and not particularly effective. Immobilisation of the chest by strapping is apt to produce atelectasis and is not recommended. Mild analgesics, such as acetylsalicylic acid, 0·6-0·9 g. (10-15 gr.), or codeine compound tablets (B.P.C.), 2-3, are adequate in most cases but a few patients may require pethidine, 50-100 mg. by mouth or intramuscular injection, or, when the pain is very severe, morphine, 10-15 mg. ($\frac{1}{6}$-$\frac{1}{4}$ gr.) subcutaneously.

The pain of acute tracheitis usually responds to the application of heat to the front of the chest, combined with inhalations of steam medicated with benzoin (p. 326). Pain due to the invasion of the chest wall by a malignant tumour usually demands a powerful analgesic such as methadone, 5-10 mg., pethidine or morphine, given by injection. In advanced cases these drugs may become ineffective and it may be necessary to block the sensory nerve roots by extradural injections of phenol at the appropriate levels.

DISEASES OF THE UPPER RESPIRATORY TRACT

VIRAL INFECTION OF THE RESPIRATORY TRACT

The number of viruses known to cause respiratory infection is continually increasing. They are universally distributed, of high infectivity, and thus of great economic importance.

Infection with these 'respiratory viruses' may cause four groups of symptoms and signs:

1. *Non-specific toxaemia*: malaise, fever, headache, shivering, muscular pain, prostration.
2. *Upper respiratory infection* (*U.R.I.*): rhinorrhoea, pharyngitis, laryngitis, 'croup' in children.
3. *Lower respiratory infection* (*L.R.I.*): bronchitis, bronchiolitis, pneumonia.
4. *Specific features*, e.g. keratoconjunctivitis and follicular conjunctivitis in adenovirus infections, herpangina in infections with Coxsackie A virus.

In general, infants and children are more severely affected than adults, with a higher incidence of L.R.I.; adults are partly immune because of previous infection. However, even adults may suffer severe and even fatal lower respiratory infections, and it is now believed that exacerbations of chronic bronchitis are often caused by viruses. The types of virus so far classified are as follows:

1. *Adenovirus*, first isolated from degenerating adenoids. A connection with mesenteric adenitis and intussusception has been suspected.

2. *Respiratory syncytial* (*RS*) *virus*, isolated from respiratory infections and forming syncytia or giant cells in tissue culture.

3. *Picornaviruses*, named because of their very small size and RNA constitution. Those causing respiratory infection are (a) *rhinoviruses*, a frequent (but perhaps not definitive) cause of the common cold (U.R.I.). (b) *Coxsackie A*, or Coe virus, related to the enteroviruses and sometimes causing gastrointestinal as well as respiratory symptoms. In children, Coxsackie A virus causes *herpangina*, a self-limiting, febrile illness marked by tiny petechiae or papules which appear on the soft palate and faucial pillars during the first two days and rapidly ulcerate.

4. *Myxoviruses*: (*a*) Influenza and (*b*) parainfluenza viruses.

5. *Psittacosis*. Man is infected by birds, notably parrots and pigeons. A patchy lobular pneumonia ensues, with high pyrexia, sometimes haemoptysis, and a tendency to relapse. The virus may be sensitive to tetracycline.

Organisms intermediate in size between bacteria and viruses may cause a type of pneumonia similar to that produced by viruses. The most important of these are: *Rickettsia* (*Coxiella*) *burneti* and *Mycoplasma pneumoniae*, the second of which may also be a cause of upper respiratory infection. The type of pneumonia for which these organisms are responsible is described on p. 353.

In some instances the virus, rickettsia or mycoplasma can be isolated and identified by special methods involving the inoculation with respiratory secretions of tissue culture, embryonated hen's eggs or animals. More frequently, however, the diagnosis is made serologically by observing a rising titre of specific antibodies in the patient's serum. With both methods there is a considerable delay before the results become available and it is often difficult to evaluate their significance. For these reasons diagnostic virology is at present only of limited value in clinical practice.

ACUTE CORYZA (COMMON COLD)

Aetiology. Primary infection of the nose and nasopharynx by any of several viruses (p. 324) produces the early features. Subsequent bacterial infection, especially by *Strept. pneumoniae*, *Strept. pyogenes* and staphylococci, is usual. Infection is favoured by aggregation in public places, and resistance may be lowered by debility and sudden changes in environmental temperature. Immunity is specific for each viral strain and is short-lived.

Clinical Features. The onset is usually sudden with a tickling sensation in the nose accompanied by sneezing. The throat often feels dry and sore, the head feels 'stuffed', the eyes smart and there is a profuse, watery, nasal discharge. These symptoms last for one to two days, after which, with secondary infection, the secretion becomes thick and purulent, and impedes nasal breathing. There may be slight fever at the beginning.

Complications. It is hard to say whether variations in course represent complication of a standard illness or the primary effects of different viruses; probably both factors are involved, as well as resistance of the host.

1. *Sinusitis*. There is usually more systemic upset than in uncomplicated coryza. Headache is often present and may be severe, and there may be pain or discomfort over the face. Localised tenderness on palpation over the maxillary and frontal sinuses may be elicited.

For anatomical reasons already discussed (p. 300) sinus infection is liable to become chronic, particularly in the maxillary sinuses. The chief symptom of chronic sinusitis is persistent purulent discharge from the front and back of the nose, often accompanied by nasal obstruction and recurrent headaches. Local tenderness is not usually as marked as in the acute stage.

2. *Eustachian catarrh*, causing deafness, and *otitis media*, causing fever and aural pain.

3. *Lower respiratory infection*—tracheitis, bronchitis, bronchiolitis and lobular pneumonia.

Diagnosis. If conjunctivitis is present in a child, *measles* must be considered. Frequent attacks of sneezing and watery rhinorrhoea, without systemic upset, suggest paroxysmal rhinorrhoea (p. 326) rather than virus infection.

Prevention. Much can be done to prevent the spread of coryza to others by voluntary isolation of patients for two to three days during the early, highly infectious stage.

In persons who are liable to frequent colds the nose and throat should be examined for enlarged adenoids, polypi, infected sinuses and deflected septum, and any such abnormality corrected. The value of mixed catarrhal vaccines in the prevention of coryza has not been conclusively proved and their use is not recommended.

Treatment. No curative treatment for the common cold is known. The congestion and excessive secretion of the nasal mucous membrane may be reduced by the periodic use of 1 per cent. ephedrine in normal saline either sprayed or dropped into the nose (proprietary preparations commonly contain a mild antiseptic in addition), or by the inhalation of amphetamine sulphate. Steam medicated with benzoin inhalation (B.P.C.) or menthol and benzoin inhalation (B.P.C.), 1 teaspoonful to 1 pint of boiling water, is beneficial, especially if the nasal sinuses are involved or if there is obstruction of the Eustachian tubes.

PAROXYSMAL RHINORRHOEA

This is a disorder in which there are episodes of nasal congestion, nasal discharge and sneezing. It may be *seasonal* (hay fever) or *perinnial* (vasomotor rhinorrhoea).

Aetiology. Seasonal paroxysmal rhinorrhoea (hay fever) is apparently due to an antigen-antibody reaction in the nasal mucosa. The usual antigens are pollens from grasses, flowers, weeds or trees, and as grass pollen is the most common cause of hay fever in Great Britain the disorder is at its peak between May and July.

Although perennial paroxysmal rhinorrhoea may sometimes be due to hypersensitivity to moulds or animal emanations it is more often a non-specific reaction to a variety of agents including dust, irritating odours or fumes, sudden changes in temperature and humidity and, in a different category, emotional tension.

Clinical Features. In the seasonal type there are frequent sudden attacks of sneezing with profuse watery nasal discharge and nasal obstruction. These attacks last for a few hours and are often accompanied by smarting and watering of the eyes and conjunctival injection. In the perennial type the symptoms are similar but as a rule less severe.

Diagnosis. In seasonal paroxysmal rhinorrhoea the diagnosis is usually easy because the attacks occur only during the pollen season. In the perennial type it may be more difficult because the symptoms of paroxysmal rhinorrhoea may be indistinguishable from the initial symptoms of coryza. In coryza, however, the persistence of symptoms and the appearance later of pus in the nasal discharge usually make the diagnosis clear.

In the seasonal type skin tests often show hypersensitivity to one or other of the pollens, but such reactions are seldom observed in the perennial type.

Prognosis. The symptoms of both types of paroxysmal rhinorrhoea, particularly the seasonal type, can be controlled by drugs, but a permanent cure is seldom obtained. In some cases, however, the condition subsides spontaneously. It is to be regarded more as a serious inconvenience than as a disease.

Prevention. In the seasonal type an attempt should be made to avoid exposure to pollen or at least reduce it to a minimum, for example, by avoiding country districts and keeping indoors as much as possible, with the windows closed, during the pollen season.

An antihistamine drug taken daily throughout the pollen season will often prevent attacks of hay fever, but some patients will require pre-seasonal desensitisation with pollen extracts (Bencard or Dome).

The prevention of paroxysmal perennial rhinorrhoea consists of avoiding, as far as possible, exposure to the mechanical, physical and emotional causes mentioned above.

Treatment. The following symptomatic measures are applicable to both seasonal and perennial rhinorrhoea:

1. Antihistamine drugs, such as chlorpheniramine maleate (Piriton), 4-8 mg. thrice daily, often provide considerable or even complete relief of symptoms.

2. Local measures which may be of value are (*a*) decongestant nasal sprays, using a 1 per cent. solution of ephedrine hydrochloride in saline and (*b*) instillations of 1-2 drops of 1 per cent. ephedrine in saline into the conjunctival sac.

3. Patients failing to respond to these measures may obtain considerable symptomatic relief from the use of a hydrocortisone or betamathasone nasal spray.

INFLUENZA

Influenza is an acute infectious disease due to a filterable virus. It is characterised by a general febrile illness, often accompanied by inflammatory changes in the respiratory tract.

Aetiology. Three distinct viruses, A, B and C, with subgroups, have been isolated. Virus A is most commonly implicated and appears to be responsible for the influenza pandemics which occur every few years. Virus B causes more limited outbreaks, while C is rare. Influenza is highly infectious, most prevalent during the winter and affects patients of all ages. Type-specific immunity follows an attack but lasts for only a few months.

Pathology. The majority of cases show only a mild catarrhal inflammation of the upper respiratory tract. At the other extreme, the virus may rapidly invade the whole respiratory system, leading to death from fulminating pneumonia and toxaemia. All intermediate grades occur. When the disease lasts for more than a day or two, secondary bacterial invasion (*Staph. pyogenes*, *Strept, pyogenes*, *Strept. pneumoniae*, *H. influenzae*) plays a major part. causing bronchitis, lobular pneumonia and empyema.

Clinical Features. The incubation period is one or two days. The illness starts suddenly, with malaise, headache, pain in the back and limbs, anorexia and sometimes nausea and vomiting. Pyrexia to 39° C. (103° F.) remits for two or three days, with chills and shivering but seldom rigor. The face is flushed, conjunctivae suffused and fauces hyperaemic with prominent lymphoid follicles. The pulse is rapid. There is often leucopenia (2,000-4,000 per c.mm.). There may be a harsh unproductive cough, without signs over the lungs. At this stage the case is indistinguishable clinically from a severe upper respiratory infection due to other respiratory viruses (p. 324).

Course and Complications. In many cases no further symptoms develop and recovery ensues within three to five days. In a considerable number of cases the disease progresses to lower respiratory infection (p. 324) in which, in all but the most rapidly fatal cases, bacterial invasion is prominent, with a polymorph leucocytosis.

Toxic *cardiomyopathy* may cause sudden death, especially in patients with pre-existent cardiac disease. *Encephalitis* and *post-influenzal demyelinating encephalopathy* are rare complications. *Post-influenzal asthenia and depression* are common, often marked, and may last for a week or two.

Diagnosis. During epidemics the diagnosis is usually easy. Most sporadic cases are identifiable only as respiratory viral infections unless serological tests for specific antibodies are carried out, and one can usually be sure of a viral origin only in retrospect, after the disease has run its course.

Prevention. Carefully controlled studies have shown that influenza virus vaccines, given in two or three doses for the first year and then annually, protect some 80 per cent. of persons inoculated.

Treatment. There is, as yet, no specific treatment for the viral infection itself. The patient should be kept in bed until the pyrexia has subsided. A mild analgesic such as codeine compound tablets (B.P.C.), 1-3, usually relieves the headache and backache. A linctus containing pholcodine or methadone (p. 323) may be used to suppress unproductive cough. The treatment of the respiratory complications of influenza due to secondary bacterial infection is dealt with later.

ACUTE CATARRHAL LARYNGITIS

Aetiology. Acute catarrhal laryngitis usually occurs either as a complication of coryza or as a manifestation of one of the infectious fevers, e.g. measles. It may also be caused by the inhalation of irritant gases.

Pathology. The laryngeal mucous membrane is swollen, congested and coated with mucus. Microscopically it is infiltrated with inflammatory cells. Rarely, in children, there may be a membranous exudate resembling diphtheria.

Clinical Features. The throat is dry and sore. The voice is at first hoarse and then reduced to a whisper. Speaking may be painful. There is an irritating, non-productive cough, but the general upset is usually mild.

In children the laryngeal opening is small and may be obstructed by viscid secretion and spasm. This may produce paroxysms of barking cough sometimes accompanied by vomiting, crowing inspiration, stridor, dyspnoea and cyanosis. The child may become unconscious. This relaxes the spasm and recovery usually follows, but if laryngeal oedema is also present the child may develop progressive respiratory obstruction similar to that seen in laryngeal diphtheria.

Treatment. The patient must be put to bed in a warm room and, to rest the larynx, he must not raise his voice above a whisper and must not smoke. Inhalations of medicated steam (p. 326) should be given three or four times a day, along with a linctus containing pholcodine or methadone (p. 323).

A child with acute laryngitis should be placed in a steam tent, and given a sedative such as triclofos syrup in a dosage ranging from 0·2 g. for a child of 1 year to 1·0 g. for a child of 12 or older. If there is no improvement within 24 hours an antibiotic, such as penicillin or tetracycline, should be prescribed. A careful watch should be maintained for laryngeal obstruction (p. 333).

Prognosis. Acute laryngitis usually clears up entirely in a few days, but if frequently repeated it may predispose to chronic laryngitis. Downward spread of the infection may cause tracheitis, bronchitis, or even pneumonia.

CHRONIC LARYNGITIS

Aetiology. Chronic laryngitis occurs as a result of:

1. Repeated attacks of acute laryngitis.
2. Improper use of the voice, especially in dusty atmospheres, e.g. in auctioneers.
3. Excessive smoking.
4. Mouth breathing from nasal obstruction.
5. Chronic nasal and oral sepsis.

Pathology. The surface of the mucous membrane is dry and covered with small papillary projections. The vocal cords are thickened and opaque. Microscopically the submucosa is infiltrated with chronic inflammatory cells.

Clinical Features. The chief symptom is hoarseness and the voice may be entirely lost. There is irritation of the throat and spasmodic cough with a little mucoid sputum.

Diagnosis. As chronic and progressive hoarseness may also be caused by tuberculosis, syphilis and tumours of the larynx and by laryngeal paralysis, these conditions must be considered in the differential diagnosis if the hoarseness does not improve within a few weeks. In some cases a chest radiograph may bring to light unsuspected pulmonary tuberculosis or a bronchial carcinoma. If no such abnormality is found the patient should be referred to a specialist for laryngoscopic examination.

Treatment. The voice must be rested completely. This is particularly important in the case of public speakers. Smoking should be prohibited. Some benefit may be obtained from frequent inhalations of steam medicated with benzoin or menthol. Predisposing conditions such as nasal and oral sepsis must be remedied.

Course and Prognosis. The disease pursues a chronic course frequently uninfluenced by treatment, and in long-standing cases the voice is often permanently impaired.

LARYNGEAL PARALYSIS

Aetiology. Laryngeal paralysis may be organic or functional. *Organic paralysis* is due to interference with the motor nerve supply of the larynx and may be caused by:

1. Lesions of the brain stem, e.g. bulbar paralysis due to vascular lesions, motor neurone disease or poliomyelitis.

2. Toxic and infective lesions of the vagus nerve or its recurrent laryngeal branch, e.g. polyneuritis, diphtheritic or lead neuropathy.

3. Interruption of the recurrent laryngeal nerve, or of the vagus trunk above the origin of that nerve, by tumour, aneurysm or trauma (p. 300). This is the most common way in which laryngeal paralysis is produced. The paralysis is nearly always unilateral and, by reason of the intrathoracic course of the left recurrent laryngeal nerve, usually left-sided. Accidental division of one or both recurrent laryngeal nerves is one of the hazards of thyroidectomy.

Functional paralysis of the larynx occurs as a manifestation of hysteria.

Clinical Features

1. *Hoarseness* always accompanies laryngeal paralysis whatever its cause. Paralysis of organic origin is seldom reversible, but when only one vocal cord is affected the hoarseness may improve or even disappear after a few weeks as a result of a compensatory adjustment whereby the unparalysed cord crosses the mid-line and approximates with the paralysed cord on phonation.

2. '*Bovine*' *cough*, which is a characteristic feature of organic laryngeal paralysis, results from the loss of the explosive phase of normal coughing consequent upon the failure of the cords to close the glottis. The difficulty in bringing up sputum which some of these patients experience can be explained on the same basis. 'Bovine' cough does not occur with hysterical paralysis.

3. *Dyspnoea* and *stridor* are occasionally present but are seldom severe except with bilateral laryngeal paralysis of organic origin.

4. *Laryngoscopy* is necessary to establish the diagnosis of laryngeal paralysis with certainty. In organic paralysis the abductors of the vocal cord are first affected and subsequently the

adductors. When the paralysis is complete the cord lies in the so-called 'cadaveric' position, midway between abduction and adduction. In hysterical paralysis only the adductors are paralysed.

Treatment. The treatment is that of the underlying disease. Psychological treatment is often necessary in hysteria. In bilateral paralysis of organic origin the passage of an endotracheal tube or even tracheostomy may be required for the relief of laryngeal obstruction (p. 334). Eventually, in these cases, it may be necessary to perform a plastic operation on the larynx in order to secure permanent restoration of the airway.

LARYNGEAL OBSTRUCTION

Aetiology

1. *Obstruction by Exudate and Oedema.*

(*a*) Laryngeal diphtheria.

(*b*) Acute laryngitis, including non-diphtheritic membranous laryngitis.

(*c*) Inhalation of poisonous gases.

(*d*) Swallowing of corrosive liquids.

2. *Obstruction by Oedema alone.*

(*a*) From inflammation in adjacent tissues, e.g. burns or cellulitis of the neck, insect stings.

(*b*) Angioneurotic oedema and drug hypersensitivity.

3. *Mechanical Obstruction.*

(*a*) Foreign body or tumour.

(*b*) Laryngeal spasm.

(*c*) Bilateral recurrent laryngeal nerve paralysis.

(*d*) Arthritis of the crico-arytenoid joints in patients with rheumatoid arthritis.

N.B. Laryngeal obstruction is much more liable to occur in children than in adults owing to the smaller size of the glottis.

Clinical Features. These depend on whether the obstruction is complete or incomplete and on the rapidity of its onset.

Sudden complete laryngeal obstruction by a foreign body produces the clinical picture of acute asphyxia—violent but ineffective inspiratory efforts with indrawing of the intercostal spaces and the unsupported lower ribs, accompanied by deep cyanosis. Unrelieved, the condition progresses rapidly to coma, and death ensues within 5-10 minutes. When, as in most cases, the obstruction is incomplete at first, the main clinical features are progressive dyspnoea and cyanosis, stridor and indrawing of the intercostal spaces and lower ribs on both sides. The great danger in these cases is that the obstruction may *at any time* become complete and result in sudden death.

Treatment

Transient attacks of laryngeal obstruction due to exudate and spasm, which may occur with acute laryngitis in children (p. 330) and with whooping-cough, are potentially dangerous but can usually be relieved by the inhalation of steam.

Laryngeal obstruction from all other causes carries a high mortality and demands prompt treatment. The following measures may have to be employed:

1. *The relief of obstruction by mechanical means.* This is necessary when the obstruction is complete or when it is incomplete but rapidly progressive. When a foreign body is known to be the cause of the obstruction it can often be dislodged by turning the patient head downwards and thumping his back vigorously. In other circumstances the nature of the obstruction should be ascertained whenever possible by direct laryngoscopy, which may also permit the removal of a foreign body or the insertion of a rigid rubber tube past the obstruction into the trachea.

Tracheostomy must be performed without delay if these procedures cannot be undertaken, or if they fail, but except in a very acute emergency the operation is best done in the operating theatre by a surgeon.

2. *Other local measures.* The application of an ice-bag to the front of the neck and spraying of the larynx with adrenaline may be tried in all cases in which oedema is suspected but these measures are not particularly effective.

3. *Treatment of the cause.* In cases of diphtheria, antitoxin should be administered and for other infections the appropriate antibiotic should be given. In angioneurotic oedema the patient should receive adrenaline, 0·5-1·0 ml. of 1:1000 solution subcutaneously and hydrocortisone hemisuccinate, 100 mg., or

betamethasone disodium phosphate, 4 mg. intravenously. It must be remembered that these remedies take time to act and tracheostomy may be required in the intervening period.

* * * * * *

ACUTE TRACHEITIS AND BRONCHITIS

Aetiology. This condition is an acute inflammation of the trachea and bronchi caused by pyogenic organisms such as *Strept. pneumoniae*, *H. influenzae* and, less frequently, *Staph. pyogenes*. Infection by these organisms is a common sequel to coryza, influenza, measles and whooping-cough, and is particularly prone to develop in patients with chronic bronchitis.

Other factors predisposing to the development of infection include cold, damp, foggy and dusty atmospheres, and chronic mouth breathing which allows unfiltered and unwarmed air to enter the bronchi.

Clinical Features. The first symptom is an irritating, unproductive cough accompanied by upper retrosternal discomfort or pain caused by tracheitis. When the bronchi become involved there is also a sensation of tightness in the chest, and dyspnoea with wheezing respiration may be present. When acute bronchitis complicates chronic bronchitis and emphysema, respiratory distress may become particularly severe. The sputum is at first scanty, mucoid, viscid and difficult to bring up, and occasionally may be streaked with blood. A day or two later it becomes mucopurulent and more copious. As the infection extends down the bronchial tree there is a general febrile disturbance, with a temperature of 38-39° C. (100-103° F.) and a neutrophil leucocytosis. In the vast majority of cases recovery takes place gradually over the next four to eight days without the patient ever becoming seriously ill. Occasionally the dyspnoea and general symptoms increase in severity, cyanosis appears, and if the infection reaches the smallest bronchi and bronchioles ('bronchiolitis') the condition virtually becomes a lobular pneumonia.

Physical Signs in the Chest. Tracheitis without bronchitis produces no abnormal physical signs. In bronchitis there is no impairment of chest wall movement or percussion note. The breath sounds are vesicular, or vesicular with prolonged expiration, and are accompanied by *bilateral* rhonchi and, occasionally, coarse crepitations. The further down the bronchial tree the infection extends, the more high-pitched are the rhonchi and the finer the crepitations.

Course and Prognosis. The disease is usually mild and of short duration, the patient recovering in two to three days if a suitable antibiotic is given. In severe cases it lasts longer, especially if bronchiolitis and lobular pneumonia develop.

Diagnosis. The diagnosis is usually easy, but it must not be forgotten that acute bronchitis may be an early and prominent manifestation of some underlying disease, such as measles or whooping-cough. When signs simulating those of acute bronchitis are confined to one part of the chest, pulmonary tuberculosis, bronchial carcinoma and bronchiectasis should be considered.

Treatment. The patient should be confined to bed. If the attack is mild, penicillin should be given orally (p. 362). When the illness is more severe, tetracycline or ampicillin, 250-500 mg. four times daily, should be substituted for penicillin. In the early stages, when cough is painful and unproductive, the tough viscid secretion should be loosened by the inhalation three or four times a day of steam medicated with benzoin or menthol. A steam kettle or steam tent may be even more effective, particularly for children or elderly patients. The cough should be controlled at night by the use of a sedative linctus containing pholcodine or methadone (p. 323). If retrosternal discomfort is troublesome, heat may be helpful, applied to the chest by means of a hot bottle or an electric pad. If symptoms or signs of airways obstruction are present a bronchodilator drug (p. 345) may be of some value.

CHRONIC BRONCHITIS

Aetiology. Chronic bronchitis is the name given to the clinical syndrome which certain individuals develop in response to the long-continued action of various types of irritant on the bronchial mucosa. The most important of these is tobacco smoke, but they also include dust, smoke and fumes, occurring as specific occupational hazards or as part of a general atmospheric pollution in industrial cities and towns. Infection is sometimes a precipitating factor in the onset of chronic bronchitis, but its main role is in aggravating the established condition. Exposure to dampness, to sudden changes in temperature and to fog may also be responsible for exacerbations of chronic bronchitis.

The disorder occurs most commonly in middle and late adult life. More males are affected than females and there may be a familial predisposition. As might be expected, it is more common in smokers than in non-smokers, and in urban than in rural districts.

Culture of the sputum may yield merely a mixture of naso-pharyngeal commensals, but pathogens such as *Strept. pneumoniae* and *H. influenzae* are often isolated. These organisms become more numerous during acute exacerbations of infection.

Pathology. In all cases there is overactivity of the mucus-secreting glands and goblet cells in the bronchi and bronchioles. The vast excess of mucus so produced coats the bronchial walls and clogs the bronchioles. Mucosal oedema further reduces the calibre of the air passages and as the degree of obstruction is greater during expiration air is 'trapped' in the alveoli. With the passage of time the alveoli become permanently overdistended and there is extensive rupture of their walls. Sooner or later, infection supervenes and this leads to widespread destruction of the bronchioles and pulmonary lobules by what is in effect a low-grade suppurative bronchopneumonia. Compensatory over-distension of the surviving alveoli adds to the disorganisation of pulmonary structure. These changes, which are responsible for the clinical syndrome of 'emphysema', are more fully described on p. 388.

Clinical Features. The disease usually starts with repeated attacks of 'winter cough', which show a steady increase in severity and duration with successive years, until cough is present all the year round. Wheezing and tightness in the chest are common complaints, especially in the morning before the bronchial secretions are cleared, often with difficulty, by coughing. The sputum may be scanty, tenacious, mucoid, and occasionally streaked with blood, or copious and watery. A frankly purulent sputum is indicative of respiratory infection, which supervenes from time to time in most cases of chronic bronchitis.

Dyspnoea in chronic bronchitis is in most cases a direct consequence of the destruction and disorganisation of pulmonary tissue. It may, however, be aggravated by airways obstruction, caused by infection or by an increase in mucosal oedema which may be produced by adverse atmospheric conditions.

Variable numbers of inspiratory and expiratory rhonchi, mainly low and medium pitched, are present in most cases of chronic bronchitis and there may also be some coarse crepitations. The physical signs found in more advanced cases are described in the section on Emphysema (p. 390).

Radiological Examination. Chronic bronchitis produces no characteristic abnormality in the radiograph, but bronchography shows various irregularities of bronchial calibre, outline and branching. The features of emphysema are present in some cases (p. 390).

Diagnosis. It is necessary to exclude other conditions, which may be associated with chronic cough, such as:

1. Chronic pulmonary tuberculosis, by repeated examination of the sputum for acid-fast bacilli and by radiological examination.
2. Cardiac failure, especially that due to mitral disease (p. 200) or hypertension (p. 230).
3. Bronchiectasis (p. 370).
4. Bronchial carcinoma (p. 375).

Course and Prognosis. Chronic bronchitis is usually a progressive disease, punctuated by acute exacerbations and remissions, and eventually causing ventilatory and cardiac failure (p. 308). Some patients die within five years of the onset of symptoms, while others survive for 20 to 30 years, with a steadily diminishing respiratory reserve. In some cases, however, chronic bronchitis is a relatively benign condition which remains static for many years.

Prophylaxis. The control of atmospheric pollution in urban areas and the increased use of measures to prevent the inhalation of dust by industrial workers would undoubtedly reduce the prevalence of chronic bronchitis. In individual cases the abandonment of tobacco smoking and the prompt treatment of acute respiratory infections are important preventive measures.

Treatment

1. *Bronchial irritation* must be reduced to a minimum. If a tobacco smoker, the patient should be urged to give up the habit completely and permanently. Dusty and smoke-laden atmospheres should be avoided. This may require a change of occupation or environment, often involving a reduction of income. Most patients find it difficult to accept this advice, but in a condition as potentially serious as chronic bronchitis it is important to point out that if exposure to dust or smoke continues the patient may become totally incapacitated long before he reaches retiring age.

2. *Respiratory infection* must be promptly controlled as every such episode causes further permanent damage to the lungs. The patient should be instructed to observe the colour of his sputum every morning and to consult his doctor at once if it becomes green or yellow. In that event he should be given either tetracycline or ampicillin in a dose of 250 mg. four times daily for five to seven days. Phenoxymethylpenicillin by mouth is seldom effective in the treatment of infective exacerbations of chronic bronchitis.

If the sputum remains consistently purulent except while antibiotics are being administered or if episodes of infection occur with extreme frequency, antibiotic therapy may have to be given on a long-term basis, possibly for the rest of the patient's life, despite the potential dangers (p. 80). Tetracycline and ampicillin are suitable drugs for this purpose. Either drug should be prescribed initially in a dose of 250 mg. four times daily, but when the sputum becomes mucoid the dose can be reduced to 750 mg. or even 500 mg. daily, provided this is sufficient to keep the sputum free of pus. In some cases it is possible to prevent episodes of infection by giving continuous treatment with an antibiotic only during the winter months, when the liability to infection is greatest. The results with tetracycline and ampicillin are broadly similar but at present tetracycline is to be preferred on grounds of cost.

3. *Symptomatic measures* may be required to control unproductive cough during the night, to enable sputum to be coughed up more easily and to relieve breathlessness and wheeze. Nocturnal unproductive cough will often be less troublesome if the patient sleeps in a heated bedroom, but pholcodine or methadone (p. 323) may be required to control it. A hot drink or the inhalation of steam helps to liquefy sputum and make it easier to bring up. So-called expectorant cough mixtures are of little or no value in this

respect. Measures for the relief of asthmatic symptoms are described on p. 343.

4. *Ventilatory failure* must be promptly treated (p. 320).

BRONCHIAL ASTHMA

Bronchial asthma is characterised by paroxysms of dyspnoea accompanied by wheezing, resulting from temporary narrowing of the bronchi by muscle spasm, mucosal swelling or viscid secretion. The bronchial narrowing interferes with pulmonary ventilation and increases the work of breathing by raising the resistance to air flow within the bronchi. Being more marked during expiration it also causes air to be 'trapped' in the lungs.

The narrowed bronchi can no longer be effectively cleared of mucus by the act of coughing and obstruction of many of the smaller bronchi by inspissated and often very tenacious secretion adds to the respiratory embarrassment. In fatal cases this is usually the most conspicuous finding at autopsy.

Aetiology. Asthma may begin at any age, but in most cases it starts in childhood, adolescence or early adult life.

Predisposing Factor

Constitution. There appears to be some basic constitutional defect which renders these patients liable to develop asthma. A family history of asthma or some other manifestation of allergy is often obtained, especially when the condition develops in childhood. The asthmatic patient tends to be highly strung, emotional and overconscientious.

Exciting Factors

In the majority of patients with bronchial asthma the agent or agents responsible for producing attacks cannot be identified. This is the main reason why treatment is so unsatisfactory. There are, however, some cases in which one or more of the following factors seem to excite attacks:

1. *Allergy.* Asthmatic attacks may occur as a manifestation of hypersensitivity to certain foreign substances (p. 20). This type of asthma generally starts in childhood or adolescence and there is

often a liability to other allergic manifestations such as hay fever, eczema and urticaria.

The more common substances to which hypersensitivity may develop are:

(*a*) *Inhalants*: dusts, moulds, grass and flower pollens, feathers, animal dander, face powder.
(*b*) *Ingestants*: wheat, egg, milk, chocolate, beans, potato, pig products, beef, shell-fish.

The presence of hypersensitivity to these substances can sometimes be detected by skin tests. A superficial scratch is made on the anterior aspect of the forearm and a drop of a specially prepared solution of the substance to be tested is smeared over it. A positive reaction is indicated by the development of a wheal 10-15 minutes after inoculation. The relationship between skin hypersensitivity and asthma is seldom clear-cut, and in practice skin tests are of limited value in the management of cases of asthma.

Asthma may also occur as a manifestation of anaphylaxis after injections of foreign protein, e.g. antitoxic serum, or of idiosyncrasy to certain drugs, e.g. aspirin, morphine and iodides.

2. *Bronchial irritation and infection*. Asthma may be induced by the inhalation of cold air, dust or acrid fumes. Respiratory infection may also precipitate an attack of asthma which may continue until the infection is controlled. In many cases, however, infection seems to develop, as a complication, after the start of an attack. This is a particularly common sequence of events in chronic asthma.

3. *Psychological disturbance*. Anxiety, worry and protracted nervous or emotional strain (p. 1259) seem to be of importance both in promoting the first attack and in perpetuating the condition.

4. *Other factors*. Occasionally asthmatic attacks are associated with the operation of conditioned reflexes. For example, in a patient whose attacks are caused by contact with the pollen of, say, roses, the sight of artificial roses may induce a paroxysm. In some cases the exciting factor is exertion, while in others it is gastric distension after a meal.

Clinical Features. In typical cases of *episodic bronchial asthma* the paroyxsms are of sudden onset, but may be preceded by a feeling of tightness in the chest. The dyspnoea, which may be intense, is chiefly expiratory in character. Expiration becomes a conscious and exhausting muscular effort, in contrast to inspiration which is short and gasping. The patient adopts an upright position, fixing the shoulder-girdle to assist the accessory muscles of expiration. Wheezing, chiefly expiratory, is heard and there may be an unproductive cough which aggravates the dyspnoea. Cyanosis or, in severe cases, pallor may be present and the pulse is rapid.

The attack may end abruptly within an hour or two, sometimes with the coughing up of tough viscid sputum, but a less intense degree of expiratory wheeze may persist for many hours or even for several days before subsiding gradually. The term *status asthmaticus* is applied when a state of intense dyspnoea persists for many hours or days.

The sputum, usually scanty, may contain numerous eosinophil leucocytes and, occasionally, gelatinous casts of small bronchi. The blood may show an eosinophilia during paroxysms, particularly in allergic cases.

In *chronic bronchial asthma* the paroxysmal character of the asthma is usually less conspicuous, the chief clinical features being chronic low-grade wheeze and breathlessness on exertion. Cough and mucoid sputum, with recurrent episodes of frank respiratory infection, are manifestations of chronic bronchitis, which often complicates this type of asthma.

Physical Signs in the Chest

1. *During a paroxysm* the chest is held near the position of full inspiration. The percussion note may be hyperresonant. The breath sounds, which are obscured by numerous high-pitched, musical rhonchi, are vesicular in character with prolonged expiration. Vocal resonance is normal or diminished.

2. *Between paroxysms* there are usually no abnormal physical signs except in patients with chronic asthma, who are seldom without rhonchi. Severe asthma starting in childhood usually causes a 'pigeon chest' deformity.

Radiological Examination of the chest in uncomplicated bronchial asthma shows no abnormality. In long-standing cases the signs of emphysema (p. 390) may be present.

In a small number of patients with asthma, transient radiological opacities appear in different parts of the lungs over a period of months or years in association with a marked degree of eosinophilia in the peripheral blood and in the sputum. The term '*pulmonary eosinophilia*' is applied to this syndrome, which seems to be an allergic response to a variety of agents including intestinal parasites and drugs (Loeffler's syndrome), microfilaria (tropical eosinophilia) and aspergillus fumigatus (p. 365).

Diagnosis

1. Paroxysmal nocturnal dyspnoea ('cardiac asthma') due to left heart failure (p. 170) must be distinguished from bronchial asthma.

2. Intense dyspnoea may develop rapidly when the trachea or a main bronchus is obstructed by a tumour or foreign body, but the stridor present in these cases is usually readily distinguishable from the characteristic asthmatic wheeze.

3. Chronic bronchitis with asthmatic features may be difficult to distinguish from chronic asthma; there is indeed no sharp dividing line between these two conditions.

Course and Prognosis. The prognosis of the individual attack is good except in severe status asthmaticus, where there is occasionally a fatal outcome. Asthma is, however, often a lifelong disorder and in the more severe cases, especially those of chronic asthma, emphysema eventually develops. Many patients, however, live to old age without serious disability. In children with episodic asthma there is a tendency for the attacks to become fewer and less severe, and even to cease spontaneously at or soon after puberty. In many cases a series of attacks may occur nightly for a few nights, after which there is freedom perhaps for months. A seasonal incidence may be observed, paroxysms occurring during the summer in those patients allergic to pollens, etc., and during the winter in those in whom respiratory infection is a precipitating factor.

Treatment

1. CONTROL OF A PAROXYSM. The patient should be allowed to take up the position which he finds most comfortable, either propped up in bed or sitting in a chair. If there is obvious cyanosis oxygen should be administered.

A paroxysm is often relieved by sympathomimetic drugs, which should always be tried in the first instance. In mild cases ephedrine, 30-60 mg. by mouth, or isoprenaline sulphate, 20 mg. sublingually, may be sufficient to abort a paroxysm. Isoprenaline may also be inhaled in the form of an aerosol (1 per cent. solution) produced by a hand nebuliser, or one of the efficient but expensive devices specially designed for this purpose, e.g. Medihaler-iso, Pressurised Iso-brovon, may be used. This method of administration is, in general, more effective than sublingual administration. In more severe cases a subcutaneous injection of adrenaline, 1 : 1000 solution, is needed. An injection of 0·5 ml., repeated if necessary 30 minutes later, should be sufficient. In some cases the patient may be taught to administer this himself. The earlier these drugs are given in an attack the more effective they are likely to be.

In very severe cases which have failed to respond to adrenaline, aminophylline, 0·25-0·5 g. in 10-20 ml. sterile water, should be slowly injected intravenously.

A patient in *status asthmaticus* who does not respond to adrenaline or aminophylline is usually relieved by the administration of one of the corticosteroid group of drugs, and in some instances this may be the only means of averting a fatal outcome. In a case of average severity prednisolone should be given by mouth in a dose of 15 mg. six-hourly on the first day, 10 mg. six-hourly on the second, and 5 mg. six-hourly thereafter. Patients who are gravely ill should receive 100 mg. of prednisolone by mouth in the first 12 hours, along with hydrocortisone hemisuccinate intravenously in a dose of 100-200 mg. four-hourly. Dehydration, which increases the viscosity of the sputum, must be corrected, if necesssary by giving fluids intravenously. If in spite of this treatment the patient's condition continues to deteriorate, and particularly if the arterial P_{CO_2} rises above 50 mm. Hg, the measures recommended for the treatment of acute ventilatory failure (p. 320) should be instituted.

Unless the patient is being artificially ventilated, hypnotics should be used with caution and opiates must never be given. Chlorpromazine, 25-50 mg. intravenously, is relatively safe, and may promote relaxation and sleep. As status asthmaticus is often complicated by respiratory infection, which may not always be readily recognisable in the early stages, a suitable antibiotic (p. 317) should be administered in every case.

The usual procedure after the patient begins to recover is to continue treatment with prednisolone in diminishing dosage for 10-14 days. Corticosteroids have, however, only a temporary suppressive effect, and asthma frequently recurs a few weeks or even a few days after treatment is stopped.

2. TREATMENT OF CHRONIC ASTHMA. Patients who have frequent recurrences of episodic bronchial asthma and those with chronic asthma (p. 342) present a special problem in treatment as many of them are incapacitated for prolonged periods by breathlessness on exertion. The first essential in these cases is to treat any respiratory infection present with an antibiotic (p. 339). Thereafter an attempt should be made to keep the asthmatic symptoms under control by prescribing relatively long-acting bronchodilator drugs such as ephedrine, 30-60 mg. thrice daily, or choline theophyllinate, 200 mg. four times daily. A combination of these two drugs with phenobarbitone is considered by some physicians to be particularly effective. In addition the patient should be provided with the means to suppress any sudden increase in symptoms. In some cases tablets of isoprenaline sulphate (20 mg.) are adequate for this purpose, but the inhalation of isoprenaline (p. 344) is usually more effective. The patient should however, be warned that the excessive use of isoprenaline inhalers may be dangerous.

In a few cases, if these measures are ineffective, it may be necessary to give prednisolone as a long-term suppressive measure. Such treatment, owing to the danger of side effects (p. 722), should be reserved for particularly intractable cases. A substantial measure of relief can be obtained by giving prednisolone on only three consecutive days per week in a dose of 5 mg. four times daily. With this method of administration the total dose is relatively small and the danger of serious side-effects slight. Occasionally, however, the symptoms can be controlled only by giving prednisolone continuously in a dose of 5-15 mg. daily. In such cases the risk of serious side-effects must be weighed against the dangers of uncontrolled asthma and the degree of disability it is causing.

3. MANAGEMENT OF FACTORS OF AETIOLOGICAL IMPORTANCE. It is essential to decide at the outset whether emotional disturbance, infection or allergy is of aetiological importance and to direct treatment accordingly.

(*a*) *Allergy*. When asthma appears to be due to hypersensitivity to an inhalant or an ingestant an attempt should be made to remove the suspected substance from the patient's environment. If skin tests show hypersensitivity, hyposensitisation may be of value. An antihistamine drug (p. 328) may be helpful when hay fever accompanies the asthma.

It must be remembered that in all asthmatic subjects there is an increased danger of anaphylactic reactions (p. 26) when serum of any kind is administered. An enquiry must be made regarding previous reactions to injections of serum and the asthmatic patient should always be tested for hypersensitivity by the injection of 0·1 ml. of the serum intradermally. If a positive reaction is obtained desensitisation should be carried out before the full dose of serum is administered.

(*b*) *Infection*. Where the attacks of asthma are clearly related to the development of respiratory infection, they can often be prevented if the infection is controlled promptly by an antibiotic (p. 336). Any chronic infection in the upper respiratory tract, such as sinusitis, must also be dealt with.

(*c*) *Emotional disturbance*. Sedation is indicated if emotional stress appears to be present. For this purpose phenobarbitone in a dose of 30-60 mg. thrice daily should be prescribed. Causes of friction and anxiety must be removed or reduced to a minimum. This can often be done by the family doctor but may require the assistance of a specialist in psychology (p. 1259). Great benefit may be obtained by having asthmatic children attend a child guidance clinic when emotional difficulties are suspected.

4. Breathing and Postural Exercises. The main object of these exercises is to prevent chest deformity and defective posture which are prone to develop in all patients with asthma, especially children.

THE PNEUMONIAS

Pneumonia is the term used to describe inflammation of the lung. There are many different kinds of pneumonia, some common, others rare. Aetiologically they can be divided into two broad groups:

1. *The Specific Pneumonias*, in which the disease is caused by a specific pathogenic organism.

2. *The Aspiration Pneumonias*, in which some abnormality in the respiratory system predisposes to the invasion of the lung by

organisms of relatively low virulence such as *H. influenzae*, some types of *Strept. pneumoniae* and certain of the bacteria forming the normal flora of the upper respiratory tract and mouth. In this group of pneumonias, as the term implies, infection generally reaches the alveoli by aspiration from other parts of the respiratory tract.

In certain types of specific pneumonia and in some forms of aspiration pneumonia suppuration is the dominant pathological abnormality and the term '*suppurative pneumonia*' has been applied to this group of cases. The features which distinguish suppurative pneumonia from most other types of bacterial pneumonia include destruction of lung parenchyma by the inflammatory process, a high incidence of abscess formation and the subsequent development of pulmonary fibrosis and bronchiectasis. The condition is considered a sufficiently important entity to warrant separate description outwith the two main aetiological groups.

THE SPECIFIC PNEUMONIAS

This group may be further subdivided into *Bacterial* and *Viral* Pneumonias.

The bacteria known to produce specific types of pneumonia are *Strept. pneumoniae*, *Staph. pyogenes*, *Klebsiella pneumoniae* and *Mycobacterium tuberculosis*.

A large number of viruses, including most of those described on p. 324, and perhaps others as yet unidentified, may produce a specific viral pneumonia. A similar illness may also result from infection with *Rickettsia* (*Coxiella*) *burneti* (Q-fever) and *Mycoplasma pneumoniae* (p. 353).

Pneumonia due to the pneumococcus, sometimes referred to as 'acute lobar pneumonia' but more accurately as 'pneumococcal pneumonia', constitutes a large proportion of all specific pneumonias and will be described in detail. Shorter accounts will be given of the other types.

PNEUMOCOCCAL PNEUMONIA
(Syn.: ACUTE LOBAR PNEUMONIA)

Pneumococcal pneumonia is characterised by homogeneous consolidation of one or more lobes or segments.

Aetiology. The disease occurs at all ages but most frequently in early and middle adult life. The highest incidence is in winter. It is usually a sporadic disease, the mode of spread being by droplet infection.

Pathology. The pneumonic process usually affects only one lobe or segment but the infection may spread to other lobes or segments in the same or opposite lung. There is coincident inflammation of the overlying pleura. The affected lobes or segments undergo consolidation in which there is exudation of fibrin, red blood cells and later white blood cells into the alveoli. Resolution is achieved first by liquefaction of the exudate by macrophages and then by its absorption or expectoration. Resolution is usually complete, fibrosis and bronchiectasis seldom following this type of pneumonia.

Clinical Features. The onset is sudden, with rigor, or with vomiting or a convulsion in children. The temperature rises in a few hours to 39-40° C. (102-104° F.). Malaise, loss of appetite, headache, and aching pains in the body and limbs accompany the pyrexia. Localised pain of the pleuritic type (p. 310) develops at an early stage in the illness. It is generally referred to the chest wall but may on occasion be referred to the shoulder or to the abdominal wall, when it may be difficult to determine whether the primary lesion is in the chest or abdomen. There is a short, painful cough, dry at first but later productive of tenacious sputum which is often rust-coloured and occasionally frankly blood-stained. Respiration is rapid (30-40 per minute in adults, 50-60 in children), shallow and painful, and there may be dilatation of the alae nasi with each inspiration. The pulse is rapid, and in severe cases the blood pressure tends to fall. The skin is hot and dry, the face is flushed, and cyanosis may occur early. Herpes labialis is often present. A marked neutrophil leucocytosis, 15,000 to 30,000 per c.mm., is characteristic. The causative pneumococcus can usually be isolated from the sputum, and a positive blood culture may be obtained in severe cases.

Course. Most cases respond promptly to the administration of an antibiotic. Within 24 to 48 hours of the start of treatment the temperature falls to 37° C. (97-99° F.), the pulse and respiratory rates drop sharply, cyanosis disappears and the systemic disturbance is dramatically relieved. The cough, sputum and pleuritic pain take rather longer to subside but seldom remain for more than a few days, and within a week the patient is well again. Delayed recovery suggests either that some complication has developed (e.g. empyema) or that the diagnosis of pneumococcal pneumonia is incorrect.

Occasionally in old or debilitated persons the response to treatment is unsatisfactory. The symptoms rapidly become worse, there is increasing weakness, dyspnoea, cyanosis and delirium, and death takes place within a few days from hypoxia or peripheral circulatory failure. A fatal outcome is more liable to occur if there has been a delay in starting specific treatment.

Physical Signs in the Chest

For the first 24 to 48 hours of the illness there is diminution of respiratory movement, slight impairment of the percussion note, and often a pleural rub on the affected side. The breath sounds are diminished vesicular, and fine crepitations may be heard at the end of inspiration. At a variable time after the onset, generally within two days, signs of consolidation appear (p. 320), the breath sounds being of the high-pitched bronchial type. When resolution begins, these breath sounds are replaced by low-pitched bronchial breath sounds, which later revert gradually to normal vesicular. Numerous coarse crepitations are heard, indicating liquefaction of the exudate.

The physical signs may be modified in the following circumstances: (1) if the pneumonic process does not extend to the periphery of the lung, there may be no abnormal physical signs throughout the illness; (2) if a bronchus is blocked by secretions, signs suggestive of atelectasis may be found (p. 320), but mediastinal displacement is usually absent, as a consolidated lobe cannot shrink to the same degree as a healthy lobe; (3) if a sterile or purulent effusion develops, the physical signs of fluid in the pleural space are usually found (p. 320), but often bronchial breath sounds persist and the presence of an effusion may be suspected only from the stony dullness of the percussion note.

Radiological Examination. This shows a homogeneous opacity localised to the affected lobe or segment, appearing within 12 to 18 hours of the onset of the illness. Radiological examination is particularly helpful when the diagnosis is in doubt or if a complication such as empyema is suspected.

Complications

1. *Pulmonary*

(*a*) Spread to other lobes. This may occur but is uncommon.

(*b*) Delayed resolution. The time taken for the abnormal physical signs and the radiological opacity to disappear varies considerably from case to case. For example, resolution is less rapid in older patients, in those with chronic bronchitis and emphysema, and in cases where the consolidation has originally been very extensive. In 85 per cent. of all cases the abnormal physical signs disappear within two weeks and the radiological opacity within four weeks. Although resolution is occasionally delayed for longer periods in uncomplicated pneumococcal pneumonia, such delay is often due to the presence of some underlying lesion such as bronchiectasis or bronchial carcinoma. This possibility must always be kept in mind when a pneumonia is slow to resolve.

2. *Pleural*

(*a*) Sterile pleural effusion (p. 398). The occurrence of a small serous effusion during the course of pneumonia is not uncommon, causes no symptoms and requires no treatment. A larger effusion should be aspirated in order to prevent pleural thickening.

(*b*) Empyema (p. 400). Recurrence of fever a few days after the initial pyrexia has settled, uninfluenced by the continued administration of an antibiotic, is strongly suggestive of empyema.

3. *Cardiovascular*

(*a*) Peripheral circulatory failure.

(*b*) Acute pneumococcal pericarditis and endocarditis. (Rare).

(*c*) Venous thrombosis in the lower limbs (p. 291).

4. *Neurological*

(*a*) Meningism. This is not uncommon in children, and lumbar puncture may be required to distinguish it from meningitis (p. 1158).

(*b*) Pneumococcal meningitis. (Rare.)

Diagnosis. The characteristic features of pneumococcal pneumonia are the initial rigor, herpes labialis, the physical signs of consolidation, a high neutrophil leucocyte count, pneumococci in the sputum, a lobar or segmental radiological opacity and a rapid and complete response to treatment with an antibiotic.

The following conditions may be difficult to distinguish from pneumococcal pneumonia:

1. *Other types of acute specific and aspiration pneumonia* (pp. 352-362).

2. *Pulmonary infarction* (p. 253) in which pyrexia is less marked and is uninfluenced by antibiotics, frank haemoptysis is common, cough is inconspicuous and the site of origin of the embolus can usually be identified.

3. *Tuberculous pleurisy with effusion*, in which the correct diagnosis can usually be suspected from the insidious onset, the virtual absence of cough and sputum, the physical signs of pleural effusion, the absence of leucocytosis and the failure of the pyrexia to respond to antibiotics. The diagnosis may be supported by the radiological findings and by the aspiration of serous fluid, in which lymphocytes predominate, from the pleural space.

4. *Pulmonary tuberculosis*, acute cases of which may simulate pneumonia. The patient is, however, seldom as acutely ill as in pneumococcal pneumonia; it is uncommon for the respiratory rate to be markedly increased and the white blood count is seldom raised above 12,000 per c.mm. The diagnosis can usually be made by radiological examination, and the isolation of tubercle bacilli from the sputum puts it beyond doubt.

5. *Atelectasis*, in which the diagnostic difficulty is usually caused by the presence of infection (aspiration pneumonia) in the collapsed lung tissue. If the breath sounds are reduced or absent and there are signs of mediastinal displacement to the same side, atelectasis is probably present, but often the symptoms and signs are indistinguishable from those of pneumococcal pneumonia and the correct diagnosis can be made only by radiological examination.

6. *Acute bronchitis*, in which the onset is less abrupt and the systemic disturbance less severe than in pneumococcal pneumonia. Pleuritic pain is not present and the physical signs and radiological appearances of pneumonic consolidation are not found.

7. *Inflammatory conditions below the diaphragm*, such as cholecystitis, perforated duodenal ulcer, acute appendicitis, subphrenic

abscess, generalised peritonitis and hepatic amoebiasis, may occasionally be mistaken for pneumococcal pneumonia. A carefully taken history is one of the most valuable means of determining the site and nature of the primary disease. A high temperature and a very rapid respiratory rate favour a diagnosis of pneumonia, whereas tenderness of the abdominal wall suggests that the primary lesion is below the diaphragm. A leucocyte count may help in some cases. Sometimes radiological examination of the chest is necessary before the presence of pneumonia can be confirmed or excluded.

Prognosis. The prognosis depends on the virulence of the infecting pneumococcus, the age of the patient (the mortality rises above the age of 60), the general state of health (the mortality is increased when pneumonia complicates some other serious disease or develops in a chronic alcoholic), and the stage of the illness at which specific treatment is instituted. The prognosis is less favourable in the absence of a brisk temperature response or when there is a poor leucocytosis, marked cyanosis, delirium or peripheral circulatory failure, or extension of the disease to other lobes.

Other Types of Specific Pneumonia

1. **Staphylococcal Pneumonia.** Pneumonia due to *Staph. pyogenes* may occur either as a primary respiratory infection or as a blood-borne infection from a staphylococcal lesion elsewhere in the body, e.g. osteomyelitis. The second condition is essentially one of pyaemic abscess formation in the lungs. Unless an empyema is produced by rupture of one of these abscesses into the pleura, the pulmonary lesions may pass unnoticed, being overshadowed by the severe general illness.

Primary staphylococcal pneumonia, although it occurs much less frequently than pneumococcal pneumonia, is a relatively common illness, especially as a complication of influenza. It may present as a lobar or segmental pneumonia, which may be difficult to distinguish clinically from a severe pneumococcal infection, or as a suppurative pneumonia (p. 359) with multiple lung abscesses which may persist as thin-walled cysts after the acute infection has subsided. Culture of the sputum yields a growth of coagulase-positive staphylococci which are frequently resistant to penicillin, streptomycin, tetracycline and chloramphenicol. At the present time few strains of staphylococci causing pneumonia are resistant to erythromycin, methicillin, cloxacillin, cephaloridine or fusidic acid, but this relatively favourable situation may alter if these drugs are prescribed on a larger scale in future.

2. **Klebsiellar Pneumonia (Friedländer's Pneumonia).** Pneumonia due to *Klebsiella pneumoniae* is a rare disease. There is usually massive consolidation and excavation of one or more lobes, the upper lobes being most often involved, with profound systemic disturbance, the expectoration of large amounts of purulent, sometimes chocolate-coloured, sputum and a high mortality. The diagnosis is made by the radiological appearances and the isolation of the causative organism from the sputum. The choice of antibiotic should be guided by the results of sensitivity tests. Streptomycin, chloramphenicol, ampicillin and kanamycin are those most likely to prove effective.

Permanent lung damage is usually produced by this type of pneumonia. Fibrosis and bronchiectasis are therefore common sequelae, the latter occasionally requiring surgical treatment (p. 374).

3. **Tuberculous Pneumonia** (p. 421).

4. **Viral Pneumonias.** A distinctive form of pneumonia may be produced by certain viruses and by other organisms which exhibit a similar pathogenicity to lung tissue:

(*a*) *Viruses of the psittacosis-ornithosis group.* This infection is endemic in birds such as parrots and pigeons. The disease may be contracted from infected birds, but sometimes it is transmitted from man to man by droplet spread.

(*b*) *Respiratory syncytial* (*RS*) *virus* and, occasionally, *adenoviruses* (p. 324).

(*c*) *Mycoplasma pneumoniae* ('*Eaton agent*'). Infection with this organism may give rise to the production of cold haemagglutinins or *Streptococcus* MG agglutinins, which can be detected in the serum.

(*d*) *Rickettsia* (*Coxiella*) *burneti.* This organism is the cause of Q-fever, which is known to be responsible for a few cases of pneumonia in Britain, the usual source of infection being cattle or sheep.

The pneumonia caused by each of these organisms gives rise to a similar clinical picture, which differs from that of the bacterial pneumonias in that fever and toxaemia usually precede the respiratory symptoms by several days. Severe headache and anorexia are characteristic features in the early stages. The physical signs in the chest appear later and are seldom gross, and the existence of a pulmonary lesion may not be recognised unless a radiograph is taken. The spleen is often palpable during the first week. The white blood count is generally normal, and the pyrexia does not respond to penicillin. If facilities for virological investigation are available the diagnosis can often be confirmed either by virus isolation or by serological tests (p. 325).

The disease is usually self-limiting. The pyrexia subsides by lysis after 5 to 10 days, and complete clinical recovery and radiological resolution follow. Very rarely, death takes place from widespread extension of the pneumonia or from an associated encephalitis.

The *influenza virus* seldom produces a specific pneumonia. Pneumonia complicating influenza is usually due to secondary bacterial invasion, e.g. by staphylococci, pneumococci or *H. influenzae*.

The term '*primary atypical pneumonia*' which is sometimes used to describe virus pneumonia is unfortunately also applied to another type of pneumonia with an entirely different aetiology, namely benign aspiration pneumonia (p. 357). It is therefore an ambiguous and confusing term and its use is not recommended.

THE ASPIRATION PNEUMONIAS

Aetiology. This group, sometimes described as the non-specific pneumonias, comprises a large number of different conditions, their common features being the absence of any specific pathogenic organism in the sputum and the existence of some abnormality of the respiratory system which predisposes to the invasion of the lungs by relatively avirulent organisms derived from the upper respiratory tract or from the mouth, e.g. streptococci, certain types of pneumococci, *H. influenzae*, Vincent's spirochaetes and fusiform bacilli.

Infection may reach the lungs in various ways. Pus may be aspirated from an infected nasal sinus or septic matter may be inhaled during tonsillectomy or dental extraction under general anaesthesia. Vomitus or the contents of a dilated oesophagus may enter the larynx during general anaesthesia, coma or even sleep. Infected secretion in the bronchi and pus from bronchiectatic cavities or from a lung abscess may also be carried into the alveoli by the air stream or by gravity.

Inefficient coughing caused by post-operative or post-traumatic thoracic or abdominal pain, by debility or immobility, or by laryngeal paralysis may also predispose to the development of aspiration pneumonia.

Bronchial obstruction, partial or complete, as for example by a carcinoma, is another potential cause of aspiration pneumonia, as it allows infection derived from the upper air passages to become established in the inadequately ventilated portion of lung beyond the obstruction.

There are *four* types of aspiration pneumonia with fairly well-defined clinical and pathological features: (1) acute lobular pneumonia, (2) benign aspiration pneumonia, (3) hypostatic pneumonia and (4) post-operative pneumonia.

Acute Lobular Pneumonia
(Syn.: Acute Bronchopneumonia)

This type of pneumonia is invariably preceded by bronchial infection, which accounts for the widespread, lobular distribution of the lesions. It occurs most frequently in children and in elderly people. In children it is often a complication of measles or whooping-cough, in adults of acute bronchitis or influenza. It is particularly common in patients with chronic bronchitis and emphysema.

Pathology. There is acute inflammation of the bronchi, especially the terminal bronchioles, which are filled with pus. Collapse and consolidation of the associated groups of alveoli follow. The lesions are distributed bilaterally in small patches which tend to become larger by confluence and are often more extensive in the lower lobes. The alveolar exudate consists of neutrophil leucocytes with a small amount of fibrin. There is interstitial oedema and cellular proliferation in the alveolar walls, and compensatory emphysema around the collapsed alveoli. Sometimes a large bronchus is blocked by secretion, and atelectasis of a whole lobe or segment follows.

Resolution of lobular pneumonia may be incomplete, and in such cases pulmonary fibrosis and bronchiectasis are common sequelae.

Clinical Features. The patient first exhibits for two or three days the clinical features of acute bronchitis and then, as lobular pneumonia develops, the temperature rises to a higher level, the pulse and respiratory rates increase, and dyspnoea and cyanosis appear. There is generally a severe cough with purulent sputum which may be blood-stained or, occasionally, rusty. Pleuritic pain is relatively uncommon and herpes labialis is seldom present, in contrast to pneumococcal pneumonia. Blood examination usually shows a neutrophil leucocytosis.

Physical Signs in the Chest during the early stages are those of acute bronchitis (p. 335), and in many cases no signs of consolidation appear. These signs (p. 320) may, however, develop over areas of confluent bronchopneumonic consolidation. If a large bronchus becomes obstructed by exudate the signs of atelectasis (p. 320) will be found.

Radiological Examination shows scattered areas of increased density in both lungs, chiefly in the lower lobes.

Course and Complications. The disease tends to run a more protracted course than pneumococcal pneumonia. The onset is less dramatic and recovery is less rapid. Penicillin, if given alone, is relatively ineffective but good results are usually obtained by combining it with streptomycin, or by substituting tetracycline or ampicillin. Serious early complications, such as lung abscess and empyema, are now rare, but incomplete resolution, which may lead to bronchiectasis, is still seen more frequently in lobular pneumonia than in pneumococcal pneumonia. The actual number of patients developing bronchiectasis in this way has, however, fallen dramatically since antibiotics became available.

Patients with chronic bronchitis and emphysema who contract lobular pneumonia are liable to develop ventilatory failure (p. 308).

Diagnosis. Except in infants and in the massive confluent forms, there is seldom much difficulty in distinguishing lobular pneumonia from *pneumococcal pneumonia*, owing to its insidious onset with preceding bronchitis, irregularity of fever and course, the frequent absence of signs of frank consolidation, the infrequency of pleurisy, herpes and rusty sputum, and the mixed nature of the organisms in the sputum.

When the illness runs a prolonged course an acute tuberculous infection must be considered in the differential diagnosis and the sputum examined repeatedly for tubercle bacilli.

Prognosis. The mortality is higher at the extremes of life, especially if the disease is associated with malnutrition or if it supervenes on chronic bronchitis and emphysema, chronic nephritis or heart disease. The more widespread the involvement of the lungs and the greater the systemic upset, the worse is the prognosis.

Prophylaxis. The incidence of lobular pneumonia can be reduced by careful attention to apparently benign upper respiratory infections such as coryza and acute bronchitis, especially when they occur at the extremes of life and in patients with chronic bronchitis. Measures to prevent whooping-cough and measles, and adequate treatment of those diseases, are also important in prophylaxis (pp. 44, 52).

Benign Aspiration Pneumonia

This type of pneumonia is due to the aspiration of infective secretion into the lungs during the course of an upper respiratory infection such as coryza or sinusitis. It is thus often associated with segmental atelectasis. The organisms causing the pneumonia, being derived from the upper respiratory tract, are generally of low virulence and the degree of systemic disturbance is usually slight. In fact, the symptoms are often no more severe than would be expected with an uncomplicated upper respiratory infection and the existence of a pneumonia may be discovered only by radiological examination. As a rule, however, the condition manifests itself by cough, purulent sputum, low-grade pyrexia and sometimes pleuritic pain, in association with a frank upper respiratory infection. Localised coarse crepitations are often the only abnormal physical signs. Leucocytosis is absent or slight. The radiological lesions are usually *unilateral*, the characteristic appearance being a mottled opacity involving a single lobe or segment, which in some cases may be atelectatic.

The condition is liable to be confused with viral pneumonia because of the paucity of pulmonary symptoms and signs and the normal white blood count, but the co-existent upper respiratory infection and the minimal systemic upset are useful distinguishing features.

Recovery generally takes place rapidly if specific treatment is given. As suppuration is not a feature of this type of pneumonia, permanent lung damage and bronchiectasis rarely occur.

Hypostatic Pneumonia

This type of aspiration pneumonia occurs in elderly or debilitated people and is a common cause of death. These patients, being physically weak and immobilised in bed, have difficulty in expectorating bronchial mucus and the alveolar transudate which tends to form as a result of hypostatic pulmonary congestion (p. 257). These secretions gravitate to the lung bases where infection, usually with upper respiratory commensal organisms, frequently supervenes. The lobular pneumonia which results is a relatively mild process but is sufficient to cause death in patients enfeebled by old age, heart failure or toxaemia.

The onset of symptoms in hypostatic pneumonia is insidious, often almost imperceptible at first. A slight cough accompanied by an increase in pulse and respiratory rates is usually the earliest manifestation. Pyrexia and leucocytosis may occur but are seldom marked. Physical signs in the chest are usually bilateral and confined to the lower lobes. Frank signs of consolidation may be present, but numerous coarse crepitations at both long bases without signs of consolidation are a more common finding.

Once the condition is established it pursues a rapidly fatal course, usually with little apparent discomfort to the patient.

Preventive measures are all-important. Elderly people should not be confined to bed unless this is absolutely necessary. Patients who have to be kept in bed should have their position changed frequently and be given deep breathing exercises.

Post-operative Pneumonia

Primarily this condition is not pneumonia but atelectasis due to obstruction of a large bronchus by viscid secretion which cannot be expectorated owing to post-operative pain. Infection may occur secondarily with the production of an aspiration pneumonia. The condition is fully described on p. 368.

Suppurative Pneumonia
(*including Pulmonary Abscess*)

Suppurative pneumonia is the term used to describe a form of pneumonic consolidation in which there is destruction of lung parenchyma by the inflammatory process. Although abscess formation is a characteristic histological feature of suppurative pneumonia, it is usual to restrict the term 'pulmonary abscess' to lesions in which there is a fairly large localised collection of pus, or a cavity lined by chronic inflammatory tissue, from which pus has been evacuated.

Aetiology. Suppurative pneumonia and pulmonary abscess may be produced by infection of previously healthy lung tissue with *Staph. pyogenes* or *Klebs. pneumoniae.* These are, in effect, specific bacterial pneumonias associated with pulmonary suppuration.

More frequently, suppurative pneumonia and pulmonary abscess are forms of aspiration pneumonia. They may develop after the inhalation of septic material during operations on the nose, mouth or throat under general anaesthesia, or of vomitus during anaesthesia or coma. In such circumstances gross oral sepsis is an important predisposing factor. Bacterial infection of a pulmonary infarct or of an atelectatic lobe may also produce a suppurative pneumonia or a pulmonary abscess. The organisms isolated from the sputum may include *Strept. pneumoniae, Staph. pyogenes, Strept. pyogenes, H. influenzae* and, in a few cases, anaerobic streptococci and other anaerobes such as Vincent's spirochaetes and fusiform bacilli. In some cases, however, no pathogens can be identified and the illness remains entirely unexplained.

Pathology. Descriptions have already been given of staphylococcal pneumonia (p. 352) and of klebsiellar pneumonia (p. 353). When suppurative pneumonia follows the inhalation of infective material from the upper air passages, it is more often unilateral than bilateral, and is usually situated in the axillary part of either upper lobe or in the apex of a lower lobe, these being the most dependent areas when the patient is lying on his side or on his back respectively. In other cases the site depends on the nature and situation of the primary pathological lesion. For example, when the abscess is secondary to bronchial obstruction by a carcinoma its site is determined by the position of the tumour in the bronchial tree.

In suppurative pneumonia the lung parenchyma is destroyed by the inflammatory process and replaced by fibrous tissue. Usually the suppurative process is localised but occasionally it spreads by direct continuity until a whole lung is irreparably damaged. Abscesses, when present, may be single or multiple. In some cases they may become very large as a result of inflation caused by a 'check valve' mechanism at the junction of the cavity and the draining bronchus.

Although antibiotic therapy controls the infection it cannot restore lung tissue damaged by suppuration. The affected parts of lung become shrunken and of rubbery consistence, and the bronchi, which are also involved in the inflammatory process, often become dilated—a condition known as bronchiectasis (p. 370).

Clinical Features. These depend to a large extent on the pathogenesis of the lesion. The onset of the illness may be either insidious or acute, but cough with purulent sputum, usually large in amount, sometimes foetid and occasionally blood-stained, is present from an early stage. There is high, remittent pyrexia with shivering and sweating, and a neutrophil leucocytosis in the region of 15,000-25,000 per c.mm. Pleuritic pain is common and clubbing of the fingers may develop as early as 10 to 14 days after the onset of the illness. Progressive deterioration in general health with marked loss of weight ensues if the case remains untreated. The rupture of a large localised abscess into a bronchus can be assumed when a large quantity of pus is suddenly expectorated. Such an incident is often preceded by blood-staining of the sputum and followed by remission of the pyrexia.

Physical Signs in the Chest. These also depend on the nature of the primary pathological process. Signs of consolidation (p. 320) are the most frequent finding, but those of atelectasis are also quite common. Frank signs of cavitation are rarely found.

Localised coarse crepitations may be the only abnormality. A pleural rub is sometimes present.

Radiological Examination. There may be a homogeneous lobar or segmental opacity consistent with consolidation or atelectasis. Alternatively, if the lesions are of lobular distribution, multiple coarse, mottled opacities may be found. A large homogeneous opacity, which may later cavitate and show a fluid level within it, is the characteristic finding when a frank pulmonary abscess is present.

Diagnosis. This cannot be considered complete unless the primary aetiological factor or factors are identified. Sputum should be sent for bacteriological examination, and if a pathogenic organism is isolated its sensitivity to the various antibiotics should be determined.

Suppurative pneumonia must be distinguished from:

1. Pulmonary tuberculosis by examination of the sputum for tubercle bacilli.
2. Bronchial carcinoma, by bronchoscopy.

Pulmonary abscess must be distinguished from:

1. Pulmonary tuberculosis with cavitation, by examination of the sputum for tubercle bacilli.
2. A cavitated malignant growth, by the radiological appearances and, if necessary, by bronchoscopy.
3. Empyema, which gives the physical signs of fluid in the pleural space and from which pus can be obtained by paracentesis.

Course and Prognosis. Untreated, the disease carries a high mortality; those who survive are liable to recurrences of infection and some develop bronchiectasis. Empyema is a not uncommon early complication. Metastatic cerebral abscess may occur.

Since the introduction of antibiotics the mortality has fallen sharply and many cases now escape with relatively little lung damage and bronchiectasis.

Prophylaxis. Every precaution should be taken during operations on the mouth, nose and throat to prevent the inhalation of blood, tonsillar fragments, etc. In view of its depressant action on the cough reflex morphine should be used cautiously after any general anaesthetic.

Oral sepsis should be eradicated, especially if a general anaesthetic is contemplated.

Bronchial obstruction should be treated whenever possible. When the obstructing agent is tenacious secretion, this can readily be removed by postural coughing or bronchoscopic aspiration. When the obstruction is due to a bronchial carcinoma, resection of the lung or lobe containing the growth is the only effective treatment.

THE TREATMENT OF PNEUMONIA

1. Chemotherapy

The principles governing the specific treatment of bacteria infections of the respiratory tract have already been stated (p. 317) When a clinical diagnosis of pneumonia is made, provided the patient is not gravely ill, the initial treatment should consist of benzylpenicillin, 0·5-1 mega unit twice daily by intramuscular injection. Where the pneumonia has developed in a patient with chronic bronchitis, tetracycline or ampicillin, 250 mg. four times daily, should be substituted for penicillin in order to control the infection with *H. influenzae* frequently present in such cases. Patients who are gravely ill and in whom a staphylococcal infection is suspected should receive, in addition to penicillin, tetracycline or ampicillin, an antibiotic to which such an organism is unlikely to be resistant, e.g. erythromycin, 500 mg. six-hourly by mouth, or cloxacillin, 500 ng. six-hourly by mouth or 250 mg. six-hourly by intramuscular injection. Methicillin is also an effective antibiotic in these circumstances but has now been superseded by cloxacillin as it is more expensive and cannot be given by mouth.

As soon as the results of bacteriological examination of the sputum are available and the drug sensitivity of the organism is known, usually 48 hours after treatment is started, the choice of antibiotic must be reviewed:

(*a*) If *Strept. pneumoniae*, *Strept. pyogenes* or an anaerobic streptococcus is isolated, or no pathogenic organisms are obtained on culture, and the patient appears to be making satisfactory clinical progress, parenteral therapy with benzylpenicillin may be stopped and phenoxymethylpenicillin, 250 mg., four times daily, given by mouth. In patients with chronic bronchitis, treatment with tetracycline or ampicillin, 250 mg. four times daily by mouth, should be maintained.

(*b*) If *Staph. pyogenes* is isolated, treatment must be modified in accordance with the results of sensitivity tests. In the unlikely event of the organism being sensitive to benzylpenicillin, no change in antibiotic need be made. If it is resistant to penicillin, treatment with streptomycin, tetracycline or chloramphenicol is seldom effective, even if *in vitro* sensitivity to these antibiotics is reported, and one of the following antibiotics will usually be required: erythromycin, 250-500 mg. four times daily, cloxacillin, 500 mg. four times daily, fusidic acid (Fucidin), 500 mg. thrice daily (all by mouth), or cephaloridine, 500 mg. twice daily by intramuscular injection. The last two preparations are very expensive and there are few occasions on which they have to be prescribed.

(*c*) If *Klebs. pneumoniae* is isolated, sensitivity tests will indicate which antibiotic is likely to prove most effective. Those to which this organism is most frequently sensitive are streptomycin, chloramphenicol, ampicillin and kanamycin. The antibiotic selected should be given initially in twice the standard dosage.

(*d*) If bacteriological examination is uninformative and a viral infection is suspected, it is usually advisable to give an antibiotic to prevent or control secondary bacterial infection. In these circumstances tetracycline is the drug of choice as it has the advantage of possessing some degree of activity against certain viruses, e.g. psittacosis, and virus-like organisms, such as *Rickettsia burneti* and *Mycoplasma pneumoniae*. A dose of 500 mg. four times daily is recommended.

It is important to take into account the clinical progress in addition to the bacteriological findings before changing from one antibiotic to another. If, for example, recovery is taking place satisfactorily, the isolation of an organism showing *in vitro* resistance to the antibiotic in use is not necessarily an indication for a change in treatment. If, however, the patient is not improving and is still febrile when such an organism is isolated, an appropriate change in antibiotic is imperative.

The impulse to substitute another antibiotic, *where there is no bacteriological indication for doing so* should be resisted. The failure of patients to respond to treatment may be due to a complicating factor such as plueral infection, tuberculosis or bronchial obstruction by a tumour, and these conditions must be carefully excluded before the antibiotic is changed.

No hard and fast rule can be laid down for the *duration* of chemotherapy. In most cases of uncomplicated pneumococcal pneumonia a seven-day course of treatment is usually adequate but this may have to be extended if the response to treatment is slow. In staphylococcal and klebsiellar pneumonia, and in other forms of suppurative pneumonia, chemotherapy should be continued for a minimum of two weeks and should not be stopped until the causative organism has been eliminated from the sputum.

2. General Measures

The usual regime of treatment for an acute infection (p. 18) should be instituted. If respiratory distress is marked the patient should be propped up comfortably with pillows or a backrest.

Cough, when distressing and unproductive, should be controlled by the measures described on p. 323. When secretions are present in the bronchi the patient should be firmly encouraged to cough them up, even if the effort to do so causes pleural pain. In these circumstances a mild analgesic (p. 323) and the support of a nurse's hand on the painful side of the chest may relieve the distress of coughing. Postural drainage (p. 373) may be of value if the sputum is difficult to bring up, particularly if it is copious, as in suppurative pneumonia, or when pneumonia complicates bronchiectasis.

Pleural pain should be treated with local heat and analgesics (p. 323). It is, however, dangerous to prescribe morphine if even a milddegree of ventilatory insufficiency is present, and the safest policy is not to use this drug at all in the treatment of pneumonia.

Hypoxia demands oxygen therapy (p. 318).

Delirium, which in the early stages is caused mainly by the high temperature, and later by cerebral hypoxia, may have to be controlled by sedation. The safest drugs to use are chlorpromazine, 50 mg., or paraldehyde, 5-10 ml., both by intramuscular injection.

Peripheral circulatory failure occurring in the course of pneumonia is seldom reversible when it has become established, but the administration of metaraminol hydrogen tartrate (Aramine) by intramuscular injection or by continuous intravenous infusion may be a life-saving measure. This treatment should be combined with intravenous hydrocortisone or prednisolone. Efficient oxygen and antibiotic therapy is essential in such cases.

Abscess formation. Suppurative pneumonia is not in itself a reason for any departure from standard antibiotic policy. When an abscess cavity is present, however, it must be kept empty by regular postural drainage. Medical treatment is almost invariably successful and surgical measures nowadays are seldom required. In occasional instances, however, a large abscess may have to be drained externally or residual bronchiectasis resected.

FUNGAL INFECTIONS OF THE BRONCHI AND LUNGS

Pulmonary actinomycosis is usually caused by infection with the anaerobic fungus, *Actinomyces israeli*, which exists as a commensal in the human mouth. It presumably gains access to the lungs by aspiration, and may produce a widespread suppurative lobular pneumonia. Empyema, often bilateral and associated with persistent chest wall sinuses, may develop at a later stage or occasionally *de novo*. The infection usually responds to benzylpenicillin, given by intramuscular injection in very large doses, e.g. 2 mega units eight-hourly for six weeks.

Bronchopulmonary aspergillosis is usually caused by infection with *Aspergillus fumigatus*. This fungus produces conidia or spores, which are ubiquitous in the atmosphere. Three main forms of the disease have been described:

1. Colonisation by the fungus of pulmonary cavities or cysts, and of lung tissue damaged by infarction or suppuration. A large mass of mycelium in a pulmonary cavity, often described as an 'aspergilloma' may simulate a tumour on radiological examination. This 'saprophytic' form of pulmonary aspergillosis seldom gives rise to symptoms, but in almost every case antibodies of the precipitin type can be detected in the serum.

2. Rarely, in debilitated subjects, there is a direct extension of infection from devitalised to healthy lung tissue. This condition has a bad prognosis and death may occur from septicaemia.

3. Some patients develop manifestations of hypersensitivity to *Aspergillus fumigatus*, including bronchial asthma, an increased eosinophil count in the peripheral blood and allergic lesions in the

bronchi and/or lungs (a form of 'pulmonary eosinophilia'). The bronchial lesions, which consist of firm plugs of mucin coated with eosinophils and containing fungal mycelium may cause lobar or segmental atelectasis. The pulmonary lesions, consisting of localised eosinophilic infiltrations, are typically transient and migratory. Most patients with allergic bronchopulmonary aspergillosis exhibit skin sensitivity to an extract of *Aspergillus fumigatus*, precipitins can often be detected in the serum, and the organism can usually be cultured from the sputum.

Treatment of bronchopulmonary aspergillosis is, in general, unsatisfactory. Aqueous suspensions of the antifungal antibiotics, nystatin and pimaricin, administered by inhalation, may be of value in some cases. Amphotericin B, which must be given intravenously, is rather more effective, but toxic effects are frequent and severe. Corticosteroids may be highly effective in allergic forms of the disorder, but the results of hyposensitisation are disappointing. A large aspergilloma may require resection.

Bronchopulmonary moniliasis is caused by *Candida albicans* which, like *Aspergillus fumigatus*, is liable to colonise devitalised lung tissue, particularly in debilitated subjects who have been treated with wide-spectrum antibiotics, and in patients dying of leukaemia or reticulosis who have been treated with corticosteroids and cytotoxic drugs. Infection of healthy lung tissue is almost unknown. The condition may show some response to treatment with nystatin, pimaricin or amphotericin B.

Other fungal infections. Histoplasmosis, caused by *Histoplasma capsulatum*, coccidioidomycosis, caused by *Coccidioides immitis*, and blastomycosis, caused by *Blastomyces dermatitidis*, are endemic in certain areas of North America, but are seldom, if ever, contracted in Britain. For further information about these diseases the reader should refer to a more specialised textbook.

PULMONARY ATELECTASIS

When a bronchus is obstructed, as for example by a growth or by a foreign body, inspired air can no longer reach the lung beyond the obstruction and the air already present in the alveoli is absorbed into the blood. The lung, lobe or segment supplied by the obstructed bronchus then shrinks, by virtue of its unopposed elastic recoil, to a fraction of its normal size. This is referred to as *atelectasis* or *absorption collapse*. Certain mechanical readjustments take place within the thorax to fill the space left by the atelectatic lung. These are:

1. Overexpansion of the lung tissue that is still aerated (*compensatory emphysema*).
2. Depression of the ribs on the affected side.
3. Elevation of the hemidiaphragm.
4. Traction of the mediastinum towards the side of the atelectasis.

The extent to which these changes occur depends on the extent of the atelectasis. If a whole lung is involved the mediastinal displacement may be so great that the heart comes to lie against the lateral chest wall (Fig. 45).

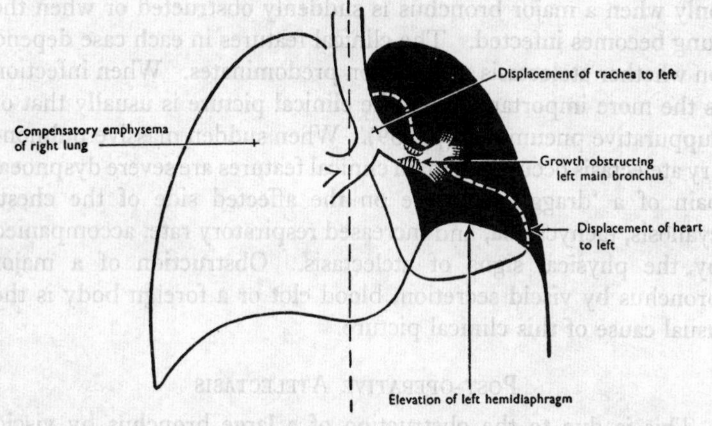

FIG. 45
THE EFFECTS ON NEIGHBOURING STRUCTURES OF ATELECTASIS OF THE LEFT LUNG

Aetiology. Bronchial obstruction leading to atelectasis may be caused by:

1. *Viscid secretion*, e.g. following surgical operations and in association with bronchiectasis, whooping-cough and sometimes acute bronchitis and bronchial asthma.
2. *Tumour*, e.g. bronchial carcinoma, bronchial adenoma.

3. *Enlarged hilar lymph nodes*, e.g. from secondary carcinoma, tuberculosis or reticulosis.

4. *Foreign body*, e.g. a fragment of tooth inhaled during dental extraction under general anaesthesia.

5. *Cardiovascular lesions*, e.g. aortic aneurysm, aneurysmal dilatation of left atrium, pericardial effusion.

Depending on the site of the bronchial obstruction, atelectasis of a lung may be total, lobar or segmental. Obstruction of the smallest bronchi or bronchioles by secretion causes lobular atelectasis, which is a characteristic histological feature of lobular pneumonia (p. 355).

Clinical Features. Atelectasis is usually an incident in the course of some other disease, and in such circumstances its occurrence may cause no new symptoms except, perhaps, increased dyspnoea on exertion. As a rule, acute symptoms are produced only when a major bronchus is suddenly obstructed or when the lung becomes infected. The clinical features in each case depend on whether atelectasis or infection predominates. When infection is the more important factor the clinical picture is usually that of suppurative pneumonia (p. 359). When sudden massive pulmonary atelectasis occurs,the main clinical features are severe dyspnoea, pain of a 'dragging' nature on the affected side of the chest, cyanosis, tachycardia, and increased respiratory rate, accompanied by the physical signs of atelectasis. Obstruction of a major bronchus by viscid secretion, blood clot or a foreign body is the usual cause of this clinical picture.

Post-operative Atelectasis

This is due to the obstruction of a large bronchus by viscid mucus which cannot be expectorated owing to post-operative pain. It occurs most commonly after upper abdominal and thoracic operations, especially in patients with chronic bronchitis, The atelectatic lobe is apt to become infected if the bronchial obstruction is not promptly relieved. The pneumonic process is usually mild but occasionally, if virulent organisms are present, the condition may proceed to suppuration with the formation of a lung abscess or an empyema.

Clinical Features. The illness generally begins 12 to 24 hours after operation, sometimes later with dyspnoea or, less commonly, pain as the presenting symptom. There is a sharp elevation of temperature, pulse and respiratory rates, and it is usually obvious from the patient's noisy respiration and from the rattle in his chest when he attempts to cough that secretion is being retained in the trachea and bronchi. The physical signs of atelectasis (p. 320) are usually present. Breath sounds are absent at first while secretion occupies the larger bronchi, but later, when the secretion has been aspirated into the peripheral bronchi, bronchial breath sounds are heard.

Prophylaxis. It is possible to reduce the incidence of post-operative atelectasis by five simple measures:

1. Forbidding the patient to smoke for at least a week before operation.
2. Teaching the patient breathing exercises pre-operatively.
3. Treating any pre-operative respiratory infection with an antibiotic.
4. Ensuring that the patient sits up as soon as possible after the operation.
5. Encouraging the patient to cough up sputum after the operation. The pain produced by coughing can be minimised by small doses of morphine, 10 mg. for an adult, and by having a doctor or nurse support the wound with a hand each time the patient coughs.

Diagnosis. The development of acute respiratory symptoms within 48 hours of a thoracic or abdominal operation is in itself almost diagnostic of pulmonary atelectasis. Pulmonary embolism and infarction tend to occur at a later stage and can usually be recognised from the history and physical signs, and by the demonstration of a source for the embolus. Radiological examination may be helpful in doubtful cases.

Pneumococcal pneumonia and pulmonary tuberculosis should always be kept in mind in the differential diagnosis of post-operative respiratory illness.

Treatment. If atelectasis occurs despite preventive measures, steps must immediately be taken to clear the bronchi of the obstructing secretion by vigorous postural coughing (p. 373) and, if that fails, by aspiration of the secretion through a bronchoscope.

Oxygen must be given continuously if cyanosis is present. A course of tetracycline or ampicillin, or of penicillin and streptomycin (p. 362), should be started as soon as the diagnosis is made, in order to prevent or control infection in the atelectatic lobe.

Atelectasis due to the Inhalation of a Foreign Body or Blood Clot

The accidental inhalation of a small foreign body is not uncommon in childhood, but most cases follow operations on the mouth or throat under general anaesthesia. The aspirated material is often more highly infective than in the usual type of post-operative atelectasis, and pulmonary suppuration is thus a more frequent complication. Bronchoscopic removal of the obstructing agent should be the first step in treatment, which is otherwise the same as for post-operative atelectasis.

BRONCHIECTASIS

Aetiology and Pathogenesis. Bronchiectasis, which is the term used to describe abnormal dilatation of the bronchi, may be produced in three different ways:

1. When atelectasis occurs following obstruction of groups of *small* bronchi by secretion, the shrinkage of the affected portion of lung exerts outward traction on the walls of the medium-sized bronchi, which become dilated. Bronchiectasis arising in this way may be reversible if the obstructed bronchi can be cleared of secretion before the walls of the dilated bronchi are seriously damaged by infection. When the bronchial obstruction is itself the result of severe bronchopulmonary infection the bronchiectasis is liable to become permanent. It is probable that damage to the deeper layers of the bronchial walls, such as occurs in all types of suppurative pneumonia and lung abscess, and in some cases of pulmonary tuberculosis and acute bronchopneumonia, is much more important in this respect than the relatively superficial lesions of acute bronchitis.

2. It may be due to bronchial distension resulting from the formation of pus beyond a lesion obstructing a major bronchus, such as a bronchial carcinoma, a tuberculous hilar lymph node or an inhaled foreign body.

3. Rarely, it may be the result of congenital maldevelopment of the bronchi.

Bronchial dilatation by itself does not necessarily cause symptoms, which are usually due to infection in the dilated bronchi and in the adjacent lung tissue.

Because of the many different causes of bronchiectasis no precise age and sex incidence can be stated. When it occurs following acute pulmonary infections or secondary to obstruction of a bronchus by tuberculous lymph nodes (the two most common causes), the disease usually starts in childhood but may not produce severe symptoms until some years later.

Pathology. The bronchial dilatations may be cylindrical, fusiform or saccular in shape. Although bronchiectasis may involve any part of the lungs, depending on the site of the primary pathological process, the lower lobes are more frequently affected than the upper and middle. In addition, the more efficient drainage by gravity of the upper lobes renders bronchiectasis there less liable to produce serious symptoms than when it involves the lower lobes. The bronchiectatic cavities may be lined by granulation tissue, squamous epithelium or normal ciliated epithelium, depending on the degree of infection present. There may also be inflammatory changes in the deeper layers of the bronchial walls and chronic inflammatory and fibrotic changes in the surrounding lung tissue.

Clinical Features. Three groups of clinical features occur in bronchiectasis:

1. *Those due to the accumulation of pus in the bronchiectatic cavities:*

(*a*) *Chronic cough*, usually worse in the mornings and often induced by changes in posture.

(*b*) *Purulent sputum*, which in advanced cases is copious and sometimes foetid.

2. *Those due to inflammatory changes in the surrounding lung tissue and pleura:*

(*a*) *Febrile episodes*, commonly ascribed to influenza or pneumonia, which often follow an upper respiratory infection and usually last for a few days but occasionally for weeks. Malaise, shivering and night sweating accompany the pyrexia, and there is almost always an increase in the amount of cough and sputum. A polymorphonuclear leucocytosis is usually present.

(*b*) *Dry pleurisy*, which frequently accompanies the febrile episodes.

(*c*) *Empyema*, which is a not uncommon complication of bronchiectasis.

3. *Those due to haemoptysis*, caused by bleeding from thin-walled anastomatic vessels connecting the pulmonary and bronchial arteries, and situated in the walls of the bronchiectatic cavities. It ranges in amount from blood-stained sputum to massive haemorrhage. It may be present in association with the first two groups of symptoms, but recurrent haemoptysis may also occur as an isolated symptom in the absence of cough and sputum ('dry' bronchiectasis).

When suppuration, either in the dilated bronchi or in the lungs, is a marked feature it causes a decline in the patient's general health, with lassitude, anorexia, loss of weight, night sweating and clubbing of the fingers and toes. In many cases, however, symptoms are slight, consisting merely of recurrent episodes of cough and purulent sputum with no symptoms in the intervening periods and no deterioration in general health.

Physical Signs in the Chest. These may be unilateral or bilateral and are usually basal. If the bronchiectatic cavities are dry and there is no atelectasis, there may be *no* abnormal physical signs. If a large amount of secretion is present, numerous coarse crepitations are heard over the affected areas. When atelectasis is present the character of the physical signs depends on whether or not the major bronchi in the collapsed lobe are patent. The signs found in both circumstances are described on p. 320.

Radiological Examination. In ordinary radiographs the dilated bronchi themselves are seldom visible, but radiological changes may be produced by associated pulmonary inflammation or atelectasis. A diagnosis of bronchiectasis can be made with certainty only from radiographs taken after the introduction into the trachea of a radio-opaque iodised oil such as propyliodone (Dionosil), which outlines the bronchi and demonstrates any bronchial dilatation that is present, its position and its extent. This procedure is known as *bronchography*.

Diagnosis. When bronchograms are available the diagnosis of bronchiectasis is self-evident, but it should not be forgotten that other conditions, notably chronic bronchitis and active pulmonary tuberculosis, may co-exist. It is of particular importance, when surgical treatment for bronchiectasis is contemplated, to consider whether the symptoms may not be principally due to chronic bronchitis. This should always be suspected when dyspnoea, wheeze and rhonchi are prominent features.

Bacteriological examination of the sputum is necessary in every case to exclude tuberculosis and to identify the predominant pyogenic bacteria. The sensitivity of these organisms to antibiotics should always be determined as the efficacy of the treatment employed may largely depend on this information.

Course and Prognosis. With modern antibiotic therapy the prognosis, even of advanced cases, has greatly improved and the incidence of complications such as pneumonia, empyema, cerebral abscess and amyloidosis has fallen considerably. A fatal outcome is usually due to a combination of infection, hypoxia and congestive cardiac failure secondary to emphysema.

Prophylaxis. As bronchiectasis commonly starts in childhood following measles, whooping-cough or a primary tuberculous infection, it is essential that these conditions receive adequate treatment. The early recognition and treatment of pulmonary atelectasis is particularly important in this respect (p. 369).

Treatment

Postural Drainage. The purpose of this measure is to keep the dilated bronchi emptied of secretion. Efficiently performed it is of great value both in reducing the amount of cough and sputum and in preventing the 'toxaemia' caused by retained sputum and associated bronchopulmonary infection.

When a lower lobe is involved the patient lies over the edge of the bed or over a chair with his hands on the floor, so that the head is below the level of the body with the base of the affected lung uppermost. He must cough while in this position and expel as much sputum as possible. The procedure should be carried out for 5 to 10 minutes three times a day before meals. If drainage is effective the quantity of sputum steadily diminishes and the cough and systemic disturbance are lessened. Eventually a regular regimen of postural drainage should be established which enables the patient to drain his bronchi effectively every morning and, if necessary, at night also. The time required will, of course, vary from case to case. In some patients the amount of sputum may become so small that postural drainage need be carried out only during exacerbations of infection.

When an upper lobe is involved, postural drainage is carried out first in the upright position and then in the lateral position with the side to be drained uppermost. For the right middle lobe the patient lies on his back with a pillow under the right side and the foot of the bed slightly raised. If more than one lobe is involved, postural drainage should be carried out in the appropriate position for each lobe in turn.

Bronchoscopic aspiration is used to supplement postural drainage only when viscid secretion obstructs a major bronchus and causes atelectasis.

CHEMOTHERAPY. The policy governing the use of antibiotics in bronchiectasis is the same as that in chronic bronchitis (p. 339).

SURGICAL TREATMENT. Before a decision can be made for or against surgical treatment it is essential to obtain bronchograms demonstrating exactly the extent of the bronchiectasis. For this purpose the bronchi of all segments of *both* lungs must be outlined with a radio-opaque contrast medium. Pulmonary function should also be assessed.

The use of antibiotics has greatly reduced the need for surgical treatment. Unfortunately many of the cases in which medical treatment has been unsuccessful are also unsuitable for surgical treatment either because the bronchiectasis is too extensive or because most of the symptoms are due to co-existing emphysema and chronic bronchitis. Emphysema of even moderate severity is a contraindication to surgical treatment, as the increase in exertional dyspnoea which inevitably results is more distressing to the patient than the symptoms of bronchiectasis. The most favourable cases for surgery are children and young adults in whom the bronchiectasis is confined to a single lobe or part of a lobe. Lobar or segmental resection in these patients is a highly satisfactory operation, carrying little risk.

In all cases treated surgically the risks of operation are materially increased by the presence of a large amount of sputum. Efficient pre-operative treatment with postural drainage and chemotherapy is thus of great importance.

OTHER MEASURES. Chronic sepsis in the nose, mouth and pharynx should be treated, and anaemia should be corrected.

INTRATHORACIC TUMOURS

TUMOURS OF BRONCHUS AND LUNG

Primary

Benign: Bronchial adenoma. (Rare.)

Malignant: Bronchial carcinoma. (Common.)

Secondary

Carcinoma: Breast, kidney, uterus, ovary, testis and thyroid are common sites of the primary tumour, but a carcinoma in any situation may produce pulmonary metastases.

Sarcoma in any site may produce pulmonary metastases.

BRONCHIAL CARCINOMA

This is the most common of all primary intrathoracic tumours. Its prevalence is about eight times as great in males as in females and it occurs most frequently between the ages of 50 and 70. It is more common in cigarette smokers than in non-smokers and the increased risk is directly proportionate to the amount smoked. For example, the death rate from bronchial carcinoma in heavy cigarette smokers is 30 times that in non-smokers. The death rate is slightly higher in urban than in rural dwellers, presumably because of the effects of atmospheric pollution.

Pathology. The tumour, which may be a squamous or 'oat-cell' (undifferentiated) carcinoma or, occasionally, an adeno-carcinoma, arises from bronchial epithelium or mucous glands and at an early stage occludes the bronchial lumen. It also invades the deeper layers of the bronchial wall and the surrounding lung tissue. When the tumour obstructs a major bronchus it causes atelectasis of the lung or lobe distal to the obstruction. Infection in the collapsed area may produce pneumonia, pulmonary suppuration or bronchiectasis, and extension of the infection to the pleura may cause pleurisy or empyema. A tumour arising from a peripheral bronchus may attain a very large size without producing a significant degree of atelectasis. Necrosis in a tumour of this type may give rise to a 'carcinomatous lung abscess'.

The tumour may involve the pleura either directly or by lymphatic spread, causing a pleural effusion which is often blood-stained. It may also invade the chest wall and cause severe pain by irritation of the intercostal nerves or the brachial plexus. The tumour or its lymph node metastases may extend into the mediastinum, involving the phrenic and recurrent laryngeal nerves, the sympathetic trunk, the superior vena cava, the pericardium and myocardium, the trachea and the oesophagus.

Lymphatic spread may occur to the supraclavicular and occasionally to the axillary lymph nodes as well as to the mediastinal lymph nodes and pleura. Blood-borne metastases occur most commonly in liver, bone, brain, suprarenals, skin and kidneys. Even a small primary tumour may cause widespread metastases.

Clinical Features. The onset is usually insidious. Cough is the most common early symptom. The amount and character of the sputum depend on the degree of secondary infection present. Repeated slight haemoptysis is a common and characteristic feature. Dyspnoea may occur early when atelectasis is present, but in other circumstances is a late symptom unless the patient is coincidentally suffering from chronic bronchitis and emphysema. Pulmonary infection beyond an obstructing tumour gives rise to a febrile illness accompanied by the clinical features of pneumonia, pulmonary suppuration or bronchiectasis. Pleuritic pain is a frequent symptom and may be due either to infective pleurisy or to malignant invasion of the pleura. A small pleural effusion in a patient with a bronchial carcinoma is often due to infection but a massive blood-stained effusion is always due to invasion of pleura by tumour. Pain in the chest wall or in an upper limb with a nerve root distribution may be present if the tumour involves intercostal nerves or the brachial plexus. Rib destruction by tumour almost invariably accompanies both these lesions.

The symptoms and signs which may occur when the tumour invades the mediastinum are described in the section on mediastinal tumours (p. 380).

Occasionally the presenting symptom is due to a metastatic deposit, e.g. epileptiform fits or personality change (cerebral metastasis), pathological fracture (skeletal metastasis), haematuria (renal metastasis), skin nodules, usually tender (cutaneous metastases). Clubbing of the fingers is often seen and a few patients present the features of hypertrophic pulmonary osteoarthropathy, peripheral neuropathy (p. 1218), cerebellar degeneration or endocrine dysfunction, none of these manifestations necessarily being related to the presence of metastatic tumour. Lassitude, anorexia and loss of weight are *late* symptoms except when pulmonary suppuration is an early development.

Physical Signs in the Chest. These depend on the size of the tumour, but even more on the nature and extent of its secondary effects on lung and pleura.

1. In the early stages a tumour may produce no abnormal physical signs whatever.
2. A tumour obstructing a large bronchus gives rise to the signs of atelectasis (p. 320).
3. A massive tumour may give rise to signs resembling those of a pleural effusion.
4. Involvement of the pleura either by infection or by tumour may produce signs of dry pleurisy (p. 320) or of a pleural effusion (p. 320).

Radiological Examination. A bronchial carcinoma may cause any of the following radiological abnormalities:

1. A dense, irregular, hilar opacity.
2. A dense, fairly well circumscribed, peripheral pulmonary opacity, usually large when first discovered, sometimes irregularly cavitated.
3. An opacity consistent with atelectasis of a whole lung, a lobe or a segment. This may or may not be associated with a dense, irregular, hilar opacity due to the tumour itself.

In some cases radiological examination may also show a pleural effusion (indicating either infection or secondary tumour in the pleura), broadening of the mediastinal shadow (due to lymph node metastases), osteolytic lesions of the ribs (indicating either direct invasion by tumour or blood-borne metastases) or unilateral diaphragmatic paralysis (indicating involvement of the phrenic nerve). A paralysed hemidiaphragm is usually raised and on fluoroscopy moves 'paradoxically' when the patient sniffs, i.e. it moves upwards instead of downwards.

Bronchoscopy. Inspection of the intrabronchial portion of the tumour and removal of tissue for histological examination is possible in about 65 per cent. of cases. In this way the diagnosis can be established with certainty, often at an early and curable stage.

Diagnosis. The diagnosis of bronchial carcinoma should be considered in every middle-aged or elderly person who complains of respiratory symptoms of recent onset which do not clear up completely within a period of two to three weeks, particularly if haemoptysis or pleural pain is present, *even if there are no abnormal physical signs.* Radiological examination should be carried out in all such cases, and bronchoscopy whenever the history or radiological appearances are at all suggestive of tumour. Examination of the sputum for cancer cells has not so far proved to be a reliable means of confirming or excluding a diagnosis of bronchial carcinoma.

The differential diagnosis includes chronic bronchitis, bronchiectasis, slowly resolving pneumonia, pulmonary tuberculosis, aspergilloma (p. 365), primary mediastinal tumour and metastatic pulmonary tumour. Sputum examination is essential in all cases to exclude tuberculosis.

Course and Prognosis. Unless surgical treatment is practicable the average period of survival after the diagnosis is made is less than one year.

Treatment. Resection of the lung (pneumonectomy) or, in selected cases, of the lobe containing the tumour (lobectomy) affords the only prospect of survival. The operation can be performed only on the small number of cases (about 20 per cent.) in which the tumour is discovered at an early and relatively localised stage and pulmonary function is adequate. Recurrence of the tumour is liable to take place even after an apparently satisfactory operation, and only 30 per cent. of such patients survive for more than five years. Earlier diagnosis would probably lead to better results.

Radiotherapy may prolong life, and occasionally cures a proven case. It may also provide temporary symptomatic improvement, particularly in patients with obstruction of the superior vena cava or of the trachea and main bronchi.

Cytotoxic drugs, such as mustine, are less effective than modern techniques of radiotherapy and are more liable to depress the bone marrow. They may, however, be of limited in value the symptomatic treatment of malignant pleural effusion (p. 399), tracheal and superior vena caval obstruction and bone metastases.

Bronchial Adenoma

This is an uncommon tumour occurring in a younger age group than carcinoma and affecting females as often as males. Although classified as a benign tumour it possesses some of the properties of a malignant growth and may eventually give rise to metastases. A bronchial adenoma of the 'carcinoid' type may secrete 5-hydroxytryptamine. The usual pathological lesion is a small, vascular tumour within the bronchial lumen with a large encapsulated extrabronchial extension.

The main clinical features, which may have a duration of several years, are recurrent haemoptysis, due to the vascularity of the tumour, recurrent pulmonary infection resulting from bronchial obstruction and, in rare cases, the carcinoid syndrome. The physical signs most frequently found are those of atelectasis. The diagnosis from bronchial carcinoma can be made only by bronchoscopy and histological examination of a portion of the tumour.

Treatment consists of resection of the pulmonary lobe or segment containing the tumour along with the bronchus from which it arises.

Secondary Tumours of the Lung

Blood-borne metastatic deposits in the lungs may be derived from malignant disease anywhere in the body. The usual sites of the primary tumour have already been stated (p. 375). Tumours of breast, kidney, thyroid, testis and bone are particularly liable to produce pulmonary metastases. The lung tumours are usually multiple and bilateral. Haemoptysis occurs in some cases but often there are no respiratory symptoms and the diagnosis can be made only by radiological examination.

Extensive infiltration of the pulmonary lymphatics by tumour may develop in patients with carcinoma of breast, stomach, pancreas or bronchus. This condition, known as *pulmonary lymphatic carcinomatosis*, causes severe and rapidly progressive dyspnoea.

TUMOURS OF THE MEDIASTINUM

Classification

Tumours of the Lymph Nodes:

1. Secondary carcinoma, usually from bronchus or breast.
2. Lymphadenoma (Hodgkin's disease).
3. Lymphosarcoma.
4. Leukaemia.

Thymic Tumours, e.g. malignant thymoma.

Connective Tissue Tumours, e.g. fibroma, lipoma (benign); sarcoma (malignant).

Neural Tumours, e.g. neurofibroma.

Developmental Tumours and Cysts, e.g. teratoma; dermoid, bronchial and pleuro-pericardial cysts.

Other Lesions presenting as Mediastinal Tumours, e.g. aortic aneurysm, aneurysmal dilatation of left atrium, intrathoracic goitre, sarcoidosis involving lymph nodes.

Pathology and Clinical Features

Benign Tumours

The conditions in this category include neural tumours, teratoma, developmental cysts and intrathoracic goitre. All of them are rare. The effects produced by a benign tumour are related mainly to its size, and symptoms are present only when it compresses vital structures The diagnosis of benign tumour is usually made by chance, when radiological examination of the chest is undertaken for some other reason. Many of the cases are found by mass radiography. If a tumour becomes very large it may cause dyspnoea by compression of lung tissue, or occasionally by narrowing the trachea. A benign tumour in the upper part of the thorax occasionally compresses the superior vena cava (p. 381). *Invasion* of mediastinal structures, bronchi or lungs never occurs.

Malignant Tumours

Included in this category are mediastinal lymph node metastases, lymphadenoma, lymphosarcoma, leukaemia, malignant thymic tumours, mediastinal sarcoma and, in addition, aortic and innominate aneurysms which have certain features in common with malignant mediastinal tumours. All of these conditions, except lymph node metastases, are uncommon.

The distinguishing feature of this group of tumours is their power to invade as well as to compress mediastinal structures, bronchi and lungs. As a result of this property even a small malignant tumour can produce symptoms, although as a rule the tumour has attained a considerable size before this happens.

The structures which may be invaded or compressed and the symptoms and signs produced in each case are:

(*a*) *Trachea*: dyspnoea, stridor, brassy cough.
(*b*) *Main bronchus*: pulmonary atelectasis, dyspnoea.
(*c*) *Oesophagus*: dysphagia.
(*d*) *Phrenic nerve*: diaphragmatic paralysis (p. 377).
(*e*) *Left recurrent laryngeal nerve*: paralysis of left vocal cord, hoarseness.
(*f*) *Sympathetic trunk*: 'Horner's syndrome' (p. 1112).
(*g*) *Pericardium*: pericarditis, either *dry* with pericardial rub, or *with effusion*.
(*h*) *Superior vena cava*: oedema and cyanosis of head and neck, and sometimes of upper limbs also, with distension of external jugular veins and dilated anastomotic veins on anterior chest wall and in axillary regions.

Radiological Examination

A *benign mediastinal tumour* generally appears as a large, round, sharply circumscribed opacity, situated mainly in the mediastinum but often encroaching on one or both lung fields.

A *malignant mediastinal tumour* seldom has a clearly defined margin and often presents as a general broadening of the mediastinal shadow.

Diagnosis. The only common mediastinal tumour is that produced by lymph node metastases from a bronchial carcinoma. An aortic aneurysm and an intrathoracic goitre can often be recognised from the other clinical features, and leukaemia from the blood picture, but the diagnosis of sarcoidosis, lymphadenoma and lymphosarcoma may be difficult unless there is involvement of superficial lymph nodes on which biopsy can be performed. The known radiosensitivity of the last two conditions is sometimes used as a diagnostic test, rapid shrinkage of the tumour following radiotherapy being a typical feature.

As bronchial carcinoma is such a common primary cause of mediastinal tumour, bronchoscopy should be carried out in all cases. In some an exact diagnosis cannot be made without surgical exploration of the chest and removal of the tumour or a portion of it for histological examination.

Treatment

Benign Mediastinal Tumours. These should be removed surgically as soon as they are discovered because (*a*) they tend to produce symptoms sooner or later and (*b*) some of them, particularly cysts, may become infected while others, especially neural tumours, may undergo malignant change. The operative mortality is very small.

Malignant Mediastinal Tumours. In lymphadenoma, lymphosarcoma, leukaemia and malignant thymoma, radiotherapy often produces a remarkable clinical improvement by reducing the size of the tumour. The improvement, although only temporary, may last for months or even years. Lymph node metastases from bronchial carcinoma sometimes respond fairly well to radiotherapy, which may provide valuable symptomatic relief. Complications such as superior vena caval and tracheal obstruction can often be relieved in this way.

PULMONARY FIBROSIS

Aetiology. There are three main types of pulmonary fibrosis:

1. *Replacement fibrosis*, in which the fibrous tissue replaces lung parenchyma damaged by infection or by some other destructive process (e.g. infarction). Fibrosis of this type is a common feature of pulmonary tuberculosis and of all types of pulmonary suppuration (pp. 414, 359).

2. *Focal fibrosis*, which is a reaction to the presence in the lungs of certain types of dust (*pneumoconiosis*).

3. *Interstitial fibrosis* (fibrosing alveolitis) an uncommon condition in which the fibrous tissue is confined to the alveolar walls. Fibrosis of this type which, as a rule, diffusely involves both lungs may develop in sarcoidosis, in certain of the connective tissue disorders and after the

application of deep X-rays to the thorax. Progressive interstitial fibrosis may also occur as a 'primary' disease, the cause of which has not yet been discovered.

Replacement Fibrosis

The fibrosis may be localised or diffuse, depending on the nature and distribution of the primary lesion. In tuberculosis and suppurative pneumonia there may be dense fibrosis confined to a lobe or segment. If the lungs are otherwise healthy, localised fibrosis does not produce any symptoms, but the physical signs described on p. 320 may be found and a radiograph of the lungs will show dense homogeneous or striate shadowing in the lobe or segment affected, with displacement of the mediastinum to the same side. Bronchiectasis may be demonstrated in the fibrotic lobe or segment by bronchographic examination.

Diffuse replacement fibrosis is a feature of some advanced cases of chronic bronchitis. Such patients are usually dyspnoeic on mild exertion, and radiographic examination shows a pattern of coarse reticular shadowing throughout both lungs. Generally, however, the fibrosis itself does not produce any specific physical signs.

Pneumoconiosis

This type of fibrosis is due to the inhalation of certain kinds of dust. The severity of the fibrosis depends not only on the concentration of the dust and the duration of exposure to it but also on the chemical composition and size of the dust particles and on certain other factors such as superadded tuberculous infection, which is particularly liable to develop in some types of pneumoconiosis.

The dust particles after inhalation are conveyed by macrophages from the bronchial mucosa to minute foci of lymphoid tissue scattered throughout the lungs. There, the irritation produced by the solution of the particles in tissue fluid causes, over the course of many years, widespread pulmonary fibrosis.

The two most common types of pneumoconiosis in Britain are *silicosis* and *coal-workers' pneumoconiosis*. Silicosis, the importance of which was first recognised in Rand gold-miners at the beginning of this century, is caused by the inhalation of dust containing a high proportion of silica particles 3μ or less in size.

It occurs in miners who are principally employed in rock-drilling, and also in metal grinders, stone masons and quarry-workers. It causes a severe, progressive type of fibrosis which in many cases is complicated by tuberculosis. Numerically, however, it is much less important than coal-workers' pneumoconiosis, which is due to the inhalation of coal dust and is particularly prevalent in South Wales. Although the presence of a certain amount of silica in the coal may be a factor in the production of this type of pneumoconiosis, its clinical course differs from that of true silicosis. In a high proportion of cases the condition, although it can be recognised radiologically, is not progressive and causes few if any symptoms. Some cases, however, after long exposure to coal dust with a high silica content, or perhaps as a result of intercurrent infection, proceed to massive fibrosis and death from emphysema and congestive cardiac failure. A few patients may develop 'open' pulmonary tuberculosis, with cavity formation and a positive sputum.

Less common types of pneumoconiosis are *asbestosis* and *siderosis*. Asbestosis, which produces a clinical picture similar to that of silicosis, is due to the inhalation of asbestos fibres, which can be recognised microscopically in the fibrotic areas of lung and as 'asbestos bodies' in the sputum. Siderosis is due to the inhalation of iron oxide and occurs in iron-foundry workers and electric-arc welders. It seldom causes serious symptoms unless there is coexistent silicosis, as in iron-foundry workers.

It must be emphasised that in most types of pneumoconiosis a long period of exposure to the dust is necessary before radiological changes appear and an even longer period before symptoms arise. Silicosis and coal-workers' pneumoconiosis can seldom be recognised radiologically until there has been at least 10 years' exposure, and in most cases 15 to 25 years' exposure is required.

Clinical Features. Dyspnoea on exertion, which is slowly progressive over a period of 10 to 15 years and which may eventually become severe and incapacitating, is the characteristic symptom of established pneumoconiosis of all types. Cough and sputum due to associated chronic bronchitis are frequently present. The sputum in coal-workers' pneumoconiosis is often black. Clubbing of the fingers may be present in asbestosis. There may be polycythaemia in advanced cases. If frank pulmonary tuberculosis develops as a complication, additional symptoms such as tiredness, loss of weight, sleep sweats, haemoptysis and pleural pain may occur. Congestive cardiac failure often supervenes as a terminal event.

Physical Signs in the Chest. In the early stages there are no physical signs directly due to pneumoconiosis, but those of associated chronic bronchitis and emphysema are often present. In the later stages the physical signs of pulmonary fibrosis may be found but they are often difficult to recognise. Even when tuberculosis develops, the signs may not be clear-cut owing to the co-existing bronchitis and emphysema.

Radiological Examination. The earliest abnormality is a fine 'nodulation' distributed uniformly throughout both lungs. Later these nodular opacities which at first are small and discrete, resembling the lesions of miliary tuberculosis, become larger and more dense. In coal-workers' pneumoconiosis very large opacities due to massive fibrosis may be present. These lesions sometimes break down and form cavities. Cavitation may also occur if frank tuberculous infection supervenes.

Diagnosis. Pneumoconiosis should be suspected in any person who has chronic respiratory symptoms and has been exposed for many years to dust known to produce the disease. Radiological examination is necessary to confirm the diagnosis and should never be omitted in any suspected case, as pneumoconiosis is a disease scheduled under the National Insurance (Industrial Injuries) Acts. The sputum must always be examined for tubercle bacilli.

Course and Prognosis. In silicosis and asbestosis the disease pursues a slowly progressive course over 10 to 20 years towards complete invalidism and death from respiratory and cardiac failure. Tuberculosis is a fairly common complication of silicosis but, if adequately treated, it should not worsen the prognosis. In asbestosis, malignant tumours of the lung or pleura may develop and cause early death. In cases of coal-workers' pneumoconiosis in which the radiological changes have not progressed beyond the stage of fine nodulation the symptoms may remain mild for an indefinite period, but once progressive massive fibrosis develops the course of the disease differs little from that of silicosis.

Prophylaxis. Pneumoconiosis can be prevented by the wearing of masks, by damping the dust, and by efficient ventilation systems. These precautions are now compulsory by law wherever there is a recognised risk of pneumoconiosis.

Treatment. When a diagnosis is made of silicosis or asbestosis, or of coal-workers' pneumoconiosis at the stage of progressive fibrosis, the patient must change his occupation. In cases of coal-workers' pneumoconiosis in which no symptoms are present and the radiological changes have not progressed beyond the stage of 'fine nodulation,' work in the pits may be permitted provided that the dust concentration is low and regular clinical and radiological supervision can be undertaken.

In the later stages the treatment is that of chronic bronchitis, ventilatory failure (p. 308) and cardiac failure. If pulmonary tuberculosis supervenes it must be treated with specific chemotherapy (p. 425).

Vegetable Dust Diseases. Occupational lung disease may also be caused by the inhalation of vegetable dust, e.g. from cotton (byssinosis), sugar cane (bagassosis) and mouldy hay or straw (farmer's lung). All these conditions may be associated with dyspnoea of rapid onset but this usually subsides soon after the patient ceases to be exposed to the dust. In byssinosis the initial lesion is a bronchiolitis. In farmer's lung and bagassosis there is an interstitial cellular reaction throughout the lungs ('allergic alveolitis') which impairs the uptake of oxygen by the blood in the pulmonary capillaries, and the chest radiograph may show diffuse pulmonary shadowing of a micronodular type.

In all these conditions it is essential to prevent any further inhalation of the dust as if this is not done permanent lung damage may result. In severe cases of farmer's lung and bagassosis, treatment with corticosteroids may be required.

Interstitial Fibrosis (Fibrosing Alveolitis)

As interstitial fibrosis, the causes of which have already been stated (p. 382), usually involves both lungs diffusely, it produces dyspnoea by increasing ventilatory demand (p. 311) and hypoxia by impairing the uptake of oxygen by the blood in the pulmonary capillaries. Even in advanced cases, however, interstitial fibrosis does not lead to hypercapnia since carbon dioxide, unlike oxygen, can readily diffuse through thickened alveolar walls.

The most severe degrees of dyspnoea and hypoxia are seen in patients in whom a diffusion defect follows the application of deep X-rays to the thorax and those in whom the interstitial fibrosis occurs as a primary disease. Interstitial oedema and cellular infiltration precede the development of fibrosis in both these conditions and may cause an acute form of the disorder, which can in some cases be relieved by one of the corticosteroid drugs. Such treatment may have to be maintained for a year or more to prevent relapse.

The clinical features of diffuse interstitial pulmonary fibrosis include progressive dyspnoea, cyanosis, persistent generalised coarse crepitations and, in primary cases, gross clubbing of the fingers. Unless there is a prompt response to corticosteroid therapy the outlook is serious, many of these patients dying within a few years of the onset of symptoms.

* * * * * *

PULMONARY EMPHYSEMA

Aetiology. The word 'emphysema' means 'inflation', in the sense of unnatural distension with air. Distension of the pulmonary air spaces may result from different pathological processes by mechanisms which are poorly understood. Morbid anatomical classifications have little precise correspondence with clinical groupings based on presentation and course.

Classification of Pulmonary Emphysema

Acute

1. *Obstructive*
   (*a*) Localised: results from partial obstruction of a main or lobar bronchus.
   (*b*) Diffuse: develops during acute attacks of bronchial asthma or bronchiolitis.
2. *Compensatory*
   Occurs adjacent to regions of acute atelectasis.

3. *Interstitial*
   Follows rupture of alveoli or bronchi due to trauma or violent coughing, and may lead to mediastinal and subcutaneous emphysema.

Chronic

1. *Diffuse atrophic emphysema*
   'Senile emphysema.'
2. *Focal emphysema*
   (*a*) Post-fibrotic.
   (*b*) Compensatory for atelectasis or surgical removal.
3. *Diffuse vesicular emphysema*
   (*a*) With chronic bronchitis.
   (*b*) Without chronic bronchitis.
4. *Diffuse lobular emphysema*
   With chronic bronchitis and bronchiolitis.

Acute Emphysema

Most of the conditions responsible for acute emphysema are described elsewhere.

Localised Obstructive Emphysema, however, warrants more detailed consideration. This uncommon type of acute emphysema results from *partial* obstruction of a large bronchus, which prevents as much air from leaving the alveoli during expiration as has entered them during inspiration. Obstructive emphysema may be produced by a bronchial carcinoma or adenoma, a tuberculous hilar lymph node or an intrabronchial foreign body. The emphysema affects a single lung, lobe or segment depending on the position of the bronchial lesion. The condition may be difficult to distinguish clinically from spontaneous pneumothorax. It can readily be recognised radiologically by an abnormal degree of transluscency in the affected area of lung, without evidence of pneumothorax but with displacement of the mediastinum to the opposite side, more marked during expiration.

Chronic Emphysema

Pathology. *Diffuse atrophic emphysema* seems to be a degenerative condition seen in elderly patients as part of the ageing process; it also occurs prematurely from the age of 30 onwards, merging in this age-group with diffuse vesicular emphysema without bronchitis. As bronchi become distorted, infection is liable to supervene.

Pulmonary fibrosis may cause widespread *focal emphysema* by obstructing bronchioles during expiration or as compensation for regions of shrunken lung. Lobar or segmental atelectasis, or removal of portions of lung, cause adjacent regions of lung to expand.

The condition underlying clinical 'emphysema' is usually *diffuse vesicular or lobular emphysema.* In vesicular emphysema the respiratory bronchioles are normal but the alveolar ducts and alveoli are distended, with breakdown and disappearance of alveolar septa. There is a history of chronic bronchitis in most cases, with appropriate pathological changes; in some, however, bronchitis does not precede the emphysema. In lobular emphysema the respiratory bronchioles are dilated as well as the ducts and alveoli; bronchitis and bronchiolitis are always present. These cases seem often to represent a more advanced phase of diffuse vesicular emphysema; obstruction of terminal bronchioles is probably the decisive factor in their production, and this group is often referred to as 'chronic obstructive emphysema'. Loss of elastic fibres in the destroyed alveolar septa leads to kinking and further obstruction of bronchioles, already narrowed by oedema and perhaps spasm of bronchiolar muscle.

Bullae, single or multiple, large or small, may develop in any of these types of chronic pulmonary emphysema, but there seems to be no direct relationship between the incidence of bullae and the degree of emphysema. Bullae are thin-walled sacs, lined by alveolar epithelium, formed by coalescence of pulmonary lobules and subsequent distension, and are commonly found along the anterior borders of the lungs. A small bulla may rupture, causing spontaneous pneumothorax. In other circumstances bullae may increase progressively in size and eventually become so large that they interfere seriously with pulmonary ventilation. Provided extensive bullous changes are not present elsewhere the surgical ablation of one or more of these 'giant' bullae always warrants serious consideration.

Pathophysiology

1. *Respiratory work.* The resting position of the chest

approaches the inspiratory position, with flat diaphragm and raised ribs; inspiration becomes more difficult. Bronchiolar oedema and kinking increase expiratory resistance, leading to forceful expiration which collapses bronchi still further, with 'trapping' of inspired air. The non-elastic work of breathing is increased (p. 306).

2. *Distribution* of blood and gas to the lungs becomes markedly uneven, with the results described on pp. 304 to 306. Diffusion is impaired by loss of alveolar surface area, aggravating hypoxia (p. 306).

3. *Pulmonary capillaries* are lost when alveolar walls are destroyed, and constricted by hypoxia. The pulmonary vascular resistance rises; there follow pulmonary hypertension, hypertrophy of the right ventricle and cardiac failure (p. 259).

Clinical Features. The patients are usually men. The only direct symptom of diffuse emphysema is dyspnoea, at first on exercise and later at rest. A history of progressive dyspnoea for which there is no cardiac cause, accompanied by chronic bronchitis, is practically diagnostic of emphysema even without confirmatory clinical signs (p. 320). In advanced cases, however, these signs are always present. A history of chronic bronchitis can be obtained in the vast majority of cases.

Four broad types of presentation are seen. Young patients (30 to 45) with a short history often progress rapidly to respiratory and cardiac failure. A later onset (45 to 60), with a longer history of chronic bronchitis, is more common; these patients deteriorate more slowly, worsening a little with each attack of acute bronchitis. In the later stages acute respiratory infection is a serious event which often precipitates ventilatory and cardiac failure. Cyanosis on slight exercise or even at rest is often seen, together with polycythaemia in a minority of cases. A third group is made up of patients over 60 who may suffer little inconvenience from emphysema because of its slow progress and their increasingly sedentary habits. Lastly, in middle age, some patients present with rapidly progressive dyspnoea, loss of weight, and pallor rather than cyanosis. They have a persistent cough but little sputum, attacks of wheezing, moderate hypoxia becoming severe on exercise, and little or no hypercapnia.

The pathological and pathophysiological basis for these different clinical pictures is not well understood, and intermediate types are often seen.

Prognosis. The patient may live, from the onset of dyspnoea, for from 5 to 20 years. Death is usually due to acute respiratory infection with ventilatory and cardiac failure. Patients seldom survive more than three such severe episodes.

Radiological Examination. There are no unequivocal radiological signs of emphysema, but the following findings suggest that it *may* be present:

1. Unusually clear lung fields *or* coarse, irregular reticular shadowing throughout both lung fields, the nature of the changes depending on the relative degrees of emphysema and fibrosis.

2. Unusually low and flat diaphragmatic shadows, which move poorly (2 cm. or less).

3. Abnormal prominence of the pulmonary arterial shadows at both hila.

4. Enlargement of the main pulmonary artery and right ventricle, indicating cor pulmonale.

Diagnosis. This can usually be made from the history. Less easy is the exclusion of independent or remediable causes of dyspnoea in a patient who has emphysema. These are (1) *left-sided cardiac failure* due to hypertension or to valvular or ischaemic heart disease, in which crepitations from pulmonary oedema may be wrongly ascribed to bronchitis; (2) *spontaneous pneumothorax*, the physical signs of which may pass unnoticed in presence of emphysema; and (3) *giant bullae*, which may be the chief cause of dyspnoea in a patient with only a mild or moderate degree of generalised emphysema. In order to exclude these conditions, radiological examination should be advised whenever an emphysematous patient experiences a rapid increase in dyspnoea. *Bronchial carcinoma*, *pneumoconiosis* and *pulmonary tuberculosis* can be excluded by radiography and bacteriological examination. Pneumoconiosis confers certain pensions rights, and in any suspected case a detailed occupational history should always be taken.

Treatment

1. As the symptoms of emphysema are markedly aggravated by respiratory infection, every effort should be made to prevent

such infection occurring by the avoidance of overheated, crowded places. If a respiratory infection develops it should be treated promptly with an antibiotic (p. 317).

2. Obesity must be prevented or corrected, as excess weight is an intolerable burden on the reduced cardiorespiratory reserve.

3. Breathing exercises of the traditional type, encouraging the patient to force the air out of his lungs, are of no value; indeed, by increasing air trapping, they may even be harmful. If physiotherapy in emphysema has any purpose at all, it should be to induce relaxation of the cervical muscles and to show the patient how to expire slowly and steadily through pursed lips.

4. The surgical ablation of giant bullae, where this is feasible, may produce a dramatic improvement in pulmonary function.

5. Associated chronic bronchitis and bronchial asthma should be treated on the lines recommended on p. 339 and p. 343 respectively.

6. Ventilatory failure should be treated as described on p. 320.

7. Congestive heart failure should receive appropriate treatment (p. 184).

DISEASES OF THE PLEURA

PLEURISY

Inflammation of the pleura manifests itself in three ways, as a fibrinous or 'dry' pleurisy, as a pleural effusion or as an empyema. Although these conditions differ clinically they have a common background and may occur in sequence.

Aetiology. Pleurisy usually occurs as a result of infection. The primary infection is most commonly in the lung, e.g. pneumonia or tuberculosis, less commonly in the chest wall, e.g. an infected wound, or below the diaphragm, e.g. subphrenic abscess, and rarely in the mediastinum. Dry pleurisy and pleural effusion may also occur in the absence of infection in pulmonary infarction and in malignant disease invading the pleura by direct spread from a bronchial carcinoma or by metastasis.

Pathology. As a result of infection or irritation of the pleura there is vascular congestion and the formation of a fibrinous exudate on the pleural surfaces, which lose their normal glossy appearance. The subsequent course of the pleurisy varies from case to case.

1. The fibrinous exudate may be absorbed, leaving the pleura normal.

2. It may undergo organisation with the formation of adhesions between the visceral and parietal layers.

3. There may be an effusion of liquid into the pleural space. The effusion may consist of clear liquid (*serous effusion*) or of pus (*empyema thoracis*). Absorption or mechanical removal of the liquid may allow the two pleural layers to approximate and eventually to adhere. A variable degree of pleural thickening results from this process, which is the natural mode of healing of most types of pleural inflammation.

The course of events in pleurisy depends mainly on the cause. In the pleurisy which accompanies pneumococcal pneumonia, for example, the disease usually does not progress beyond the stage of fibrinous exudation, but sometimes a serous effusion forms and occasionally an empyema develops. In tuberculous pleurisy, on the other hand, the formation of a large serous effusion is common. Such an effusion is usually absorbed spontaneously, unlike a malignant effusion which may continue to re-accumulate for the rest of the patient's life despite repeated paracentesis.

Fibrinous ('Dry') Pleurisy

This term is used to describe cases of pleurisy at the stage of fibrinous exudation when there is no significant degree of effusion. It may be produced by any of the aetiological conditions mentioned above. It may also occur in association with a viral infection (Coxsackie B), which primarily involves the intercostal muscles and is known as 'Bornholm disease'.

Clinical Features. The characteristic symptom of dry pleurisy is *pleuritic pain* (p. 310). On examination, rib movement is restricted and the breath sounds, though vesicular, are diminished on the affected side. A *pleural rub* is heard in a high proportion of cases. This may take the form of a coarse grating or creaking sound or merely of a faint crackling sound audible only towards the end of inspiration, resembling crepitations but unaltered by coughing. In all cases the rub is increased by deep breathing and is never heard when the patient is holding his breath except near the pericardium, where a so-called *pleuro-pericardial rub* may be heard. In the acute stage of dry pleurisy respiration may be so painful that the limited range of movement of the chest wall may be insufficient to produce an audible rub.

The other clinical features depend on the nature of the lesion causing the pleurisy.

Diagnosis. 'Dry pleurisy' is not a complete diagnosis. An attempt must always be made to find a primary cause such as tuberculosis, carcinoma or bronchiectasis. To this end radiological examination must be performed in every case. A negative radiograph does not necessarily exclude a pulmonary cause for the pleurisy. A preceding history of a few days' cough, purulent sputum and pyrexia is presumptive evidence of a pulmonary infection which may not have been severe enough to produce a radiographic abnormality or which may have resolved before the film was taken. Recurrent attacks of dry pleurisy over a number of years, especially if they occur on the same side, are suggestive of underlying bronchiectasis.

Dry pleurisy must be distinguished from intercostal myalgia (pleurodynia), fractured rib, costochondritis, herpes zoster, spontaneous pneumothorax and acute upper abdominal disease.

Course. Depending on the cause, complete clinical recovery may ensue or an effusion may develop, either serous or purulent.

Treatment. The primary cause of the pleurisy must be treated. The symptomatic treatment of pleural pain is described on p. 323.

Pleural Effusion

This term, by general consent, is applied only to serous effusion. The condition of purulent effusion or empyema is described separately on p. 400. The passive transudation of fluid into the pleural cavity, as occurs in congestive cardiac failure, etc., causes the condition called *hydrothorax* to which reference is made on pp. 258 and 302.

Four conditions, viz. pneumonia, tuberculosis, malignant disease and pulmonary infarction, account for the great majority of cases of serous pleural effusion.

Clinical Features. The symptoms and signs of dry pleurisy often precede the development of effusion, but the onset in other cases may be insidious, with little or no pleuritic pain. Pyrexia occurs in most cases, whatever the primary cause, but is more severe in the presence of infection, and more protracted when the infection is tuberculous.

The principal symptom related to the effusion itself is dyspnoea. The severity of the dyspnoea depends on the size of the effusion and on the rate at which it accumulates. A rapidly accumulating effusion of moderate size may cause more severe dyspnoea than a large effusion accumulating slowly.

Physical Signs in the Chest are those of fluid in the pleural space (p. 320).

Radiological Examination shows a dense uniform opacity in the lower and lateral parts of the hemithorax shading off above and medially into the translucency of the lung. When the effusion is loculated, e.g. in an interlobar fissure, a localised opacity is seen.

Diagnosis. The presence of a pleural effusion can usually be recognised from the physical signs, but in some cases it may not be suspected until radiological examination is carried out. Absolute proof that an effusion is present can be obtained only by the aspiration of fluid. A needle should be inserted through an intercostal space over the area of maximum dullness on percussion. or, ideally, at the site of maximum radiological opacity as shown by postero-anterior and lateral films or by fluoroscopy. At least 50 ml. of fluid should be withdrawn, 20 ml. or more being placed in a sterile container for bacteriological examination, 20 ml. in a citrated container for cytological examination and 10 ml. in a chemically clean container for biochemical examination. The second investigation can normally be performed by the clinician, but if malignant disease is suspected a specimen should be sent to a pathologist for examination by a special technique for cancer cells. The appearance and composition of the fluid in the various types of pleural effusion will be referred to later.

Failure to obtain fluid in a suspected case of pleural effusion is often due to faulty localisation, but if aspiration with a wide-bore needle is repeatedly unsuccessful, it is unlikely that a significant amount is present. The clinical features and radiological appearances should then be reviewed with four possibilities in mind: pneumonia, pulmonary infarction, atelectasis and pleural thickening.

Pleural thickening, fibrinous or fibrous, which may follow a pleural effusion, produces similar physical signs except that the mediastinum is either central or displaced *towards* the side of the lesion. Thickening of the pleura can often be recognised by a sensation of resistance transmitted from the point of the needle to the hand manipulating the aspirating syringe when the pleura is penetrated.

Many investigations, apart from diagnostic aspiration, may be required to determine the primary cause of a pleural effusion. Estimation of the total and differential leucocyte count in the peripheral blood and examination of the sputum for tubercle bacilli should never be omitted. Radiological examination of the chest, which should also be performed in all cases, may disclose underlying pulmonary disease and indicate its nature. The aspiration of 500-1,500 ml. (1-3 pints) of fluid immediately before examination may be desirable when the lung is obscured by a massive effusion. Pleural biopsy (p. 317) may provide a histological diagnosis in effusions due to tuberculosis or malignant disease. Bronchoscopy, thoracoscopy and supraclavicular lymph node biopsy are other investigations which may be of value in determining the cause of a pleural effusion.

Individual Types of Pleural Effusion

1. Tuberculous Pleural Effusion. This type of effusion may develop in the course of post-primary pulmonary tuberculosis, but many cases occur in the absence of recognisable pulmonary disease. The pleural infection is always secondary to tuberculosis elsewhere, usually in the underlying lung or in the mediastinal lymph nodes, reaching the pleura by direct extension, by lymphatic spread or, occasionally, by haematogenous dissemination. When a pleural effusion occurs in the absence of radiologically apparent pulmonary tuberculosis it is usually the sequel to a primary tuberculous infection three to six months previously. In these cases, which commonly occur in adolescence and early adult life, and less often in childhood, the pleural infection is presumably derived either from a minute subpleural primary pulmonary focus or by lymphatic spread from caseous mediastinal lymph nodes.

Although a pleural effusion of this type cannot occur in the absence of tubercle bacilli, the number of bacilli may be small and the disproportionately severe pleural reaction may be due mainly to the hypersensitivity of the pleural tissues ('allergy') which develops after the primary tuberculous infection (p. 413).

The onset of a tuberculous pleural effusion may in some cases be sudden, with severe pleuritic pain preceding the physical signs of effusion for several days. In others the only complaints may be of vague ill-health and loss of weight for a period of weeks or even months before the effusion is discovered. In untreated cases, pyrexia of the remittent type, rising to 39° C. (101-103° F.), is generally present for the first three to six weeks of the illness, and sleep sweats are a common feature. The patient, however, never appears as seriously ill as one with acute pneumonia. There is usually a considerable degree of tachycardia, but the respiratory rate is not markedly increased and dyspnoea at rest is present only if the effusion is very large. Unless frank pulmonary tuberculosis co-exists, cough is not a prominent symptom and tubercle bacilli can seldom be isolated from sputum or gastric juice. These tests, however, should be performed in all cases, in conjunction with radiological examination of the chest, to determine whether or not there is an active tuberculous lesion in the lungs.

The total white blood count, which is usually within normal limits in tuberculous pleural effusion, is often a useful diagnostic aid in the early stages of the illness when the differential diagnosis from pneumococcal pneumonia may be difficult.

The pleural fluid in tuberculous effusions is amber or straw-coloured, with a specific gravity of 1·016 or more and a total protein content of over 4 g. per 100 ml. It usually clots on standing. The cells, which are relatively few, are chiefly lymphocytes. The fluid is sterile on ordinary methods of culture, but tubercle bacilli can often be isolated on culture or by guinea-pig inoculation. In such cases the sensitivity of the organism to streptomycin, PAS and isoniazid (p. 426) should always be ascertained.

Normal lung fields on radiological examination with negative bacteriological findings in sputum and pleural fluid do *not* exclude tuberculosis as the cause of the effusion, and in young adults a tuberculous aetiology should be assumed unless the tuberculin reaction (p. 417) is negative or some other cause can be clearly established. Now that a simple and effective method of pleural biopsy is available (p. 317) it is possible in many cases to confirm the diagnosis of tuberculous pleurisy histologically.

Treatment. The patient should be kept in bed until the temperature has returned to normal and the pleural fluid has stopped accumulating. Antituberculosis chemotherapy (p. 426) should be started as soon as the diagnosis is made and continued for at least 12 months. If there is an associated tuberculous lesion in the lung, treatment must be maintained for 18 months. As much pleural fluid as can be obtained should be aspirated with a large two-way syringe and needle twice a week until the effusion ceases to reaccumulate. There seems to be no advantage in giving streptomycin intrapleurally in preference to the systemic route.

Very rapid absorption of pleural fluid can sometimes be obtained by giving a corticosteroid drug, such as prednisolone by mouth, in addition to antituberculosis chemotherapy.

The patient can be allowed to resume work about four weeks after he starts to get up and provided he takes antituberculosis drugs with complete regularity, no restrictions need be placed on his activities. His chest should, however, be examined radiologically every six months for the next two years and every year for the following three years so that in the now unlikely event of a pulmonary lesion developing it can be detected and treated at an early stage.

2. Post-pneumonic Serous Effusion. A serous pleural effusion may be a complication of any type of pneumonia, but is particularly common with pneumococcal pneumonia. The effusion is usually small and, apart occasionally from a slight recrudescence of pyrexia, seldom produces clinical features distinct from those of the pneumonia itself. In a few cases the effusion becomes purulent; such an outcome was common before the advent of specific treatment.

The pleural fluid is clear, amber or straw-coloured, the cells it contains are predominantly polymorphonuclear leucocytes, and it is usually sterile on culture.

A serous effusion can safely be regarded as 'post-pneumonic,' and therefore non-tuberculous, only if there is a preceding history typical of pneumonia, a polymorphonuclear leucocytosis in the blood of over 12,000 and a predominance of these cells in the pleural fluid.

Treatment. Specific treatment for the pneumonia should be continued until after the pyrexia subsides and the effusion should be aspirated every two or three days until it stops reaccumulating. This usually occurs within 7 to 10 days and if it takes longer the diagnosis should be reviewed, with particular regard to the possibilities of tuberculous pleural effusion and empyema.

3. MALIGNANT PLEURAL EFFUSION. The most common cause of pleural effusion over the age of 40 is malignant disease. A primary pleural tumour (mesothelioma) is rare, and a malignant effusion is usually secondary to a bronchial carcinoma or to a primary tumour elsewhere. Pleural effusion, often bilateral, may also occur in patients with reticulosis. A malignant pleural effusion is usually large, and dyspnoea is an early and prominent symptom. Pyrexia may be present but is not as common as with effusions of inflammatory origin.

The pleural fluid may be serous or blood-stained. Inflammatory cells are seldom numerous, but clumps of malignant cells may be found by special staining methods.

In many cases bronchoscopy demonstrates a primary bronchial growth, but in females the breasts should previously have been examined with care in order to exclude a primary tumour there. When bronchoscopy is negative and the primary tumour is thought to be extrapulmonary, the stomach, kidneys and pelvic organs should be investigated. In most cases, especially if a primary lesion cannot be located, an attempt should be made to obtain histological confirmation of the diagnosis by means of a needle biopsy of the parietal pleura (p. 317) or by removing with biopsy forceps a specimen of any suspicious tissue seen on the pleural surfaces at thoracoscopy (p. 317). In some advanced cases the same information may be obtained more readily from histological examination of an enlarged supraclavicular lymph node.

Treatment. No curative treatment is known and the effusion tends to re-accumulate with increasing rapidity, despite frequent aspiration for the relief of dyspnoea. In some cases the exudation of fluid can be slowed down or even halted temporarily by the intrapleural administration of the cytotoxic drug, mustine hydrochloride, which is given as a single injection of 30 mg. in 60 ml. of normal saline.

4. Pulmonary Infarction. This is a common cause of a small effusion, which may be bloodstained and which often contains large numbers of eosinophil leucocytes. The diagnosis can usually be made from this feature and from the other clinical and radiological manifestations.

Treatment. This is described on p. 256.

Empyema Thoracis

This is the term used to describe the presence of pus in the pleural space. The pus may be as thin as serous fluid, or so thick that it is difficult to aspirate through even a wide-bore needle. Microscopically, leucocytes are present in large numbers, with polymorphs predominating. The causative organism may or may not be isolated from the pus. An empyema may involve the whole pleural space ('total' empyema) or only part of it ('loculated' or 'encysted' empyema). It is almost always unilateral.

Aetiology. Empyema is always secondary to infection in a neighbouring structure, usually the lung. The principal pulmonary infections liable to produce empyema are the specific and suppurative pneumonias and tuberculosis. Extrapulmonary causes of empyema are less common, but this condition may follow an infected penetrating wound of the chest wall. A haemothorax may become infected or a subphrenic abscess may rupture through the diaphragm. Empyema has become a relatively rare disease because pulmonary infection can now be so readily controlled.

Pathology. The infection reaches the pleura either by lymphatic spread or by direct extension from the primary focus, e.g. following the rupture of a small subpleural lung abscess or tuberculous cavity. Both layers of the pleura are covered with a thick, shaggy, inflammatory exudate. In the course of time the exudate becomes converted into fibrous tissue which, in the case of the visceral pleura, may encase the collapsed lung so rigidly that it cannot re-expand when the pus is removed by aspiration or by an external drainage operation. The pus in the pleural space is often under considerable pressure and if the condition is not adequately treated it may rupture into a bronchus, from which it is expectorated, or through an intercostal space with the formation of a subcutaneous abscess or a sinus. When an empyema ruptures into a bronchus, a bronchopleural fistula is produced. This allows air to enter the pleural space, and a pyopneumothorax is formed.

The only way in which an empyema can heal is by apposition of the visceral and parietal layers of the pleura with obliteration of the empyema space by organisation of the intervening exudate. This cannot occur unless re-expansion of the collapsed lung is secured *at an early stage* by removal of all the pus from the pleural space. Re-expansion of the lung cannot take place if, through delay in treatment or inadequate drainage, the visceral pleura becomes grossly thickened and rigid, if the pleural layers are kept apart by air entering the pleura through a bronchopleural fistula, or if disease in the lung itself, such as bronchiectasis, bronchial carcinoma or pulmonary tuberculosis, renders it incapable of re-expansion. In all these circumstances an empyema tends to become chronic and healing may not take place without recourse to major thoracic surgery.

Clinical Features. An empyema is usually preceded by the symptoms and signs of the primary infective lesion in the lung or elsewhere. In the case of pneumococcal pneumonia the development of an empyema usually becomes apparent a few days after the acute stage of the pneumonia has subsided. Empyema should always be suspected in such cases if there is a recurrence of pyrexia which fails to respond or responds only partially to the continued administration of a suitable antibiotic. Occasionally, failure of the initial pneumonic illness to respond to these drugs is due to the co-existence of an empyema.

In other cases the illness produced by the primary infective lesion may be so slight that it passes unrecognised and the first definite clinical features are due to the empyema itself.

In the fully developed case two separate groups of clinical features are found:

1. Those due to toxic absorption from undrained pus:

(*a*) Pyrexia, usually high and remittent but sometimes slight.
(*b*) Rigors and sweating.
(*c*) Malaise, anorexia and loss of weight.
(*d*) Tachycardia.
(*e*) Polymorphonuclear leucocytosis.

2. THOSE DUE TO THE LOCAL EFFECTS WITHIN THE THORAX OF THE EMPYEMA:

(*a*) *Dyspnoea.* This is marked only when the empyema is very large and producing mediastinal displacement. An empyema by the time it is recognised is usually walled off by dense pleural adhesions and is incapable of producing progressive mediastinal displacement.

(*b*) *Pleuritic pain.* This may be severe in the early stages but usually subsides later when the pleura becomes rigid and immobile.

(*c*) *Cough and sputum* are usually related to the underlying lung disease, but the expectoration of large amounts of pus may be due to the rupture of an empyema into a bronchus.

Sometimes an empyema produces no symptoms referable to the respiratory system. It must therefore be considered as a possible diagnosis in all cases of pyrexia with polymorphonuclear leucocytosis for which no other cause can be found.

Physical Signs in the Chest. An empyema usually produces the typical signs of fluid in the pleural space (p. 314), but occasionally, as with a serous effusion, the breath sounds may be bronchial instead of diminished or absent. In these cases, however, the presence of fluid can usually be suspected from the 'stony' dullness of the percussion note.

A small localised empyema, particularly when situated in an interlobar fissure, may produce no abnormal physical signs.

Radiological Examination. The appearances are indistinguishable from those of serous pleural effusion (p. 395). When air is present in addition to pus (pyopneumothorax), a horizontal 'fluid level' marks the junction of the fluid and the air if the film is taken in the erect position.

Diagnosis. Although the clinical features suggest the diagnosis in most cases, final confirmation of the presence of an empyema depends on the aspiration of pus. A wide-bore needle should be inserted through an intercostal space over the area of maximal dullness on percussion. Whenever possible the position of the empyema should have previously been confirmed by postero-anterior and lateral radiographs. Bacteriological examination of the pus may help to determine the cause of the empyema.

In post-pneumonic cases where intensive treatment with antibiotics has been given the pus is frequently sterile. Sterile pus is also found in some cases of tuberculous empyema, but the distinction between tuberculous and non-tuberculous cases can usually be made from the radiological changes in the lungs or by the isolation of tubercle bacilli from the sputum.

Course and Prognosis. If an acute empyema is unrecognised or inadequately treated the patient may die as a result of toxic absorption from the undrained pus. Alternatively, the empyema may pass on to the chronic stage and cause general ill-health, recurrent episodes of pyrexia, clubbing of the fingers and sometimes amyloid disease. A small empyema occasionally heals spontaneously, partly by absorption of the pus but mainly by organisation of the exudate, which produces gross thickening and sometimes calcification of the pleura.

The mortality from empyema depends mainly on the nature of the infecting organism and on the patient's resistance. It has fallen sharply since the introduction of penicillin and the newer antibiotics. The duration of the illness, on the other hand, depends on mechanical factors, particularly on the ability of the lung to re-expand.

A non-tuberculous empyema, treated early, usually heals quickly; one which is drained at a late stage seldom heals without further surgical intervention. Tuberculous empyema is potentially a serious condition, difficult to treat and slow to heal.

Treatment

Non-tuberculous Empyema

1. *Early stage*: i.e. when the patient is acutely ill, and the pus is thin in consistence:

(*a*) *All* the pus that can be withdrawn should be aspirated daily or on alternate days.

(*b*) An antibiotic to which the organism causing the empyema is sensitive should be given by intramuscular injection or by mouth.

(*c*) If the organism isolated from the pus is sensitive to penicillin, cloxacillin or streptomycin, the appropriate antibiotic should also be given intrapleurally after each aspiration. For this purpose a dose of 1 mega unit of benzylpenicillin, 0·5-1·0 g. of cloxacillin, or 1 g. of streptomycin sulphate should be used.

(*d*) When the pus is sterile but the infection is likely to have been pneumococcal the patient should be treated with benzylpenicillin, given both intramuscularly and intrapleurally.

If treatment is started early enough and the organisms are drug-sensitive, an empyema can often be aborted by these measures. It is, however, useless and possibly dangerous to continue treatment on these lines if the pus becomes thick and difficult to aspirate or if the amount of pus obtained does not become progressively smaller with each aspiration. Occasionally this form of treatment does not relieve the systemic disturbance and the patient becomes gravely ill. This is particularly liable to occur with drug-resistant infections. In such cases it may be necessary to institute continuous 'closed' drainage by means of an intercostal tube, connected to a water-seal drain (p. 408) to prevent air entering the pleural space.

2. *Later stage*: i.e. when the patient is usually less acutely ill and the pus is thick in consistence. Many cases are first seen at this stage; others may have had preliminary treatment with pleural aspiration and antibiotics.

(*a*) If the patient is in fairly good general condition and if, on full investigation, no evidence is found of any associated pulmonary disease such as bronchiectasis or bronchial carcinoma, the most effective treatment may be resection of the empyema sac *in toto*.

(*b*) In other circumstances, particularly if there is any doubt as to the patient's fitness to withstand a major operation, rib resection and drainage of the empyema should be performed instead, and breathing exercises given to encourage re-expansion of the lung.

3. *Chronic stage*. At this stage, whether or not a drainage operation has been performed, it is unlikely that the lung will be able to re-expand sufficiently to bring about obliteration of the empyema space. Treatment therefore must consist of resection of the empyema with decortication of the lung, supplemented if necessary by thoracoplasty to reduce the size of the pleural space.

Tuberculous Empyema

Pus should be aspirated repeatedly and streptomycin instilled intrapleurally in an attempt to secure obliteration of the empyema space. Effective antituberculosis chemotherapy (p. 427) should be maintained by the systemic route. It may be necessary later to resect the empyema sac *en bloc* but this must not be undertaken until the pulmonary lesion has been controlled by chemotherapy.

When secondary pyogenic infection is present an initial drainage operation is usually required.

SPONTANEOUS PNEUMOTHORAX

Aetiology. The two chief causes of spontaneous pneumothorax are:

1. Rupture of a subpleural emphysematous bulla or of the pulmonary end of a pleural adhesion.
2. Rupture of a subpleural tuberculous focus into the pleural space.

In Britain the first cause is very much more common than the second. Active pulmonary tuberculosis is, in fact, responsible for very few cases of spontaneous pneumothorax, a finding which is in sharp conflict with the experience of thirty years ago.

Certain other conditions such as staphylococcal lung abscess, pulmonary infarction and bronchial carcinoma may, in rare instances, give rise to spontaneous pneumothorax. As with tuberculosis, the pneumothorax in all these conditions results from the rupture of a pulmonary lesion situated close to the pleural surface.

Pathology. There are three types of spontaneous pneumothorax:

1. *Closed* (Fig. 48*a*). The communication between pleura and lung seals off as the lung collapses, and does not reopen. In this type of case the air is gradually absorbed and the lung re-expands.

2. *Open* (Fig. 48*b*). The communication is generally with a bronchus ('bronchopleural fistula') and does not seal off when the lung collapses. The air pressure in the pleural space thus approximates to atmospheric pressure throughout both inspiration and expiration and the lung cannot re-expand. Moreover, the large bronchial communication facilitates the transmission of infection from the air passages into the pleural space and empyema is a common complication.

3. *Valvular* (Fig. 46*c*). The communication between pleura and lung persists but is small and acts as a one-way valve which allows air to enter the pleura during inspiration but prevents it from escaping during expiration. Very large amounts of air may be 'trapped' in the pleural space during bouts of coughing and the intrapleural pressure may rise to well above atmospheric level. This results not only in complete collapse of the underlying lung but also in gross mediastinal displacement towards the opposite side with compression of the opposite lung. This type of pneumothorax is usually referred to as a 'tension pneumothorax'.

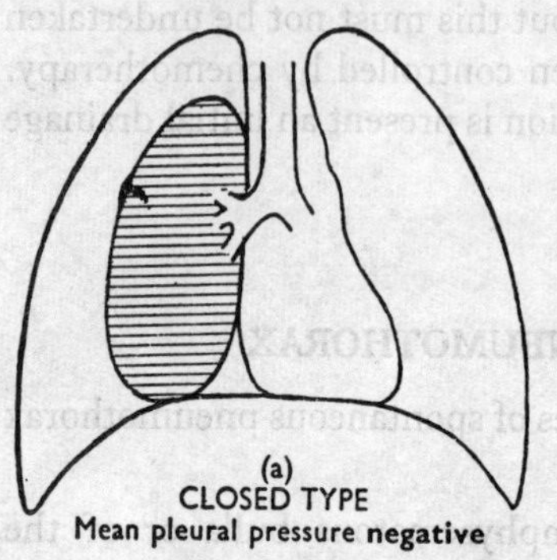

(a)
CLOSED TYPE
Mean pleural pressure **negative**

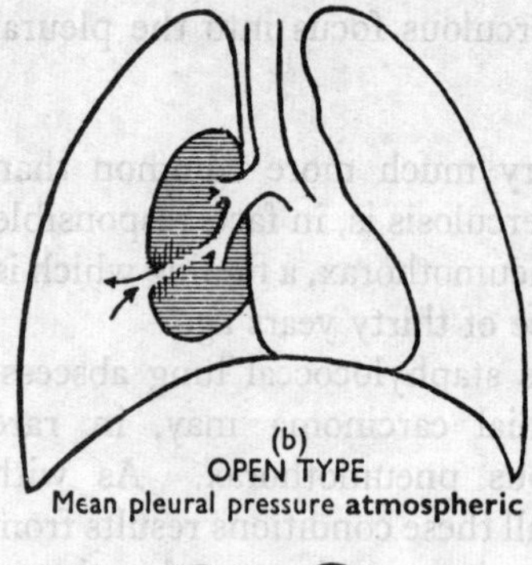

(b)
OPEN TYPE
Mean pleural pressure **atmospheric**

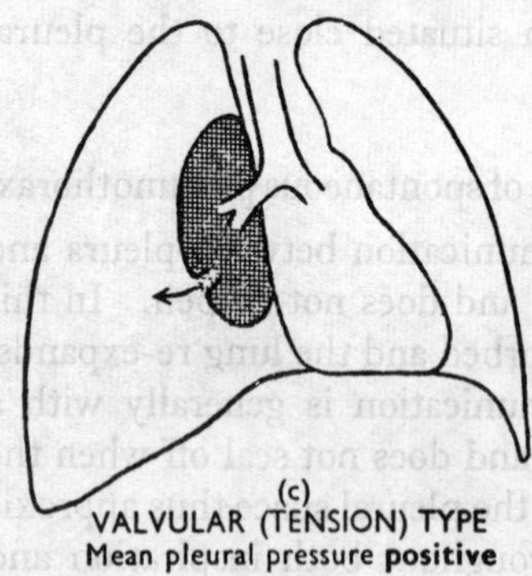

(c)
VALVULAR (TENSION) TYPE
Mean pleural pressure **positive**

FIG. 46
THE MECHANISMS OF SPONTANEOUS PNEUMOTHORAX

Clinical Features. The onset is usually sudden, with pain or a feeling of 'tightness' on the affected side of the chest, which may be aggravated by deep inspiration.

The patient then becomes increasingly breathless and in severe cases cyanosis appears, sometimes of a marked degree. The physical signs in the chest are those of air in the pleural space (p. 320). When the pneumothorax is small and localised there may be no abnormal signs, and the condition may be revealed only by radiological examination.

With the *closed* type of spontaneous pneumothorax the

dyspnoea, which is seldom severe, gradually subsides over the course of 24 hours. Thereafter, progressive spontaneous absorption of the air takes place and re-expansion of the lung is complete between two and six weeks later, depending on the initial size of the pneumothorax. Pleural infection is uncommon in this type of pneumothorax, even when it has a tuberculous basis.

The *open* type of spontaneous pneumothorax is usually of tuberculous origin. The onset is similar to that of the closed type, but the dyspnoea, although it is not rapidly progressive, does not improve and within a few days the appearance of pyrexia and systemic disturbance, accompanied by physical and radiological signs of air and fluid in the pleural space, indicate the development of a pyopneumothorax. In tuberculous cases acid-fast bacilli can be isolated from the pleural fluid at an early stage.

The *valvular* type of pneumothorax ('tension pneumothorax') produces the most dramatic clinical picture of all. The dyspnoea is rapidly progressive from the start and is accompanied by deep cyanosis. The patient may die from asphyxia within a few minutes, but usually the course of events is less rapid and medical attention can be obtained in time to avert a fatal outcome. Occasionally, a valvular type of spontaneous pneumothorax is maintained for months, or even for a few years, by the nature of the pleuro-pulmonary communication. In this condition, which is called *chronic spontaneous pneumothorax*, there may be an initial acute episode of severe respiratory distress, but eventually the only symptom is dyspnoea on exertion.

Recurrent spontaneous pneumothorax is not uncommon, especially in cases with emphysematous bullae. Subsequent incidents usually occur on the same side as the first but may also occur on the opposite side.

Radiological Examination shows the sharp edge of the collapsed lung, and between this and the chest wall there is complete translucency with no lung markings. The degree of pulmonary collapse varies from case to case.

Diagnosis. The diagnosis of spontaneous pneumothorax can usually be made on the history and physical signs but should, whenever possible, be confirmed by radiological examination. This also shows the size of the pneumothorax and the degree of mediastinal displacement, and gives information regarding the presence or absence of pleural effusion and underlying pulmonary tuberculosis. Bacteriological examination of the sputum and pleural fluid is of great importance in distinguishing tuberculous from non-tuberculous cases.

Treatment

1. In *closed spontaneous pneumothorax* the air is gradually absorbed and the lung re-expands slowly during the next few

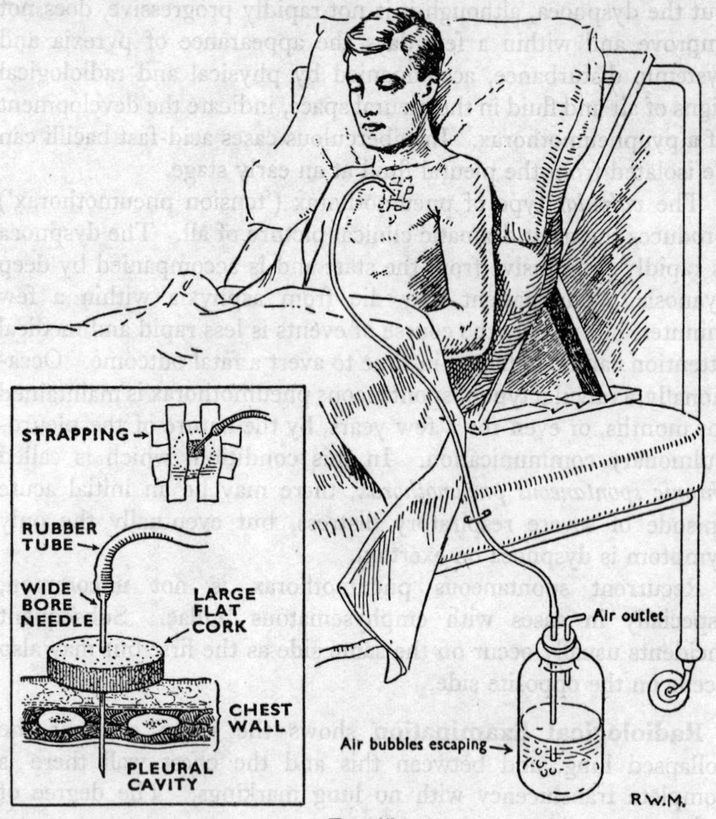

FIG. 47

THE RELIEF OF TENSION PNEUMOTHORAX BY 'WATER-SEAL' DECOMPRESSION

The water seal allows air to leave the pleural space but prevents it from re-entering. This reduces the intrapleural pressure and encourages re-expansion of the lung.

The wide-bore needle shown on the illustration, although of great value in an emergency, is apt to be dislodged and readily becomes blocked. It should therefore be replaced by a rubber catheter as soon as possible.

weeks. When the pneumothorax is small and the patient is not dyspnoeic no treatment is required but observation should be continued until re-expansion of the lung is complete. If, however, the pneumothorax is large and causing dyspnoea, it is preferable to employ more active measures. Immediate and complete re-expansion of the lung can be obtained by inserting a rubber catheter into the pleural cavity through an intercostal space and connecting it to a water-seal drainage system (Fig. 47). The catheter is left in place for five or six days. This form of treatment considerably shortens the period of incapacity and has the additional advantage that it may produce pleural adhesions and prevent further incidents of spontaneous pneumothorax.

If a tuberculous aetiology is suspected, specific chemotherapy (p. 426) should be started immediately. If a pleural effusion develops, the fluid may be drained through the catheter by suitable posturing or aspirated with a needle and syringe.

2. In *open spontaneous pneumothorax*, which can be recognised by the presence of an atmospheric intrapleural pressure in contrast to a negative pressure in closed cases, there is a frank broncho-pleural fistula, and pleural infection rapidly supervenes. Such cases are seldom amenable to medical treatment and, whether tuberculous or non-tuberculous, should be referred to a thoracic surgeon for treatment of the resulting pyopneumothorax.

3. *Tension pneumothorax* constitutes an acute medical emergency. A wide-bore needle should be inserted immediately and connected to a water-seal drainage system, as shown in Figure 47. Symptomatic relief is immediate and dramatic. As soon as possible the needle should be replaced by a catheter, and suction applied by connecting the air outlet to an electric pump.

4. The treatment of *recurrent spontaneous pneumothorax* and of *chronic spontaneous pneumothorax* should be undertaken by a thoracic surgeon.

* * * * * *

TUBERCULOSIS

Although tuberculosis is a problem of rapidly diminishing proportions in Western Europe and North America, it remains, in the words of a World Health Organization Report, 'the most important specific communicable disease in the world'. It is by far the largest single cause of death in the developing countries, and although the death rate in Britain has fallen to an almost negligible figure, no less than 17,273 new cases of tuberculosis were notified during 1966. These are considered good and sufficient reasons for retaining in this book a detailed account of this dangerous but now eminently curable disease.

The Aetiology of Tuberculosis. The fact that tuberculosis is a specific infective disease was first proved by Koch's discovery of the tubercle bacillus in 1882. Tuberculosis is unlike other infections in that while many members of the population become infected in early life only a relatively small number develop clinically recognisable evidence of disease, either at the time of the first ('primary') infection or in later years. It is possible by means of the tuberculin skin sensitivity test (p. 417) to determine whether or not a person has at any time contracted a tuberculous infection. Periodic surveys of the proportion of positive tuberculin reactors in a community may thus provide a valuable long-term indication of the efficacy of the measures employed to control the disease. In Scotland, for example, the number of positive reactors amongst 13-year-old children fell from 56 per cent. in 1952 to 16·4 per cent. in 1966. Comparable figures for older age groups are not available as vaccination with BCG (*Bacille Calmette Guérin*), which renders the tuberculin test positive, is now offered to all negative reactors before they leave school.

THE TUBERCLE BACILLUS. There are two types of tubercle bacillus responsible for the disease in man:

(*a*) the *human* type—endemic in man.
(*b*) the *bovine* type—endemic in cattle.

In Britain considerably less than one per cent. of tuberculosis in man is now caused by the bovine bacillus, which is transmitted by milk. The rapid decline in this type of infection during the past 20 years is accounted for by the energetic efforts which have been made to render milk safe by pasteurisation or by increasing the number of tuberculosis-free dairy herds. All milk produced on registered farms in Britain is now safeguarded in one or both of these two ways. The bovine bacillus is more liable to cause tuberculosis of the tonsils and alimentary tract, and of the related cervical and abdominal lymph nodes respectively, whereas the human bacillus, which is spread mainly by droplet infection, is responsible for almost all cases of pulmonary tuberculosis.

Immunity and Susceptibility. Entry of the tubercle bacillus into the body, by the alimentary or respiratory tract, is not necessarily followed by a clinical illness, the development of which is dependent on several other factors:

1. *Natural resistance.* Susceptibility to tuberculosis is not inherited in the strict sense of the word, but the fact that certain races, such as Africans and Indians, and even certain regional groups, such as the inhabitants of the Western Isles of Scotland and of Ireland, are more prone to develop tuberculosis suggests that natural resistance varies from race to race and even from region to region.

2. *Acquired immunity.* The nature and effects of acquired immunity in tuberculosis are not fully understood. It has, however, been proved that if a person contracts and recovers from a primary tuberculous infection he is less likely to develop active tuberculosis on subsequent exposure to the tubercle bacillus than a patient who has not previously been infected. The use of a vaccine containing an attenuated bovine bacillus (BCG) to induce a controlled and innocuous primary infection is based on this observation.

3. *Allergy.* After the primary infection has become established the tissues react to the tubercle bacillus in a way that differs from their initial reaction. This altered response, referred to as *allergy* (p. 20), takes the form of hypersensitivity to tuberculin, a complex protein constituent of the tubercle bacillus, and can be recognised by the finding of a positive tuberculin reaction (p. 417).

The effect of hypersensitivity to tuberculoprotein, which is maximal during the months following the primary infection, is to fix and destroy tubercle bacilli in the tissues. It is, therefore, one of the processes which help to localise the infection at or near its point of entry, and in that sense can be regarded as a defence mechanism. On the other hand, hypersensitivity through its power to produce caseation and liquefaction in the primary lesion and in the regional lymph nodes may exert an unfavourable influence on the course of the disease. The fortuitous discharge into a blood vessel of the contents of a caseous lymph node leads to wide dissemination of tuberculosis to other organs and is a well recognised hazard of every severe primary infection.

4. *Massive infection and re-infection.* The gravity of a tuberculous illness bears some relationship, although not a constant one, to the size of the infection. The danger is greatest when a young child is exposed to a massive infection from an open case of pulmonary tuberculosis (i.e. a patient whose sputum contains tubercle bacilli).

The degree of immunity conferred by a primary infection, which varies considerably in different individuals, affords no certain protection against re-infection, particularly the massive re-infection which results from close contact with an open case of tuberculosis.

5. *Housing conditions.* Overcrowding increases the risk of massive infection or re-infection occurring if one of the occupants happens to be suffering from open tuberculosis. When housing conditions are bad it is not uncommon to find several members of one household suffering from tuberculosis. Overcrowding is one of the most important factors in the spread of the disease.

6. *Diet.* Only a diet grossly deficient in protein and vitamins can logically be blamed for lowering resistance to tuberculosis. In Britain at the present time dietary deficiency of this degree is very uncommon but in the developing countries of Asia and Africa it may be an important aetiological factor.

7. *Occupation.* Occupation has seldom any direct bearing on the prevalence of tuberculosis. A higher or lower tuberculosis rate in any particular occupation is usually determined not by the nature of the occupation itself but by the social and economic status of those who are engaged in it and by the opportunities it provides for the transmission of infection from one person to another.

The only two occupations in which there is a direct causal relationship to tuberculosis are mining, where pneumoconiosis is the determining factor in the higher prevalence, and nursing, where massive infection is the chief factor. The increased risk in nurses is, however, mainly confined to those with a negative tuberculin reaction, and BCG vaccination of all such subjects (p. 431) is a valuable preventive measure.

8. *Conditions affecting individual patients.* Diabetes mellitus and congenital heart disease both predispose to the development of tuberculosis, but tuberculous infection in such subjects responds normally to antituberculosis chemotherapy.

Pregnancy may have an unfavourable influence on the course of untreated pulmonary tuberculosis but has no adverse effect on patients under correct supervision and treatment.

The Pathology of Tuberculosis. The characteristic lesion of tuberculosis is the *tubercle*. This consists of a microscopic nodular collection of epithelioid cells surrounded by zones of lymphocytes and fibroblasts. There may be giant cells and a few bacilli in the centre. Adjacent tubercles enlarge and coalesce at an early stage, and this is followed by central necrosis or 'caseation' which may advance rapidly with widespread tissue destruction. The lesions tend to heal by fibrosis and calcification, but destructive and reparative processes frequently co-exist.

The initial or 'primary' tuberculous infection usually occurs in the lung but occasionally in the tonsil or in the alimentary tract, especially the ileo-caecal region. The primary infection differs from later infections in that the primary focus in lung, tonsil or bowel is almost invariably accompanied by a caseous lesion in the regional lymph nodes, i.e. in the mediastinal, cervical or mesenteric groups respectively.

In most people the primary lesion and the associated lymph node lesion heal and calcify. In a few, healing (particularly of the lymph node lesion) is incomplete and surviving tubercle bacilli may under certain circumstances, such as a lowering of the general health or an alteration of the balance between allergy and immunity, be discharged into the blood stream. Such patients may in consequence develop tuberculous lesions elsewhere in the body. The most common sites for 'haematogenous' lesions of this kind are the lungs, bones, joints and kidneys. Such lesions may develop months or even years after the primary infection.

The primary infection may in some cases fail to heal. A primary pulmonary lesion, particularly when it occurs during adolescence or early adult life, may lead to progressive pulmonary tuberculosis. A tuberculous mediastinal lymph node, in children especially, may compress a large bronchus and produce *atelectasis*, or ulcerate through the bronchial wall, discharge caseous material into the lumen and produce an extensive lesion in the related lobe or segment. Infection may also be carried by lymphatics from tuberculous mediastinal glands to the pleura or pericardium with the production of *tuberculous pleurisy* or *pericarditis*. Comparable complications may occur when the primary lesion is in the tonsil or gut, e.g. 'cold abscess' of the neck, tuberculous peritonitis.

Rarely, a caseous tuberculous focus either at the site of the primary infection or, more commonly, in an associated lymph node ruptures into a vein and produces acute dissemination of the disease throughout the body, a condition known as *acute miliary tuberculosis*. *Tuberculous meningitis* often accompanies this condition.

Progressive pulmonary tuberculosis may develop directly from a primary lesion or it may occur later, following reactivation of an incompletely healed primary focus in the lung or as a result of haematogenous dissemination from an unhealed lymph node lesion. Alternatively it may be the result of re-infection from an outside source after the primary focus has healed completely. All these forms of pulmonary tuberculosis, although differing in pathogenesis, have similar pathological features and can be grouped together under the term *post-primary pulmonary tuberculosis* or *adult phthisis*. The characteristic pathological feature of this condition is the *tuberculous cavity*, which forms when the caseated and liquefied centre of a tuberculous pulmonary lesion is discharged into a bronchus. The walls of cavities harbour large numbers of tubercle bacilli, and the persistence of cavitation, which is determined chiefly by mechanical circumstances, is the most important single factor preventing recovery from the disease. There is, however, a strong tendency for the lesions to be localised by fibrous tissue, and provided that gross cavitation is not present the disease is frequently self-limiting, although complete healing by fibrosis and calcification is a slow process. Extension of the disease to other parts of the same lung or to the opposite lung is a common consequence of cavitation and is caused either by direct spread of the disease or by aspiration, via the bronchi, of infected secretions from the cavity.

Extension of the infection to the pleura either by direct or lymphatic spread causes *tuberculous pleurisy*, which is sometimes accompanied by effusion and is occasionally followed by the development of a *tuberculous empyema*. Blood-borne dissemination to other organs of the body is uncommon in this form of pulmonary tuberculosis.

Clinical Features. There are two groups of clinical features in tuberculosis:

1. Those due to the systemic effects of the disease, which

include lassitude and malaise, lack of appetite, loss of weight, anaemia, sleep sweats, pyrexia and tachycardia. The pyrexia is usually most marked in the late afternoon or evening and sometimes occurs only at these times.

2. Those caused by the local effects of the tuberculous lesions, which are summarised below according to anatomical site.

Lungs and bronchi: cough, sputum, haemoptysis, dyspnoea.
Pleura: pleuritic pain, dyspnoea due to pleural effusion.
Larynx: hoarseness, with dysphagia at a later stage from involvement of pharynx.
Tongue: ulceration. (Rare.)
Intestine: diarrhoea, malabsorption or intestinal obstruction.
Peritoneum: ascites, attacks of intestinal obstruction due to plastic peritonitis.
Pericardium: pericardial effusion, constrictive pericarditis later.
Kidneys and bladder: haematuria, increased frequency of micturition. (These are relatively late developments, early renal lesions being symptomless.)
Epididymis: painless swelling, sinus formation later.
Brain: tuberculoma.
Meninges: symptoms and signs of meningitis.
Lymph nodes: enlargement of nodes, often with 'cold' abscess and sinus formation later.
Suprarenal glands: symptoms and signs of Addison's disease.
Bones and joints: osteitis, synovitis, 'cold' abscesses.
Skin: lupus vulgaris, erythema nodosum.
Eyes: phlyctenular keratoconjunctivitis, iridocyclitis, choroiditis.

In the sections which follow an account is given of those manifestations of tuberculosis which involve the lungs, viz. primary pulmonary tuberculosis, acute miliary tuberculosis and post-primary pulmonary tuberculosis. Tuberculous pleurisy is described on p. 396. For information regarding other manifestations of tuberculosis the reader should refer to the appropriate section of the book. The treatment and prevention of tuberculosis are dealt with on pp. 424-432.

PRIMARY PULMONARY TUBERCULOSIS

The pathological features of this type of tuberculosis have already been described (p. 413). The primary infection usually occurs in childhood but is sometimes delayed until adult life. A history of contact with a case of active pulmonary tuberculosis is obtained in many instances.

Clinical Features

1. In the vast majority of cases the primary infection produces no symptoms or signs and passes unnoticed unless routine radiological examination of the chest happens to be carried out at the appropriate moment or serial tuberculin tests show conversion from negative to positive. Such close observation is seldom undertaken unless there is a particular liability to tuberculous infection, e.g. in children or nurses exposed to open cases of tuberculosis.

2. In a few cases the primary infection produces a febrile illness. It is generally mild and lasts for no more than 7 to 14 days, but it may be accompanied by other clinical features of tuberculous toxaemia. It is unusual for gross focal symptoms or signs to develop in an uncomplicated case, but a slight dry cough is occasionally present. The leucocyte count is usually normal but the erythrocyte sedimentation rate is invariably raised.

3. The primary infection may be accompanied by *erythema nodosum*. This condition is characterised by bluish-red, raised, tender cutaneous lesions on both shins and, less commonly, on the thighs, and is associated in some cases with pyrexia and polyarthralgia. The lesions of erythema nodosum do not exhibit the histological features of tuberculosis and tubercle bacilli cannot be isolated from them. They are thus assumed to be non-specific focal manifestations of allergy. Erythema nodosum may, however, be the first clinical indication of a tuberculous infection. In such cases the tuberculin reaction (p. 417) is always strongly positive and evidence of primary tuberculosis can usually be detected on the chest radiograph.

Erythema nodosum may be seen in conditions other than primary tuberculosis, e.g. sarcoidosis, streptococcal infections and, rarely, following the administration of a sulphonamide drug. It may also occur as an isolated phenomenon without apparent cause. In countries where tuberculosis is no longer prevalent sarcoidosis (p. 433) is the condition with which erythema nodosum is most frequently associated. In such cases the tuberculin reaction is negative or only weakly positive and the chest radiograph usually shows *bilateral* enlargement of the hilar lymph nodes without at this stage any pulmonary abnormalities.

4. Occasionally the primary pulmonary infection pursues a progressive course (p. 413). Symptoms and signs due to its complications may appear either during the course of the initial illness or after a latent interval of weeks or months. Such complications include dry pleurisy or pleural effusion (p. 396), lobar or segmental atelectasis (p. 366), acute miliary tuberculosis (p. 418), tuberculous meningitis (p. 1159), and post-primary pulmonary tuberculosis (p. 414).

Diagnosis. The three most valuable diagnostic investigations in primary pulmonary tuberculosis are:

1. *Radiological examination of the chest.* In children this usually shows unilateral enlargement of the hilar lymph nodes and demonstrates the primary intrapulmonary lesion if it is large enough to be visible radiologically. In adolescents and young adults the lymph node component of the primary complex is usually less conspicuous than in children and the pulmonary lesion more prominent. Complications such as pleural effusion, atelectasis and acute pneumonic tuberculosis may be superimposed.

2. *Tuberculin test.* With the Mantoux technique a solution of Old Tuberculin or purified protein derivative (P.P.D.) tuberculin is injected intradermally on the flexor aspect of the forearm. The test is regarded as positive if, two to four days after injection, there is a reaction consisting of a raised area of inflammatory oedema not less than 5 mm. in diameter, with surrounding erythema. The test is regarded as negative if there is no reaction at all or if there is an immediate (non-specific) reaction which disappears completely within 48 hours. The test should first be carried out with 1 tuberculin unit (T.U.) in 0·1 ml. of normal saline. If there is no reaction it should be repeated with 10 T.U. in the same volume of saline. In order to obtain accurate results it is essential to use freshly prepared dilutions of tuberculin.

The significance of the tuberculin test in relation to tuberculous infection has already been discussed (p. 411). The younger the patient the greater the diagnostic significance of a positive test. A repeatedly negative test over a period of six weeks from the onset of symptoms practically rules out a diagnosis of tuberculosis.

Tuberculin testing is an essential part of the examination of the family contacts of cases of tuberculosis. Apart from its value as a diagnostic measure it indicates which of the contacts should be vaccinated with BCG. When large numbers are being tested, particularly of children, the Heaf multiple puncture tuberculin test is preferable to the Mantoux technique as it is more rapidly performed and is less painful. For this test a solution containing 100,000 T.U. of P.P.D. tuberculin per ml., to which adrenaline has been added, should be used.

3. *Bacteriological examination.* Sputum is seldom available in cases of primary pulmonary tuberculosis, but tubercle bacilli can sometimes be isolated by culture of fasting gastric juice or of secretion obtained by swabbing the larynx. At least three specimens should be examined. The isolation of tubercle bacilli is absolute proof of the diagnosis, but a negative result does not exclude it.

Primary pulmonary tuberculosis must be distinguished from other febrile illnesses such as influenza and infectious mononucleosis, from acute respiratory infections such as acute bronchitis and pneumonia and from other causes of hilar lymph node enlargement such as the reticuloses (p. 654) and sarcoidosis (p. 433).

Prognosis. Since primary pulmonary tuberculosis and its complications respond satisfactorily to antituberculosis chemotherapy (p. 426), which should be given in every case, the prognosis is excellent.

ACUTE MILIARY TUBERCULOSIS

The pathogenesis of this condition has already been discussed (p. 414). It occurs chiefly in children and young adults. Before the introduction of streptomycin and isoniazid it was invariably fatal but most cases now recover completely. The lesions, which are minute tuberculous foci, are scattered throughout the body and with the aid of radiological examination their presence can be readily recognised in the lungs during life.

Clinical Features. The disease may start suddenly or may be preceded by a few weeks of vague ill-health. The systemic disturbance rapidly becomes profound. In particular, there is high remittent or intermittent pyrexia with drenching sweats during sleep, marked tachycardia and usually a progressive secondary anaemia. Cough and dyspnoea are occasionally present. There may be no abnormal physical signs in the lungs, although widespread fine crepitations are not infrequently heard at some stage of the disease. The spleen is often palpable and sometimes tender. Choroidal tubercles may be visible in the retina on ophthalmoscopy. Leucocytosis is usually absent or slight, but the erythrocyte sedimentation rate is very high. If chemotherapy is not given the patient's condition deteriorates rapidly and death takes place from exhaustion or from tuberculous meningitis within four to eight weeks.

Diagnosis. The diagnosis of acute miliary tuberculosis can be made with certainty only when radiological examination of the chest shows a fine, 'miliary' mottling symmetrically distributed throughout both lung fields. These changes may take a few weeks to develop, but the diagnosis can often be suspected at an earlier stage by the finding of splenomegaly or choroidal tubercles in a patient whose symptoms and temperature chart are consistent with acute tuberculous toxaemia. Although the tuberculin reaction (p. 417) is usually positive, a negative result does not always exclude acute miliary tuberculosis, as tuberculin sensitivity is occasionally depressed in the acute phase of the illness.

Acute miliary tuberculosis must be distinguished from other causes of severe pyrexia without obvious localising symptoms or signs, such as enteric fever (p. 28), bacterial endocarditis (p. 213), staphylococcal septicaemia (p. 41), empyema (p. 400), subphrenic abscess, acute pulmonary tuberculosis (p. 413) and Hodgkin's disease (p. 655).

Prognosis. Antituberculosis chemotherapy (p. 426) has reduced the mortality of acute miliary tuberculosis from 100 per cent. to less than 5 per cent. The cause of death is almost always tuberculous meningitis, although many patients who develop this complication make a complete recovery, provided there has been no delay in starting treatment.

POST-PRIMARY PULMONARY TUBERCULOSIS

(Syn: Adult phthisis)

Most of the morbidity and mortality from tuberculosis is caused by this form of the disease. Although in the developing countries it is most prevalent in adolescence and early adult life, the majority of cases in Western Europe and North America now occur in middle-aged and elderly subjects, particulary males.

The nature of the pathological lesions has already been described (p. 413). They are most commonly situated in the upper lobes. Another common site is the apex of a lower lobe. The disease is frequently bilateral; usually it starts in one lung and spreads via the bronchi to the other; less commonly it develops in both lungs at the same time. Occasionally, when the disease takes an acute form, the initial lesion is pneumonic or bronchopneumonic.

Clinical Features. The onset of post-primary pulmonary tuberculosis is usually insidious, with the gradual development of general symptoms (p. 414) or of cough and sputum. Sometimes a dramatic incident such as a haemoptysis, an attack of pleurisy or a spontaneous pneumothorax marks the onset of the disease, but with the increasing use of mass radiography the diagnosis is now frequently made before any symptoms have appeared.

The local respiratory symptoms which may occur during the course of the illness are:

1. *Cough*, which may be one of the earliest symptoms or which may not be troublesome until a late stage. Its absence does *not* exclude a diagnosis of pulmonary tuberculosis.

2. *Sputum*, which, like cough, may not become a prominent feature until the disease has reached an advanced stage. It is usually mucoid at first but later becomes purulent. It is rarely foetid.

3. *Haemoptysis*. In the early stages it is due to the erosion of a small vessel in a caseating lesion and the bleeding is usually slight. In the late stages it originates from a large vessel in the wall of a cavity and the haemorrhage may be large, occasionally fatal.

4. *Dyspnoea on exertion*, usually a late symptom, but may develop acutely when due to a spontaneous pneumothorax or to a rapidly developing pleural effusion.

5. *Pleuritic pain*, which is usually due to dry pleurisy but occasionally to spontaneous pneumothorax.

Physical Signs in the Chest. In the early stages no abnormal physical signs may be elicited, but, despite this, quite an extensive lesion may be visible radiologically. The earliest physical signs consist of a few medium or coarse crepitations, usually situated over one or other lung apex posteriorly. These crepitations may be present only after coughing.

As the disease advances the percussion note over the site of the lesion loses its normal resonance and there is a change in the character of the breath sounds, which may become either diminished in intensity or harsh vesicular with prolonged expiration. The crepitations become more numerous and more coarse. Ultimately the physical signs of consolidation (p. 320), cavitation (p. 320) and fibrosis (p. 320) may appear.

Pleurisy, with or without effusion, and spontaneous pneumothorax may modify the pulmonary signs.

Radiological Examination. This is of paramount importance for diagnosis in the early stages before physical signs appear and for assessment of the extent and progress of the disease. The earliest radiological change is an ill-defined opacity or opacities, usually situated in one of the upper lobes. In more advanced cases the opacities are larger and more widespread, and may be bilateral. Occasionally there is a dense, homogeneous shadow involving a whole lobe ('pneumonic tuberculosis').

An area or areas of translucency within the opacities indicates cavitation. Very large cavities may be visible in some cases. If there is progress towards healing the opacities shrink, become more clearly defined, and may later show calcification. When fibrosis is marked the trachea and heart shadow are displaced towards the side of the lesion.

In any case of tuberculosis it is common for lesions at different stages of development to co-exist. Thus in one area there may be cavitation, in a second evidence of fibrosis and in a third an opacity due to recent disease.

The presence of cavitation in an untreated case usually indicates that the disease is active. When cavitation is absent, however, it may sometimes be difficult to assess the activity of a tuberculous lesion from a single radiograph. Observation of the lesion over a period of time may be necessary in doubtful cases.

The radiological appearances of pleural effusion and pneumothorax, which may accompany those of pulmonary tuberculosis, have already been described (pp. 395 and 407).

Diagnosis. The general principles governing the diagnosis of tuberculosis have already been stated (p. 417). The grounds on which pulmonary tuberculosis should be suspected are:

1. Unexplained cough persisting for more than three weeks.
2. Haemoptysis.
3. Pleuritic pain not associated with an acute illness.
4. Spontaneous pneumothorax (although most cases are *not* tuberculous).
5. Unexplained tiredness or loss of weight, even in the absence of respiratory symptoms.

The presence of any of these symptoms demands immediate radiological examination of the lungs and, if any abnormality is found, the examination of at least three specimens of sputum for tubercle bacilli.

When bacilli are numerous, the diagnosis can readily be made by microscopical examination of sputum smears stained by the Ziehl-Neelson method, but culture of the sputum (or of fasting gastric juice or laryngeal swabs, if no sputum can be obtained) is essential for the isolation of bacilli present in small numbers and for the detection of drug resistance (p. 425). Cultural methods are thus of great practical value and should be used in the examination of every specimen, if facilities permit.

The conditions with which pulmonary tuberculosis may be confused include pneumonia (p. 347), bronchial carcinoma (p. 375), bronchiectasis (p. 370), chronic bronchitis (p. 336), subacute bacterial endocarditis (p. 213), diabetes mellitus (p. 738) and thyrotoxicosis (p. 695).

In the vast majority of cases the diagnosis of pulmonary tuberculosis can be made with certainty by radiological examination of the chest, bacteriological examination of the sputum for tubercle bacilli, or a combination of the two. In some cases it is necessary to carry out further radiological examination after a course of penicillin in order to exclude an acute inflammatory cause for an abnormal shadow.

Pulmonary tuberculosis must be regarded as active and requiring treatment if one or more of the following features is present:

1. Local or general symptoms, particularly haemoptysis or pleural pain.

2. A radiological opacity known or suspected to be of recent

development, or one which has increased in extent during a period of observation.

3. Radiological evidence of cavitation.

4. Tubercle bacilli in the sputum, gastric juice, or laryngeal swabs.

Complications

1. *Pleurisy with or without effusion.* This common complication is described on pp. 396-398.

2. *Spontaneous pneumothorax*, due to rupture of a tuberculous lesion into the pleural space (p. 405).

3. *Tuberculous empyema or pyopneumothorax* (p. 400), which may complicate spontaneous pneumothorax.

4. *Tuberculous laryngitis.* The larynx becomes infected by the lodgement of sputum containing tubercle bacilli. It usually occurs as a complication of advanced pulmonary disease.

5. *Tuberculous enteritis* (p. 937). This is practically confined to advanced cases. It is due to the swallowing of heavily infected sputum.

6. *Ischio-rectal abscess and fistula-in-ano.* The abscess forms as a result of tubercle bacilli passing through an abrasion in the rectal mucosa. Secondary pyogenic infection invariably occurs, and a fistula may form when the abscess is incised or if it ruptures spontaneously.

7. *Dissemination of tuberculosis via the blood stream* is very unusual in post-primary pulmonary tuberculosis, but may occur in advanced cases with the production of renal tuberculosis or tuberculous meningitis.

Prognosis. With the advent of effective chemotherapy there has been a remarkable decline in the mortality from pulmonary tuberculosis. Provided the tubercle bacilli are not initially drug-resistant and chemotherapy is used correctly, a fatal outcome is indeed extremely uncommon, even if the disease has reached a fairly advanced stage when it is first recognised. If, however, the bacilli have become resistant to two, or to all three, of the standard antituberculosis drugs (streptomycin, PAS and isoniazid) the outlook for the patient is much less favourable, as the drugs which have to be substituted are less effective and are often poorly tolerated because of side-effects.

If pulmonary tuberculosis has reached an advanced stage before treatment is started, extensive areas of lung tissue may be completely destroyed. Although the tuberculous infection itself can be controlled, the residual pulmonary damage, and the fibrosis and emphysema with which it is invariably associated, may leave the patient seriously disabled by exertional dyspnoea. Ventilatory failure (p. 308) and pulmonary heart disease (p. 259) which eventually develop in many of these cases are nowadays more common causes of death than tuberculous infection itself. Secondary infection of extensively damaged lungs with pyogenic bacteria or with fungi, such as *Aspergillus fumigatus* (p. 365), may lead to chronic ill-health. Occasionally the rupture of a large blood vessel in the wall of a pulmonary cavity or a dilated bronchus may result in a massive or even fatal haemoptysis long after the tuberculous infection has been eradicated. These serious late complications can all be prevented if pulmonary tuberculosis is diagnosed at a reasonably early stage and is efficiently treated.

THE TREATMENT OF TUBERCULOSIS

General Principles

1. *Antituberculosis chemotherapy* is by far the most important measure in the treatment of all forms of tuberculosis and should be given to every patient with active disease.

2. *Rest* is now regarded as of secondary importance. The current practice is to keep patients in bed only until symptoms have subsided and then to allow gradually increasing amounts of activity, provided there is continuing evidence that the local lesion is responding satisfactorily to chemotherapy.

3. Patients from whom tubercle bacilli have been isolated and who are therefore potentially infectious should be admitted to hospital without delay and should not be discharged until bacteriological examination is consistently negative. An exception may be made to this rule only if adequate isolation and nursing care can be provided elsewhere. Patients who are not infectious and in whom the disease is discovered at an early stage can be treated satisfactorily at home, often without any restriction of their activities. If, however, a patient cannot be relied upon to take antituberculosis drugs regularly, an initial period of treatment in hospital should be advised.

4. Immobilisation of a tuberculous lesion is still an important therapeutic measure when the disease involves bones or joints, but 'collapse therapy', in which an attempt is made to immobilise and relax a tuberculous lung by measures such as artificial pneumothorax and thoracoplasty, has no place in the modern treatment of pulmonary tuberculosis.

5. As tuberculosis is seldom a sharply localised disease, attempts to eradicate it by surgical resection have not been uniformly successful. Recent advances in the chemotherapy of tuberculosis have drastically curtailed the indications for surgical treatment but it is still occasionally necessary to resect a lung or part of a lung, a joint, a kidney or a group of superficial lymph nodes in order to accelerate recovery or prevent relapse, particularly in cases with drug-resistant bacilli (see below). An irreparably damaged organ may also have to be resected if it becomes secondarily infected with pyogenic bacteria or fungi. A tuberculous cold abscess, which may develop as a complication of cervical lymph node tuberculosis despite adequate chemotherapy, may have to be drained and a similar procedure may be required in the treatment of tuberculous empyema.

Chemotherapy

Apart from a few minor variations in dosage and duration of treatment (p. 428) the policy governing the use of antituberculosis drugs is the same for all manifestations of the disease.

Drugs. The three most effective drugs in the treatment of tuberculosis are streptomycin, *para*-aminosalicylic acid (PAS) and isoniazid. If any one of these drugs is given alone the bacilli soon become resistant to it and its therapeutic effect is lost, probably for ever. A combination of any two of the drugs is, however, capable of preventing the development of resistance and thus of providing effective treatment for an indefinite period, usually until the disease has healed.

Because in the past chemotherapy was often used incorrectly by present standards, the sputum of some patients with chronic pulmonary tuberculosis contains drug-resistant organisms. Persons coming into contact with such patients may contract infection with bacilli resistant to one or more of the chemotherapeutic agents. This may have serious consequences to the victim, who in certain circumstances may be completely deprived of the benefits of chemotherapy. In Britain at present the tubercle bacillus in about 5 per cent. of new cases is resistant to one of the three standard drugs but fortunately it is very seldom resistant to two drugs (0·4 per cent.) or to all three drugs (0·1 per cent.). In the developing countries where, for economic reasons, isoniazid is often given alone, resistance to this drug is very common.

The selection of a suitable combination of drugs for a patient with tuberculosis depends on many different factors, such as the results of *in vitro* sensitivity tests, the nature of any previous chemotherapy and the risk of side effects. It is also important to consider in what form the treatment can be most conveniently and reliably administered. Although in most cases drugs which can be given by mouth are to be preferred, particularly for out-patient treatment, it may be necessary to employ methods whereby patients who cannot be trusted to take antituberculosis chemotherapy regularly are given one drug (streptomycin) by injection while the whole daily dose of a second drug (e.g. isoniazid) is administered by mouth at the same time under strict supervision.

When the diagnosis is first made, information regarding the drug sensitivity of the tubercle bacillus is not usually available as the results of *in vitro* sensitivity tests are not obtainable for 6 to 12 weeks. Treatment clearly cannot be deferred for this length of time, and a combination of drugs must therefore be selected which takes into account the possibility of infection with a drug-resistant organism.

Ideally, all newly diagnosed cases of tuberculosis should be treated with streptomycin, PAS and isoniazid in the following doses:

Streptomycin sulphate: 1 g. daily by intramuscular injection.
PAS (sodium salt): 5 g. thrice daily by mouth.
Isoniazid: 100 mg. twice daily by mouth (200 mg. twice daily in acute miliary tuberculosis).

This triple drug regimen ensures that the patient receives two drugs in full therapeutic dosage even if he has been infected by a strain of tubercle bacillus which is resistant to the third.

Some patients may, however, be unable to tolerate full doses of streptomycin and PAS:

(*a*) If streptomycin causes vestibular side-effects the dose should be reduced to 0·75 g. daily, and patients over the age of 40, who are particularly prone to develop vestibular damage, should be given this dose from the outset. If side-effects persist when the lower dose is given, streptomycin may have to be withdrawn completely.

(*b*) If PAS causes intractable vomiting or diarrhoea the dose should be reduced to 5 g. twice daily. If severe side-effects still persist PAS may have to be withdrawn completely. Vomiting can sometimes be prevented by giving the drug in the form of enteric-coated granules ('Bactylan').

The original triple drug regimen should be modified when the sensitivity of the tubercle bacilli to the three drugs is known:

(*a*) If the organism is fully sensitive to streptomycin, PAS and isoniazid one of these drugs may be withdrawn. If the patient is being treated in hospital the usual practice is to omit PAS, which is less potent that the other two and more liable to cause side-effects, and to continue treatment with streptomycin and isoniazid. When treatment is being given at home it is more convenient to omit streptomycin, as daily injections are difficult to arrange, particularly when the patient is working. The dose of isoniazid should be maintained at 100 mg. twice daily but that of PAS can at this stage be reduced to 5 g. twice daily. In order to eliminate the possibility of one drug being taken without the other, PAS and isoniazid should be dispensed together in rice-paper cachets. The following preparations provide the correct daily doses of the two drugs:

Sodium Aminosalicylate and Isoniazid Cachets, N.F., 4 cachets twice daily.
Pycasix (Smith and Nephew) or Pasinah 6PH (Wander), 3 cachets twice daily.

(*b*) If the organism is resistant to *one* of the three drugs, treatment should be continued with the other two in one of the following combinations:

Streptomycin, 0·75-1 g. daily, *plus* isoniazid, 100 mg. twice daily.
PAS 5 g. twice daily, *plus* isoniazid, 100 mg. twice daily.
Streptomycin, 0·75-1 g. daily, *plus* PAS 5 g. *thrice* daily.

(*c*) If the organism is resistant to *two* or to all *three* drugs the chemotherapeutic regimen will have to include one or, more commonly, two of the newer antituberculosis agents named below in descending order of potency:

Ethambutol, 15-25 mg./kg.	given in a single daily dose by mouth
Pyrazinamide, 2-3 g.	
Ethionamide, 1 g.	
Thiacetazone, 150 mg.	

With the exception of ethambutol these drugs are somewhat less effective and more toxic than the 'standard' drugs, but if they are correctly used, preferably in combination with any 'standard' drug to which the tubercle bacilli are still sensitive, control of the tuberculous infection can be achieved in almost every case.

Information on drug sensitivity cannot of course be obtained if attempts to culture tubercle bacilli are unsuccessful. In these circumstances it is the usual practice to assume that the organism is fully sensitive to streptomycin, PAS and isoniazid and to advise treatment accordingly.

Side-effects. *Streptomycin* and *PAS*, and occasionally *isoniazid*, may produce a reaction of hypersensitivity, consisting of pyrexia and an erythematous skin eruption, which usually develops two to four weeks after treatment is started. If this occurs the patient must be desensitised by giving small but increasing doses of the drug until the full dose is tolerated. An antihistamine drug (p. 328) may be given at the same time. Occasionally the hypersensitivity is so severe that corticosteroids have to be used to control it and to allow desensitisation to be undertaken.

Other side-effects include:

Streptomycin: vertigo (common); deafness (rare).

PAS: anorexia, nausea, vomiting, diarrhoea (common); goitre and hypothyroidism (rare); hepatitis, usually associated with hypersensitivity (rare); hypokalaemia (rare); haemolytic anaemia (rare).

Isoniazid: polyneuropathy (rare); pellagra (rare).

Duration of Treatment. The duration of treatment should *never* be less than 15 months. In most cases a period of 18 months' treatment is adequate but when the disease is advanced this must be extended to two years. A minimum of two years' treatment should be given to all patients with tuberculosis involving lymph nodes, bones and joints, in which there is a greater tendency for the infection to relapse.

RESPONSE TO TREATMENT. If the bacilli at the start of treatment are fully sensitive to the drugs in use it is most unusual, even in advanced cases, for cultures of sputum, gastric washings, laryngeal swabs or urine to remain positive for more than six months. The persistence of tubercle bacilli for a longer period is in most instances due either to drug resistance or to irregular treatment. In such cases surgical measures (p. 425) may be required.

When PAS has been prescribed an impression of the patient's reliability in regard to treatment can be obtained by testing specimens of urine occasionally for the presence of PAS. This is done by adding a few drops of a 10 per cent. solution of ferric chloride to 1 ml. of acidified urine. If PAS is present a purple colour is produced. A negative result indicates that no PAS or any chemically related substance, such as aspirin, has been taken for at least 18 hours. The test can be performed more conveniently by the use of Phenistix (Ames Company).

Dosage of Antituberculosis Drugs in Children.

Streptomycin sulphate: 30 mg. per kg. body weight, to a maximum of 1 g. daily.

PAS (sodium salt): 0·35-0·5 g. per kg. body weight, to a maximum of 10-15 g. daily, given in two or three divided doses.

Isoniazid: 3-5 mg. per kg. body weight, to a maximum of 200 mg. daily, given in two divided doses.

In acute miliary tuberculosis and tuberculous meningitis the daily dose of isoniazid should be increased to 10 mg. per kg. body weight, to a maximum of 400 mg.

Inexpensive Treatment Regimens. In the developing countries it will usually be impossible for economic reasons to adhere to the recommended chemotherapeutic regimens. The following inexpensive forms of treatment are reasonably effective if given for a year or longer:

(*a*) Isoniazid (300 mg.) *plus* thiacetazone (150 mg.) given in a single daily dose by mouth.

(*b*) Streptomycin (1 g.) by intramuscular injection *plus* isoniazid (14 mg. per kg. body weight) by mouth, given together on two days per week, along with pyridoxine (10 mg.) by mouth to prevent toxic effects from the large doses of isoniazid.

Corticosteroid Drugs

These agents suppress the inflammatory reaction excited by the tubercle bacillus and by interfering with tissue defence mechanisms may promote a rapid dissemination of infection throughout the body. If, however, a corticosteroid drug is given in conjunction with effective antituberculosis chemotherapy it may exert a *favourable* influence on the course of the disease by reducing the severity both of the local inflammatory reaction and of the associated systemic disturbance. In acute cases of pulmonary tuberculosis such treatment will rapidly relieve pyrexia, and will often produce a dramatic improvement in the radiological appearances. The effect is temporary and ceases when the corticosteroid drug is withdrawn, but it may save the lives of patients with fulminating tuberculous infection by permitting them to survive until antituberculosis chemotherapy has had time to exert its influence. Prednisolone, the drug most frequently used in these cases, is given in a dose of 15-20 mg. daily for about three months.

Corticosteroid drugs may also be of value in tuberculous pleural effusion and in tuberculosis involving the hilar, mediastinal or cervical lymph nodes.

Symptomatic Treatment

(*a*) *Cough.* (p. 322.)

(*b*) *Haemoptysis.* Morphine, which depresses the cough reflex, may have the effect of allowing blood clot to accumulate in the bronchi and should seldom be prescribed. A barbiturate may be given if required to allay anxiety, e.g. phenobarbitone, 60 mg. twice daily. Haemoptysis nearly always stops spontaneously, and firm reassurance to this effect lessens the strain of what, to the patient and his relatives, is a most alarming experience.

If the haemorrhage is very severe a blood transfusion should be given and, if respiratory obstruction develops, the blood must be removed from the bronchi by aspiration through a bronchoscope. Control of the bleeding by surgical measures is occasionally required.

(*c*) *Pain in the Chest.* The treatment of pain due to dry pleurisy or spontaneous pneumothorax has been described on p. 323.

(*d*) *Fever and Sweating.* These symptoms usually subside soon after chemotherapy is started. When persistent and excessive they should be treated by repeated tepid sponging.

(*e*) *Hoarseness.* Hoarseness is usually due to tuberculous laryngitis, which responds rapidly to specific chemotherapy provided the organisms are not drug-resistant.

(*f*) *Diarrhoea.* Severe and continued diarrhoea in a patient with pulmonary tuberculosis is usually due to tuberculous enteritis. In most cases it can be rapidly controlled by chemotherapy. It must be remembered, however, that diarrhoea may also be caused by PAS.

THE PREVENTION OF TUBERCULOSIS

A great deal has already been achieved in the control of tuberculosis, but the number of new notifications is still high. The three most important preventive measures are:

1. Raising the resistance of the population to the disease by:

(*a*) *Good social conditions*, including satisfactory housing and adequate diet.

(*b*) *BCG Vaccination.*

Intracutaneous vaccination with BCG (p. 411) of persons showing a *negative* reaction to the tuberculin test affords a degree of protection against the disease similar to that conferred by a primary tuberculous infection, while avoiding the risks of such an infection. It is thus of great value in persons with a negative tuberculin reaction who are liable to be in close contact with infectious cases of tuberculosis, such as the family contacts of a tuberculous subject and the medical, nursing and domestic staff of hospitals and sanatoria. In Britain, BCG vaccination is given in all these special cases but its more general use is limited to adolescents, whose liability to develop tuberculosis is greater than that of the rest of the community and in whom the results are highly satisfactory.

The criterion of successful vaccination is the development of a positive tuberculin reaction six weeks later.

2. Reduction of the incidence of human infection by:

(*a*) *The admission to hospital of infectious cases of pulmonary tuberculosis.* Under this category must be included every patient in whom tubercle bacilli are isolated from the sputum by the direct or concentration method. Those with no sputum or from whom tubercle bacilli are obtained only on culture are usually regarded as non-infectious, although they may not necessarily remain so. Any infectious or potentially infectious patient treated at home should be isolated in a well-ventilated room. He should have his own eating and drinking utensils which should if possible be sterilised after use. Waxed cardboard sputum containers and paper handkerchiefs should be provided, these being burned after use. He should avoid contact with children, in whom tuberculous infection is particularly liable to have grave consequences.

(*b*) *The detection and isolation of the maximum number of cases*, if possible before tubercle bacilli are present in the sputum. Persons who have been in contact with active cases of tuberculosis are much more liable to develop the disease than other members of the community and must always be offered clinical and radiological examination at a chest clinic as soon as the primary case is diagnosed. Mass miniature radiography enables case-finding to be pursued on a very much larger scale but priority should be given to the examination of persons most likely to be suffering from pulmonary tuberculosis, e.g. those with suspicious symptoms, and groups of people who, if they should develop the disease, would by reason of their occupation be particularly liable to infect others, e.g. teachers, hairdressers and bus conductors.

(*c*) *The elimination of conditions favouring the spread of infection*, such as bad housing, overcrowding, inadequate ventilation of houses, shops, factories and places of entertainment.

3. THE ELIMINATION OF TUBERCULOUS INFECTION IN MILK.

Tuberculosis in dairy cattle has been virtually eradicated in Britain and as, in addition, most of the milk on sale is now pasteurised, bovine tuberculosis in man has almost completely disappeared. Pasteurisation kills the tubercle bacillus by heat while preserving the nutritive components of the milk with the exception of vitamin C. It also sterilises milk infected with pathogenic organisms such as streptococci, typhoid bacilli and *Brucella abortus*. Unpasteurised milk produced under strictly controlled hygienic conditions ('Certified' or 'Tuberculin-tested') is still obtainable but is more expensive than ordinary pasteurised milk and potentially less safe.

SARCOIDOSIS

Sarcoidosis is a systemic granulomatous disease of unknown cause. Apart from the absence of caseation and tubercle bacilli, the lesions are histologically similar to tuberculous follicles, but there is no convincing evidence to support the view that the two diseases are related. Chronic beryllium poisoning produces a disease which mimics sarcoidosis both pathologically and clinically, but as exposure to beryllium is extremely uncommon few cases of sarcoidosis can be caused in this way. Histological changes resembling those of sarcoidosis are occasionally seen in individual organs, such as lymph nodes, in conditions such as carcinoma, reticulosis and fungal infections, but these localised 'sarcoid reactions' are not associated with systemic sarcoidosis.

Pathology. The mediastinal and superficial lymph nodes, lungs, liver, spleen, skin, eyes, parotid glands and phalangeal bones are the organs most frequently involved. The characteristic histological feature consists of non-caseating epithelioid follicles. These lesions usually resolve spontaneously but in some cases they stimulate the production of fibrous tissue, which may have grave effects on the structure and function of the organs involved. The disease is seldom fatal, and then only when it affects vital organs such as the lungs, the heart or the central nervous system. An increase in serum calcium, which occurs in rare instances, may produce renal calcinosis and uraemia.

Clinical Features. Sarcoidosis may present in a subacute or a chronic form. Subacute sarcoidosis is usually a benign and self-limiting disorder. One of its most common manifestations is bilateral enlargement of the hilar lymph nodes, which is often accompanied at the outset by erythema nodosum, pyrexia and polyarthralgia. Later, transient pulmonary changes may be seen on radiological examination in addition to the lymph node enlargement. Other cases of subacute sarcoidosis may present with bilateral parotid swelling, which often persists for several weeks. Neurological manifestations, which are uncommon, include arachnoiditis, cranial nerve lesions and polyneuropathy.

Chronic sarcoidosis is a more serious condition, which is less likely to resolve spontaneously and is more liable to cause permanent damage to the structures it involves. Chronic pulmonary sarcoidosis may lead to the development of interstitial fibrosis, pulmonary hypertension and cor pulmonale. Myocardial sarcoidosis may produce arrhythmias and cardiac failure. The commonest ocular lesion is bilateral iridocyclitis which, if untreated, may cause blindness. Various types of skin lesion may be seen, such as cutaneous 'sarcoids' (reddish-brown papules) or lupus pernio (raised purple plaques, usually on the face, resembling chilblains). Cystic lesions may develop in the phalangeal bones of the hands or feet.

Diagnosis. In most cases skin sensitivity to tuberculin is depressed or absent, and the Mantoux reaction (p. 417) is therefore a useful 'screening' test, a strongly positive reaction to 1 TU. virtually excluding sarcoidosis. Although the diagnosis can often be made with a fair measure of confidence from the clinical and radiological features and the tuberculin test, it should, if possible, be confirmed histologically by biopsy of a superficial lymph node or of a skin lesion, when these are present. The Kveim test is also a useful diagnostic procedure, provided a potent antigen can be obtained from human sarcoid tissue. The antigen is injected intradermally and when the test is positive a small nodule develops about four weeks later, biopsy of which reveals typical sarcoid follicles.

Treatment. As subacute sarcoidosis usually resolves spontaneously treatment is seldom required but, occasionally, patients with persistent erythema nodosum, pyrexia, or parotid swelling may have to be given one of the corticosteroid drugs for a short period. Patients with chronic sarcoidosis, particularly if it involves the lungs, eyes or other vital organs, are much more likely to require treatment with corticosteroids, which may have to be continued for several years. The dose should be kept to the minimum required to suppress the manifestations of the disease. Some physicians who believe that sarcoidosis is a form of tuberculosis advise that antituberculosis chemotherapy should be given at the same time, but this is probably unnecessary.

THE PREVENTION OF RESPIRATORY DISEASE

The main causes of respiratory disease are: infection, mechanical derangements of the bronchi, lungs or pleura, vascular lesions in the pulmonary circulation, allergic phenomena, the inhalation of noxious agents (such as dusts and gases), and tumours.

The preventive measures applicable to each cause will be discussed in turn.

Infection

The following are the most important factors in the prevention of respiratory infection:

1. *The avoidance of contact with persons suffering from a specific respiratory infection*

The strict application of this principle may be unnecessary in diseases of low infectivity such as pneumococcal pneumonia or impracticable in the case of ubiquitous diseases such as coryza or influenza. It has its most important application in the infectious 'fevers', such as measles and whooping-cough, and in tuberculosis, particularly when the subject at risk is a child. In all infective diseases, however, the improvement of housing conditions with the eradication of overcrowding must be regarded as an essential preventive measure. Improved ventilation of public transport vehicles, factories, shops and places of entertainment would also help to limit the spread of respiratory infection.

The wearing of face masks by persons suffering from acute upper respiratory infections in order to prevent dissemination of disease is hardly feasible in ordinary circumstances, but this precaution should always be taken by members of the medical, nursing and domestic staff of hospitals, especially children's hospitals, if they have to remain on duty while suffering from such an infection.

2. *Natural and acquired immunity to infection*

Natural immunity, although of importance in determining the outcome of an exposure to infection, has little practical bearing on the prevention of respiratory infection, except possibly in the case of tuberculosis (p. 411). The artificial production of acquired immunity is, however, of considerable value in the prevention of tuberculosis (p. 431) and of diseases such as diphtheria, whooping-cough, influenza and measles, which are liable to have serious respiratory complications. The use of vaccines prepared from autogenous pyogenic bacteria for the prevention of coryza and bronchitis is now considered to be of no value.

Mechanical Derangements of the Bronchi, Lungs or Pleura

Suitable pre-operative measures can do much to prevent bronchial obstruction by tenacious secretion, which is liable to complicate thoracic and abdominal operations (p. 369). The proper supervision of children reduces the risks of the accidental inhalation of a foreign body, and adequate protection of the larynx during operations on the mouth and throat under general anaesthesia will virtually eliminate the possibility of the inhalation of teeth, tissue fragments or blood clot. Bronchiectasis can to a large extent be prevented by the early and adequate treatment of pulmonary infection and by the prompt relief of bronchial obstruction, where that is possible.

As the cause of emphysema is not known no measure is available to prevent it, but the prophylaxis and early treatment of bronchial and pulmonary infections can undoubtedly mitigate the effects of the disease. Pulmonary fibrosis occurring as a sequel to pulmonary infection may be prevented by the early and adequate control of such infection.

There are no known means of preventing the initial episode of spontaneous pneumothorax, but the risks of a recurrence can be eliminated by the induction of an artificial pleurisy which obliterates the pleural space.

Allergic Phenomena. Hay fever can usually be prevented by the routine use of an antihistamine drug during the flowering season or by pre-seasonal desensitisation with the causal antigen. The complex problems involved in the prevention of bronchial asthma have been discussed on p. 341.

The Inhalation of Noxious Agents. There now seems to be no doubt that pollution of the atmosphere in urban areas by smoke containing large amounts of irritant substances, such as sulphur dioxide, is an important aetiological factor in chronic bronchitis, and a nation-wide drive to control this menace to public health is urgently needed. Measures to reduce the inhalation of dust and fumes in certain occupations are also important in the prevention of chronic bronchitis and the specific industrial lung diseases (pp. 336 and 383).

Tumours. It has now been established beyond reasonable doubt that the smoking of tobacco (especially cigarettes) is the most important factor in the production of bronchial carcinoma. The presence of carcinogens in the polluted atmosphere of our cities and towns also contributes to the high incidence of the disease. These two observations suggest that bronchial carcinoma is, to some extent at least, a preventable disease and it is the duty of the medical profession actively to discourage the habit of smoking and to support vigorously the drive for 'clean air'.

I. W. B. GRANT.
E. A. HARRIS.

Books recommended:

Bates, D. V. & Christie, R. V. (1964). *Respiratory Function in Disease: An Introduction to the Integrated Study of the Lung.* Philadelphia: Saunders.

Comroe, J. H., Forster, R. E., Dubois, A. B., Briscoe, W. A. & Carlson, E. (1962). *The Lung. Clinical Physiology and Pulmonary Function Tests*, 2nd ed. (1962). Chicago: Year Book Medical Publishers.

Hinshaw, H. C. & Garland, L. H. (1963). *Diseases of the Chest*, 2nd ed. Philadelphia: Saunders.

NUTRITIONAL DISORDERS

Introduction. At the beginning of the present century medical thought was dominated by the brilliant achievements of bacteriology. Within the span of the professional life of a single doctor one after another of the great human diseases had been added to the impressive list of those in which a causative infecting organism was positively identified.

That disease might be due to lack of some essential factor had little place in the thinking of 50 years ago. Consequently the concept of *deficiency diseases*, nutritional and endocrine, grew slowly in the present century. As the deficiency diseases came to be recognised and understood, the next step was the realisation that lack of nutritional and endocrine factors affects primarily the chemistry of the body; disease may result from a 'biochemical lesion', and the structural changes demonstrated by the morbid anatomist are late effects, secondary to this change in function. Thus was born the science of chemical pathology.

This revolution in medical thought had profound practical consequences. The great nutritional diseases that flourished within the lifetime of many doctors still in practice have now vanished wherever medical knowledge has been linked with proper administration of food supplies. Florid rickets is now a clinical curiosity in Britain, yet in the streets of our big cities we still see elderly people, bandy-legged, stunted and pigeon-chested, who carry the scars of it. Pellagra, prior to 1940, affected tens of thousands of poor country people in the southern states of the U.S.A.; better knowledge of nutritional needs and above all, improved economic circumstances, have swept it away. The classic nutritional diseases now only occur in situations where there is a failure both of food supplies and medical care.

Even in times of severe food shortage, proper application of medical knowledge can do much to overcome the worst effects of *qualitative* dietary deficiencies; medicine can deal with beriberi, scurvy and pellagra, but has no direct means of treating the effects of underfeeding—subnutrition. Consequently lack of sufficient food continues to be a most serious cause of ill-health in many underdeveloped countries.

The present world population is estimated to be more than 3,000 million and is increasing by 70 million per year. In the absence of major catastrophies by the year 2000 there will probably be twice as many inhabitants in the world as there are today. The greatest threat to the well-being of mankind is this explosive population growth rate. Agricultural production in many parts of the world has remained practically static over the past 10 years; one-third of the world's population now receives less than 2,000 Cal./head/day. Agricultural production is hampered by bad climates, soil erosion, poor soil, lack of fertilisers, antiquated farming methods and war. Serious subnutrition is fortunately rare in Britain today, but in many other countries doctors are faced with the problem of dealing with large numbers of underfed patients. This situation will steadily deteriorate unless national programmes of population control are evolved and effectively put into operation.

Aetiology and Definition. There are three essential causes of nutritional disorders:

1. Not enough food (quantitative dietary deficiency) results in *subnutrition* (underfeeding) or *frank starvation.*
2. Wrong food (qualitative dietary deficiency) results in *malnutrition.* The term 'malnutrition' should be restricted to those nutritional disorders, e.g. rickets, scurvy, which are due to lack of specific chemical components (nutrients) of a proper diet.
3. Too much food (overfeeding) results in *obesity.*

Social and Economic Causes of Nutritional Disorders. Even in countries where food, ample in quantity and quality, can be purchased, nutritional disorders arise because of poverty, prejudice, ignorance or bad housekeeping often caused by bad housing. The old, the solitary and the young are most often affected.

Pathological Causes of Nutritional Disorders. Even with an ample income, an adequate home and an expert knowledge of dietetics, a patient may develop a nutritional disorder through some other disease which 'conditions' (facilitates) it in one or more of the following ways.

DEFECTIVE INTAKE OF FOOD. (*a*) *Loss of appetite* (anorexia) may be an important symptom of organic disease, e.g. cancer of the stomach, and also of psychogenic disease, e.g. anorexia nervosa. Deficiency of thiamine may present with anorexia. (*b*) *Persistent vomiting* from any cause. (*c*) *Foods fads*. (*d*) *Alcohol* provides calories but no essential nutrients. Chronic alcoholics suffer from malnutrition more often than subnutrition. (*e*) *Unbalanced therapeutic diets*, e.g. diets for digestive diseases may lack ascorbic acid unless care is taken to provide it. (*f*) *Prolonged parenteral feeding* with intravenous glucose after surgical operations may precipitate acute deficiencies of the vitamin B complex.

DEFECTIVE DIGESTION AND ABSORPTION. (*a*) *Achlorhydria* is a contributory factor in the causation of iron deficiency aneamia. (*b*) *Steatorrhoea* limits the absorption of calcium and fat-soluble vitamins. (*c*) *Intestinal hurry* due to surgical short circuits, etc. may impair digestion. In starving people the ingestion of unsuitable food often causes intestinal hurry and intensifies their plight. (*d*) *Antibiotics*, if their administration is prolonged, may interfere with the production of certain vitamins synthesised by intestinal bacteria (p. 479).

DEFECTIVE UTILISATION. (*a*) *Cirrhosis* of the liver may interfere with the proper utilisation of ingested nutrients, e.g. of protein and vitamin K. (*b*) *Malignancy*, in some unknown way, may produce a state of subnutrition despite an adequate diet. The same may be true of tuberculosis and other prolonged infections.

LOSS OF NUTRIENTS FROM THE BODY. (*a*) In the *nephrotic syndrome* there is the continuing loss of protein in the urine. (*b*) In *diabetes mellitus* uncontrolled glycosuria causes subnutrition. (*c*) In *excessive menstrual bleeding* (menorrhagia) secondary iron deficiency anaemia is common.

INCREASED NUTRITIONAL NEEDS. (*a*) In pregnancy, lactation and adolescence (especially after an illness in the last named), and for those engaged in hard physical work, particularly in cold climates, a 'normal' diet may be insufficient. (*b*) In fevers and hyperthyroidism hypermetabolism calls for more calories. (*c*) After burns, fractures and major surgery, there is an increased catabolism of protein and ascorbic acid which cannot be replaced until later, i.e. when convalescence begins.

Although nutritional disorders are often precipitated and sometimes caused by such conditioning factors, the prime cause is usually a diet deficient in one or more nutrients. It is therefore poor practice to prescribe a single nutrient (e.g. a vitamin) without first looking for evidence of other deficiencies and thereafter taking all possible measures to improve the diet.

QUANTITATIVE ASPECTS OF NUTRITION

Requirements for calories vary widely, even among apparently similar individuals. 'Recommended Allowances' provide only a rough standard for assessing the adequacy of a diet for an individual patient.

An international committee of authorities on nutrition, sponsored by the Food and Agriculture Organization of the United Nations, recommended in 1957 as suitable allowances:

3,200 Cal./day for a man aged 25, weighing 65 kg., doing light physical work for eight hours daily in a temperate climate;
2,300 Cal./day for his wife aged 25, weighing 55 kg., with children to tend.

Reductions in these allowances are made for people who are (*a*) older, (*b*) less heavy, (*c*) less active or (*d*) live in warmer surroundings.

The population of Britain, including infants, children and adults, probably needs an overall average *intake* of 2,500 Cal./head/day. In order that the population may actually consume this amount, the food retailed in the shops must provide more to allow for household wastage. The food supplies of Britain ordinarily provide 3,000 *retail* Cal./head/day. It is this shop-value of our food supplies that is sometimes discussed in Press and Parliament and often confused with average physiological requirements.

Subnutrition and Starvation

Starvation may conveniently be defined as subnutrition of sufficient severity to warrant in-patient treatment in hospital. In starvation the body weight may be reduced by 25 per cent. or more.

Subnutrition and starvation arise (1) when there is not enough food to eat, for instance in times of famine, (2) when there is severe disease of the digestive tract, preventing the absorption of nutrients, as in the malabsorption syndrome and cancer of the oesophagus or (3) when there is a toxaemia which prevents the normal metabolism of the nutrients by the tissues; such a toxaemia might be metabolic in origin (i.e. in renal or hepatic failure) or due to severe and long-continued infection. In all these circumstances there is wasting of the body with much loss of both muscle and fat. This gives rise to a clinical picture with an underlying morbid anatomy and chemical pathology which is essentially similar whatever the primary cause.

Clinical Features. When the caloric value of the diet is inadequate, children cease to grow or even lose weight. Adults also lose weight. The loss may be rapid at first, but tends to slow down and become stabilised at a lower level because the body is able to adapt itself, at least partly, to an insufficient intake of food. This adaptation is possible because (*a*) the bulk of the muscles and glands is reduced in size, requiring less energy for their maintenance, (*b*) the basal metabolism of the tissues is reduced, (*c*) the body, being lighter, requires less mechanical work to move it about, and (*d*) all unnecessary voluntary movements are curtailed.

The patient becomes thin and the skin lax, most noticeably over the upper arm and abdomen. The skin is thin, dry, inelastic and often cyanosed at the extremities. The hair becomes dull, dry and inflexible ('staring' hair). The eyes are dull and sunken, yet the wasting of orbital tissues may give them an unusual prominence. The heart is reduced in size and there is often bradycardia and a reduced systolic blood pressure. Atrophy of the small intestine is always present in starvation and may be severe; in which case the inability to digest and absorb nutrients will greatly prejudice the chances of recovery. In addition, once diarrhoea has begun, the loss of fluid in the stools causes grave disturbances in water and salt balance. Eventually, in severe cases, dependent 'famine' oedema begins to appear.

This results from prolonged consumption of a diet providing less than 1,000 Cal. and 50 g. protein/day. It is often preceded by a period of nocturnal polyuria. The oedema is not necessarily associated with any fall in the level of plasma proteins, but is due rather to wasting of tissues without a corresponding loss of body water; hence it has been called 'isohydric' famine oedema. A mild to moderate normocytic, normochromic anaemia is common, due to a reduction in the red cell population without corresponding alteration in the plasma volume.

Seriously underfed patients are weak and sometimes suffer from attacks of syncope. Psychological symptoms frequently occur in starving people. Mental restlessness, irritability and indifference to the troubles of others may be combined with physical apathy.

Diagnosis. In times of famine the signs of starvation may be all too obvious, so much so that other causes of emaciation can be overlooked. However, a similar clinical picture may be produced by the cachexia of advanced cancer, tuberculosis, dysentery or other severe chronic infections. It is also seen in the protein calorie malnutrition syndrome.

Famine oedema must be distinguished from other primary causes of oedema—cardiac, renal or hepatic. The diagnosis of subnutrition depends on (*a*) careful enquiry into the social, economic and dietary history and a knowledge of local food conditions, and (*b*) evidence of recent weight loss and the other clinical features mentioned above.

Treatment. In simple subnutrition, all that is needed is suitable food. Its management is more an administrative than a medical problem. When the patient suffering from starvation is seriously ill the nature of the treatment depends essentially on the facilities available.

Most famine victims, because of some alimentary dysfunction, cannot deal with large quantities of food. The patient's desire for food may be immense and no guide to his digestive capacities. Limitation of the food intake is often necessary. This is essential if there is nutritional diarrhoea or a severe degree of nutritional cachexia.

The choice of food is difficult. Only bland foods can be tolerated by the thin-walled intestines lacking essential digestive enzymes. Probably the best food of all is skimmed milk, fresh or reconstituted from dried milk powder. Frequent small feeds of skimmed milk, 100 ml. or so at a time (as often as the patient is willing and able to take them) is the best way of averting death from starvation. This requires constant personal attention and nursing care. A variety of mild flavouring essences may be useful for improving the appetite and a compound vitamin syrup may be added. As the patient begins to recover he should be encouraged gradually to take semi-solid foods, along the lines followed in weaning a baby. With re-feeding there may be some increase in oedema, especially if unlimited table salt is allowed; in which event the supply of salt should be temporarily restricted.

There may come a time when a patient with severe starvation refuses all food, although fully rational. The outlook is then very grave. Feeding of milk and other fluids through a tube passed into the stomach via the mouth or nose then provides the only hope. Spectacular improvement may follow this measure, but some patients are beyond recovery.

Prognosis. Physical and psychological recovery is usually complete if sufficient calories are provided for cases of primary subnutrition. When irreversible changes have developed in the heart and small intestine, as occurs in severe starvation, the prognosis is poor.

Prevention. This rests with the social, economic and agricultural legislators and executives.

OBESITY

Obesity is the most common nutritional disorder at the present time in North America, Australia, New Zealand, Britain and most European countries and gives rise to more ill-health than all the vitamin deficiencies put together.

While it is easy to define obesity as an excessive accumulation of fat in the storage areas of the body, it is difficult to state in individual instances the point at which this accumulation may be considered to be excessive. Gradual change in weight commonly occurs as age advances. Most individuals gain a few pounds in weight during the years from 25 to 40, while an even greater gain may take place in the succeeding decade. After the age of 50 to 60 there is usually a decline in weight. Obesity as a condition requiring treatment can be taken to be present when fat deposition has raised the body weight 10 per cent. or more above the standards for people of the same age, sex and race (pp. 1304 and 1305).

Age and Sex. Obesity may occur at any age and in either sex. In children both sexes are equally affected, but after puberty it is more common in women than in men. It is especially liable to arise after pregnancy and at the menopause.

Economic Status. In Britain obesity is probably more common among the poor than among the rich, perhaps because foods rich in fat and protein, which satisfy appetite more readily than carbohydrates, are more expensive than foods with a high starch content which provide the bulk of cheap meals.

Physical Activity. In all countries obesity is seldom found in those who lead active lives or follow occupations or recreations demanding hard physical exercise. The amount of energy expended when walking is of great interest to all of middle age or older. If a man weighing 160 lb. walks at the rate of 3½ miles an hour he will expend 5 Calories per minute. If he walks for an hour he will expend 300 Calories, which represents approximately the caloric value of 1 oz. of fat. This may seem a very small amount, but an intake of 1 oz. of fat daily, if *additional* to one's maintenance requirements, could mean an increase of weight of over 20 lb. in a year.

With the mechanisation of industry and the widespread use of motor vehicles, the proportion of people who take adequate exercise has declined and the number of sedentary workers, has increased. Hence, inactivity may be an important factor explaining the frequency of what has been described as 'creeping' overweight in modern Western societies. Although it is fashionable to decry exercise as a means of reducing weight, a combination of exercise and diet is strongly recommended.

Psychological Factors. There can be no doubt that some women often over-eat for emotional reasons. Naturally, this is a happy hunting ground for the deductive speculations of the Freudians. For the practising physician it is perhaps sufficient to know that some women over-eat because they are unhappy. They find solace in scones and cream cookies, for the same reasons that may drive their husbands to seek relief in alcohol.

Eating Habits. The eating habits of obese people are variable. In some, continual nibbling seems to be an important cause of the excess food intake. These include many housewives and also others who work in kitchens.

Genetic Factors. It is a matter of common observation that obesity runs in families. The nature of the genetic factors responsible is certainly not simple and probably several genes are involved. Moreover it is difficult to distinguish their influence from environmental factors such as family custom and eating habits.

Endocrine Factors. These are often blamed for obesity, though seldom on any good evidence. Many obese patients make the excuse that 'My doctor says it's glands'. In reality, defective secretion by the thyroid, pituitary or sex glands is seldom the cause of obesity.

Pregnancy. A healthy woman may be expected to gain about 12·5 kg. (27·5 lb.) during pregnancy. About half of this represents the weight of the foetus, placenta and uterus. Water retention in the tissues may account for 1-2 kg. The remainder can be attributed to an increase in adipose tissue, which serves as a store against the future demands of lactation. Many women gain more and retain this extra weight after the termination of lactation, thus becoming progressively more obese with each succeeding child.

Comment. Interest in all the above factors should not distract attention from the primary basic fact that obesity is always due to a greater consumption of food than the individual requires. Adipose tissue cannot come out of the air; it can only come from food. A consistent excess intake of as little as 50 Cal./day can lead to a gain of 4 lb. in a year. Fifty calories can be obtained from the following small amounts of food or drink: 1 oz. of lean meat or chicken; 2 oz. potato; $\frac{3}{4}$ oz. bread; $\frac{1}{4}$ oz. butter; $\frac{1}{2}$ oz. of sugar; a quarter of a glass of milk; or quarter of a pint of beer. A similar result could occur from a small reduction in physical activity even if the daily calorie intake remained constant. In other words, the cause of obesity is too much food, too little exercise, or both.

Metabolism in obesity. There is certainly no reduction of energy expenditure by obese patients, though repeated efforts have been made to prove the contrary. Their basal metabolic rate is usually within normal limits and there is no reduction in the specific dynamic action of foodstuffs. There is no possibility that they succeed in extracting more calories from their food, because the absorption of food is about 95 per cent. efficient in normal thin people. Obese patients do not conserve energy by doing physical work with greater metabolic efficiency than normal; in fact they have an expenditure of energy greater than normal, to move their weight about in day-to-day activities.

It has been suggested that normal people manage to keep their weight within normal limits by virtue of some special ability for burning off any excess calories, perhaps during the night. Failure of this mechanism might account for obesity. However, there is no good evidence that such a 'luxus Konsumption' mechanism exists.

In conclusion it must be admitted that at the present time it is not possible to define precisely a metabolic disorder causing human obesity. Nevertheless there may be, in addition to over-eating and underexercising, as yet unknown physiological mechanisms which regulate the metabolism of the tissues.

Clinical Features. The diagnosis should be made on the clinician's observation that there is too much adipose tissue in some part of the body. The distribution of this tissue is variable and attempts have been made to distinguish different types of obesity on this basis, but it is doubtful if they serve any useful purpose.

Complications. Apart from aesthetic considerations, obesity leads to mechanical disabilities, predisposes to metabolic and cardiovascular disorders and so reduces the expectancy of life.

PSYCHOLOGICAL. Aesthetic considerations are sufficient to make many people aware of the threat of obesity and anxious to avoid it; those who do not succeed may become unhappy. Thus obesity creates psychiatric problems in addition to any that may have been partly responsible for it.

MECHANICAL DISABILITY. The structure of the human skeleton is not well adapted to carry an extra load, consequently flat feet and osteoarthritis of the knees, hips and lumbar spine are more common in obese people than in those of normal weight. The abdominal muscles that support the viscera, and those in the legs which help by their contractions the venous return of blood to the heart, are infiltrated with fat. Hence their normal mechanical action is impaired, with consequent abdominal hernias and varicose veins. A close association has been demonstrated between obesity and the frequency with which hiatus hernia occurs. Adipose tissue around the chest and under the diaphragm interferes with the mechanics of respiration and predisposes to bronchitis.

Metabolic. Obesity is associated with a number of metabolic disturbances. Diabetes mellitus arising for the first time in middle life occurs most commonly in obese people; fortunately, however, the majority of obese people escape it. Obesity is often associated with an elevated level of cholesterol in the blood plasma; perhaps in consequence, obese people develop stones in the gall-bladder more frequently than those of normal weight. Another site where cholesterol is deposited is the intima of the arteries, producing atherosclerosis (p. 278). Gout is a rare disease that afflicts the obese more commonly than others.

Cardiovascular. Apart from atherosclerosis, obese people suffer from hypertension more commonly than those of normal weight. It is usually of a benign kind, and since the patient is often unaware of its existence, he is best left in ignorance of its presence. The work of the heart is increased by the extra mechanical effort needed in moving the overweight body and by an increased peripheral vascular resistance in patients with hypertension. This extra load on the heart, coupled with the tendency to atherosclerosis in the coronary arteries, no doubt accounts for the liability to angina pectoris and cardiac failure among obese people in middle life. The exceptional incidence of varicose veins has already been mentioned.

Skin. The excessive deposit of subcutaneous fat predisposes to skin infections in the obese, particularly at the flexures, e.g. intertrigo below the breasts.

Accidents. Obese people are often slow and ungainly and therefore liable to accidents. At work they have difficulty in avoiding the moving parts of machinery and in the street cannot quickly escape the traffic. At home they may trip over the carpet and spill kettles of boiling water over themselves.

Life Expectancy. In view of these manifold complications it is not surprising that obese people are poor risks from the standpoint of life insurance. The statistics of the Metropolitan Life Insurance Co. (U.S.A.) have shown that for a man of 45, an increase of 25 lb. above standard weight reduces his life expectancy by 25 per cent. In other words he is likely to die at 60 when he might otherwise have lived to 80 had he not been obese. The risks of obesity in women are somewhat less.

Diagnosis. This apparently obvious disorder is frequently overlooked because the doctor is often preoccupied with one of its many complications. In addition many consulting rooms and hospital wards are still not equipped with reliable balances for weighing patients, and even when they are available they may not be used sufficiently. A regular practice of weighing patients and examining them for evidence of excessive fat deposits would prevent this. People with small hands, small feet and small bones may appear to be of normal weight as judged by accepted standards, and yet may be obese; their obesity—often concentrated in the abdomen—will be missed unless they are examined. But a combination of weighing and physical examination is sufficient to make the diagnosis.

Obesity should be distinguished from normal causes of an increase in weight. Occasionally the diagnosis of pregnancy is missed, and this creates embarrassment. Athletes in training are sometimes considerably overweight as judged by normal standards; their extra weight is due to muscular hypertrophy.

Another important cause of gain in weight is oedema resulting from cardiac, renal or hepatic failure. It does not generally become manifest until the extracellular fluid is increased by 10 per cent. or more, so that the initial gain in weight may be mistaken for obesity, if the patient is not properly examined for evidence of the underlying causative disease.

In myxoedema there may be a sufficient accumulation of myxoedematous tissue to cause excessive weight. The material in this tissue is not fat, but a protein which biochemically resembles collagen.

Treatment

General. The obese person will look fitter, feel better and have a better chance of keeping well and living longer if she reduces her weight to the standard for her age, sex, height and occupation (pp. 1304, 1305).

The *first essential* is for the patient to understand the reasons why she should reduce her weight. She must be convinced that she must give up permanently those habits which have led to obesity; otherwise the reduction in weight which she can expect to obtain from an anti-obesity diet will not be maintained when dietary restrictions are somewhat relaxed. In every case of obesity, income exceeds expenditure, and rational treatment must correct the balance. False knowledge about treatment, often acquired from popular papers and books must be eradicated.

The *second essential* is to instruct the patient in some elementary physiological principles in regard to appetite, exercise and the expenditure of energy.

The *third essential* is to teach the patient about the caloric value of different foods. It must be made clear that there are no 'slimming foods' and no successful 'slimming diets' which do not depend on a reduced intake of calories. *The essence of treatment is to reduce the quantity of food eaten.*

The patient should know at the outset the kinds of foods which she is likely to eat in excess and which therefore may contribute largely to the obesity. These are often bread, cakes, pastry, thick soups and fried foods. She should also learn that snacks, chocolate, sweets, cocktail 'pieces', apéritifs, beer, stout and other alcoholic drinks all add to the caloric intake and hence cannot be permitted unless the patient is prepared to make a corresponding caloric reduction in her diet.

The successful treatment of obesity requires a strict regimen. This is often difficult for people with irregular habits with regard to both food and exercise, such as many doctors, commercial travellers and company directors. An evening with friends, a business lunch, a banquet or a holiday, if care is not taken, may undo the good habits established by weeks of conscientious dieting.

The essential regimen for the treatment of obesity is to regulate the daily intake of calories. It is therefore wise that patients should at first make a practice of weighing what they are about to eat. This must be continued for a few weeks until they become accustomed to judging correctly quantities of food. A suitable balance for this purpose, on the sideboard or kitchen table, is needed. Adherence to an exact diet necessitates good discipline.

Diets must not depart too much from established food habits. It would be absurd to advise an obese rice-eating Indian to take for breakfast one thin slice of wheaten bread. He may not take any breakfast, and wheaten bread may be unavailable. This is where the art of the trained dietitian comes in—to provide a diet of proper composition suitable to the needs and habits of the particular patient. A printed diet sheet, handed out to a patient at a single interview, seldom achieves results. It may however be profitably employed to keep the patient's attention concentrated on the important points, provided this is preceded by adequate discussion and explanation.

The Weighed Diet. Energy output has been determined with great accuracy for people undertaking various activities. To keep in caloric balance a person doing sedentary clerical work will require about 2,000-2,500 Cal. daily, a person doing light work 2,500-3,000 Cal., while a person doing heavy work, such as felling trees, may need 4,000 Cal. or even more. Dietary requirements therefore vary greatly according to occupation and a business executive might require only about half the caloric intake of a manual worker doing heavy work.

An obese middle-aged housewife will usually lose weight satisfactorily on a diet providing about 1,000 Cal./day, such as Diet No. 3. This is based on sound physiological principles. If her daily energy expenditure is 2,200 Cal./day the negative balance will be 1,200 Cal. The caloric value of obese tissue is about 7·5 Cal./g. The weekly negative caloric balance is therefore equivalent to $\frac{1200 \times 7}{7 \cdot 5}$ g. or 1·1 kg. (2·4 lb.). A weekly weight loss of 2-3 lb. should be the general aim. An obese man engaged in active physical work cannot tolerate a diet as low as 1,000 Cal./day. A satisfactory weight loss can be expected from a diet containing 1,500 Cal./day.

Protein. The protein content of the diet should be sufficient to maintain nitrogenous equilibrium (p. 462). Usually 60 g./day (or even less) is sufficient for this purpose. Some weight-reducing regimens (e.g. that of Banting) have been based on the principle of eating mostly meat and other foods rich in protein. Some scientific support was given to this principle by the knowledge that proteins stimulate specific dynamic action and should encourage the dissipation of surplus calories. High protein diets may readily satisfy appetite more effectively than carbohydrate, but are very expensive and so seldom practical.

Carbohydrate. The intake of foods rich in carbohydrate should be drastically reduced since over-indulgence in such foods is the most common cause of obesity. There have been unfounded fears that too drastic reduction of the carbohydrate intake may lead to ketosis and that this ketosis is responsible for numerous complaints such as headache, weakness and nausea, sometimes made by obese patients when first faced with the necessity of dietary restriction. In fact, obese people seldom develop more than a trace of ketosis on any diet and never sufficient to cause symptoms.

In a diet of 1,000 Cal./day, 100 g. of carbohydrate is a suitable allowance.

FAT. A diet providing 1,000 Cal. and containing 100 g. of carbohydrate and 60 g. of protein, cannot include more than 40 g. of fat. This allowance of fat, though small, is sufficient to make the diet palatable and acceptable to the patient.

Recently popular books and newspaper articles have stated that there is no need to restrict the intake of fat in obese patients. Eat fat and get slim is advice which has an obvious appeal. In clinical practice this advice is of no therapeutic value since patients could not be expected to tolerate for more than a short time a bizarre diet which is rich in fat and low in carbohydrate and one which ultimately fails to cause a greater loss of weight than the properly balanced diet described above. It can be said with confidence that the aphorism 'fad diets are bad diets' is true because they are ineffective in the long run and are based on faulty nutritional foundations.

Continuous reduction of weight can only be achieved by a continuous restriction of total caloric intake below the level of energy expenditure.

THE UNWEIGHED DIET. For patients who are only moderately overweight (less than 15 per cent. above standard) and for those who have already reduced themselves substantially, careful weighing of the food is unnecessary. It is also impractical for persons with severe visual defects and sometimes because of mental or physical incapacity. Others may be unable or unwilling to co-operate in the accurate regulation of the calorie intake by means of a weighed diet. In such circumstances an unweighed diet is recommended. It is similar to that used in the treatment of diabetes (p. 754). The patient is given a list of foods which are classified into three groups (p. 1303).

1. Foods which must be avoided. These include especially the carbohydrate-rich foods.

2. Foods which can be taken in moderation.
3. Foods which can be taken without restriction.

For the treatment of obesity meat and fish should be included in group 2. All visible fat should be removed from meat, and fish and eggs should not be fried. The daily ration of milk (½ pint) and butter or margarine (½ oz.) must be clearly stated.

As in the case of the weighed diet, the patient must receive instruction on the rationale of treatment. In the opinion of the writer, the regime of the weighed diet is the method of choice for all patients who are moderately (*i.e.*, more than 15 per cent.) or markedly overweight, because it is a more scientific and accurate method of ensuring that the desired reduction in weight is achieved. It also affords a better means of inculcating the patient at the start of treatment with the vital importance of strict discipline if a satisfactory loss of weight is to be obtained and maintained.

VITAMINS. A properly constructed reducing diet should contain plenty of green vegetables and fruits, since they contain few calories, while their bulk helps to fill the stomach and relieve hunger; they also help to relieve constipation which is a common trouble on a low food intake. Their vitamin A and vitamin C activity will be sufficient to meet the body's needs. With meat, fish and eggs in the diet and little or no refined cereals and sugar, it is improbable that deficiency of any component of the vitamin B complex will arise. A good reducing diet will meet the patient's needs for vitamins. Multivitamin tablets are unnecessary for most patients. Any doctor who has doubt about the vitamin intake of a particular patient should recommend in the first instance some natural source of the vitamin B complex such as yeast extract (e.g. Marmite) or wheat germ (e.g. Bemax).

MINERALS. The only minerals that need serious consideration are calcium and iron. Provided that the diet includes half a pint of skimmed milk, there is little likelihood of a negative calcium balance in an adult. The supply of iron is less sure. In the treatment of obese patients—as indeed of all others—the doctor must be constantly on the alert for the earliest signs of anaemia.

WATER AND SALT. At one time patients were often advised to restrict their intake of water, but there is no logical reason for keeping fat patients thirsty by denying their ordinary desires for fluids. Plain water or unsweetened tea can be taken but not sweetened 'juices'. Alcoholic drinks are a source of calories and hence are best avoided, but if taken, a corresponding reduction in the diet is necessary.

In obese patients with oedema from congestive heart failure or other causes, there will be both water and sodium retention. For all such patients, salt restriction is necessary and suitable diuretics should be given (p. 189).

Diet No. 3 (p. 1287) is in general suitable for the treatment of an overweight middle-aged housewife in Britain. But it may be unsuitable in other circumstances and in other climates. Dietitians with knowledge of local eating habits can achieve a great deal of good by devising diets, suitable to established customs which also provide about 1000 Cal. made up from about 60 g. protein, 100 g. carbohydrate and 40 g. fat. An obese man engaged in active work cannot tolerate so little and will lose weight on about 1500 Cal.

PROPRIETARY POWDERED FOOD PRODUCTS. Vigorous advertising campaigns by various firms recommend their products for the treatment of obesity. These products contain a balanced mixture of protein, carbohydrate and fat with the addition of essential vitamins and minerals. Half a pound (230 g.) of one proprietary preparation is stated to provide 900 calories daily. It is mixed with 2 pints of water and taken in divided quantities at four, five or six feeds in the day. On such a diet the loss of weight will be similar to that achieved by a patient partaking of a 900-1,000 Cal. diet made up of natural foods, as recommended in Diet No. 3. Since these proprietary food products are relatively expensive and less palatable and more monotonous than this diet, they are not recommended for the routine treatment of obesity. If, however, patients are unable or unwilling to learn the basis of the caloric value of the different foods or will not take the trouble to weigh articles of food, or if experience shows that the patient has not the will power to take only the amounts of food prescribed for him, then a trial of one of the proprietary powdered food products is justified.

Exercise. The value of physical exercise has probably been underestimated. It is sometimes stated (but without evidence) that exercise promotes appetite in excess of caloric needs and so may aggravate obesity. But there is evidence from experiments of animals that the reverse is true. A certain minimum amount of exercise may be necessary if the accurate regulation of food intake by the appetite is to be achieved.

Most obese patients lead sedentary lives and the full extent to which urban and industrial life restricts activity is only now being realised. There is little doubt that most obese people would be improved by exercise, e.g. walking, swimming, gardening, provided it does not exceed their cardiovascular capacity. All obese patients, whose occupation is sedentary, should be advised to walk for at least an hour a day, always provided they are fit to do so. Regular *daily* exercise is much more valuable than spurts of activity at the week-end.

The benefits of exercise must not distract attention from the diet. Treatment often involves changes in both the diet and manner of life.

Intensive Treatment. The regimen of dietary restriction and physical activities, already described, aims at achieving a rate of weight loss of just over 1 kg. or 2 lb. a week. Very fat patients would have to persist with such a regimen for many months before achieving a satisfactory weight loss. Such slow progress may be disheartening and lead to the abandonment of treatment. Provided there are no orthopaedic or cardiovascular complications, it is possible to increase the physical activities and reduce the diet still further. Patients have been kept for up to six weeks on diets providing only 400 Cal./day, whilst they walked 10 miles daily. This regimen involved negative balances of the order of 3,000 Cal./day. The patients lost weight at rates of up to 3 kg. or 7 lb. a week, yet they remained well and were able to carry out the exercise.

A period of several weeks of starvation in hospital, only water and non-caloric drinks being allowed, has been recommended for very obese patients who have failed to respond to orthodox anti-obesity treatment. Although the initial loss of weight may be marked the long-term results are usually unsatisfactory since many patients regain most of the weight lost when this strict regimen is discontinued. However it may be of value for selected patients, particularly as a demonstration of what can be achieved with sufficient discipline. Such a regimen is clearly contraindicated for elderly patients, especially if they have cardiovascular complications.

The majority of obese patients will do well if they persist in a regimen of one hour's walk and a diet of 1,000 Cal./day, and this is the regimen recommended.

Other Physical Measures. Turkish baths, massage and even colonic lavage have had their popularity as a means of reducing weight. Though they achieve a temporary success, this is due solely to loss of body water which is very soon replaced. They provide no escape from the inevitable necessity of dietary restriction.

Drugs. ANORECTIC DRUGS. During the past 100 years a great many drugs have been recommended as 'slimming agents'. Modern criticism has disposed of the claims made on behalf of most of them except a group known as the 'anorectic drugs', which are related chemically to amphetamine. The anorectic drugs most frequently prescribed are amphetamine and phenmetrazine.

The amphetamine drugs stimulate the higher cortical centres. In this way they may overcome depression and create a sense of well-being which may help the patient to persevere with an unwelcome dietary regimen. They may also stimulate the satiety centre in the hypothalamus and thus have a depressive effect on appetite. There are serious disadvantages to their use. They may cause insomnia, irritability and serious disturbances of behaviour and also lead to an increased heart rate, raised blood pressure and other evidence of excessive activity of the nervous system. Patients rapidly become habituated to them. Hence the danger of their developing dependence or even addiction. To overcome some of these disadvantages several proprietary preparations have been introduced which contain an anorectic drug together with a sedative or tranquilliser. In such a compound preparation it is impossible to alter the dose of either constituent independently of the other, and this is unsatisfactory. If it is desired to counteract the stimulating effects of anorectic drugs, it is advisable to prescribe sedatives separately.

The anorectic drug should be prescribed for periods not exceeding two to three months, since its effect in suppressing appetite seldom lasts for more than a few weeks. With the possible exception of fenfluramine it is doubtful if any of the relatively expensive and much advertised recent proprietary anorectic drugs are more effective than the B.P. tablets of amphetamine or dexamphetamine. However the dangers of addiction may be less. The usual dose of amphetamine is one tablet (5 mg.) two or three times a day before meals. If insomnia results, this may be overcome by giving a suitable barbiturate at bed-time.

Anorectic drugs are no substitute for a dietary regimen and the radical alteration of the patient's food habits. At best they are an aid which may help some patients to adhere more strictly to their diets. It is never justified to use these drugs at the beginning of treatment. If an obese person has failed to adhere to a diet despite efforts to do so, then the use of an anorectic may be advised but only after the serious disadvantages discussed above have been carefully considered.

THYROXINE. The administration of the thyroid hormone to euthyroid obese patients is not only useless but is potentially dangerous, especially if degenerative disease of the myocardium is present. Only if hypothyroidism co-exists with obesity should thyroxine be prescribed and then it should be given cautiously.

METHYL CELLULOSE. This is an indigestible substance which adds bulk to the diet. It distends the stomach and so may help to allay hunger. In clinical trials it has been shown to have little if any effect in promoting weight loss, and it is very doubtful if this product is of any value as an adjunct to dietary therapy. However, it is quite harmless.

SEDATIVES AND TRANQUILLISERS. These drugs should only be used in the treatment of obesity if the patient also has the associated features of the anxiety state (p. 1248) which require sedation. They are no substitute for careful explanation by the doctor of the aims of treatment and instruction in the proper way it should be carried out.

DIURETICS. Unless oedema is present as a result of cardiac, renal or hepatic disease, diuretics are of no value in the treatment of obesity.

Prognosis. It is easy for an obese person to lose up to 10 lb. in weight. This accounts for the temporary successes of numerous popular 'slimming cures'. How difficult it is to achieve further losses is not generally realised. In Edinburgh, Rose reported in 1959 a large number of failures. In a six months follow-up of 407 patients treated at the Obesity Clinic in the Royal Infirmary 148

(36 per cent.) did not report again after the first interview and only 15 per cent. were discharged after having achieved the desired loss of weight. The published records of seven obesity clinics in the U.S.A. showed that satisfactory results ranged from 12 to 28 per cent. if the index of success was the loss of 25 lb. or more.

Experience in many clinics has shown that it is difficult for patients to maintain their reduced weight after successful treatment.

The reasons for these poor results are not clear. Perhaps the failure of doctors to appreciate the complicated and difficult problems concerned with the aetiology and treatment of obesity as presented by each obese patient is a contributory factor. Hence it is most important that doctors, assisted by dietitians where possible, should supervise carefully and persistently the details of the management of each patient. The best way of reducing the number of failures is to encourage patients to persevere with the reducing regimen and to report to their medical adviser or dietitian at regular intervals as described below.

Management. With proper dietetic advice and regular interviews the majority of obese patients should lose weight satisfactorily provided they carry out conscientiously the instructions in regard to diet and exercise.

No known drug provides an easy alternative to the discipline of a strict dietary regimen. The patient should weigh herself at weekly intervals; day-to-day variations in weight are not important; they may be due to retention of urine or faeces, or to the increase in body water that frequently precedes menstruation. The patient needs to be seen at regular intervals. After a weight-reducing diet has been prescribed, she should attend at first perhaps every fortnight and later every month or so. The object of these visits is threefold.

First, to check progress. At each visit the patient should be weighed. A good balance is necessary. Spring balances are unreliable and need frequent checking. Lever balances are good and need checking only once a year. If the weight loss has exceeded 3 lb./week some addition to the diet may be permitted, such as an additional thin slice of bread (1 oz., 15 g. of carbohydrate, 70 Cal.). The initial weight loss is often dramatic and frequently mainly due to loss of water, but it impresses the patient. Thereafter it often slows up, due sometimes to waning interest, but perhaps also to the same physiological adjustments to a lower caloric intake as happens in underfed people (p. 441).

Secondly, to encourage the patient. If the weight loss has been satisfactory, simple assurance of the need to persevere is all that is necessary. If it is not, then every art of persuasion may be needed -reasoning, begging and even mild bullying.

Thirdly, to check the patient's general health. If weight loss is not proceeding satisfactorily, a constant watch for the complications of obesity must be maintained. If any complications, orthopaedic, metabolic or cardiovascular, are present, regular supervision is necessary. If the patient suffers from one of these, persuasion to persevere with the regimen is easier—for promise of relief from the distressing symptom can be given only if the patient will lose weight.

It is difficult sometimes to decide how long to continue a regimen.

The nearer a middle-aged woman can get back to her desirable weight (p. 1305), the better chance she has for a healthy and happy future. Once a satisfactory weight has been achieved, discipline can be only partially relaxed. Many unfortunate people exist for whom the slightest dietary relaxation results immediately in a rapid gain in weight; for them there is no alternative but life-long attention to a restricted food intake, and it is here that the advice and encouragement of a doctor or dietitian can be most helpful.

Finally, there are those who fail to lose weight despite regular encouragement and the best dietetic advice. Anorectic drugs (p. 456) may be helpful in such cases. In the last resort, admission to hospital or nursing home may be the best advice, with the attentions of a skilled dietitian who will prove to the patient that loss of weight is possible with proper regulation of the food intake. A period of complete starvation or a diet providing as little as 400 Cal./day can be used with success for this purpose, and with proper care no harmful effects will follow.

Prevention. Prevention of obesity rests with the doctor who early discerns when his patients are beginning to put on too much weight. Young mothers especially are apt to do so during and after a confinement. One of the most useful records that a doctor can keep about his patients is that of their weight, measured at regular intervals. Sudden, unexplained changes may not only warn of the threat of obesity but, in the opposite direction, can be the first indication of other diseases in their earliest stage.

It is a guiding principle in medicine that prevention is better than cure. Accordingly the following points for the prevention of obesity should be made clear to all who are liable to become overweight.

(*a*) *Remember* that under-exercising and over-eating are the causes of obesity. Regular exercise should be an essential part of the reducing regimen not only because it burns up fat but because exercise is of great value in keeping the body healthy. The motor vehicle is at the same time a great boon and one of the great medical dangers to modern man. Always walk as much as possible every day.

(*b*) *Remember* that calories are the key to the weight problem.

(*c*) *Remember* that you can eat what you like and grow thin provided you make sure that your caloric intake is less than your caloric expenditure.

(*d*) *Remember* that mental work does not require additional calories.

(*e*) *Remember* that alcohol may be an important factor in the causation of obesity. Alcohol is used by the body solely as a source of energy and thus it frees an equivalent number of food calories which are then stored as fat. Few people realise that a large whisky or gin, or a pint of beer, is the caloric equivalent of two medium-sized eggs, or one glass of milk, or a medium-sized slice of bread and butter, or an average helping of potatoes.

(*f*) *Remember* to weigh yourself regularly, say once a week. This is essential if you are to find out in good time that you are putting on weight—and it will show how successful are your efforts to reduce overweight. Use the same scales and always weigh yourself either naked or in approximately the same clothes.

(*g*) *Remember* to put into operation immediately the necessary measures to reduce weight—increasing expenditure of energy by added exercise and reducing caloric intake by cutting to the minimum the intake of butter and foods rich in fat and the carbohydrate-rich foods such as bread, cakes, potatoes, sugar and thick soups. Feed mainly on foods low in calories such as clear soups, lean meat, chicken, white fish, green and yellow vegetables and fresh fruits. By making small but essential adjustments in one's eating habits, obesity can usually be prevented. No diet sheet is required but some knowledge of the caloric value of different foods is necessary and instruction by a dietitian may be helpful. The longer the delay in taking the necessary steps to prevent the development of obesity, the more unpleasant, lengthy and strict will be the dietary restrictions required for its correction. Hence the need for regular weighing so as to be warned of what may be occurring insidiously.

Conclusion. It is foolish for people to attempt to 'slim' on their own initiative without proper advice. A qualified dietitian can provide one of the most useful ancillary services to medicine by giving her time and her knowledge of nutrition to the practical problems of treating obesity. The relief of so many common ailments, such as backache, sore knees, coughs and even angina of effort are all part of the rewards of a dietitian's skill. But it is clearly sensible that she should always work in collaboration with a doctor. Everyone should know of the undesirable and potentially dangerous complications of overweight. Everyone must decide for himself whether he wishes to take these risks or not. Since the immediate causes of obesity are over-eating and under-exercising, the remedies are available to all, but many patients require much help in using them.

QUALITATIVE ASPECTS OF NUTRITION

ENERGY-YIELDING NUTRIENTS ('PROXIMATE PRINCIPLES')

Carbohydrates. These usually provide the greater part of the calories in a normal diet, but no individual carbohydrate is an absolute dietary necessity in the sense that the body needs it but cannot make it for itself from other nutrients.

Fats. With their high caloric value, fats are useful to people with a large energy expenditure; moreover they are helpful in cooking and making food appetising. Though rats need certain essential unsaturated fatty acids in their diet, as yet there is no certain evidence that they are necessary nutrients for man.

The possible role of cholesterol, fats and essential fatty acids in the pathogenesis of atherosclerosis and coronary thrombosis is discussed in detail on page 278.

Proteins. Proteins provide amino acids, of which eight are essential for normal protein synthesis and for maintaining a positive nitrogen balance in adults. These are termed *essential amino acids* because the body cannot make them for itself and so must obtain them from the diet. The eight essential amino acids are lysine, tryptophan, phenylalanine, leucine, isoleucine, threonine, methionine and valine. There is evidence that histidine and perhaps arginine are needed to maintain growth in infants.

The 'biological value' of different proteins depends on the relative proportions of essential amino acids they contain. Proteins of animal origin, particularly from milk, eggs, meat, liver and kidney, are generally of higher biological value than the proteins of vegetable origin. Certain vegetable proteins are deficient in some of the essential amino acids; but a mixed vegetable diet, including pulses (peas, beans, etc.) can supply enough of all.

The usual recommended allowance for an adequate protein intake is 11-14 per cent. of the total calories.

PATHOLOGY OF PROTEIN DEFICIENCY. A deficient intake of protein leads to (*a*) negative nitrogen balance; (*b*) wasting of tissues; and (*c*) fall in plasma albumin. For further information see Pathology of Kwashiorkor (p. 463).

PROTEIN-CALORIE DEFICIENCY DISEASE

The concept has recently been advanced that protein-calorie malnutrition, especially in early childhood, should be regarded as a spectrum of disease. At one end there is kwashiorkor in which the essential feature is a qualitative and quantitative deficiency of protein. Calories are often restricted but may even be in excess of requirements. At the other end is nutritional marasmus (p. 470) which is a total inanition of the infant and is due to a severe and continuous restriction of calories and protein as well as other nutrients. In the middle of the spectrum is marasmic kwashiorkor in which children have the clinical features of both disorders.

Kwashiorkor

With the possible exception of iron deficiency anaemia and deficiency of calories it is the most important dietary deficiency disease of childhood in the world and hence will be described in considerable detail.

History and Geographic Distribution. Cicely Williams in 1933 was the first to record that 'some amino acid or protein deficiency' might be an aetiological factor in kwashiorkor, the name given to this disease by the Ga tribe living in and around Accra, the capital of the Gold Coast (now Ghana). She noted that the same condition had been described in 1906 in Germany, in 1924 in Indo-China, in 1926 in Mexico and in 1928 in East Africa. In fact, the disease may occur in any part of the world if the dietary conditions described below are present.

Aetiology and Incidence. As with other deficiency diseases all the clinical features cannot be attributed to a single dietary defect; but there is little doubt that the predominant features are due to a deficiency of protein, either absolute or relative to energy requirements. The importance of the caloric value of a diet to ensure optimum protein utilisation is well recognised. When there is great need for both protein and energy to meet the demands of growth, as in infancy, childhood and at puberty, or during pregnancy and lactation, dietary restriction of either protein or calories, or both as is most often the case, will precipitate the development of kwashiorkor. If the customary diet of a population is limited in protein and calories to around the levels of minimal requirements, the disease may be precipitated in epidemic proportions by outbreaks of febrile illnesses such as malaria, measles or whooping-cough or by helminthic infection.

The syndrome has been described at all ages and in both sexes. It is most common in infants and in toddlers between 1 and 4 years whose mothers wean their children from the breast on to diets which are mainly composed of starchy gruels containing too little protein and providing too little energy. This may be on account of ignorance of good nutritional practices, seasonal food shortages or lack of money to buy better foods.

Kwashiorkor is a rare disease in countries in which literacy, education and developed food-processing industries have made it possible for all classes of the population to obtain and consume diets which provide sufficient energy and nutrients.

Pathology. The inadequate supply of amino acids leads to a failure of protein synthesis in the tissues, which prevents the normal development of all the organs of the body.

The total protein content of the body may be reduced to one-third of normal while the water content is greatly increased. The failure to synthesise serum albumin reduces the concentration to a figure which may be as low as 1·5 g./100 ml. By contrast the serum globulin is usually well maintained. A failure to synthesise digestive enzymes is frequently present, including those secreted by mucosa of the small intestine (especially lactase) and by the pancreas. This may be partially responsible for the gastro-intestinal upsets and diarrhoea which are so commonly present and which cause marked electrolyte disturbances due to loss of potassium and magnesium in the stools. Dietary deficiency of protein results in a failure to maintain the normal structure of the liver and muscles. The protein content of the liver is greatly reduced, while the fat content is much increased.

Clinical Features. Failure to grow is a constant and essential feature of the disease. The child's weight is usually much below standard for his age, but real weight may be masked by oedema which may be very extensive. The muscles are always wasted and this is particularly noticeable around the chest and the upper arm; the wasting of the legs and around the hips is frequently concealed by oedema. If the disease has resulted from a dietary restriction of both calories and protein, muscle wasting and an almost complete lack of subcutaneous fat is the most striking feature, but the feet are oedematous ('marasmic kwashiorkor'). Subcutaneous fat is often plentiful in children whose diets have provided ample calories but little protein. The child is apathetic, miserable and anorexic. The hair is nearly always affected in African children; in Asiatics the changes are less frequent and less marked. There is an alteration in texture. The hair becomes fine, straight and soft, it loses its curl and lustre and is often sparse. The hair of African children may show a variety of pigmentary changes. Shades range from brownish-black and brown to a pale greyish-brown or even a straw colour. The extent of these changes in the hair is not an indication of the severity of the disease. They are sometimes pronounced in children who have been unwell for a long time but never seriously ill. Alterations in the skin are often present, especially in severe cases. These include pigmentation, depigmentation, desquamation and ulceration. The legs, buttocks and perineal areas are most frequently involved, but any region may be affected. This is in contrast to pellagra in which the dermatosis occurs mainly on the exposed surfaces. The skin lesions may be determined in part by associated vitamin deficiencies. The liver may be greatly enlarged and it may extend down to the umbilicus. When associated with splenomegaly the possibility of co-existing malaria should be remembered. Anorexia and vomiting occur and there is usually diarrhoea, with the passage of stools containing much undigested food. This feature may be secondary to the failure of the pancreas to secrete digestive juices or to an associated gastro-enteritis. Important losses of potassium and magnesium may result from the diarrhoea. Anaemia, sometimes severe, is frequently present. The blood and bone marrow changes are discussed on page 535. Both the degree of anaemia and its nature are largely determined by associated infections and other dietary deficiencies, including especially vitamins A and the B complex.

Prolonged mild to moderate protein-calorie malnutrition may result in a syndrome called *nutritional dwarfing*, in which the children are light in weight and short in stature with relatively normal body proportions and subcutaneous fat. This is a form of pre-clinical kwashiorkor and marasmus and since it occurs in millions of children in underdeveloped countries its clinical recognition is very important.

Differential Diagnosis. A variety of diseases may be confused with kwashiorkor. Chronic dysentery, abdominal tuberculosis, coeliac disease, infantile pellagra, fibrocystic disease of the pancreas and nephritis are diseases which have clinical features in common with kwashiorkor. The age of onset, the dietary history and the response to protein therapy should help to distinguish them.

Hookworm infection with anaemia and oedema may resemble kwashiorkor in many respects.

Prevention. Ignorance and poverty are the two main factors responsible for kwashiorkor. Obviously these causes must be removed. Education in nutrition, the introduction of improved farming methods and the development of food industries whereby protective foods may be made available at a reasonable cost to the consumer, are all important. In each country careful thought must be given to the provision of protein-rich foods made from local crops which are suitable both for infant feeding and for supplementing diets low in protein. For this purpose concentrates of vegetable protein made from oil-seed cakes and from flours made from edible pulses are valuable supplements to cereals such as wheat, sorghum and the millets.

Even small amounts of food of animal origin, such as dried milk or concentrates of fish protein, are of great value when mixed with high protein vegetable foods. A mixture of one part of casein and 10 parts of groundnut flour is effective in the prevention and treatment of kwashiorkor.

Education of parents, particularly mothers, in regard to the value of foods and the best methods of preparing them, especially at the time of weaning, is invaluable. Much could be done to alleviate this disorder by the establishment or extension of Child Welfare Clinics and Health Centres where free or subsidised skimmed milk powder is supplied, advice on diet is given, and where diseases which are liable to lead to kwashiorkor can be prevented or properly treated.

Treatment

General Measures. An easily digested diet which provides sufficient calories and adequate amounts of protein of good biological value, together with sufficient minerals and vitamins, is essential. Dried skimmed milk is of particular value as a source of first-class protein and should be used in treating serious cases in the early stages. Calcium caseinate is also of value for this purpose but is more expensive than dried skimmed milk powder. If neither of these preparations is available or the cost of maintaining the supply of milk becomes prohibitive, protein-rich preparations such as one of those described above should be used.

Severely ill children are often unable to maintain their body temperature even in warm climates. Hence heated rooms or electric blankets or heat cradles are essential for such cases. Vitamin A and ascorbic acid should be given and therapeutic doses of iron administered. If dermatosis is severe the skin should be cleaned and carefully protected. The child's weight may fall during the first days of treatment due to loss of oedema fluid. The initiation of cure is indicated by increasing appetite and a gain in weight.

Diets for Severe Cases. For the first day or two, if the child is unable to feed from a spoon, a polythene tube passed into the stomach through the nose will be necessary. The following recipe for a baby food based on skimmed milk powder has been widely used in Jamaica.

Ingredients: 60 g. (2 oz.) skimmed milk powder
15 g. (1½ teaspoons) butter
20 g. (2 teaspoons) flour
250 ml. (½ pint) water

250 ml. (½ pint) of this mixture contains about 22 g. protein and 250 Cal.

This recipe was constructed after it had been demonstrated that skimmed milk powder alone is unable to meet a child's needs for growth and moreover is liable in excessive amounts to cause diarrhoea. It must therefore only be used as a supplement. The mixture should be given in divided doses four to six times a day so as to provide the patient with approximately 5 g. of protein for each kilogram of the ideal weight of a child of the same age. On the second or third day it should be possible to start on a banana/milk or cereal/milk diet. In countries such as Uganda and Jamaica where bananas are a staple article of diet, they should be used because they mix better with skimmed milk powder than do flours made from cereals or roots (cassava) and the mixture is very palatable.

The following recipe is widely used in Uganda:

Mash 400 g. of peeled sweet bananas and mix thoroughly with 200 g. of dried skimmed milk powder in 500 ml. of water which has been brought to the boil and allowed to cool. Divide the mixture, which represents one day's ration, into six equal parts. Feed with a spoon.

This diet, which provides in one day's ration about 75 g. of protein and 1,200 Cal., will lead to an improvement in appetite, digestion and strength.

Where bananas are not available, as is the case in many countries where kwashiorkor is endemic, a flour made from semolina, rice, cassava, cereals, Bengal gram or other pulses will have to be used. In this case it is strongly recommended that an ounce of some fat (butter or margarine) or an edible oil such as that made from sunflower seeds, should be added as it makes the mixing of the flour and milk powder easier and the mixture is more palatable and digestible and of higher caloric value.

Anorexia may be serious, but often can be overcome by feeding the child very slowly in the mother's lap and not in bed. Food may be taken better cold than hot. Sometimes Marmite or Bovril as flavouring may be acceptable.

As the clinical condition improves the food consumption should be increased gradually. Whole milk powder can be substituted for skimmed milk powder; eggs, fish and bean flour can be added to the diet until the child is eating a satisfactory diet of local pattern, including adequate amounts of easily digested protein-rich foods.

Infants may lose 1-4 g. of potassium chloride (13-52 m.Eq/kg.) in the stools in one day if there is severe diarrhoea. The effect of the resulting potassium depletion on the myocardium may cause sudden death. Potassium should be given by mouth as a routine to all infants admitted with kwashiorkor. Depending on the age and weight of the child and the severity of the diarrhoea, the dose should be from 0·5-1 g. of potassium chloride dissolved in water and added to three or four feeds each day. There is little or no danger of potassium intoxication when the mixture is given by mouth in the doses recommended.

Parental Therapy. It is a common experience that children with kwashiorkor, especially when oedematous, tolerate intravenous infusions poorly.

For very ill patients treated in a well equipped and well staffed hospital, who are suffering from marked dehydration and shock, or very severe anaemia from any cause, repeated slow transfusions of packed erythrocytes may be a life-saving measure.

Vitamins. Therapeutic diets based on skimmed milk and plant proteins are unlikely to be seriously lacking in any of the B group of vitamins and it should be necessary to prescribe them only in exceptional circumstances. Such diets are more likely to be deficient in vitamin A and ascorbic acid, which are present in insignificant amounts in dried skimmed milk powder. The treatment and prevention of these deficiencies are discussed on pages 485 and 508. Large doses should be avoided, 400 i.u. of vitamin A and 20 mg. ascorbic acid being sufficient. There appears to be no satisfactory evidence that vitamin B_{12} has any beneficial effect on the disease, except when a megaloblastic anaemia is present.

Infections and Infestations. The treatment of these is important. If a respiratory infection or skin sepsis is present, a course of penicillin is advisable. Tetracycline or some other suitable antibiotic should be given for infections of the gastro-intestinal tract. Most of these children suffer from infection with worms and require treatment (p. 595). However, all anthelmintics are potentially toxic and must be used with due care in patients who are seriously ill. If anaemia from hookworm is so severe as to endanger life, blood transfusions should be given and will probably restore the child's condition sufficiently to permit appropriate treatment later. Iron deficiency anaemia, which is frequently present due to dietary deficiency of protein and iron and as a consequence of infections and infestations, requires appropriate treatment (p. 616). Much more rarely a megaloblastic anaemia is present which responds excellently to folic acid (p. 625). Anti-malarial drugs in both prophylactic and therapeutic doses are well tolerated. The possibility of tuberculosis being present should always be considered, particularly if the child does not make the expected progress to recovery. Tuberculosis, if not too far advanced, responds well to streptomycin combined with other antituberculous drugs (p. 425).

Mild Kwashiorkor and follow-up Cases. Such cases can be treated as out-patients and milk in any form can be recommended, but preferably dried skimmed milk sprinkled over the food, rather than reconstituted with water with the resulting liability to infection in hot climates where facilities for sterilisation are poor. It is essential that the mothers of such patients should be given instruction in regard to hygiene, cooking and methods of feeding.

Prognosis. Kwashiorkor is often a severe malady with a fatal termination, but it exists in a great variety of forms and may be so mild as to escape attention; in such cases complete recovery is the rule. The name 'pre-kwashiorkor' has been suggested for the state of subclinical protein deficiency in children in which a failure in growth, a reduction in the serum albumin and an increased liability to diarrhoea and respiratory infections are the salient clinical features. There is good reason to believe that pre-kwashiorkor is extremely common in regions where the fully developed syndrome is found. When early, adequate and sufficient treatment is given, the fatty degeneration of the liver which is always present in infants with kwashiorkor does not progress to cirrhosis of the liver, a condition which is common in many parts of the tropics. It is probable that prolonged *untreated* cases whose fatty livers are also subjected to infections and other poisons, may develop progressive hepatic disease. The usual causes of death are intercurrent infections and severe malnutrition, including potassium deficiency. The availability of medical care is another important factor influencing prognosis. Many children who suffer from kwashiorkor pass through their formative years with their physical and mental faculties partially impaired by their inadequate diet. The importance of this in the educational and physical development of people in countries in which kwashiorkor is endemic, is not always fully appreciated.

Nutritional Marasmus

The importance of nutritional marasmus as a cause of mortality and morbidity in infants at the present time has not been adequately appreciated. In parts of some underdeveloped countries marasmus is of greater clinical importance than kwashiorkor. It affects principally infants under 1 year of age in contrast to kwashiorkor which is chiefly encountered in the pre-school child (1-4 years). Marasmus is more likely to occur in poor people in underdeveloped countries who live in cities, while kwashiorkor occurs more frequently in people living under traditional tribal conditions in rural areas. The urban influences which predispose to marasmus are a rapid succession of pregnancies, and early and often abrupt weaning, followed by dirty and unsound artificial feeding of the infants with very dilute milk or milk products which are given in inadequate amounts to avoid expense. Thus the diet is low in both calories and protein. In addition unsatisfactory home conditions make the preparation of uncontaminated feeds almost impossible. Repeated infections therefore develop, especially of the gastro-intestinal tract, which the mother often treats by starvation for long periods, the infant receiving water, rice water or some other non-nutritious fluid.

The most important cause of marasmus, namely early weaning, is in contrast to the late weaning, often extending over two years, which is characteristic of kwashiorkor. The mother may be induced to stop breast feeding for various reasons, including the presence of infections in herself or in the infant. Unfortunately she may have been influenced unwisely by advertisements in the press or on the radio which advocate, for commercial reasons, the advantages of artificial food products. The most frequent reason for stopping breast feeding is the beginning of another pregnancy. There appears to be a widespread belief among poor, uneducated women in underdeveloped countries that the milk of a pregnant woman is bad for her child.

Clinical Features. The two constant features of marasmus are (1) retardation of growth and reduction of weight which is much more marked than that of length, and (2) wasting of muscles and subcutaneous fat which gives the infant a wizened, old appearance. In contrast to kwashiorkor, oedema is absent and the characteristic changes in the hair and skin, apathy and anorexia are seldom encountered. The features of associated vitamin disorders such as angular stomatitis or keratomalacia, may develop, as may a deficiency of minerals, especially potassium and magnesium. Dehydration frequently results as a consequence of gastro-intestinal infection.

Prevention and Treatment. This is a complex and difficult problem. Education of mothers so that they will continue breast feeding for as long as possible is of the greatest importance. Further research is urgently needed into improved methods of feeding both healthy and ill infants in underdeveloped countries. The epidemiology of the failure of lactation and the control of infection in infants are other important matters requiring further investigation. In the acute stage of marasmus survival depends primarily on the efficiency with which measures can be applied to combat dehydration and restore electrolyte balance. In addition the child must be given a satisfactory diet such as the skimmed milk diet described on p. 467 and a supplement of vitamins if necessary. Even when these objectives have been successfully accomplished the death rate may be higher and the morbidity greater than in equivalently severe cases of kwashiorkor.

In summary, it is probable that in the future marasmus will become of increasing clinical importance in underdeveloped countries as a consequence of a continuing decline in breast feeding and the urbanisation of uneducated families, socially insecure and living in poor, insanitary houses and with insufficient money to buy adequate supplements of milk or milk substitutes.

WATER AND ELECTROLYTES

The normal concentrations of ions, both in the intracellular and extracellular fluids, is preserved by a balance between the intake of water and electrolytes in the diet and the output in the excretions.

Water. The water intake comprises the fluid drunk and the water in the food eaten. The metabolic water formed by the oxidation of carbohydrate, protein and fat is also available. The output consists of the urine, the water in the faeces and the water evaporated from the skin and lungs.

The water and other fluids drunk are approximately equal to the urine output. It is this fact that makes the 'fluid balance chart' (kept by the nursing staff) a useful practical procedure. It is particularly valuable in the care of febrile patients in the tropics, who are liable to become dehydrated unless carefully supervised.

Salt. Man's need for sodium chloride has been a subject of dispute since the beginnings of medical practice. Wars have been fought over its sources, and for centuries its trade was more important than that of any other material. Yet a separate supply of salt in addition to that present in the foods is not essential for man. There are primitive people who do not use it.

Most people suffering from congestive cardiac failure and hypertension benefit if the salt in their diet is restricted.

These considerations make recommendations for human needs for salt difficult. It is certainly true that life can proceed without the deliberate addition of salt to food; yet for civilised man salt appears to be an indispensable adjunct to life. In Britain a healthy adult takes from 1½ to 2½ litres of fluid and 10 to 15 g. NaCl daily.

The normal distribution of water and electrolytes in the body and the disturbances which result when their intake or output is diminished or increased are discussed in detail on p. 839.

MINERALS

The following physiologically important elements occur in the human body:

sodium, chlorine, calcium, sulphur, iron, iodine, fluorine

(phosphorus, potassium, magnesium, copper, cobalt, manganese, zinc).

Deficiencies of those bracketed are not known to occur in man *solely* as the result of an inadequate dietary intake.

Sulphur. This is mainly supplied by the S-containing amino acids in the diet—methionine and cysteine; effects of its deficiency are therefore inseparable from those of protein.

Phosphorus. The normal human body contains 600-900 g. of phosphorus, 80-85 per cent. of which is present in the bones where, in combination with calcium, it goes to provide their hard structure. The remainder is chiefly in the cells.

Phosphorus is present in all natural foods, though in refined and processed foods the phosphorus content may be greatly reduced. The best sources are those foods that also contain good amounts of calcium and protein. Phosphorus normally presents no problem for the dietitian. A useful working rule is 'take care of the calcium and the phosphorus will look after itself'. Phosphate is essential for most metabolic processes; perhaps for these reasons dietary deficiency of phosphorus is not known to occur in man.

For further information see sodium (p. 841), potassium (p. 845), iron (p. 604), copper (p. 617), cobalt (p. 473) and magnesium (p. 850).

Elements of Importance in Human Dietetics

Calcium. The body of an adult normally contains about 1,200 g. of calcium. At least 99 per cent. of this amount is present in the skeleton, where calcium salts (chiefly phosphate) held in a cellular matrix provide the hard structure of the bones and teeth. Obviously all of this calcium comes from the diet. Among common foods, the calcium-containing protein of milk (caseinogen) is much the richest source, which is one reason why milk and cheese are especially valuable for growing children. Half a litre (just under a pint) of cow's milk contains about 0·6 g. of calcium. Most other foods contribute much smaller amounts. However, peas, beans, other vegetables and particularly cereal grains are frequently the chief contributors because of the large amounts eaten. By contrast, there are certain foods that are extraordinarily rich in calcium, yet which are eaten so rarely or in such small amounts that they contribute little to the regular intake.

Drinking water can provide significant amounts of calcium. In Britain the average intake from this source is about 75 mg. Ca/day; but the variations are large: from none in water from peaty, acidic hill lochs in Scotland to 200 mg. or even more in water obtained from wells sunk in chalk or limestone.

Absorption. The problem of calcium absorption is extremely complicated. There can be no clear answer that will explain why as much as 70 per cent. of the calcium in the food is normally excreted in the faeces. Calcium absorption is not just a simple matter of the passage through the intestinal mucosa of free calcium ions, kept in solution by the influence of gastric juice. Other factors are involved.

Calcium absorption may be impaired either by lack of vitamin D, by any conditions causing small intestinal hurry, e.g. diarrhoea, by the combination of calcium with excess fatty acids to form insoluble soaps, e.g. steatorrhoea, or by certain substances in the diet which can form insoluble salts with it. These include foods rich in oxalic acid (e.g. spinach) and, of much greater importance, phytic acid. Phytic acid is present in the outer layers of cereal grains. Hence bread made from 'high extraction' flour ('wholemeal' bread) contains more phytic acid than 'white' bread. To overcome the influence of phytic acid, calcium carbonate has been added to flour in Britain.

Daily Calcium Requirements. The allowances recommended by the National Research Council in the U.S.A. and accepted by the Committee on Nutrition of the British Medical Association in 1950 are as follows: adults 0·5-0·8 g.; children 1 g. rising to 1·4 g. during adolescence; pregnancy (latter half) 1·5 g.; lactation 2 g.

In many parts of Africa and Asia children develop healthy bones and adults remain in calcium balance despite calcium intakes which may be no more than half the above recommendations. The possible role of unlimited sunshine in producing this effect should be remembered. Hence an intake of 500-600 mg. daily will be suitable for infants, children, adolescents and adults in tropical countries, but 1,000 mg. should be taken during pregnancy and lactation.

Deficiency of calcium and vitamin D go hand in hand and are best considered together (p. 487).

Iron. A good mixed diet with an average helping of meat and vegetables and an egg daily will contain about 12-15 mg. of iron. Cheap monotonous high carbohydrate diets based on refined wheaten flour will contain much less. An account of the foodstuffs rich in iron, of the factors increasing the need for iron and facilitating its absorption and of the measures for the prevention and treatment of iron deficiency anaemia is given on pp. 616 to 619. Next to obesity iron deficiency anaemia is the most important nutritional cause of ill-health in Britain and other prosperous countries.

Iodine. Simple enlargement of the thyroid gland attributed to lack of iodine in the food and drinking water occurs sporadically in every country. In certain parts of the world, however, generally speaking mountainous regions far removed from the sea (the Alps, Himalayas, Central States of America, New Guinea, the Peak District of Derbyshire in England) it is much more frequent (endemic goitre).

There are certainly factors other than the lack of iodine in the diet which can contribute to the causation of simple goitre (p. 692).

SOURCES. Iodine in small amounts is widely distributed in living matter. Fish, vegetables and milk are the most useful sources in the diet.

Much attention has been directed in the past to the iodine content of drinking waters in areas where goitre occurs, as compared with the waters in goitre-free districts. As a result there has been a tendency to regard drinking water as an important source of iodine. But, in fact, fresh water usually contains only small amounts of iodine, e.g. 1 to 50 $\mu g./l.$ in Britain, so that it contributes little to the needs of the body. The iodine content of the water in a locality is more important as an index of the amount of iodine that is likely to be provided by the cereals and vegetables that grow in the soil which the water irrigates.

PROPHYLACTIC AND THERAPEUTIC USES. The Medical Research Council has recommended the addition of potassium iodide (p. 693) to all table salt in Britain as this has been proved to be highly successful in reducing the incidence of simple goitre in Switzerland, the U.S.A. and other parts of the world. Unfortunately the legislation required to enforce this recommendation in Britain has not been enacted.

Small doses of potassium iodide may be of value in the treatment of endemic goitre at least in its earliest stages. Larger doses have a temporary value in the preparation of patients with hyperthyroidism for surgical operation.

Fluorine. Fluorine has not yet been proved to be an indispensable nutrient for any species of animal. However, its regular presence in minute amounts in human bones and teeth and its influence on the prevention of dental caries justifies its inclusion as an element of importance in human dietetics.

SOURCES. Most human adults ingest between 2 and 3 mg. of fluorine daily. The chief source is usually drinking water, which, if it contains 1 part per million (p.p.m.) of fluorine, will supply 1-2 mg./day. Soft waters may contain no fluorine, whilst very hard waters may contain over 10 p.p.m. Compared with this source, the fluorine in foodstuffs is of little importance. Very few foods contain more than 1 p.p.m.; the exception is sea-fish which may contain relatively large amounts of the order of 5-10 p.p.m. Another significant source is tea. In Britain and Australia, where people drink tea frequently, the adult intake from this source may be as much as 1 mg. daily.

USE OF FLUORINE IN THE PREVENTION OF DENTAL CARIES. Epidemiological studies in many parts of the world have established beyond doubt that where the natural water supply contains fluorine in amounts of 1 p.p.m. or more, the incidence of dental caries is lower than in comparable areas where the water contains only traces of the element.

Fluorides become deposited in the enamel surface of the developing teeth of children. Such fluorotic teeth are unusually resistant to caries for reasons not yet fully understood; it may be that traces of fluorine in the enamel discourage the growth of acid-forming bacteria. Alternatively, the calcium phosphate of the enamel may be rendered more resistant to organic acids by combination with traces of the element. It should be noted that fluorine is not deposited in fully developed adult teeth, so that no benefit to adults can be expected when they begin for the first time to drink water containing traces of fluorine.

The deliberate addition of traces of fluorine to those public water supplies which are deficient in fluorine is now a widespread practice throughout North America. In at least 17 other countries similar projects have been started.

In view of the widespread incidence of caries throughout Britain, the case for the addition of fluorine up to 1 p.p.m. to the water supplies of those areas where it is lacking, has been strongly supported by carefully controlled trials. Accordingly, the announcement by the British Government in 1965 that official action may be taken to implement the fluoridation of water, is very welcome. Unfortunately, many local authorities still refuse to add fluorine to their water supplies.

FLUOROSIS IN MAN. In many parts of the world where the fluorine content of the water is high (over three to five parts per million) mottling of the teeth is common. The enamel loses its lustre and becomes rough. Bands of brown pigmentation separate patches as white as chalk. Small pits may be present on the surface. All the teeth may be affected, but mottling is usually best seen on the incisors of the upper jaw. Dental fluorosis is not usually associated with any evidence of skeleton fluorosis, as occurs in chronic fluorine poisoning, or indeed with any impairment of health.

CHRONIC FLUORINE POISONING. This has been reported in several localities in India, China, Argentina and the Transvaal, where the water supply contains over 10 p.p.m. fluorine. Fluorine poisoning has also occurred as an industrial hazard among workers handling fluorine-containing minerals such as cryolite, used in smelting aluminium. The main clinical features are referable to the skeleton which shows sclerosis of bone, especially of the spine, pelvis and limbs, and calcification of ligaments and tendinous insertions of muscles.

Magnesium Deficiency and Intoxication. See p. 850.

THE VITAMINS

Although gross vitamin deficiency disorders are now rare in Britain they deserve consideration in some detail because they are still widespread in many parts of the world, wherever the proper foods are scarce and medical knowledge is not applied for their relief. Moreover the history of the identification, isolation and final synthesis of several vitamins and their application to medicine offers such a striking instance of the impact of science on medicine during this century that the vitamin deficiency disorders deserve consideration even in Britain, though chiefly today as an exercise in medical education.

Definition. Vitamins are organic substances which the body requires in small amounts for its normal metabolism and yet cannot synthesise for itself (at least in adequate quantities). They are therefore needed in the diet. A large number of substances conforming to this definition have been recognised by feeding tests on animals, but deficiencies of only 10 vitamins have, so far, been demonstrated to have clinical effects in man. These 10 are:

Fat-soluble	*Water-soluble*	
Vitamin A	Ascorbic acid	
Vitamin D	Thiamine	included in the vitamin B complex.
	Nicotinic acid	
Vitamin K	Riboflavine	
	Pyridoxine	
	Cyanocobalamin	
	Folic acid	

The vitamins of the B complex are grouped together (although unrelated chemically) because they are found together in the same kinds of food. These foods are rich in cellular material with an active metabolism (e.g. yeast, liver). The reason why the vitamins of the B complex are found in active cells is that they are essential parts of specific enzyme systems on which cellular metabolism depends. Thus thiamine pyrophosphate is cocarboxylase, which is concerned with the removal of pyruvic acid in the catabolism of carbohydrate. Riboflavine is an important component of the flavoproteins which play an essential role in tissue oxidation. Nicotinic acid amide is part of the nucleotides, Co-enzymes I and II, which are also concerned in tissue oxidation.

Other components of the vitamin B complex needed by certain animals (e.g. pantothenic acid, biotin) also have enzymic properties and certainly take part in the metabolism of human tissues, but there is no evidence that any clinical disorder results from their deficiency except when highly artificial diets have been given for experimental purposes.

Vitamin E is another vitamin present in human tissues, yet not proved essential for human needs. It has the interesting property of reducing tissue oxidation and has been recommended for therapeutic use in many human diseases, mostly quite unconnected with dietary deficiencies. So far, however, it has no proven therapeutic value.

Factors influencing the Utilisation of Vitamins

1. **Availability.** Not all of a vitamin may be in absorbable form. For instance some of the nicotinic acid in maize is bound in such a way that it is not absorbed from the gut. Fat-soluble vitamins may fail to be absorbed if the digestion or absorption of fat is impaired.

2. **Antivitamins.** These are known to be present in some natural foods. Several synthetic analogues of vitamins have proved to be highly poisonous (e.g. aminopterin, desoxypyridoxine), presumably because they block the enzymes with which the true vitamins are concerned.

3. **Provitamins.** Substances occur in foods which are not themselves vitamins but are capable of conversion into vitamins in the course of digestion. Thus the carotenes are the provitamin of vitamin A and, to some extent at least, the amino acid tryptophan can be converted to nicotinic acid.

4. **Biosynthesis in the Gut.** The normal bacterial flora of the gut is capable of synthesising significant amounts of certain vitamins (e.g. vitamin K, nicotinic acid, riboflavine, vitamin B_{12}, folic acid). Bacteria are also capable of extracting vitamins from the ingested food and retaining them until excreted in the faeces. It is unlikely that bacterial activity significantly affects the amounts of vitamins available to a *healthy* human body with the exception of vitamin K (p. 503). Bacteria are more likely to reduce than to increase the amounts of vitamins available for absorption, as is clearly demonstrated in the blind loop syndrome (p. 940).

These considerations indicate how difficult it may be in practice to define the nutritive value of a diet in respect of a given vitamin by simple reference to a chemical analysis of its vitamin content, and that the true requirements for a given vitamin are likely to vary very much from one individual to another.

CLINICAL DISORDERS DUE TO VITAMIN DEFICIENCIES

RECOMMENDED INTAKES OF VITAMINS

There has been much confusion in the use of terms to define the amounts of vitamins required in the diet to maintain health, e.g. minimum requirements, optimum requirements, recommended allowances, etc. Hence the importance of the World Health Organization Technical Report Series, No. 362, published in 1967. This contains the recommendations of a joint FAO/WHO group of nutritional experts on the requirements of vitamin A, thiamine, riboflavine and nicotinic acid. 'Recommended intake', which was chosen as the most suitable term for this purpose, was defined as 'the amount of the vitamin considered sufficient for the maintenance of health in nearly all people'. It was not expected to cover additional needs which may result from such conditions as infections, malabsorption or metabolic abnormalities. In addition the recommended intake is only applicable when the requirements for calories and other nutrients are met. The Committee states that in view of the well recognised roles of thiamine, riboflavine and nicotinic acid in energy expenditure, it seems reasonable to relate these requirements to energy expenditure. Therefore the recommended daily intakes should be expressed in terms of mg./1,000 Cal. Vitamin requirements vary with factors such as body weight, physical activity and the presence of infections, but only to the extent that calorie expenditure is related to these factors. Hence the advantage of expressing vitamin requirements in terms of milligrams per 1,000 calories ingested as this enables the same value to be used for adults (male and female), pregnant and lactating women and children.

The recommended daily intake per 1,000 calories ingested is 0·4 mg. for thiamine, 0·55 mg. for riboflavine and 6·6 nicotinic acid equivalents for nicotinic acid. The term 'nicotinic acid equivalents' is used because it enables the calculation of the combined effects of nicotinic acid and tryptophan in preventing the symptoms of pellagra (p. 524). One nicotinic acid equivalent is defined as being equal to either 1 mg. of nicotinic acid or 60 mg. of tryptophan.

The Committee states that in view of the availability of crystalline vitamin A_1 alcohol (retinol) as a reference standard, the practice of expressing vitamin A values in terms of international units (i.u.) is no longer necessary or desirable. Hence recommended intakes should be described in units of weights, namely micrograms (μg.) of retinol. The conversion factor is 1 i.u. = 0·3 μg. of retinol or, in the case of the provitamin, 0·6 μg. of β carotene. The term 'retinol' should be used to mean vitamin A_1 alcohol, while the term 'vitamin A' should be used to include all compounds with vitamin A activity. The recommended intake per day of retinol for adults and adolescents and pregnant women is 750 μg., for lactating women 1,200 μg., for children from 7 to 13 years of age 400-575 μg. and from 1 to 6 years of age 250-300 μg. according to age.

The recommendation of the Joint FAO/WHO Committee are likely to receive universal acceptance in the near future.

Vitamin A (Retinol)

Chemistry and Physiological Action. Retinol is found only in foods of animal origin. Animals obtain the vitamin from its precursor or provitamin—the pigment, carotene. The conversion of β carotene into retinol in the human body is not complete and involves considerable losses (see below). It takes place largely, if not entirely in the walls of the small intestine. The absorption of both retinol and carotene is facilitated by fats and bile salts.

It seems likely that retinol has a place in the metabolism of all human cells, but the precise way that it behaves is not yet explained in biochemical terms except in one situation—the retina of the eye (see below).

Pathology. Deficiency of the vitamin results in morphological changes in the epithelial surfaces of all parts of the body. The cells undergo *squamous metaplasia* whereby they become flattened and heaped one upon another. The sebaceous glands and hair follicles of the skin and the tear glands of the eye become blocked with horny plugs of keratin so that their secretions diminish. The lack of tears and the heaping up of epithelium on the scleral conjunctiva and cornea produce the condition of *xerophthalmia*. When softening, ulceration and necrosis of the cornea develop, the condition is referred to as keratomalacia (p. 484). Squamous metaplasia in the urinary tract of dogs results in the formation of urinary calculi, but there is no good evidence that vitamin A deficiency is a cause of renal stones in man.

Dietary Sources. Retinol is chiefly found in milk, butter, cheese, egg yolk, liver and some of the fatty fish. The liver oils of fish are the richest natural sources but these are used as nutritional supplements rather than foods.

Carotene is widely distributed among plant foods. It is found chiefly in green vegetables in association with chlorophyll, so that the green outer leaves of vegetables like cabbage and lettuce are good sources of carotene, while the white inner leaves contain little or none. Other useful sources are yellow and red fruits and vegetables. All vegetable oils are devoid of vitamin A activity with the exception of red palm oil which is extensively produced in West Africa, Indonesia and Brazil. This oil is a rich source of carotene. In Britain and some other countries retinol is added artificially to margarine to provide the same concentration as that of good quality summer butter.

Losses in the Preparation and Handling of Food. Both retinol and carotene are stable to ordinary cooking methods, though some loss may occur at temperatures above 100° C. as when butter or palm oil is used for frying. Fruits and other foods that are dried in the sun lose much of their vitamin A potency. The stability of carotene in tinned foods was dramatically shown by Drummond in 1939 who found that cooked carrots that had been sealed in air-tight containers in 1824 for the Arctic voyage of H.M.S. *Hecla* had much the same carotene content as fresh carrots when the containers were finally opened in 1939.

Recommended Intakes. Owing to the large stores in the liver, it is difficult to determine how much of the vitamin or its precursors should be taken from day to day in order to maintain this reserve. A further difficulty arises when a large part of the dietary needs are supplied by carotenes from vegetables, for the conversion of carotenes to retinol is always incomplete. Having regard to this fact, a satisfactory daily intake would be 3,000 i.u. made up from 250 μg. of retinol (750 i.u.) and 1,400 μg. of carotene (2,350 i.u.).

Therapeutic Uses. A dietary deficiency of vitamin A arises only when there is an insufficient supply of dairy produce, fish and vegetables.

Retinol is invaluable in the treatment of xerophthalmia, keratomalacia and of night blindness—when this is due to dietary failure. It should also be given to malnourished people who show evidence of follicular keratosis. Treatment and prevention are discussed on p. 485.

Where vitamin A deficiency is prevalent, minor disorders of the eyes and skin often recover more rapidly in children receiving regular prophylactic doses of the vitamin. There is also the clinical impression that it often improves their growth and well-being.

The prescription of retinol for the prevention of the common cold and other infections in people taking a good mixed diet is not justified by any reliable clinical evidence.

Night Blindness (Hemeralopia)

Retinol is an essential component of the pigment rhodopsin (visual purple) on which vision in dim light depends. Hence lack of retinol may result in impairment of 'dark adaptation' which can be measured by means of an adaptometer. Night blindness is common, as also is vitamin A deficiency, in poor people living in underdeveloped countries; in which case it responds excellently to retinol. Fatigue and anxiety states may cause persons to complain of night blindness. It may also result from organic disease of the eye such as retinitis pigmentosa. The diagnosis can only be made with certainty when it has been shown that there has been a marked improvement in dark adaptation following a therapeutic dose of the vitamin.

Xerosis Conjunctivae, Bitôt's Spots and Xerophthalmia

The earliest sign of xerosis conjunctivae is a dry, thickened and pigmented bulbar conjunctiva. The pigmentation gives the conjunctiva a peculiar smoky appearance. Bitot's spots are glistening white plaques formed of desquamated thickened conjunctival epithelium, usually triangular in shape and firmly adherent to the underlying conjunctiva. Xerosis conjunctivae and Bitôt's spots are certainly common in children whose diet is deficient in vitamin A but they also occur in children whose intake of the vitamins is satisfactory. When dryness spreads to the cornea it takes on a dull, hazy, lacklustre appearance due to keratinisation, and xerophthalmia is said to be present.

In young children, xerophthalmia is almost always attributable to recent vitamin A deficiency. In older children and in adults its interpretation is less simple. Exposure to dust and glare may produce similar changes. They should, however, always call attention to the diet. Xerophthalmia by itself may not cause any disability unless associated with night blindness. The condition is important since it may precede the development of keratomalacia.

Keratomalacia

This disease causes blindness among Indians, Chinese, Indonesians and other rice-eating people of Asia; it also occurs in parts of Africa, Arabia and Latin America. In Europe and North America it is very rare. Children between the ages of 1 and 5 years are most commonly affected. It only occurs in persons who have been living for long periods on diets almost entirely devoid of vitamin A. Early cases respond promptly to the administration of fish-liver oils rich in the vitamin. The disease is frequently associated with kwashiorkor and also with riboflavine deficiency.

The earliest manifestations are night blindness and xerophthalmia. Later the cornea undergoes necrosis and ulceration. Unless early and adequate treatment is given, there is a grave risk of blindness or death from associated diseases. In many Eastern countries keratomalacia is at least as important as smallpox, syphilis and gonorrhoea in destroying the sight of children.

Follicular Keratosis (Phrynoderma, 'Toad Skin')

In this condition the hair follicles are blocked with horny plugs of keratin, rendering the skin surface rough and dry. The typical distribution is over the backs of the upper arms and the fronts of the thighs. Therapeutic trials in Africa have repeatedly shown a striking clinical improvement in follicular keratosis when patients are given halibut liver oil or red palm oil. Nevertheless, it is not a specific sign of vitamin A deficiency, since it occurs not uncommonly in people who, by every other criterion, are adequately nourished in respect of vitamin A. It differs in appearance from the folliculosis of scurvy (p. 506).

Treatment and Prevention of Diseases due to Deficiency of Vitamin A

Treatment. A good all round diet and attention to any associated infection is essential for the treatment of the above disorders. In severe adult cases of night blindness or xerophthalmia 25,000 μg. of retinol (75,000 i.u.) daily, in the form of halibut liver oil or some equally potent preparation, e.g. concentrated solution of vitamin A, B.P., of which 0·6 ml. contains about 8,000 μg. of retinol (25,000 i.u.) by mouth for one or two weeks is usually sufficient to bring about a rapid and marked improvement, while in early mild cases 3,000 to 7,000 μg. of retinol (10,000 to 20,000 i.u.) daily is a satisfactory dose. For follicular keratosis and keratomalacia treatment with large doses of retinol should be continued for some weeks. Riboflavine, 5 mg. three times a day by mouth should also be given for xerophthalmia and keratomalacia. Some authorities instill into the eye drops of a solution containing retinol. This is not recommended. An antibiotic should be instilled for the prevention or treatment of secondary infection.

Prevention. The essential needs for prevention are the education of mothers, better social services and an improvement in food production. The prime objective is to make sure that infants and young children obtain adequate amounts of vitamin A in their diet or as a supplement. In countries where vitamin A deficiency is endemic the distribution of a national concentrated source of vitamin A is desirable, especially for children. For this purpose cod-liver, shark-liver or red palm oil can usefully be given according to which is most easily available locally. A satisfactory prophylactic dose of retinol is 300 μg. (1,000 i.u.) for infants and young children, 500-600 μg. of retinal (1500-2000 i.u.) for children of 9 to 15 years and 750 μg. of retinol (2,250 i.u.) for adolescents and adults daily.

Blindness

It has been estimated that there are more than 10 million blind people in the world and that most of these become blind before the age of 5 years. The situation is all the more tragic because probably about two-thirds of the cases of blindness are preventable if energetic Public Health measures were introduced and good ophthalmic clinics were available in adequate numbers. Vitamin A deficiency is one of the seven most common causes of blindness, the others being trachoma, smallpox, onchocercosis, venereal disease, accidents, cataract and glaucoma.

VITAMIN D

Although cod-liver oil has been used in the treatment of rickets for more than 100 years it was not till 1918 that Sir Edward Mellanby clearly showed by his classical studies on puppies that rickets is a nutritional disease responding to a fat soluble vitamin in cod-liver oil. This vitamin was finally prepared in pure form in 1931.

Chemistry and Physiological Action. A number of distinct but closely related compounds possess rickets-preventing (antirachitic) properties. These are all sterols, chemically related to cholesterol and to the hormones of the adrenal cortex and sex glands. Certain sterols on exposure to ultraviolet irradiation undergo a small structural change which makes them antirachitic. Only two 'activated' sterols are of importance in nutrition and therapeutics. These were first described as vitamin D_2 and D_3 and are still known as such. The material originally described as vitamin D_1 was subsequently shown to be an impure mixture of sterols.

Calciferol (Vitamin D_2). Calciferol is manufactured by exposing ergosterol, a sterol found in fungi and yeasts, to the action of ultraviolet light.

Although calciferol is widely used in therapeutics, it occurs very rarely in nature.

Vitamin D_3. This substance is the natural form of vitamin D found in egg yolk, milk and fish liver oils. It is produced by the ultraviolet irradiation of 7-dehydrocholesterol, a sterol widely distributed in animal fats, such as the oily secretions of mammalian skin and the oil of the preen glands of birds.

Activation of 7-dehydrocholesterol takes place when the surface of the body is exposed to sunlight. In man the vitamin so formed enters the body directly by way of the skin. In other mammals and birds the entry is by ingestion through the gut, as a result of licking the fur or preening the feathers.

The liver oils of fish are very rich in vitamin D_3, probably from the ingestion of microscopic plankton that live near the surface of the sea and are hence exposed to the sun's rays.

Ingested vitamin D requires the presence of bile and probably fatty acids for its absorption from the gut. It is stored mainly in the liver.

Vitamin D is necessary for the formation of normal bone and the calcification of rachitic bone. It probably has a direct effect on bone but the mechanism underlying this action is uncertain. In addition it promotes the absorption of calcium and phosphate from the gut, thus ensuring a sufficient supply of these minerals at the growing points of the bones where the calcium comes in contact with inorganic phosphates liberated from organic phosphates under the influence of the enzyme phosphatase. Thus calcium phosphate is formed and used by the osteoblasts to make new bone.

Dietary Sources. The sources of the natural vitamin are all fat-containing animal products. The richest sources are fatty fish and their oils, some of which contain many thousands of international units of vitamin D per 100 g. edible portion. Vitamin D is also present in dairy products such as milk, eggs, butter and in vitaminised margarine in much smaller quantities. It is important to remember that milk has a very small content of vitamin D. Cereals, vegetables and fruit grown in temperate climates contain no vitamin D and meat and white fish insignificant amounts.

Recommended Intakes. See p. 491.

RICKETS

Infantile rickets is a disease of calcium and phosphorus metabolism which occurs when infants obtain insufficient vitamin D. In addition, the intake of calcium is usually low because of an insufficiency of milk in the diet.

Rickets is still an important clinical problem in some underdeveloped countries, especially in large towns and cities. In such countries infants in their first year are mainly affected due to an inadequate intake of vitamin D because of the low content of this vitamin in both human and animal milk. In addition for various social and cultural reasons, e.g. to prevent their infants acquiring a dark complexion, their mothers wrap them up in swaddling clothes thus preventing their exposure to sunlight. Lack of exposure to ultraviolet light in slums and old walled cities, particularly if the mothers are living in purdah, is another cause of vitamin D deficiency. By the second year the infant is able to crawl about in the sunshine and spontaneous healing usually occurs. In contrast the age group mainly affected in Britain and other wealthy countries is from 1 to 3 years and the disease is now very rare. This is the result of a variety of measures which have been introduced during the last 60 years and which have led to greatly improved standards of nutrition and housing. Of particular importance are the various schemes which have resulted in a satisfactory supply of milk, the distribution of cod-liver oil and other sources of vitamin D and the fortification with vitamin D of preparations of dried milk, margarine and some proprietary cereal foods. That it would be rash to suggest that any of these measures is now redundant is clearly indicated by recent reports of limited outbreaks of clinical rickets in coloured immigrant children in Glasgow, London and Birmingham and occasionally in underprivileged white children living in slum areas in Glasgow. Rickets has been characteristically a disease of the poor rather than the rich. Milk (providing calcium) and cream, butter and eggs are the only common foods providing a satisfactory dietary source of vitamin D and calcium. They may be too expensive for poor urban families, and in addition the amount of vitamin D they contain in the quantities eaten by infants is insufficient to prevent rickets. Wealthier families, on the other hand, not only enjoy these foods but usually also have access to gardens in which the children may benefit from sunlight. If the diet of poor families consists predominantly of cereals the inhibitory effect of phytic acid in the cereals on the absorption of calcium may be rachitogenic. A plentiful supply of cereals provides calories which may enable growth to take place faster than the skeleton can be properly formed if calcium absorption is inadequate. Indeed it used to be a commonplace that the fat, flabby child, who won the prize at the local baby show by virtue of being so much heavier than his competitors, was usually rachitic. The disease is liable to occur in premature babies who grow rapidly.

Chemical Pathology. With the deficiency of calcium in the body, the calcium in the blood serum tends to fall from its normal level of about 10 mg./100 ml. of which approximately 50 per cent is available in the ionised form. It may fall as low as 5 mg. or even less, which usually causes tetany (pp. 715, 718). More commonly the serum inorganic phosphorus falls from the normal level of about 3·5 mg./100 ml. to 3 mg. or less. This is thought to be due to the activity of the parathyroid glands which respond to a slight reduction in serum calcium by increasing the excretion of phosphorus in the urine, with consequent reduction in the level of inorganic phosphorus in the blood.

Clinical rickets may occur when the levels of calcium and phosphorus in the serum are still within normal limits. A diagnostic change is an increase in serum alkaline phosphatase. This enzyme is formed by the osteoblasts which accumulate in the osteoid tissue at the growing points of the bones. These cells, unable to make bone without a sufficient supply of calcium, probably liberate into the circulation the excess of this enzyme which they cannot use. The normal range of serum alkaline phosphate in the first three years of life is up to 12 King-Armstrong units per 100 ml. Even in early cases of rickets 30 to 40 units are frequently found.

The reduction in circulating ionised calcium makes the motor nerves over-susceptible to stimuli which may result in tetany, while muscles lose tone and become flaccid. The bones are especially affected, leading to characteristic rachitic deformities.

Clinical Features. The infant with rickets has often received sufficient calories and may appear well nourished, but he is restless, fretful and pale, with flabby and toneless muscles. Excessive sweating of the head is common. The abdomen is distended as a result of the flabby abdominal muscles, the atony of the intestinal musculature and the intestinal fermentation that may arise from excessive carbohydrates in the diet. Gastrointestinal upsets with diarrhoea are common. The infant is prone to respiratory infections, although these are probably due not so much to the disease itself as to the other unhealthy aspects of the environment. Development is delayed so that the teeth often erupt late and there is failure to sit up, stand, crawl and walk at the normal ages.

The bony changes are the most characteristic and easily identifiable signs of rickets. There is extension and widening of the epiphyses at the growing points, where cartilage meets bone. The earliest bony lesion is often craniotabes—small round unossified areas in the membranous bones of the skull, yielding to the pressure of the finger, with a crackling feeling, like parchment. This sign is of particular value in the diagnosis of rickets in underdeveloped countries where the disease is common in infants under 1 year of age. Another early sign is enlargement of the epiphyses at the lower end of the radius and at the costochondral junctions of the ribs, the latter producing the clinical sign known as 'beading' of the ribs or 'rickety rosary'. Craniotabes usually disappears after six months, but later there may be 'bossing' of the frontal and parietal bones and delayed closure of the anterior fontanelle. Later too, there may be deformities of the chest such as undue prominence of the sternum ('pigeon chest') and 'Harrison's sulcus'—the latter apparently caused by the indrawing of the softened ribs on inspiration during whooping-cough or other respiratory infections to which rachitic children are prone.

If rickets continues into the second year of life, these signs may persist or be magnified. Deformities such as kyphosis of the spine develop as a result of the new gravitational and muscular strains, caused by sitting up and crawling. At the same time there may be enlargement of the lower ends of the femur, tibia and fibula. When the rachitic child begins to walk, deformities of the shafts of the leg bones develop, so that 'knock knees' or 'bow legs' are added to the clinical picture. The spinal kyphosis is often replaced by lordosis. Pelvic deformities may follow and lead many years later to serious difficulties at childbirth in women who have suffered from rickets in childhood.

When there is a reduction in the level of ionised serum calcium infantile tetany may result, with spasm of the hands and feet and of the vocal cords. The latter causes a high-pitched, distressing cry and great difficulty in breathing. In bygone days—when florid rickets was common—tetany was sometimes associated with alarming general convulsions. The treatment of tetany is discussed on page 717.

Diagnosis. In a fully developed case this is easy, but in countries where the disease is now rare, there is an increasing likelihood that mild cases will be missed. A flabby baby towards the end of its first year, unable to pull itself up, fretful and easily irritated, with too few teeth showing and liable to profuse sweats, should always be suspected of rickets. The diagnosis may be supported by the dietary history and the finding of craniotabes. Early evidence of rickets may be overlooked in a child ill with bronchopneumonia or diarrhoea. If there is any doubt or suspicion, radiological examination of the wrist will show characteristic changes at the epiphyses; the outline of the joint is blurred and hazy, and the epiphyseal line becomes broadened. Later, in older children, as a result of decalcification of the metaphysis and the effects of movements and stresses the classical concave 'saucer' deformity is clearly shown radiographically. The opinion of an experienced radiologist may be needed to distinguish the picture from that of infantile scurvy. A raised level of serum alkaline phosphatase gives the best objective support to the initial clinical diagnosis.

It is sometimes necessary to distinguish rickets from other rare disorders involving the bones, such as congenital syphilis, achondroplasia and osteogenesis imperfecta. Radiological examination of the bones is helpful in differentiating these disorders.

Treatment. The two essentials of treatment are the provision of a supplement of vitamin D and an ample intake of calcium. A therapeutic dose of vitamin D will vary from 1,000-5,000 i.u. daily, depending on the severity of the disease. In contrast, the prophylactic dose is 400 i.u. or less daily. A British Pharmacopoeial (B.P.) preparation of cod-liver oil contains not less than 340 i.u. per teaspoonful (about 4 ml.). Children who find cod-liver oil unpalatable can be given halibut-liver oil in a very small dose (6 drops) since its concentration of vitamins A and D is three to four times that of cod-liver oil. Alternatively various proprietary preparations are available which contain standard amounts of vitamins A and D dispensed as palatable syrups, but they are more expensive. For severe cases needing 5,000 i.u. daily, synthetic calciferol is useful because the volume of cod-liver oil required to provide this dose is excessive. For such patients the B.P. solution of calciferol is satisfactory. One ml. contains about 3,000 i.u. of vitamin D. In times of social upheaval, such as may be occasioned by war, floods or pestilence, when an infant or young child may be seen once by an emergency medical service and perhaps not again for months, a single massive dose of vitamin D, e.g. 150,000 i.u. (3 B.P. calciferol tablets), can be given by mouth with reasonable safety and curative effects. The single dose can be given by intramuscular injection but this has no proved advantage over the oral route. The daily administration of small doses is the method recommended for normal practice, because of the danger of overdosage (p. 494).

In addition to vitamin D, rachitic infants and children require an ample supply of calcium, the best source of which is milk. At least one pint (about 0·5 *l.*) should be taken daily by a young child with mild rickets. For a severe case a supplement of calcium lactate should also be given orally. The diet after weaning can include with advantage an egg daily and some butter. An adequate intake of iron and ascorbic acid is also needed.

Vitamin D and diet are not the whole solution to the treatment of rickets. An attempt must be made to improve the hygienic environment of the child. This often requires the tactful education of the mother in better feeding practices and general care. Unnecessary clothing should be removed and, if the child was previously confined indoors, he should be allowed out as much as possible to enjoy the sunshine. This is particularly important in countries where supplements of vitamin D are not provided.

The earliest evidence of healing in rickets is provided by radiological examination of the growing ends of the bones. The levels of calcium and phosphorus in the serum provide an inconstant and unreliable guide. A more constant change is a decrease in the raised serum alkaline phosphatase level (p. 489) but this does not usually occur for several weeks after treatment is initiated; the therapeutic dose of vitamin D should be continued so long as the phosphatase level remains elevated; thereafter it may gradually be reduced to the prophylactic dose of 400 i.u. daily.

Occasionally cases of rickets are encountered which are resistant to ordinary therapeutic doses of vitamin D. The disease persists into late childhood ('late rickets') or even adult life, producing the clinical appearance of osteomalacia, unless adequately treated. The cause of this resistance is not understood, though perhaps it is due to excessive loss of phosphates in the urine. A similar state may sometimes arise as a conditioned deficiency resulting from malabsorption or renal failure. Whatever the cause, treatment consists in giving large doses of vitamin D by mouth in the form of calciferol, together with calcium salts, e.g. calcium lactate in pill or powder form, 5 g. three times daily or 2 calcium Sandoz effervescent tablets, each containing 380 mg. of elemental calcium, three times daily. The dose of calciferol will vary from 50,000 to 150,000 i.u. (1-3 B.P. calciferol tablets) daily but it should be reduced at the first suspicion of toxic symptoms.

Prognosis. Rickets is not a fatal disease *per se*, but the untreated rachitic child is always a weakling owing to the risk of infections, notably bronchopneumonia. For some unknown reason the skeletal changes, if mild in degree, usually tend to heal spontaneously as the child gets older, but in severe cases pigeon chest, spinal curvature, knock knees, bow legs or pelvic deformities may persist. With early and sufficient treatment these changes are entirely avoided.

Prophylaxis. The provision of adequate milk for children, the clearing of industrial city slums, the building of new housing estates and the attack on the smoke nuisance are basic prophylactic measures which must be continued at all costs. If a young child can have one pint of cow's milk, an egg and some butter daily, and has free access to a garden in which he can run about in the sun, the administration of a supplement of vitamin D is probably not essential for his future health. Nevertheless practical experience shows that the majority of children who do not enjoy these advantages regularly, or who live in a climate where sunshine is scanty, benefit by receiving a daily supplement of about 400 i.u. of vitamin D, preferably in the form of some natural source such as cod-liver oil, which also provides useful amounts of vitamin A. This is also advisable in sunny tropical countries if the mothers insist on keeping their infants wrapped in swaddling clothes during the first year of life. It seems reasonable that the supplement should be started within two weeks of birth because human and animal milk has a negligible content of vitamin D. In some countries it is necessary to remember that fish oils may be adulterated by the addition of vegetable oils; the label on the bottle should clearly state the vitamin D content of the oil, as attested by some reliable agency.

Before deciding on the prophylactic dose of cod-liver oil or other fish oil, it is necessary to consider how much vitamin D the infant is getting from other sources. Thus, if he is being brought up on a preparation of dried milk 'fortified' with vitamin D (e.g. British National Dried Milk which contains 100 i.u. per oz. of powder) the supplement of cod-liver oil should be small. Furthermore, it should be remembered that some proprietary cereal foods for infants are 'fortified' with vitamin D by the manufacturers.

All brands of British margarine are fortified with vitamin D and contain about twice as much vitamin D as butter. This may help to secure good calcification of the bones during the growth of older children.

Not only is there no advantage in giving infants and young children more than 400 i.u. of vitamin D daily *from all sources* for prophylactic purposes, but there is a distinct possibility that higher doses given over a long period may have harmful effects. The potential dangers of overdosage with vitamin D have been emphasised by the discovery that infantile hypercalcaemia is not such a rare condition as was formerly believed. The toxic effects of overdosage include nausea, vomiting, diarrhoea, drowsiness and signs of renal failure; metastatic calcification in the arteries, kidneys and other tissues may occur.

It should be noted, however, that the prophylactic dose of vitamin D for premature infants should be twice that for full-term infants and the supplement should be started within two weeks of birth. There has been divergence of view among paediatricians in the past about the length of time that the prophylactic administration of vitamin D should be continued. Obviously such features as the social and economic status of the parents and the climate in which the family lives are matters of importance. It seems reasonable to suggest that in temperate climates at least, a daily intake of about 400 i.u. should be continued summer and winter for the first five years of life.

OSTEOMALACIA AND OSTEOPOROSIS

These are two chronic diseases of the skeleton. Although they have a similar effect on the mechanical function of bone because they weaken the parts affected, their pathology, chemistry and treatment are different. For reasons given below it is possible that the distinction may not be so sharp, since calcium deficiency may be of aetiological importance in both diseases.

Osteomalacia, which means softening of bone, is primarily due to a deficiency of vitamin D, and to a lesser extent of calcium, or both. This results in a failure to lay down calcium and phosphorus in the organic matrix of bone. Hence the ratio of calcium phosphate to matrix is reduced.

Osteoporosis, which is an atrophy of bone, is believed to be due to defective formation of bone matrix which leads to a reduction in the total mass of bone. In other words osteoporosis may be defined as a disorder of too little bone of normal composition. In contrast to osteomalacia the ratio of calcium phosphate to matrix is normal. It may arise from a variety of causes. Both osteoporosis and osteomalacia occur in old people in all countries and cause much suffering.

Osteomalacia

Aetiology and Geographic Distribution. Osteomalacia is the adult counterpart of rickets. In its fully developed form as it occurs in women in purdah in oriental countries, it causes great deformity and suffering. Such women are of the child-bearing age who live on poor cereal diets devoid of milk, who are kept indoors all day and seldom see the sun, and who by repeated pregnancies become depleted of calcium. In oriental countries the onset often coincides with the first pregnancy, a remission occurring after delivery, but symptoms return with each succeeding pregnancy. It has recently been shown in Scotland that osteomalacia is a relatively common disease in old people, especially women, and that it occurs much more frequently than scurvy or rickets. The disease may be due to malabsorption from any cause, including previous operations on the gastrointestinal tract, or to direct dietary deficiency of vitamin D. Chronic renal disorders (p. 497) are a less important cause of the disease.

Pathology. The changes in the blood are essentially the same as those in rickets. The progressive decalcification of the bones leads to the replacement of bony substance with soft osteoid tissue. This process goes on all over the skeleton, but the effects are greatest in the spine, ribs, shoulder girdle, pelvis and lower limbs. A combination of osteomalacia and osteoporosis is not uncommon.

Clinical Features. Pain is usually present and ranges from a dull ache to severe pain. Sites frequently affected are the ribs, sacrum, lower lumbar vertebrae, pelvis and legs. Bone tenderness on pressure is common. Muscular weakness is often present and the patient may find difficulty in climbing stairs or getting out of a chair. A waddling gait is not unusual. Tetany may be manifested by carpopedal spasm and facial twitching. Spontaneous fractures may occur, independent of the pseudo-fractures described below.

Diagnosis. The early symptoms may be mistaken for those present in osteoporosis or rheumatic disorders. The clinical examination must be supported by a careful enquiry into adverse social, economic and dietary factors which may be present. In addition biochemical tests, including calcium, phosphorus and alkaline phosphatase determinations and radiological examination of the skeleton should be undertaken, and histological examination of bone obtained by biopsy may be required. Radiological examination shows rarefaction of bone and commonly translucent bands (pseudofractures, Looser's zones), often symmetrical, at points submitted to great compression stress. Common sites are the ribs, the axillary borders of the scapula, the pubic rami and the medial cortex of the upper femur. Looser's zones are diagnostic of osteomalacia. Correct diagnosis is essential as the results of treatment with vitamin D are excellent if undertaken prior to the establishment of gross deformities and it is also necessary for the assessment of dosage of vitamin D.

Treatment. This is essentially the same as for rickets when osteomalacia is primarily due to a defective intake of vitamin D, namely 1,000 to 5,000 i.u. daily (p. 491). If there is evidence of malabsorption (p. 497) the dose should be 50,000 i.u. daily and it may have to be given intramuscularly at weekly intervals. If the disease is secondary to renal disorders the dose may be 100,000 i.u. or more (p. 497). Maintenance treatment with vitamin D will be required for all cases of osteomalacia in which the cause cannot be removed. In addition a good diet should be given which includes milk, eggs, butter or margarine. This may be difficult or impossible under the conditions in which the disease arises in the East. In all cases of osteomalacia and especially when both osteoporosis and osteomalacia are present a supplement of calcium should be given orally, namely 1-2 g. in the form of calcium lactate or preferably 1 to 2 calcium Sandoz effervescent tablets each containing 0·38 g. of elemental calcium three times a day. Within four to eight weeks of starting treatment the pain and weakness has usually disappeared. The decision to reduce or discontinue the dose of vitamin D and calcium is based on the improvement in the clinical features and the disappearance of biochemical and radiological abnormalities. The dangers of vitamin D intoxication should be kept in mind.

Prevention. Once major deformities are established they cannot be corrected by diet or drugs but only by an orthopaedic surgeon. Hence the great importance of early and correct diagnosis and proper treatment. Free access to sunshine and an adequate intake of dairy produce, supplemented when necessary with fish-liver oil, will prevent nutritional osteomalacia. With improved education and better standards of living the disease is now much rarer in many Asian towns where previously it was common.

LATE RICKETS AND OSTEOMALACIA

Osteomalacia may occur in children whose diet is exceedingly poor in vitamin D and calcium and who are deprived of sunshine as a result of living in purdah. It also occurs in children of Indian or African parents who are brought up in northern sunless climates.

SECONDARY RICKETS AND OSTEOMALACIA

The clinical picture of rickets or osteomalacia is occasionally seen as a result of other diseases which 'condition' the calcium deficiency. These diseases are of two kinds.

1. **The Malabsorption Syndrome** (p. 939). If the intestinal absorption of fat, and therefore of fat soluble vitamin D, is impaired, the body is deprived of a sufficiency of this vitamin to promote the normal absorption of calcium. In the adult secondary osteomalacia may result. Of particular interest is the frequency with which osteomalacia alone or in combination with osteoporosis has been reported as a sequel to partial gastrectomy. Treatment should include both vitamin D and calcium in the doses recommended on page 496.

2. **Renal Disorders.** In renal failure with uraemia and in a variety of disorders of the kidney with disturbances in tubular

function, including the Fanconi syndrome, renal rickets may occur in children and osteomalacia in adults. These disorders are probably due to defective absorption of calcium secondary to the development of resistance to the action of vitamin D on the absorption of calcium and on the metabolism of bone.

Treatment. In addition to the treatment of the causal condition, vitamin D and calcium should be given in large doses (p. 496).

OSTEOPOROSIS

Osteoporosis is the disease of bone most frequently encountered in clinical practice. It may be a localised or generalised disease.

Local Osteoporosis. The most common cause is immobilisation but it may also arise as a result of inflammation or neoplasm of bone. Disuse removes the stresses and strains which stimulate the osteoblasts to lay down new bone, whilst the osteoclasts continue to remove calcium salts. This happens when movement is restricted by splinting, by inflammation or by pain, or when a patient is confined to bed. Extra provision of nutrients in the diet cannot prevent this process.

Generalised Osteoporosis. Osteoporosis represents a non-specific reaction of the skeleton to a wide variety of stimuli. It is, however, a clinico-pathological entity since it can be differentiated from other generalised diseases of bone such as osteomalacia and osteitis fibrosa cystica by its characteristic clinical, radiological and pathological features.

Aetiology, Incidence and Classification. The incidence of osteoporosis steadily increases in both sexes with advancing age. The density of the bones has been shown to decline in all people from the age of 20 onwards, the process accelerating after middle age. This physiological atrophy of bone makes it difficult to decide on the value of any form of treatment and the validity of the terms used to describe the various types of osteoporosis, e.g. idiopathic, secondary, post-menopausal, senile, etc. However it seems probable that those patients who develop the clinical features of osteoporosis before the age of 50 to 60 have had the physiological ageing process *accelerated* by factors known or unknown.

Such factors may cause 'acute' attacks of osteoporosis, often accompanied by a marked temporary increase in negative calcium balance.

HORMONAL DEFICIENCY. The frequency with which osteoporosis develops in women after the menopause and the fact that it is much more common in women than in men has led to the belief that a failure of sex hormone secretion may be one of the factors concerned with the production of this type of osteoporosis. The similar condition in men often described as senile osteoporosis, is thought to be related to diminished androgen formation.

CALCIUM DEFICIENCY. A high faecal content of calcium and a low calcium absorption has been reported in osteoporosis by some workers. This suggests that a failure in calcium absorption or a failure in the normal compensating ability of the kidneys to decrease urinary excretion of calcium may be of aetiological importance, especially if the intake of calcium in the diet has been low for many years. However, other authorities deny that there is a negative calcium balance in most cases. In addition they are doubtful if dietary deficiency of calcium plays any significant role in the causation of the human disease. Studies with the isotopes of calcium and strontium have failed to unravel the mystery of the aetiology of osteoporosis, nor have they helped in its diagnosis or treatment.

Types of Osteoporosis.

IDIOPATHIC OSTEOPOROSIS. Osteoporosis may occur rarely in juveniles and in adults between 20 and 40 years without any apparent cause. A period of increased osteoporotic activity develops and may last for many months with the production of features identical to those occurring in classical osteoporosis in old people. This activity usually remits eventually and clinical and radiological improvement occurs even without treatment.

The age group of 60 years and over is the one in which most of the cases of osteoporosis are seen in practice. Such cases are usually the end-result of the physiological ageing process but in some of them self-limiting acute exacerbations of the disease occur with marked negative calcium balances for which no adequate explanation is available.

OSTEOPOROSIS DUE TO CAUSES KNOWN OR SUSPECTED. The most important of these causes are (1) hypogonadism in both males and females, (2) hyperadrenalcorticism as occurs in Cushing's syndrome or after prolonged treatment with adrenal corticosteroids, (3) acromegaly, (4) prolonged calcium deficiency.

Other disorders which are less frequently associated with osteoporosis are scurvy, rheumatoid arthritis, protein malnutrition, hepatic disease of long standing, uncontrolled diabetes, thyrotoxicosis and chronic alcoholism.

Symptoms and Signs. There may be no symptoms despite clear-cut radiological changes or there may be much disability. Episodes of severe bone pain are usually due to fractures of the brittle bones and may occur after minimal trauma. The pain is usually relieved by complete immobilisation and made worse by movement. Pain due to fractures of the vertebrae may radiate round the trunk, to the buttocks or down the legs. Spinal cord compression rarely occurs. Healing of fractures is not impaired in osteoporosis and pain usually subsides spontaneously as healing takes place. More persistent backache, often described as lumbago, is a secondary and frequently late feature of osteoporosis and is due in part to progressive vertebral collapse resulting in osteoarthritis. Pain occurs much more rarely in the sternum, pelvis, ribs and long bones; persistent pain elsewhere in the skeleton is not a feature of osteoporosis, but is more characteristic of osteomalacia, Paget's disease or skeletal metastases. Pathological fracture of the neck of the femur is common in senile osteoporosis. Patients with osteoporosis do not show the proximal myopathy which is so common in most cases of severe osteomalacia. The persistent nagging continuous pain in osteomalacia which is due to strain on tender soft bone, contrasts with the intermittent severe attacks of pain followed by periods of improvement which are so characteristic of osteoporosis. Patients with osteoporosis are usually surprisingly well and lack the features of a serious systemic disease.

The most important physical sign in osteoporosis is loss of stature due to shortening of the trunk consequent on vertebral collapse. Later a deformed shrunken thoracic cage may result. Involvement of the long bones will produce obvious signs of deformity secondary to fractures.

Biochemistry and Histology. Plasma calcium, phosphorus and alkaline phosphates levels are normal, hence plasma biochemistry is of value only in the differential diagnosis of osteoporosis from other generalised disorders of bone.

The histological appearance of osteoporotic bone is qualitatively normal in contrast to osteomalacia where there is a failure of mineralisation of bone matrix and evidence of abnormally large amounts of osteoid tissue.

Radiological Appearances. These play an important part in diagnosis. The principal radiological findings are (1) loss of bone density, (2) reduction in number and size of trabeculae, (3) thinning of the bone cortex and (4) changes in shape of the vertebral bodies due to the impaction of fractures of the brittle bones. These occur at irregular time intervals and have an irregular distribution. The vertebral bodies first become biconcave at the upper and lower surfaces. Later collapse of whole vertebrae produces a wedge-shaped appearance. In contrast, all the vertebrae in osteomalacia. being softer than normal, are uniformly involved so that there is an increase in the size of the intervertebral disc spaces with biconcavity of all vertebral bodies, while wedging of vertebrae is very uncommon. Radiological evidence of osteoporosis may be found in other bones as well as the spine. Thinning of the cortex is the most important sign.

Differential Diagnosis. See p. 496 for differential diagnosis from osteomalacia.

Treatment. Treatment remains unsatisfactory, especially in those cases in which the cause is uncertain or unknown. All that can be expected is an arrest of the progress of the disease. The most favoured method of treatment at the present time is either the prescription of sex hormones or the administration of a high intake of calcium. The value of treatment with strontium or fluoride is much more doubtful. The natural history of the disease makes it difficult to evaluate any method of treatment because the patient often seeks medical advice on account of pain resulting from a fracture and this spontaneously remits following rest. Any drug prescribed at that time is likely to be given the credit for achieving this result.

If treatment with sex hormones is advised for women because of pain and frequency of fractures, stilboestrol is recommended in a dose of 1-3 mg. a day for courses of four to five weeks with intervals of one week between courses.

For senile osteoporosis in males methyltestosterone may be given continuously in a dose of 25-50 mg. a day sublingually. Both are often followed by relief of pain; whether they have any effect on the mineralisation of bone is uncertain. It is also advisable to make sure that the dietary intake of calcium and vitamin D is satisfactory.

Anabolic agents such as norethandrolone (Nilevar) or nandrolone phenylpropionate (Durabolin) have also been recommended for the relief of pain and as a source of well being. Their value for these purposes is doubtful and the mechanism by which they achieve such effects is far from clear.

For those who believe that a marked improvement in the calcium balance can be obtained by dietary means, a high calcium intake, supplemented with large amounts of calcium, is advised (calcium lactate 5 g. or 2 calcium effervescent tablets three times a day). In addition, to ensure adequate absorption, a physiological dose of vitamin D (p. 491) should be prescribed.

It is essential to get the patient up and about as much as possible. Fortunately the majority of osteoporotic fractures do not require to be treated by prolonged bed rest or immobilisation which might aggravate their bone atrophy. If there is much backache a light spinal brace may help. Whatever one's views about the aetiology of the disease, a good mixed diet is desirable. One pint of milk, which will provide 20 g. of protein and 700 mg. of calcium, should be given daily.

Prognosis. Despite the disappointing effects of all forms of treatment the prognosis for length of life is good and few persons die of the disease. Most patients keep well despite intermittent attacks of severe pain due to fractures or chronic pain from secondary osteoarthritis. Many patients, particularly in the younger age groups, pass through a phase lasting several years in which several fractures may occur, but subsequently stabilise and have little further trouble.

Prevention. Since the cause of osteoporosis is uncertain and since demineralisation of the skeleton is known to begin at the age of 20 although symptoms may not appear for many years, its prevention is obviously a formidable task. An active life and a well-balanced diet containing a pint of milk daily to ensure an adequate intake of protein and calcium, are certainly worthwhile preventive measures. It is most important that middle-aged and elderly persons with chronic diseases do not allow their ill-health to immobilise them. All such patients must be encouraged to take exercise as much as their disability permits.

A programme of hormonal prophylaxis which would have to be continued over decades in apparently healthy people is impractical.

VITAMIN K AND RELATED SUBSTANCES

Vitamin K is required for the formation in the liver of prothrombin, which is necessary for the normal clotting of blood. It exists in nature in two forms, vitamin K_1 and vitamin K_2. Since the latter is not important in medical practice it need not be discussed further. Vitamin K is an essential factor in the formation of prothrombin in the liver. It can be synthesised by bacteria in the gut and it also occurs in various vegetables.

Natural vitamin K_1 is a yellow oil, soluble in fat solvents, but only slightly in water.

Dietary Sources. Vitamin K is present in fresh dark-green vegetables, such as kale, spinach, nettles and lucerne. Cauliflower is a good source and also extract of pine needles. All foods of animal origin, including fish-liver oils, are poor sources unless they have undergone extensive bacterial putrefaction. Fortunately, however, there are no indications for prescribing a diet rich in vitamin K.

Therapeutic Uses. Vitamin K is indicated for the following purposes: (1) In bleeding diseases of the newborn (p. 667); (2) in biliary obstruction and fistula (p. 667); (3) in malabsorption (p. 939); and (4) in anticoagulant therapy (p. 668).

ASCORBIC ACID—VITAMIN C

Chemistry and Physiological Action. Ascorbic acid (AA) is a simple sugar. It is the most active reducing agent found in living tissues and is easily and reversibly oxidised to dehydroascorbic acid (DHA). Its highest concentration in the body is in the adrenal cortex (from which it was first isolated). Burns and severe injuries lead to a loss of ascorbic acid from the cortex, as does the injection of corticotrophin. Ascorbic acid is catabolised excessively in rheumatoid arthritis and some infections. The presumption therefore is that ascorbic acid is intimately concerned in bodily reactions to stress, though in a manner as yet obscure.

Ascorbic acid is a white crystalline substance, stable, when dry, in air and light. It is very easily destroyed by (1) heat, (2) alkalis, (3) traces of copper, (4) an oxidase liberated by damage to plant tissues. It is very soluble in water. For these reasons many traditional methods of cooking reduce or completely eliminate it from the diet. A satisfactory daily allowance is 30 mg.

Dietary Sources. Ascorbic acid is present in insignificant amounts in foods of animal origin. Especially good sources are: blackcurrants, oranges, tomatoes, brussels sprouts, watercress and extracts of rose hips and pine needles. The importance of a particular food as a source of a vitamin depends on the amount eaten. Thus in Britain potatoes are more important than watercress even though they have a much lower content of vitamin C.

Pathology of Ascorbic Acid Deficiency. Ascorbic acid deficiency results in defective formation of collagen in connective tissue, defective intercellular cement, defective dentine in teeth, and defective osteoid tissue in bone. Capillary haemorrhages, delayed healing of wounds and (during growth) defective formation of teeth and bones result. In adults the teeth may become loose. Anaemia may be a prominent feature of scurvy (p. 628).

Scurvy

History and Epidemiology. In 1497 Vasco da Gama sailed round the Cape of Good Hope and established a trading centre on the Malabar coast. Scurvy broke out among his crew on the voyage and 100 out of his 160 men died. For the next 300 years scurvy was a major factor determining the success or failure of all sea ventures.

In 1753 Lind, a Scots naval surgeon, published *A Treatise of the Scurvy*, in which he showed by a carefully controlled clinical experiment not only that the disease could be cured by fresh oranges and lemons but that it could be prevented by adequate dietary and other hygienic measures.

Although scurvy ceased to be an important disease of sailors, it continued to afflict the garrisons and civil populations of besieged towns and those confined to prisons. It also developed in another section of the community, namely infants fed on preserved and artificial milks. These provided an adequate substitute for the protein, fat and carbohydrate in human milk but contained little or no ascorbic acid, so scurvy in infants became an important disease. The hey-day of infantile scurvy was in the last 20 years of the nineteenth century. At a later date, cases of scurvy used to arise among adult patients treated for peptic ulcer by severe and prolonged dietary restriction. When knowledge of the importance of the vitamin was established early in this century scurvy soon became a rare disease in Britain and other highly developed countries. It still occurs however as a result of ignorance, poverty and maternal neglect as is clearly indicated by recent reports from Australia, Canada and the U.S.A. Sporadic cases of the disease continue to arise, though chiefly at the other extreme of age, amongst old people, especially males. There are now in our cities an increasing number of old people who live alone and have neither the opportunity nor the aptitude to feed themselves properly; accordingly they sometimes develop scurvy. The social problem of ensuring the satisfactory nutrition of old and solitary people has yet to be solved.

Scurvy appears to be a rare disease in infants and children in most subtropical and tropical countries. It is more likely to occur in arid regions of the world in times of drought, as in Arabia and parts of India for instance, after a failure of the monsoon rains.

Aetiology. Scurvy results from the prolonged consumption of a diet devoid of fresh fruit and vegetables. The principal deficiency in such a diet is the lack of ascorbic acid which is responsible for the characteristic features of the disease. Nevertheless such diets are likely to be deficient also in other nutrients such as iron, vitamin A and sometimes protein. Thus, although ascorbic acid will relieve the predominant signs of the disease, it does not always cure the patient.

Clinical Features. The best clinical account of scurvy is that given in 1753 by Lind who had greater experience of the disease than any modern physician and described his observations with the clarity and elegance characteristic of his time. He said that the pathognomonic sign of the disease was the appearance of the gums, and certainly the characteristic gingivitis often first suggests the diagnosis. The gums are swollen, particularly in the region of the papillae between the teeth, sometimes producing the appearance of 'scurvy buds'. These may be so extensive that they project beyond the biting surface of the teeth and almost completely conceal them. The swollen gums are livid in colour and bleed on the slightest touch. There is always some infection; indeed this seems necessary for the production of the scorbutic gingival appearances since human volunteers suffering from ascorbic acid deficiency did not develop it if their gums were previously healthy. Associated with the infection there is a strikingly offensive foetor. In patients without teeth the gums appear normal.

The first sign of cutaneous bleeding is often to be found on the lower thighs, just above the knees. These haemorrhages are *perifollicular*—tiny points of bleeding around the orifice of a hair follicle. For some time beforehand the follicle can be seen to be raised above the general surface of the skin, giving the appearance of *folliculosis*, which is quite commonly seen in varying degrees in people apparently well supplied with ascorbic acid. The condition in scurvy can be distinguished by its appearance from the *follicular keratosis* sometimes associated with vitamin A deficiency. In the latter condition there is usually a horny plug of keratin projecting from the orifice of the hair follicle. In scurvy there is a heaping-up of keratin-like material on the surface around the mouth of the follicle, through which a deformed 'corkscrew' hair characteristically projects. Such perifollicular haemorrhages may subsequently appear on the buttocks, abdomen, legs and arms; they are often followed by petechial haemorrhages, developing independently of the hair follicles, due to rupture of capillary vessels. Such purpuric spots are usually first seen on the feet and ankles. Thereafter large spontaneous bruises (ecchymoses) may arise almost anywhere in the body, but usually first in the lower extremities, producing the characteristic 'woody leg'.

Before the changes in the gums and skin appear, the patient has usually felt feeble and listless for some weeks or months. If hard work is expected of him, he may have been suspected of malingering, through absence of clinical signs suggesting disease. Unlike pellagra, in scurvy there is usually no loss of weight through subnutrition.

By the time the disease is fully developed the patient is often anaemic (p. 628). In a large series of cases, about one-third had severe anaemia, a third moderate anaemia, and the remaining third no anaemia at all.

Examination of an adult patient with scurvy usually reveals no abnormal physical signs of disease except gingivitis and cutaneous haemorrhages and hence the gravity of his condition may not be appreciated. Yet in fact he may die suddenly and without warning, apparently from cardiac failure. Lind himself described how a sailor afflicted with scurvy fell dead while working at a windlass.

The main clinical features of infantile scurvy are lassitude, anaemia, painful limbs and enlargement of the costochondral junctions.

Until the teeth have erupted, scorbutic infants do not develop gingivitis. When this occurs the gums have the classical appearance of 'scurvy buds' (p. 506), a feature of considerable diagnostic importance. The first sign of bleeding is usually a large subperiosteal haemorrhage immediately overlying one of the long bones—frequently the femur—producing the characteristic 'frog-legs' position. This gives rise to intense pain, especially on movement. The infant may cry continuously and agonisingly, and scream even louder when lifted.

Diagnosis. The distinctive appearance of the gums must be distinguished from other causes of gingivitis, the most common of which is periodontal disease (pyorrhoea alveolaris). In this disorder there are usually accumulations of tartar on the teeth, with retraction of the gum margin. The inflamed rim of the gums is bright red in colour, in contrast to the cyanotic appearance in scurvy, and there is usually much less swelling. In Vincent's angina the gums are acutely inflamed, ulcerated and painful, but here again the bright red appearance of the lesions is distinctive. Poisoning with heavy metals, particularly lead and mercury, produces a gingivitis in which the gum margin is stained blue; but there is usually little swelling and the appearance is easily distinguished from scurvy. Hydantoin derivatives used in the treatment of epilepsy may cause marked swelling and hypertrophy of the gums, but they preserve their normal colour and do not bleed.

The perifollicular haemorrhages of scurvy are distinctive in appearance. But if only petechiae are visible, other causes of purpura must be excluded, e.g. blood dyscrasias, drug poisoning or prothrombin deficiency. If ecchymoses are the chief manifestation, the patient may be seen first by a surgeon, on the suspicion of some undisclosed traumatic accident.

Scurvy in infants and children may sometimes be mistaken for rheumatic fever or osteomyelitis, because of the pain caused by a subperiosteal haemorrhage in immediate relation to one of the long bones. The refusal of the child to use one leg may cause the disease to be mistaken for poliomyelitis.

The dietary and social history is invaluable in establishing the diagnosis in doubtful cases. Old solitary people may insist that they fend very well for themselves, but careful questioning will reveal that they do not bother to purchase fresh fruit or vegetables. In other instances the proper foods may be purchased but they are so badly cooked that in fact the diet is made scorbutic.

Special Investigations. Capillary fragility, as shown by the Hess test, may be increased, but this is not a specific test for scurvy; it may be positive in any of the many states in which capillary fragility is greater than normal.

Ascorbic acid can be estimated with relative ease either in blood plasma or whole blood. This is useful only in excluding the diagnosis since, if any measurable amount of ascorbic acid can be detected in the blood, the case is not one of scurvy. The absence of detectable ascorbic acid, however, does not necessarily indicate that the patient has scurvy, since the blood level of the vitamin falls to unmeasurable levels long before the disease develops.

A better index of the body reserves of the vitamin is its concentration in the white blood corpuscles. If none can be measured, the diagnosis of scurvy is practically certain.

Treatment. Because of the danger of sudden death, synthetic ascorbic acid should be given at once in adequate amounts. Parenteral treatment has no advantage over oral administration. The aim should be to saturate the body with ascorbic acid with as little delay as possible. The fully saturated body contains about 5 g. of the vitamin, so that a dose of 250 mg. by mouth four times daily should achieve this within a week, despite a considerable loss in the urine which quickly follows each dose.

Scurvy sometimes occurs among people far removed from supplies of synthetic ascorbic acid (e.g. among prisoners of war); in such situations valuable therapeutic effects are obtained by the use of natural sources of the vitamin such as fresh fruit and vegetables, sprouting peas or extract of pine needles (p. 510).

Once the danger of sudden death is averted, attention should be paid to correcting the general deficiencies of the patient's former diet. A liberal diet, including fresh fruit and as much properly cooked vegetables as are available and the patient will accept, should be given. If the patient is anaemic, ferrous sulphate tablets by mouth are indicated.

Finally the doctor must do what he can to correct the social, agricultural and economic circumstances that originally deprived his patient of foods providing ascorbic acid.

Prognosis. With adequate treatment no patient dies of scurvy and recovery is usually rapid and complete.

Prevention. It has already been said that in Britain at least, scurvy tends to occur at the two extremes of age: infancy and old age. The prevention of scurvy in infants has been accomplished by the better education of mothers and helped by the distribution of cheap, concentrated orange juice of standard ascorbic acid content, through the Welfare Food Service. Fruit juice should be given, especially to bottle-fed infants, for the first two years of life.

So far, however, the Welfare State has failed to find any simple administrative means of preventing scurvy among the old and solitary, who are largely unresponsive to education. Should the physician be unsuccessful in achieving the dietetic aims discussed above, he should at least insist on the patient taking one 25 mg. tablet of synthetic ascorbic acid daily. Alternatively a massive dose can be given at longer intervals—say 0.5 g. on the first day of every month. This method is justified only by the fact that patients who are careless about diet are nearly always defaulters when daily medication is called for.

Special provision against scurvy is desirable for any group of people living on packed, preserved rations for any length of time such as the explorers of inaccessible lands and oceans, or armed forces defending a barren territory. Synthetic ascorbic acid tablets are invaluable under such conditions. In default of such supplies antiscorbutic remedies can often be prepared from green herbs on the spot. Scurvy grass (*Cochleatia officinalis*), which grows on seashores, and infusions of pine or spruce needles are traditional remedies.

In times of drought and famine when fresh vegetables are not available many lives have been saved, particularly in India, by the organised distribution of sprouting peas and beans. The germination is produced by spreading the dried pulses under wet cloths.

THIAMINE (VITAMIN B_1, ANEURINE)

Chemistry and Physiology Action. Thiamine hydrochloride is a white crystalline substance which is readily soluble in water but not in most fat solvents nor in fats. It is specially concerned with a stage in the breakdown of carbohydrate, namely the removal of pyruvic acid. Since the energy requirements of the brain and the nerves are derived solely from the oxidation of carbohydrate, a deficiency of thiamine rapidly leads to a biochemical lesion in the nervous system of experimental animals and in human beings.

Dietary Sources. Peas, beans and other pulses, the germ of cereals and in addition yeast, are the only rich sources. All green vegetables, roots, fruits, flesh foods and dairy produce (except butter) contain significant amounts of the vitamin, but none are rich sources. As the vitamin is not soluble in fats, it is not found in butter or in any separated vegetable or animal oil. In the refining of sugar and many cereal products (wheat, millet, rice) nearly all the naturally occurring vitamin may be removed; there is also none in distilled spirits. Rich sources of thiamine used in the treatment of beriberi are dried brewer's yeast, yeast extract (Marmite) and the bran of rice and wheat.

As thiamine is readily soluble in water, considerable amounts may be lost when vegetables are cooked in an excess of water which is afterwards discarded. It is relatively stable to temperatures up to boiling point, provided that the medium is slightly acid, as in baking with yeast. But if baking powder is used, or if soda is added in the cooking of vegetables, almost all the vitamin may be destroyed. The loss of thiamine in the cooking of an ordinary mixed diet is usually about 25 per cent. Modern processes for freezing, canning and dehydrating food result in only small losses. Unlike vitamin A, thiamine is not stored in the body to any appreciable extent; hence symptoms due to deficiency may develop within a few weeks.

Therapeutic Uses. Thiamine is life-saving in the treatment of cardiovascular and infantile beriberi and Wernicke's encephalopathy as discussed below. It may be given, though without expectation of dramatic results, in cases of nutritional neuropathy. There is no reliable evidence that it is useful in any other disorder of the nervous system. The value of synthetic thiamine, either alone or in combination with other vitamins, as a general tonic or appetiser, is supported by no good scientific evidence.

BERIBERI

Beriberi is a nutritional disorder encountered especially in South and East Asia where it still constitutes a public health problem. The frequency with which absence of knee jerks and the presence of tenderness of the calf muscles has been noted in nutritional surveys undertaken in regions where the disease is endemic, suggests that a mild to moderate deficiency of thiamine is common. Beriberi is caused by eating diets in which most of the calories are derived from highly milled rice. The disorder is often precipitated by infections, hard physical labour or pregnancy and lactation. The clinical picture usually suggests the presence of a multiple nutritional disorder, although lack of thiamine produces the predominant clinical changes.

Three forms are described: (1) wet beriberi in which oedema and cardiac failure occur, (2) dry beriberi, a nutritional polyneuropathy, and (3) infantile beriberi. Thiamine promptly relieves the oedema and circulatory distress, but has no clear-cut effect on the neuropathy (p. 519). Wet and dry beriberi differ greatly in their clinical features, yet they are closely associated epidemiologically. Though caused by the same types of diet, the biochemical lesions responsible may differ in degree or in kind.

History and Aetiology. A Japanese naval surgeon, Takaki was the first to demonstrate that beriberi is essentially a nutritional disease arising when the proportion of polished rice in the diet is excessive. By replacing part of the rice in the ration by wheaten bread and by increasing the allowance of vegetables and milk the disease was eliminated from the Japanese Navy.

Further observations in the Far East also showed that beriberi was associated with the consumption of rice that had been polished (highly milled) in the raw state and that it could be prevented either by adding other foods, as Takaki had done, or by substituting parboiled rice for highly milled rice. A striking example of the disease afflicting wheat-eaters occurred in 1916 when the 3rd Indian Division was besieged by the Turks at Kut-el-Amara. During the siege the Indian sepoys ate whole-wheat chapattis and did not develop beriberi. The British troops ate white bread made from refined wheat flour and beriberi broke out amongst them.

Chemical Pathology. Owing to a lack of thiamine carbohydrates are incompletely metabolised and there is an accumulation of lactic acid and pyruvic acid in the tissues and body fluids. The local accumulation of these metabolites causes dilatation of peripheral blood vessels, as in normal subjects. In beriberi this vasodilatation may be extreme, so that fluid leaks out through the capillaries, producing oedema. At the same time the blood flows rapidly through the dilated peripheral circulation. The heart, which is already embarrassed through lack of thiamine needed for the normal metabolism of carbohydrate in the heart muscle, dilates and eventually a 'high output' type of congestive heart failure results, which further accentuates the oedema. Sudden death may result from acute myocardial exhaustion.

In dry beriberi these biochemical changes have seldom been reported and the level of blood pyruvate is usually within normal limits.

Morbid Anatomy. In wet beriberi the heart at autopsy is found greatly dilated, especially on the right side; there is general oedema of the tissues and serous effusions into the body cavities, often most marked in the pericardium. Microscopic examination usually shows loss of striation of myocardial fibres, which are also finely vacuolated and often fragmented and separated by oedema.

In dry beriberi there is severe wasting of soft tissues. In long-standing cases there is degeneration and demyelination of both sensory and motor nerves. The vagus and other autonomic nerves may be affected. Degenerative changes both in the tracts and in grey matter of the cord are found, but these are usually not so marked as in the peripheral nerves.

Clinical Features. The *early* symptoms and signs are common to wet and dry beriberi. The onset is usually insidious, though sometimes precipitated by unwonted exertion or a minor febrile illness. At first there is anorexia and ill-defined malaise, associated with heaviness and weakness of the legs. This may cause some difficulty in walking. There may be a little oedema of the legs or face and the patient may complain of precordial pain and palpitations. The pulse is usually full and moderately increased in rate. There may be complaints of 'pins and needles' and numbness in the legs. The tendon jerks are usually sluggish, and the calf muscles may be slightly tender on pressure. Hypo-aesthesia or anaesthesia of the skin, especially over the tibiae, is common. Such a condition may persist for months or even years with only minor alterations in the symptoms. In areas where beriberi is endemic it is often extremely common. The patients are only mildly incapacitated and many continue to earn their living even as manual labourers, but at a very low level of efficiency. At any time this chronic malady may develop into either of the severe forms.

Wet Beriberi

The patient often appears well fed. Wet beriberi seldom occurs in underfed people. A diet relatively sufficient in calories and carbohydrate and lacking in thiamine is the essential cause. Oedema is the most notable feature which may develop very rapidly and involve not only the legs but also the face, trunk and serous cavities. Palpitations and breathlessness are marked. There may be pain in the legs after walking. This pain is probably due to the accumulation of lactic acid and other carbohydrate catabolites. It is similar to that which occurs physiologically in the muscles of a runner and pathologically as a result of an insufficient blood supply as occurs in angina pectoris and intermittent claudication. The veins of the neck become distended and show visible pulsations. The apex beat of the heart is displaced outwards. In the arteries there is often a lowered diastolic pressure and a proportionally higher systolic pressure. The pulse is generally fast and bounding as in aortic regurgitation.

If the circulation is well maintained, the skin is warm to the touch owing to the associated vasodilation: when the heart begins to fail it becomes cold and cyanotic, particularly on the face. Electrocardiograms show no consistent changes. The volume of the urine is diminished, but there is no albuminuria. The mind is usually clear. The patient is constantly in danger of a sudden increase in the oedema, and acute circulatory failure, extreme dyspnoea and death.

Dry Beriberi

The essential feature is a polyneuropathy (p. 519). The early symptoms and signs are described on p. 512. The muscles become progressively more wasted and weak, and walking becomes increasingly difficult. The thin, even emaciated patient needs at first one stick, then two, and may finally become bedridden. The disease is essentially a chronic malady, which may be arrested at any stage by improving the diet. Bedridden patients and those with severe cachexia are very susceptible to infections. When bacillary dysentery or tuberculosis accompanies dry beriberi, a fatal result may rapidly occur unless prompt and efficient treatment is given. Patients with dry beriberi are always liable to a sudden onset of oedema which may be due to a variety of dietary causes, e.g. lack of protein, calories or thiamine.

The older accounts of beriberi record that cerebral manifestations are uncommon. However, amongst the British prisoners of war in Japanese camps, where beriberi was endemic, there were cases of a cerebral disorder, which usually responded quickly to thiamine therapy. This disorder has been called 'cerebral beriberi' or Wernicke's encephalopathy (p. 1215); either designation would appear to be correct.

Infantile Beriberi

This is a special form of beriberi, common in endemic areas. It occurs in breast-fed infants, usually between the second and fifth months. Although the mothers of such infants must have been eating a diet and secreting milk with a low thiamine content, classical signs of beriberi are stated to be absent in 50 per cent. of them. The illness usually starts acutely and is rapidly fatal, from cardiac failure, if not promptly treated; the mother may have noticed that the infant is restless, cries a lot, is passing less urine than normal and shows signs of puffiness. The infant then may suddenly become cyanosed with dyspnoea and tachycardia and die within 24-48 hours. Other serious signs are convulsions and coma. One characteristic sign, usually encountered only in severe cases, is partial or complete aphonia usually preceded by the infant's cry becoming thin with a plaintive whine. In the chronic form a state of marasmus develops due to a general failure of nutrition often associated with anorexia, vomiting and diarrhoea, but there is little evidence of structural disease in the nervous system.

Infantile beriberi remains an important problem, especially in isolated rural areas in South-East Asia. It has been proved that the most important cause of a high death rate in infants between the ages of 2 and 6 months in such areas is beriberi.

Differential Diagnosis. In endemic areas the diagnosis is usually not difficult.

In mild and chronic cases there may be few or no physical signs and the diagnosis may have to depend on the interpretation of symptoms and the dietary history, often inaccurately described. In prisons and labour forces, such patients may be accused of malingering. The symptoms also closely resemble the manifestations of anxiety states common amongst Europeans.

The oedema of wet beriberi must be distinguished from that associated with hepatic and renal disease and congestive cardiac failure. The hot extremities in cardiac beriberi and the absence of protein in the urine are useful diagnostic points. Famine oedema should seldom be a diagnostic difficulty if a proper dietary history is taken. Wet beriberi and famine oedema seldom occur together in adults.

Cardiovascular beriberi must be distinguished from other causes of high output cardiac failure, notably hyperthyroidism and severe anaemia, both of which may produce many of the same clinical features. In all doubtful cases of wet beriberi the therapeutic response to thiamine will settle the diagnosis.

Cardiovascular beriberi is by no means the only nutritional cause of heart failure. Cardiomyopathies occurring in tropical and subtropical countries may be due to nutritional deficiencies (p. 242).

The features of dry beriberi are sometimes indistinguishable on clinical examination from other forms of nutritional, infective and toxic polyneuropathy (p. 1217). The differential diagnosis is accordingly based on the presence or absence of a history of nutritional deficiency and of such aetiological factors as alcoholism, the ingestion of toxic substances or an infective illness. In endemic areas the disease may be confused with neuritic leprosy.

The diagnosis of infantile beriberi may be difficult. Neither oedema nor paralysis is an early sign and sudden death may occur before either is present. In cases of doubt the presence of minimal signs or symptoms of beriberi in the mother may decide the issue. A history of the sudden death of a previous child between the ages of 2 and 5 months is highly suggestive. In public health practice among a rice-eating community, a rise in death-rate of infants should suggest the possibility that infantile beriberi has become endemic.

Laboratory Diagnosis. The most useful laboratory test is the estimation of pyruvic acid in the blood. The test is made more sensitive if it is carried out after exercise or after the administration of glucose. Since there are other causes of elevated blood pyruvic acid the test is not specific and must be interpreted in connection with an accompanying therapeutic trial.

Treatment

WET BERIBERI. Treatment must be started as soon as the diagnosis is made, because fatal heart failure may occur with great suddenness. Complete rest is essential and thiamine should be given at once to correct the causative biochemical lesion. For a case of average severity thiamine should be given intramuscularly in amounts of 25 mg. daily for three days. In critically ill patients the initial dose should be increased to 50 or even 100 mg. and should be administered intravenously very slowly; a dose of 50 mg. should be given intramuscularly for the next two or three days. Thereafter oral treatment with thiamine should be given in a dose of 10 mg. two or three times a day and continued until convalescence is established.

To ensure that in such a dangerous disorder as cardiovascular beriberi the body's depleted stores of thiamine are rapidly and completely made good, the large doses mentioned above are recommended by many authorities today because the drug is in plentiful supply and is cheap and non-toxic. It is probable that much smaller amounts are adequate since many prisoners-of-war in Malaya during the Second World War responded excellently to a daily dose of thiamine as low as 5 mg. which was all that could be allotted in view of the severe shortage of supply.

The prompt response of a patient with cardiovascular beriberi to thiamine is one of the most dramatic events of medicine. Within a few hours the breathing is easier, the pulse-rate slower, the extremities cooler and a rapid diuresis begins to dispose of the oedema. Within a few days the size of the heart is restored to normal. Muscular pain and tenderness are also dramatically improved.

With relief of the cardiac emergency, the patient may still be incapacitated as a result of other deficiencies in his former diet. These may include protein, vitamin A, nicotinic acid and riboflavine. A good mixed diet with less emphasis on rice is needed. Whole wheat, millet or some other cereal should, if possible, be substituted for part of the rice in the diet. Pulses have a well-deserved reputation for curing and preventing beriberi; 120 g. (4 oz.) of beans or lentils are a useful daily addition to the diet. Any foods of animal origin that are available should be included. The diet can be supplemented usefully by natural sources of the entire vitamin B complex such as yeast or yeast extract, wheat germ or rice polishings. Half an ounce or more of dried yeast daily is a valuable remedy for aiding recovery.

In both wet and dry beriberi, preoccupation with dietary treatment should not divert attention from the necessity of good nursing, management of associated infections, physiotherapy and subsequent rehabilitation.

Dry Beriberi. The treatment of dry beriberi is described on p. 519.

Infantile Beriberi. The simplest way to treat infantile beriberi is via the mother's milk. The mother should receive 10 mg. thiamine hydrochloride twice daily—in severe cases by injection. Thereafter the mother should receive a good diet, supplemented if possible by yeast or rice bran. In addition the infant must be given thiamine. In cases of mild to moderate severity 10 to 20 mg. of thiamine should be given intramuscularly once a day for three days, followed by oral treatment with 5 to 10 mg. of thiamine twice a day for several weeks. For cases critically ill with severe heart failure or convulsions and coma the initial dose of thiamine should be increased to 25 mg. or even 50 mg. given intravenously very slowly. Thereafter treatment is by intramuscular injection followed by oral therapy as described above.

Prevention. In principle this is easy. All that is necessary in endemic areas is to prevent the production of over-milled rice or wheat. In practice, however, there are many difficulties in the control of milling processes and in persuading people to change their customary diet.

Wherever possible, it is desirable to reduce the proportion of rice in the diet and encourage the growth of alternative crops and protective foods. Much can sometimes be done with small gardens properly cultivated. The substitution of parboiled rice for highly milled rice will also greatly reduce the incidence of beriberi. Ignorance of the relative nutritional values of different foods is usually a contributory factor and this can only be overcome by better education.

NUTRITIONAL NEUROPATHIES

It has long been realised that the nervous system is susceptible to damage from dietary causes. This is scarcely surprising since the nutritional welfare of this system is dependent on a finely adjusted mechanism requiring a source of energy derived only from carbohydrate of which it has no immediate store, and a variety of highly complicated enzyme systems which govern and control the use of this energy.

The various nutritional neuropathies arise only when there is either a definite history of a gross defect in the quality or quantity of the food or clear evidence of a digestive disturbance leading to failure of absorption. They are mostly chronic conditions and as such present a strong contrast to the clinical features of certain other nutritional disorders, such as the heart failure of wet beriberi and the haemorrhagic manifestations of scurvy, which usually respond dramatically to treatment with the appropriate vitamin. Nerve cells, however, have limited powers of recovery compared with other cells; hence no sudden or striking diminution of symptoms or signs in any chronic disease of the nervous system with structural changes can be expected to follow dietary or vitamin therapy.

Classification

Group I—where the lesion is predominantly in the peripheral nerves. This group includes:

(*a*) The polyneuropathies of beriberi, alcoholism and pregnancy.

(*b*) The burning feet syndrome.

Group II—where the lesion is predominantly in the central nervous system. This group includes:

(*a*) Wernicke's encephalopathy.

(*b*) Nutritional amblyopia.

(*c*) The cord syndromes—spinal ataxia; spastic paraplegia and lathyrism; vitamin B_{12} neuropathy (subacute combined degeneration of the cord).

Nutritional Polyneuropathy

The polyneuropathy of dry Oriental beriberi is the classic example. It arises from the consumption of a poor diet composed chiefly of polished rice, but is not due to lack of any one single dietary nutrient. Nutritional neuropathies occur most frequently in thin, underfed people. In countries outside the tropics an essentially similar disease occurs not infrequently in chronic alcoholics and rarely during pregnancy when vomiting is a prominent feature, and in the malabsorption syndrome.

These disorders have been described in the past as 'multiple nutritional polyneuritis', but since there is no evidence of an infective or toxic inflammation, the term 'polyneuropathy' is preferable.

The morbid anatomy and clinical features of the polyneuropathy of dry beriberi have already been described (p. 512) and these are similar to those of the polyneuropathies arising from the other causes mentioned above.

Treatment. This demands first, attention to the patient's diet both in quantity and quality. The neurological lesions will not improve until the patient regains his strength, so every effort should be made to restore him to his original body weight. Plenty of protein—milk, eggs, meat, fish—is desirable, supplemented by natural sources of the vitamin B complex—yeast or yeast extract (e.g. Marmite), rice bran or wheat germ. This may be difficult to provide for poor, rice-eating sufferers from beriberi and unacceptable to alcoholic patients with gastritis or pregnant women who have been vomiting after every meal. The physician's art must be adapted to find the best means of supplying the needs of the individual patient.

The value of synthetic thiamine is disputed. There is no satisfactory evidence that its administration has improved in any striking way the objective signs of nutritional polyneuropathy. Nevertheless many physicians prescribe it in the same dosage, given orally, as for wet beriberi.

Burning Feet Syndrome

Outbreaks of this clinical syndrome have occurred in Europe, Central America, Africa and India among people living on very poor diets. It became very troublesome among European prisoners in the Far East during the Second World War.

The earliest symptom is aching, burning or throbbing in the feet. This becomes more intense and is followed by sharp, stabbing, shooting pains, which may spread up as far as the knee like an electric shock, causing excruciating agony. They come on in paroxysms and are usually worse at night. Repeated pain and loss of sleep produce a thin, exhausted, red-eyed, irritable patient.

In contrast to the striking symptoms, objective signs of neuropathy are seldom marked unless the polyneuropathy of beriberi co-exists. The tendon jerks are usually normal but may be exaggerated. In the great majority of cases there is no demonstrable sensory change.

The syndrome results from the prolonged consumption of a diet deficient in protein and the B group of vitamins. Patients who suffer from it may also develop the orogenital syndrome p. 530) or nutritional amblyopia (p. 521), but rarely frank beriberi. Patients improve when given yeast, Marmite, rice polishings, soya beans and other foods rich in the vitamin B complex and a good diet rich in protein.

Wernicke's Encephalopathy

This disease is caused by an acute biochemical lesion in the brain through lack of essential nutrients to maintain normal metabolism. The principal deficiency concerned is almost certainly lack of thiamine. The majority of cases described in Europe and the U.S.A. have been in alcoholics, although it occasionally occurs as a result of carcinoma of the stomach, pregnancy toxaemia, prolonged vomiting, diarrhoea or other causes of gross digestive failure. The syndrome occurred in European prisoners of war in Singapore, associated with outbreaks of beriberi. The clinical features and treatment are discussed on p. 1215.

Nutritional Amblyopia

A progressive failure of vision attributable to a retrobulbar neuropathy occurred amongst prisoners of war in the Far East in the Second World War. Similar amblyopias occasionally occur in beriberi, pellagra, subacute combined degeneration of the spinal cord and the orogenital syndrome. Many cases were reported in Nigeria between 1930 and 1940.

All the patients appear to have had one feature in common, a period of many months on diets grossly deficient in respect of many essential nutrients. It would appear unlikely that a deficiency of any single nutrient or of any constant association of nutrients is responsible.

A typical history is that in over a period of three weeks or so there is a growing inability to see the colours of small objects. A mist obscures the central field of vision and gradually becomes so intense that it becomes impossible to recognise acquaintances. There is usually no pain, but sometimes the eyes smart. Tinnitus, deafness and dizziness—apparently due to associated involvement of the eighth nerve—sometimes coexist. In the Japanese camps no prisoners became completely blind, but several were severely incapacitated.

On examination of the visual fields a central or paracentral scotoma is always present. The visual acuity varies greatly.

When the symptoms are not severe they are relieved rapidly by a good diet supplemented by some natural source of the entire vitamin B complex, but when vision is markedly affected little or no improvement results from any form of treatment.

NUTRITIONAL SYNDROMES INVOLVING THE SPINAL CORD

Spinal Ataxia

Patients who have been living for long periods on diets deficient in the B group of vitamins occasionally develop neurological signs that indicate that the principal lesion is in the posterior columns of the spinal cord, involving particularly proprioceptive sensation. The gait is unsteady and the patient is unable to stand upright without swaying when the eyes are closed (Romberg's test). Vibration sense in the legs is often lost. The condition has been described in association with nutritional amblyopia.

Lesions of the spinal cord sometimes occur in pellagra (p. 526). They appear most often in very chronic cases, late in the disease. The dorsal and lateral columns are often both affected. Probably the essential dietary deficiency is lack of vitamin B_{12}, which occurs only in foods of animal origin or in foods fermented by microorganisms. In other words, the disease may be a form of subacute combined degeneration of the cord, but due to a *direct* dietary deficiency of vitamin B_{12}, in contrast to the *conditioned* deficiency that occurs in Addisonian anaemia. Nutritional spinal ataxia is seldom associated with significant macrocytic anaemia, presumably because a vegetable diet generally supplies sufficient folic acid.

Vitamin B_{12} Neuropathy

(Subacute Combined Degeneration of the Cord—SCD)

This disease is a form of spinal ataxia characterised by degenerative changes in the posterior and lateral columns of the spinal cord occurring usually in association with Addisonian anaemia (p. 621). The essential cause is a deficiency of vitamin B_{12} due either to a failure in absorption of the vitamin or very rarely to a deficiency in the diet. The clinical features and treatment are discussed on pp. 1213-1215.

Spastic Paraplegia

Lathyrism. *Lathyrus sativus* is a drought-resistant pulse, widely grown in parts of Asia, Africa and Southern Europe. If eaten in excessive amounts, it gives rise to lathyrism.

Epidemic lathyrism is essentially a disease of famine since the pulse is only eaten in large quantities when the main crops have failed. It would appear that long periods on an inadequate diet, deficient in calories, proteins and vitamins, predispose to nutritional spastic paraplegia. Plant toxins may be a precipitating factor. There is no evidence to suggest a virus or other infective agent.

The onset is usually sudden and is often preceded by exertion or exposure to cold. Sometimes backache and stiffness of the legs antedate the onset of the paralysis by a few days. The condition is a spastic paralysis of the lower limbs, due to a localised lesion of the lower parts of the pyramidal tracts. The motor nerves to the muscles of the trunk, upper limbs and sphincters are spared. The sensory nervous system is not involved. In severe cases the disease progresses to a paraplegia on flexion, but in mild cases there is only stiffness and weakness of the legs and exaggerated knee and ankle jerks.

There is no specific treatment. All patients need a good diet. Minor cases may make a complete recovery following satisfactory dietary and physical rehabilitation. In most cases the pathological changes are irreversible and, as already stated, the patients readily drift into beggary and become an important social problem.

Other Forms of Spastic Paraplegia. Spastic paraplegia of uncertain origin occurring in adults is not infrequently seen in various parts of Asia and Africa and in Jamaica. Spastic paraplegias, very similar to lathyrism, were reported amongst prisoners of war both in the Far East and in Egypt. The great majority of these patients had never at any time of their life eaten lathyrus, but had subsisted for many months on an inadequate diet. Whether these cases of spastic paraplegia are due directly to dietary deficiency of some food factor or whether they are due to a toxic dietary factor, e.g. 'bush teas', as has been suggested as the cause of a spastic disorder in Jamaica, is still a matter of controversy.

NICOTINIC ACID (NIACIN) AND NICOTINAMIDE

Chemistry and Physiological Action. Nicotinic acid is a simple derivative of pyridine. Its essential activity is concerned with tissue oxidation. Although related chemically to nicotine, it possesses very different physiological properties and is non-toxic, even in large doses. It is a white crystalline substance readily soluble in water and resistant to heat, oxidation and alkalis; it is in fact one of the most stable of the vitamins. Nicotinic acid is synthesised on a large scale commercially.

Dietary Sources. Nicotinic acid is widely distributed in plant and animal foods, but only in relatively small amounts, except in meat (especially the organs), fish, wholemeal cereals and pulses. In a normal Western European diet about half the nicotinic acid content is provided by meat and fish.

Cooking causes little actual destruction of nicotinic acid but considerable amounts may be lost in the cooking water and 'drippings' from cooked meat if these are discarded. In a mixed diet, from 15 to 25 per cent. of the nicotinic acid of the cooked foodstuffs may be lost in this way. Commercial processing and storage of foodstuffs cause little loss.

As a result of the wide distribution of nicotinic acid among foodstuffs and its stability to heat and storage, even a moderately good diet normally contains satisfactory amounts. Yeast and bran are good natural sources of the vitamin, but the removal of the bran in the milling of wheat and rice can reduce their nicotinic acid content to a low level.

PELLAGRA

Pellagra is a nutritional disease endemic among poor peasants who subsist chiefly on maize (Indian corn). The greater part of the nicotinic acid in maize may be in a bound unabsorbable form. Moreover maize is poor in the essential amino acid tryptophan, the 'provitamin' from which nicotinic acid can be synthesised in the body. Pellagra has been called the disease of the three Ds: dermatitis, diarrhoea and dementia.

History and Geographical Distribution. Pellagra is a relatively new disease, unknown to classical and mediaeval physicians, and first described as a clinical entity by Casal in Spain in 1730.

It has occurred all over the world, wherever maize has become the staple cereal. It is still endemic in some countries of the Near East, Africa and South-East Europe and also occurs in India, Asia and Latin America. Isolated cases of pellagra occur among people who are not dependent on maize. It is a well-recognised complication of chronic alcoholism in the U.S.A., though curiously rare among similar patients in Europe. A generation ago it was frequently reported among the inmates of lunatic asylums in Britain. The poor diet given to mental patients at that period, their frequent unwillingness to eat, coupled with recurrent outbreaks of infectious diarrhoea in the asylums, all contributed to its development. Certainly any chronic disease of the gastro-intestinal tract, leading to malabsorption, may result in the development of one or more of the clinical features of the disease.

Chemical Pathology. The metabolic disturbances in the body that produce the clinical features of pellagra result in no easily detectable chemical abnormality in the blood or urine, like the accumulation of pyruvic acid in thiamine deficiency. Examination of the blood may reveal anaemia and hypoproteinaemia, due to the associated dietary deficiencies. The anaemia may be macrocytic or microcytic, depending on the predominant associated deficiency.

Morbid Anatomy. There are no pathognomonic changes to be seen at autopsy, though subsequent microscopic sections of the spinal cord may show the degenerative changes in the posterior and lateral tracts that account for the neurological signs observed in life.

Clinical Features. GENERAL. The patient is often underweight, and presents the general features of subnutrition.

SKIN. The diagnosis is generally first suggested by the appearance of the skin. Characteristically, there is an erythema resembling severe sunburn, appearing symmetrically over the parts of the body exposed to sunlight, especially the backs of the hands, the wrists and forearms, face and neck. Exposure to trauma or mechanical irritation of the skin may also determine the site of the lesion. The skin in the affected areas is at first red and slightly swollen; it itches and burns. In acute cases the skin lesions may progress to vesiculation, cracking, exudation and crusting with ulceration and sometimes secondary infection; but in chronic cases the dermatitis occurs as a roughening and thickening of the skin with dryness, scaling and a brown pigmentation.

DIGESTIVE SYSTEM. Complaints of digestive upset are usual, and diarrhoea is common but not always present. There may be nausea, a burning sensation in the epigastrium and sometimes constipation in chronic cases. These symptoms may be aggravated by the presence of intestinal parasites. The mouth is sore and often shows angular stomatitis and cheilosis (p. 530). The tongue characteristically has a 'raw beef' appearance—red, swollen and painful, though usually without loss of papillae. Secondary infection of the mouth with Vincent's organisms is common. It is probable that a non-infective inflammation extends throughout the gastrointestinal tract and accounts for the diarrhoea; certainly the rectum and anus are frequently inflamed. The diarrhoea is characteristically profuse and watery, sometimes with blood and mucus in the stools, and accompanied by tenesmus.

NERVOUS SYSTEM. In the milder cases the symptoms consist chiefly of weakness, anxiety, depression, irritability and failure of concentration; in severe cases delirium is the most common mental disturbance in the acute form of the disease and amentia in the chronic form. Because of these changes, chronic pellagrins may be admitted to mental hospitals. In chronic cases there may be signs of degenerative changes in the posterior and lateral columns of the spinal cord—decreased sensation to touch and loss of vibration and position sense are often accompanied by hyperaesthesia and paraesthesia in the feet. The loss of position sense may give rise to ataxia. Spasticity and exaggerated tendon reflexes give evidence of involvement of the pyramidal tracts. Alternatively there may be foot-drop, and impairment of tendon reflexes, indicating a peripheral nerve lesion.

Diagnosis. The classical case in an endemic area should present no diagnostic difficulties if a careful dietary and social history is taken and the typical clinical signs are present. It is the occasional case in a non-maize eater that may present difficulties. A variety of erythemas and exfoliative skin lesions may mimic pellagra. The two characteristic features of cutaneous pellagra are its symmetrical distribution, determined by the clothes of the patient and exposure to sunlight, and the therapeutic response to nicotinic acid. A nutritional glossitis identical with the tongue changes seen in pellagra may occur without the other signs of the disease. Pellagra may closely resemble sprue and, if the skin changes are minimal, the distinction between the diseases may be difficult. The neurological signs may sometimes occur without any apparent involvement of the skin and digestive tract. If unexplained delirium or amentia or disease of the peripheral nerves or spinal cord is found in a person who has been taking a poor diet for a prolonged period, the possibility of a pellagrous origin should be remembered.

Treatment. SPECIFIC VITAMIN THERAPY. For quick relief of symptoms nicotinic acid or, preferably, nicotinamide is invaluable.

Nicotinamide is to be preferred, partly for the theoretical reason that it is the form in which the vitamin is actually utilised in the body, but also because it does not cause the unpleasant flushing and burning sensations that often result from taking nicotinic acid. These sensations are harmless and transitory, but may alarm the patient. A suitable dose for either nicotinamide or nicotinic acid is 100 mg. every 4-6 hours by mouth, although a smaller dose is likely to be effective. The vitamin is very rapidly absorbed from the stomach, despite the most severe digestive disorders. There is therefore no indication for giving it parenterally, although preparations can be obtained for this purpose. The immediate response to nicotinamide is usually dramatic; within 24 hours the erythema of the skin diminishes, the tongue becomes paler and less painful and the diarrhoea ceases. Often there is also striking improvement in the patient's mental attitude. Although the three outstanding clinical features usually respond rapidly to nicotinic acid, there are others that respond less readily, or not at all. The improvement in the mental state is sometimes disappointing. The orogenital and spinal cord changes, the anaemia and hypoproteinaemia, which are all recognised features of the syndrome, are clearly due to deficiencies other than that of nicotinic acid. The administration of yeast or yeast extract is a valuable aid to treatment, supplemented if necessary by riboflavine, thiamine and vitamin B_{12}.

Diet. If possible, the food should provide 100 to 150 g. of good protein, supplied by milk, eggs, meat or fish. Plenty of carbohydrate and fat is also desirable, sufficient to provide up to 3,500 Cal./day, to restore the patient to normal weight. The food should be low in roughage at first in order to avoid further irritation to the inflamed intestines and consequent continued diarrhoea. The diet may be poorly tolerated at first, because the mental state of the patient may result in rebellion against the unaccustomed food. Furthermore, the sore mouth may make eating difficult, and extra food may temporarily intensify the diarrhoea.

General Measures. Rest in bed and sedation are necessary for severely ill pellagrins, especially those with marked mental symptoms; they are often troublesome patients, so their behaviour must be tolerated with objective understanding of its cause. If the dermatitis is associated with much crusting or secondary infection, gentle washing with a dilute disinfectant solution is indicated. If the diarrhoea is severe enough to interfere with sleep or to cause electrolyte disturbances, treatment with tincture of opium should be given until it is brought under control with nicotinamide.

Prognosis. In the endemic areas the majority of patients are mild cases, improving in the winter and relapsing with the increased sunshine in the spring. In long standing cases there may be persistent mental, spinal cord and digestive disorders.

Occasionally a fulminating form develops, with fever and severe prostration which may be fatal. In the past most of the deaths arose from secondary infections (notably tuberculosis and dysentery) or from emaciation due to general dietary failure, intensified by the diarrhoea.

Prevention. The remarkable fact that pellagra has vanished from the Southern States of America, whereas before the Second World War it afflicted tens of thousands of poor country folk, demonstrates in a dramatic way that the disease is preventable. Its disappearance has sometimes been attributed to the fortification of bread with nicotinic acid, but this is only one of several factors which have produced this satisfactory result. The most likely reason is the general improvement in the economic state, education and nutrition of the population.

From the standpoint of agricultural policy, it is clearly wise to avoid too much dependence on a single cereal crop, such as maize, or to devote too great an acreage of fertile land to the cultivation of cash-crops, such as cotton or tobacco. Animal husbandry should be encouraged in all areas where pellagra is endemic.

For the medical practitioner in such an area, without direct influence in matters of agricultural policy, the best advice that he can give to his patients is to take as much milk, eggs and meat as they can afford. He will also do well to prescribe yeast extract for the families of his pellagrous patients.

RIBOFLAVINE

Chemistry and Physiological Action. Riboflavine is a yellow crystalline substance slightly soluble in water, but not in fats. Though stable to boiling in acid solution, in alkaline solution it is decomposed by heat. It is also destroyed by exposure to light.

Riboflavine is a constituent of the flavoproteins which are concerned with tissue oxidation.

Dietary Sources. The best sources of riboflavine are liver, beef, mutton, pork and eggs. Milk and green vegetables are moderate sources. It differs from other components of the vitamin B complex in that it occurs in good amounts in dairy produce, but is relatively lacking in cereal grains, especially when highly milled. It is also present in beer. Ordinary methods of cooking do not destroy the vitamin apart from losses that occur when the water in which green vegetables have been boiled is discarded. If foods, especially milk, are left exposed to sunshine, large losses may occur. Particularly good sources of the natural vitamin are yeast extract (e.g. Marmite) and meat extract (e.g. Bovril).

Therapeutic Uses. Synthetic riboflavine, both for oral and parenteral administration, is readily available. Its therapeutic uses and the clinical features of deficiency have been a subject of controversy for many years. There is, however, little doubt on the basis of experimental studies, nutritional surveys and therapeutic trials, that deficiency of riboflavine is of frequent occurrence in underdeveloped countries in many parts of the world. Riboflavine may be tried in cases of corneal vascularisation, angular stomatitis, cheilosis, the orogenital syndrome and nutritional glossitis, as discussed below, and in pellagra and the malabsorption syndrome if there are reasons for thinking that the absorption of riboflavine is impaired.

DISORDERS DUE TO RIBOFLAVINE DEFICIENCY

Corneal Vascularisation

The essential lesion in this condition is an invasion of the normally avascular *cornea* by capillary blood vessels. These vessels cannot be seen with the naked eye, nor with an ordinary hand lens. A slit-lamp microscope in the hands of an experienced observer is needed for positive identification. Small greyish-white opacities may also be seen on the surface of the cornea. The patient usually complains of a burning sensation in the eyes, misty vision, lachrymation and photophobia. Associated with the condition there is often injection of the conjunctiva with dilated blood vessels. Other factors besides lack of riboflavine can produce a keratitis identical in appearance, some of which are unconnected with malnutrition. Corneal vascularisation may be associated with the orogenital syndrome and with keratomalacia (p. 484).

Angular Stomatitis

This is an affection of the skin at the angles of the mouth, characterised by heaping-up of greyish-white sodden epithelium into ridges, giving the appearance of fissures radiating outwards from the mouth. It may extend across the mucocutaneous boundary and produce whitish patches on the mucous membrane lining the cheeks. In differential diagnosis it must be distinguished from other lesions in the same site, notably syphilitic rhagades, herpes labialis and lichen planus.

Angular stomatitis often responds rapidly to large doses of riboflavine. Yet undoubtedly riboflavine deficiency is not always the main cause. Other patients have responded to pyridoxine. Angular stomatitis occurs in association with iron deficiency anaemia and other debilitating diseases. The most common cause in Britain is ill-fitting dentures.

Cheilosis

This is the name given to a zone of red, denuded epithelium at the line of closure of the lips. It is frequently seen in pellagrins and is often associated with angular stomatitis. Both lesions may have a seasonal incidence and only appear during periods of drought and lack of fresh foods; but it is unlikely that lack of any one specific vitamin or other nutrient is usually the sole cause.

Orogenital Syndrome

In this condition, a lesion resembling angular stomatitis (which is always present and a feature of the syndrome) affects other mucocutaneous junctions. Soggy, whitish patches may appear at the outer angles of the eyes, within the ears, at the vulva or prepuce of the penis and around the anus. Associated with these changes there is often corneal vascularisation (p. 529) and a scaly, greasy eczema at the angles of the nose, on the lips, chin and behind the ears. A dry, intensely itching, erythematous eczema, with a well-defined edge, may appear on the genitalia—the scrotum or mons pubis, over the perineum and down the inner sides of the thighs. If this eczema becomes secondarily infected, or invaded by maggots, the results may be terrible. The syndrome caused much distress among British prisoners of war in Japanese hands.

Associated with the above disorders there may be a glossitis of an unusual colour—the magenta tongue.

Treatment. When such disorders are found the first step in treatment is the investigation and correction of any dietary error. Synthetic riboflavine may be tried, e.g. 5 mg. three times a day by mouth. It should always be supplemented with a natural preparation of the vitamin B complex such as yeast extract (Marmite), rice polishings, etc., and a well balanced diet.

PYRIDOXINE (VITAMIN B_6)

Chemistry and Physiological Action. Vitamin B_6 is not a single substance but consists of three closely related chemical compounds with similar physiological actions.

Pyridoxal phosphate is the coenzyme of the enzyme transaminase which plays a decisive part in the metabolism of the amino acids.

Dietary Sources. Vitamin B_6 is widely distributed both in plants and animal tissues which reflects its importance in the metabolism of many kinds of cell. Meat, liver, pulses, egg yolk, vegetables and the outer 'coats' (bran) of cereal grains are all good sources.

DISORDERS DUE TO PYRIDOXINE (VITAMIN B_6) DEFICIENCY

Although pyridoxine plays an important role in the metabolism of amino acids, and although a series of pathological changes in the skin, liver, blood vessels, nervous tissue and bone marrow have been produced experimentally in various animals such as the monkey, dog, pig, rat and chicken, nevertheless disorders due to deficiency of pyridoxine rarely occur in man, and then very seldom as a result of dietary deficiency. Convulsions, which respond to pyridoxine, have been reported to occur in infants on artificial feeds of powdered milk deficient in pyridoxine. In adults dermatitis, cheilosis, glossitis and angular stomatitis have been produced by means of the pyridoxine inhibitor, 4-desoxy-pyridoxine. The peripheral neuritis associated with isoniazid therapy is due to a conditioned pyridoxine deficiency. A hypochromic microcytic anaemia can be produced in pigs by a diet deficient in pyridoxine. During the past few years a small number of well documented cases of hypochromic anaemia have been reported which were refractory to treatment with iron given orally or parenterally, but which responded dramatically to the oral administration of 10 mg. of pyridoxine hydrochloride. Folic acid may also be required. In contrast to the classical case of iron deficiency anaemia, the level of serum iron is normal or high and there is a great increase in stainable iron (sideroblastic anaemia, p. 640). The diagnosis is established by excluding other types of anaemia with high levels of iron in the serum and tissues, e.g. the haemolytic anaemias and especially thalassaemia, and by the therapeutic response to pyridoxine. The mechanism of production of the naturally occurring pyridoxine deficiency anaemia in man is not understood. Neither dietary deficiency nor malabsorption was present in most of the reported cases. It is possible that some defect in the intermediary metabolism of pyridoxine is responsible.

NUTRITIONAL DISORDERS OF THE SKIN, HAIR, NAILS, MOUTH AND EYES

Follicular keratosis (p. 484), folliculosis (p. 506), xeroderma (dryness of the skin, crackled skin, crazy paving skin), pachyderma (elephant skin), atrophy of the skin, pigmentary changes of the skin, tropical ulcers and the orogenital syndrome are disorders of the skin and mucous membranes which are frequently seen in persons subsisting for long periods on unsatisfactory diets. In such individuals there may also be changes in the texture and colour of the hair (p. 464), and the finger nails may be thin, brittle or spoon-shaped (p. 612). Disorders of the eye may also be present (p. 483), and deficiency of nicotinic acid, riboflavine, vitamin B_{12}, folic acid or iron may give rise to a nutritional glossitis and stomatitis. Until more is known about the chemical pathology of the skin, hair, nails and eyes it will continue to be difficult to assess the significance of certain clinical changes in these structures which are not infrequently seen in examination of underfed or malnourished people. Hence it would be unwise always to attribute these disorders solely to dietary deficiency. Undoubtedly exposure to dirt, heat, moisture, trauma and infection can contribute to their causation. The practical importance of these stigmata is that their presence in either an individual or a community should at once draw attention to the diet.

The Anaemia-Preventing Vitamins

Vitamin B_{12}—Cyanocobalamin and Related Substances

Dietary Sources. The cobalamins are present only in foodstuffs of animal origin and in micro-organisms—bacteria and moulds—which alone seem capable of synthesising them and are probably the sole original source. The common vegetables in human diets contain insignificant traces of vitamin B_{12}.

Therapeutic Uses. The cobalamins, given by injection, provides complete and satisfactory treatment in cases of Addisonian pernicious anaemia and certain other megaloblastic anaemias (p. 620). They have also been used as the 'animal' protein factor in farm husbandry for accelerating the growth of pigs and fowls. Controlled trials in malnourished children living on little or no protein in various parts of the world showed that vitamin B_{12} has no beneficial effect on growth or nutrition.

Folic Acid—Pteroylglutamic Acid (PGA) and Related Substances

Dietary Sources. Fresh, dark-green vegetables and liver are the best sources, with other green vegetables, cauliflower and kidney the next best. Beef, fresh fruits, root vegetables and wheaten flour contain a little, whilst milk, eggs and poultry are poor in folic acid. Considerable losses may occur in the process of cooking.

Therapeutic Uses. Pteroylglutamic acid is used in the treatment of nutritional megaloblastic anaemia (p. 625), the megaloblastic anaemias of pregnancy and infancy (p. 627), and in some cases of the malabsorption syndrome (p. 626). It is also of value in the treatment of megaloblastic anaemia complicating haemolytic disease and due to anticonvulsant drugs. A daily dose of 5-10 mg. by mouth is usually sufficient. It should never be used in

Addisonian anaemia because it does not prevent or cure the neurological features of that disease.

NUTRITIONAL ANAEMIAS

The life of a red blood corpuscle is about 120 days. The bone marrow is continually making replacements at a rate which enables the total red cell population to be renewed every three to four months. This renewal requires the daily synthesis of 7-10 g. of haemoglobin and the construction of the corpuscles to carry the pigment. For this synthesis a variety of materials is needed by the bone marrow, particularly certain minerals (especially iron and also copper and cobalt in very small amounts), vitamins (vitamin B_{12}, folic acid, ascorbic acid, pyridoxine) and protein required for the production of the protein portion of the stroma of the red corpuscles and the synthesis of globin. Since these materials must be obtained from food it is not surprising that nutritional anaemias are common wherever the diet is unsatisfactory or when additional demands for nutrients have to be met. The nutritional hypochromic and megaloblastic anaemias are discussed on pp. 612 and 625.

Anaemia due to Subnutrition and Starvation

Patients who have lost weight from a simple insufficiency of food are often mildly anaemic. One effect of weight loss from lack of calories is a smaller red cell population in a normal plasma volume. If the patient has lost 25 per cent. of his normal lean body weight, the haemoglobin concentration in his blood is likely to be 75 per cent. of normal.

Nutritional Anaemia in Tropical Countries

It is certain that anaemia, especially the type due to iron deficiency, is extremely common and causes a vast amount of ill-health and a great loss of working capacity and economic efficiency in all temperate climates even when the economic state of the people is good. In underdeveloped tropical countries nutritional anaemias occur even more frequently and are more severe in degree. The basic causes of the different types of anaemia in tropical countries, their clinical features and their treatment, are similar to those occurring in temperate climates (p. 611). There are, however, certain factors in tropical countries which are not present in temperate climates and which require consideration. Thus, in some tropical countries the demands for iron may be greatly increased by the loss of haemoglobin in the faeces resulting from haemorrhage due to hookworm infection. In addition significant amounts of iron may be lost daily in the sweat and shed epithelial skin cells when work is undertaken in hot climates. When these additional factors operate in persons who are already partaking of diets which may be gravely deficient in iron and protein, it is not surprising that iron deficiency anaemia in tropical countries is both frequent and severe.

The nutritional megaloblastic anaemias of tropical climates are always associated with diets poor in animal protein and rich in carbohydrate, and hence low in vitamin B_{12} and especially in folic acid. The role of *protein malnutrition* in the causation of tropical nutritional anaemia has been extensively studied in the disease kwashiorkor (p. 462). The anaemia is usually moderate in degree and is normocytic or slightly macrocytic with a normoblastic bone marrow. However, when parasitic infections are present, as is frequently the case, or when protein deficiency in the diet is augmented by a failure in protein synthesis by a diseased liver, or when the intake of essential haematinics such as iron, ascorbic acid, vitamin B_{12} and folic acid, is poor, the resultant anaemia in kwashiorkor may be severe in degree and may be of the hypochromic type, the megaloblastic type or a mixed type, giving the peripheral blood picture described as dimorphic. For information about anaemia in the tropics the reader is referred to *Tropical Diseases*, by Wright and Baird, a Supplement to this book.

COMMENT ON VITAMIN DEFICIENCY DISORDERS

Although the presenting clinical features may suggest a predominant deficiency of one particular nutrient, careful search will generally show that others also are lacking. It follows that pure synthetic nutrients, e.g. vitamins, have a limited place in therapy. The first line of treatment is to correct the diet, and to provide extra amounts of the nutrient indicated, especially from natural sources (e.g. cod-liver oil, yeast, fruit juice) which may contain other essential nutrients as yet unknown and still unsynthesised.

The indiscriminate prescribing of synthetic vitamins as general non-specific tonics is poor and slipshod practice. Pills and capsules containing various mixtures of pure synthetic vitamins are no substitute for food. The shot-gun prescription of such preparations is deplorable; for one thing it is unnecessarily expensive; further, it lulls the physician into a complacent sense of having done all that is necessary to safeguard his patient's nutrition.

'Subclinical' Deficiency Disorders. It is often suggested that many people in Britain suffer from 'subclinical' disorders due to deficiency of vitamins in their diet. Vague symptoms of fatigue, lassitude, loss of appetite or irritability are frequently attributed to this cause and treated with vitamin pills. Unfortunately the certain diagnosis of subclinical disorders is difficult and laboratory aids are unhelpful. But if the dietetic and social history is satisfactory, and physical examination provides no evidence of any disorder causing a conditioned deficiency, it is very unlikely that the symptoms are due to a subclinical nutritional disorder. In any case, the proper treatment of such a disorder consists, in the first instance, in helping patients to choose and prepare a better diet. Vitamin pills may bring psychological benefit, but are no substitute for a well-balanced diet.

Vitamins as Drugs. Since pure synthetic vitamins became available there has been an understandable tendency to try them empirically in a great variety of diseases, abandoning all pretence of correcting a non-existing dietary deficiency, but using them with the knowledge that they are biologically active substances and presumably fairly harmless. There is no justification for this attitude, with the exception of giving massive doses of calciferol in the treatment of lupus vulgaris (tuberculosis of the skin).

PREVENTION OF NUTRITIONAL DISORDERS

The medical profession can do little, relatively, towards preventing nutritional disorders. The economic, social and agricultural issues involved are primarily the concern of statesmen, administrators and farmers. In addition, effective national programmes of population control must be evolved in many underdeveloped countries (p. 439).

The problem of the present world shortage of calories is unlikely to be improved except by international action, involving the proper agricultural development of fertile, but at present unproductive, parts of the world and by effective family planning.

At the national level, individual countries that are short of food can do much towards making the best use of their limited supplies by ensuring the equitable distribution of essential foodstuffs through a sound system of rationing, and by preventing black market operations. In Britain, since 1940, there has been a great achievement in making special provision for 'vulnerable groups' (mothers and children). School meals, school milk, a guaranteed milk supply and supplements of cod-liver oil and orange juice for these groups are, without doubt, a most important contribution to the present and future health of the country. Since osteomalacia and minor degrees of scurvy are now known to be much more common in old people than was formerly recognised, especially if they are living alone and are confined to the house by infirmity, it is suggested that they should be classified as a 'vulnerable group' and that a free supplement of cod liver oil and orange juice should be provided by the National Health Service. The fortification of foods, such as the addition of calcium carbonate to bread and of fat-soluble vitamins to margarine, is also a nation-wide contribution to better mutrition. The development of proper Maternity and Child Welfare Services provides a means for better education in sound nutrition.

At the community level, the individual doctor has a chance to help by giving advice to the housewife on what foods to select and how to make the best use of them. In a more general way, doctors have an important responsibility in keeping their patients properly informed about the importance to health of good nutrition. The food policies of the future can be influenced decisively for good, if those responsible for them have a proper understanding of the medical problems involved.

STANLEY DAVIDSON.

Book recommended:

Davidson, Sir Stanley & Passmore, R. (1966). *Human Nutrition and Dietetics* 3rd ed. Edinburgh : Livingstone.

THE CHRONIC RHEUMATIC DISEASES

THE chronic rheumatic diseases differ from each other in regard to aetiology, pathology and clinical course. All of them cause symptoms in relation to the locomotor system, and the term 'rheumatism' has been applied to all conditions causing pain and stiffness of the muscles and joints. The principal members of the group are rheumatoid arthritis, osteoarthritis, ankylosing spondylitis and non-articular rheumatism. Gout is a metabolic disease but is grouped with the chronic rheumatic diseases because the joints are involved. Non-articular rheumatism, so called because no underlying pathology of the joints can be demonstrated in the majority of cases, affects the soft tissues and includes a large number of miscellaneous conditions of obscure aetiology but of great prevalence. The collagen diseases, or diseases of connective tissue, are considered briefly as they not infrequently present with symptoms referable to the muscles or joints.

The chronic rheumatic diseases account for an important proportion of temporary or permanent disablement in temperate climates. These diseases are second only to bronchitis in men and hold first place among women as a reason for seeking medical advice. A survey in 1961 suggested that approximately 1,740,000 of the population of Britain were affected by rheumatoid arthritis, and that some 3,700,000 persons over the age of 65 were disabled by osteoarthritis. From the Ministry of Pensions and National Insurance Digest of Statistics for the year 1953-54 it has been calculated that approximately 730,000 persons claim sickness benefit annually on account of rheumatic complaints, leading to a loss of more than 27,000,000 working days, equivalent to over £32 million in terms of wages. In general practice it has been estimated that about 10 per cent. of practitioners' work is devoted to the diagnosis and treatment of various forms of rheumatism.

RHEUMATOID ARTHRITIS

Definition. Rheumatoid arthritis can be defined as a chronic polyarthritis affecting mainly the more peripheral joints, running a prolonged course with exacerbations and remissions, and accompanied by a general systemic disturbance. The disease is characterised by swelling of the synovial membrane and periarticular tissues, subchondral osteoporosis, erosion of cartilage and bone and wasting of the associated muscles.

Aetiology

1. *Age.* The average age at onset is about 40, but the disease may occur at all ages. It is less common before puberty.
2. *Sex.* Females are affected two to three times as frequently as males.
3. *Climate.* In the past it was believed that the disease was most common in temperate zones and particularly associated with cold and damp. Whilst the incidence is less in tropical countries a recent survey of the population of a subtropical region has shown that rheumatoid arthritis is as common there as in temperate climates, although it tends to be less severe.
4. *Heredity.* Although the influence of heredity is not known, a family history of the disease is not infrequently obtained.
5. *Bodily Constitution.* It is commonly stated that rheumatoid arthritis occurs most often in persons of asthenic build. This is particularly noticeable when the disease starts in women between the ages of 20 and 40, but when the disease starts at a later age constitutional factors are less apparent.
6. *Infection.* It can be stated that rheumatoid arthritis is not due to invasion of the joints by any organism which can be demonstrated regularly by methods available at the present time.

   The belief that foci of infection are important aetiologic factors has largely been discarded. Such foci occur as frequently in the general population as they do in patients with rheumatoid arthritis.

   The presence in the serum of abnormal globulins with the characteristics of antibodies in a high proportion of patients has led to the idea that rheumatoid arthritis may be associated with a derangement of the immune response to exogenous antigens or to antigens derived in part at least from the patient's own tissues. The presence of these antibodies, which can in certain conditions react with material derived from a human source, suggests that they may play some part in the production of tissue damage, although there is as yet no direct evidence in support of this hypothesis.

7. *Endocrine Factors.* It has been suggested that rheumatoid arthritis may arise as a result of an abnormal response to stress, characterised by the production of a relative excess of mineralocorticoid hormones by the adrenal glands. This view has received no support from studies of the output of aldosterone, the main naturally-occurring, salt-retaining hormone. No other abnormality of pituitary-adrenal function has been demonstrated by the methods available at present. It is now recognised that suppression of the symptoms and signs of inflammation by cortisone, hydrocortisone and their synthetic analogues is non-specific in nature and due to a pharmacological rather than a physiological effect.

8. *Psychological Factors.* Rheumatoid arthritis is sometimes precipitated and often aggravated by emotional disturbances or excessive and long-continued worry and overwork, but the incidence of such psychological factors has been found to be no greater amongst patients with rheumatoid arthritis than it is amongst individuals of similar age, sex and social circumstances who do not suffer from the disease.

9. *Nutrition.* There is no evidence that the dietetic habits of patients suffering from rheumatoid arthritis differ in any way from the normal. The fact that these patients are often underweight is a result rather than a cause of the disease.

In summary, the aetiology of the disease remains obscure, but it may well arise as a result of the interplay of a number of factors, some of which may be genetically determined and others may be of environmental origin.

Pathology. The earliest change is swelling and congestion of the synovial membrane and the overlying connective tissue, which become infiltrated with polymorphs, lymphocytes and macrophages. At this stage the pathological process is still reversible and no permanent damage to the joint has taken place. Subsequently, hypertrophy of the synovial membrane occurs. The external capsular layer becomes thickened. Inflammatory granulation tissue or pannus is formed, which spreads over and under the articular cartilage with patchy destruction of the cartilage. Later fibrous adhesions may form between the layers of pannus across the joint space. The changes are no longer reversible and permanent damage to the joint has taken place. Owing to the irregular contraction of fibrous tissue in the capsule and to the adoption of a position of flexion for the relief of the pain, deformities of alignment develop. Later still, fibrous and even bony ankylosis may occur. In disorganised joints, in which movement is still possible, secondary osteoarthritic changes appear. Effusion of synovial fluid into the joint space takes place during the active phase of the disease. Along with these changes osteoporosis occurs in the parts of the bones adjacent to the joint margins and there is atrophy of associated muscles with round-cell infiltration. Later the osteoporosis becomes generalised. Subcutaneous nodules have a characteristic histological appearance. There is a central area of fibrinoid material consisting of swollen and fragmented collagen fibres, fibrinous exudate and cellular debris, surrounded by a palisade of radially arranged proliferating mononuclear cells. The nodule is surrounded by a loose capsule of fibrous tissue.

Clinical Features. In the majority of cases the onset is insidious. For a period of weeks or months before the joints become involved the patient may complain of tiredness, general malaise, fatigue, numbness and tingling in the extremities, loss of weight, vasomotor disturbances and general debility. Not infrequently there is transient articular or muscular pain. In less than 10 per cent. of cases the onset may be acute with fever and rapid involvement of many joints. In the typical case the small joints of the fingers and toes are the first to become affected. As the disease progresses it spreads to involve the wrists, elbows, shoulders, ankles and knees. Only in more severe cases are the hips affected. The temporo-mandibular and sternoclavicular joints are not infrequently involved. Muscular stiffness is a prominent symptom, and it is particularly marked in the morning or after periods of inactivity. It is frequently present before the joints become affected. Swelling of the proximal interphalangeal joints gives rise to the typical spindled appearance of the fingers. As the disease progresses, joint pain and swelling increase and muscular stiffness becomes more marked. Muscular atrophy takes place early and becomes a very prominent feature. During the active stage of the disease signs of a systemic disturbance are present. Low-grade pyrexia, tachycardia, hypochromic anaemia, mild polymorph leucocytosis, raised erythrocyte sedimentation rate (ESR) and altered plasma protein pattern (increased globulin and fibrinogen; decreased albumin) are commonly found. In more advanced cases pain and muscle spasm give rise to flexion deformities in the joints. At first these deformities are correctable, but later permanent contractures develop and the joints may become completely disorganised. The characteristic deformity in the hands is anterior subluxation of the metacarpophalangeal joints and ulnar deviation of the fingers.

In the early phase the disease is characterised by remissions and relapses. At this time radiological examination of the affected joints will show only demineralisation of the bone ends. Later, as the pathological process progresses to involve the articular cartilage, there is narrowing of the joint space and marginal erosions appear. In the late stages, in joints which are still capable of some movement, radiological examination will show the appearance of osteoarthritis, which arises as a secondary manifestation in the damaged joints. In joints which have been immobilised by pain and muscular spasm, fibrous or bony ankylosis may take place. Subcutaneous nodules appear in from 10 to 20 per cent. of patients. The most common site is the extensor surface of the forearm about 1 or 2 inches below the elbow joint. They may also occur over the patella, scapula, sacrum, scalp and along the tendons of the fingers and toes. In severe cases amyloidosis may complicate the later stages of the disease.

Diagnosis. In the average case of rheumatoid arthritis there is usually little difficulty in reaching a diagnosis, but when the disease starts in an atypical manner it will have to be distinguished from the following conditions:

1. *Rheumatic Fever*. In rheumatic fever the joint pain is of a flitting character. The fever is usually higher and spindling of finger joints is rare. Occasionally subacute rheumatic fever may

be difficult to distinguish from rheumatoid arthritis with a febrile onset, but the articular symptoms of rheumatic fever are more likely to be suppressed by full doses of salicylates.

2. *Gonorrhoeal Arthritis.* An acute arthritis with fever may follow a gonorrhoeal infection, but since the advent of antibiotics this complication has become much less frequent. It can be distinguished from rheumatoid arthritis by a history of urethritis preceding the joint symptoms by two or three weeks. In the majority of cases demonstration of the gonococcus in smears from the urethra, prostate or cervix uteri will confirm the diagnosis. In only about 25 per cent., however, can the gonococcus be cultured from the synovial fluid. The gonococcal complement fixation test is positive in about 80 per cent. of cases.

3. *Reiter's Syndrome.* Reiter's syndrome is characterised by acute urethritis, conjunctivitis and arthritis. The condition may occasionally be difficult to distinguish from rheumatoid arthritis. Urethritis and conjunctivitis, however, are rare complications of rheumatoid arthritis. The joint symptoms in Reiter's syndrome usually clear up completely, but in a small proportion of cases the disease becomes chronic and the radiological changes in the joints may be indistinguishable from those in rheumatoid arthritis.

4. *Acute Pyogenic Arthritis.* Acute pyogenic arthritis is usually monarticular. The joint is acutely inflamed and painful. The signs of a generalised infection, including high fever, are present. Both blood and synovial fluid should be cultured.

5. *Gout.* Gouty arthritis in its earlier stages may be confused with rheumatoid arthritis. In the classical case the first joint to be affected is the metatarso-phalangeal joint of the big toe. The onset is very sudden, the pain extremely acute, but the attack usually clears up completely, leaving no residual changes in the joint. A high blood uric acid will usually be found in this disease. The response to the administration of colchicine is dramatic.

6. *Tuberculous Arthritis.* Tuberculous arthritis may at times be mistaken for rheumatoid arthritis. The onset is insidious. Usually only one joint is involved, but occasionally several are affected. Involvement of three or more joints is a point against the diagnosis of tuberculous arthritis. The condition is most common in children. In adults tuberculosis of the spine is the most common form. The radiological appearances, demonstration of the organisms in the synovial fluid or biopsy of the synovial

membrane will differentiate this condition from rheumatoid arthritis.

7. *Osteoarthritis*. Osteoarthritis usually affects the larger joints such as the knees, hips and spine. In middle-aged women, however, osteoarthritic changes not uncommonly affect the fingers, and care should be taken to distinguish this condition from rheumatoid arthritis. In a typical case Heberden's nodes (p. 561) appear in relationship to the terminal interphalangeal joints. At first these nodes may be painful, but later they subside to leave a firm hard nodule which frequently causes deformity of the distal interphalangeal joint. The ESR is usually within normal limits.

8. *Psoriatic Arthritis*. It is now accepted that an erosive arthritis distinct from rheumatoid arthritis may complicate psoriasis. It is characterised by early involvement of the terminal interphalangeal joints, ridging, thickening, cracking and pitting of the nails, and the absence of subcutaneous nodules. The spine and sacro-iliac joints are not infrequently affected. The sensitised sheep cell test is negative.

In cases of doubt, examination of synovial fluid may provide valuable information. When infection is suspected fluid should be cultured and inoculated into guinea-pigs. In gout, uric acid crystals may be seen on microscopic examination. Fluid from traumatic or degenerative forms of arthritis is clear, viscid, does not clot and contains few cells. In rheumatoid arthritis or pyogenic infection the fluid is of low viscosity, turbid, clots on standing and contains many cells.

Sensitised Sheep Cell Test. A serological test has become available which has proved valuable in the diagnosis of atypical forms of rheumatoid arthritis. It is known as the Rose-Waaler or sensitised sheep cell test and is positive in 65 to 70 per cent. of cases of rheumatoid arthritis. It depends on the presence in the sera of a factor which agglutinates sheep erythrocytes sensitised with anti-sheep cell antibody produced in the rabbit. The test is also positive in 25 to 30 per cent. of patients with disseminated lupus erythematosus and in 15 to 20 per cent. of cases of juvenile rheumatoid arthritis (Still's disease). Latex particles coated with human gamma globulin form the basis of a simplified test (latex fixation test).

Treatment

As the aetiology of the disease is unknown, treatment must be directed towards the relief of symptoms, the improvement of the patient's general health and the conservation and restoration of function in the joints damaged by the disease process.

Acute Phase

1. General Measures. When many joints are swollen and painful and when signs of severe constitutional disturbance, such as fever, anaemia and rapid ESR are present, the patient should be confined to bed until these signs and symptoms begin to subside. This period of general rest may last for several weeks and certain measures must be adopted to prevent unnecessary deterioration in physical efficiency. Attention should be directed to the maintenance of good posture. The mattress should be firm or fracture boards should be inserted beneath it. A firm back rest with the minimum number of pillows should be in position during the day. A roomy cage with a padded footrest should be placed over the legs and feet; pillows behind knees should be forbidden; at night only one firm pillow should be allowed; after the midday meal the patient should spend an hour resting flat with a small pillow under the lumbar spine. A further 15 minutes should be spent in the prone position with a pillow under the abdomen. Foot exercises should be performed daily by all patients confined to bed. The general level of physical efficiency should be maintained by the use of suitable exercises. These exercises are designed to have their effect on the groups of muscles in the thoracic, gluteal and abdominal regions. Rest in bed, by the cessation of weight-bearing on the inflamed joints, will go far towards fulfilling the first principle of treatment—the relief of symptoms, as pain and spasm are largely conditioned by movement and weight-bearing. Most patients in the acute phase of the disease will have lost weight and the diet should be of high caloric value with ample protein. Additional vitamin concentrates have been prescribed although their value is doubtful if a well-balanced diet containing milk, eggs and fruit is eaten. A liberal supply of milk should be given to ensure an adequate intake of calcium and first-class protein.

2. Local Measures. Experience has shown that the correct treatment of the inflamed joints may be of fundamental importance

in controlling both local and systemic symptoms in rheumatoid arthritis. Painful joints should be immobilised in skin-tight plaster of Paris splints. These splints should be maintained in position until the more acute symptoms have subsided. In the past undue emphasis may have been placed on the use of daily active and passive movements at this stage. The symptoms of inflammation subside more quickly if the joints are left at complete rest for a period of one to two weeks. The danger of joints becoming ankylosed if immobilised for any length of time has been exaggerated. The principle of a period of complete rest is of particular importance in the treatment of weight-bearing joints. When pain and swelling have subsided the splints are removed for active non-weight-bearing exercises. The patient should be taught these exercises and instructed to perform them frequently throughout the day. The application of heat before the sessions of exercise is useful in relieving stiffness. When the constitutional symptoms have begun to subside and power has been restored to wasted muscles, the patient is allowed up for increasing periods. Physiotherapy is used to supplement active forms of treatment. Wax baths are beneficial in reducing stiffness in the joints of the hands and feet. Faradic foot baths may be helpful in initiating activity in the intrinsic muscles of the feet. Residual pain may be eased by radiant heat, infra-red rays or short wave diathermy.

Radiotherapy. When all other measures fail to alleviate pain in a single joint radiotherapy may be tried but the results are seldom as good in the peripheral joints in rheumatoid arthritis as they are in the spine in ankylosing spondylitis (p. 555).

Occupational therapy is of considerable value in restoring manual dexterity and conditioning the patient for a return to productive employment.

3. Drugs

Analgesics. Aspirin, undoubtedly the most valuable drug for the control of symptoms, should be given to the limit of the patient's tolerance. The dose will range from 4-6 g. (gr. 60-90) daily. Calcium aspirin should be used when ordinary aspirin is not well tolerated. When pain is severe, tab. codeine. phos. (B.P.) 1 tablet two to three times daily should be prescribed. Aspirin may cause gastro-intestinal bleeding, but rarely in amounts greater than 2-3 ml. daily. Dyspepsia may be troublesome, in which case enteric coated tablets should be prescribed. Paracetamol is less effective in controlling symptoms, but may be used when aspirin is poorly tolerated. The dose is 6-8 g. daily. The long-term use of preparations containing phenacetin should be avoided on account of the danger of renal damage.

Phenylbutazone (Butazolidin) is an effective analgesic but like aspirin it has no curative action. The initial dose should be 200 mg. daily. It may be increased, but should not exceed 600 mg. daily. Toxic effects occur in 20 to 40 per cent. of patients. Most common are nausea, vomiting, skin rashes and oedema due to sodium retention. More serious complications in the form of haematemesis, perforation of peptic ulcers, agranulocytosis, thrombocytopenia, aplasia of the bone marrow, haematuria and anuria have been reported. The drug should only be used when the response to aspirin and the conservative measures described has been unsatisfactory. It should not be prescribed if there is evidence of gastrointestinal, renal or cardiovascular disease.

Oxyphenbutazone (Tanderil) is a derivative of phenylbutazone. It is equally effective and can occasionally be taken by patients intolerant of phenylbutazone. The dose is 300-400 mg. daily.

Indomethacin (Indocid) is claimed to possess powerful anti-inflammatory and analgesic properties. The drug is available in capsules containing 25 mg. The recommended dose is one capsule daily for three to four days, increasing thereafter by one capsule daily until symptoms are controlled. The total daily dose should not exceed 150 mg., the average maintenance dose being 75 to 100 mg. The main side effects are severe headache, vertigo, depression, nausea, vomiting and, more rarely, peptic ulceration and haemorrhage. This drug should be used with caution and be reserved for those patients with no history of dyspepsia who are intolerant of other analgesics.

CORTICOSTEROIDS

Cortisone. In Britain controlled clinical trials were conducted under the auspices of the Medical Research Council, the Nuffield Foundation and the Arthritis and Rheumatism Council, designed to compare the value of cortisone and aspirin in the long-term treatment of the disease. The conclusion was reached that cortisone in tolerable doses was no more effective than aspirin when results were compared at the end of one, two and three years. Its use in rheumatoid arthritis is therefore no longer recommended.

Hydrocortisone (*Cortisol*). Hydrocortisone is the natural hormone secreted by the adrenal gland. It is of particular value for intra-articular injection (p. 549).

Synthetic Corticosteroids. It has been shown that the synthetic corticosteroids produced by alterations in the steroid molecule may be, weight for weight, several times more potent than either cortisone or hydrocortisone. The introduction of a second double bond in the first carbon ring of cortisone produces prednisone. A similar modification of hydrocortisone results in prednisolone. Clinical trials with these new corticosteroids have shown that symptoms can be controlled by daily doses ranging from 5-15 mg. The reduction in dosage as compared with cortisone is not accompanied by a corresponding reduction in the incidence of troublesome side-effects. The incidence of dyspepsia and peptic ulceration may be actually greater.

The results of clinical trials showed that at the end of two and three years patients on prednisolone had maintained a significantly greater degree of improvement in all respects, than patients receiving aspirin or other analgesics and that radiological evidence of progression of arthritis was less. The optimal daily dose of prednisolone is 10 mg. or less. Major side-effects are only likely to occur in patients receiving 20 mg. or more daily. To reduce the incidence of dyspepsia and peptic ulceration the tablets should be crushed and taken along with food. Enteric coated tablets are now available which markedly reduce the incidence of gastric symptoms, and are as effective as uncoated tablets. They are worthy of trial in patients with dyspepsia or a previous history of peptic ulcer.

A number of other synthetic corticosteroids have been produced. Methyl prednisolone and triamcinolone (9α-fluoro-16α-hydroxyprednisolone) are a little more potent than prednisolone on a weight for weight basis, but do not appear to differ in their overall effects. Dexamethasone (9α-fluoro-16α-methylprednisolone) and betamethasone (16α-beta-methyl-9-alpha-fluoro-prednisolone) are the most potent additions to this group of synthetic products. Both are between five and eight times as potent as prednisolone. There is no evidence to date that they have any other advantage. The daily dose should not exceed 2 mg.

These powerful hormones should still be used with great

caution and only in patients who have failed to respond to an adequate trial of more conservative measures and in whom the disease is running a progressive downhill course. They should be used with care in patients with active peptic ulceration, diabetes mellitus, hypertension, or marked osteoporosis. Infections will not be masked by moderate doses, but the additional stress of illness, injury or operation may make necessary a temporary increase in dosage (p. 723). All patients on corticosteroids should carry a card indicating the name of the preparation being used, its daily dose, and the address of the physician or hospital responsible for their supervision. Should withdrawal of corticosteroids become necessary, this must be done very slowly, the dose being reduced by not more than 2·5 mg. weekly of prednisolone or an equivalent amount of other preparations.

Corticotrophin (*ACTH*). Stimulation of the patient's own adrenal gland by the injection of corticotrophin is as effective as the administration of corticosteroids by mouth. Stable, long-acting preparations are available, which need only be injected once daily. Side-effects are similar to those which may complicate treatment with corticosteroids, but fluid retention and hypertension are more common. On the other hand, dyspepsia and peptic ulceration occur less frequently. The initial dose is 20 units daily. In most cases a satisfactory response is maintained by a dose between 20 and 30 units daily. Patients can be taught to inject themselves. It is claimed by the advocates of this form of treatment that a remission of the disease occurs in a significant number of patients (15 of 78 patients in a recent report) which is maintained after the slow withdrawal of the hormone. This can rarely be achieved in patients who have been on oral corticosteroids for any length of time. The disadvantage of daily injection and the development of resistance to the hormone limits the value of corticotrophin, but it may have a place in the treatment of severe and progressive cases who cannot tolerate corticosteroids.

Local Use of Corticosteroids. The intra-articular injection of a suspension of hydrocortisone acetate is followed by a reduction of pain and swelling. Duration of relief varies from a few days to two to three weeks in individual patients, but is worthwhile in over half the cases treated. The dose used varies from 5 mg. in the small joints of the fingers to 50 mg. in the case of the hip or knee.

It has been claimed that delayed absorption from the joint with more prolonged relief of symptoms follows the use of less soluble compounds such as hydrocortisone tertiary butylacetate and prednisolone trimethylacetate but these compounds are more expensive and it is doubtful if their routine use is justified at the present time.

Repeated injections of corticosteroids at short intervals should be avoided, particularly in the case of weight-bearing joints, as rapid deterioration of the radiological appearances have been noted in the absence of a recurrence of symptoms.

Extra-articular lesions can be treated by local injection of the three corticosteroids mentioned above. The method is of value in painful ligamentous attachments, tenosynovitis around the wrist and ankle, and nodules in tendons leading to limitation of movement.

Eye drops of hydrocortisone (1 per cent. solution) are valuable in controlling inflammatory conditions of the eye which occur not infrequently in the more severe cases of rheumatoid arthritis.

Hypnotics. When sleep is disturbed a sedative such as amylobarbitone (amytal), 0·2 g., should be prescribed at night.

Iron. If anaemia is present, it is usually resistant to oral iron, but in the majority of cases improvement follows the administration of iron by intramuscular or intravenous injection. Suitable preparations are now available (p. 617). A total of 2 g. should be given in divided doses over a period of two weeks.

Gold Salts. Gold salts have been used in the treatment of rheumatoid arthritis for over 30 years, but only recently has evidence of their value been provided by the results of a controlled clinical trial conducted under the auspices of the Arthritis and Rheumatism Council. A water-soluble preparation such as Myocrisin, a 50 per cent. solution of sodium aurothiomalate, is recommended. Intramuscular injections are given at weekly intervals. The first four doses are each of 10 mg. If no toxic symptoms appear the dose is raised to 50 mg. and maintained at this level until a total of 1 g. has been given. If signs of activity persist a second course may be given after an interval of three months. It has been suggested that the best effects may be achieved by the continued administration of small maintenance doses of gold after completion of the first course; 50 mg. is given every three to four weeks over a period of many months. Toxic reactions may occur at any time during treatment. Pruritic rashes may precede the development of exfoliative dermatitis.

Thrombocytopenia, agranulocytosis and anaemia may result from depression of bone marrow. Only rarely has evidence of renal or hepatic damage been recorded.

It is essential that all patients receiving injections of gold salts should have the urine and skin examined before each injection. The most important measure, however, is to impress on the patient the necessity of reporting immediately any untoward symptoms appearing during the administration of gold.

TREATMENT OF TOXIC REACTIONS. Dimercaprol (BAL, British Anti-Lewisite) has greatly reduced the danger of toxic reactions. The drug combines with heavy metals to form a stable compound which is rapidly excreted in the urine. Dimercaprol is given by intramuscular injection in doses of 3 mg./kg. body weight every six hours for three to four days. The drug is marketed in 2 ml. ampoules each containing 100 mg. in solution in oil. It should be used if signs of toxicity persist for more than a few days after injections of gold have been stopped. Should agranulocytosis develop, antibiotics should be given in full doses (p. 644). For more severe reactions prednisolone 15-20 mg. daily has proved valuable in controlling symptoms.

Chloroquine and Hydroxychloroquine. The antimalarial drug, mepacrine, was first reported to have a beneficial effect on rheumatoid arthritis in 1951. Since then many reports on the value of chloroquine and hydroxychloroquine in the long-term treatment of rheumatoid arthritis have been published. Some authors claim that a satisfactory response occurs in between 70 and 80 per cent. of patients. The results of controlled trials certainly suggest that these drugs possess some anti-rheumatic effect, but the incidence of side-effects is considerable. Some 50 per cent. of patients experience moderate or mild toxic symptoms including skin rashes, pruritus, gastrointestinal upsets, headache, mental disturbance, and depression of the white cell count. Visual disturbances from deposition of the drug in the cornea may occur, but disappear on its withdrawal. Much more rarely permanent impairment of sight follows the development of retinopathy. Annual examination of the eyes of patients on these drugs should be carried out. The first signs of improvement may not become evident for several weeks. The dose of chloroquine is 200-250 mg. daily. Hydroxychloroquine is claimed to be less toxic and a maintenance dose of 400 mg. daily is recommended.

Treatment of Mild Cases or during Remissions. Many patients suffering from rheumatoid arthritis never become severely incapacitated, as the disease frequently runs a mild subacute course These patients should be under periodic clinical observation Splints should be fitted to the affected joints and always worn at night. Physiotherapy and remedial exercises on an out-patient basis may do a great deal towards maintaining these patients at a good functional level. The measures detailed for the active stage should be started if symptoms become acute.

When the patient cannot return to a former occupation it will be necessary to suggest a change of employment where less strain will be thrown on the damaged joints. Training schemes are available under the auspices of the Ministry of Labour. Rehabilitation and vocational training constitute an essential part of any scheme for the treatment of the chronic rheumatic diseases. It cannot be too strongly emphasised that the attitude of hopeless resignation to rheumatoid arthritis which has been adopted by the lay public and the medical profession is unjustified, since adequate treatment initiated in the early stages enables many patients to return to some form of wage-earning activity. Hopeless crippling can be prevented even in the 25 per cent. of cases running a progressive course.

Surgery. It has become clear that the orthopaedic surgeon, working in collaboration with the physician, has an important contribution to make to treatment. Early clearance of proliferating synovial tissue from tendon sheaths results in relief of pain, improvement in function, and prevention of rupture. Ulnar deviation of the fingers can be corrected and much can be done to relieve pain in the feet. Early synovectomy of both large and small joints appears to arrest the progress of the disease locally for prolonged periods. When deformity is already present much can be done to restore both alignment and function. By a combination of skilled medical and surgical care many severely crippled patients can be restored to a remarkable degree of independence.

Prognosis. Rheumatoid arthritis usually runs a subacute or chronic course over a period of years. Its progress may be interrupted at any stage, so that no patient with rheumatoid arthritis should be considered as being beyond medical aid. In severe cases the disease progresses by a series of exacerbations and remissions. Each acute attack causes further damage to the joints, deformity and disability increase, and the patient may become completely bedridden. Relapses may be precipitated by a variety of factors such as intercurrent infection, cold, damp, worry, overwork, or excessive use of the affected joints. The outlook so far as life is concerned is good. In some 300 patients admitted to hospital over a period of three years and followed up for an average of nine years, 24 per cent. remained fit for all normal activities, 40 per cent. suffered only moderate impairment of function, 26 per cent. were more severely disabled, but only 10 per cent. had become helpless cripples. The earlier treatment is instituted, the better will be the prognosis in the individual case.

Summary

The successful treatment of rheumatoid arthritis depends on the co-ordinated efforts of the physician, orthopaedic surgeon, physiotherapist, occupational therapist and social service worker. The programme of treatment must be co-ordinated to meet the needs of each case. Factors likely to have an adverse influence on the patient must be dealt with, and recommendations as to future activity must be based on an accurate knowledge of functional capacity. These ends can best be achieved in special units devoted to the study and treatment of the chronic rheumatic diseases. Ambulatory patients should be instructed in the use of simple forms of physiotherapy which can be employed at home, such as wax baths, radiant heat lamps, contrast baths, hot fomentations and remedial exercises. Regular attendance at a follow-up clinic is essential if improvement is to be maintained and exacerbations of the disease controlled by appropriate adjustments in treatment.

SJÖGREN'S SYNDROME

Sjögren in 1933 described a group of patients in whom dryness of the eyes and mouth was associated with polyarthritis of the rheumatoid type. Kerato-conjunctivitis sicca develops as a result of reduction in the secretion of tears, and xerostoma follows involvement of the salivary glands. Mucus secreting glands of the upper respiratory and gastro-intestinal tracts are commonly affected, resulting in recurrent respiratory infections and achlorhydria. Not infrequently there is loss of hair and atrophic changes in the nails. The diagnosis depends on the demonstration of diminished lacrymal secretion and the presence of ulcers on the cornea. The sheep cell test is positive in the majority of cases. Treatment is essentially the same as that outlined for rheumatoid arthritis. Topical application of hydrocortisone eye drops (0·5 to 2 per cent) has proved useful in controlling local inflammation in the eye. Artificial tears (methycellulose drops) may also be required in more severe cases and may be combined with sealing of the lacrymal puncta.

STILL'S DISEASE

This is the name applied to a chronic polyarthritis which occurs in children. The clinical and pathological features are the same as those of rheumatoid arthritis, with the addition of enlarged lymph glands and splenomegaly. The disease often runs a progressive course and crippling deformities of the joints are common. The joints of the cervical spine are frequently involved. Skeletal growth may be much retarded. The treatment is that of rheumatoid arthritis. Corticotrophin and cortisone are effective but their use in treatment is limited by the same considerations already discussed in relationship to rheumatoid arthritis (p. 547).

ANKYLOSING SPONDYLITIS

Aetiology. The disease, a progressive inflammatory arthritis of the spinal articulations, affects persons between the ages of 20 and 40. Males are affected about ten times more commonly than females. The victims are often young men of excellent physique. In a small proportion of cases the onset of the disease is said to have been precipitated by an injury to the back. The disease presents many of the features of an infective process. The ESR may be rapid and low-grade pyrexia is not uncommon in the active phase. However, no specific organism has been isolated and the aetiology of the disease is unknown. The sensitised sheep cell test is negative in 80 per cent. of cases.

Pathology. Biopsy material from cases in which the peripheral joints have been affected shows changes similar to those found in rheumatoid arthritis. Bony ankylosis, however, occurs more frequently in ankylosing spondylitis.

Radiological Examination. The earliest changes are seen in the sacro-iliac joints, which show irregularity of the joint margins and osteoporosis. There is an increase in density of the bone adjacent to the joints. Later the sacro-iliac joints become ankylosed and the vertebral ligaments show progressive ossification (bamboo spine).

Clinical Features. The onset is often insidious. A history of repeated attacks of lumbago in a healthy young male should always suggest the possibility of ankylosing spondylitis. Radiological examination of the lumbar spine and sacro-iliac regions should never be omitted in such cases. As the disease progresses there is increasing stiffness of the whole spine. Involvement of the costo-vertebral joints gives rise to marked limitation in chest expansion. In milder cases the spine may become rigid without much deformity. In more severe cases kyphosis involving the cervical, dorsal and lumbar spine is not uncommon. Such patients are severely incapacitated, and if the hips become affected they may be rendered completely helpless. In a small proportion of cases the disease involves the peripheral joints, in which the changes closely resemble those found in rheumatoid arthritis. Iritis occurs in between 25 and 30 per cent. of cases and may occasionally be the first sign of the disease. In 2 per cent. of patients aortic incompetence develops, usually in the later stages of the disease.

Differential Diagnosis. Osteoarthritis of the spine may give rise to pain and limitation of movement. This disease seldom gives rise to symptoms before the age of 50. It is not accompanied by signs of systemic disturbance and the two conditions are readily differentiated by radiological appearances. In osteoarthritis the sacro-iliac joints are rarely involved, the intervertebral spaces are commonly diminished due to degenerative changes in the discs, and exostoses develop at the edges of the vertebral bodies. Another condition to be differentiated from ankylosing spondylitis is protrusion of the nucleus pulposus of an intervertebral disc since both conditions can affect young men and present with backache. Scoliosis and sciatic pain are common in protrusion of intervertebral discs (p. 1223) and rare in ankylosing spondylitis.

Treatment. The treatment of choice in the active phase of ankylosing spondylitis is radiotherapy. In early cases the results are excellent. The disease process is apparently arrested. Even in more advanced cases with fixed deformities much benefit may result. The incidence of leukaemia is significantly increased following radiotherapy (3 per 1,000 cases treated); but in active cases this risk is outweighed by the good results obtained. In all cases exercises for strengthening the spinal muscles and mobilising the costo-vertebral joints should be prescribed. In the more advanced cases a spinal support may be required to maintain reasonable posture. Deformity of the spine may be corrected by the use of serial plaster shells. Where such correction is not possible and where the deformity is marked, spinal osteotomy may allow the patient to regain a reasonable posture. Where the hips have become affected, vitallium cup arthroplasty has proved useful. The general measures described in the treatment of rheumatoid arthritis should be used in the acute phase, but prolonged immobilisation should be avoided. Corticotrophin and corticosteroids are effective in ankylosing spondylitis, but their use in treatment is limited by the same considerations already discussed in relationship to rheumatoid arthritis (p. 547).

Phenylbutazone is particularly effective in relieving the symptoms of this disease. It is worthy of trial in those patients who fail to respond satisfactorily to radiotherapy and where pain cannot be controlled by other analgesics. The dose should not exceed 300 mg. daily. Close supervision is required in view of the possibility of toxic effects (p. 547).

Prognosis. In early active cases treated by radiotherapy the prognosis is good. Even in more advanced cases the combination of general measures, radiotherapy and orthopaedic procedures can do much to restore these patients to a reasonable level of function.

THE COLLAGEN DISEASES

Diseases of connective tissue

The idea that a number of clinical conditions, otherwise apparently unrelated, should be grouped under the term diseases of collagen was introduced by Klemperer and his colleagues in 1942. The basis for this classification was the demonstration of a typical pathological change arising from a disintegration of collagen fibres in connective tissue and the deposition of material rich in polysaccharides. This lesion, designated as fibrinoid change, is found widely distributed in a number of diseases, and on this basis these conditions have been called diseases of collagen. As all elements of connective tissue are affected, a more accurate definition would be diseases of connective tissue. Commonly included are rheumatic fever, rheumatoid arthritis, systemic lupus erythematosus, dermatomyositis, scleroderma and polyarteritis nodosa.

The aetiology of these conditions is unknown.

The clinical features of these diseases differ widely but all tend to be characterised by evidence of severe systemic disturbance in the form of recurring fever and raised ESR. Joint pain and swelling may be present at some time in all members of the group, and all, with the exception of acute rheumatic fever, tend to run a subacute or chronic course.

Rheumatic fever, polyarteritis nodosa and rheumatoid arthritis have been dealt with elsewhere.

Systemic Lupus Erythematosus

This disease is now recognised as a diffuse disorder involving connective tissue in many parts of the body. Although fulminating cases occur, the disease usually runs a more chronic course, periods of activity alternating with remissions of varying length. It predominantly affects young women. The incidence is considerably higher than was thought in the past, due largely to more accurate diagnosis since the test for the L.E. (lupus erythematosus) factor became generally available.

A number of factors appear to precipitate the onset, or precede exacerbations. These include exposure to sunlight, infection, the administration of drugs such as sulphonamides or penicillin, and periods of emotional tension. The appearance in the blood of proteins with some of the characteristics of antibodies has given rise to the idea that the disease may be due to an immune response to antigens derived from the patient's own tissue. The L.E. test depends on the presence of an abnormal globulin with an affinity for the nuclei of cells. Normal leucocytes, incubated in serum of patients with this disease, extrude nuclear material which is phagocytosed by other leucocytes. These cells, containing amorphous inclusion bodies of altered nuclear material, present a typical appearance on staining (L.E. cells).

The most common presenting features are fever and an acute migratory arthralgia resembling rheumatic fever, erythematous eruptions on the face and hands, excessive fatigue, malaise, weight loss, anorexia and rapid ESR; anaemia, often haemolytic in type, is frequently present with leucopenia and, more rarely, thrombocytopenia accompanied by bruising and haemorrhage. The occurrence of pleural effusion, proteinuria, retinal exudates, pneumonitis, pericarditis or endocarditis indicates the diffuse nature of the disease. A proportion of patients present with an erosive arthritis of the rheumatoid type. Diffuse or local alopecia often develops. The diagnosis should always be considered in any patient with arthralgia or arthritis associated with a rash of 'butterfly' distribution on the face, especially if fever and signs of visceral involvement are present. The L.E. factor can be demonstrated in the serum of the majority of cases in the active phase of the disease. An antibody to nuclear material, demonstrable by immuno-fluorescence techniques, is present in the great majority of cases, and failure to demonstrate its presence is against the diagnosis of systemic lupus erythematosus.

Renal failure is the most common cause of death. The presence of proteinuria early in the course of the illness is of serious prognostic significance.

Treatment. In the presence of acute manifestations corticosteroids are the treatment of choice. Severe symptoms can be controlled but large doses may be required (prednisolone 40-60 mg. daily). At this dosage the incidence of serious side effects is high. Useful control however can often be attained and maintained by lower doses (10-20 mg. daily). Care must be exercised in the use of corticosteroids in the presence of renal or myocardial involvement, as hypertension not uncommonly develops. Although of great value in controlling acute symptoms, there is little evidence that corticosteroids prolong the duration of life in this disease.

In the subacute or chronic forms many observers have reported good results from the use of chloroquine in doses of 250-300 mg. daily.

Dermatomyositis

This rare disease is characterised by focal or segmental necrosis of voluntary muscles, which may be accompanied by increase in fibrous connective tissue between the muscle fibres. Clinically, two forms of the condition have been described: (1) Acute dermatomyositis, most common among children, in which oedema, tenderness, swelling and weakness of the proximal muscles of the limbs are accompanied by fever, leucocytosis and an erythematous skin eruption. Involvement of the respiratory muscles may rapidly lead to a fatal termination, but in other cases the acute phase subsides, leaving deformity of the limbs due to contracture of fibrous tissue in the muscles. (2) Chronic polymyositis, which runs a more prolonged course, and involves especially the peripheral muscles; lesions of the skin are not always present, but occasionally changes resembling scleroderma occur. This is the type most commonly seen in adults. All grades between these two forms are seen. A common clinical manifestation is oedema of the eyelids with a characteristic heliotrope discolouration. In acute cases the response to corticosteroid therapy may be dramatic and even life-saving. Large doses may be required initially (60 mg. prednisolone daily) which are then slowly reduced. In the self-limiting form of the disease, complete withdrawal may be possible. In others maintenance therapy is required (10 mg. prednisolone daily). Response in the more chronic cases is usually unsatisfactory. A combination of splints and physiotherapy is used to prevent or correct deformity.

Scleroderma

In this disease the collagen fibres of the dermis first become swollen, then dense and sclerotic, giving rise to contractures and deformities of the joints. The pathology is not confined to the skin. In progressive cases the alimentary tract, lungs, myocardium and kidneys may be affected. Blood vessels in the skin and viscera show marked intimal thickening. Intercurrent infection, and cardiac or renal failure are common causes of death. Treatment is unsatisfactory. The corticosteroids are of little value. Every effort must be made to prevent crippling deformities of the peripheral joints by the use of splints and physiotherapy, but care must be exercised in the use of all forms of heat due to the marked impairment of the circulation to the skin.

OSTEOARTHRITIS

Osteoarthritis is characterised by degeneration of the articular cartilage and the formation of bony outgrowths at the edges of the affected joints. A generalised form of the disease occurs commonly in middle-aged women in whom the small joints of the fingers, the carpometacarpal joint of the thumb and the interfacetal joints of the spine are particularly affected. The more localised form, where only one or two of the larger joints are involved occurs amongst elderly people of both sexes. The condition may appear at any age in a joint which has been damaged by disease or injury.

Aetiology. Osteoarthritis arises as a result of an exaggeration of the normal ageing process in the joints. When one joint is particularly affected a history is frequently elicited of an injury to that joint some years before. Malalignment, following fractures of the long bones, frequently gives rise to osteoarthritis in adjacent joints. Symptoms are prone to develop in weight-bearing joints and in those joints subjected to excessive strain. Thus, osteoarthritis of the hips, spine or knees is particularly common in those engaged in heavy labour, and in obese subjects. It is a disease associated with advancing years, and in most patients symptoms do not appear before the age of 50 Males and females are both affected, but when the small peripheral joints are involved the incidence is far higher in women. It has been suggested that in those cases with many joints affected there may be an inherited defect of the articular cartilage.

Pathology. There is patchy degeneration and splitting of the articular cartilage at the points of maximum weight-bearing, with exposure of the underlying bone, which tends to become denser and harder. New bone is laid down at the edges of the joints, resulting in the formation of osteophytes. Bony ankylosis never occurs, although limitation of movement may be very marked.

Clinical Features. The joints most frequently involved are those of the spine, the hips, knees, elbows, and in women the terminal joints of the fingers. The symptoms are gradual in onset. Pain is at first intermittent and of an aching character, appearing especially after the joint has been used, and relieved by rest. As the disease progresses, movement in the affected joints becomes increasingly limited, at first by muscular spasm and later by the loss of joint cartilage and the formation of osteophytes. There may be repeated effusions into the joints, especially after minor twists or injuries. Crepitus may be felt or even heard. Muscular wasting is always present to a greater or lesser extent. This is an important factor in conditioning the progress of the disease, as in the absence of normal muscular control the joint becomes more prone to injury. In the majority of male patients the disease is confined to one or two joints, especially the hips or the knees. In middle-aged women the generalised form of the disease affecting many joints is much more common, and it is in these that a hereditary defect in articular cartilage may be the important factor. The terminal interphalangeal joints of the fingers are commonly affected. Cartilaginous or bony outgrowths usually appear on the dorsal aspect of these joints (Heberden's nodes) and may give rise to considerable deformity of the joint but little local disability. General health is usually excellent and the ESR is within normal limits.

Diagnosis. There is usually little difficulty in distinguishing the condition from rheumatoid arthritis, in which there is evidence of a general systemic disturbance and characteristically the small peripheral joints are involved. It must be borne in mind, however, that in long-standing cases of rheumatoid arthritis osteoarthritic changes may appear in the affected joints. Degenerative changes not uncommonly appear in the joints in gout. A history of attacks of acute pain over a period of many years will usually distinguish gout from osteoarthritis.

Radiological Examination. There is characteristically a loss of joint space, and some sclerosis of the articular margins. In more advanced cases osteophytes appear at the bone edges.

Course and Prognosis. The disease is progressive. The rate of progress will depend on the amount of use to which the affected joints are put. It must be borne in mind that degenerative changes are present in the joints of most people over the age of 50 years, but only a few complain of any symptoms. The pain in osteoarthritis is probably due to changes in the joint capsule and periarticular tissues.

Treatment. The pathological changes in osteoarthritis are irreversible, but much may still be done to alleviate symptoms, especially in the early stages of the disease. A good deal will depend on the social circumstances of the case and whether undue stresses and strains can be removed from the affected joints by a change of occupation or a transfer to lighter work. The institution of rest periods during the day may greatly alleviate pain and stiffness. The patient may require to give up the unduly strenuous pursuit of such hobbies as golf, mountaineering or fishing. The fitting of rubber heels to the footwear may help by reducing jarring and minimising the risk of slipping. In obese patients the most important single form of treatment is to obtain a substantial reduction in weight, especially in cases where the hips or knees are affected. When pain is a prominent symptom rest in bed is required, combined with local heat and gentle active exercises. Full doses of analgesics such as aspirin, and codeine should be given. Phenylbutazone may be effective in relieving pain where other measures have failed (p. 547). It should be used with caution in elderly patients. The use of hot mud or wax packs may be beneficial. Hydrotherapy is of benefit in cases of osteoarthritis. Gentle movement of the joint under water relaxes spasm of muscles, diminishes pain and increases the range of movement. In cases where one hip or one knee is dominantly affected, arthrodesis of the joint will provide a stable pain-free joint. Vitallium cup arthroplasty has been used with success in osteoarthritis of the hip. The presence of a loose body may give rise to repeated locking of the joint and surgical removal may become necessary. In cases which fail to gain relief from the methods of treatment described, radiotherapy may be worth a trial. In about 50 per cent. of cases relief of pain may follow.

The intra-articular injection of corticosteroids (p. 549) has been followed by improvement in a high proportion of cases. Results are most favourable in the knee, but less satisfactory in the hip. Improvement may be maintained by injections given at intervals of one to three months. Patients should be warned to avoid excessive use of weight-bearing joints during the period following injection.

NON-ARTICULAR RHEUMATISM

Non-articular rheumatism, muscular rheumatism and fibrositis are terms which have been used to describe a number of conditions characterised by pain and stiffness, often of sudden onset, affecting mainly the neck, shoulders, back and gluteal regions. Usually no cause can be found, and radiological examination of related articular structures shows no abnormality. Areas of acute tenderness can often be demonstrated in the soft tissues. Pressure on these reproduces the pain felt by the patient and they have been described as 'trigger' areas or 'myalgic' lesions. Systemic symptoms are usually absent and the ESR is within normal limits. The symptomatology varies according to the structures involved.

Aetiology. The aetiology is obscure, but there are several predisposing and precipitating factors which may be of importance.

1. *Cold.* Exposure to cold and damp has traditionally been regarded as a common cause of 'muscular' rheumatism. Local chilling of the affected area appears to be of more importance than general exposure to cold.

2. *Fatigue.* Unaccustomed muscular activity is followed by pain and stiffness, which disappear in a few days. Undue prolongation of such symptoms may occur in susceptible individuals. In occupations involving strenuous muscular work, 'muscular rheumatism' is very common. Excessive muscular activity followed by chilling seems to precipitate symptoms more readily than fatigue or cold alone.

3. *Trauma.* Following injury to muscle or tears at musculotendinous junctions, scar tissue may be laid down. The subsequent loss of elasticity may give rise to pain on use.

4. *Posture.* Poor posture is frequently a cause of persistent aching pain, particularly in the cervical, dorsal and lumbar regions, where muscular and ligamentous strain can readily result. Symptoms arising from this cause are common in obese people and in thin, underdeveloped subjects with dorsal kyphosis and lumbar lordosis. Marked degrees of flat foot, or congenital short leg may be remote causes of low back pain.

5. *Infection.* Muscular aching is common in acute infections such as tonsillitis, influenza or meningitis. It has been suggested that this is due to local inflammatory lesions in the muscles which may persist and form the basis for further attacks of pain and stiffness later.

Mention must be made of *epidemic myalgia or Bornholm disease.* This condition is due to a virus infection. Diagnostic features are the sudden onset of fever accompanied by intercostal or abdominal pain. The illness usually lasts from 5 to 10 days, but occasionally may continue for several weeks. Epidemic stiff neck is another condition believed to be due to a virus infection.

6. *Metabolic Disorders*. Complaints of pain in relationship to muscles and joints are common in obese patients, particularly in women after the menopause. In rare instances a raised blood uric acid has been found in patients complaining of pain and stiffness without clinical evidence of joint involvement. Such cases respond to the measures used in the treatment of gout (p. 570).

7. *Endocrine Disorders*. In hypothyroidism, hypoadrenalism and hypopituitarism painful tender areas in muscles and subcutaneous tissues are common.

8. *Psychogenic Causes*. In a proportion of patients complaining of muscular pain and stiffness symptoms are psychogenic in origin. Excessive muscular tension is often seen in cases of anxiety neurosis and may cause aching and fatigue. In others the symptoms are diffuse and variable and are manifestations of emotional conflict. It is of fundamental importance to distinguish these cases from those with a physical basis.

Pathology. The use of the term 'fibrositis' to indicate inflammation of fibrous tissue in non-articular rheumatism is not justified. Reports on biopsy material obtained from 'fibrositic' nodules have not confirmed the claims of earlier observers who described hyperplasia of connective tissue, sero-fibrinous exudate, and the formation of new blood vessels.

Biopsy of 'nodules' in the thoracic and lumbar regions has shown in some cases herniation of fat through gaps in the fibrous septa. It is claimed that surgical removal of these 'nodules' has relieved symptoms, but this is seldom done at the present time.

Muscular pain and spasm arise most commonly as a result of strain or injury to related ligamentous or articular structures. It is recognised that the majority of cases of brachial neuralgia, lumbago and sciatica result from degenerative changes in the intervertebral disc. Loss of resilience in these structures renders the ligaments and interfacetal joints of the spine more prone to injury, even before radiological evidence of narrowing of disc spaces appears. Attacks of backache follow unusual physical activity or heavy lifts. Injury to spinal ligaments and joints is often accompanied by muscle spasm and referred pain. When more marked degenerative changes in the intervertebral discs have taken place, prolapse of the nucleus pulposus or narrowing of the intervertebral foramina causes pressure on nerve roots.

Clinical Features. The presenting symptoms are most commonly pain and stiffness, which are often of acute onset. The patient may be severely incapacitated. In the more chronic stage, pain is felt most acutely after rest and improves with moderate activity. Acutely tender points, sometimes referred to as myalgic lesions, may be located, pressure on which reproduces the pain complained of by the patient. Muscular spasm may be marked and movement limited. The features in each case will depend on the site of the lesion. Involvement of the structures in the cervical region may give rise to occipital headache or pain radiating to the shoulder and arm. Structures around the shoulder joint are affected in the condition known as 'frozen shoulder', where progressive limitation of movement follows the acute phase. The dorsal region of the spine is less commonly affected, but in the more mobile lumbar spine episodes of acute pain and stiffness, sometimes called acute lumbago, are a frequent cause of incapacity in middle-aged people, often with no radiological evidence of disc degeneration.

Tender pads of fatty subcutaneous tissue are frequently found in obese women over the dorsal spine, in the gluteal regions, and over the inner aspects of the knees. The skin is often tacked down over these areas giving a 'peau d'orange' appearance. The condition is sometimes referred to as panniculitis.

Differential Diagnosis. It is essential to distinguish by careful clinical examination the many other possible causes of pain. It is important to differentiate muscular pain and stiffness of psychogenic origin, as the treatment of this condition by physiotherapy is strongly contraindicated. The main features in these cases are the long history, insidious onset, the variability of the site of pain, the exaggerated description of the suffering endured and the overreaction to physical examination. Tenderness is usually diffuse and poorly localised, and although movement may be limited by voluntary contraction of muscles at times, it is always possible to show that there is a full range of movement.

Treatment. *Acute Stage.* Although there is no systemic upset, pain in the acute stage may be severe, and complete rest in bed with full doses of analgesics may be necessary. Local symptoms are greatly eased by the application of some simple form of heat—a hot-water bottle, electric blanket or poultice. Relief may be obtained by the application of a belladonna plaster, elastoplast or a sling. The search for 'trigger' points should be delayed until these general measures have had their effect. When located these spots should be injected with 2-3 ml. of local anaesthetic (1 per cent. solution of procaine). The proof of accurate location is the immediate amelioration of symptoms. Injection may have to be repeated once or twice to obtain the maximum benefit. Infiltration should be followed by heat, massage and active exercises. Local pain throws the musculature out of balance, and if this is not corrected postural changes may be produced, causing a recurrence of symptoms.

In certain more chronic cases hydrotherapy provides heat combined with active movement, and this is often effective when other measures have failed. The benefits of spa treatment are due to a combination of the physical and psychological effects which result when a patient is removed from the cares associated with his home or his work, given a holiday in pleasant surroundings and submitted daily for several weeks to a carefully planned course of physical medicine in the widest sense of this term.

In the obese patient the most important measure is to secure a reduction in weight. An endeavour should be made to prevent further attacks by correcting faulty posture and by giving advice regarding the avoidance of chilling and excessive physical fatigue. In some cases a change of occupation may be necessary. The vast majority of patients will make a good recovery if treatment is adequate, but inaccurate diagnosis may lead to prolonged incapacity.

In severe cases, with signs of root pressure due to lesions of the intervertebral discs, a more prolonged period of rest in bed, combined with graduated exercises for the extensor muscles of the spine, may be required. In recurrent cases a spinal brace may control symptoms. In others, with persistent evidence of root involvement, surgery may be indicated (p. 1231).

Prognosis. Most cases run a short acute course and are symptom-free in one to two weeks. A proportion of cases become chronic, especially if treatment of the initial attack has been inadequate.

Polymyalgia Rheumatica

This descriptive term has been applied to a syndrome which has certain features in common with other forms of non-articular rheumatism. It is characterised by severe pain and stiffness affecting mainly the muscles of the shoulder and pelvic girdles. It is accompanied by marked systemic disturbance in the form of mild fever, greatly increased ESR and moderate anaemia. It affects the middle-aged to elderly and women more often than men. In some cases there is evidence of temporal arteritis and intracranial vessels may be affected. The aetiology is unknown and biopsy of muscles has revealed no consistent abnormality. Symptoms may persist for many months but usually subside without residual disability.

Treatment. This should follow the lines used in other forms of non-articular rheumatism, i.e. rest, full doses of analgesics and graduated physiotherapy. Should improvement not occur within a week or 10 days, and particularly when systemic symptoms are marked, 15-20 mg. of prednisolone should be given daily in divided doses. When symptoms are controlled the dose should be gradually reduced, first by 2½ mg. every few days, then by 1 mg. weekly. Complete withdrawal is possible within 4-6 months in the majority of cases. When signs of arteritis are present prednisolone should be given at once in doses of 30-40 mg. daily and maintained until symptoms are fully controlled. Withdrawal should be even more gradual in these patients.

GOUT

Definition. Gout is a disease characterised by recurrent attacks of acute pain and swelling at first affecting only one joint, usually the metatarso-phalangeal joint of the big toe, later becoming polyarticular. Although gout is the result of an inborn error of purine metabolism, it is described in this section because its principal clinical features are connected with the locomotor system.

Aetiology

1. *Hereditary Factors.* Gout is undoubtedly a hereditary disorder. A family history of the disease is obtained in from 50-80 per cent. of cases.
2. *Age.* The disease is infrequent before the age of 40.
3. *Sex.* Gout is a very rare disease in women.
4. *Climate.* Gout occurs most commonly in temperate climates.
5. *Diet.* In the past it was believed that an excessive intake of foods high in purines was the primary and essential cause of gout. This view is not generally accepted at the present time, although there is some evidence to suggest that an acute attack can be induced by high purine diet in patients predisposed to gout.
6. *Secondary gout* may occur as a complication of haematological disorders such as *polycythaemia*, *leukaemia* and *myelofibrosis*, and following administration of drugs of the chlorthiazide group.

Precipitating Factors. An acute attack may be precipitated by dietary indiscretions including over-indulgence in alcohol and an idiosyncrasy to certain foods. An attack may also be precipitated by injury, excessive exercise, intercurrent infection and surgical operations.

Pathology. Urates are deposited in the articular and periarticular tissues, the extra-articular cartilages (especially in the ears) and the kidneys. The deposits in cartilage and bone lead to absorption of bone and give rise to the cyst-like appearances or punched-out areas seen in radiographs. There is an inflammatory reaction in the synovial membrane. As the disease progresses the articular cartilage becomes eroded and thinned. Urates are deposited in the subchondral bone and synovial membrane. Finally the changes of osteoarthritis appear.

Clinical Features

Acute Form. The acute attack may be heralded by some gastrointestinal upset, such as nausea, flatulence or vague abdominal pain. In others polyuria and frequency occur. The big toe is the first joint to be affected in over 90 per cent. of cases. The onset is sudden; the patient is commonly awakened through the night by excruciating pain; the joint becomes red, swollen and exquisitely tender. The neighbouring veins are distended. The appearance of the joint may suggest a pyogenic infection or local cellulitis. Gout should always be borne in mind when these symptoms appear for the first time in a middle-aged male. Pyrexia, sweating, loss of appetite, constipation and scanty highly coloured urine are common accompaniments of the acute attack. Blood, examination may reveal a polymorph leucocytosis and a rapid ESR. After a few days the pain begins to decrease. The skin over the affected joint becomes scaly and itchy. In the early stages of the disease the attacks occur at long intervals. Between attacks the patient is free from symptoms and radiological examination reveals no change in the affected joint. During the acute attack the plasma uric acid is raised, but may return to normal between attacks. The normal value of the plasma uric acid in the male is 2-6 mg./100 ml. In women it is slightly lower.

Chronic Form. Attacks occur more often and are of longer duration. Finally a stage is reached where remissions between the attacks are incomplete and there is persistent pain and stiffness with deformity of the affected joint. The arthritis becomes polyarticular, the ankles, hands and wrists being first affected, then the knees, elbows, shoulders and hips. Tophi begin to appear in the periarticular tissues and the cartilages of the ears. These consist of deposits of urates of chalky consistency.

Complications. In the late stages signs of progressive renal failure may appear, and examination of the urine reveals protein, casts and red blood cells. Excessive excretion of urates may lead to calculus formation and attacks of renal colic. These calculi are not radio-opaque. Arteriosclerosis and hypertension may complicate the picture, and death from coronary thrombosis or cerebral thrombosis may occur. In the chronic form the plasma uric acid is continuously high.

Diagnosis. The diagnosis may be made on a history of acute recurring attacks of arthritis with complete remissions, usually occurring in a male between 30 and 50 years of age. A family history of gout is frequently obtained. In early cases the plasma uric acid may be normal between attacks and radiological examination negative. In later cases a high plasma uric acid combined with typical radiological findings will clinch the diagnosis.

It is important to bear in mind the fact that gout may be the first manifestation of the myeloproliferative disorders already mentioned.

Treatment

ACUTE ATTACK. The patient should be put to bed and the affected joints protected by a cage. Hot or cold compresses should be applied and analgesics given in adequate doses (codeine 65 mg. or pethidine hydrochloride 50-100 mg.). Diet should be of a vegetarian type and ample fluids should be given. Until recent years colchicine was the most effective drug available for controlling the acute attack of gout, but in the doses required frequently caused severe gastrointestinal upset. It has been shown that phenylbutazone is even more effective and it is now the drug of choice. Phenylbutazone is very effective in relieving acute symptoms. It should be prescribed in doses of 500-800 mg. on the first day. The dose should then be reduced to 200-300 mg. daily until the symptoms are controlled. Corticotrophin or corticosteroids will be required only in exceptional cases of gout which fail to respond to the administration of phenylbutazone. Indomethacin is also effective but is liable to cause severe headache and gastrointestinal symptoms in the doses necessary to suppress symptoms.

CHRONIC GOUTY ARTHRITIS. Although diet plays a minor role in the treatment of gout, nevertheless certain articles of food rich in purine should be excluded (sweetbreads, liver, kidney, brain, heart, small fatty fish, fish roe, meat extracts). It is wise to restrict the intake of fat in patients who are obese. It has been suggested that an idiosyncrasy to certain articles of food is of more importance in precipitating an attack of gout than is the purine content of the foodstuff. On this basis dietary restrictions should be founded on the results of a careful investigation in each patient with particular reference to the liability of individual foods and drinks to produce an attack of gout. Moderate exercise should be encouraged, but strenuous exercise avoided. Prolonged administration of drugs which increase the excretion of uric acid leads to a diminution in the number of acute attacks, a lowering of the blood uric acid, a decrease in the size of tophi, and may diminish the incidence of renal damage. The drugs of choice are probenecid (Benemid) in doses of 0·5 g. three or four times daily and sulphinpyrazone (Anturan) in doses of 200-400 mg. daily. Experience has shown that acute attacks may become more frequent during the first few months of uricosuric treatment, but their incidence can be reduced by the administration of colchicine 0·5 mg. two or three times daily. Ample fluids should be taken to prevent the deposition of urates in the kidney, and the urine should be kept alkaline. Since salicylates antagonise the uricosuric action of these drugs, their coincidental use must be forbidden. If surgical operation becomes necessary in a patient suffering from gout, 0·5 mg. colchicine should be given thrice daily for three days before and for three days after the operation. In cases with damaged or deformed joints the physiotherapeutic measures described for the treatment of rheumatoid arthritis should be applied. An annual visit to a spa may be of considerable value in patients suffering from chronic gout. When tophi have become large or have ulcerated through the skin, they should be removed surgically.

A new approach to the treatment of chronic gout has now become possible by the introduction of a drug, allopurinol, which inhibits the enzyme xanthine oxidase responsible for the conversion of xanthine and hypoxanthine to uric acid. Thus the level of serum uric acid falls and the excretion of its precursors is increased. These are more soluble and have a higher renal clearance rate than uric acid. The level of serum uric acid can be reduced to normal levels by a dose of 300 mg. daily. As is the case with all drugs which markedly reduce the level of serum uric acid, fluctuations, particularly a rapidly falling level, may be associated with acute attacks of gout. Accordingly, colchicine 0·5 mg. three times a day should be prescribed along with allopurinol during the first two or three months of treatment. Allopurinol has already been shown to be remarkably free from toxic effects, mild skin rashes being the most common.

PREVENTION OF THE CHRONIC RHEUMATIC DISEASES

Methods for controlling the incidence of the chronic rheumatic diseases are limited by a lack of precise knowledge of their aetiology. Nevertheless the harmful effects of cold and damp in initiating rheumatic diseases are accepted even if the mechanism by which they act is not understood. There are two methods by which these effects can be minimised. The first is by taking suitable precautions with regard to clothing and footwear so as to prevent chilling. Suits and overcoats should be adjusted to the prevailing working and weather conditions. Footwear should be strong enough to avoid getting the feet wet, with subsequent chilling of the body. The second preventive measure which must be mentioned is the planning of dwelling-houses and factories, to make them free from draughts and damp, and have them adequately ventilated and heated. By these means undue humidity, chilling and excessive variations in temperature can be reduced to the minimum. Other important aetiological factors believed to be important in the chronic rheumatic diseases are excessive muscular fatigue and the undertaking of frequent repetitive movements, especially if performed in cramped and unnatural positions, as occurs in many heavy industries. For prophylactic purposes much can be done by the intelligent use of devices designed to reduce fatigue and to prevent excessive strain falling on the muscles and joints.

The adverse effects of certain occupational factors are shown in the report by the Department of Health for Scotland published in 1945. The highest incidence of the chronic rheumatic diseases occurred in miners, general labourers, transport workers and metal workers. It is clear that much might be done to reduce the incidence of the chronic rheumatic diseases by the planning of devices to reduce fatigue and make repetitive movements less common; also benefits can be expected from improved construction and air-conditioning of homes and factories so as to limit the ill effects of variations in temperature and humidity. Certain prophylactic measures are important in osteoarthritis, namely the correct treatment of fractures as this will obviate the mechanical stresses which follow union in bad position, and the control of obesity which should lessen the development of arthritis in weight-bearing joints.

Finally, in regard to the prevention of gout, while it is not possible to alter the inherited metabolic defect it is possible to control the aetiological factors, discussed on p. 568, which play a part in precipitating attacks of the disease.

J. J. R. Duthie.

Books recommended:

Copeman, W. S. C. (1967). *Textbook of Rheumatic Diseases*, 4th ed. Edinburgh: Livingstone.

Hollander, J. L. (1966). *Arthritis and Allied Conditions*, 7th ed. London: Kimpton.

TROPICAL DISEASES AND HELMINTHIC INFECTIONS

THE immensity of the problem of tropical diseases is seldom fully appreciated by those who have not visited tropical or subtropical countries. Well over one-half of the world's population live in areas where tropical diseases and malnutrition still undermine the health of a large proportion of the people. Some diseases are strictly tropical because the vectors, such as the tsetse flies, which convey the trypanosomes causing African sleeping sickness, are limited to the tropics, but many prevail because of poor hygiene.

The method of attack on tropical diseases should, therefore, be preventive rather than curative. In the tropics this depends largely on the institution and maintenance of effective sanitation, drainage and a safe water supply. Education of the people in ways of cleanliness is essential to ensure that the available sanitary facilities are properly used. As a first step in underdeveloped areas health visitors, practical men and women living in the villages, known and liked by the villagers, can do much to educate these people in simple but effective measures against disease. A little money used on these lines will do far more good than large sums spent on expensive drugs for the treatment of preventable diseases. When the co-operation of the people has been secured, such measures as mass spraying with insecticides or large-scale immunisation may be very successful in reducing the incidence of malaria, yellow fever, smallpox and other killing diseases.

Many of the inhabitants of tropical countries are so weakened by disease and malnutrition that they are unable to produce sufficient food even for their own needs. By controlling tropical illnesses the health of the people will be so greatly benefited that production of food and raw materials may reach and even exceed local requirements, the surplus then becoming available for export. With these improved conditions there will inevitably be an increase in the birthrate and a fall in infant mortality. Instead of only 3 out of 10 children surviving to reach adult life

7 or 8 of the 10 may grow up. The resulting swelling of the population creates new economic and social problems and in some countries instruction in family planning has become an urgent necessity. The World Health Organization and other public bodies are providing valuable aid to developing countries by financing projects which must, however, become an integral part in the overall national effort. The execution of these plans entails great capital outlay as well as the provision of many experts in medicine, agriculture, engineering and science. The maintenance of improved health is dependent on a sound economy and political harmony.

HISTORICAL ASPECTS

The history of many of the tropical diseases goes back to the earliest days. The story of malaria is an interesting one. The cardinal signs of the disease were described by Hippocrates. The Romans thought that malaria was due to bad air rising from the marshes, and by draining them they reduced unwittingly the breeding-places of the mosquitoes and so had less malaria. Effective treatment with cinchona bark was known long before the malaria parasite was first demonstrated by Laveran in 1880. Then in 1897 Ronald Ross, encouraged by Manson's discovery of the transmission of *W. bancrofti* by the mosquito, searched for and found oöcysts in the stomach wall of anopheline mosquitoes which had previously fed on persons suffering from malaria. The following year, working in Calcutta with sparrows infected with bird malaria, he found that culicine mosquitoes fed on these sparrows developed similar cysts in the stomach wall; these eventually burst and liberated bodies which reached the salivary glands of the mosquito. He next showed that these mosquitoes conveyed the infection to healthy sparrows. From this he deduced that human malaria was conveyed from man to man by infected mosquitoes, and this was shortly afterwards confirmed by Italian workers.

Despite this knowledge of the method of spread of the disease there was little improvement in the malaria situation until the Second World War when the urgent need to maintain a non-immune population in highly malarious areas stimulated research into methods of personal protection. It was established that a daily dose of mepacrine enabled soldiers to serve in highly malarious areas and to remain free from symptoms. Since then antimalarials with fewer side-effects have replaced mepacrine. Except where strains of parasites resistant to the antimalarial in use have emerged, non-immune persons taking the drug remain free from malaria. Perhaps of even greater importance, huge areas, such as much of India, formerly endemic for malaria, have been virtually freed from infection chiefly by the widespread application of insecticides such as dicophane (DDT), sometimes in combination initially with chemoprophylaxis. Such eradication campaigns, usually initiated by WHO, require careful planning and subsequent vigilance to ensure that malaria does not return.

Another disease, kala azar, was long considered to be a form of chronic malaria until Leishman in 1903 discovered the causal protozoon in the spleen of a soldier from Calcutta, and in the following year Rogers cultured it and found that it then assumed a flagellate form. Before the discovery of the curative properties of intravenous antimony, kala azar decimated rich populous tracts of Bengal and Assam. It is still a prevalent disease in certain tropical and subtropical countries and is liable also to attack visitors who may develop fever and hepatosplenomegaly after leaving the endemic area.

The use of emetine and other drugs in the treatment of amoebiasis has enormously reduced the incidence of liver abscess, its most important complication, although amoebiasis is still a common disease in many parts of the world.

For centuries epidemics of louse-borne typhus have occurred when men are brought together under poor hygienic conditions and become verminous. By protective vaccination and the use of DDT as a lousicide it is now possible to prevent this disease. The success of chloramphenicol and tetracycline in the treatment of louse-borne, mite-borne and tick-borne typhus has also completely altered the outlook in these diseases. Recovery can now be expected even when treatment has been much delayed. A protective vaccine is also available for Rocky Mountain spotted fever, a variety of tick-borne typhus.

De Lesseps, who built the Suez Canal, was defeated by malaria and yellow fever in his attempt to construct the Panama Canal in 1880. The American Yellow Fever Commission in 1901 proved that urban yellow fever was transmitted by the bite of the mosquito

Aedes aegypti. Gorgas, by applying this knowledge, eradicated the disease from the Panama area in 1905 by the destruction of this vector. Although yellow fever persists in primates and mosquitoes in some forest areas, vaccination with 17D attenuated yellow fever virus now provides a sure protection against the disease.

The havoc wrought by plague is recorded in the Old Testament. The great plague of London in 1664-65 killed 70,000 of London's 460,000 inhabitants. Now the disease is largely prevented by antirodent measures and insecticides and is also successfully treated with antibiotics.

Cholera has disappeared from Europe although formerly it recurred in epidemics every 10 years or less. It remains endemic in parts of India, and epidemics are still liable to afflict pilgrims and others living under conditions of great overcrowding and poor sanitation in tropical and subtropical countries. In 1947 there was a large epidemic in Egypt and since 1961 cholera due to the *Vibrio eltor* has spread widely in the Far East and South East Asia and in 1965 occurred in the Middle East.

Trypanosomiasis of man and animals is due to a variety of trypanosomes. African sleeping sickness, its most serious human manifestation, formerly occurred in devastating epidemics. Animal trypanosomiasis is also of great importance to human health and economy as it reduces the areas where cattle can be kept. All forms of trypanosomiasis except the South American type, Chagas' disease, are spread by tsetse flies. By studying their habits and applying appropriate control measures and by using potent drugs for human protection and treatment the incidence of the disease has been greatly reduced.

Leprosy was described in ancient Egypt in 1350 B.C., in the time of Rameses II. The disease still affects about 15 million people mainly living in tropical and subtropical countries. The establishment of colonies for patients with leprosy in the infectious stage has helped to limit the spread of the disease. Prolonged treatment with sulphone drugs has proved effective in the treatment and control of the disease where the co-operation of the patients and their relatives has been secured. B.C.G. vaccination and specific drugs given to children at risk are new promising measures in prophylaxis.

Egyptian medical papyri record that haematuria was common, and calcified ova of *Schistosoma haematobium* have been demonstrated in the kidneys of Egyptian mummies of the twentieth dynasty, 1250 to 1000 B.C. Bilharz in 1851 described the adult worm found in the portal vein of man. The intermediate host was proved by Japanese workers to be a freshwater snail. In 1915 Leiper, working in Egypt, observed that the development of *S. haematobium* and *S. mansoni* took place in different freshwater snails. He showed that these were two distinct species of parasitic worms. In 1917 Christopherson introduced effective treatment with antimony salts given intravenously.

Diagnosis. In addition to a careful history and clinical examination, a microscopic investigation is usually essential for the diagnosis of tropical diseases. A wet film of the blood may reveal the actively moving microfilariae which are larval forms of the filarial worms responsible for causing elephantiasis and other lesions in man. It may also show the trypanosomes of African sleeping sickness though these are found more readily in fluid obtained from puncture of an enlarged lymph node. A well-stained blood film will reveal malaria parasites and the spirochaetes which cause relapsing fever. Absence of a leucocytosis in a patient with pyrexia who is, or has recently been, in the tropics will suggest the possibility of malaria, brucellosis or typhoid fever. Leucopenia is profound in kala azar. A leucocytosis may indicate leptospirosis or hepatic amoebiasis. An eosinophilia will suggest a recent intestinal helminthic infection, filariasis or schistosomiasis. Microscopic examination of the faeces may reveal *Entamoeba histolytica* or ova of the roundworm, hookworm, schistosome or other helminth.

Air travel increases the likelihood of tropical diseases being encountered outside the tropics. There are specific remedies for most of these diseases, but delay in diagnosis and in treatment may have the gravest consequences for the patient. Every medical man should, therefore, have a reasonable knowledge of the more common tropical diseases even though he may not intend to practise in the tropics.

Only rabies, malaria, amoebic dysentery and the more common helminthic infections are described here. Shortly after arriving in Britain a person may hear that a dog with which he had recently been in contact has died of rabies; under these circumstances no time must be lost in instituting preventive treatment. The other infections have been chosen because of their frequency in this country. Tables 6 and 7 (pp. 580-583) summarise other important tropical diseases. For further information the tropical diseases supplement to this book should be consulted. When the diagnosis is in doubt, patients should be referred without delay to a centre specialising in this field.

RABIES

Owing to strict quarantine regulations there has been no rabies in Britain in animals since 1922 except in a few dogs under observation in quarantine kennels. Rabies is a virus infection affecting a variety of animals and is endemic in many countries. It is spread to man by bites or the licking of an abrasion or mucous membrane, especially by dogs, cats, jackals or vampire bats. The length of the incubation period depends chiefly on the site and severity of the bites. In man it is usually between 30 and 70 days, but it may be as short as 10 days or extend to many months.

Clinical Features. At the onset there may be insidious fever or paraesthesia at the site of the bite. Shortly afterwards spasm of the muscles of deglutition appears and irritability progresses until the slightest stimulus, such as the sound, sight or even mention of water, activates spasm of these muscles; hence the alternative name, hydrophobia. The respiratory muscles and others are also affected; delusions and hallucinations develop, with lucid intervals in which the patient is acutely anxious. Paralysis ensues and the patient invariably dies within a week of the onset of symptoms. In some the disease takes the form of an ascending myelitis without other symptoms.

Treatment and Prevention. After the symptoms of rabies have appeared only palliative treatment with sedatives is possible, but adequate treatment early in the *incubation period* will prevent this calamity, as was shown by Pasteur in 1885. If possible an animal suspected of having rabies should not be killed; it should be kept in isolation under restraint. If it does not die within 10 days it was not infective for rabies at the time of biting. If it dies, demonstration of Negri bodies in the brain confirms the diagnosis. If the victim has been severely bitten a single dose of

5,000 units of hyperimmune serum should be given intramuscularly and, if possible, 5,000 units infiltrated around the wound. In addition, in all probable or definite cases, after cleansing the wound, a course of vaccine should be given (see below). In very doubtful cases, especially with only a superficial bite on the leg, the giving of vaccine may be deferred until the dog has died, as the incubation period is over a month after such a bite. If a person is bitten severely or on the face, the incubation period is shorter and treatment must be given at once. Sometimes, especially after inadequate doses of vaccine, the incubation period may be prolonged for many months.

The Semple-type vaccine, which has to be preserved in a refrigerator, is given by deep subcutaneous injection, usually in the anterior abdominal wall. The dose varies from 2 to 10 ml. daily for 7 to 14 days, according to the severity of the bite, the time of instituting treatment and the age of the patient. Directions accompany the vaccine which should be kept available in administrative centres.

Rarely, serious and even fatal neuroparalytic disorders have resulted from the vaccine, due to sensitivity to its content of animal neural tissue but this risk must be taken if there is reason to believe that the animal was rabid. A vaccine grown in duck embryo is largely free from danger but probably less efficient. Two doses are given, on the 10th and 20th days, after completing the course of Semple vaccine. Duck embryo vaccine may be used alone for minor exposure or licks where risk of infection is low, or in an individual who has been given a Semple vaccine on a previous occasion. Local allergic reactions are reduced by the use of antihistamines, and corticosteroids may ameliorate the neuropathic sequelae.

Vaccine treatment should be stopped immediately if the suspected animal survives for 10 days, as this proves it did not have rabies.

MALARIA

Malaria occurs wherever there are human hosts and a sufficiency of malaria-transmitting anopheline mosquitoes together with conditions of temperature and humidity which permit the complete development of the parasite in the infected mosquito. Malaria

TABLE 6

TROPICAL DISEASES

This Table sets out the salient features of the more important tropical diseases not detailed elsewhere in this book. For further information see Supplement to this book.

DISEASE	CAUSATIVE ORGANISM	METHOD OF SPREAD	MAIN SYMPTOMS AND SIGNS	TREATMENT
African Trypanosomiasis (Sleeping Sickness).	*Trypanosoma gambiense.* *T. rhodesiense.*	Tsetse flies.	Fever, lymphadenopathy, circinate rashes, finally paralyses and coma.	Suramin, pentamidine, melarsoprol, trimelarsan.
Visceral Leishmaniasis (Kala azar).	*Leishmania donovani.*	Sandflies. (In Mediterranean, dogs are reservoir hosts.)	Prolonged fever, hepatosplenomegaly, granulocytopenia.	Pentavalent antimony or pentamidine.
Plague.	*Pasteurella pestis.*	Fleas from rats dying of plague. Droplet infection from man in pneumonic plague.	1. *Bubonic.* High fever, painful swollen lymphatic glandular mass regional to bite. 2. *Septicaemic.* High fever, leucocytosis, no bubo. 3. *Pneumonic.* Virulent pneumonitis.	Streptomycin or tetracycline in large doses.
Cholera.	*Vibrio cholerae.* *V. eltor.*	From vomit or faeces of patient or convalescent.	Violent diarrhoea. Vomiting. Rice water stools. Rapid dehydration. Cramps.	Intensive intravenous replacement of water and electrolyte losses.
Leprosy.	*Mycobacterium leprae.*	Close contact with lepromatous patient, relative or children's nurse.	1. *Tuberculoid.* Asymmetrical hypopigmented anaesthetic patches; thickened nerves; mutilating complications of peripheral neuritis. *M. leprae* scanty or absent. 2. *Lepromatous.* Initial faint macules, then nodules on ears, face and elsewhere. Many *M. leprae* in skin and nasal mucosa.	Good food, exercise. Dapsone for years. Thiambutosine is an initial alternative. Tuberculoid form indicates a good resistance and is more easily cured.

TABLE 6—*continued*

Typhus Fevers:				
1. Epidemic typhus.	*Rickettsia prowazeki.*	Faeces of body lice from infected man.	Prolonged high fever, severe toxaemia, macular rash.	Tetracycline.
2. Scrub typhus.	*R. tsutsugamushi.*	Larval mites from infected rodent.	Fever often with eschar at site of bite, and a rash, pneumonitis.	Ditto.
3. Tick typhus.	*R. conori.*	Ticks from dogs, rodents or marsupials.	Fever, varying toxaemia, eschar, lymphadenopathy and rash.	Ditto.
Many other varieties due also to rickettsiae.				
Yaws.	*Treponema pertenue.*	Non-venereal spread from early lesions through the abraded skin of children.	Early papillomatous proliferative lesions, swelling of bones. Late destructive lesions resembling tertiary syphilis. No visceral or neurological complications. Never congenital.	Long-acting penicillin in a single dose, e.g. P.A.M. (procaine penicillin in 2% aluminium monostearate) 1·2 mega units.
Relapsing Fevers:				
1. Louse-borne.	*Borrelia recurrentis.*	Body lice from man to man.	Fever, lasting 5 days, with 1 or 2 relapses after short intervals. Jaundice. Epidemic.	Tetracycline.
2. Tick-borne.	*Bor. duttoni.*	Infected soft ticks (e.g. in mud huts)	As above, but repeated relapses, neuropathies as sequelae. Endemic.	Ditto.
Yellow Fever.	Arbovirus.	Aedes mosquitoes infected from man (or monkey in jungle yellow fever).	Fever, jaundice, bradycardia, increasing proteinuria. Black vomit. High mortality. Mild cases also occur.	Symptomatic. Vaccination with 17D virus protects for 10 years.
Dengue.	Arbovirus.	Aedes mosquitoes.	Fever, pains in bones, rash.	Analgesics.
Sandfly Fever.	Arbovirus.	Sandflies.	Resembles dengue without a rash.	Analgesics.

Table 7

COMMON TROPICAL HELMINTHS

Name of Helminth	Intermediate Hosts	Method of Acquisition Main Symptoms and Signs.	Laboratory Diagnosis	Treatment
Schistosoma spp.	Fresh water snails.	Acquired by wading in infected water.		For all three species trivalent antimony salts, e.g. antimonyl sodium tartrate intravenously or Astiban intramuscularly are used.
1. *S. haematobium.*	1. *Bulinus spp.*	1. Haematuria, ulceration and papilloma of bladder. Complications, obstruction of ureters, pyonephrosis, carcinoma of bladder, cor pulmonale.	1. Ovum with terminal spine, in urine and stool.	
2. *S. mansoni.*	2. *Biomphalaria spp.*	2. Preliminary fever, urticaria and eosinophilia, subsequent mild dysentery. Complications: rectal polypi, cirrhosis of liver, splenomegaly.	2. Ovum with lateral spine, in stool.	Lucanthone orally is moderately successful for *S. haematobium.*
3. *S. japonicum* (adults, also in mice, dogs, sheep, etc.).	3. *Oncomelania spp.*	3. Clinical features same as 2. Also cerebral granuloma, fits.	3. Ovum with small knob, in stool.	Niridazole (Ambilhar) orally under trial.
Hookworms: 1. *Ancylostoma duodenale.* 2. *Necator americanus.*	None.	Acquired by walking barefoot on infected soil. Epigastric pain. Complication: severe anaemia.	Ova in stools.	Tetrachloroethylene or bephenium hydroxynaphthoate.
Strongyloides stercoralis.	None.	Acquired in same manner as hookworms. Minimal intestinal symptoms. Erythematous linear cutaneous eruptions (larva currens).	Motile larvae in stool.	Dithiazanine iodide or thiabendazole

TABLE 7—*continued*

Filariidae 1. *Wuchereria bancrofti* *Brugia malayi*	1. Mosquitoes, esp. *Culex fatigans.* Esp. *Mansonioides spp.*	1. Mosquito-borne. Recurrent lymphangitis, with fever and eosinophilia. Complications: Lymph scrotum, elephantiasis. Chyluria.	1. Microfilariae in blood at night.	1. Diethylcarbamazine.
2. *Loa loa.*	2. *Chrysops spp.*	2. Bites of chrysops flies. Calabar swellings. Worm may cross eye.	2. Microfilariae in blood at mid-day.	2. Ditto.
3. *Onchocerca volvulus.*	3. *Simulium spp.*	3. Bites of simulium flies. Chronic irritating erythematous maculopapular rash. Subcutaneous nodules containing adult worms. Complication, corneal opacities, 'African river blindness'.	3. Microfilariae in skin snips. A group complement fixation test for 1, 2 and 3.	3. Ditto and antihistamines, nodulectomy. Also suramin for persisting infections.
Dracunculus medinensis (Guinea worm).	*Cyclops* (Water flea).	Swallowing cyclops in well water. Urticaria; later vesicle through which adult female extrudes and discharges fluid containing larvae. Complications: Pyogenic infection of track after death of worm.	Detection of larvae in opalescent exudate.	Slow extraction of adult under sterile conditions. Niridazole (Ambilhar) aids extraction.
Clonorchis sinensis.	1. Snails. 2. Cyprinoid fish.	Eating uncooked fish. Often symptomless. Cholangitis.	Ova in stool.	Dithiazanine iodide.
Paragonimus westermani.	1. Snails. 2. Crabs and crayfish.	Eating uncooked crustacea. Fever, cough, 'endemic haemoptysis'. Epilepsy.	Ova in sputum or stool.	Bithionol.

may also be transmitted by a blood transfusion from an apparently healthy donor from whom the parasites have not been fully eradicated.

The Parasite. The four recognised species of malaria parasites pathogenic to man are *Plasmodium falciparum*, *P. vivax*, *P. malariae* and *P. ovale*. *P. vivax* and *P. ovale* produce a clinically similar 'tertian' fever, the temperature rising on the first and third days and continuing with this periodicity; *P. malariae* produces a quartan type of fever with apyrexial intervals of two days; *P. falciparum* causes a more continuous fever, the so-called subtertian fever. When a female anopheles feeds on infective human blood, the sexual forms of the parasite reach the mosquito's stomach. The female macrogametocyte is fertilised by the male microgametocyte. The resultant fertilised cell penetrates the stomach wall of the mosquito and there forms the oöcyst. Within this cyst sporozoites are developed, and in 7 to 20 days, depending on the temperature, these are liberated and travel to the salivary glands of the mosquito. When this infected mosquito bites man, sporozoites are introduced. These sporozoites soon disappear from the circulating blood and enter the liver cells, where pre-erythrocytic development takes place. After 6½ days from infection with *P. falciparum* and between 8½ and 11 days with the other species the infected liver cells rupture and liberate numerous merozoites which then infect the red blood corpuscles. In *P. falciparum* infection all the parasites in the liver mature about the same time and all are discharged into the circulation, while in the other malarial infections exoerythrocytic forms persist for months in the liver cells where they cannot be reached by most antimalarial drugs. This accounts for the frequency of relapses in these forms of malaria and the absence of relapses in falciparum infection after stopping drugs which have removed the parasites from the circulating blood. On entering the red cells the young parasite appears as a ring form, and its development thereafter is shown in Plate VI (p. 602). When the schizont is mature, the red cell ruptures and liberates a new generation of merozoites which enter other red blood cells and develop into either asexual or sexual forms. The sexual forms begin to appear about 7 to 10 days after the asexual forms; they cause no symptoms but make the individual harbouring them a reservoir of infection.

Clinical Features. The incubation period varies but is often about a week or 10 days for *P. falciparum* infections and somewhat longer for vivax and malariae malaria. Occasionally an apparent primary attack of malaria occurs months after the patient has left the tropics, and suppressive drugs may delay the onset for as long as a year after stopping the drug. In many cases vivax malaria starts with a period of several days of continued fever before the development of classical bouts of fever every other day. The attack has three clinical stages: first a cold stage, followed by a hot stage, which ends in a sweating stage. In the cold stage or rigor the patient feels intensely cold and shivers, and frequently his teeth chatter. The temperature is already elevated and rapidly reaches its height, e.g. 40° C. (105° F.). Vomiting is often troublesome and headache severe. After half an hour or so, the hot stage is reached; the patient feels burning hot and may be delirious—vomiting often continues into this stage. After one to six hours, profuse perspiration starts, the temperature drops and the patient becomes comfortable and falls asleep. He will feel reasonably well on the next day, but fever subsequently recurs with a periodicity characteristic for the infecting species. Usually the spleen and, especially in children, the liver become palpable and tender, but the absence of detectable splenic enlargement does not exclude malaria. Herpes simplex, usually round the mouth, is a common accompaniment of malaria.

P. falciparum infections, especially primary attacks, are more insidious and dangerous than other forms of malaria. The fever in this variety is prolonged and irregular and does not usually rise to quite so high a level as in vivax or malariae malaria. Sometimes the patient, although very ill, remains afebrile with a heavy *P. falciparum* infection. The cold, hot and sweating stages are seldom found in this form of malaria, but vomiting and severe headaches are common. A severe haemolytic anaemia develops. In uncomplicated cases only the ring stage of the parasites and later the gametocytes are found in the peripheral blood, whereas in vivax, ovale and malariae malaria all stages of the parasites occur in the circulating blood. A patient with falciparum malaria, apparently not seriously ill, may suddenly develop complications which render his condition very grave.

A mixed infection with more than one species of malaria parasite may occur—therefore the demonstration of *P. vivax* does not exclude the possibility of a *P. falciparum* infection.

P. malariae malaria is usually associated with mild symptoms and bouts of fever every fourth day. With this infection parasitaemia may persist for many years without producing any symptoms.

Complications of Falciparum Malaria. These are due to interference with the capillary circulation, destruction of erythrocytes, or toxaemia. The symptoms and signs associated with impaired capillary circulation depend on the situation and extent of the vessels involved. In cerebral malaria the cerebral capillaries are affected causing the rapid onset of coma, hyperpyrexia or mental changes and, exceptionally, signs of a focal lesion such as aphasia, hemiplegia or monoplegia. With intestinal capillary blockage there may be severe gastric symptoms or intense diarrhoea resembling bacillary dysentery. Acute renal failure may occur.

Blackwater Fever. This is brought about by a rapid intravascular haemolysis and is invariably associated with a chronic falciparum malaria, most commonly in those who have taken antimalarial treatment irregularly. This haemolysis may be quite unexpected and very extensive, destroying many uninfected as well as parasitized red cells. The attack is not infrequently provoked by injudiciously administered quinine or by fatigue. The colour of the urine varies from dark red to almost black, depending on the amount of intravascular haemolysis. Acute renal failure may follow.

Relapses. These are characteristic of vivax and malariae malaria and are due to persistence of the exoerythrocytic form of the parasite in the liver. Immunity eventually overcomes the infection, and relapses seldom occur longer than two years after the patient has left the malarious area.

Endemic Malaria. The manifestations of malaria in unprotected indigenous residents show considerable variation according to the degree of endemicity and the age of the patient. In areas of hypoendemicity little immunity is acquired, epidemics of malaria are liable to occur and the disease does not differ materially from that in non-immunes. In mesoendemic areas malaria is frequent but only seasonal. Repeated infections lead to anaemia, considerable enlargement of spleen with the danger of rupture from a minor blow to it, and chronic ill health with bouts of fever. The growth and development of children may be retarded and *P. malariae* infections may cause nephrosis. Where malarial transmission takes place throughout the year, but with seasonal increases, the zone is termed hyperendemic, and adults show considerable immunity. Although adults will have palpable spleens and occasional parasitaemia, in them malaria causes only occasional short bouts of fever. In holoendemic areas malarial transmission is intense throughout the year and adults possess almost complete tolerance for the infection, a condition called 'premunity', and enlargement of the spleen in them is uncommon. In hyperendemic and in holoendemic areas malaria takes a toll of older infants and young children. The regular taking of antimalarial drugs prevents the manifestations of chronic malaria.

Malaria in Pregnancy and Childhood. Parasitisation of the placenta frequently causes abortion. The mother may be very ill and have a severe macrocytic anaemia. Indigenous babies in hyperendemic areas have some inherited immunity for the first few months but other infants and young children are very susceptible and in them the onset may be insidious with only gastro-intestinal or pulmonary symptoms. Convulsions, coma and death may quickly supervene if adequate treatment is not promptly given or the child may become dangerously anaemic.

Diagnosis. If a patient is in a malarious locality or has recently left such an area, malaria should be considered. A history of periodic fever, perhaps associated with an enlarged spleen and anaemia, is very suspicious. Well-stained blood films, thick and thin, should be examined, at frequent intervals if necessary. *P. falciparum* parasites may be very scanty and only present in the peripheral circulation for a short period. In those who have recently taken ineffective doses of an antimalarial drug parasites may be difficult to find. Where the clinical condition of the patient makes a diagnosis of malaria very probable, it is justifiable to give antimalarial treatment even though parasites have not been found.

Treatment. GENERAL. The patient should be put to bed and encouraged to drink fluid freely. Aspirin or paracetamol is useful for the relief of headache. During the cold stage hot-water bottles and extra blankets are required. When dehydration is marked and vomiting troublesome, intravenous infusion of saline and glucose may be necessary.

Specific Treatment. This should be started as early as possible, especially in falciparum malaria. The drugs of choice are the 4-aminoquinolines, chloroquine or amodiaquine. The usual chloroquine tablet contains 150 mg. base and amodiaquine 200 mg. of the base. A course of treatment consists of 4 tablets followed by 2 tablets in six hours and 2 tablets daily for three more days. In a few areas patients have been found infected with a *Plasmodium falciparum* resistant to 4-aminoquinolines; such require treatment by quinine dihydrochloride 600 mg. three times daily for 10 days. A combination of sulphormethoxine (Fanasil) 1 g. and pyrimethamine 50 mg. in a single dose has also been employed successfully. None of these drugs, however, ensures that there will be no relapse in vivax, ovale and malariae malaria from exoerythrocytic parasites in the liver cells invading the circulating erythrocytes. Proguanil and pyrimethamine are both too slow in action for effective use alone in the treatment of an acute attack of malaria in non-immune subjects. Small doses of antimalarials may be adequate to curtail fever in indigenous residents in endemic areas.

Treatment of Complicated P. falciparum Infections. Patients severely ill with falciparum malaria must be treated as medical emergencies. The immediate intravenous administration of chloroquine or quinine is indicated, the drug being given very slowly to avoid collapse, taking at least 10 minutes to give the full dose, repeated, if necessary, after four to six hours. Ampoules of chloroquine in aqueous solution containing 200 mg. in 5 ml. are available and 200 mg. to 300 mg. should be given; the dose for quinine dihydrochloride is 500 mg. dissolved in at least 10 ml. of isotonic saline. Such severely ill patients usually require intravenous saline, and the antimalarial drug may be injected into the delivery tube of the infusion. The results of prompt treatment are very gratifying. Blood transfusions may be required to combat severe anaemia. In less fulminating cases, chloroquine may be given intramuscularly with excellent results. The dosage for small children must not exceed 5 mg. per kg. body weight, as fatal collapse may occur with larger doses and intravenous or even intramuscular quinine may be safer. If, in the treatment of the comatose patient, return to consciousness is delayed, lumbar puncture is indicated to exclude concomitant meningitis. Oral therapy should replace parenteral treatment as soon as the patient's condition allows. A liberal supply of fluid should be given by mouth as soon as the patient can take and retain this, and a normal diet should be provided as soon as acceptable to the patient.

BLACKWATER FEVER. The treatment of blackwater fever depends on the amount of blood which has been destroyed. When there has been severe haemolysis leading to a marked degree of anaemia, circulatory and renal failure may ensue and blood transfusion is urgently needed to replace the destroyed red blood cells and to restore the circulation. Corticosteroids are of value in preventing further haemolysis. It is very important that physical and mental rest should be secured; good nursing and sedatives are of great value. The renal output must be watched carefully. Sufficient fluid must be given by mouth, or intravenously if necessary, to ensure a urinary output of more than a litre in 24 hours. Careful records of fluid intake and output must be kept and appropriate treatment should be instituted if features of acute renal failure develop (p. 824).

RADICAL CURE OF MALARIA DUE TO *P. vivax*, *P. malariae* and *P. ovale*. While relapses can usually be prevented by taking one of the antimalarial drugs in suppressive doses over a period of months, radical cure can only be ensured by a course of one of the 8-aminoquinolines, which destroy these parasites in their exoerythrocytic phase in the liver; chloroquine or amodiaquine for four days should precede the beginning of the course. Primaquine is probably the least toxic of the 8-aminoquinolines; each tablet contains 7·5 mg. of base; a course of two or three such tablets taken daily for 14 days produces a high percentage of cures. The patient must, however, be under medical supervision for this period as haemolysis may develop. This is relatively frequent in coloured races, affecting those whose erythrocytes are deficient in glucose-6-phosphate dehydrogenase. Cyanosis due to the formation of methaemoglobin in the red cells, 'methaemoglobincythaemia', is frequent but not dangerous.

Causal Prophylaxis and Suppression. So far no drug is known which will destroy the sporozoites injected by the mosquito. Clinical attacks of malaria can, however, be prevented by drugs which attack the pre-erythrocytic form ('causal prophylaxis'), or by drugs which act on the parasite after it has entered the erythrocyte ('suppression'). Both proguanil and pyrimethamine destroy the pre-erythrocytic stage of *P. falciparum*; they also act on the asexual erythrocytic forms of all species of human malaria parasites. Consequently they give reliable protection against clinical attacks of malaria if started on entering a malarious region. These two drugs also prevent further development of the falciparum gametocytes in the mosquito. The adult dose of pyrimethamine is one tablet (25 mg. base) once a week; for a child up to six years ¼ tablet (6·25 mg.) and from six to twelve years ½ tablet (12·5 mg.) weekly is adequate. It has an attractive flavour, and some children who have obtained access to the drug have died from an overdose. The suppressive dose of proguanil for adults is 1 or 2 tablets (each containing 87 mg. base) daily; children aged one to five years require ½ tablet and under one year ¼ tablet. Proguanil is a valuable drug for preventing clinical attacks of malaria as it is almost free from side-effects. In addition, since it is taken daily, the routine is unlikely to be forgotten.

Local strains of *P. falciparum* resistant to these two drugs are occasionally encountered; the higher dose of proguanil, namely 2 tablets, can then with advantage be employed, or chloroquine prophylaxis can be substituted. Although chloroquine and amodiaquine are usually effective as suppressants, in some countries where they have been widely used for this purpose strains of *P. falciparum* resistant to these drugs have emerged and constitute a serious hazard. For this reason 4-aminoquinolines should only be used for prophylaxis if local strains are known to be resistant to proguanil and pyrimethamine.

The adult dose of 4-aminoquinolines is 2 tablets once a week. Children aged 6 to 12 years require 1 tablet and under 6 years ½ tablet. A syrup is also available. Alternatively half doses can be given twice weekly or for adults a small 50 mg. tablet of chloroquine daily. Occasional toxic side effects include slight visual disturbance. This makes chloroquine unsuitable for aeroplane pilots.

Prophylactic drugs are ineffective unless taken in the required dose with the utmost regularity. These drugs should be begun on the day of arrival in a malarious area and to ensure eradication of *P. falciparum* infection should be continued for four weeks after departure.

Personal Protection against Malaria. Control of anopheline mosquitoes (p. 575) especially by the spraying of houses with an insecticide such as DDT, has greatly reduced or abolished the risk of malaria in many areas. However, unless eradication is complete, all visitors and non-immune residents should take regular prophylactic or suppressive drugs as detailed above. Sleeping under a mosquito net at night will give freedom from the nuisance of those mosquitoes which only bite in the dark and may also reduce the likelihood of acquiring some mosquito-borne viral infections. The use of protective clothing and mosquito boots is becoming archaic. However, only complete protection from the bites of infected anopheline mosquitoes will ensure that there will be no late relapse of *P. vivax* or *P. malariae* malaria after leaving endemic areas, even although suppressive drugs have been given for four weeks after departure.

AMOEBIC DYSENTERY

Amoebic dysentery is typically a subacute or chronic afebrile disease, thus differing from bacillary dysentery which is an acute disease with a sudden onset often associated with pyrexia. Symptoms of amoebic dysentery may not appear for months or even years after the infection has been acquired.

The *Entamoeba histolytica*, which is responsible for the disease, is found in two phases: a vegetative form, 'trophozoite', actively motile and more easily recognised under the microscope in a fresh warm specimen of faecal blood and mucus, and a resting cystic phase. These cysts are found only in the lumen of the bowel and in the faeces. The vegetative forms invade the mucous membrane of the large intestine. The lesions are usually maximal in the caecum. They may, however, be found as far down as the anal canal. Tiny elevations are produced in the mucosa. These soon break down, producing flask-shaped ulcers varying greatly in size and surrounded by healthy mucosa. Amoebae may find their way into a vein and be carried to the liver where they multiply and cause hepatocellular necrosis ('amoebic abscess'). Amoebic ulcers only rarely penetrate through the muscular coat of the colon. A large vessel may sometimes be eroded, and severe intestinal haemorrhage may result. A localised granuloma, 'amoeboma', presenting as a palpable local thickening of the bowel wall and causing a filling defect on radiography, is a rare complication. It responds well to anti-amoebic treatment; it is therefore important that it should not be mistaken for a carcinoma.

Cysts of *Entamoeba histolytica* may continue to be passed in the faeces when the disease is inactive. These, not the vegetative forms, are responsible for the spread of the disease.

Clinical Course. The disease usually runs a chronic course with grumbling pains in the abdomen and two or more rather loose stools a day. The symptoms sometimes resemble those of a duodenal ulcer. Periods of diarrhoea alternating with constipation are a frequent feature. Mucus is usually passed and the motions often have a very offensive odour. On palpation of the abdomen there may be tenderness along the line of the colon, usually more marked over the caecum and pelvic colon. The right iliac pain may simulate acute appendicitis, and if an operation is performed the amoebae may cause ulceration of the wound and surrounding tissue. Perforation, when it occurs, is usually in the region of the caecum. Superadded pyogenic infection of the ulcers may lead to more acute bowel symptoms, with very frequent motions and the passage of considerable quantities of blood and mucus, thus simulating bacillary dysentery. Bacillary and amoebic dysentery may occur together, the bacillary infection probably lighting up latent amoebiasis. Macrophages seen microscopically in the stool of patients with bacillary dysentery are sometimes mistaken for amoebae.

Hepatic amoebiasis is a common complication of the bowel infection, and the possibility of this condition must always be remembered in any one who has lived in the tropics or subtropics. Early symptoms may be local discomfort and intolerance of fatty foods; later a swinging temperature, sweating and an enlarged tender liver are characteristic, but symptoms may remain vague and signs minimal. In particular, the less common abscess in the left lobe may remain hidden. There is usually some increase in the total leucocytes and radiology is invaluable in demonstrating a raised diaphragm with diminished movement on the right side.

When hepatic amoebiasis is diagnosed early, before appreciable abscess formation, the response to emetine or chloroquine is very rapid and gratifying. Delay in recognition may, however, allow a large abscess to form, making the prognosis serious unless adequate treatment is promptly instituted. An untreated liver abscess may invade neighbouring structures or organs, most frequently the lung from where its contents may be expectorated. Rupture into the peritoneal cavity or pericardial sac is usually fatal unless promptly treated surgically.

Diagnosis. The signs and symptoms of amoebic dysentery are often vague and may amount only to some degree of ill-health and abdominal discomfort with irregularity of the bowels, perhaps looseness alternating with constipation. A careful naked-eye examination of a freshly passed motion should be made. If mucus is found, a small piece should be selected and examined at once under the microscope. It should be kept at about body temperature with some heating device so that the *E. histolytica* may retain its motility. Such active amoebae are readily recognised; they are up to 30 μ in diameter or even larger, with a clear ectoplasm and a granular endoplasm, and usually contain red blood cells. Pseudopodia containing clear ectoplasm are protruded and retracted. Movements cease very soon if conditions are not favourable. Sigmoidoscopy may reveal typical ulcers. A scraping from one of these should be examined for *E. histolytica*. Ulcers may, however, be present in the bowel only above the reach of the sigmoidoscope and so escape detection. In chronic amoebiasis a number of stools may need to be examined before cysts are found.

Treatment. Emetine has a specific action in controlling the symptoms of active amoebic dysentery. Three to five days' treatment with emetine hydrochloride, 60 mg. daily, given subcutaneously, relieves acute symptoms, but to effect a radical cure this must be followed by emetine bismuth iodide (EBI) or diloxanide furoate. EBI, 200 mg. as a powder in a capsule, is given on each of eight successive evenings with a draught of water, four hours after the last meal and preceded by sodium amytal, 200 mg. No further food or fluids should be taken before morning. Given in this way the EBI is less likely to be lost by the vomiting which it is liable to induce. Particularly for those who are malnourished tetracycline for five to seven days preceding the specific treatment appears to be beneficial. During emetine treatment the patient must be kept in bed because of the toxic action of the drug on the heart. Dehydroemetine is claimed to be less toxic than emetine hydrochloride and in the same dosage is equally effective. It may not be available in Britain. Diloxanide furoate (Furamide) is non-toxic and in a dose of 500 mg. three times daily for 10 days appears to be a satisfactory substitute for EBI. Following a course of EBI or diloxanide furoate the patient should be instructed to report four weeks later for tests of cure. These consist of a sigmoidoscopy and at least six consecutive stool examinations and further stool examinations at monthly intervals for three to six months.

For the treatment of hepatic amoebiasis there are two drugs, emetine hydrochloride and chloroquine. Emetine is the slightly more potent and 60 mg. subcutaneously daily for 10 days gives excellent results. Chloroquine is effective because it is highly concentrated in the liver. If the patient has any myocardial damage chloroquine is preferable to emetine. The dose is 4 tablets, each of 150 mg. base orally, daily for two days then 2 tablets daily for 21 days. Many cases are satisfactorily treated by a combination of three or four injections of emetine followed by oral chloroquine. If the liver contains a sizeable abscess, it will also be necessary to evacuate its contents. Should local signs indicate easy accessibility it should be aspirated under local anaesthesia on alternate days until no further fluid accumulates. In other cases, aspiration should be carried out under general anaesthesia in an operating theatre; if the abscess cannot be found, immediate laparotomy should be performed. If one or more abscesses are then located, their contents should be removed. When the lesion is located in a site which can easily be re-aspirated through the chest wall, this practice should subsequently be followed with aseptic precautions, but under modern conditions the insertion of a drainage tube, with an underwater seal and antibiotic cover for a few days has proved to be fully satisfactory. Formerly, such drainage was reserved for abscesses found to be secondarily infected by bacteria. If emetine has been used for the treatment of the hepatic amoebiasis there should be an interval of one week before starting EBI—chloroquine has the advantage of making an interval unnecessary.

Recent investigations indicate that metronidazole (Flagyl) in the large dose of 40 mg./kg. body weight daily, in three divided doses, for five days, is effective in the treatment of intestinal and hepatic amoebiasis and is unaccompanied by serious toxic effects.

Personal precautions against contracting amoebiasis in the tropics and subtropics consist of not eating fresh uncooked vegetables or drinking unboiled water.

HELMINTHIC INFECTIONS

Helminthic infections are very common in the tropics and are often the cause of much ill-health. The more important tropical helminths are described in the *Supplement on Tropical Diseases.*

NEMATODES

Enterobius vermicularis (Threadworm)

This helminth is common throughout the world, including Britain. It affects children especially. The sexes are separate, the male being 2 to 5 mm. long and the female 8 to 13 mm. The ovum is flattened on one side and is about half the size of the ascaris egg. After the ovum is swallowed, development takes place in the small intestine, but the adult worm is found chiefly in the large gut. The mature gravid female worm lays fully developed ova around the anal orifice, and her movements in this region are responsible for intense itching, especially at night. The ova are often carried to the mouth on the fingers of the child and so re-infection takes place. In female patients the genitalia may be invaded. The adult worms may be seen moving on the buttocks or in the stool. Ova are detected by applying the adhesive surface of celophane tape to the perianal skin in the morning. This is then examined on a glass slide under the microscope.

Treatment. Prevention of re-infection is most important. Nails should be kept short and the hands washed carefully, especially before meals. Piperazine salts are effective remedies. A convenient form is piperazine phosphate administered with senna (Pripsen). The adult dose is 10 g. containing 4 g. of piperazine phosphate; children under six years are given 5 to 7·5 g. The drug is given in a single dose but should be repeated if the infection persists. An alternative single dose treatment is viprynium embonate (Vanquin), 5 mg. base/kg. body weight. Success is more likely to be achieved if the whole family is treated simultaneously, particularly as symptomless infections may be present in adults.

Ascaris lumbricoides (Roundworm)

This is a large, pale yellow worm 20-35 cm. long, something like an earthworm, but not segmented. The sexes are separate and the ovum is easily recognised under the 2/3 inch lens.

Man is infected by ova containing developed embryos gaining access to the mouth via contaminated fingers or food. The larvae escape from the ova in the duodenum and find their way to the lungs where they develop further. After invading the alveoli they then ascend the bronchi and trachea and are swallowed, thus entering the intestine where they reach maturity. In heavy infections, such as occur in the tropics, migration of many larvae through the lung may cause a helminthic pneumonitis, with cough, haemoptyses, urticaria and eosinophilia (Loeffler's syndrome). Adult worms live in the lumen of the small intestine. Symptoms may be absent or consist of nausea, colicky abdominal pain and irregular motions. Sometimes a worm is vomited or passed *per rectum*. In children with heavy infections a tangled mass of worms may cause intestinal obstruction. Other complications due to migration of adult worms include blockage of the bile or pancreatic duct and obstruction of the appendix. The diagnosis is made by finding ova in the faeces or by observing an adult worm. A solely male infection is usually revealed only after the giving of an anthelmintic to a patient with an unexplained eosinophilia. Occasionally the worms are demonstrated by radiography.

Treatment. Piperazine salts are easily administered and effective and should be given as recommended for threadworms (p. 595). The worms may not be passed until several days later.

Toxocara canis

This is a common intestinal ascarid of dogs. The eggs are passed in the animal's faeces. Children who are in close contact with infected dogs are particularly liable to ingest ova of *Toxocara canis*. Larvae, liberated in the stomach, then migrate through the body and may cause allergic phenomena such as asthma, hepatosplenomegaly and eosinophilia. The worms do not usually mature in the human host although they may do so and reach the intestinal lumen. Occasionally a granuloma develops around a dead larva in the eye and causes an obstruction to vision, resembling a neoplasm.

A skin test, using an antigen derived from *T. canis* is employed for diagnosis. There is evidence to suggest that larvae of *T. canis* may be an occasional cause of epilepsy and might convey the virus of poliomyelitis from the intestine to the nervous system. The larval worms can be killed by diethylcarbamazine (9-12 mg./kg. body weight daily for three weeks) and the adult worms expelled by giving piperazine salts as recommended for threadworms (p. 595). Granulomata may require surgical treatment.

Trichuris trichiura (Whipworm)

Under unhygienic conditions infection with whipworms is common and they are occasionally acquired in rural districts in Britain. Man is the only host. The ova are passed in stools and infection takes place by the ingestion of earth or food contaminated with ova which have become infective after lying for three weeks or more in moist soil. The adult worm is 3-5 cm. long and has a coiled anterior end resembling a whip. Whipworms inhabit chiefly the caecum but occasionally also the lower ileum, appendix and colon. There are usually no symptoms, but heavy infections in children may cause persistent diarrhoea. The diagnosis is readily made by examining the stools under the low power of the microscope, when the ova $50 \times 22\ \mu$ are seen resembling miniature beer barrels. Treatment is by oral dithiazanine iodide in doses of 20-40 mg./kg. body weight daily, in three divided doses for 21 days.

Trichinella spiralis

This parasite of rats and pigs is transmitted to man by eating partially cooked infected pork, usually as sausage or ham. Symptoms result from invasion of the body by larvae produced by the adult female worm in the small intestine and from their encystment in striated muscles.

The clinical course of trichinosis depends largely on the number of larvae which enter the tissues; light infections may be symptomless. In heavy infections after 24 to 48 hours the adult worms may irritate the bowel and cause nausea and severe diarrhoea. Soon, however, these symptoms are overshadowed by those associated with larval invasion, namely pyrexia, rapid pulse, and oedema of the face, eyelids and conjunctivae. Invasion of the diaphragm may lead to pain, cough and dyspnoea; involvement of the muscles of the limbs, chest and mouth causes stiffness, pain and tenderness in the affected muscle groups. Pyrexia may reach 40° C. (104-105° F.), with daily remissions. Larval migration may cause acute myocarditis and encephalitis. A leucocytosis with an eosinophilia is usually found after the second week. A heavy infection may prove fatal, but in those who survive complete recovery is the rule.

Diagnosis. This may be difficult but the disease may be suspected from the clinical picture. It is not uncommon for a group of persons who have eaten infected pork from a common source to develop symptoms about the same time. When suspected, biopsy from the deltoid or gastrocnemius may reveal encysted larvae. A positive biopsy result can be expected from the fourth week after the onset of symptoms. Precipitin and intradermal tests are also helpful.

If diagnosed very early anthelmintics and purgation may remove some of the adult female worms from the gut. Corticosteroids are of considerable value in controlling urgent symptoms. Recently thiabendazole, 50 mg./kg. body weight, on two successive days has been used successfully to relieve persistent pain in muscles. It is believed to act as a larvicide.

Prevention. Pigsties should be kept free from rats. Efficient food inspection or thorough cooking of pork and sausages prevents the disease.

CESTODES
(Tapeworms)

Cestodes are ribbon-shaped worms which inhabit the human intestinal tract. They have no alimentary system and absorb nutrition through the surface. The anterior end, or scolex, is provided with suckers for attachment to the host. From the scolex arises a series of progressively developing segments, the proglottides, which when shed may continue to show active movements for some time. Ova, present in large numbers in mature proglottides, remain viable for weeks and during this period they may be consumed by the intermediate host. The larvae liberated from the ova pass into the tissues of the intermediate host, and the human disease is acquired by eating undercooked beef infected with *Cysticercus bovis*, the larval stage of *Taenia saginata* (beef tapeworm), undercooked pork containing *Cysticercus cellulosae*, the larval stage of *T. solium* (pork tapeworm), or undercooked fresh water fish containing larvae of *Diphyllobothrium latum* (fish tapeworm). The adult cestode may produce little or no intestinal upset in human beings, but knowledge of its presence, by noting segments of the worm in the faeces or on underclothing, may distress the patient. Infection with a tapeworm is easily proved by the finding of segments or, less commonly, ova on microscopic examination of the stool.

Taenia saginata

This worm may be several metres long. The scolex, the size of a pin head, has four suckers; mature segments contain a central-stemmed uterus with 15 to 20 lateral branches which are easily seen if the segments are left in water for 24 hours. The ova of both *T. saginata* and *T. solium* are spherical and indistinguishable microscopically. The thick outer shell has radial striations and the ovum contains 6 hooklets. It is about the size of a threadworm ovum.

Infection with *T. saginata* occurs in all parts of the world, including the United Kingdom.

Prevention. This depends on efficient meat inspection or the thorough cooking of beef.

Treatment. The drug of choice for *T. saginata* and *D. latum* is niclosamide. No preparation of the patient is required other than to ensure that the bowels have been opened on the day preceding treatment. Before any food is taken in the morning, 2 tablets of the drug, each containing 0·5 g., are chewed and swallowed with a little water. One hour later a further 2 tablets are similarly taken. There are no side-effects and the worm is nearly always successfully destroyed.

Taenia solium and Cysticercosis

T. solium, the pork tapeworm, was formerly cosmopolitan in distribution but is now rare except in Central Europe, Ethiopia, South Africa and in certain regions of Asia. It is not so large as *T. saginata*, and the uterus has less than 14 lateral branches. The scolex has, in addition to suckers, two circular rows of hooklets anterior to the suckers. The adult worm is found only in man, but the larval cysticercus stage, which normally occurs in the pig, may occasionally develop in man as the result of the ova having gained access to the human stomach by contaminated food or fingers or by regurgitation of ova from the intestine. In the stomach the shells of the ova are digested and the larvae, liberated from the eggs, penetrate the intestinal mucosa and are carried to many parts of the body where they develop and form cysticerci. The most common locations are the subcutaneous tissue and skeletal muscles; when superficially placed they can be palpated under the skin or mucosa as pea-like ovoid bodies. Here they cause few or no symptoms; however cysts may also develop in the brain. About five years later the larvae die; in the brain the tissue reaction may cause epileptic fits, obscure neurological disorders, personality changes and occasionally internal hydrocephalus. After death of the larvae in muscles the cysts calcify and this enables them to be recognised radiologically. In the brain, however, much less calcification takes place and in this situation calcified larvae are only occasionally demonstrated radiologically. Epileptic fits starting in adult life should suggest the possibility of cysticercosis if the patient has lived in an endemic area. The subcutaneous tissue should be palpated and radiological examination of the skeletal muscles for calcified cysts must be made and repeated after intervals of six months if at first negative.

Treatment. *T. solium* can be removed by filix mas administered as follows. After a 48 hours period of bowel preparation by fluid diet and saline aperients morning and evening 2·5 ml. (38 min.) of a fresh extract of filix mas in capsules or as an emulsion is given at 6 a.m. and again at 6.15 a.m. and 6.30 a.m.; an appropriately smaller dose is given to a child. The patient takes only sips of water until 7 a.m. when for an adult 60 ml. (2 oz.) of saturated sodium sulphate solution is given. If the scolex is not passed by 9 a.m. a soap and water enema is administered. Food can be offered as soon as the scolex is seen or by 9.30 a.m. in any case. All motions are scrutinised to detect the scolex. Further experience is required before niclosamide can be confidently recommended for *T. solium* as disintegration of a segment might possibly release viable ova with the risk of cysticercosis.

Treatment of cysticercosis of the brain is essentially the same as for idiopathic epilepsy; sedatives and anticonvulsants should be given to tide the patient over the period until the reaction in the brain has subsided. Most patients treated on these lines make a good recovery. Operative intervention is seldom indicated.

Prevention. Prevention of *T. solium* infection consists in having pork well cooked before consumption. Cysticercosis is avoided if food is not contaminated by ova or segments and if there is no regurgitation of gravid segments or ova from the duodenum into the stomach as may occur when a patient harbouring an adult *T. solium* vomits. Great care must be taken by nurses and others to avoid contaminating the hands with ova from the patient.

Echinococcus granulosus (Taenia echinococcus)

This is the smallest tapeworm of medical importance. The larval stage, a hydatid cyst, usually occurs in sheep and cattle. Dog, by ingesting these cysts, is the most important definitive host, and a man, after handling a dog, may swallow ova excreted by the dog. The embryo is liberated from the ovum in the small intestine and gains access to the blood stream; it develops most frequently in the liver, but sometimes in the lung or elsewhere. The resultant cyst grows very slowly.

In man a hydatid cyst is typically acquired in childhood and it may, after growing for some years, cause pressure symptoms. These will vary, depending on the organ or tissues involved. In nearly 75 per cent. of patients with hydatid disease the right lobe of the liver is invaded and contains a single cyst. In others a cyst may be found in the lung, brain, orbit or elsewhere. The diagnosis depends on the clinical and radiological findings in a patient who has lived in close contact with dogs. Intradermal (Casoni) and complement fixation tests may give useful support to the diagnosis.

Treatment. When the cyst is causing pressure symptoms, surgical removal of the cyst and its laminated membrane is required, care being taken to avoid spilling the fluid containing scolices which may develop into further cysts later. Cysts in a long bone usually necessitate amputation.

F. J. Wright.

J. P. Baird.

Books recommended:

Wright, F. J. & Baird, J. P. (1968). *Tropical Diseases* 3rd ed.: Supplement to *The Principles and Practice of Medicine*, 9th ed., ed. Davidson, S. Edinburgh: Livingstone.

Hargreaves, W. H. & Morrison, R. J. G. (1965). *The Practice of Tropical Medicine*. London: Staples.

Macfarlane, L. R. S. (1960). *A Short Synopsis of Human Protozoology and Helminthology*. Edinburgh: Livingstone.

Manson-Bahr, Sir Philip (1966). *Manson's Tropical Diseases*, 16th ed. London: Cassell.

FALCIPARUM MALARIA (*Plasmodium falciparum*)

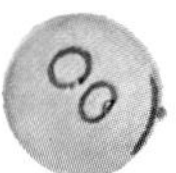
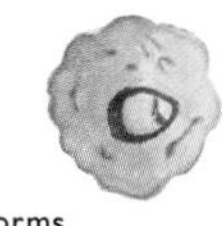
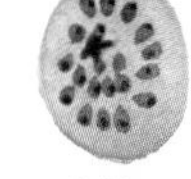
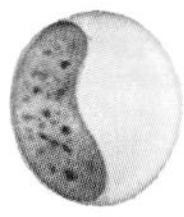
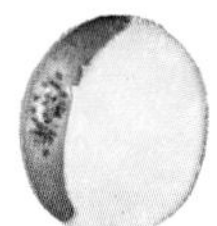

Ring Forms — Schizont — male — female
gametocytes

VIVAX MALARIA (*Plasmodium vivax*)

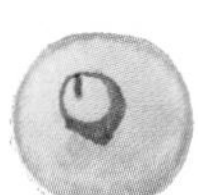
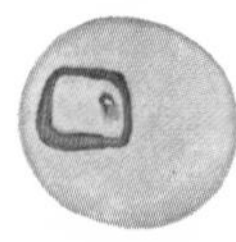
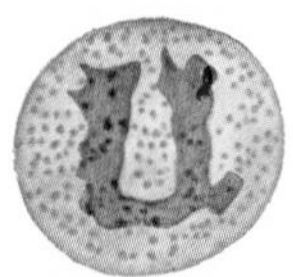
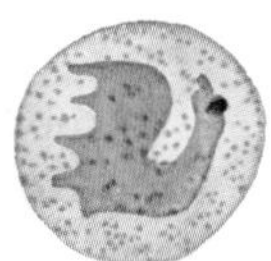

Ring forms — Amoeboid forms

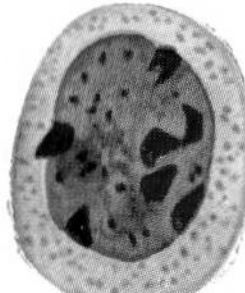
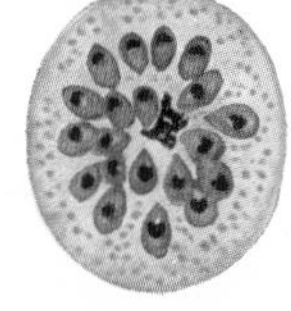
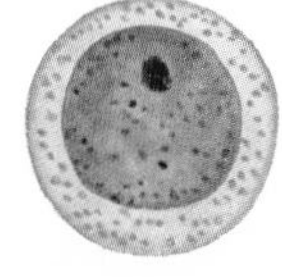
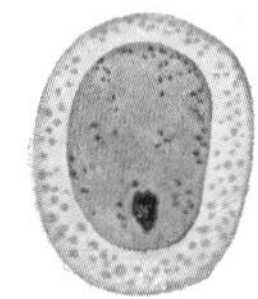

Schizont — male — female
gametocytes

MALARIAE MALARIA (*Plasmodium malariae*)

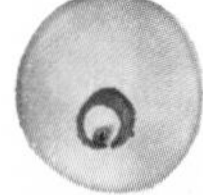
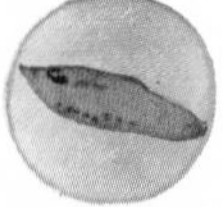
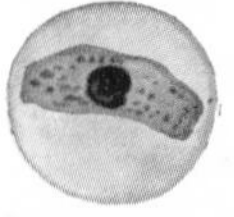
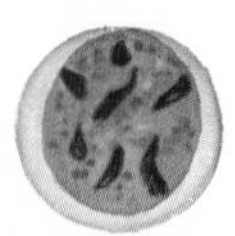

Ring forms — Band forms

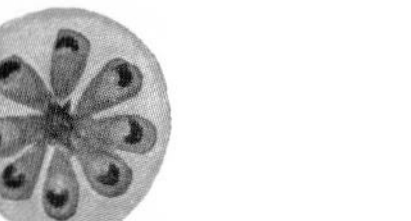
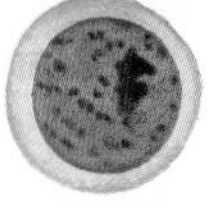
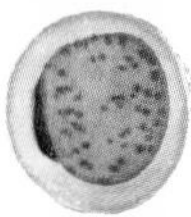

Schizont — male — female — Normal sized red cell
gametocytes

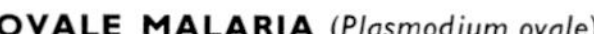

OVALE MALARIA (*Plasmodium ovale*)

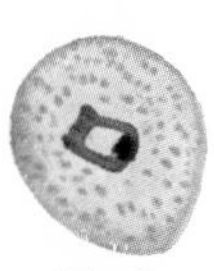
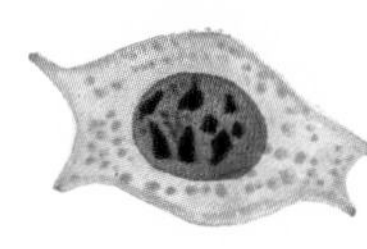
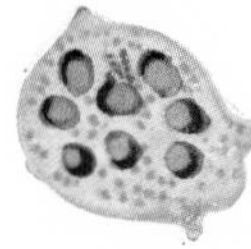
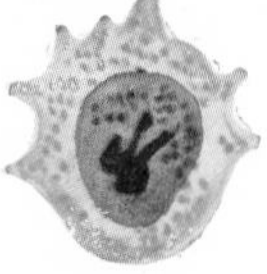
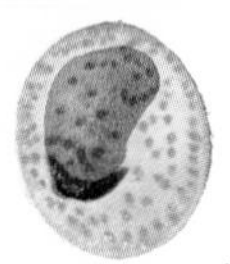

Ring form — Schizont — male — female
gametocytes

PLATE VI—MALARIA PARASITES

(Modified from 'Manson's Tropical Diseases'. London. Cassell. Drawings by Sir Philip Manson-Bahr.)

[*Facing page* 602

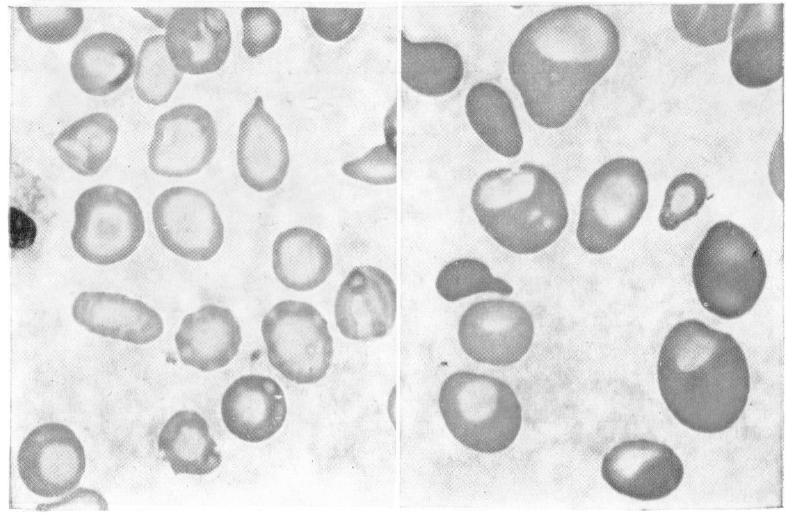

A B

A. Blood film. Iron deficiency anaemia, showing marked hypochromia.

B. Blood film. Pernicious anaemia, showing macrocytosis, anisocytosis and poikilocytosis. The cells are well haemoglobinised.

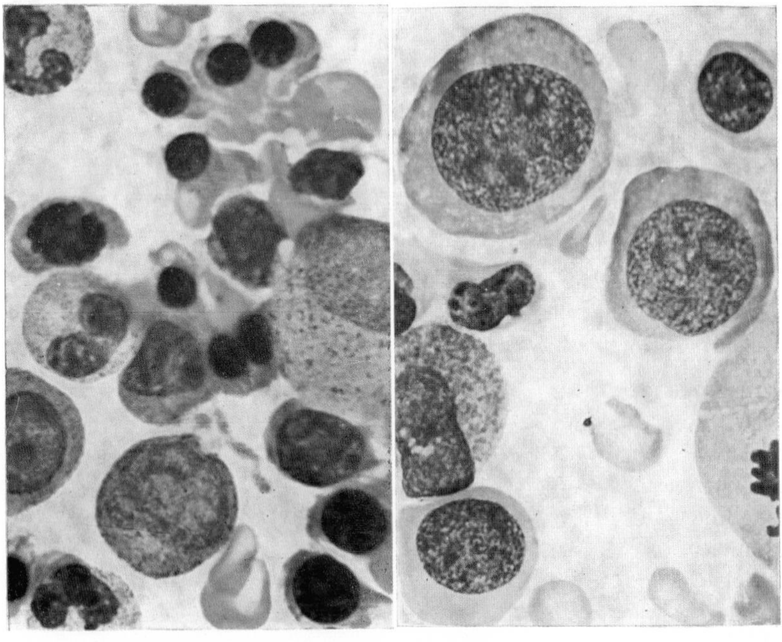

C D

C. Marrow film. Iron deficiency anaemia, showing hypochromic intermediate and late normoblasts.

D. Marrow film. Pernicious anaemia, showing a promegaloblast with nucleoli, an early and an intermediate megaloblast, and a lymphocyte in the upper right hand corner.

PLATE VII

By kind permission of McDonald, G. A.; Dodds, T. C., and Cruickshank, B. *Atlas of Haematology*. Edinburgh: Livingstone.

DISORDERS OF THE BLOOD AND BLOOD-FORMING ORGANS

BLOOD FORMATION

In early embryonic life blood cells are formed in the liver and spleen. By the fifth month, blood formation in the foetus begins in the medullary cavities of bones, which thereafter gradually supersede the liver and spleen in this function. From birth onwards normal haemopoiesis is restricted to the marrow of both flat and long bones. During childhood and adolescence there is a progressive diminution of red (haemopoietic) marrow in the long bones until in the young adult haemopoiesis is restricted to the heads of the femora and humeri and to the flat bones such as the sternum, ribs and vertebrae. An increased demand for blood formation results in an extension of red marrow into the shafts of the long bones.

The progenitor of all blood cells is the fixed reticulo-endothelial cell. From this are derived (1) the red cells, (2) the granular series of white cells, (3) the lymphocytes, (4) the monocytes, (5) the blood platelets.

1. The Red Blood Corpuscles

The primitive cell, the proerythroblast, is large with deeply basophilic cytoplasm, no haemoglobin, and a finely reticulated nucleus containing nucleoli. From this cell, by division, and under the influence of certain haemopoietic factors, is derived the early normoblast, which is smaller and has a denser nucleus and basophilic cytoplasm. Maturation proceeds by condensation of the nucleus and the development of haemoglobin as indicated by the polychromatic character of the cytoplasm. Complete maturation of the normoblast is reached when the cell is fully haemoglobinised and contains a dense and pyknotic nucleus. The disappearance of the nucleus then completes the formation of the erythrocyte. The young erythrocyte is slightly larger than the mature erythrocyte and stains faintly bluish (polychromasia) with the Romanowsky stains (e.g. Leishman). With supravital staining (cresyl blue) the polychromatic material appears as a fine reticulum (reticulocyte). The mature erythrocyte is eosinophilic in staining and contains no reticular material. It is a circular biconcave disc with remarkable uniformity of size, the diameter of the great majority being 7·2 μ. In the healthy adult only mature erythrocytes and a few (less than 1 per cent.) reticulocytes are to be found in the peripheral blood. Nucleated red cells do not normally appear in the peripheral blood and their presence indicates excessive or abnormal blood formation or irritation of the bone marrow. An excessive number of reticulocytes may occur for the same reasons. The megaloblast, an abnormal red cell precursor, is considered on page 619.

Haemoglobin is formed in the bone marrow in the maturing red cell. It is a conjugate of a red pigment (haem) and a protein (globin). Haem consists of a porphyrin combined with ferrous iron. Haemoglobin is the compound which enables the erythrocytes to transport oxygen and it also plays a role in the buffering of carbonic acid (p. 861).

Iron is absorbed from the upper small intestine according to the requirements of the individual, the usual amount in the adult being 0·5-1·0 mg. from a daily dietetic intake of 10-15 mg. Women of the child-bearing age require to absorb about a further 1 mg. daily to cover menstrual blood loss and the requirements are greater during pregnancy and lactation. The body conserves its iron content so that almost all of that liberated by the breakdown of effete red cells is utilised for fresh haemoglobin synthesis. Hence only about 1 mg. daily is lost from the skin and alimentary and urinary tracts. In men this small iron loss is easily replaced by the iron in the food, but balance is more difficult to maintain in women and especially so during pregnancy and lactation. Foods which are particularly rich in iron are liver, meat, eggs, wholemeal cereals, oatmeal, peas, beans and lentils. Where there is iron deficiency it is possible that the absorption of iron from the food is greater if there is hydrochloric acid in the stomach.

The iron content of the body gradually increases from 0·5 g. at birth to about 5 g. in the average adult. Of this some 60 per cent. is in the erythrocytes and a reserve is held in the liver, spleen and bone marrow for the replacement of about 25 per cent. of the circulating haemoglobin following haemorrhage. This reserve is stored in the body in two forms, ferritin and haemosiderin. There is iron in myoglobin and certain enzymes, such as cytochrome.

Vitamin B_{12} and Folic Acid (members of the vitamin B complex) are required for the maturation of the nuclei of primitive erythroblasts to the normoblastic state. In addition protein, iron, vitamin C, thyroxine and possibly some trace elements such as copper and manganese are necessary for the continuation of normal erythropoiesis. Lastly there is increasing evidence to suggest that the natural controlling stimulus of erythropoiesis is a hormone-like substance called erythropoietin which is produced mainly by the kidney.

Vitamin B_{12}. The name vitamin B_{12} is used in a general sense to include various forms of cobalamins that occur in foodstuffs and play a vital role in certain metabolic processes, possibly in coenzyme forms. The role of gastric intrinsic factor is to facilitate the assimilation of vitamin B_{12} from the alimentary tract. If the bone marrow receives an inadequate supply, normoblastic blood formation changes to an abnormal type characterised by the presence of megaloblasts (p. 619). Two alternative forms are used in treatment: cyanocobalamin, which is the true vitamin B_{12}, and hydroxobalamin or vitamin B_{12b}. The latter is less rapidly excreted in the urine and is therefore more effective in therapy. It is probable that neither form is the one that is metabolically active at the cellular level in the body.

Folic acid (pteroylglutamic acid) also appears to be essential for the continuation of normoblastic blood formation. It occurs in conjugated forms in varying concentrations in many natural foods. A deficiency of folic acid resulting in anaemia may arise directly or indirectly as discussed on page 620.

Vitamin B_{12} and folic acid play an essential but little understood role in the metabolism of nucleic acid and are required for the continuation of normoblastic blood formation and for many other metabolic processes in the body.

2. The White Blood Corpuscles

(*a*) *The Granular Series*. The primitive cell is the myeloblast with basophilic non-granular cytoplasm and a nucleus with fine reticular structure and several nucleoli. About 2 per cent. of white cells in the bone marrow are myeloblasts. Mitotic division of the myeloblast leads to the formation of the myelocyte, which is the progenitor of the polymorph leucocyte. About 30 per cent. of white cells in the bone marrow are myelocytes. They are smaller cells than the myeloblasts with a coarser nuclear reticulum, no nucleoli and a round nucleus. As they mature, myelocytes acquire granules in the cytoplasm which, according to their staining reactions, are neutrophil, eosinophil or basophil. As maturation proceeds the nucleus becomes condensed, kidney-shaped (metamyelocyte) and then lobulated (polymorphonuclear leucocyte or granulocyte). The older the cell the more lobes there are to the nucleus. Granulocytes are classified as neutrophil, eosinophil and basophil according to the staining reactions of the granules. Metamyelocytes and polymorph leucocytes are the only cells of this series normally to be found in the peripheral blood. The presence of myeloblasts or myelocytes in the peripheral blood in the absence of severe infection usually indicates a primary disease of the bone marrow (e.g. leukaemia). Myelocytes, however, may be found in the peripheral blood in myelofibrosis (p. 660), or when the bone marrow is stimulated by severe pyogenic infections or irritated by metastatic deposits of malignant disease. The simultaneous presence of myelocytes and normoblasts in the peripheral blood of an anaemic patient, as a result of bone marrow irritation in malignant disease (p. 640, 648) or myelofibrosis (p. 660) is frequently referred to as a leucoerythroblastic blood picture.

(*b*) *The Lymphocyte Series*. The primitive cell is the *lymphoblast*, which arises from endothelial cells lining the sinusoids of the germ-centres of lymphatic tissue throughout the body, especially lymph nodes. Some lymphoblasts develop in the bone marrow. The lymphoblast closely resembles the myeloblast in appearance. From the lymphoblast are derived *large and small lymphocytes*. The former have abundant clear blue cytoplasm and a moderately dense nucleus while the latter are small cells with very little cytoplasm and a small dense nucleus. The peripheral blood contains both large and small lymphocytes. Recent evidence suggests that the small lymphocytes have a very long life span and that they play an important part in immunological processes.

(*c*) *The Monocyte Series*. The primitive cell, the *monoblast*, is derived from reticulum cells mainly in the spleen. This cell resembles the myeloblast. From it develops the *monocyte* which appears in the peripheral blood. It has a cloudy blue cytoplasm with a few minute red granules, and a kidney or basket-shaped nucleus with finely reticulated chromatin.

The primary function of the white blood corpuscles is the defence of the body against infection by phagocytosis and probably by the production of antibodies.

3. The Platelets (Thrombocytes)

These are derived in the bone marrow from megakaryocytes, which are very large cells containing multilobulated nuclei and granular cytoplasm from which the platelets are formed. Platelets are small (2-4 μ) hyaline non-nucleated bodies with blue or purple granules.

RANGE OF NORMAL VALUES

Examination of the peripheral blood of normal healthy adults gives the following *approximate* range of values for these blood constituents:

Haemoglobin—Men, 14·6-16·0 g. per 100 ml.; Women 13·6-15 g. per 100 ml. (100 per cent = 14·6 g. per 100 ml.).

Red Cells—Men, 5-6 million per c.mm.; Women, 4·5-5·5 million per c.mm.

There has been a tendency in recent years for red cell counts not to be done because of their inaccuracy, but there would still appear to be a value in such estimations when accurate electronic counters are employed.

Reticulocytes— < 1 per cent.

Colour Index

$$= \frac{\text{Haemoglobin per cent.}}{\text{Red cell count (millions per c.mm.)} \times 20} = 0{\cdot}9\text{-}1{\cdot}09$$

Packed Cell Volume (PCV)—Men, 40-54 per cent.; Women, 36-47 per cent.

$$\text{Mean Cell Volume (MCV)} = \frac{\text{PCV} \times 10}{\text{Red cell count in millions}}$$

$$= 75\text{-}95 \text{ cu.microns } (\text{c.}\mu).$$

Mean Corpuscular Haemoglobin Concentration (MCHC)

$$= \frac{\text{Hb. concentration (in g./100 ml.)} \times 100}{\text{PCV}}$$

$= 32\text{-}38$ per cent.

Mean Corpuscular Haemoglobin (MCH)

$$= \frac{\text{Hb. g. per 1000 ml.}}{\text{Red cell count (millions per c.mm.)}}$$

= 27-32 micromicrograms (μμg.).

Mean Cell Diameter—7·2 μ.

Total White Cells—4,000-10,000 per c.mm.

Metamyelocytes—4 per cent. (160-400 per c.mm.)

Neutrophil Granulocytes—60-70 per cent. (2,500-7,000 per c.mm.)

Basophil Granulocytes—0-1 per cent. (0-100 per c.mm.)

Eosinophil Granulocytes—1-4 per cent. (40-400 per c.mm.)

Lymphocytes—25-35 per cent. (1,000-3,500 per c.mm.)

Monocytes—4-8 per cent. (160-800 per c.mm.)

Platelets—150,000-400,000 per c.mm.

Bleeding time—2-5 minutes (p. 661).

Whole blood clotting time—4-10 minutes (p. 662).

Erythrocyte Sedimentation Rate (ESR)— <15 mm. in 1 hour (Westergren).

BLOOD DESTRUCTION

The mature red cell probably exists in the peripheral blood for as long as 120 days. Old cells disintegrate in the blood stream, the fragments being taken up by the reticulo-endothelial cells, chiefly in the spleen. There the haemoglobin is broken down. The iron-free pigment, bilirubin, is carried by the plasma to the liver for excretion. Some of the iron is carried to the bone marrow for the formation of new haemoglobin, and the remainder is stored in the body, especially in the liver and spleen.

While the length of life of the erythrocytes is known and that of the platelets has been measured as 9-11 days, there is much more doubt about the length of life of the leucocytes. The granulocytes probably last three to four days but the life of the monocytes and lymphocytes is uncertain.

Destruction of all formed elements of the blood finally occurs in the cells of the reticulo-endothelial system.

Common Abnormalities of the Blood Cells

(*a*) *Anaemia* is said to be present when the number of red cells or their content of haemoglobin or both are reduced.

(*b*) *Microcytosis*. The average diameter of the red cells is reduced. This is commonly found in iron deficiency anaemia.

(*c*) *Macrocytosis.* Here the average diameter of the red cells is greater than normal. This is seen, for instance, in pernicious anaemia and is depicted in Plate VIIB (p. 603).

(*d*) *Hypochromia* exists when the red cells contain less than the normal amount of haemoglobin. They stain less deeply and show central pallor and the MCHC is lower than normal. Hypochromia is commonly associated with microcytosis and is the characteristic feature of iron deficiency anaemia. It is seen in Plate VIIA (p. 603).

(*e*) *Anisocytosis* is the name given to inequality in the size of the red cells. It is found in many forms of anaemia but is most prominent in pernicious anaemia. It is an indication of abnormal activity of the bone marrow.

(*f*) *Poikilocytosis* is the name given to irregularity in the shape of the red cells and has the same significance as anisocytosis.

(*g*) *Polychromasia and Reticulocytosis.* Young red cells when stained by the ordinary Romanowsky method appear bluish. This phenomenon is called *polychromasia.* When stained by vital staining methods (cresyl blue) they appear as reticulocytes. Increased numbers of polychromatic and reticulated erythrocytes in the peripheral blood indicate very active production of new red cells by the bone marrow.

(*h*) *Punctate basophilia.* Pathologically damaged young red cells may show several deep blue dots in the cytoplasm when stained by Romanowsky stains. Punctate basophilia may be found in any severe anaemia, but the presence of many cells affected in this way is most commonly seen in chronic lead poisoning, where it may occur when anaemia is slight.

(*i*) *Nucleated red cells*, usually normoblasts, are occasionally found when erythropoiesis is very vigorous or more often where there is irritation of the bone marrow, as in leukaemia.

(*j*) *Leucocytosis* means an increase in the total number of white blood cells to over 10,000 per c.mm. This may take the form of a polymorphonuclear leucocytosis in which the increase is due to the outpouring of many young neutrophil granulocytes, as occurs in the presence of pyogenic infections such as tonsillitis or pneumonia. Alternatively it may take the form of a lymphocytosis, as is frequently found, for example, in whooping-cough. Infants commonly respond to infections by producing a lymphocytosis.

(*k*) *Leucopenia* means a decrease in the total number of white cells below 4,000 per c.mm. This usually involves a reduction only of the granulocytes (granulopenia) with, therefore, a *relative* lymphocytosis. *Leucopenia* with relative lymphocytosis is found in tuberculosis, enteric fever, influenza, undulant fever, etc. Occasionally a leucopenia is found in overwhelming infections and is then a bad prognostic sign.

(*l*) *Eosinophilia* is the term used when the proportion of eosinophil granulocytes exceeds 4 per cent. Eosinophilia is found most commonly in infection with worms, in allergic diseases such as asthma, hay fever, urticaria, and in certain skin diseases.

(*m*) *Monocytosis* (over 8 per cent.) is found in, for example, infectious mononucleosis, advancing tuberculosis, subacute bacterial endocarditis and malaria.

(*n*) *Thrombocytopenia* means a diminution in the number of blood platelets (normal figure 150,000-400,000 per c.mm.). Bleeding tends to occur when the platelet count falls to below 40,000 per c.mm., but there is no exact relationship between the platelet level and a bleeding tendency.

CLINICAL FEATURES OF ANAEMIA

Anaemic patients have clinical features which are the direct consequence of the diminished oxygen-carrying power of the blood on the tissues and organs of the body. Their occurrence and severity depend on the degree of anaemia, and especially on the rapidity of its development, but are independent of its type. It is therefore essential to realise that the diagnosis of the type of anaemia cannot be made on the clinical features alone. They are:

1. General fatigue and lassitude.
2. Breathlessness on exertion.
3. Dizziness, giddiness, dimness of vision, headache, insomnia.
4. Pallor of the skin, and much more important, of mucous membranes.
5. Palpitation, tachycardia, cardiac dilatation, functional systolic murmurs.
6. Anorexia and dyspepsia.
7. Tingling and 'pins and needles' in the fingers and toes (paraesthesiae). This occurs particularly in pernicious anaemia.

8. In severe cases there may be some oedema of the ankles and crepitations at the bases of the lungs.
9. Angina pectoris (due to myocardial anoxaemia), especially in older patients with coronary artery disease.

CLASSIFICATION OF THE ANAEMIAS

I. Anaemias Due to Deficiency of Factors Essential for Normal Blood Formation

A. Iron.

(1) Chronic nutritional hypochromic anaemia.
(2) Post-haemorrhagic anaemia.
(3) Hypochromic anaemia due to malabsorption of iron.

B. Vitamin B_{12} and Folic Acid.

(1) Addisonian pernicious anaemia.
(2) Nutritional megaloblastic anaemia.
(3) Megaloblastic anaemia complicating pathological conditions of the gastrointestinal tract.
(4) Megaloblastic anaemia of pregnancy.
(5) Megaloblastic anaemia of infancy.
(6) Megaloblastic anaemia due to anticonvulsant drugs.
(7) Megaloblastic anaemia complicating haemolytic anaemia or leukaemia.

C. Vitamin C. The anaemia of scurvy.

D. Thyroxine. The anaemia of myxoedema.

II. Anaemias Due to Excessive Blood Destruction (Haemolytic Anaemias)

(1) Due to congenital abnormalities of the erythrocyte.
(2) Due to infective, toxic or allergic factors.
(3) Due to erythrocyte antibodies.

III. Anaemias Due to Aplasia or Hypoplasia of the Bone Marrow

Aplastic and Hypoplastic Anaemia.

(1) Idiopathic.
(2) Secondary.

IV. Anaemias of Uncertain Origin.

Due to chronic infection, uraemia, rheumatoid arthritis, liver disease or widespread malignant disease. Sideroblastic anaemia (p. 640) also may be included under this heading.

N.B.—It must be remembered that the iron deficiency anaemias constitute by far the most important group of anaemias. Hundreds of such patients are encountered for every case of megaloblastic anaemia, haemolytic anaemia or aplastic anaemia.

ANAEMIAS DUE TO DEFICIENCY OF FACTORS ESSENTIAL FOR NORMAL BLOOD FORMATION

ANAEMIA DUE TO DEFICIENCY OF IRON
CHRONIC NUTRITIONAL HYPOCHROMIC ANAEMIA

Aetiology. This is the most common type of anaemia not only in Britain but in every country of the world. It occurs mainly in women of the child-bearing age because of (*a*) the enhanced demands for iron resulting from blood loss from menstruation, and the increased nutritional requirements of pregnancy and lactation; (*b*) insufficient intake of iron in the diet; (*c*) achlorhydria or marked hypochlorhydria which is frequently present and diminishes the absorption of ingested iron. To meet these increased demands women of the child-bearing age would need to absorb two or three times the amount of iron required by women past the menopause or by men (p. 604).

Clinical Features. The symptoms are of gradual onset. In addition to the general features of anaemia described on p. 610 there are other features of nutritional deficiency, particularly glossitis, angular stomatitis, koilonychia and atrophy of the mucosa of the pharynx and stomach, giving rise to dysphagia and impairment of gastric secretory function. The glossitis is usually referred to as chronic atrophic glossitis because atrophy of the papillae and mucous membrane gives the tongue a smooth glazed appearance. The atrophy begins at the edges and later affects the whole tongue. As a result the tongue appears moist and exceptionally clean. Koilonychia is the name given to certain changes in the nails first evidenced by brittleness and dryness.

Later there is flattening and thinning and finally concavity (spoon-shaped nails). In a small proportion of severe long-standing cases the spleen may be palpable. In anaemia due to deficiency of iron the combination of dysphagia, glossitis and anaemia is commonly known by the British name of Kelly-Paterson syndrome or the American name of Plummer-Vinson syndrome (p. 886).

While paraesthesiae may occur, objective signs of disease of the central nervous system are never found in anaemia due solely to iron deficiency. Blood examination shows a hypochromic, microcytic anaemia. The haemoglobin commonly lies between 4 and 8 g. per 100 ml., and the red count between 3 and 4·5 million, with an MCHC of 26-30 per cent. Anisocytosis and poikilocytosis are present but not marked. The total and differential white counts show little change from normal. The bone marrow shows a normoblastic reaction (Plate VIIc, p. 603).

Diagnosis. The differential diagnosis from other types of anaemia depends on accurate blood examination. When the presence of hypochromic anaemia has been established a search for possible causative conditions must be undertaken. These include bad diet, haemorrhage, obvious or occult from any site, malignant disease, especially of the alimentary tract, tuberculosis and other infections, etc., and the appropriate examination and investigations must be carried out.

Prognosis. The anaemia is often well advanced, e.g. haemoglobin level 7-8 g. per 100 ml., before significant symptoms are apparent. If untreated the condition follows a chronic course. The importance of the syndrome is not that it is dangerous to life but that it leads to a loss of efficiency and lowered resistance to infection.

Hypochromic Anaemia in Infancy and Childhood

Aetiology. The following aetiological factors are of importance in explaining the great frequency of anaemia in infants.

(*a*) *Prolonged Milk Feeding.* Breast-fed infants and particularly artificially fed infants who are kept too long on milk alone without supplements of iron-containing foods become anaemic.

(*b*) *Low Birth Weight.* At birth the full-term baby has about 300 mg. of iron stored mainly in the liver and largely accumulated in the last trimester *in utero.* Hence infants born prematurely have low iron stores. The haemoglobin at birth is around 18 g. per 100 ml., falling to about 11 g. at three months due to a decreased rate of red cell production with a consequently reduced demand for iron. Excess iron from red cell destruction forms a valuable addition to the iron stores at this time. Premature infants or infants of low birth weight (e.g. twins) are at a disadvantage as they have a small circulating red cell mass and derive a reduced amount of iron from red cell destruction. It follows that premature infants will inevitably become anaemic by about the tenth week unless prophylactic iron therapy is given.

(*c*) *Nutritional Anaemia in the Mother*. When a mother is suffering from nutritional iron deficiency anaemia her child's ante-natal stores of iron may be inadequate.

(*d*) *Infections* in infants readily suppress erythropoiesis.

(*e*) *Intestinal malabsorption* as in gluten enteropathy is an occasional cause of hypochromic anaemia in infants or children.

Clinical Features. In infants the symptoms of anaemia are in general much less easy to recognise than in adults; undoubtedly anaemia leads to impairment of general health and vitality and an increased incidence of infections.

Hypochromic Anaemia in Pregnancy

Anaemia is commonly found during pregnancy. The fall in the haemoglobin value is due to one or a combination of the following three causes.

(*a*) Iron deficiency anaemia present before pregnancy but exaggerated by (*b*) and (*c*); (*b*) the relative increase of the plasma volume compared to the red cell mass which usually occurs in pregnancy; and (*c*) a deficient intake of iron in relation to the increased demands of the growing foetus. This may be aggravated by anorexia or vomiting.

ANAEMIA DUE TO LOSS OF BLOOD

Post-haemorrhagic anaemia may be acute or chronic.

Acute Post-haemorrhagic Anaemia. The sudden loss of a large volume of blood, 1 litre or more, from, for example, trauma or intestinal bleeding, produces the features of peripheral circulatory failure (shock, p. 176).

The rapid loss of 2-3 litres of blood is usually fatal, whereas an even greater quantity may be lost without causing death if it is spread over a period of 24-48 hours. During this period restoration of the circulating blood volume is proceeding by the withdrawal into the blood of tissue fluid. This haemo-dilution, which takes some hours to develop, is reflected by a fall in the haemoglobin level and red cell count. Hence, *immediately* after a haemorrhage of, for example, 1 litre in a previously normal person, the blood count will show normal figures, e.g. haemoglobin 14·6 g. per 100 ml., r.b.c. 5,000,000 per c.mm., but when dilution has occurred the figures may have fallen, giving a haemoglobin level of 11·7 g. per 100 ml., r.b.c. 4,000,000 per c.mm. When the circulating blood volume is partially restored, the acute symptoms of shock subside. During convalescence the general symptoms and signs of anaemia may be present. During recovery, red cells are formed more rapidly than haemoglobin and the MCHC falls. New red cell formation is reflected by the appearance of a temporary reticulocytosis of 5-10 per cent. and there is anisocytosis, poikilocytosis and a leucocytosis of 10-15,000 per c.mm. The platelet count may be increased.

Chronic Post-haemorrhagic Anaemia results from persistent or repeated loss of small amounts of blood. The most frequent causes are menorrhagia, and bleeding from haemorrhoids, alimentary carcinoma and peptic ulcer. Alimentary bleeding from the taking of aspirin must be remembered. Such persistent blood loss causes a progressive fall in haemoglobin. The clinical and haematological features are similar to those found in chronic nutritional hypochromic anaemia (p. 612). In addition, the clinical features of the causative disorder will be present.

Diagnosis depends upon the finding of a blood picture of hypochromic anaemia and the discovery of a source of chronic haemorrhage. It is frequently important to test the faeces for occult blood, look for haemorrhoids and perform a full radiographic examination of the alimentary tract.

PROPHYLAXIS AND TREATMENT OF IRON DEFICIENCY ANAEMIA

Prophylaxis. There are two main principles in the prevention of nutritional iron deficiency anaemia in women.

1. The regular consumption of a well-balanced diet containing an adequate quantity of the iron-rich foods.
2. The periodic administration of medicinal iron to women during times of increased physiological demands, e.g. pregnancy, lactation and when menstruation is excessive.

In the prevention of iron deficiency anaemia in infants the maintenance of a normal blood level in the mother is desirable. Premature and unduly small infants should be given medicinal iron as a routine. Iron-containing foods should be introduced into the infant's diet by the third to fourth month and thereafter be progressively increased. Following the control of infection, iron should be given to all infants if the haemoglobin level is reduced.

Treatment.

ADULTS. While a diet rich in iron should be prescribed, medicinal iron must also be given. In iron deficiency anaemia unlike pernicious anaemia and the haemolytic anaemias, there is a depletion of the body's usually considerable iron reserves. In consequence the absorption of iron through the intestinal wall is greatly increased in such patients. The ferrous salts of iron are for more effective in treatment than the ferric salts. A very satisfactory preparation is ferrous sulphate, which should be given in the form of tablets of 200 mg., 1 to 2 tablets being taken thrice daily *after* food. Alternative preparations of iron in pill or tablet form are ferrous gluconate, ferrous succinate and ferrous fumarate. All these preparations are equally effective in treatment, but ferrous sulphate is much less expensive. A slow release preparation of ferrous sulphate is available (Ferro-Gradumet) but the cost does not justify its routine use. Intolerance to oral preparations of iron is infrequent if the drug is taken only after meals and if the patients are reassured that undesirable side-effects are uncommon. If ferrous salts are given in a mixture they must be dispensed in a 50 per cent. solution of glucose to prevent oxidation to the ferric state. Proprietary liquid preparations are more palatable but more expensive. They include Fersamal Syrup, Plesmet Syrup and Sytron. A rise in haemoglobin of at least 1 per cent. per day is to be expected, and in the average case the blood level is restored to normal in four to eight weeks. In general, synthetic vitamin preparations need not be prescribed if iron medication is supplemented by a well-balanced diet. In particular, expensive preparations containing iron and folic acid should not be used. The addition of trace elements such as copper manganese and cobalt is of no clinical value. Attention should be paid to sites of *gross* focal infection, and any source of abnormal blood loss controlled. Apparent lack of response to iron therapy usually means that the patient is not taking the iron.

When the haemoglobin is below 5 g. per 100 ml. it is usually advisable for the patient to be kept in bed. The decision to transfuse should be based more on the clinical state of the patient than on the haemoglobin level.

After restoration of the blood to normal in a patient who has a chronic iron deficiency anaemia it is desirable to continue iron therapy for some eight weeks in order to replenish the depleted body stores. Thereafter relapse can usually be prevented by an iron-rich diet. The periodic administration of iron may, however, be required in women of the child-bearing age.

Parenteral Iron Therapy. Commercial preparations of iron for injection are saccharated oxide of iron for intravenous use (Ferrivenin) and preparations that can be given intramuscularly. The latter include an iron-dextran complex (Imferon) and an iron-sorbitol-citric acid complex (Jectofer). As a general rule such preparations should not be used except when one or other of the oral preparations of iron mentioned above cannot be tolerated or is found to be ineffective. The parenteral route of administration is suitable for the few patients who are genuinely unable to take iron by mouth because of pain, vomiting and diarrhoea, or who are unable to absorb iron because of some disorder of the gastro-intestinal tract, e.g. in the malabsorptive disorders (p. 939). Iron given by injection has been recommended for the treatment of the anaemia of rheumatoid arthritis and for the correction of severe anaemia in the late stages of pregnancy and following major operations.

Ferrivenin is now being withdrawn from the market. In 5 ml. there are 100 mg. of elemental iron and this amount is sufficient to increase the haemoglobin level by approximately 4 per cent. It is usual to give a test dose of 25 mg. of elemental iron at the first injection and thereafter 100-200 mg. every second or third day until a satisfactory haemoglobin level is reached. Reactions such as nausea, backache and collapse are uncommon, but as they may occur the patient should be observed for an hour or so after each injection and the material should be injected slowly and in amounts not exceeding 200 mg. of iron at any one injection. The total dosage of iron given in a course of injections should not exceed 2·5 g., and courses should not be repeated for at least three months. The latter precautions are necessary because of the high degree of retention in the body of the injected metal.

The use of the iron-dextran complex (Imferon) has been called into question because intramuscular injections of this preparation in rats have been followed by the development of sarcomata. While there is no evidence that similar changes will necessarily occur in humans it would seem wise to reserve intramuscular iron for the very few cases in which parenteral therapy is essential and the intravenous route of administration is impossible. Imferon must be given by deep intramuscular injection to avoid staining of the skin, and a test dose of 1 ml. equivalent to 50 mg. of elemental iron is first administered. Thereafter 2 to 5 ml. doses are given every second or third day until a total adult dosage of 20 to 40 ml. has been reached, depending on the severity of the anaemia. Recently the total iron requirements have been given in a single dose by one intravenous infusion of Imferon over a period of 4-10 minutes. Alarming general reactions may occur. The iron-sorbitol-citric acid complex Jectofer causes less staining of the skin and has not been shown to cause sarcomata in animals. Its iron content is 50 mg. per ml. and it is administered like Imferon by deep intramuscular injection in a dosage of 1·5 mg. per kg. of body weight. The administration of iron by mouth should cease while Jectofer is being given and for a few days beforehand, since toxic effects may occur. The urine sometimes turns black on standing.

INFANTS. The treatment of iron deficiency anaemia in infants requires the administration of medicinal iron as well as the introduction of iron-containing food into the diet. The dose of liquid iron preparations should give about 6 mg. iron per kg. body weight daily or 2·5 mg. iron per lb. per day. The British National Formulary ferrous sulphate mixture for infants is unpalatable and attacks dental enamel. A proprietary preparation such as ferrous fumarate syrup (Fersamal Syrup) costs little more. Only when parental iron therapy is essential and intravenous injection is impossible should iron, e.g. Jectofer, be given intramuscularly.

Treatment of Post-haemorrhagic Anaemia.

ACUTE. Treatment consists of bed rest, the administration of sedatives and the correction of the peripheral circulatory failure by the transfusion of sufficient quantities of whole blood or whole blood substitutes to restore the blood volume. The cause of the blood loss should be sought and treated. Thereafter iron should be given.

CHRONIC. Treatment involves the arrest of the haemorrhage by appropriate means where possible and the administration of iron and a good diet.

HYPOCHROMIC ANAEMIA DUE TO MALABSORPTION OF IRON

Iron deficiency anaemia commonly occurs in patients with gluten enteropathy, idiopathic steatorrhoea or tropical sprue, or with organic disease of the small intestine, e.g. regional enteritis or tuberculosis. It also occurs subsequent to partial gastrectomy or resection or short-circuiting of the small intestine because of failure of absorption of food iron. Months or years may elapse before the anaemia becomes manifest. Hence the patient will have left the charge of the specialist and be under the care of the general practitioner, who should be on the lookout for this development.

THE MEGALOBLASTIC ANAEMIAS

The continuation of normal blood formation is dependent on the supply of various factors to the bone marrow. Mention has already been made of iron, ascorbic acid, thyroxine and proteins. Vitamin B_{12} and folic acid are also required, and a deficiency of these vitamins will result in a change of normal erythropoiesis to a pathological type of blood formation (Plate VIID, p. 603).

The megaloblastic marrow is characterised by the presence of pathological nucleated red cells which differ from normoblasts. Early megaloblasts are larger than early normoblasts. While the cytoplasm is deeply basophilic in both, the nucleus of the megaloblast has a much more loosely woven network of chromatin. This essential character is seen in megaloblasts even when haemoglobinisation is taking place. Thereafter disintegration and disappearance of the nucleus occurs. The resulting erythrocyte, called a macrocyte, is larger than a normal erythrocyte, has a full complement of haemoglobin, and hence stains uniformly pink; it tends to be more oval than round in shape. Since a certain amount of normoblastic blood formation is proceeding simultaneously in a megaloblastic marrow, the peripheral blood shows a wide variety of cells of different shapes and sizes. Another feature that is often noted is the presence of giant metamyelocytes in the bone marrow. Megaloblastic anaemia may arise in several ways:

1. By a failure in assimilation of vitamin B_{12} consequent on defective production of intrinsic factor by the stomach. This is the cause of Addisonian pernicious anaemia, which is by far the most important type of megaloblastic anaemia in temperate climates. A similar result occurs after total gastrectomy and may occur after partial gastrectomy or, very rarely, gastroenterostomy. Very rarely there may be an inborn deficiency of intrinsic factor secretion, giving rise to so-called juvenile pernicious anaemia.

2. By an intake of a diet deficient in folic acid, vitamin B_{12}, or both, leading to nutritional megaloblastic anaemia.

3. By a failure of absorption of folic acid or vitamin B_{12} as a result of dysfunction, disease, resection or short-circuiting of the small intestine (p. 626).

4. Where there is a blind or stagnant loop of small intestine containing bacteria which apparently utilise vitamin B_{12}, thus rendering it unavailable to the host. The same may occur in jejunal diverticulosis.

5. In pregnancy and infancy. Sometimes in pregnancy, and exceptionally in infancy, there develops a megaloblastic anaemia which invariably responds to folic acid but may be partially or completely refractory to a cobalamin.

6. Infection with the fish tapeworm, *Diphyllobothrium latum*, a condition found chiefly in Finland, may lead to megaloblastic anaemia particularly in those predisposed to pernicious anaemia because the worm ingests vitamin B_{12} in the alimentary tract of the host.

7. From the administration of anticonvulsant drugs, particularly phenytoin sodium or primidone for prolonged periods.

The cause is uncertain, but it is possible that the drugs concerned interfere with folic acid metabolism.

8. Where there is a haemolytic or leukaemic process, the rapidly dividing cells may have an increased utilisation of folic acid.

In Britain six out of seven cases of megaloblastic anaemia are due to intrinsic factor deficiency (Addisonian pernicious anaemia). Of the remainder the megaloblastic anaemias associated with pregnancy or with diseases and disorders of the gastro-intestinal tract are the most important. In tropical countries malnutrition and pregnancy are the two main factors concerned in the aetiology of the megaloblastic anaemias.

ADDISONIAN PERNICIOUS ANAEMIA

The name Addisonian pernicious anaemia should be limited to the group of megaloblastic anaemias which is due to a failure in secretion of intrinsic factor by the stomach other than from surgery.

Aetiology. This disease is rare before the age of 30 and affects females more than males between 45 and 65 years of age. Achylia gastrica is invariably present. The condition is often familial. The gastric mucosa fails to produce a substance (intrinsic factor) required for the absorption of vitamin B_{12} from the alimentary tract and there is evidence from the finding of gastric antibodies that an autoimmune mechanism may be responsible for initiating the process.

Pathology. In the stage of relapse there is extension of red bone marrow into the shafts of the long bones. This marrow shows a 'megaloblastic reaction,' i.e. the presence of many megaloblasts and a great reduction in the number of normoblasts. Polymorphonuclear leucocytes and megakaryocytes are also diminished in number. There is evidence of increased blood destruction—enlargement of the spleen, hyperbilirubinaemia and increased deposition of iron (haemosiderin) in the liver, spleen, kidneys and bone marrow. The gastric mucosa is thin and atrophic. In untreated or inadequately treated cases degenerative changes in the posterior and lateral tracts of the spinal cord may be found.

Clinical Features. The onset is insidious and the degree of anaemia is often great before the patient consults the doctor. In addition to the general symptoms of anaemia (p. 610) there may be intermittent soreness of the tongue and occasionally periodic diarrhoea.

On examination the patient generally appears well nourished despite the fact that weight loss is a common feature. The skin and mucous membranes are pale, and in severely anaemic cases the skin may show a faint lemon-yellow tint. When the tongue is painful it often has a red, raw appearance, sometimes with ulcers; later the mucous membrane becomes smooth and atrophic. The spleen is seldom palpable. Gastric analysis invariably shows histamine-fast achlorhydria. The urine is found to contain excess of urobilinogen in the relapse stage. In about 80 per cent. of cases in relapse paraesthesiae occur in fingers and toes—numbness, tingling, 'pins and needles.' Occasionally there are objective signs of involvement of the posterior and lateral columns of the spinal cord (subacute combined degeneration (p. 1212)), which may rarely occur before the anaemia.

Examination of the stained blood film shows a macrocytic anaemia. The mean corpuscular volume is raised and the macrocytes appear fully stained. There is marked anisocytosis and poikilocytosis and many cells are oval in shape. Occasionally in severe cases a few nucleated red cells or haemoglobinised megaloblasts are seen in the peripheral blood. Reticulocytes number less than 1 per cent. (except during the commencement of remission). There is leucopenia, the reduction involving only the granulocytes, which are mature, some having an increased number of lobes (more than five) in the nuclei. There is thrombocytopenia, which is usually moderate but can be marked and associated with purpura (p. 670). The serum bilirubin level is raised.

Diagnosis. It should be realised that the term macrocytic anaemia merely signifies that the number of large red cells in the peripheral blood is increased and hence the MCV is greater than normal. Macrocytic anaemia can arise from many causes and the bone marrow may be megaloblastic (as in the conditions mentioned on p. 620 or normoblastic (as in some cases of haemolytic anaemia, aplastic anaemia, hepatic cirrhosis, myxoedema, leukaemia). The term megaloblastic should be reserved for cases in which megaloblasts can be demonstrated in the bone marrow or in the 'buffy coat' of the blood after centrifugation. The differential diagnosis of pernicious anaemia from other forms of megaloblastic anaemia depends upon the age of the patient, the finding of histamine-fast achlorhydria, and upon the absence of pregnancy and the lack of evidence of malnutrition, malabsorption or structural change in the small intestine. Inquiry should also be made about the taking of anticonvulsant drugs. In complex cases of megaloblastic anaemia additional methods of investigation may be required, e.g. measurement of the serum vitamin B_{12} or folate levels and estimation of the absorption from the alimentary tract of folic acid or of cyanocobalamin labelled with radioactive cobalt (e.g. the Schilling test).

Treatment. *General.* The patient should be kept in bed until the haemoglobin is about 7 g. per 100 ml. The diet should be light and easily digested and should be rich in protein, iron and vitamin C. The decision to give a blood transfusion is based on general principles concerning the clinical state of the patient. When the haemoglobin level is so low as to endanger life, e.g. under 4 g. per 100 ml. it should always be carefully considered. In all types of chronic anaemia of sufficient severity to require transfusion the blood must be carefully matched and should be given very slowly because of the danger of producing sudden cardiac failure.

Specific. Parenteral injection of a cobalamin should be given as soon as the diagnosis is established. Folic acid should ***never*** be used in the treatment of Addisonian pernicious anaemia as it does not prevent the development of neurological complications, and may possibly precipitate them. Hydroxocobalamin is better retained in the body than the cyano form, and hence is the preparation of choice. It should be given in a dosage of 1,000 micrograms twice during the first week, then 250 micrograms weekly until the blood count is normal.

Within 48 hours of the first injection of a hydroxocobalamin the bone marrow shows a striking change from a megaloblastic to a normoblastic state. Within two to three days the reticulocyte count begins to rise, reaching a maximum about the fifth to seventh day. The maximum rise tends to vary inversely with the initial red cell count, e.g. initial red cell count 1,000,000 per c.mm.—maximum reticulocyte count about 40 per cent.; initial red cell count 2,500,000 per c.mm.—reticulocyte count about 15 per cent. About 12-14 days after treatment has started the reticulocyte count returns to 1 per cent. or less. Shortly before the reticulocyte peak the red cell count and haemoglobin level begin to show a sharp rise, and this rise is steadily maintained till normal figures are attained. An increase of 500,000 red cells and 1 g. per 100 ml. haemoglobin per week can be expected. The mean corpuscular volume progressively approaches normality, and macrocytosis, anisocytosis and poikilocytosis disappear. There is also a rise to normal in white cell and platelet counts.

In some cases the rapid regeneration of the blood depletes the iron reserves of the body so that the haemoglobin fails to rise above 10-11 g. per 100 ml. and the MCHC falls below normal. To prevent this occurring ferrous sulphate 200 mg. thrice daily should be given in addition to hydroxocobalamin soon after the commencement of treatment. A combined deficiency of vitamin B_{12} and iron is recognised by the presence of macrocytosis and hypochromia. It is sometimes referred to as a dimorphic blood picture.

When subacute combined degeneration of the cord is present the dose of hydroxocobalamin should be 250 micrograms twice weekly and continued at this high level for at least six months.

If a patient diagnosed as having pernicious anaemia fails to respond to the parenteral administration of adequate dosage of hydroxocobalamin, then it means that the diagnosis is wrong, the preparation used is not potent, or alternatively the patient is suffering from one of the other types of megaloblastic anaemia, e.g. megaloblastic anaemia of pregnancy or of idiopathic steatorrhoea, which may be partially or completely refractory to hydroxocobalamin. Such cases respond to folic acid.

Maintenance. It is vital that the patient suffering from pernicious anaemia should continue to receive regular doses of a cobalamin for the rest of his life. The dose must be so regulated that the haemoglobin level is maintained at approximately 14·6 g. per 100 ml. and the red cell count at 5,000,000. The dose of hydroxocobalamin usually given is 1,000 micrograms by intramuscular injection every four to six weeks. Theoretically the interval between doses may be longer than this but there is no merit in seeking the minimal effective dose. Indeed, regular blood counts should be done every six months and the assessment should never be made solely on clinical impression or on the haemoglobin level alone. Only thus can the appearance or progression of subacute combined degeneration of the cord be prevented. The oral administration of large doses of vitamin B_{12} alone or in combination with intrinsic factor concentrate has not proved satisfactory. When a relative of a patient with pernicious anaemia becomes ill, it is important to remember that he or she may have the same disease.

Prognosis. In the untreated case the disease runs a course which is progressive and usually insidious. Death occurs from anaemia with or without the complication of subacute combined degeneration of the cord, or from intercurrent infection. With the maintenance of a normal blood count by adequate specific treatment the patient remains healthy and has a normal expectancy of life. In cases already suffering from subacute combined degeneration of the cord before treatment is started, adequate therapy restores the blood to normal, prevents further deterioration in the cord changes, and may produce considerable functional improvement if the process is not too far advanced.

NUTRITIONAL MEGALOBLASTIC ANAEMIA

This type of megaloblastic anaemia is directly due to the prolonged ingestion of a diet which is deficient in folic acid, and perhaps vitamin B_{12} and other unknown factors. Such diets are gravely deficient in many nutrients but especially in protein foods, fruit and vegetables. It is of common occurrence in tropical countries, and is very rarely encountered in Britain.

Achlorhydria is not a characteristic feature and lesions of the central nervous system are extremely rare. The peripheral blood shows a macrocytic anaemia unless there is a complicating iron deficiency. The bone marrow is megaloblastic.

Treatment consists of the administration of a well-balanced high protein diet together with folic acid 5-10 mg. daily. Injections of hydroxocobalamin alone are frequently ineffective, but it is reasonable to supplement folic acid therapy with injections of hydroxocobalamin. Other vitamins and iron may be required in addition. Maintenance treatment with folic acid is not required if the patient takes an adequate diet.

MEGALOBLASTIC ANAEMIA ASSOCIATED WITH DEFECTIVE INTESTINAL ABSORPTION

Megaloblastic anaemia is commonly seen in tropical sprue and idiopathic steatorrhoea (a condition which is frequently a form of gluten enteropathy). It is due to failure of absorption of folic acid, of vitamin B_{12} or of both.

Megaloblastic anaemia may occur subsequent to resection or short-circuiting of a large segment of the small intestine. Normally folic acid is absorbed readily throughout the small intestine, but vitamin B_{12} only from the lower ileum. There is sometimes a complicating defect in the absorption of iron and other vitamins, in which case a dimorphic blood picture results (p. 624). Gluten enteropathy in childhood is seldom associated with megaloblastic anaemia.

The clinical features are those of the underlying alimentary disease together with the general symptoms of anaemia. In addition symptoms and signs of various vitamin and mineral deficiencies are also frequently present (p. 942). Histamine-fast achlorhydria is uncommon and subacute combined degeneration of the cord is very rare. Jejunal biopsy by the oral route and other investigations referred to on p. 623 may be of great help if the diagnosis is in doubt.

In tropical sprue and idiopathic steatorrhoea there is usually an excellent response to folic acid, which should be given intramuscularly for the first two or three days and orally in a dosage of 20 mg. a day thereafter. It is wise to supplement this with 1,000 micrograms of hydroxocobalamin by injection every four to six weeks and, particularly in the tropics, iron by mouth may also be required. When there has been resection or short circuiting of the ileum, the primary deficiency will be of vitamin B_{12}. It is generally agreed that a child with gluten enteropathy must be given a gluten free diet and that in the adult with idiopathic steatorrhoea, which is frequently a form of gluten sensitivity, a gluten free diet should be tried for at least six months and continued thereafter if there is benefit. Other aspects of treatment are considered on p. 945.

MEGALOBLASTIC ANAEMIA ASSOCIATED WITH BLIND OR STAGNANT LOOPS OF SMALL INTESTINE

In this condition which is mentioned on p. 620, there is likely to be a response to hydroxocobalamin therapy, but surgical correction of the causal lesion is usually required if a permanent cure is to be achieved. The effects of gastrectomy and gastroenterostomy are also referred to on p. 620.

MEGALOBLASTIC ANAEMIA OF PREGNANCY

A temporary macrocytic anaemia with megaloblastic reaction in the bone marrow may occur during pregnancy or the puerperium. The clinical features are the same as those of Addisonian pernicious anaemia except that free hydrochloric acid is commonly present in the gastric juice, and subacute combined degeneration does not occur. The factors involved in its causation include increased demands and dietary deficiency, especially of folic acid and more rarely of vitamin B_{12}.

Prior to modern treatment with blood transfusions and folic acid, there was a mortality of 50-75 per cent., death occurring from shock and anaemia aggravated by haemorrhage at childbirth. With modern treatment the prognosis is excellent.

Cases of megaloblastic anaemia of pregnancy usually respond dramatically to the oral ingestion of 10 mg. of folic acid daily. If the anaemia is very severe and is not discovered until close to full term, transfusion of compatible blood is indicated in addition. Folic acid therapy should be stopped after the puerperium when the blood level has reached normal, since the disease is self-terminating. Megaloblastic anaemia may recur in subsequent pregnancies. A coexisting deficiency of iron is frequent, and this leads to a dimorphic blood picture. Iron therapy is indicated in such cases. Since there is biochemical evidence of folic acid depletion in about 20 per cent. of pregnant women in the United Kingdom and because Addisonian pernicious anaemia is rare in this age group, it is reasonable to give folic acid as a prophylactic in pregnancy. This is even more important in tropical countries. In Britain it is convenient to give 2 tablets of Pregamal (Glaxo) daily for prophylaxis. These contain 100 micrograms of folic acid and 200 mg. of ferrous fumarate in each tablet.

MEGALOBLASTIC ANAEMIA IN INFANCY

This type of anaemia occurs infrequently in infants whose diets are markedly deficient in protein, folic acid and ascorbic acid, and who in addition are suffering from infections and diarrhoea. Although the disease is very rare in the United Kingdom it is being recognised in underdeveloped countries as a complication of kwashiorkor (p. 462). The anaemia responds to treatment with folic acid and ascorbic acid. In gluten enteropathy, anaemia is almost invariably due to iron deficiency, but the occasional case with a megaloblastic anaemia will respond to folic acid therapy. Juvenile pernicious anaemia is a rare disease in which there is lack of intrinsic factor, usually without achlorhydria.

MEGALOBLASTIC ANAEMIA ASSOCIATED WITH HAEMOLYTIC ANAEMIA OR WITH LEUKAEMIA

Patients with haemolytic anaemia may develop megaloblastic change in the marrow if for some reason, particularly malnutrition, they are deficient in folic acid. In acute leukaemia or in the chronic myeloid form the rapidly dividing white cell precursors may deplete the red cell precursors of folic acid. Folic acid therapy is necessary in megaloblastic anaemia if it is a complication of haemolytic anaemia, but such therapy may cause an exacerbation of a leukaemic process which may therefore require more intensive treatment.

MEGALOBLASTIC ANAEMIA ASSOCIATED WITH THE ADMINISTRATION OF ANTICONVULSANTS

This form of anaemia, described on p. 620, responds to folic acid therapy even if treatment with the anticonvulsant drugs is continued.

ANAEMIA DUE TO DEFICIENCY OF VITAMIN C

Anaemia may be found in association with scurvy, a nutritional disease in which there is usually a defective intake of protein and minerals as well as ascorbic acid. The anaemia may be normocytic or macrocytic in type but the bone marrow is not megaloblastic unless there is coincidental deficiency of folic acid or vitamin B_{12}. The cause of the anaemia of scurvy has usually been attributed either to (*a*) loss of blood from the alimentary tract or into the tissues, or (*b*) defective blood formation as a result of ascorbic acid deficiency. It has recently been shown by radio-isotope studies that a haemolytic element may be present and this can be corrected by the administration of ascorbic acid. The administration of vitamin C alone may produce a reticulocyte crisis and a rapid increase of erythrocytes. When associated with an iron deficiency, iron must also be given.

Although frank scurvy is rare in Britain, subscorbutic levels of vitamin C are not infrequently present in cases of nutritional iron deficiency anaemia, especially in elderly men living alone. The giving of ascorbic acid is however generally unnecessary if a well-balanced diet containing fruit and vegetables is prescribed.

ANAEMIA DUE TO DEFICIENCY OF THYROXINE

The anaemia of myxoedema is usually moderate in degree and normocytic or macrocytic in type. Accompanying iron deficiency is not uncommon. The clinical picture may strongly suggest pernicious anaemia, but treatment with hydroxocobalamin is ineffective, except in the rare cases with co-existing pernicious anaemia. It is recognised that pernicious anaemia occurs more commonly in patients with myxoedema and that in both conditions there may be evidence of an autoimmune process. In the true anaemia of myxoedema, administration of thyroid extract produces a slow improvement in the blood level. Associated iron deficiency must be appropriately corrected.

ANAEMIAS DUE TO EXCESSIVE BLOOD DESTRUCTION (HAEMOLYTIC ANAEMIAS)

Definition. Destruction of red blood corpuscles either by the cells of the reticulo-endothelial system (intracellular) or within the circulating blood (intravascular) causes anaemia if the degree of haemolysis exceeds the regenerative ability of the bone marrow. The excessive destruction of red cells results in hyperbilirubin-aemia with latent or manifest jaundice but without bilirubinuria, hence the name acholuric jaundice. There is, however, excess of urobilinogen in the urine. In some rare types there is free haemoglobin in the plasma and in the urine. The continuous demand for new red cells results in a constant reticulocytosis, often over 10 per cent. Thus the essential features of any haemolytic anaemia are persistent anaemia, persistent reticulocytosis, hyperbilirubinaemia and excess urobilinogen in the urine and the faeces.

HAEMOLYTIC ANAEMIA DUE TO CONGENITAL ABNORMALITIES OF THE ERYTHROCYTE

(*a*) Congenital Spherocytosis (Acholuric Jaundice)

This is a familial disease transmitted and inherited by both sexes. The underlying cause is unknown but many of the red cells produced are abnormal in shape, being more nearly spherical than biconcave (microspherocytes). Such cells are unduly fragile and therefore more easily destroyed. This is the fundamental abnormality which is responsible for the clinical and haematological features of the disease.

The symptoms usually appear in childhood but they are often insufficient to cause the patient discomfort. Moderate pallor and a slight yellow tint in the skin are however noticeable. Anaemia and jaundice are mild to moderate in degree, while the spleen is invariably enlarged.

Crises may occur at variable intervals with severe anaemia and jaundice and increased splenic enlargement. At such times the patient complains of weakness and breathlessness, which, in severe cases, may be very marked and associated with rigors, fever and vomiting. The mechanism of the crisis is not fully understood, but it may be precipitated by infection.

Between the crises, blood examination shows a moderate normochromic anaemia, e.g. haemoglobin 10 g. per 100 ml., red cells 3,500,000 per c.mm. The reticulocyte count is persistently raised —5-20 per cent. Stained filmsshow well-filled red cells, the diameter of which is less than normal, but the thickness of which is increased—microspherocytosis. The red cells are unduly fragile in hypotonic salt solution, laking beginning at 0·5-0·75 per cent. saline and being complete at 0·4 per cent. (normal 0·45 per cent. and 0·3 per cent. respectively); the serum bilirubin level is usually from 2-4 mg. per 100 ml. The urine contains excess urobilinogen but no bilirubin. During a haemolytic crisis the red blood count falls rapidly to a level of 1,000,000-2,000,000 per c.mm. and subsequently the reticulocyte count rises sharply to 40-60 per cent. or even more. A leucocytosis also occurs. Normoblastic hyperplasia of the bone marrow is found.

The recognition of the existence of a haemolytic anaemia is made on the finding of the characteristic blood picture as described above. The differentiation from other types of haemolytic anaemia depends upon the demonstration of increased fragility of red cells, microspherocytosis, splenomegaly, and especially on the family history of other cases of anaemia and jaundice. Spherocytes may be found in other forms of haemolytic anaemia. If red cells are tagged with ^{51}Chromate and returned to the patient's circulation, their time of survival will be found to be reduced. The Coombs' test (p. 636) is negative in congenital spherocytosis.

While many patients lead a normal life and die of old age, others suffer from severe episodes of haemolytic anaemia or cholecystitis secondary to the development of pigment stones in the gall-bladder. Such episodes may end fatally.

Treatment. Splenectomy results in striking and usually permanent improvement both in the symptoms and in the anaemia. All authorities are agreed that operation should be advised when the anaemia causes persistent impairment of health, when severe haemolytic crises have occurred, when other members of the family have died from the disease, or where evidence of cholecystitis and cholelithiasis is present. Opinion differs as to the desirability of operation in mild cases with no resulting disability. The operation should be carried out during a period of remission, and in young children should be deferred until school age. Severe haemolytic crises require treatment by blood transfusion. Blood must be matched very carefully and administered by very slow drip, as gross haemolytic transfusion reactions are common in this disease. Iron and other haematinics are of no value. In this type of haemolytic anaemia treatment with steroids is not indicated.

(*b*) Hereditary Haemoglobinopathies

The hereditary haemoglobinopathies include a wide range of haematological disorders in which, as a result of genetic mutations, there is a disorder of haemoglobin synthesis and the red cells contain a proportion of one or more abnormal haemoglobins. In some cases the haemolytic anaemia may be so severe as to lead to fatal results, while in others it may be so mild as to cause little or no inconvenience. Examples are thalassaemia (Cooley's anaemia), in which haemoglobin-F may persist in post-natal life, and sickle cell disease, a condition most commonly found in negroes, in which haemoglobin-S occurs. There is no specific treatment and splenectomy is contraindicated.

The increase of immigration into Britain in recent years of racial groups in whom the haemoglobinopathies are common, and the introduction of relatively simple techniques for identifying abnormal haemoglobins have led to the recognition of considerable numbers of persons suffering from haemoglobinopathies. Very occasionally, refractory iron deficiency anaemia in British subjects without known Mediterranean ancestry may be due to thalassaemia minor.

HAEMOLYTIC ANAEMIA DUE TO INFECTIVE OR TOXIC FACTORS

Haemolytic streptococci, staphylococci and *Clostridium welchii* are the most important micro-organisms which can produce a haemolytic anaemia in man, although such an occurrence is very rare. Malaria is the most important protozoal infection leading to a haemolytic anaemia in the tropics. In blackwater fever (p. 589) a complication of falciparum malaria, severe intravascular haemolysis with haemoglobinuria occurs.

Of the numerous agents which on occasion have been reported to cause haemolytic anaemia, mention should be made of the following: arsenic and its derivatives, lead, sulphonamides, potassium chlorate, naphthalene, phenylhydrazine, methyldopa and nitrofurantoin.

The red cells in some people are deficient in gluco e-6-phosphate dehydrogenase activity. Such individuals may develop haemolytic anaemia from contact with beans of the plant, *Vicia faba*, or with its pollen, or from taking certain drugs, particularly primaquine. Some of the agents mentioned above may cause haemolysis by this mechanism.

HAEMOLYTIC ANAEMIA DUE TO ERYTHROCYTE ANTIBODIES

The most important examples of anaemia in this group are:

Haemolytic disease of the newborn.
Idiopathic (acquired) haemolytic anaemia.
Symptomatic haemolytic anaemia.
Paroxysmal haemoglobinuria.

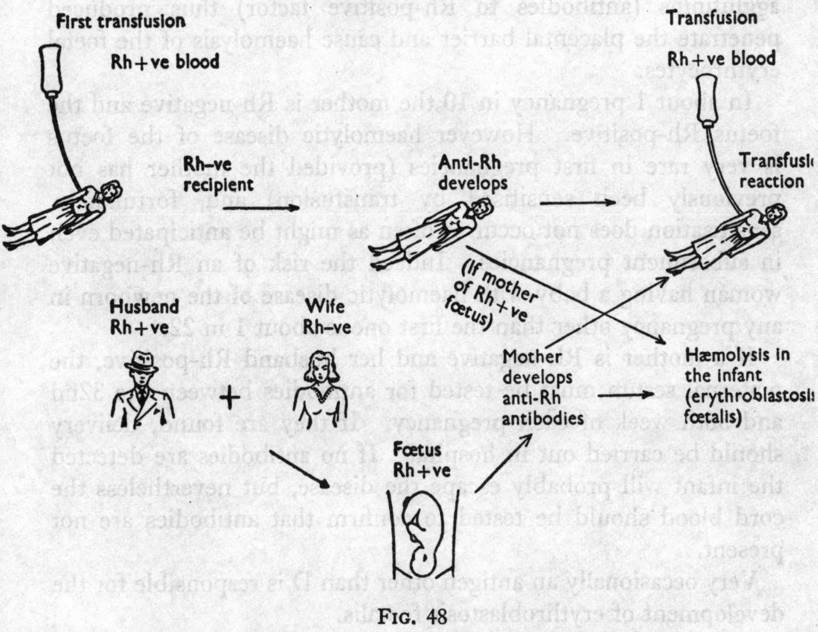

Fig. 48

Common Examples of Rh Incompatibility

Haemolytic Disease of the Newborn

This disease, sometimes called erythroblastosis foetalis, occurs in either sex at birth or within the first two to three days. The first-born child in the family is usually healthy, but in successive children the severity of the disease increases and later children may be born dead. Hydrops foetalis is the most severe form, death occurring *in utero*; icterus gravis neonatorum is a dangerous illness but compatible with survival; congenital anaemia of the newborn is the mildest form.

It appears that in most cases the rhesus (Rh) factor is the sensitising agent or antigen. The majority (85 per cent.) of people, men and women, have red cells which contain the Rh antigen, D, and these people are said to be Rh-positive. Some of the children of an Rh-positive father and an Rh-negative mother are Rh-positive, since the factor is inherited as a Mendelian dominant. The Rh-negative mother becomes sensitised by the Rh-positive substance contained in the foetal red cells. The maternal agglutinins (antibodies to Rh-positive factor) thus produced penetrate the placental barrier and cause haemolysis of the foetal erythrocytes.

In about 1 pregnancy in 10 the mother is Rh-negative and the foetus Rh-positive. However haemolytic disease of the foetus is very rare in first pregnancies (provided the mother has not previously been sensitised by transfusion) and, fortunately, sensitisation does not occur as often as might be anticipated even in subsequent pregnancies. Indeed the risk of an Rh-negative woman having a baby with haemolytic disease of the newborn in any pregnancy other than the first one is about 1 in 22.

If a mother is Rh-negative and her husband Rh-positive, the maternal serum must be tested for antibodies between the 32nd and 36th week of each pregnancy. If they are found, delivery should be carried out in hospital. If no antibodies are detected the infant will probably escape the disease, but nevertheless the cord blood should be tested to confirm that antibodies are not present.

Very occasionally an antigen other than D is responsible for the development of erythroblastosis foetalis.

It must be remembered that an Rh-negative mother who has had an Rh-positive foetus may be sensitised to Rh-positive blood. If she receives a transfusion and Rh-positive blood is given a haemolytic reaction may occur. Consequently all women of child-bearing age or under and all pregnant women who may require transfusion must have their blood typed for Rh factors as well as for the main blood groups.

Clinical Features. The clinical features of haemolytic anaemia of the newborn are those of severe haemolytic anaemia with oedema and enlargement of the liver and spleen. Clinical jaundice is usually absent for 24 hours after birth. Thereafter deep jaundice leading to kernicterus may occur (p. 1196). The severity of the jaundice is largely due to the immaturity of the foetal liver which is unable to conjugate the large amounts of bilirubin with which it has to deal. The blood picture is very striking. The haemoglobin level which should normally be about 18 g. per 100 ml. at birth, falls rapidly. Enormous numbers of nucleated red cells (50,000 per c.mm. or more) and reticulocytes 10-50 per cent. are found in the peripheral blood.

In the severe cases the mortality is 70-80 per cent. without treatment, death occurring within two weeks, but with exchange transfusion the mortality is low. Spontaneous recovery occurs in the mild cases.

Treatment. Exchange transfusion should be given to all severely affected infants, as this is the only method of treatment that will overcome heart failure in the very anaemic infant and prevent deep jaundice and kernicterus in others. Delay of even a day may prove fatal and hence early diagnosis is essential. Antenatal prediction from tests of the maternal serum for antibodies gives the infant his best chance. In mild cases simple transfusion will be sufficient, and in some instances no treatment is required. It is now believed that the most common cause of primary Rh immunisation may be transplacental haemorrhage during labour, and that if an Rh-negative mother has an Rh-positive baby as judged by examination of the cord blood, the development of Rh antibodies may be prevented by giving potent anti-D γ-globulin to the mother immediately after pregnancy. This may be most important in the prevention of this distressing disorder in later babies.

Idiopathic (Acquired) Haemolytic Anaemia

In this form of haemolytic anaemia no family history can be obtained and the fault is believed to lie in the production of auto-agglutinins and auto-haemolysins which injure the red blood corpuscles.

The clinical features are the same as those described for the congenital type, but the crises are more severe and more frequent and the residual anaemia during remissions of greater degree, e.g. red cell count persistently at or below 3,000,000 per c.mm. Microspherocytosis is usually but not always absent, and the fragility of the red cells is either normal or but slightly increased. A serological test for immune globulin (the Coombs' test) is frequently positive in idiopathic acquired haemolytic anaemia, but negative in the congenital form. It should, however, be realised that the test is not a specific one for the former condition.

The prognosis is more serious than in the congenital from, death in haemolytic crises being more frequent.

The treatment of idiopathic (acquired) haemolytic anaemia is initially by the repeated transfusion of carefully typed blood. The risks of reactions to blood transfusion are even greater than in the congenital form. It would appear reasonable to try the effect of prednisone in a dosage of 60 mg. daily by mouth for two to three weeks, and if a remission is induced the dose should be reduced to the lowest that will maintain the patient in a partial or complete remission without inducing toxic effects. Should steroids fail initially or in maintenance treatment, splenectomy should be carried out, especially if excessive blood destruction by the spleen can be shown to be present by radioactive isotope studies. The final results of this operation are not as satisfactory as in congenital haemolytic anaemia and when splenectomy fails, steroids may have to be tried again.

Symptomatic Haemolytic Anaemia and Paroxysmal Haemoglobinuria

Mention need only be made of these rare forms of haemolytic anaemia. Haemolytic anaemia occurs occasionally in association with a variety of diseases such as chronic leukaemia, lymphadenoma, malignant disease, cirrhosis of the liver and infections such as syphilis and tuberculosis. The underlying mechanism is obscure. A cold-antibody type of haemolytic anaemia sometimes occurs as a complication about the third week of an attack of virus pneumonia and may be associated with Raynaud's phenomenon (p. 295).

Paroxysmal haemoglobinuria caused by intravascular haemolysis is found occasionally in association with syphilis, evertion, and also without any known cause.

Treatment of these groups of haemolytic anaemias consists of treatment of the underlying condition where possible, and blood transfusions as required. Splenectomy is contraindicated but steroid therapy is sometimes beneficial.

TRANSFUSION WITH INCOMPATIBLE BLOOD

Transfusion with incompatible blood results in the haemolysis of the infused red cells. Such a situation may arise: (1) when the infused red cells are of the wrong main blood group due to careless typing of the bloods; (2) when the bloods of recipient and donor are of compatible main groups but incompatible sub-groups. Direct cross-matching of recipient's serum against donor's cells greatly reduces this risk; (3) from the transfusion of Rh-positive blood to a sensitised Rh-negative recipient.

Symptoms usually begin after only a few millilitres of blood have been given, and if the transfusion is immediatly stopped there may be no serious consequences. The patient complains of shivering and restlessness, nausea and vomiting, praecordial and lumbar pain. There is a cold, clammy skin with cyanosis. The pulse and respiration rates increase and the temperature rises to 38-40° C. (101-105° F.). The blood pressure falls and the patient passes into a state of shock. There is haemoglobinaemia, and possibly even haemoglobinuria; oliguria and even anuria may occur with nitrogen retention due to acute tubular necrosis. Jaundice appears after a few hours. In severe cases the anuria persists and uraemia develops, from which the patient may die. In others diuresis occurs even after several days and the patient recovers. In the majority the acute features subside in 24-48 hours.

Prophylaxis involves great care in the typing of blood and direct cross-matching before administration. The first 50-100 ml. of any transfusion should be given very slowly and the transfusion stopped at once if any untoward symptoms develop. The patient should be under continuous observation during transfusion.

Treatment of the established reaction involves giving 100 mg. of hydrocortisone hemisuccinate intravenously, and initiating the general treatment of peripheral circulatory failure. When oliguria occurs the measures recommended for its treatment on p. 824 must be instituted at once.

ANAEMIAS DUE TO HYPOPLASIA OR APLASIA OF THE ERYTHROPOIETIC TISSUE IN THE BONE MARROW

PRIMARY (IDIOPATHIC) APLASTIC ANAEMIA

This is a rare disease of unknown aetiology. The bone marrow shows a great reduction in all formative elements, and the sample obtained by sternal puncture contains only a few scattered cells in a gelatinous and fatty matrix. The disease may occur at any age but is most common in young adults, or in the elderly.

The clinical features are those of a steadily progressive anaemia with haemorrhage into the skin or from the mucous membranes (due to thrombocytopenia) and fever and necrotic ulcers in the mouth and throat (due to granulopenia). The blood picture is that of a normocytic normochromic anaemia, e.g. haemoglobin 6 g. per 100 ml., red cell count 2,000,000 per c.mm,, MCHC 32 per cent. The reticulocyte count is persistently low. There is leucopenia (2,000-1,000 per c.mm.) with progressive diminution in the proportions of granulocytes. The platelet count also falls progressively to figures less than 10,000 per c.mm. The term 'pancytopenia' is frequently used when all the formed elements of the peripheral blood are diminished in this way. The disease is usually fatal within three to nine months, but complete recovery can occur.

SECONDARY HYPOPLASTIC OR APLASTIC ANAEMIA

This may be due to:

1. Idiosyncrasy to certain drugs such as chloramphenicol, phenylbutazone, organic arsenicals, troxidone, dinitrophenol, gold, thiouracil, potassium perchlorate, or certain industrial chemicals, chiefly benzol and its derivatives such as trinitrophenol, trinitrotoluene. It may also result from the use of antimetabolites and cytotoxic drugs which are employed in the treatment of malignant disease.
2. Exposure to X-rays and radioactive substances.

There is no direct correlation between the dose of a toxic agent and the occurrence or degree of anaemia. Some persons are unduly sensitive. Aplastic anaemia may develop weeks or months after the cessation of administration of such drugs as chloramphenicol, gold or organic arsenicals, or exposure to benzol or other industrial poisons, a point of legal importance in claims for compensation.

Clinical Features. The clinical features and blood changes are similar to those of primary aplastic anaemia (p. 638).

The course varies from that of a rapidly progressive fatal aplastic anaemia to a chronic hypoplastic process in which an anaemia of 6-9 g. haemoglobin per 100 ml. may persist for months or years. Complete recovery occasionally occurs, but is rare when chloramphenicol is the causative agent.

Diagnosis of Aplastic Anaemia. The essential haematological findings which serve to distinguish this from other types of anaemia are: a normochromic anaemia with little anisocytosis and poikilocytosis, absence of reticulocytes or other signs of blood regeneration, granulopenia and thrombocytopenia. A failure to respond to the administration of iron, cobalamin, folic acid and vitamin C strongly supports the diagnosis.

The diagnosis from aleukaemic leukaemia may be extremely difficult unless the bone marrow is examined. Other blood diseases which should be considered are idiopathic thrombocytopenic purpura and agranulocytosis (pp. 669, 643).

Treatment. Since the cause of idiopathic aplastic anaemia is unknown, all that can be done is to support life by repeated blood transfusions and give the patient ample amounts of all known haemopoietic factors such as a cobalamin, folic acid, iron and vitamin C. A course of treatment with prednisone, e.g. 40 mg. daily for three weeks, may also be given a trial. Marrow grafting has been employed, but without success. Treatment with repeated blood transfusions, oral antibiotics and haematinics must be continued for at least six months before being abandoned as recovery occurs in a small proportion of cases. If the cause of secondary aplastic anaemia can be found and removed the patient may recover provided the bone marrow has not been irretrievably damaged. Injections of dimercaprol should be tried if aplastic anaemia is due to gold or organic arsenicals. In other respects treatment is the same as for primary aplastic anaemia. Recently attempts have been made to treat aplastic anaemia with phytohaemagglutinin derived from the seeds of *Phaseolus vulgaris* but the value of this remains to be proved.

ANAEMIAS OF UNCERTAIN ORIGIN

Infection. Anaemia, which is mild or moderate in degree and normochromic in type may develop secondary to a severe chronic infection, particularly if fever is present. A mild degree of iron deficiency may be found. The response to iron therapy, both oral and parenteral, is usually unsatisfactory unless the primary cause of the anaemia is removed.

Uraemia. In chronic renal disease anaemia is common but the bone marrow remains cellular until nitrogen retention is very marked, when hypoplasia may be found. It is possible that in advanced renal damage there may be a deficiency of erythropoietin (p. 605). The anaemia may be normocytic, microcytic or even macrocytic, and hypochromia may be present.

Hepatic Cirrhosis. Here the anaemia is usually macrocytic or normocytic and the marrow macronormoblastic. If megaloblastic anaemia occurs this is probably due to primary malnutrition, and is found particularly in chronic alcoholics with cirrhosis. The occurrence of iron deficiency anaemia suggests gastric or oesophageal haemorrhage.

Malignant Disease. The causes of anaemia in widespread malignant disease are numerous. They include impaired appetite, malabsorption or blood loss from the alimentary tract, multiple deposits in the bone marrow, and occasionally increased haemolysis.

Sideroblastic Anaemia. Abnormal utilisation of iron by the marrow may cause a refractory anaemia. Some cases respond to pyridoxine therapy (p. 531).

POLYCYTHAEMIA

Polycythaemia may be defined as an increase in the number of the circulating red blood cells.

RELATIVE POLYCYTHAEMIA

An increase in the haemoglobin percentage and the red cell count is found in the presence of marked dehydration and haemoconcentration, e.g. after persistent vomiting or diarrhoea, traumatic shock, or extensive burns. There is a decrease in plasma volume and in total circulating blood volume, and the haemoglobin and red cell count fall when the dehydration is overcome.

Secondary Polycythaemia (Erythrocytosis)

This is a compensatory mechanism on the part of the erythropoietic tissue in response to the stimulus of anoxaemia. Hence it is found in:

1. Persons living at altitudes over 10,000 feet;
2. Chronic pulmonary disease, e.g. emphysema, or chronic pulmonary fibrosis, or chronic pulmonary congestion in mitral stenosis;
3. Congenital cardiac disease, especially with a veno-arterial shunt.

The clinical picture is that of the underlying condition. In contradistinction to what occurs in polycythaemia vera, splenomegaly is rarely present. Blood examination shows haemoglobin 16-20 g. per 100 ml., red cell count 6,000,000-8,000,000 (occasionally up to 10,000,000-12,000,000) per c.mm. Leucocytosis and thrombocytosis are usually absent. The total blood volume is increased.

The polycythaemia is beneficial to the course of the underlying condition and requires no treatment.

Polycythaemia also may occur in association with cysts or tumours of the kidney, hydronephrosis and Cushing's syndrome.

Polycythaemia Vera (Erythraemia)

This is a rare disease occurring in both sexes mostly about middle age. The cause is unknown. There is overactivity of the haemopoietic tissue, with extension of red marrow throughout the long bones. Microscopically the marrow is hyperplastic, with an increase of normoblasts, myelocytes and megakaryocytes. It is believed that the disease represents a proliferative disorder of the marrow which occasionally progresses to myelofibrosis (p. 660) or to chronic myeloid leukaemia (p. 650).

Clinical Features. The onset is insidious and the patient complains of throbbing headache, dizziness, tinnitus, dyspepsia and fatigue.

In the later stages of the disease hypertension occurs in about 50 per cent. of cases and arterial degeneration is even more common. Owing to the increased viscosity of the blood, there is liability to thrombosis. Thus symptoms of peripheral occlusive vascular disease, and vascular accidents, such as coronary thrombosis and cerebral thrombosis, or congestive cardiac failure, may occur. There is also a tendency to haemorrhage from the stomach, urinary tract or uterus.

Examination shows a dusky red and cyanotic facies. The spleen is palpably enlarged and firm in about 75 per cent. of cases.

Examination of the blood shows haemoglobin 16-20 g. per 100 ml., red cell count 7,000,000-13,000,000 per c.mm., PCV 60-70 per cent. The granular white cell count is elevated, and the platelet count is often much increased. The red cells are usually slightly smaller than normal and there may be a relative deficiency of haemoglobin giving a low MCHC. There is a marked increase in blood viscosity due to increase in red mass.

Diagnosis depends upon (1) the finding of an increased red cell count and mass, with leucocytosis, (2) the presence of splenomegaly and (3) the absence of conditions described above leading to secondary polycythaemia.

It is wise to carry out an intravenous pyelogram, and to estimate the P_{O_2} as it is more likely to be low in secondary polycythaemia of cardiac or respiratory origin.

If a blood count is not carried out the disease may be confused with essential hypertension, psychoneurosis, thrombophlebitis, leukaemia and the various causes of gastrointestinal or urinary haemorrhage.

With modern treatment the course may be a prolonged one, with normal expectation of life, but death may occur in a few years from one of the complications, such as the various thrombotic or haemorrhagic episodes mentioned above, or from heart failure. Some cases develop chronic myelogenous leukaemia terminally.

Treatment

1. Venesection. This gives temporary relief, and removal of 500 ml. of blood once or even twice weekly can be done to bring the haematocrit level down to about 54 per cent.

2. Irradiation. A satisfactory method of reducing erythrocyte

production is by irradiation of the bone marrow. This may be achieved by the administration of radioactive phosphorus (^{32}P), a single dose of 3-7 millicuries of ^{32}P being given by intravenous injection. Further treatment of this nature will depend upon the response to the first dose.

3. Chemotherapy. Busulphan (p. 652) in an initial dosage of 2-4 mg. daily followed by a maintenance dose of 2 mg. once or twice weekly has been found effective. It has been suggested that patients treated in this way are less likely to develop acute myelogenous leukaemia than after treatment with radioactive phosphorus. The antimalarial drug pyrimethamine, has also been used. It is a folic acid antagonist.

AGRANULOCYTOSIS

Agranulocytosis is a serious disease characterised by marked leucopenia with great reduction in, or absence of, polymorphonuclear leucocytes.

Aetiology. The disease occurs more often in women than in men, and is more common at and after middle age.

1. In most cases the cause is an idiosyncrasy or sensitisation to, or poisoning by, a variety of drugs. Among these the most important are amidopyrine (Pyramidon), gold salts, sulphonamides, organic arsenicals, methyl and propyl thiouracil, isoniazid, chlorpropamide, phenylbutazone, quinidine and certain benzol derivatives.

2. In some cases there is no discoverable cause—idiopathic agranulocytosis.

3. It may follow excessive irradiation or the use of cytotoxic drugs or antimetabolites.

4. Agranulocytosis is found as an integral part of aplastic anaemia (p. 638), leukaemia and some cases of hypersplenism (p. 659).

5. It occurs, rarely, in severe infections.

Pathology. In most cases the bone marrow shows a virtual disappearance of the granular cells and their precursors. In some the marrow contains many early myelocytes, with few mature forms—an arrest of maturation. In the cases in group 4 the appearance of the bone marrow is that of the underlying blood disease. The pathology of hypersplenism is uncertain.

Clinical Features. There may be a history of exposure to one of the noxious agents mentioned above. The onset may be either sudden or gradual. In the acute and severe cases the condition begins with sore throat, fever and often rigors which are followed by great prostration. There is rapidly advancing necrotic ulceration in the throat and mouth, with little evidence of pus formation. In fulminating cases the patient dies in a few days from toxaemia and septicaemia. In less acute cases there may be a preliminary period of general malaise and weakness.

Blood examination may show little alteration in the haemoglobin or red cell count. There is marked leucopenia, usually below 2,000 per c.mm., and falling to 500 per c.mm. or less. The percentage of granulocytes falls rapidly until none may be found.

A chronic type has been described in which there is a persistent or recurring leucopenia with granulopenia (e.g. white cell count 2,000-2,500 per c.mm., granulocytes 20-30 per cent.). Rarely the neutropenia occurs in cycles of three weeks (cyclic neutropenia). In such cases the symptoms are chiefly malaise, low grade fever and sore throat often without ulceration.

Diagnosis. This depends upon the examination of the blood. The condition may be confused with diphtheria and Vincent's angina. Whenever necrotic ulcers are found in the mouth or throat, it is important to carry out an examination of the blood and bone marrow to eliminate primary blood diseases like aplastic anaemia and leukaemia. Enquiry must be made to determine whether or not there has been exposure to one of the drugs listed above.

Prophylaxis. All the drugs mentioned at the beginning of this section should be regarded as potentially dangerous and should be carefully employed. A white cell count should be performed before treatment and the patient warned to report to his doctor if he feels unwell and feverish or if he develops a sore throat.

Treatment. On the first appearance of sore throat and fever the administration of any of these drugs should be stopped and a white cell count carried out. Antibiotics should be administered preferably by the oral route, e.g. ampicillin (p. 73), and fresh blood should be transfused. Even the fulminating cases may be saved by these means, but no cure will result unless the formation of granulocytes is resumed. This usually occurs within two to three days if infection is controlled and the cause has been removed. Should improvement not occur, the patient should be given blood transfusions. Careful nursing in isolation is required with adequate diet and extra vitamins. Regular toilet of the mouth will contribute greatly to the patient's comfort. Dimercaprol injections should be given if agranulocytosis follows the administration of gold salts or organic arsenicals.

Prognosis. In severe cases the mortality is very high, but in chronic or recurring cases recovery is common. Spontaneous resumption of granulocyte formation frequently occurs, especially if the leucotoxic drug is withdrawn, and this gives rise to difficulty in assessing the value of 'specific' therapy.

INFECTIOUS MONONUCLEOSIS (GLANDULAR FEVER)

This is a benign acute infective disease of unknown origin. It occurs chiefly in children and young adults of either sex both sporadically or in epidemics. The condition is mildly infectious, the agent probably being a virus. The incubation period is probably 5-10 days.

Clinical Features. The most common presenting features are tiredness, malaise and generalised pains in muscles, headache, pyrexia and enlargement of superficial lymph nodes. These are frequently followed by sore throat with or without exudate. The glandular enlargement may not occur until the third week. A maculopapular rash often appears during the first 10 days in adults. The spleen may be enlarged but seldom extends much below the costal margin. It is soft and not tender.

Blood examination shows no characteristic abnormality in regard to the red cells or the haemoglobin. There is usually a leucocytosis of 10,000-30,000 per c.mm. but occasionally the white cell count is normal or low. In the first few days there may be an increase in the proportion of granulocytes, but thereafter the characteristic increase in non-granular white cells appears, amounting to 60-80 per cent. of the total white cell count. These include ordinary lymphocytes, ordinary monocytes and 'atypical' lymphocytes (large cells with blue-staining often foamy cytoplasm and nuclei with coarse chromatin), which may be oval, kidney-shaped or have a pseudopodial appearance. The proportions of these cells vary greatly in different cases but immature leucocytes are not present.

The Paul-Bunnell test for heterophile antibodies becomes positive in titres of 1 in 200 or more, usually in the first 10 days and nearly always in the first three weeks in cases occurring sporadically. High titres may persist for many weeks. The Wassermann reaction may be positive. In epidemics the Paul-Bunnell test is frequently negative, which suggests that a different virus is concerned.

Diagnosis. During the invasive phase, especially in children, the disease may be confused with the various exanthemata, tonsillitis and diphtheria. Distinction must be made from leukaemia in which there is persistence of the clinical features, including lymph node enlargement, and in which the marrow biopsy is characteristic and the Paul-Bunnell test is negative; and from lymphadenoma in which the lymph node enlargement is persistent and progressive and the peripheral blood does not show the characteristic 'atypical' lymphocytes. The secondary stage of syphilis must also be excluded.

Treatment is symptomatic, the patient being kept in bed during the febrile period.

Prognosis. Although recovery is invariable, some patients may be ill for weeks or months with intermittent fever, sweats and debility. Very occasionally hepatitis or rupture of the spleen may occur. Sometimes there is thrombocytopenia or haemolytic anaemia of the autoimmune type.

THE LEUKAEMIAS

The name leukaemia is given to a group of diseases characterised by an abnormal and excessive proliferation of leucopoietic tissues throughout the body, and usually associated with an increase in the total number of circulating white blood corpuscles, among which immature forms occur. Though the course of the disorder may vary considerably from a few weeks to several years, the leukaemias are all invariably fatal, death being due to progressive anaemia, haemorrhage or inter-current infection.

The cause of leukaemia is not known. In some ways the condition behaves as a neoplastic process, as there is uncontrolled proliferation of cells and the development of foci of leucocyte formation in organs other than the bone marrow and lymph nodes. However, the process appears to start simultaneously throughout the leucopoietic tissue and the cells show no truly invasive properties as do malignant tumour cells. These features are more suggestive of a generalised humoral disturbance. Cytogenetic studies have shown that chromosomal abnormalities are present in some leukaemic cells. Furthermore it is recognised that exposure to ionising irradiation may produce chromosome damage and that such irradiation may in some instances be an aetiological factor in the initiation of leukaemic change. The possibility of a viral aetiology of leukaemia continues to attract widespread attention.

The formation of granulocytes, lymphocytes or monocytes may be affected by the leukaemic process, but in any one patient the condition only involves one series. Further, each type of leukaemia may occur as an acute or as a chronic disease. Thus there are: acute and chronic myeloid leukaemia, acute and chronic lymphatic leukaemia and monocytic leukaemia which is nearly always acute. The term subleukaemic leukaemia (sometimes called aleukaemic leukaemia) is applied to any form of leukaemia in which the total white cell count in the peripheral blood is not increased, though the differential blood count may show the presence of immature circulating leucocytes.

ACUTE LEUKAEMIA

Owing to the similarity in the clinical picture, it is convenient to consider all forms of acute leukaemia together. Acute lymphatic leukaemia is in general the most common variety, and is the most frequent type of leukaemia in children, occurring often in the subleukaemic form. It is the most common cause of death from malignant disease in childhood. Acute myeloid leukaemia and the least common variety, monocytic leukaemia, occur at all ages. Both sexes are affected. The pathological changes are similar to those found in the chronic forms (pp. 650, 652), but myeloblasts, lymphoblasts or monoblasts predominate in the respective types. The spleen and lymph nodes do not usually become as large as in the chronic forms.

Clinical Features. The disease may begin insidiously but the clinical onset is usually abrupt. There is fever, general malaise and a rapidly advancing anaemia. Epistaxis, spongy bleeding gums or other haemorrhagic manifestations, including purpura, are common and are due largely to thrombocytopenia. Sore throat and ulcers in the mouth or pharynx are frequent, due to reduction in normal polymorphonuclear leucocytes. Hypertrophy of the gums is often noted in monocytic leukaemia. Muscular and joint pains may occur. The spleen and often the liver are enlarged in the later stages. The cervical lymph nodes may be enlarged secondary to pharyngeal sepsis, but in the lymphatic form increase in size of these and other lymph nodes is common.

Blood examination shows a profound and increasing anaemia of normocytic normochromic type. Normoblasts and increased numbers of reticulocytes are frequently seen in the peripheral blood, due to disturbance of the erythropoietic tissues in the bone marrow by leukaemic infiltration. Thrombocytopenia is common with a prolonged bleeding time The white cell count may be normal or low but is usually increased to 20,000-50,000 per c.mm. Immature ('blast') cells comprise 30-90 per cent. of the white cells. The distinction between the different types of primitive white cells is often difficult, but in acute myeloid leukaemia myelocytes and granulocytes, in acute lymphatic leukaemia lymphocytes, and in monocytic leukaemia monocytes, form most of the remainder of the white cells and suggest the diagnosis.

The bone marrow shows a marked predominance of the appropriate primitive white cell to the almost complete exclusion of all normal marrow cytology.

Diagnosis. In the early stages the condition may be confused with acute infective illnesses, such as miliary tuberculosis, acute rheumatic fever, and infectious mononucleosis, which is most important in differential diagnosis. Aplastic anaemia, agranulocytosis and the haemolytic anaemias may also be simulated. The rapidly advancing anaemia, the eventual enlargement of the spleen, liver or lymph nodes and the finding of immature white cells in the peripheral blood suggest the diagnosis and this is established by marrow biopsy, which shows a large excess of primitive white cells of the appropriate type. The subleukaemic form may give particular difficulty since the total white count is normal or low, but immature cells are to be found in the peripheral blood on careful search or in buffy coat smears, and marrow biopsy reveals the typical picture of acute leukaemia.

Treatment. There is no known cure for acute leukaemia and apart from the lymphatic form in children, the outlook is so uniformly bad that only symptomatic or palliative treatment can be offered. Radiotherapy has proved of no value and is contraindicated in this condition. Chemotherapy with antimetabolites or cytotoxic agents may induce temporary remissions in some patients but their main value is in acute lymphatic leukaemia in childhood where in conjunction with steroid administration they can prolong the survival time from a few weeks to two years or more in the majority of cases. All such agents are very toxic drugs capable of producing severe haemopoietic depression and other serious side-effects. Details of dosage will vary from case to case and must be determined by repeated haematological examinations. Mercaptopurine and methotrexate are examples of antimetabolites which deprive rapidly dividing leukaemic cells of essential factors. Vincristine, a periwinkle alkaloid and cyclophosphamide, one of a large group of alkylating agents known as the nitrogen mustards, are examples of compounds which act by stopping cell mitosis. These drugs are all more effective in acute lymphatic leukaemia than in the other types, but resistance to therapy develops and relapse is inevitable. Prednisone is an important drug in all cases of acute leukaemia as its action on capillaries reduces the bleeding tendency associated with thrombocytopenia. Furthermore, its marked lympholytic effect is especially valuable in the lymphatic type where it is the drug of choice in inducing an initial remission and for subsequent use when changing from one chemotherapeutic drug to another after relapse. Blood transfusion and oral antibiotics are also important supportive measures to counteract rapidly progressive anaemia, haemorrhage and the intercurrent infection which frequently accompanies the agranulocytosis. In adults, very few cases of acute leukaemia derive other than very temporary remission from treatment and the myeloid and monocytic forms are notable unresponsive at any age.

A general approach to the treatment of a case of acute lymphatic leukaemia in a child is as follows. After transfusion, if required, an attempt is made to induce an initial remission with prednisone 40-60 mg. daily and weekly intravenous injections of vincristine, 0·05 mg. per kg. of body weight. When the blood picture has returned to normal (usually in about three to four weeks), methotrexate therapy is started to maintain the remission and is given twice weekly by intramuscular injection in a dose of 0·5 mg. per kg. of body weight. The prednisone is withdrawn over the next four to six weeks but is started again with vincristine as soon as haematological relapse appears and the methotrexate has to be stopped. After a second remission is induced a change in maintenance chemotherapy is made to mercaptopurine given orally in daily doses of 2·5 mg. per kg. of body weight and the drugs used to induce the remission are stopped until needed again after further relapse. If a third remission is obtained it can sometimes be maintained with cyclophosphamide giving 2 mg. per kg. of body weight. By this time the chances of further palliation are slender. Toxic reactions to the drugs may at any time demand modification of treatment and meningeal involvement may call for intrathecal injections of methotrexate. Methods of treatment have been reported in which intensive chemotherapy with combinations of cytotoxic drugs is given in an attempt to eradicate the leukaemic process, but such therapy is associated with profound marrow depression and requires very special facilities for nursing in pathogen-free conditions.

Prognosis. The condition is fatal and unless the course is modified by chemotherapy death occurs usually within a few weeks, due to anaemia, secondary infection or haemorrhage. Temporary short remissions may sometimes occur in the monocytic variety.

CHRONIC MYELOID LEUKAEMIA

The disease occurs chiefly between the ages of 35 and 60 years and is equally common in males and females.

Pathology. There is extension of the marrow throughout the long bones. The marrow is grey and gelatinous and is crowded with myelocytes and young polymorphonuclear leucocytes. Leukaemic infiltrations occur in the liver, spleen and lymph nodes, and in most organs throughout the body.

Clinical Features. The onset is insidious and the clinical features are very varied. There may be slowly advancing anaemia with loss of weight, dragging discomfort in the left upper quadrant of the abdomen due to the great enlargement of the spleen, and enlargement of the abdomen. Attacks of acute left upper abdominal pain may develop when infarction occurs in the spleen. Epistaxis or other haemorrhages may occur in the later stages.

The spleen is found to be much enlarged, occasionally extending across the midline and reaching below the umbilicus. It is firm and smooth and may be tender if infarction has recently occurred. The liver is also enlarged but the lymph nodes are usually of normal size.

Blood examination shows an anaemia of normocytic, normochromic type which increases as the disease progresses. Normoblasts are often found. The white cell count is greatly increased to 50,000-500,000 per c.mm. or more and consists almost entirely of young polymorphonuclear cells and myelocytes. In the later stages the appearance of an increasing number of myeloblasts indicates the approach of a terminal acute phase. The platelet count is often high initially but thrombocytopenia gradually develops.

Diagnosis. This depends upon the finding of the characteristic blood picture. The diagnosis of the infrequent subleukaemic or aleukaemic form may be extremely difficult. Marrow biopsy may be required to exclude other conditions causing a leuco-erythroblastic blood picture (p. 606). The granulocytes of chronic myeloid leukaemia are deficient in alkaline phosphatase and this is the basis of a staining reaction to differentiate them from the leucocytes found in a leukaemoid reaction. In a high proportion of cases a characteristic abnormality of the 21 chromosome, the Philadelphia chromosome, can be demonstrated in the myelocytes of the marrow and peripheral blood.

Treatment. Radiotherapy and chemotherapy are equally effective methods of palliative treatment in restoring most patients to a period of symptom-free life. Radiography, given as a course of localised splenic irradiation, reduces the size of the spleen and brings about a fall in the abnormal white cell count with a simultaneous improvement of the anaemia and general health. The dosage is controlled by frequent blood examinations and treatment is stopped when the white cell count falls to about 20,000 per c.mm. or if the platelet count drops excessively. Further irradiation is needed when relapse occurs, usually after about nine months, and thereafter courses may be required at shorter intervals. Blood transfusion may be necessary to correct increasing anaemia and in some cases, where there is evidence of haemolysis, steroids may be beneficial.

In the alternative treatment by chemotherapy the alkylating agent, busulphan (Myleran) is employed. It is given orally in a commencing dose of 4 mg. daily and can bring about a temporary but satisfactory clinical and haematological remission in a high proportion of cases. Subsequent maintenance dosage, e.g. 2 mg. daily, is continued and regulated according to the results of frequent blood examinations and the general state of the patient. It must be emphasised that all such drugs are capable of producing severe haemopoietic depression and their administration requires careful haematological supervision. The too rapid destruction of abnormal white cells may cause a rise in blood uric acid and even uric acid nephropathy.

Prognosis. The disease pursues a chronic course with increasing general features of anaemia. Irrespective of the type of treatment given, the average duration of life from the time of diagnosis is two to three years, though some patients live longer. The terminal acute stage is indicated by the appearance of an increased number of myeloblasts up to 10-15 per cent. or more, by marked anaemia and by haemorrhages.

CHRONIC LYMPHATIC LEUKAEMIA

The disease occurs much more commonly in males than in females and in the age period 45-75 years.

Pathology. There is moderate enlargement of lymph nodes and other lymphoid tissue throughout the body, the normal structure being replaced by a mass of lymphocytes. The spleen and liver are moderately enlarged and show lymphocytic infiltration. The bone marrow becomes progressively infiltrated with lymphocytes, which eventually replace the erythropoietic and myeloid tissue.

Clinical Features. The onset is very insidious and in contrast to chronic myeloid leukaemia the development of anaemia tends to be much slower and the presenting feature is usually the finding of firm rubbery, discrete and painless lymph nodes in the cervical, axillary and inguinal regions. The spleen is palpable but is usually smaller than in chronic myeloid leukaemia. The liver may also be enlarged. Haemorrhagic manifestations are much less common than in the chronic myeloid variety, but in widespread lymphoproliferative disorders there is an increased tendency to recurrent infections due possibly to altered immunity mechanisms.

Peripheral blood examination usually shows a mild but increasing anaemia, though normoblasts are rarely found. Haemolytic anaemia may occur. The white cell count is greatly increased, up to 500,000 per c.mm. Of these cells about 95 per cent. are lymphocytes, which are predominantly of the small variety. Lymphoblasts are rare except in the terminal stages. The platelet count is usually low and may fall below 100,000 per c.mm.

Diagnosis. When the white cell count is very high the recognition of the disease is easy by examination of a blood film. When the white cell count is below 30,000 per c.mm. marrow biopsy is essential. Chronic lymphatic leukaemia must be distinguished from (1) *lymphadenoma* and other forms of reticulosis in which there is no characteristic blood picture and which usually occur in a younger age group; (2) *infectious mononucleosis*, which has an acute febrile onset, in which the enlarged lymph nodes are soft and may be tender, the proportion of monocytes is increased, the lymphocytes are atypical and the Paul-Bunnell test for heterophile antibodies is frequently positive; and (3) *tuberculous cervical lymphadenitis*, which occurs in young people and in which there is usually no enlargement of lymph nodes in other areas or of the spleen.

Treatment. It should be remembered that in both varieties of chronic leukaemia and in the reticuloses it is important to treat the patient rather than the disease. In general, radiotherapy and chemotherapy should be withheld for as long as possible provided that the clinical state of the patient remains satisfactory. This is especially so in elderly patients with chronic lymphatic leukaemia who may remain in relatively good health with little or no anaemia for several years. When treatment becomes necessary, splenic irradiation or chemotherapy may be used. In general the response in chronic lymphatic leukaemia is less dramatic than in chronic myeloid leukaemia, and increasingly frequent courses of treatment are required. The most satisfactory chemotherapeutic agent at present available is the alkylating agent chlorambucil (Leukeran). The suggested dose is 0·1-0·2 mg./kg. of body weight given daily in tablet form for two to eight weeks depending on the haematological response. Steroid therapy may be of value where there is evidence that haemolysis is contributing to the anaemia.

Prognosis. The course of the disease is more slowly progressive than that of chronic myeloid leukaemia, but death usually occurs within five years of the time of diagnosis. In elderly patients it tends to progress very slowly and may not materially shorten the expectation of life. An increase in the number of lymphoblasts is a grave prognostic sign as it frequently heralds an acute terminal phase.

THE RETICULOSES

This is a group of uncommon but fatal conditions characterised by progressive widespread proliferation of the cells of the reticulo-endothelial system. Lymph node and splenic enlargement are usually present and cachexia and severe anaemia are frequent accompaniments The hyperplasia is suggestive of a neoplastic disorder, which may manifest itself initially as general involvement of the lymphoid tissue or as a localised process affecting one group of nodes. The former clinical type is usually associated with a more rapidly fatal course. On pathological grounds a large number of conditions, widely differing in their clinical features and course, could be included among the reticuloses because the cellular elements involved belong to or are derived from the reticulo-endothelial system. In clinical practice however it is customary to limit the term to a group of diseases in which lymph node and splenic enlargement are present without the peripheral blood picture of leukaemia. This group includes lymphosarcoma, reticulum cell sarcoma, giant follicular lymphoma, myelomatosis and lymphadenoma (Hodgkin's disease), this last being a common and important member of the reticuloses.

LYMPHADENOMA (HODGKIN'S DISEASE)

This disease is characterised by progressive painless enlargement of lymphoid tissue throughout the body, and anaemia.

Aetiology. The disease occurs in both sexes, chiefly in adolescence and early adult life. The pathogenesis is unknown and the condition is regarded as a form of malignant disease allied to other tumours of the reticulo-endothelial system (reticuloses).

Pathology. Microscopic examination of the enlarged discrete lymph nodes shows a replacement of the normal structure by proliferation of reticulo-endothelial cells. Giant cells with two or three nuclei are seen, and there may be many eosinophils. The fibrous stroma is later increased. Caseation and necrosis are not found. Infiltration with greyish areas of Hodgkin's tissue causes enlargement of the spleen and liver. The bone marrow, lungs, kidneys and alimentary tract are also frequently involved though deposits are very rare in the nervous system.

Clinical Features. The disease has an insidious onset, enlargement of one group of superficial nodes usually occurring first. The cervical groups are often involved earliest. The progressive enlargement includes the axillary and inguinal groups and extends to thoracic and abdominal nodes which are occasionally affected first. The nodes are usually painless, discrete and rubbery, and they vary in size from half to three inches in diameter. The skin is freely mobile over them. Pressure by the glandular masses and Hodgkin's deposits on neighbouring structures may cause a variety of features such as dysphagia, dyspnoea, venous obstruction, jaundice and paraplegia. The spleen is enlarged and usually palpable; it is firm and painless, and its enlargement may be the earliest presenting feature. Enlargement of the liver is commonly present.

General features include progressive weakness and loss of weight. Fever is often present, and in some cases is of a low grade irregular type, while in others there are recurrent bouts of pyrexia with the temperature rising to 39° C. (102-103° F.) for several days, alternating with apyrexial periods (Pel-Ebstein fever). Fever is characteristic of the cases in which the spleen and abdominal lymph nodes are primarily affected. In many cases there is no fever until the terminal stages. Pruritus is a troublesome symptom in about 10 per cent. of cases.

Anaemia is usual and progressive. It is commonly normochromic and normocytic and occasionally symptomatic haemolytic anaemia is present. There is no diagnostic change in the white cells. The count may be normal, increased or decreased, the last especially in the terminal phases when there is frequently accompanying thrombocytopenia. The proportion of granulocytes is usually increased, and 15-20 per cent. of cases show a moderate eosinophilia. Usually marrow puncture fails to reveal any diagnostic features, although occasionally and quite fortuitously the needle may penetrate a mass of Hodgkin's tissue in the sternal cavity.

Diagnosis. This involves the differential diagnosis of conditions producing enlargement of lymph nodes and of the spleen. The diseases with which Hodgkin's disease are most readily confused are: tuberculous lymphadenitis, which is usually confined to the neck, in which the nodes may become matted together, may show caseation and sinus formation, and in which there is no spenomegaly; chronic pyogenic lymphadenitis (chiefly also of the neck), in which the nodes are small and tender, in which a source of infection can be found, and in which there is no splenomegaly; lymphatic leukaemia, in which the examination of the blood and bone marrow reveals the characteristic changes; infectious mononucleosis, in which the lymph node and splenic enlargement is transient and the blood examination and a positive Paul-Bunnell test are diagnostic; lymphosarcoma and reticulum cell sarcoma, which can only be distinguished by microscopic examination of an excised node; secondary syphilis with generalised lymph node enlargement, in which the swelling is transient, a skin rash is common and the Wassermann reaction is positive; and the anaemia associated with the syndrome of portal hypertension (p. 659) in which there is splenomegaly but lymph node enlargement is absent.

In many cases the only way by which the diagnosis can be established with certainty is by biopsy of a lymph node.

Treatment. In cases where the disease appears to be localised to one area of superficial lymph nodes localised radiotherapy is unquestionably the treatment of choice. Where the disease is more widespread initially or becomes so as it progresses, chemotherapy is indicated in preference to radiotherapy. The drugs of most use are alkylating agents of the nitrogen mustard group. Cyclophosphamide may be given in an initial dose of 3·5 mg. per kg. body weight daily until the white cell count begins to fall and then in a dose of 1 mg. per kg. body weight daily. The drug tends to produce alopecia. In severely ill patients the bis form of intravenous nitrogen mustard (mustine hydrochloride), may be given in a daily dosage of 0·1-0·15 mg. per kilogram of body weight on four to six consecutive days with repetition of the course at intervals of a few weeks. Another chemotherapeutic agent of value in the generalised form of the disease is vinblastine sulphate (Velbe). This is a periwinkle alkaloid and is administered intravenously at weekly intervals in a dosage increasing from 0·1 to 0·3 mg. per kg. body weight. There is no evidence that steroids are of value in lymphadenoma other than for the treatment of a secondary haemolytic anaemia or to minimise bleeding when thrombocytopenia occurs.

Prognosis. The disease is fatal but in many cases is only slowly progressive. The five-year survival rate in patients with localised disease treated by radiotherapy may be 50 per cent., and it is not uncommon for such cases to enjoy good health for 10 to 20 years. In others the course is fairly rapid over a period of months. Unfavourable features are those due to pressure by glandular masses and progressive cachexia, fever and anaemia.

MYELOMATOSIS

This uncommon malignant reticulosis is associated with a neoplastic proliferation of abnormal plasma cells in the bone marrow. It occurs chiefly after the age of 50 years in either sex. The plasma cells produce local tumours of bone, sometimes solitary at first, but eventually becoming widespread and in this form the condition is known as multiple myeloma. A common presenting symptom is back pain due to pressure on spinal nerve roots, and pathological fracture may occur in any bone involved. Vertebral body collapse may give rise to paraplegia. Increasing plasma cell replacement of the marrow is associated with progressive normocytic anaemia, and eventually there is also granulopenia and thrombocytopenia. In the variety known as diffuse myelomatosis the clinical picture is that of progressive marrow involvement without the formation of bony lesions, and in the rare extramedullary type soft tissue tumours may occur. There is usually no enlargement of the spleen, lymph nodes or liver. Other features commonly present are a marked increase in abnormal serum globulin associated with a myeloma band on electrophoresis, an undue liability to infections, especially of the respiratory tract, a very rapid ESR and the presence of Bence-Jones protein in the urine. Renal failure may occur due to the disturbance in the serum proteins. Hypercalcaemia is commonly present.

The diagnosis is based on bone marrow examination which reveals large numbers of plasma cells with a slate-blue cytoplasm and an eccentric, sometimes double, nucleus. Plasma cells are only occasionally found in the peripheral blood. Radiological examination of the skeleton may show widespread punched-out osteolytic areas best seen in the skull, ribs, pelvis and vertebrae, and diffuse osteoporotic changes are common. In addition determination of the electrophoretic pattern of the serum proteins is important and abnormal protein may be demonstrated in the urine.

The disease is fatal, usually in two to three years. There is no curative treatment but localised irradiation will reduce the severity of bone pain and allow healing of spontaneous fractures. Palliative results may sometimes be obtained with chemotherapy. For this purpose the oral administration of the alkylating agent melphalan or cyclophosphamide has occasionally been of value. In cases with anaemia associated with marrow replacement, repeated blood transfusions may prolong life and intercurrent infections should be promptly treated with appropriate antibiotics.

DISEASES OF LIPOID STORAGE

Gaucher's Disease, Niemann-Pick's Disease and Hand-Schüller-Christian's Disease

These are very rare familial disorders occurring most frequently in children of the Jewish race. They are characterised by the abnormal storage of lipoids in the cells of the reticulo-endothelial system, with consequent anaemia and splenomegaly. Lipoid deposits may also occur in membranous bones. The conditions are slowly progressive and eventually fatal. There is no specific treatment available, although the bony lesions in Hand-Schüller-Christian's disease may be benefited by radiotherapy.

ANAEMIA ASSOCIATED WITH PORTAL HYPERTENSION (SPLENIC ANAEMIA)

Definition and Aetiology. Portal hypertension most commonly results from hepatic cirrhosis causing obstruction to the portal circulation through the liver, but occasionally the block may be extra-hepatic due to thrombosis or other lesion in the portal or splenic veins. The results of such an obstruction are splenomegaly and dilatation of veins at the lower end of the oesophagus and elsewhere to afford anastomotic communications between the portal and systemic circulations. It is loss of blood from such cardio-oesophageal varices that is responsible for the chronic iron deficiency anaemia which commonly occurs. Leucopenia and thrombocytopenia are believed to be due to depression of bone marrow function by inhibiting factors produced by the enlarged spleen, or to excessive destruction of leucocytes and platelets by this organ. The term hypersplenism is commonly used to describe the depression of granulocyte and platelet formation often encountered in a wide variety of conditions in which splenomegaly is a prominent feature.

Clinical Features. Portal hypertension may occur at any age. The aetiology and clinical features of the syndrome are described on p. 1024. Massive haematemesis or melaena may be the earliest sign of the condition or the onset may be insidious with chronic anaemia and the finding of an enlarged spleen. The latter may be symptomless or cause a dragging discomfort in the left hypochondrium, sometimes amounting to pain if perisplenitis occurs. The hypochromic anaemia is usually accompanied by leucopenia and thrombocytopenia.

Differential Diagnosis. It is necessary to exclude other diseases in which splenomegaly and anaemia occur, e.g. haemolytic anaemia, leukaemia, reticuloses such as Hodgkin's disease, and tropical infections such as malaria, kala azar, etc. Gross enlargement of the spleen with anaemia may also occur in myelofibrosis. The latter is a rare condition in which the bone marrow becomes largely replaced by fibrous tissue and the spleen and liver enlarge to provide alternative sites of haematopoiesis.

Treatment. Iron deficiency anaemia is treated on the lines indicated on p. 616, whilst more severe episodes of alimentary bleeding often require blood transfusion and other measures to combat shock (p. 178). The medical and surgical management of portal hypertension is discussed on pp. 1032 to 1034.

HAEMORRHAGIC DISEASES

Under this heading are included a large number of conditions characterised by an abnormal tendency to bleeding.

The factors concerned in the arrest of haemorrhage are many and coagulation itself is believed to involve a chain of reactions between at least ten factors.

A. *Intrinsic Factors concerned with the Coagulation of Blood*

Much of our knowledge of blood coagulation is hypothetical, but it may be said that when blood comes in contact with a foreign surface, an interaction is initiated which involves the platelets and a number of factors present in normal blood, including factors V, VII, VIII (antihaemophilic factor) and IX (Christmas factor). These interact in the presence of calcium ions to form thromboplastin, which activates prothrombin to thrombin. Prothrombin, which is believed to be produced in the liver, requires for its synthesis vitamin K. The thrombin produced reacts in turn with fibrinogen to form fibrin. The mechanism of interaction of clotting factors is a matter of great complexity, but the following scheme forms a basis for any discussion:

Platelets
Antihaemophilic factor
Christmas factor
Factor V
Calcium ions
} —— Factor VII ——→ Thromboplastin.

Prothrombin —— Thromboplastin ——→ Thrombin.

Fibrinogen —— Thrombin ——→ Fibrin.

Within the meshwork of the fibrin clot, red and white cells and platelets are enclosed. The fibrin filaments contract, the clot shrinks and becomes firmer and serum is expressed.

There is also a fibrinolytic mechanism which limits fibrin deposition by making this protein more soluble. Plasminogen activator is released from damaged tissues and leads to the production of an enzyme, plasmin, from the inactive precursor, plasminogen, in the blood thus:

$$\text{Plasminogen} \xrightarrow{\text{Plasminogen activator}} \text{Plasmin.}$$

$$\text{Fibrin} \xrightarrow{\text{Plasmin}} \text{Soluble product.}$$

B. *The Thrombocyte*

An adequate supply of normal platelets is of great importance in arresting haemorrhage. Not only do platelets take an important part in the production of thromboplastin, but they also play a mechanical role in the plugging of bleeding points in vessels. It is also possible that they may play some part in maintaining a normal resistance of capillary endothelium to injury. Even in thrombocytopenic states there are sufficient thrombocytes to initiate clotting.

C. *The Vascular Factor*

Active contraction of capillaries in response to injury constitutes an essential feature of natural haemostasis. This, together with plugging of the bleeding points by platelets, gives time for clotting to occur before the injured vessels re-open.

Definition of Purpura. Purpura, which is not itself a disease but a manifestation of disease, may be defined as bleeding into the skin or from the mucous membrane. The haemorrhagic spots do not disappear on pressure and they exhibit the progressive colour changes of a bruise before they disappear.

Tiny purpuric haemorrhages of pin-point or pin-head size are known as *petechiae*. Large purpuric haemorrhages are known as *ecchymoses*.

Simple Technical Procedures required for the Investigation of a Patient Suffering from a Haemorrhagic Disease

Bleeding Time. This is a measure of the time required for the arrest of haemorrhage from a puncture wound. A single prick is made in the lobe of the ear and a piece of filter paper applied to the drop of blood every 30 seconds, without touching the skin, until bleeding stops. *The normal bleeding time by this rough method is two to five minutes.*

Whole-blood Clotting Time (Macfarlane and Biggs' modification of the Lee and White method). Blood is removed from a vein and 1 ml. is put in each of 4 tubes ($2\frac{1}{2} \times \frac{3}{8}$ in.), and these are placed in a water bath at 37° C. The tubes are all tipped at $\frac{1}{4}$ to $\frac{1}{2}$ minute intervals until they can be inverted without the spilling of any blood. The time is recorded from the moment at which blood begins to enter the syringe until the tubes can safely be inverted, and the clotting time is expressed as an average for the four tubes. The normal range varies from 4 to 10 minutes. If a water bath is not available the test may be made at room temperature, but since coagulation is retarded by this cooling a control with known normal blood should be done at the same time.

Platelet Count. Accurate counts require considerable skill and practice. A rough indication of whether gross platelet deficiency exists can be obtained by the examination of blood films stained with cresyl blue (p. 604) on cover slips in which normally many platelets, single and in clumps, can be seen. The normal platelet count varies from 150,000-400,000 per c.mm., when the thrombocytes are counted directly in a counting chamber. Higher values are obtained if they are counted indirectly against the number of red cells in a stained film, a calculation that necessitates an erythrocyte count.

Capillary Resistance Test. The resistance of the capillary walls to increased intravascular pressure may be tested by Hess's method. A sphygmomanometer cuff is applied to the upper arm and inflated to a pressure midway between the systolic and diastolic blood pressure and kept at this level for five minutes. The cuff is then deflated and the skin over the forearm examined. Normally not more than two or three tiny haemorrhagic spots are to be seen. When capillary resistance is decreased (fragility increased) a large crop of small haemorrhagic spots is found. A circle the size of a penny may be inked on the forearm and the spots within this counted.

'Prothrombin' time. Routine laboratories throughout the world use the one-stage 'prothrombin' time to control the dosage of anti-coagulant drugs such as the coumarins and phenindione (p. 223). This is the time taken for plasma to clot under certain standard conditions, but it is a measure of the level, not only of prothrombin but also of certain other factors. Recently another test, the thrombotest, has been introduced. It measures in addition factor IX (p. 660) which may also be affected by these anticoagulants. Bleeding can occur from factor IX deficiency when the result of the prothrombin time test suggests that the dosage of phenindione is satisfactory.

CLASSIFICATION OF HAEMORRHAGIC DISEASES

The following classification is provisional, since in many forms the exact pathogenesis is not fully understood.

A. **Due to Defects in the Intrinsic Clotting Mechanism**

1. Haemophilia.
2. Christmas disease.
3. Hypoprothrombinaemia.
4. Congenital or acquired fibrinogenopenia.

B. **Due to Deficiency of Blood Platelets**

1. Idiopathic thrombocytopenic purpura.
2. Secondary or symptomatic thrombocytopenic purpura.

C. **Due to Defects of the Capillary Endothelium**

1. Infections, e.g. typhus, typhoid, meningococcal meningitis measles, bacterial endocarditis, septicaemia, smallpox.
2. Chemical agents, e.g. carbromal, atropine, ergot, iodides, phenobarbitone, phenytoin, quinidine, quinine, salicylates and snake venom.
3. Anaphylactoid purpura.
4. Senile purpura.
5. Metabolic purpura (uraemia, cholaemia).
6. Avitaminosis C.
7. Von Willebrand's disease.
8. Hereditary haemorrhagic telangiectasia.

HAEMOPHILIA (Factor VIII Deficiency)

Of the various factors in normal plasma concerned with the *intrinsic* clotting mechanism, the most important from a clinical point of view is the antihaemophilic factor, a deficiency of which leads to haemophilia. This factor is normally present in the globulin fraction of plasma.

Haemophilia is a hereditary disorder of blood coagulation characterised by a lifelong tendency to excessive haemorrhage and a greatly prolonged coagulation time.

The sons of a haemophilic man do not suffer from haemophilia and do not transmit the trait to their descendants. The daughters of a haemophilic man all conduct the trait. Some of the sons of a female conductor suffer from haemophilia. Some of the daughters of a female conductor carry the trait. There is no method of detecting whether any woman of a haemophilic family can marry with impunity. In many instances no family history can be obtained.

Clinical Features. The bleeding tendency is not apparent at birth, but is usually noticed within the first three years. Haemorrhage occurs from the nose, in the mouth or alimentary tract, from the urinary tract, from injuries to the skin, into the muscles, subcutaneous tissue or joints, or after eruption or extraction of teeth, circumcision, tonsillectomy, etc. Some trauma is necessary for the initiation of the bleeding, but often this may be so slight as to pass unnoticed. Injury may in fact cause haemorrhage in any organ, including the brain and spinal cord. The characteristic feature of the bleeding is not its profuseness but its persistence, and the total loss of blood may be very serious. In nearly every case bleeding occurs at some stage into joints, most commonly the knees, ankles and elbows. When this happens there is pain and swelling of the joints, and fever. There can be repeated haemorrhages into joints without serious after effects, but organisation of the blood clot may lead to firm ankylosis with marked deformity and crippling.

The coagulation time is usually prolonged and the bleeding time, platelet count and prothrombin time are normal. Anaemia may be a feature depending upon the extent of the bleeding.

Diagnosis. The occurrence of habitual haemorrhage in a male with a family history of bleeding in male relatives or forebears and with the haematological findings described above suggests that the diagnosis is either haemophilia or Christmas disease (p. 666). Occasionally, however, the coagulation time is normal. Such cases can now be recognised by certain recently devised but complex laboratory tests, one of the most useful of which is the thromboplastin generation test. There are haemophilia centres in all regions of Britain at which these investigations can be done.

The patient is then issued with a card giving necessary information, including the diagnosis and blood group.

Treatment. Even for the most trivial surgical intervention, such as the extraction of a tooth, the patient must be given intravenously, before and after operation, fresh plasma or plasma that has been dried or frozen when fresh, or a special preparation of the globulin fraction of human plasma containing the antihaemophilic factor. Fresh blood is required to replace blood that has been lost. The management of the case requires careful planning by the dentist or surgeon, the physician and the blood transfusion officer.

When bleeding occurs the patient should be confined to bed. It may be necessary to give many pints of fresh plasma or blood over a period of several days. The administration of antihaemophilic factor also requires to be repeated intravenously at intervals of 24 hours or less, and this is the treatment of choice, subject to availability of the factor at transfusion centres. Antihaemophilic factor from bovine or porcine sources is available commercially. It is, however, antigenic and will cause sensitivity reactions which may be fatal if it is given for more than one short course of treatment. Hence it should be reserved for use in grave emergencies such as major operations. The post-haemorrhagic anaemia should be treated with iron. Local measures consist of the application to the bleeding point (after cleaning away blood and clot) of dressings soaked in substances designed to promote haemostasis. These include Russell's viper venom, adrenaline, fresh whole blood, and preparations of thrombin. Soluble dressings such as gelatin sponge, oxidised cellulose or fibrin foam are useful. It may be necessary to give an antibiotic because of the danger of infection, particularly in the mouth, but intramuscular injections should be avoided because of the danger of haematoma formation.

A joint which is the site of bleeding should never be opened surgically but should be splinted, lightly bandaged and protected. The same applies to haematomata. Aspiration should be avoided. Most patients obtain relief from the pain due to haemorrhage into a joint if cold packs or icebags are applied. Splinting of the limb should not be continued too long or fibrous ankylosis will result. Analgesics may be required but pethidine and morphine should be avoided because of the danger of addiction and aspirin should not be given in case it leads to a haematemesis. Epistaxis may require firm packing of the nose with gauze dressings. Bleeding from tooth sockets can be controlled by packs which may be retained in position by a special dental plate.

Prognosis. In some patients the disease is a mild one, causing little inconvenience. In others it may be very severe, with recurrent joint haemorrhages and troublesome bleeding from minor cuts. Persistent haemorrhage may occur after minor surgical procedures such as circumcision, tonsillectomy or tooth extraction. The whole life of the haemophiliac is coloured by the fear of haemorrhage, particularly into the joints. With modern methods of treatment, the prognosis has improved greatly.

Prophylaxis. Since there is no known cure for haemophilia, haemophilic men, their sisters and their daughters should be strongly advised not to have children. Sterilisation should be considered. Limitation of the risks of bleeding involves the haemophiliac leading a sheltered and careful life with avoidance of trauma, but sufferers from the condition should not be encouraged to consider themselves as curiosities. Some children with mild haemophilia can attend ordinary schools, but for others education should be provided by the local authority either in the patients' homes or in a school for handicapped children. When the boy reaches the age of 14 or 15 the local Youth Employment Officer should be approached to assist in the choice of a career. Regular dental supervision is necessary as a prophylaxis against tooth extraction.

CHRISTMAS DISEASE (Factor IX Deficiency)

About one-tenth of the patients with the clinical picture of haemophilia, including a prolonged clotting time, can be shown by special laboratory tests, particularly the thromboplastin generation test, not to have haemophilia but a condition that has been named Christmas disease because the surname of the first patient investigated in Britain was Christmas. The condition is frequently less severe than haemophilia. The blood of these patients is not deficient in antihaemophilic factor, but in a different factor, the so-called Christmas factor, which is less labile than the antihaemophilic factor. Local and general treatment is the same as in haemophilia, except that preparations of antihaemophilic factor are of no value in the treatment of Christmas disease.

HYPOPROTHROMBINAEMIA

This condition is characterised by a deficiency of plasma prothrombin, a tendency to spontaneous and traumatic internal and external haemorrhage, and a prolonged coagulation time.

Prothrombin is formed in the liver from the fat-soluble vitamin K, which is ingested in certain foodstuffs such as spinach, cabbage, cauliflower, kale and tomatoes, and is also synthesised in the gut by bacterial action. The latter is the more important source in man. The absorption of vitamin K from the intestine requires the presence of bile salts.

Hypoprothrombinaemia occurs:

(*a*) In haemorrhagic disease of the newborn, which appears in about 1 in 800 births. The bleeding tendency is believed by some authorities to be due to an exaggeration of the normal hypoprothrombinaemia which occurs 24-72 hours after birth. During this time there is no bacterial formation of vitamin K in the gut. Two to four days after birth, bleeding may occur into the alimentary tract (melaena neonatorum), into the skin or subcutaneous tissue, brain, spinal cord, peritoneal cavity, etc. In some cases so-called birth injuries may be due to bleeding consequent on hypoprothrombinaemia. Spontaneous recovery usually occurs in mild cases, but death may result in severe cases. In the newborn, especially if premature, water soluble analogues of vitamin K may cause hyperbilirubinaemia and kernicterus (p. 1196). Phytomenadione (vitamin K_1) is relatively free from these effects and can be given to the affected baby in a dose of 1 mg. intramuscularly. Blood transfusion may also be required.

(*b*) In gross hepatic disease, conditions causing obstructive jaundice and chronic diarrhoeal diseases, chiefly sprue, idiopathic steatorrhoea, fistulae and ulcerative colitis.

In hepatic disease there is impaired synthesis of prothrombin; in the other conditions impaired absorption of vitamin K. Although spontaneous bleeding may occur in all these conditions, the point of greatest practical importance is the tendency to excessive haemorrhage during and after surgical operation on patients suffering from obstructive jaundice. In these cases the pre-operative administration of phytomenadione (vitamin K_1), which should be used in preference to other vitamin K analogues, reduces the prothrombin time to normal. It should be given intramuscularly in a dosage of 10-20 mg. daily for three days. When gross hepatic disease is present the liver may be unable to synthesise prothrombin from vitamin K. In such cases blood transfusion will be required.

(*c*) As a result of the administration of phenindione or the coumarin group of drugs. These are widely employed in medicine for the prevention and treatment of vascular thrombosis and pulmonary embolism (pp. 291, 256). Their activity has in the past been controlled by the test commonly referred to as the one-stage prothrombin time. Newer tests such as the thrombotest are now coming into use (p. 662). Treatment consists of the stoppage of the anticoagulant drug that has been employed, the administration of phytomenadione (vitamin K_1), 10 mg. by mouth or by intravenous injection, and the transfusion of fresh blood, especially if the bleeding has made the patient anaemic. Vitamin K preparations other than phytomenadione are not sufficiently active.

It should be noted, however, that the deficiency here is probably not only of prothrombin but also of factors VII and IX.

CONGENITAL OR ACQUIRED FIBRINOGENOPENIA

A deficiency of plasma fibrinogen, which may be complete or partial, may arise very rarely as a congenital abnormality or as a result of severe liver disease. Most often the condition occurs in the late stages of pregnancy with complications, and is believed to be due to the entry into the blood of thromboplastic substances derived fron the placenta. The condition is recognised by the coincidence of a haemorrhagic tendency with a prolonged coagulation time. The congenital form is distinguished from haemophilia by its occurrence in both sexes, the absence of a family history, and by the chemical determination of the amount of fibrinogen in the blood.

Blood transfusion may be required for the anaemia, but for the treatment of fibrinogenopenia the giving of concentrated plasma or of a preparation of the fibrinogen fraction of blood is essential.

The clotting abnormalities may be complex, and expert assistance should be sought.

IDIOPATHIC THROMBOCYTOPENIC PURPURA

This is a disease of unproved aetiology characterised by a quantitative deficiency of platelets and in some instances it may be due to an antigen-antibody reaction. The disease occurs most commonly in children and young adults. In children it may follow rubella.

Intermittent purpura and bleeding may occur in any site, most frequently from the nose, alimentary or urogenital tracts, and such bleeding may be fatal, especially should it occur in the brain or subarachnoid space. The disease is usually a chronic one with remissions and relapses, bleeding tending to occur when the platelet count falls below 40,000 per c.mm. The spleen is rarely palpably enlarged. The blood shows, in addition to the thrombocytopenia, a hypochromic microcytic anaemia, the degree depending on the amount of blood loss. The bleeding time is much prolonged, e.g. 15-20 minutes, and the capillary resistance test is strongly positive during relapse. The coagulation time is normal but the clot formed is soft, friable and retracts poorly.

Treatment. The effects of repeated transfusion of blood and large amounts of prednisone (60 mg. daily) should always be tried before surgery is contemplated. In a high proportion of cases remissions varying in degree and duration can be produced. In the majority of patients, however, cessation of steroid therapy or reduction of dosage to a level which can be tolerated by the patient is usually followed by clinical and haematological relapse. In children recovery usually occurs spontaneously or may coincide with the cessation of steroid therapy. If the bleeding tendency is not controlled or greatly improved by blood transfusion and steroids within two weeks, splenectomy should be carried out without further delay. Within a few minutes of the removal of the spleen, the prolonged bleeding time and increased capillary fragility start to improve, to be followed within 24-48 hours by a rise in thrombocytes. Although these beneficial haematological effects are not always maintained, at least 80 per cent. of cases of idiopathic thrombocytopenic purpura are greatly benefited by splenectomy.

SECONDARY OR SYMPTOMATIC THROMBOCYTOPENIC PURPURA

Secondary or symptomatic thrombocytopenic purpura occurs in aplastic anaemia, leukaemia, hypersplenism, multiple neoplastic deposits in the bone marrow, from excessive exposure to X-rays or radioactive substances, and occasionally in very severe fevers. It may be found in megaloblastic anaemia and in disseminated lupus erythematosus, and can follow massive blood transfusion.

Thrombocytopenia may be part of a general pancytopenia following drugs such as benzol, organic arsenicals, gold and chloramphenicol, in which case the treatment is that of aplastic anaemia (p. 639). In addition patients may develop thrombocytopenia because of sensitivity to certain drugs, including quinine and quinidine. It also occurred in certain individuals taking the hypnotic sedormid which is not now widely used because of this danger. Here the prognosis is much better, provided the drug is withdrawn and transfusion given as required.

THE VASCULAR PURPURAS

In this group of haemorrhagic diseases the lesion usually consists of damage to the capillary walls. The injury may be due to allergic reactions (the anaphylactoid purpuras) or to the direct toxic effect of certain infections or chemical agents (p. 663), metabolic and malignant diseases, old age and scurvy. In both the toxic and anaphylactoid types it is unusual to find qualitative or quantitative changes in the platelets and under these conditions the term non-thrombocytopenic purpura may be used. In a minority of cases of vascular purpura, however, the capillary damage is accompanied by a reduction in the number of platelets, due presumably to the combined effects of the toxic and sensitising factors mentioned above. It should be noted that some younger persons, particularly women, bruise spontaneously or from minor trauma, without any recognised disease being present.

Anaphylactoid Purpura. The various clinical forms of this rare condition are manifestations of an allergic reaction but the antigen is often unknown.

Purpura Simplex is found in association with sensitivity to certain bacterial infections, notably streptococcal. Thus it occurs in rheumatic fever, scarlet fever, etc. Small haemorrhagic spots appear on the limbs or over the whole body. The condition is usually of no significance and calls for no treatment.

Henoch Schönlein Purpura occurs in children and adolescents. Sero-haemorrhagic effusion into the wall of the gut may cause colic and melaena and intussusception may be simulated. Peri-articular effusion may cause painful swelling of joints. Mild fever is usual. Purpura of the skin may or may not be present. The prognosis is good but relapses often occur.

In anaphylactoid purpura other allergic manifestations are sometimes found in addition, such as urticaria or angio-neurotic oedema. Acute nephritis is the most dangerous complication when the purpura is secondary to streptococcal infection. The platelet count and the bleeding and coagulation times are all normal. The capillary resistance test may be positive. The diagnosis may present great difficulty if purpura of the skin or mucous membranes is not present.

Senile Purpura. This is a benign condition found in elderly people, and related to atrophic changes in the skin which permit rupture of small vessels by shearing strains. Such haemorrhages are common on the dorsum of the hand and are slowly reabsorbed without a bruise.

Metabolic Purpura. Purpura and bleeding from various mucous membranes may occur in association with late stages of renal and hepatic failure.

Scurvy. Purpura and bleeding from the gums are classical features of a fully developed case of scurvy (p. 505).

Local and General Measures for Control of Bleeding in the Purpuras

The measures described for this purpose in the treatment of haemophilia (p. 665) are applicable in purpura except that transfusions must be of fresh whole blood. When purpura is a manifestation of scurvy, ascorbic acid should be given. Splenectomy is of value only in idiopathic thrombocytopenic purpura.

In the treatment of purpura associated with infections, antibiotics may be of value. In the anaphylactoid group improvement sometimes occurs as a result of the administration of antihistamine drugs, or of steroids in the dosage recommended for idiopathic thrombocytopenic purpura (p. 669).

Von Willebrand's Disease. This is a rare disease inherited as a simple Mendelian dominant that affects both sexes. The main defect is believed to be an abnormality of the capillaries. The bleeding time is prolonged but the coagulation time and platelet count are normal. In some cases a deficiency of anti-haemophilic factor has been demonstrated. The bleeding manifestations include prolonged bleeding from minor injuries and tooth extractions, menorrhagia and bleeding from the gastro-intestinal tract. Treatment is symptomatic, namely iron and blood transfusions as required. Splenectomy is contraindicated.

Hereditary Haemorrhagic Telangiectasia. This is a rare hereditary disease transmitted as a Mendelian dominant characterised by bleeding from multiple telangiectases which consist of localised collections of non-contractile capillaries. It occurs in both sexes and the first and frequently the only symptom may be epistaxis. However haematemesis, haemoptysis or bleeding elsewhere may occur. Telangiectases are not usually prominent till the age of 20 or more and may be found on the face or hands, or in the mucous membrane of the nose or mouth. Treatment of bleeding areas is sometimes difficult, but cauterisation of the nose may be helpful.

THROMBOCYTOSIS

An increased number of platelets may be found

(*a*) after splenectomy;

(*b*) after haemorrhage and, to a lesser extent, after operation or injury;

(*c*) in chronic myeloid leukaemia

(*d*) in some cases of polycythaemia vera and of myelofibrosis.

(*e*) in a rare primary disease called haemorrhagic thrombocythaemia.

PREVENTION OF DISORDERS OF THE BLOOD

The most common blood disorder both in Britain and in other countries is chronic nutritional hypochromic anaemia in women of the child-bearing age. The essential cause of this anaemia is that the dietary intake of iron is insufficient to meet the physiological requirements. The regular consumption of a well-balanced diet containing foods rich in iron, such as liver, meat, peas, lentils, beans and green vegetables, will accomplish much in the prevention of this disorder. In addition, during pregnancy and lactation, when menstruation is heavy, and when malabsorption may follow operations on the stomach and small intestine, prophylactic administration of oral iron is indicated. It is important to make sure that sites of chronic blood loss, such as alimentary bleeding, are investigated and dealt with where possible. In countries where hookworm infection is rife, this is essential.

Attention has also been drawn to the frequency of nutritional hypochromic anaemia in infancy and childhood. Prophylactic iron should be given to infants of low birth weight and to those recovering from infections. The institution of a good mixed diet by the fourth month is also of importance in this respect.

The megaloblastic anaemias in general are not susceptible to prevention with the exception of the types due to direct dietary deficiency, most commonly encountered in the tropics and in pregnancy (p. 620). The prevention of subacute combined degeneration of the spinal cord in Addisonian pernicious anaemia by early diagnosis and efficient treatment cannot be too strongly emphasised. Expensive preparations containing iron and folic acid should not be used blindly in uninvestigated cases of anaemia. Treatment with hydroxocobalamin by injection will be necessary after total gastrectomy and the possibility of megaloblastic anaemia developing some years after partial gastrectomy or, even more rarely, gastroenterostomy, or from disease or resection of the ileum, should be borne in mind.

The aetiology of most of the other blood disorders is not known and hence prophylactic measures are not always possible. This is true of the idiopathic forms of haemolytic anaemia, aplastic anaemia, thrombocytopenic purpura and agranulocytosis. However, some types of these disorders may develop secondary to toxic or infective agents known to have deleterious effects on the bone marrow or circulating blood. Avoidance of such factors where possible, and careful observation of individuals exposed to these hazards are obvious precautions which must be carried out.

Blood transfusions may be responsible for the transmission of disease, e.g. infective hepatitis, malaria, and syphilis or for the production of severe reactions if the blood groups are incompatible. It is well recognised that women requiring blood transfusion must be given blood of the same Rh type as themselves, in order to avoid the production of antibodies liable to cause haemolytic reactions after subsequent transfusions or erythroblastosis foetalis in their future offspring. Accordingly a knowledge of the dangers associated with blood transfusions can lead to highly successful prophylactic measures for their avoidance. Measures to anticipate the development of erythroblastosis foetalis are discussed on p. 634.

In the prevention of haemorrhagic diseases mention need be made of haemophilia, Christmas disease and hypoprothrombinaemia. With regard to the former two disorders female carriers of the trait should be told that for the sake of posterity child-bearing should not be undertaken and sterilisation should be considered.

Hypoprothrombinaemia arising in obstructive jaundice, biliary fistulae, chronic diarrhoeal diseases such as sprue, and in some newborn infants can be prevented and corrected by the parenteral administration of phytomenadione (vitamin K_1). Such prophylactic treatment may be the means of avoiding a severe or fatal haemorrhagic state.

The possibility that ionising radiation may be responsible for genetic changes leading to leukaemia must be borne in mind and all unessential irradiation, whether for diagnostic or therapeutic purposes, must be avoided.

Of the miscellaneous diseases of the blood dealt with in this section, such as polycythaemia and disorders of the reticulo-endothelial system, including leukaemia, lymphadenoma, myelomatosis, Gaucher's disease, etc., all that need be said is that the causes are not at present known and hence prophylactic measures cannot be undertaken.

R. H. GIRDWOOD.
JAMES INNES.

Books recommended:

Wintrobe, M. M. (1967). *Clinical Hematology*, 6th ed. London: Kimpton.
Thompson, R. B. (1965). *A Short Textbook of Haematology*, 2nd ed. London: Pitman.

Disease	Hb. g.	Hb. %	R.B.C. Millions per c.mm.	MCHC	C.I.	MCV	Reticulocytes %	W.B.C. per c.mm.	Blood Film	Bone Marrow
Chronic Iron deficiency Anaemia	8·0	55	4·0	25	0·7	70	1	4–6,000	Hypochromia, microcytosis, moderate anisocytosis and poikilocytosis.	Normoblastic hyperplasia.
Pernicious Anaemia	5·8	40	1·5	36	1·3	105	1	2–4,000	Macrocytosis, marked anisocytosis and poikilocytosis. Oval cells present.	Megaloblastic; (normoblasts also present).
Aplastic and Hypoplastic Anaemias	5·8	40	2·0	32	1·0	90	1	500–2,000	Normal red cells, thrombocytopenia and granulocytopenia.	Hypoplasia of all elements.
Congenital Acholuric Jaundice	10·2	70	3·5	36	1·0	80	5–20	6–10,000	Microspherocytosis; reticulocytes present in excess; anisocytosis.	Normoblastic hyperplasia.
Polycythaemia Vera	19·0	130	7·0	32	0·9	85	1–4	15–30,000	Normochromia or hypochromia; normoblasts. Polymorph leucocytosis. Platelets numerous.	Hyperplasia of all elements.
Acute Myeloblastic Leukaemia	7·3	50	2·5	32	1·0	90	1–5	5–30,000	Increase of granulocytes. 'Blast' cells present.	Increase of white cells and their precursors.
Chronic Myeloid Leukaemia	10·2	70	3·5	32	1·0	90	1–5	50–500,000	Great increase of granulocytes and myelocytes. Increased numbers of platelets. Normoblasts.	Increase of white cells and their precursors.
Chronic Lymphatic Leukaemia	10·2	70	3·5	32	1·0	90	1–2	50–500,000	Great increase of lymphocytes. Platelets reduced.	Large numbers of lymphocytes present.
Infectious Mononucleosis	14·6	100	5·0	32	1·0	90	1	10–30,000	Many monocytes, lymphocytes or abnormal mononuclear cells.	Normal or some increase of mononuclears.

100% Haemoglobin=14·6 g. per 100 ml. of blood.

Table 9.—Summary of Findings in Common Haemorrhagic Diseases

	Purpura	Platelet Count	Bleeding Time	Coagulation Time	Capillary Resistance Test	'Prothrombin Time' One-Stage Method	Thromboplastin Generation Test
Thrombocytopenic purpura	present	low	prolonged	normal	positive	normal	normal
Vascular purpuras	present	normal	normal	normal	may be positive	normal	normal
Scurvy	present	normal	normal	normal	usually positive	normal	normal
Haemophilia and Christmas disease	absent	normal	normal	usually prolonged	normal	normal	abnormal
Hypoprothrombinaemia	may be present	normal	normal	usually normal	may be positive	prolonged	normal
Fibrinogenopenia	may be present	normal	normal or prolonged	prolonged	normal	prolonged	normal
Von Willebrand's disease	present	normal	prolonged	prolonged in some	may be positive	prolonged in some	normal or abnormal

TABLE 10.—ORIGIN AND DEVELOPMENT OF BLOOD CELLS

RETICULO-ENDOTHELIAL CELL

	Erythrocyte Series	Granulocyte Series			Lymphocyte Series	Monocyte Series	Thrombocyte Series
	Proerythroblast		Myeloblast		Lymphoblast	Monoblast	Megakaryoblast
	Early Normoblast		Promyelocyte				Megakaryocyte
	Intermediate Normoblast	Neutrophil Myelocyte	Eosinophil Myelocyte	Basophil Myelocyte			
	Late Normoblast						
Present in Normal Peripheral Blood	Reticulocyte Erythrocyte	Neutrophil Polymorph	Eosinophil Polymorph	Basophil Polymorph	Lymphocyte	Monocyte	Platelet

DISEASES OF THE ENDOCRINE SYSTEM

In recent years technological advances have greatly enhanced our understanding of the role of hormones in health and disease, and have thus increased the accuracy of diagnosis, and improved the management of patients.

The action of hormones may be studied by several methods. In the first place, the clinical effects of increased output of endogenous hormones may be noted, as for instance in hyperthyroidism. Secondly, when a gland fails to secrete, the results of hormonal deficiency may be seen and compared with the normal state or that due to an excess: thus hypothyroidism or myxoedema may be contrasted with hyperthyroidism. The third method is to observe the response to the administration of exogenous or synthetic hormones such as steroids or thyroxine. Laboratory methods of studying the effect of hormones in animals are especially valuable, since experiments may be designed to isolate an effect in a way that is not possible with a patient. This method is of particular importance, since deviations from the normal represent the sum of many interrelated reactions which modify each other. For example, the concentration of glucose in blood is dependent on a series of factors, including absorption from the intestine, storage and secretion by the liver, formation from body protein, utilisation by the tissues and sometimes loss in the urine. These changes of blood glucose are influenced by insulin, glucagon, adrenaline, adrenocortical hormones, the pituitary growth hormone, the activity of the hepatic cells, and the renal glucose threshold. It follows, therefore, that a fall in blood glucose concentration cannot be attributed solely to the action of insulin; any change occurring may be the result of several effects, some of which are antagonised by others.

Control of the activity of the thyroid, the adrenal cortex and the gonads is maintained through the pituitary trophic hormones. A reciprocal relationship exists between the pituitary and its end organs analogous to the 'servo' or 'feed back' mechanisms used in engineering. Thus the secretion of trophic hormones by the anterior lobe of the pituitary gland appears to be controlled in part by the concentration in the blood of the hormone from the target gland. When the ovary at the menopause fails to produce oestradiol, the amount of oestrogen in the circulation falls, and in an attempt to compensate for this the pituitary secretes an increased amount of gonadotrophic hormones. Such excessive pituitary activity, though not necessarily harmful in itself, can be controlled by the administration of exogenous hormone, for example oestradiol by injection, or more frequently and economically by giving a synthetic oestrogenic substitute, for example stilboestrol, by mouth.

It is usually found that the administration of a hormonal preparation depresses the activity of the gland whose secretion is being supplemented from exogenous sources. Thus the administration of cortisone or synthetic analogues will depress the production of the hormones of the adrenal cortex (p. 723).

Storage of hormones in the body is very limited, with the notable exception of thyroxine or its precursors in the thyroglobulin forming the colloid in the follicles of the thyroid gland. The normal thyroid gland probably contains sufficient hormone to meet the needs of the individual for two to three months. The adrenal cortex by contrast carries small stores of formed hormone, but has a large capacity to secrete hormones with great rapidity. It is known that more cortisol can be obtained from an adrenal vein in a few minutes than can be obtained by extracting the whole gland.

The species specificity of some of the protein hormones secreted by the anterior lobe of the pituitary gland contrasts with the absence of specificity in others. Thyroxine for example, extracted from the thyroid gland of a sheep, is just as effective when given to a man, as it is when used to accelerate metamorphosis in the tadpole. Growth hormone on the other hand is species specific in the sense that an effect can only be demonstrated in man when the material used has been prepared from human pituitaries or from those of apes. The administration of some hormones provokes the formation of anti-hormones, so that repeated injections are followed by progressively diminishing effects. This occurs when gonadotrophins prepared from pregnant mares' serum are used to stimulate gonadal activity in the human. Likewise para-

TABLE 11

HORMONE	SYNONYMS	SOURCE	EFFECT AND SITE OF ACTION IN MAN
Growth hormone	Somatotrophin	Anterior lobe of pituitary (Adenohypophysis)	Stimulates tissue growth (? Diabetogenic). Mobilises fat.
Adrenocorticotrophic hormone	ACTH Corticotrophin	,,	Stimulates adrenal cortex.
Thyrotrophic hormone	TSH (thyroid-stimulating hormone)	,,	Stimulates thyroxine formation and release from thyroid.
Follicle-stimulating hormone	FSH	,,	*In male*. Develops germinal epithelium of testicular tubules and so spermatogenesis. *In female*. Induces maturation of ovarian Gräafian follicle.
Interstitial cell stimulating hormone	ICSH Luteinising hormone (LH)	,,	*In male*. Stimulates interstitial (Leydig) cells of testis to produce testosterone. *In female*. Develops corpus luteum.
Luteotrophic hormone	Lactogenic hormone Prolactin	,,	*In male*. No known action. *In female*. (i) Maintains activity in fully developed corpus luteum. (ii) Induces milk secretion in 'primed' mammary gland.
Oxytocin		Posterior lobe of pituitary (Neurohypophysis)	Stimulates contraction of parturient uterus.
Vasopressin	Antidiuretin	,,	(i) Promotes water reabsorption from the distal tubule of the kidney. (ii) Stimulates smooth-muscle contraction.
Thyroxine		Thyroid	Increases metabolism of most tissues.
Triiodothyronine		Thyroid, or derivative of thyroxine	,,

TABLE 11—*continued*

HORMONE	SYNONYMS	SOURCE	EFFECT AND SITE OF ACTION
Thyro-calcitonin		Parafollicular cells of thyroid	Inhibits reabsorption of mineral from bone
Parathyroid extract	Parathormone	Parathyroids	Increases urinary phosphorus excretion. Mobilises calcium and phosphorus from bone.
Insulin		Pancreatic islets of Langerhans (β cells)	(i) Lowers blood glucose, by increasing formation of muscle and liver glycogen. (ii) Inhibits protein catabolism. (iii) Increases fat storage.
Glucagon		,, (α cells)	Mobilises liver glycogen.
Adrenocortical hormones e.g. aldosterone, cortisol	Corticosteroids	Adrenal cortex	Necessary for maintenance of life, and affect metabolism of water, electrolytes, carbohydrates, protein and fat.
Adrenaline Noradrenaline		Adrenal medulla	Widespread effects due to stimulation of adrenergic nerve endings.
Testosterone		Interstitial (Leydig) cells of testis	(i) Develops male secondary sex characters. (ii) Induces protein anabolism.
Oestrogens, e.g. oestradiol-17β oestrone oestriol		Ovary Placenta Adrenal cortex	(i) Develop female secondary sex characters. (ii) Contribute to the changes of menstrual cycle.
Progesterone		Corpus luteum of ovary Placenta Adrenal cortex	Secretion increases during 'luteal' phase of menstrual cycle and prepares uterus for implantation of fertilised ovum.
Chorionic gonadotrophin		Placenta	Similar to pituitary interstitial cell stimulating hormone.

thyroid hormone (parathormone) cannot be used for prolonged replacement therapy, since after a few days its effect rapidly diminishes.

The hypothalamus is widely accepted as of fundamental importance because it is responsible for integrating the functions of the endocrine system and the nervous system. It has numerous nervous connections with the cerebral cortex, particularly with the frontal lobes. It forms the 'head ganglion' for the autonomic nervous system (i.e. sympathetic and parasympathetic). It is known to have direct nervous connections with the posterior lobe of the pituitary; in this way the osmolality of the blood is maintained through the secretion of the antidiuretic hormone vasopressin, and in turn the excretion of water by the kidney. Part of the blood supply of the anterior lobe of the pituitary is derived from 'portal' vessels. These drain into the gland, having ramified previously in the corpora mammillaria of the hypothalamus. Stimulation of this part of the hypothalamus in animals is capable of provoking the secretion of pituitary trophic hormones through the agency of releasing factors elaborated in the hypothalamus. In this way if the hypothalamus is regarded as a relay station, it can be seen how it serves to relate cerebral cortical activity, autonomic nervous function and the production of hormones.

Table 11 on pp. 680-681 is a brief summary of the sources and actions of the more important hormones.

THE HYPOPHYSIS (PITUITARY BODY)

The anterior lobe of the pituitary gland controls the activity of many of the other endocrine glands through the trophic hormones. It affects growth, thyroid activity, sexual life, lactation, water, carbohydrate, protein and fat metabolism by regulating the secretions of the other ductless glands. It weighs about 0·5 g. only, and measures approximately $1 \times 1 \times 0{\cdot}5$ cm.

Site. The pituitary body lies in the sella turcica, bridged over by the diaphragma sellae, with the sphenoidal air sinuses below, and the optic chiasma in the subarachnoid space above.

Anatomy of the Pituitary Gland. The gland is composed of two lobes, anterior and posterior, and is connected to the base of the brain by the infundibular stalk.

The anterior lobe is composed of two cell types.

1. *Chromophobe* cells, which are usually regarded as the precursors of the secretory cells.

2. These secretory cells are either *eosinophil* (*acidophil*) or *basophil*.

The posterior lobe (*pars nervosa*) contains neuroglial fibres and, together with the supraoptic and paraventricular nuclei of the hypothalamus, forms the neurohypophysis.

Physiology of the Pituitary Gland

ANTERIOR LOBE. Six hormones have now been isolated and corticotrophin has been synthesised (Table 11, p. 680).

POSTERIOR LOBE. This secretes two hormones.

1. *Vasopressin*. The principal action of this hormone is to increase the resorption of water by the renal tubules, so that the osmolality of the blood is maintained. This action has given rise to its alternative name *antidiuretin* or antidiuretic hormone (ADH).

2. *Oxytocin* induces contraction of the parturient uterus, and is widely used in obstetrics for this purpose.

CLINICAL MANIFESTATIONS OF PITUITARY DISEASE

The clinical features of pituitary disease vary, depending on the type of lesion in the pituitary gland, and on whether both lobes are involved or only one. Destruction of the gland in part or in its entirety will be followed by hypopituitarism. Enlarging tumours of the gland may sometimes present with signs attributable to increased output of hormones, or more commonly, failure of secretion, and amenorrhoea, for example, is an early and often the only symptom in younger adult women. At other times the early symptoms may take less specific forms, such as headache or visual deterioration.

A chromophobe adenoma is much the most common tumour of the pituitary gland. It may produce evidence of raised intracranial pressure and local effects, as well as signs of hypopituitarism caused by pressure on acidophil and basophil cells. Occasionally, however, chromophobe tumours may be associated with Cushing's disease. Tumours arising from the other cells are less common. In some patients with signs of hyperfunction, only hyperplasia of one cell type at the expense of the others is found. A cyst or a neoplasm (craniopharyngioma) may occur in Rathke's pouch, from which the anterior lobe of the pituitary is derived. Symptoms from local pressure effects may follow, and the mass may destroy the pituitary or compress the posterior lobe of the gland and the hypothalamus. A craniopharyngioma frequently calcifies and may then be recognised radiologically.

A. **Clinical features due to the site and size of the tumour**

Headache is the most constant but least specific symptom Involvement of an optic nerve, the optic chiasma, or an optic tract may lead to impaired visual acuity. The patient occasionally notices a visual field defect, but more usually examination of the visual fields by confrontation or by perimetry will be required to identify the likely point of interference with the visual pathway. Optic atrophy may be apparent on ophthalmoscopy. Diplopia and strabismus may follow pressure on the third, fourth and sixth cranial nerves. Enlargement of the sella turcica and erosion of the clinoid processes may be detected on radiological examination. Some tumours expand sufficiently to interfere with vasopressin secretion and so to cause diabetes insipidus, or to press upwards on the hypothalamus, thus producing disturbances of sleep and appetite.

B. **Syndromes due to disorder of anterior pituitary function**

1. HYPERSECRETION

(*a*) *Eosinophil Cells.* If hypersecretion of growth hormone develops before the epiphyses have united, **giantism** is produced. If it occurs in adult life, after union of the epiphyses, the condition is described as **acromegaly** (large extremities). If hypersecretion begins in adolescence and persists into adult life, giantism and acromegaly may be associated. Acromegaly is characterised by an increase in the size of the bones and soft tissues of the hands, feet, supraorbital ridges, sinuses and the lower jaw. The skin becomes thick and coarse; the subcutaneous tissues increase in depth, while enlargement of the tongue, lips and ears may be conspicuous. The viscera, for example the heart, thyroid and liver, enlarge. Carbohydrate tolerance may be reduced, and glycosuria occurs in about 50 per cent. of untreated cases. As the disease progresses, the patient often develops a kyphosis and muscular weakness. Hypertension is a common complication. Mental capacity deteriorates, the patient becomes irritable and complains of persistent headache. Sweating is often a troublesome symptom. The disease tends to progress slowly over several years, but patients are frequently seen with certain features of acromegaly in whom development of the condition has apparently been arrested, or a phase of hyperpituitarism may pass into hypopituitarism. New and sensitive radio-immunological methods of assaying growth hormone in blood now make it possible to assess with precision the activity of these tumours and the results of treatment.

(*b*) *Basophil Cells.* Hypersecretion by these cells leads to *Cushing's disease* (p. 731).

2. Hyposecretion

(i) *Hyposecretion in children* causes dwarfism and pituitary infantilism. The term 'dwarfism' means that growth is retarded; 'infantilism' implies that sexual development is subnormal for the individual's age, though it is also used to indicate retention of infantile as opposed to adult proportions of the head, limbs and trunk.

These dwarfs have been likened physically to the description of 'Peter Pan'; they fail to grow or to develop sexually. Their mental development tends to keep pace with their physical development rather than their chronological age.

Fröhlich's Syndrome or *Dystrophia Adiposo-genitalis.* While this rare condition may be associated with pituitary destruction, most of its features are a sequel to associated damage to the hypothalamus. Both the gland and the hypothalamus may be damaged by an expanding tumour, for example a craniopharyngioma. Obesity and diabetes insipidus (p. 689) may then be associated with sexual infantilism, and occasionally disturbances of temperature and sleep mechanisms may occur, particularly excessive somnolence. The accumulation of fat is probably due to a combination of increased appetite and diminished energy output: these patients spend much of their time asleep between meals.

(ii) *Hyposecretion in Adults.* Hypopituitarism (Simmonds' disease) follows.

HYPOPITUITARISM (SIMMONDS' DISEASE)

Aetiology. Destruction of the anterior lobe of the hypophysis is most commonly due to infarction, and this in turn is usually a sequel to post-partum shock (*Sheehan's syndrome*). In the male the disorder is most commonly due to a *chromophobe adenoma*. Other causes include non-functioning tumours, a fractured skull, infection, granulomata (syphilis, sarcoidosis) and the presence of simple cysts. Surgical treatment of tumours of the gland is often followed by a degree of hypopituitarism calling for substitution therapy, and complete hypophysectomy is sometimes performed in the treatment of some forms of malignant disease, for example carcinoma of the breast.

Clinical Features. In Sheehan's syndrome, a history is usually obtained that several years before the onset of the presenting illness, the patient had a difficult confinement with haemorrhage and a need for blood transfusion. Lactation failed or was never established, amenorrhoea persisted indefinitely, and other changes attributable to the absence of the trophic hormones gradually made their appearance. Some of the features of hypothyroidism are usually present, but myxoedema does not develop. Absent or scanty axillary and pubic hair are characteristic findings. Symptoms of adrenal insufficiency and a low blood pressure may be noted, but the changes in serum electrolytes found in severe adrenal insufficiency do not occur in hypopituitarism. This is probably because aldosterone continues to be secreted by the glomerulosa layer of the adrenal cortex, since this function is not dependent upon corticotrophin. Cortisol production, however, falls to a minimum because the essential corticotrophic stimulus from the pituitary gland is absent or inadequate. In contrast to the pigmentation of the skin in Addison's disease (p. 724) a most striking degree of pallor is often one of the signs suggesting hypopituitarism. Although a mild degree of normochromic anaemia is usually present, this is quite insufficient to explain the remarkable pallor of the skin. Capillary vasoconstriction and the absence of melanin together account for this arresting sign. Loss of weight is unusual and when present is often due to some other disease. The term 'pituitary cachexia' is sometimes used but is unfortunate because it is ambiguous. It was originally applied to 'wasting' of the gland, and it is now occasionally employed to indicate loss of body weight erroneously attributed to destruction of the pituitary gland.

Coma in Hypopituitarism. Patients with hypopituitarism are peculiarly liable to go into coma if inadequately treated. While the onset of coma may occur for no apparent reason, it usually follows some mild infection or injury, in the same way that an Addisonian crisis may follow some relatively trivial stress (p. 726). The coma may be due to one or more disorders particularly associated with hypopituitarism. These include spontaneous or reactive hypoglycaemia, and an increased sensitivity to insulin. Hypothermia with a rectal temperature as low as 32° C. (90° F.) or less may develop. Water intoxication is another important factor, due to a disturbance of water metabolism in patients with adrenal insufficiency (p. 728). Hypothyroidism is also an important component (p. 709) in the causation of coma, and failure of ventilation with anoxia and respiratory acidosis should also be considered in treating what is frequently a lethal complication of hypopituitarism.

Diagnosis. Hypopituitarism is sometimes confused with *anorexia nervosa* (p. 983). This psychoneurosis occurs usually in young women who for various reasons refuse to eat, and in late cases become grossly emaciated. There is good evidence for suggesting that as a result of starvation functional hypopituitarism occurs, so that in this respect the two conditions may be similar. The distinguishing features lie in the history, the retention of pubic and axillary hair in anorexia nervosa, and the satisfactory response of the latter to adequate psychotherapy. In addition, anorexia nervosa is characterised by an absent appetite and gross wasting, whereas in hypopituitarism neither is striking unless some other cause is present. The excellent response of patients with hypopituitarism to treatment with corticosteroids will also help to distinguish between the two conditions.

Treatment

1. *Radical.* Whenever a tumour is sufficiently large to produce local pressure effects, particularly visual field defects, an attempt should be made to remove it. Radiotherapy is also of some value, particularly in dealing with chromophobe adenomas, and may be combined with surgery. Radioactive yttrium is sometimes used in the form of pellets inserted through a cannula into the pituitary gland, and destruction of tumours by cryosurgery is also under trial.

2. *Symptomatic Treatment of Hypopituitarism.* The aim should be to provide adequate substitution therapy, so that the patient

can lead a normal life. Cortisone should be given by mouth in doses of 12·5 mg. twice or three times daily. Thyroid hormone will usually be required and should be given orally as thyroxine 0·1-0·2 mg. daily. In some circumstances it may be helpful to add an oestrogen such as ethinyl oestradiol 50 μg. daily, and for adolescent or adult men an androgen may be required (p. 737). Depot preparations of corticotrophin which are slowly absorbed (e.g. Acthar Gel) may be given by intramuscular injection in doses of 40 i.u. twice or three times weekly to induce endogenous adrenocortical activity. Cortisone by mouth as recommended is adequate however, and more convenient. It is dangerous to give thyroid hormone to these patients until they have been protected by cortisone or a similar drug against the possibility of an Addisonian type of crisis. Should coma occur it may be dealt with in the same way as an Addisonian crisis (p. 729).

Differential Diagnosis of Dwarfism

(*a*) Infantilism Due to Malabsorption (p. 939). This disability is characterised by steatorrhoea with defective absorption, especially of fat, minerals, and vitamins. Dwarfs of this type are usually larger than the pituitary type, and may be further distinguished by a prominent abdomen due to intestinal distension, and by a history of the passage of pale, bulky, offensive stools. *Fibrocystic disease of the pancreas* may simulate malabsorption due to gluten sensitivity.

(*b*) Dwarfism of Rickets (p. 487). This may be due to a defective diet or to malabsorption; kyphosis, pigeon-chest deformity and leg-bowing are common sequelae.

(*c*) Pituitary Infantilism (p. 685).

(*d*) Achondroplasia. This hereditary disorder of endochondral ossification is characterised by failure of the long bones of the arms and legs to grow properly, while the trunk and head develop normally. Dwarfs of this type are intellectually normal and frequently find employment in circuses.

(*e*) Renal Dwarfism. This is due to renal failure arising in early childhood. It may be caused by 'achalasia' at the outlet of the bladder, which produces back-pressure and hydronephrosis, or it may be due to congenital cystic disease, congenital hypoplasia of the kidneys or most commonly, chronic pyelonephritis. Many of the characteristic features of renal failure may be found, for example hypertension, a raised blood urea and changes in the fundus of the eye (p. 808).

(*f*) Cretinism. If this condition is not recognised and treated early in childhood, stunting of growth will occur (p. 710).

DIABETES INSIPIDUS

This rare disease is characterised by the persistent excretion of excessive quantities of urine of low specific gravity, and by constant thirst.

Aetiology. The disease develops after damage to the neurohypophyseal mechanism for the production of vasopressin. It occurs with tumours of the pituitary or after operations in this region, with a craniopharyngioma, and as a sequel to encephalitis, basal meningitis, syphilis, and following fractures at the base of the skull. In some cases no cause can be identified; a rare genetic form exists due to unreponsiveness of the renal tubules to vasopressin.

Symptoms. The most marked symptoms are polyuria and polydipsia. The patient may pass 5 to 20 or more litres of urine in 24 hours. The urine is clear and the specific gravity is 1002-1004. It does not contain sugar, blood or albumin. Such patients may become markedly dehydrated if water is withheld, since they continue to secrete urine in considerable volumes.

Differential Diagnosis

1. *Diabetes Mellitus.* The volume of urine increases because of the excess of solute (glucose) present, i.e. an osmotic diuresis.

2. *Hysterical Polydipsia.* This produces *polyuria.* In such cases if fluids are withheld for 24 hours the urine is found to concentrate to a normal specific gravity. Accurate weighing of the patient will show whether she has been drinking surreptitiously meanwhile.

3. *Chronic Renal Disease.* Several forms of disease, including glomerulonephritis, pyelonephritis, polycystic disease, partial ureteric obstruction and potassium depletion, may all be marked by an increase in the volume of urine formed in order to compensate for the loss of the capacity of the kidney to secrete a concentrated urine. Nocturia may be a more prominent complaint than polyuria.

4. *Hyperparathyroidism.* Though rare, this condition may be responsible for complaints of polyuria and polydipsia (p. 713).

A positive diagnosis of diabetes insipidus depends on demonstrating that a rise of plasma osmolality induced either by withholding fluids or infusing hypertonic saline is not accompanied by a rise in the osmolality or specific gravity of the urine, but that when intravenous pitressin is given, such a rise does occur. This final test is necessary in order to show that the kidney is capable of concentrating the urine.

Treatment. The minimum amount of vasopressin required to keep the patient in water balance must be determined by controlling the fluid output and then reducing the dose of hormone without permitting polyuria or excessive thirst to recur.

The most convenient preparation for clinical use is pitressin tannate in oil, which may be given in doses of 0·5-1 ml. (2·5-5 units) subcutaneously. The larger dose may cause headache, but if tolerated will last longer than the smaller dose. Patients usually require to repeat the injection every two to three days. It is important to warm the ampoule and to shake it vigorously before use so that the active material is resuspended before the contents are drawn up into the syringe.

A solution of synthetic lysine vasopressin may also be administered in the form of a nasal spray absorbed from the mucous membrane of the nose. Although the effect persists for a few hours only the method is often preferable in children and is useful for others until it is convenient for them to have a further injection.

Chlorothiazide, an oral diuretic, has been used with some success to control the thirst and polyuria of diabetes insipidus. The mechanism of action appears to depend largely on the suppression of thirst which otherwise serves to perpetuate the polydipsia and polyuria.

Prognosis. The cause of the neurohypophyseal damage will determine the patient's progress.

THE THYROID GLAND

ANATOMY AND PHYSIOLOGY

The thyroid gland consists of an isthmus and two lateral lobes, and lies in front of and on either side of the upper part of the trachea and the laminae of the thyroid cartilage. Posteriorly it is closely related to the recurrent laryngeal nerves which lie in the space between the trachea and the oesophagus; the gland is separated from the nerves by its fibrous sheath. The thyroid gland is provided with a rich blood supply through the superior and inferior thyroid arteries. The parathyroid glands are usually to be found lying on the posterior aspect of the thyroid in its substance or in the fibrous sheath.

Thyroxine and triiodothyronine, the hormones secreted by the gland, are amino acids containing four and three atoms respectively of iodine in each molecule. Both are normally stored in the colloid vesicles of the thyroid as thyroglobulin, and they are formed and released into the circulation under the control of the thyroid stimulating hormone (TSH) secreted by the adenohypophysis. An abnormal excitor is now known to simulate the action of TSH in hyperthyroidism, namely the long-acting thyroid stimulator (LATS) described on p. 696. Triiodothyronine appears to be about five times as active, weight for weight, as thyroxine. When given to a patient, the effects of triiodothyronine become apparent in a few hours, unlike those of thyroxine which may be delayed in onset for several days. Both hormones act directly on most of the tissues of the body to increase cellular metabolism. It is possible that triiodothyronine is a derivative of thyroxine.

The rapid action of triiodothyronine may sometimes be a disadvantage, and the only clear indication for using this preparation is in the rare cases of coma associated with hypothyroidism (p. 687), when it may be given intravenously. Thyroxine is therefore normally regarded as the drug of choice when treatment with thyroid hormone is required.

GOITRE

This term merely indicates enlargement of the thyroid and does not imply any alteration of function or any particular type of histological change.

SIMPLE (COLLOID) GOITRE

This may occur sporadically, but in certain parts of the world it is found more frequently and is then referred to as endemic goitre. Generally speaking, such areas are far removed from the sea, for example the Alps, Himalayas and certain of the central states of North America. In Britain it is relatively common in the Peak District of Derbyshire, hence one of its synonyms 'Derbyshire neck'.

Aetiology. This is not fully understood, but it is generally believed to be closely related to iodine deficiency. This may arise in various ways, of which the most important is probably the first of those mentioned below.

1. An absolute iodine deficiency in the diet is more likely to occur in the mountainous areas described. The water supplies lack iodine, and sea foods like fish which contain iodine are scarce.

2. The excessive calcium in hard water supplies may interfere with iodine absorption.

3. Hereditary goitres occur rarely and are due to absence of one or more of several enzymes required by the gland in the synthesis of thyroxine. These defects are genetic and their endemic nature is therefore not environmental.

4. The iodide concentrating mechanism of the thyroid may be interfered with in such a way that the gland is no longer able to collect the element from the blood or, having done so, to synthesise the active amino acids, thyroxine and triiodothyronine. A number of substances have now been recognised which are capable of blocking this mechanism. For example, iodine deficiency is known to occur in the thyroid glands of rabbits when they are fed on a diet containing excessive amounts of vegetables of the Brassica family, such as cabbage, brussels sprouts and turnips. Similarly, goitres have developed in patients who were eating large amounts of this type of vegetable in the uncooked state. A recent epidemic of goitre in children in Tasmania has been attributed to such a goitrogen occurring in the milk of cows which had been fed on certain vegetables. It is possible that other naturally occurring substances might be implicated in the production of some goitres.

In addition to the antithyroid drugs used in the treatment of hyperthyroidism, a wide variety of other drugs is known to interfere to some extent with thyroxine synthesis; sulphonamides, resorcinol and PAS (p. 425) for example may do so when administered for long periods. Iodides taken persistently in large doses as self-medication for asthma are also known to induce considerable thyroid enlargement. In each of these examples the secretion or release of thyroid hormone is depressed. Consequently, the pituitary increases the output of TSH and the thyroid gland responds with epithelial hyperplasia. In this way the gland enlarges, often without clinical evidence of any alteration in hormone production. If an adequate amount of iodine then becomes available, the follicles of the gland fill with colloid, and the epithelium lining the follicles becomes less active and appears flattened in histological preparations. Repeated episodes of hyperplasia and involution lead eventually to permanent enlargement of the gland and may be important in the development of the nodules which are often a prominent feature of goitres of long standing.

In many countries where iodine deficiency in the diet is known to occur, legislation has been introduced to ensure that traces of iodine are added to table salt. As a result the incidence of goitre has been markedly reduced. In Britain, the Medical Research Council has recommended the addition of sufficient sodium or potassium iodide to ensure the presence of 1·5-3·0 mg. of iodine per 100 g. of domestic salt, but the legislation required to enforce this recommendation has not yet been enacted.

Clinical Features. Simple goitre often makes its appearance in childhood, and though tending to disappear about puberty in boys, goitres occurring in girls may enlarge further or appear for the first time at this age. They may also recur or appear for the first time during pregnancy. Generally speaking, no symptoms are produced, but occasionally symptoms suggesting hypothyroidism may be found. The enlarged gland may cause embarrassment because of disfigurement. If part or the whole of the swelling lies retrosternally, venous engorgement of the head and neck may occasionally occur. The swelling of the gland is usually soft, smooth and symmetrical, but nodules may appear in goitres of longer standing, so that the gland becomes irregular in outline and consistency. Bruits and thrills, which are signs of increased vascularity, do not occur in simple goitres.

Differential Diagnosis. Enlargement of the thyroid must be distinguished from swellings arising in other structures in the root of the neck. The position and shape of the mass, together with its mobility on swallowing, will usually help to identify those of thyroid origin. Simple goitre must then be differentiated further from a number of other causes of enlargement of the thyroid.

1. *Toxic goitre* (*hyperthyroidism* p. 701).

2. *Lymphadenoid goitre* (*Hashimoto's disease*). The importance of this relatively common form of goitre has only recently been fully recognised. It is now accepted that this disease is a sequel to the development of antibodies to antigens of thyroid origin, including thyroglobulin in some, and the microsome component of thyroid epithelial cells in other cases. The condition is thus one form of *auto-immunisation*, a process long regarded as impossible, but which is now believed to be responsible for several diseases.

The disease is characterised by infiltration of the thyroid gland with plasma cells and lymphocytes; with the gradual destruction of the gland hypothyroidism ultimately appears, and it is now evident that such a cycle of events is responsible for the majority of cases of hypothyroidism or myxoedema. In many cases thyroid insufficiency develops without the gland ever having been clinically enlarged. Serological studies of the disease have shown that the antibody concerned may be demonstrated by precipitin, complement fixation and fluorescent antibody tests, and by other tests depending on the agglutination of red cells hardened with tannic acid and coated with antigen. An excess of circulating gamma globulin may be found, and the erythrocyte sedimentation rate is often raised. The tests for antibody mentioned above are occasionally found to be positive in other conditions, for example hyperthyroidism and thyroid carcinoma, and lymphadenoid goitre, of course, may coexist with either. Treatment with thyroxine in full doses will usually lead to shrinkage of the goitre of Hashimoto's disease, and will relieve the symptoms of hypothyroidism when the disease has reached this stage. When patients with hyperthyroidism are treated with radioiodine or surgically, Hashimoto's disease is responsible occasionally for the subsequent appearance of thyroid insufficiency.

3. *Riedel's goitre* ('woody' or 'iron-hard' thyroiditis) is remarkable because of its hardness. This may represent one form of the later stages of Hashimoto's disease.

4. *Carcinoma of the thyroid* may arise *de novo*, or in a goitre of long standing. Fixation of the mass, or evidence of local extension or metastases may suggest the diagnosis on clinical grounds.

5. *Subacute* (*giant-cell*) *thyroiditis* and thyroiditis due either to pyogenic or more chronic granulomatous infections such as tuberculosis are all very uncommon.

In a doubtful case of goitre when thyroidectomy is not otherwise contemplated, the value of histological examination of an adequate biopsy specimen of the gland should be borne in mind.

Treatment of Simple Goitre. Potassium iodide 0·1 g. daily by mouth is worthy of trial. In cases of recent onset, particularly if associated with puberty or pregnancy, this may be sufficient to abolish the swelling. If, as rarely happens, there are signs of hypothyroidism, thyroxine should be given instead of potassium iodide, and indeed some authorities recommend the administration of thyroxine even in the absence of such signs. If the goitre is of long standing and large, neither potassium iodide nor thyroxine is likely to be of any value. Disfigurement or symptoms from pressure may justify the removal of a large portion of the gland. Hypothyroidism or frank myxoedema may follow operation, but can be readily controlled by treatment with thyroxine (p. 709).

An adequate intake of iodine, in the early years of life particularly, is the only really satisfactory way of preventing the disease.

HYPERTHYROIDISM OR THYROTOXICOSIS

This is also known as *toxic goitre*, *exophthalmic goitre*, and *Graves' disease*, *Parry's disease* and *Basedow's disease*, after those who described it early in the 19th century. Excluding exophthalmos, the features of the disorder are due to excessive secretion of thyroid hormone.

Incidence. The disorder occurs much more frequently in women than in men (8 : 1), usually in early adult life, but it is not uncommon later, when its features differ somewhat from those seen in the younger adult.

Aetiology. It used to be suggested that hyperthyroidism is induced by excessive secretion of TSH and that some of the features of the condition, particularly exophthalmos are also due to this hormone or to a closely related substance which causes exophthalmos (exophthalmos-producing substance, EPS). However, it is now known that the thyroid activator found in the plasma of most cases of hyperthyroidism is an immunoglobulin and differs from TSH of pituitary origin. Because of its behaviour in biological assays it is known as the 'long-acting thyroid stimulator' (LATS). Unlike TSH, it cannot be suppressed by the administration of thyroxine, and TSH, as might be anticipated, cannot be detected in the plasma in hyperthyroidism. The factors responsible for the formation of LATS have not yet been identified, but it may be formed as an antibody to an antigenic component of the thyroid gland in an individual genetically predisposed to auto-immunisation.

Accident, fright, emotional shock, severe illnesses or surgical procedures may precede or appear to be responsible for the onset of hyperthyroidism, but this concept is not well supported. Latent hyperthyroidism may however become obvious in these circumstances, and indeed an operation performed for an unrelated condition may precipitate a thyroid crisis (p. 699) in a patient with hyperthyroidism previously unrecognised or inadequately treated.

There is some evidence in favour of a genetic predisposition to several of the disorders of the thyroid gland, including hyperthyroidism.

Pathology. In hyperthyroidism the gland shows histological evidence of enhanced activity and the vesicles are relatively empty of colloid; the epithelium is tall and columnar in contrast to the flat cuboidal epithelium of the resting gland or the simple goitre after treatment with iodine or thyroxine. The vessels are dilated, and sometimes there is increased infiltration of the stroma by lymphocytes or even the typical changes of Hashimoto's disease. The heart is not enlarged, except when the condition is complicated by atrial fibrillation or congestive cardiac failure. In cases with much exophthalmos the retro-orbital fat is oedematous and the extrinsic muscles of the eye show degenerative changes with oedema and round cell infiltration. The liver may show fatty degeneration, and in cases of long standing the bones may appear decalcified on radiological examination, due to osteoporosis. Degenerative changes in striated muscle are also common and may be associated with marked weakness and clinical evidence of myopathy.

Clinical Features. Many of the early symptoms are similar to those found in anxiety states, from which it may be difficult sometimes to distinguish the mild case of hyperthyroidism. Nervousness, unfounded fears, restlessness, tiredness, undue sweating, emotional lability, breathlessness on exertion, tachycardia and palpitations are frequent complaints. The hyperthyroid patient will often have noticed how much more readily she can tolerate the cold, or her family, her friends or her husband may complain that they cannot tolerate the temperature that she finds acceptable. A fine rapid tremor affecting particularly the outstretched hands appears early in many cases. The skin, especially of the hands, is warm and occasionally moist in contrast to the hands of the patient with an anxiety state, which are usually cold and clammy. Many of the symptoms and signs of hyperthyroidism resemble those following an injection of adrenaline, and it has been suggested that the excess of thyroxine in the circulation sensitises the tissues to adrenaline. As the condition develops the more typical signs are found.

1. *The thyroid gland is enlarged*, though the degree of enlargement bears no relation to the severity of the disorder. Occasionally there may be no enlargement, or it may not be seen or felt because the gland is retrosternal. The swelling may be asymmetrical, affecting one lobe more than the other. The surface of the gland may be smooth or irregular. Its blood supply is increased so that it may pulsate, a 'thrill' may be palpable, and a systolic 'bruit' may be heard on auscultation over the gland.

2. *Increased Prominence of One or Both Eyes*. This may be due to two components:

(*a*) *Lid retraction*, which is significant if the sclera can be seen above and below the cornea when the patient looks straight ahead. 'Lid lag' is the term applied to the failure of the upper eyelid to follow movement of the globe when the patient looks down.

(*b*) *Exophthalmos*, or proptosis, means that the eye is pushed forward in the orbital cavity, and this is usually caused by swelling of the retro-bulbar tissues. It is important to distinguish exophthalmos from lid retraction as the latter, if present alone, will usually regress when the hyperthyroidism is relieved. Exophthalmos, however, may appear in the absence of disordered thyroid function; it may not regress and may even appear for the first time or be aggravated when hyperthyroidism has been successfully treated. Weakness of the external ocular muscles, particularly of the superior recti, is commonly associated with exophthalmos and, if the condition becomes severe, interference with the movements of the eyes may lead to diplopia. In severe cases, oedema of the conjunctivae may make it impossible to close the eyelids properly and the cornea may be damaged by exposure and drying. This condition is known as *malignant exophthalmos* or *exophthalmic ophthalmoplegia*. It is remarkable that while hyperthyroidism is so much more common in women, this type of exophthalmos and its complications are as common in men as in women.

Exophthalmos may, however, occur apart from its association with thyroid disorders. It is found when retrobulbar tumours push the eye forward. Cavernous sinus thrombosis will produce much oedema of the retro-orbital tissues. An aneurysm of the internal carotid artery or an arteriovenous aneurysm between the internal carotid artery and the cavernous sinus will be accompanied by pulsating exophthalmos, over which a 'bruit' may be heard.

In some patients with hyperthyroidism there may be considerable oedema of the eyelids. If lid retraction or exophthalmos is not marked, the presence of this oedema may be misleading and even suggest the diagnosis of myxoedema.

3. *Cardiovascular Changes*. (See also Thyrotoxic Heart Disease, p. 252).

Sinus tachycardia, persisting during sleep, is one of the earliest and most constant signs; it may be accompanied by extrasystoles. Vasodilation is usual, so that the skin feels warm. The pulse pressure is increased and capillary pulsation may be detectable. In the presence of coincident systolic hypertension a collapsing pulse may be noted. Cardiac enlargement is unusual in the absence of complications. If the disorder is allowed to persist, atrial fibrillation may follow, sometimes preceded by paroxysmal fibrillation. This is more likely to occur in the older patient, in whom eye signs are less common.

4. *Metabolic Features*. The appetite is usually increased, and if food intake is inadequate to keep pace with the increased metabolism, loss of weight will occur. In contrast, weight may be gained occasionally if the appetite and diet are greater than the metabolic demands. Weight changes during treatment should be followed closely. Arrest of weight loss suggests control of hyper-

thyroidism and a sudden increase in weight may be due to several causes, including fluid retention with myxoedema.

Slight glycosuria is sometimes found and is relieved when hyperthyroidism has been controlled. True diabetes mellitus may occasionally be complicated and aggravated by hyperthyroidism (p. 740).

5. *Other Manifestations*. Patients occasionally complain of passing loose stools, or more frequently that their bowel habit has altered from one, to two or three formed stools daily. Amenorrhoea occurs infrequently, but oligomenorrhoea is relatively common.

Thyrotoxic crises are now uncommon, as cases of hyperthyroidism are recognised and treated earlier and more effectively. They were sometimes seen immediately after thyroidectomy in severe cases who had been inadequately prepared for operation, who had been operated on for some other disability without latent hyperthyroidism having been recognised, or during some severe infection, for example pneumonia, and they even occurred spontaneously. Mental symptoms with delirium, delusions or mania are common; diarrhoea and vomiting with excessive salt and fluid loss occur, but the condition is most dangerous because of potentially fatal circulatory collapse.

Hyperthyroidism in children seldom occurs until about puberty, and even at that age it is most unusual. It occurs very rarely in the newborn infant.

Hyperthyroidism in middle-aged and elderly persons is not uncommon and is an important cause of atrial fibrillation and congestive cardiac failure. Largely because the more usual symptoms and signs of hyperthyroidism are often absent, the diagnosis is frequently overlooked. Loss of weight, an altered bowel habit, skin pigmentation and minimal thyroid enlargement may be detected incidentally in a patient presenting with symptoms due to cardiac failure. Provided the hyperthyroidism is recognised and relieved, atrial fibrillation and congestive cardiac failure can often be readily controlled or even cured.

Laboratory diagnostic procedures

(*a*) *Radioactive iodine metabolism*. By using radioactive isotopes of iodine it is possible to study the metabolism of iodine by the thyroid gland. The dose of radiation involved can be so low that the dangers in the method can be almost disregarded. As little as 5 microcuries of the isotope ^{131}I given by mouth may be sufficient to show clearly whether the thyroid is unduly active. This can be demonstrated in several ways. In the first place, the amount of the dose collected by the thyroid in a given time can be estimated by placing a suitable counter directly over the neck. An indirect measure is also obtainable by estimating the amount of radioactive iodine excreted in the urine in 24 or 48 hours: it is assumed that the remainder of the dose not excreted is almost entirely concentrated in the thyroid. The rate of secretion of radioactive thyroid hormone from the thyroid after a dose of radioiodine may also be estimated by measuring the protein bound ^{131}I at an interval of 24 or 48 hours after a suitable dose.

Radioiodine for any purpose should be avoided during pregnancy. With children, the isotope ^{132}I with a half-life of 2·3 hours may be permissible for essential diagnostic purposes, since the radiation dose is so much smaller than with ^{131}I which has a half-life of 8·1 days.

(*b*) *Serum protein-bound iodine* (PBI) *determinations* measure the amount of circulating organic iodine, largely in the form of thyroxine (normal range 3-8 μg./100 ml.). Both radioiodine tests and PBI estimations are frequently invalidated because patients have been taking drugs containing iodine or have been given preparations of iodine for diagnostic purposes, for example cholecystography.

(*c*) The *triiodothyronine* (T_3), *resin uptake* has recently been introduced and is valuable in that it can be used to identify cases of hyperthyroidism even when their plasma contains an excess of non-hormonal iodine.

(*d*) The *basal metabolic rate* is raised in hyperthyroidism, but is rarely used now for diagnosis. The plasma cholesterol concentration tends to be low in hyperthyroidism, but is quite unreliable as a test of thyroid function.

Differential Diagnosis

1. *Anxiety neurosis* may be difficult to distinguish from hyperthyroidism on clinical grounds alone, particularly in the earlier stages (p. 1248). In hyperthyroidism the pulse rate during sleep tends to remain raised, while the tachycardia often associated with an anxiety neurosis will settle. The majority of patients with

hyperthyroidism, except those requiring surgical treatment, can now be dealt with adequately without admission to hospital, but occasionally the need for closer clinical observation will justify admission.

2. A *simple* (*colloid*) *goitre* may be mistaken for the goitre of hyperthyroidism. The presence of an enlarged thyroid is no criterion of hyperthyroidism, and its size is never a measure of its secretory activity. The goitre of hyperthyroidism is firm and smooth in the young, but is often nodular and irregular in older patients (see below).

3. *Rheumatic heart disease* is sometimes diagnosed in error because a praecordial systolic murmur is found. If the possibility of hyperthyroidism is remembered under such circumstances, it is unlikely that this error will arise.

4. *Atrial fibrillation* and in some cases congestive cardiac failure, are occasionally not recognised to be complications of hyperthyroidism, particularly in older patients (p. 252).

5. Symptoms occurring with *the menopause* may sometimes be difficult to distinguish from those attributable to hyperthyroidism.

6. *Respiratory failure* in a patient with, for example, chronic bronchitis and emphysema may resemble hyperthyroidism because of tachycardia, warm extremities, tremor and prominent bright glistening eyes.

Clinico-Pathological Varieties of Hyperthyroidism. Confusion tends to arise because the clinical disorder is sometimes named according to the pathological changes in the gland. The clinical features of hyperthyroidism are due to increased secretion of thyroid hormones; the histological changes in the gland vary greatly, and may be difficult to correlate with functional activity or with possible aetiological factors, especially after medical treatment.

1. *Primary toxic goitre* (Graves' disease) is associated with smooth firm elastic enlargement of the gland.

2. *Secondary toxic goitre* is the clinical term applied when a simple goitre becomes toxic. It may be histologically indistinguishable from toxic nodular goitre.

3. *Toxic nodular goitre*. This term refers to the naked-eye and microscopic appearance of a gland which has become irregularly enlarged, probably as the result of alternating phases of hyperplasia and involution over the course of time; sooner or later 'toxic'

symptoms and signs appear. (A 'foetal' adenoma is sometimes distinguished which is believed to arise as a benign neoplasm from foetal cell rests in the inter-acinar parenchymal tissue.)

Toxic nodular goitre is often preceded by thyroid swelling for some years, and hyperthyroidism with this type of goitre usually occurs in older patients (50 years or over); eye signs and nervous symptoms are often slight or absent, and cardiac manifestations predominate. Nodular goitres of this type may also cause pressure symptoms, sometimes suddenly, if haemorrhage occurs into them; rarely they may undergo malignant change. A solitary nodule occurring in an otherwise normal gland (*toxic adenoma*) may sometimes be responsible for hyperthyroidism.

Treatment. The methods of treating hyperthyroidism may be summarised as follows:

1. Antithyroid drugs, such as carbimazole;
2. Surgery, after preparation with potassium iodide;
3. Radioactive iodine.

1. *Antithyroid drugs*

Before the introduction of the thiouracil group of drugs, surgical treatment—the removal of about five-sixths of the thyroid gland—was the therapeutic method of choice. The antithyroid drugs which act by suppressing the secretion of thyroid hormones have provided a valuable supplementary method of treatment.

Carbimazole is a suitable preparation and is given initially in full suppressive doses of 20 mg. three times daily for the first six to eight weeks of treatment. When the evidence of hyperthyroidism has disappeared, a daily dose of 10-15 mg. is usually sufficient to maintain control. This treatment should be continued for 12 months in cases of primary toxic goitre, but relapse is likely to occur in about 50 per cent. of patients and more than this in older age groups. Further courses can be given, but it is common practice to advise surgical treatment, after appropriate preparation, when relapse occurs.

If carbimazole is not tolerated methyl thiouracil may be given a trial in tenfold larger doses, before resorting to treatment by radioactive iodine or surgery. A further alternative is provided by potassium perchlorate in a total daily divided dose of 1 g. initially, and 200-400 mg. daily for maintenance.

After some weeks' treatment with these drugs the thyroid gland may enlarge, due to further hyperplasia. This in itself is not harmful unless the gland or part of it lies behind the sternum, where its presence might lead to respiratory embarrassment. In the neck it may be unsightly and, for this reason, disturbing to the patient. It may be necessary to reduce the dose of antithyroid drug further, since enlargement of the gland in these circumstances is sometimes the result of too intensive treatment. Alternatively thyroxine, 0·2 mg. daily, may be given along with antithyroid drugs, with the aim of maintaining a blood level of thyroid hormone sufficient to prevent secretion of TSH by the pituitary gland. It is also possible that used in this way thyroxine may reduce the risk of exophthalmos appearing, or of deteriorating if already present.

Carbimazole and the thiouracil group of drugs as well as potassium perchlorate are liable to produce toxic effects, of which the most serious is agranulocytosis. Others include dermatitis, nausea, vomiting and diarrhoea, jaundice, urticaria, lymph gland enlargement, drug-fever and thrombocytopenia. Routine white cell counts are of little value in the early detection of agranulocytosis, as it occurs with dramatic suddenness, usually in the first few weeks of treatment. Patients taking the drugs must be warned to report a sore throat immediately. If the diagnosis of agranulocytosis is confirmed by a white cell count and the drug is stopped, serious results can be avoided by giving penicillin until the leucocyte count returns to normal, which usually occurs after one to two weeks (p. 643).

Iodine should not be given to patients before treatment with the antithyroid group of drugs, as it will delay the response. It is, however, most valuable in the preparation of patients for operation (see below). Phenobarbitone 0·1 g. twice daily is useful in many cases of hyperthyroidism as it acts as a cerebral depressant and is also thought to diminish tissue responsiveness to thyroxine.

2. *Surgical treatment*. Operative treatment may be called for in the following circumstances:

(*a*) If the patient chooses operation after explanation of the alternatives. Some patients prefer an operation to 12 months' treatment with drugs when no assurance can be given that medical treatment will be successful.

(*b*) If the patient is thought to be unreliable and therefore unlikely to persist with treatment by drugs.

(*c*) If drug sensitivity reactions occur with more than one preparation.

(*d*) For cosmetic reasons if the gland is very large, or if it is causing pressure symptoms.

(*e*) For 'nodular' goitres, which respond less well to antithyroid drugs than 'primary' toxic goitres, and particularly since the former may cause pressure, or suddenly increase in size due to haemorrhage into their substance.

(*f*) For cases which relapse after prolonged drug therapy.

(*g*) For retrosternal goitres which may enlarge when treated with antithyroid drugs and so cause difficulty in respiration.

In recommending surgical treatment some of its potential disadvantages should be borne in mind. Partial thyroidectomy may be complicated by postoperative recurrent laryngeal palsy with hoarseness. Tetany or subclinical hypoparathyroidism may occur if some of the parathyroids are inadvertently removed. The patient will develop myxoedema if too much thyroid tissue is excised. A proportion of glands removed from patients with hyperthyroidism show the histological changes of Hashimoto's disease. Such patients will progress ultimately to a stage of thyroid insufficiency. This may account for some of the cases of hypothyroidism which occur as a late post-operative sequel. On the other hand, recurrence of hyperthyroidism will occur sooner or later in about 10 per cent. of patients treated by partial thyroidectomy. Even in the most skilful hands and with all the advantages of modern anaesthesia, deaths occasionally occur, but this should happen in considerably less than 1 per cent. of cases if they are properly prepared for operation.

If operation is decided upon, careful pre-operative treatment is essential. Hyperthyroidism should first be brought under complete control with carbimazole. Phenobarbitone 0·1 g. is given twice daily if necessary. Carbimazole is withdrawn two weeks before operation. Potassium iodide 0·1 g. is then given once daily by mouth until operation, and for a further week afterwards. This not only lessens the risk of a thyrotoxic crisis, but also reduces the vascularity of the gland. The suppressive effect of iodide is transient and if operation is delayed beyond three weeks it may be necessary to repeat the preparation with antithyroid drugs.

When atrial fibrillation or congestive cardiac failure is present this must be fully treated before operation (p. 169). In patients with atrial fibrillation spontaneous return to normal rhythm frequently follows operation. If the disorder of rhythm persists, lignocaine, quinidine or procainamide should be used as described on p. 193. Reversion to sinus rhythm can often be induced by direct current electric shock therapy. Convalescence may be necessary for some weeks before return to work.

3. *Radioactive iodine* provides an alternative method of controlling hyperthyroidism when surgical treatment is unsuitable, and control by the antithyroid drugs is impracticable. Indeed in patients past the reproductive years of life, it is the method of choice. It will control hyperthyroidism satisfactorily provided an adequate dose is used. The isotope ^{131}I is given by mouth and is rapidly accumulated in the thyroid, where it irradiates and destroys the hyperactive tissue. The effective dose is difficult to estimate. In some cases a single dose of radioactive iodine is sufficient, but in others it may have to be repeated. Special safety measures are required for handling the drug. Radioactive iodine should never be used during pregnancy, and in view of the capacity of irradiation to accelerate genetic mutation, its use should be avoided until the later years of life. The incidence of hypothyroidism after treatment with radioiodine may be as high as 50 per cent. or more, and although it is easily treated, this potential complication must be considered in planning treatment.

Radioactive iodine may also be used to locate active thyroid tissue, for example a retrosternal goitre, or occasionally metastases arising from a carcinoma of the thyroid.

Treatment of a Thyrotoxic Crisis. When this dangerous complication of hyperthyroidism occurs, it should be treated vigorously, the details depending on the features present. Potassium iodide (1 g.) should be given by mouth or if necessary intravenously. Intravenous fluids may be required if vomiting, diarrhoea or undue sweating have been responsible for excessive fluid loss. Chlorpromazine may be required for excitement or for hyperpyrexia, and intravenous corticosteroids, for example hydrocortisone sodium succinate, may be needed as for the treatment of an Addisonian crisis (p. 729). If heart failure is impending digoxin should be given and propranolol should also be considered unless congestive cardiac failure and hypotension are severe.

Treatment of Exophthalmos. Exophthalmos, an important but relatively infrequent complication of hyperthyroidism, may be so severe as to call for special consideration in the management of these patients (p. 697). If neglected, it may proceed to corneal ulceration and permanent blindness.

Several procedures are used in the treatment of this condition. It may be necessary to stitch the lateral margins of the eyelids together to prevent damage to the cornea (tarsorrhaphy). In severe cases decompression of the orbital cavity may be required. Radiotherapy to the pituitary is occasionally employed with the intention of reducing the production of EPS (p. 696). The irradiation of the tissues in the orbital cavity incidental to this procedure may be responsible for the benefit which sometimes follows.

It is important to ensure that the patient is never allowed to become hypothyroid, especially after operation, since this would tend to be followed by secretion of pituitary TSH and possibly EPS as well. Thyroxine should be given in moderate doses whenever exophthalmos is of sufficient degree to cause any anxiety, especially when the patient is being treated for hyperthyroidism with antithyroid drugs (p. 703). Guanethidine used as 5 per cent. eye drops is useful in reducing the complaint of 'grittiness' frequently offered by these patients, but because of the danger of keratitis it should only be used under supervision by an ophthalmologist.

HYPOTHYROIDISM

Myxoedema is the term used to describe patients with diminished thyroid function who appear oedematous. The word myxoedema (lit. = mucus + swelling) was invented to describe the condition because the characteristic feature is an accumulation in the skin of material which stains like mucus, and gives the appearance of oedema. Clinically it is distinguished from true oedema by its failure to pit on pressure, but the two may coexist.

The distinction between hypothyroidism and myxoedema is important because although all myxoedematous patients show diminished thyroid function, not all patients who are deficient of thyroid hormone show myxoedema. Because of this the diagnosis of hypothyroidism is readily and frequently overlooked.

Aetiology. If the cases due to radioiodine therapy and occasionally to thyroidectomy are excluded, the remainder are due almost entirely to the end-result of Hashimoto's disease (p. 694). Antibodies to thyroglobulin or thyroid cell components can usually be demonstrated, except in cases of very long standing. A secondary form of hypothyroidism is sometimes distinguished, due to failure of the pituitary gland to secrete TSH; this is usually one feature of hypopituitarism (Simmonds' disease, p. 686). The changes found, apart from those in the thyroid, are the result of lack of thyroxine and can be fully restored to normal by replacement therapy.

Hypothyroidism may be associated with some of the goitres discussed on p. 694.

Incidence. The condition is more common in women than men; the onset is usually about the age of the menopause, but it may occur at any age, including childhood.

Clinical Features. The *symptoms* are the result of lowered metabolism and slowing of physical and mental activity. The onset is gradual, and mental activity is so depressed that the patient's relatives notice the changes more readily than the patient. Questioning may elicit such symptoms as sensitivity to cold, weakness, tiredness, stiffness, gain in weight, poor appetite, constipation, loss of hair, a dry skin, disturbances of menstrual function, hoarseness, deafness, and 'rheumatism', i.e. vague muscular pains. Acroparaesthesiae may occur since these patients are predisposed to the carpal tunnel syndrome (p. 1226).

Signs. The face appears swollen, with puffy eyelids, thick lips and enlarged tongue. The skin is pale, and may be thickened by myxoedema; sometimes a moderate malar flush is found. Sweating is conspicuously absent, and in some areas the skin is rough and scaly. The hair tends to be more sparse than normal, short and lustreless. Speech is slow, monotonous and often hoarse and croaking in character. Mental impairment may be indicated by a poor memory, slowing of reaction time, apathy and drowsiness. Frank psychosis with hallucinations and delusions may occur, accompanied by phases of excitement—'myxoedematous madness.' Characteristically the pulse is slow, but if the condition has progressed to congestive cardiac failure tachycardia may be found. Commonly there is evidence of coronary artery insufficiency with angina pectoris or ECG evidence of myocardial ischaemia. On radiological examination the heart is frequently seen to be enlarged, in some cases as the result of pericardial effusion: this is usually reversible with treatment. The blood pressure in uncomplicated hypothyroidism is usually low. Since however degenerative vascular disease is common in hypothyroidism this may account for the rise in systolic pressure often found. The ankle jerks show a characteristic abnormality, namely marked slowing of the recovery phase of the reflex, due to delayed relaxation of the calf muscles. Patients with myxoëdema may occasionally pass into a state of coma similar to that which sometimes complicates hypopituitarism (p. 686).

Examination of the blood may show anaemia (p. 629). The plasma cholesterol concentration is usually raised to 300-500 mg./100 ml. (normal, 100-300 mg./100 ml.). The BMR may be as low as −40 per cent., depending on the degree of hypothyroidism. Tests with radioactive iodine will usually confirm that the thyroid concentrates little, if any, of a dose of labelled iodine. The serum PBI (p. 700) will be less than 3 μg./100 ml.

This description applies to fully developed cases; milder degrees of hypothyroidism with mental apathy, poor memory, anaemia, dry skin and 'rheumatism' are common in the menopausal or post-menopausal female, and are frequently overlooked because myxoedema is not present.

Differential Diagnosis

1. *Obesity*. Many patients with hypothyroidism are incidentally moderately obese, and it is a common error for hypothyroidism to be either incorrectly diagnosed or overlooked in obese patients. Thyroxine is frequently prescribed in obesity in the optimistic but erroneous belief that it will help to dispose of the excess fat. An interesting paradox is seen when, owing to apathy and anorexia, weight is often actually lost in the more advanced cases of myxoedema. In patients with myxoedema the administration of thyroxine is followed by a diuresis and an initial rapid and marked fall in weight at first which is not found in simple obesity; such a therapeutic test may occasionally be justifiable.

2. *Nephrotic Syndrome* (p. 805). In this condition the oedema

pits on pressure and the mental slowing and most of the other features of hypothyroidism are not present. A heavy proteinuria will be found.

3. *Pernicious or Iron Deficiency Anaemia.* Hypothyroidism may be associated with pernicious anaemia (p. 621) or with an iron deficiency anaemia (p. 612).

4. *Psychosis.* In hypothyroid patients with mental symptoms the signs of hypothyroidism will also be present. Mistakes will be avoided if the possible relationship of a psychosis with diminished thyroid function is remembered.

5. *Hypopituitarism* (*Simmonds' disease*) (p. 685). The aetiological relationship of this condition to hypothyroidism may be overlooked as the features of hypothyroidism may predominate. Adequate history-taking will frequently reveal the cause of the pituitary damage, and there may be evidence of failure of other endocrine organs. Sometimes the abnormal responsiveness of these patients to thyroxine first draws attention to their pituitary insufficiency.

6. The muscular aches and pains from which hypothyroid patients frequently suffer may be regarded in error as due to *osteoarthritis* or *muscular rheumatism*, though these may of course be found in patients with hypothyroidism.

Treatment. In uncomplicated cases treatment with thyroxine should start with 0·1 mg. daily. The dose should not be increased more frequently than every 14 days, owing to the delay of several days in eliciting a response. It may be necessary to raise the dose to 0·3 mg. daily, but rarely more, and treatment must be maintained indefinitely. Patients frequently abandon treatment when they feel better, and must therefore be seen regularly to ensure that they continue treatment. Caution in dosage is particularly desirable when coronary disease is present; such patients are best kept at a slightly lower level of metabolism than normal, and smaller initial doses should be used, for example 0·05 mg. of thyroxine or less daily. In a patient known to have ischaemic heart disease propranolol should be given along with thyroxine. The greatest care should also be taken in using thyroid hormone when hypopituitarism is suspected (p. 688).

The need for a change of dose is judged by the patient's symptoms, the resting pulse rate, and weight.

In special circumstances triiodothyronine may be used as an alternative to thyroxine (p. 691).

Other Types of Hypothyroidism

(1) *Juvenile myxoedema* is a rare condition which makes its appearance during childhood, and should be distinguished from (2) *Cretinism*, or infantile hypothyroidism. In the latter disorder there is a congenital defect of the thyroid which may fail to develop at all or may lack one of several enzymes required for the synthesis of the thyroid hormones. These genetic defects are inherited as Mendelian recessives: in the heterozygous state the child may be goitrous only, but in the homozygous state both goitrous and a cretin. The child's development, mental and somatic, is arrested or delayed. The facial features are typically coarse, with a broad flat nose, thick lips and a large tongue protruding from the mouth. The abdomen is prominent and an umbilical hernia is frequently present. The skin is dry. Mental deficiency or retardation is usual, and unless treatment is started in the early months of life imbecility will follow. If, however, treatment is begun early and maintained regularly, physical development may be indistinguishable from normal, although full mental development is rarely achieved.

Thyrocalcitonin. Recent investigations have made it clear that the parafollicular cells of the thyroid gland secrete a peptide hormone unrelated to thyroxine, and with an action mainly on calcium metabolism. Injections of the hormone are known to lower the concentration of both calcium and phosphorus in serum and to enhance the output of phosphorus in urine. It appears to act by inhibiting the reabsorption of bone, and in this sense might be regarded as a physiological antagonist of parathyroid hormone. The hormone has been shown to reduce hypercalcaemia; a few cases of hypocalcaemia have also been described with the suggestion that an excess of thyrocalcitonin might have been responsible for this finding. The clinical importance and the therapeutic value of this new hormone remain to be determined.

PARATHYROID GLANDS

These small glands each measure about 5 mm. in diameter. They may vary in number, four being the most common, and are usually situated on the posterior aspect of the thyroid gland, or in its fibrous capsule. Ectopic glands may be found in the superior mediastinum.

Function. The parathyroid glands control the concentration of calcium and inorganic phosphorus of the blood plasma, both by enhancing the removal of these substances from the skeleton, and particularly by promoting the excretion of phosphorus by the kidney.

Normal serum calcium is 9-11 mg./100 ml.

Normal serum inorganic phosphorus is 2·5-4·5 mg./100 ml.

Calcium occurs in serum in two forms: 'diffusible' and 'non-diffusible.' The diffusible calcium consists of ionised calcium, and a small amount of non-ionised calcium salts of organic acids. The non-diffusible fraction is that portion which is bound to the serum proteins. The amount of this fraction is closely related to the total serum protein concentration; if this is abnormally low, the total serum calcium might be 8 mg./100 ml. and yet the diffusible calcium could be normal. When the serum protein concentration is high, the serum calcium might be 12 mg./100 ml. or even more, but this would not necessarily constitute evidence of hyperparathyroidism. From the point of view of neuromuscular function and the occurrence of tetany, it is the 'ionised' serum calcium concentration which is important. When interpreting the serum calcium concentration it is essential to know the concentration of plasma proteins as well; an estimate of the plasma specific gravity (normally 1·027) is a suitable alternative to the chemical determination of the plasma protein concentration. Since thyrocalcitonin also affects the metabolism of calcium and phosphorus this factor must be considered in disorders of these elements.

HYPERPARATHYROIDISM

This term is used to describe the consequences of excessive secretion of parathyroid hormone, due to primary changes in the parathyroid glands, or secondary to renal disease. Primary hyperparathyroidism is uncommon and is usually due to a single parathyroid adenoma. Very occasionally it may be caused by simple hyperplasia or multiple adenomas: a functioning parathyroid carcinoma is also known to occur.

Secondary hyperparathyroidism with hypertrophy of the glands is found in advanced renal disease with acidosis and phosphate retention. The chemical pathology involved is complex because of the primary metabolic changes of renal origin, modified in turn by the increased parathyroid activity. It may also occur as a sequel to the osteomalacia associated with the malabsorption syndrome.

When hyperparathyroidism involves the bones, the condition is known as *osteitis fibrosa generalisata* or *von Recklinghausen's disease of bone.* Radiological evidence of involvement of the bones is seen only in a minority of cases, and since other systems may be affected, the term *hyperparathyroidism* is preferable.

Clinical Features. Some of the clinical findings in hyperparathyroidism are more readily understood if the action of the parathyroid hormone is recalled. In the first place the excretion of phosphorus in the urine is increased, and often that of calcium also; both phosphorus and calcium are mobilised from bone. The most significant chemical finding is an increase in the serum concentration of calcium, occasionally to as much as 20 mg./100 ml. The serum concentration of inorganic phosphorus may fall below 2·5 mg./100 ml., while the excretion of calcium in the urine may be increased. The plasma alkaline phosphatase, an index of osteoblastic activity, may be raised above the normal concentration of 3-12 (King-Armstrong) units/100 ml., depending on the degree of bone involvement.

In association with the enhanced excretion of calcium in the urine, renal calculi frequently form. While many patients with hyperparathyroidism develop symptoms due to renal calculi, relatively few presenting with renal calculi owe their disorder to increased parathyroid activity. In other cases of hyperparathyroidism deposits of calcium form in and around the renal tubular epithelium (nephrocalcinosis), so that in severe cases scattered radiological opacities may be visible within the renal outline.

Tubular reabsorption of water may be impaired as a consequence of medullary calcium deposition, secondary infection, or the direct effects of parathyroid hormone. Polyuria and thirst may be sufficiently severe to suggest diabetes insipidus. In cases of long standing, and in those with associated pyelonephritis, the renal disease may progress to uraemia in spite of the relief of the hyperparathyroidism.

Patients with hypercalcaemia frequently complain of weakness, loss of appetite, drowsiness, nausea and vomiting. Many of these patients also have a peptic ulcer, and the symptoms due to this may obscure those of hyperparathyroidism. In those with bone disease, backache is a common complaint. In some, only radiological evidence of demineralisation may be found or subperiosteal erosions may be noted in the phalanges. The 'pepperpot' appearance seen in lateral radiographs of the skull is virtually diagnostic of hyperparathyroidism. Occasionally characteristic cysts composed of fibrous tissue, osteoblasts and osteoclasts may be seen. Preoccupation with the search for bone cysts may mean that the other more widespread but less arresting changes are overlooked.

Physical examination is often unhelpful. The muscles may be hypotonic. Normochromic anaemia is common. Occasionally a parathyroid adenoma is sufficiently large and suitably placed to be palpable or even visible as a swelling in the region of the thyroid. Measurement of calcium excretion in the urine is a useful investigation in this disease. Provided the intake does not exceed 500 mg. daily, amounts of calcium in the urine persistently in excess of 200 mg. daily should be regarded as abnormal, and an indication for further study.

Much the most important single diagnostic feature of this condition is a raised serum calcium concentration, and it may be necessary to carry out a series of estimations at intervals in doubtful cases, since the hypercalcaemia may be episodic. It is important that a tourniquet should not be used in obtaining blood samples, since this may be responsible for raising the serum calcium concentration appreciably. Methods of assay for parathyroid hormone are being developed and should bring a new measure of precision to what is often a difficult diagnosis.

A parathyroid adenoma may occasionally co-exist with secreting adenomas in the pituitary gland and pancreas; hence unusual accompaniments of hyperparathyroidism may be accounted for in this way.

Treatment. Removal of a solitary adenoma is usually sufficient to produce clinical cure, provided advanced renal disease is not already present. Patients with multiple adenomas or generalised hyperplasia of all the parathyroids may be difficult to manage, especially when the glands lie in unusual situations such as the superior mediastinum, but surgical treatment offers the only prospect of amelioration.

HYPERCALCIURIA

Although balance studies may occasionally be necessary for the precise investigation of mineral metabolism, much help regarding the extent and activity of certain diseases, especially of bone, may be obtained by measuring calcium excretion in urine.

The following are some of the conditions which may be associated with hypercalciuria.

1. *Immobilisation.* This factor may be of particular importance in enhancing an existing hypercalciuria in a patient with, for example, hyperparathyroidism.
2. *Metastatic malignant disease* in bone, particularly from carcinoma of the breast.
3. *Paget's disease of bone* (p. 718), especially when the patient is confined to bed.
4. *Hyperparathyroidism* (p. 711). *Primary* and *Secondary*.
5. *Sarcoidosis* (p. 433).
6. *Overdosage with vitamin D* (p. 718).
7. *Myelomatosis* (p. 657).
8. *Renal disease with osteomalacia* (p. 497).
9. *Idiopathic hypercalciuria.* These patients usually present with renal calculi. The cause of the condition is unknown.
10. *Cushing's syndrome*, or treatment with moderate or large doses of corticosteroids.

HYPOPARATHYROIDISM

This condition is uncommon and usually follows a thyroidectomy in which the parathyroid glands have been inadvertently removed. Less often it may occur temporarily when the blood supply of the parathyroids is ligated during thyroidectomy. There may also be temporary hypoparathyroidism following removal of a parathyroid adenoma or carcinoma. It can occur as a congenital condition which may be associated with cretinism. An idiopathic variety is rarely encountered. Parathyroid insufficiency is usually associated with hypocalcaemia and a raised phosphorus concentration, but the possibility that thyrocalcitonin might be involved when these metabolic abnormalities are found must now be borne in mind.

Hypoparathyroidism is one cause of tetany.

TETANY

Definition. An increased excitability of nerves, due to a reduction in the concentration of ionised calcium in the plasma and usually accompanied by painful muscle spasm.

Aetiology. Fundamentally, there are two precipitating factors:

(A) A low plasma calcium concentration.
(B) Alkalosis.

Naturally, a combination of a lesser degree of each will suffice to produce tetany. Evidence is emerging that in the future magnesium depletion will also have to be considered as a contributing factor.

(A) Conditions associated with a Low Serum Calcium

1. *Inadequate Intake or Absorption of Calcium.* Rickets (p. 487), osteomalacia (p. 495), malabsorption syndrome (p. 939).
2. *Parathyroid Deficiency* (Hypoparathyroidism, p. 714).
3. *Chronic Renal Failure* (p. 820). In this condition however, although the serum calcium concentration is often low, coincident acidosis usually prevents the appearance of tetany.

(B) **Alkalosis.** In alkalosis the proportion of the serum calcium in the ionised form may be decreased, though the total serum calcium concentration remains unaltered. Such a change may lead to tetany. Among the causes of alkalosis, the following should be considered.

1. Repeated vomiting of acid gastric juice, as in pyloric stenosis. Persistent vomiting with carcinoma of the stomach is unlikely to produce alkalosis as the vomitus usually contains little acid.

2. Excessive quantities of alkalis given by mouth. When this is associated with repeated vomiting it may cause severe alkalosis.

3. Hyperventilation, which is most commonly due to hysteria or some emotional disturbance. Overbreathing lowers the alveolar carbon dioxide concentration, and consequently the plasma CO_2 tension.

4. Tetany may be associated with alkalosis in some cases of primary aldosteronism (p. 733).

Clinical Manifestations of Tetany

In *children* a characteristic triad of carpopedal spasm, laryngismus stridulus and convulsions may occur, though one or more of these may be found independently. The hands in carpal spasm adopt a characteristic position. The metacarpophalangeal joints are flexed and the interphalangeal joints of the fingers and thumb are extended (*main d'accoucheur*). Pedal spasm is much less frequent. Laryngismus stridulus is caused by spasm of the glottis.

In *adults* convulsions and laryngismus stridulus are rarely encountered. Carpopedal spasm is the usual finding; rarely bronchospasm simulating asthma may occur. The usual complaint is of painful cramps in the limbs and tingling in the hands and feet.

Latent tetany may be present when signs of *overt tetany* (e.g. spontaneous carpopedal spasm) are lacking. It is recognised by eliciting the following signs:

1. *Chvostek's Sign.* A tap over the facial nerve in the parotid gland stimulates the hyperexcitable nerve, and the facial muscles go into spasm. The lips twitch and the mouth is pulled to the stimulated side; a response may occasionally be elicited in normal persons.

2. *Trousseau's Sign.* Inflation of the sphygmomanometer cuff on the upper arm to more than the systolic blood pressure is followed by characteristic spasm in the forearm muscles within four minutes.

3. Increased muscular excitability can be demonstrated by electrical methods, but this is seldom necessary.

Treatment

(A) TREATMENT OF THE ATTACK. When the condition is believed to be due to a low serum calcium concentration, as in tetanic convulsions in a child with rickets, 20 ml. of a 10 per cent. solution of calcium gluconate may be injected slowly into a vein to obtain an immediate rise in the serum calcium. An intramuscular injection of 10 ml. may also be given to obtain a more prolonged effect.

In *alkalotic tetany* the serum calcium concentration is normal, but the ionised calcium is believed to be reduced by the rise in blood *p*H. In severe cases intravenous calcium gluconate often relieves the spasm, while more radical treatment of the alkalosis, which will vary with the cause, is being applied.

1. In persistent vomiting, intravenous saline is the most effective treatment.

2. When alkalis have been given to excess their withdrawal may suffice to stop the tetany, but if not, ammonium chloride 2 g. should be given four-hourly until relief has been obtained.

3. The hysterical patient who hyperventilates should be treated firmly by appropriate psychotherapy (p. 1273). The inhalation of 5 per cent. carbon dioxide in oxygen may be prescribed for the correction of the alkalosis, or more simply, the patient should be made to rebreathe her own expired air from a suitable bag. If the patient is then asked to overbreathe until tingling is again felt in the fingers (usually within five minutes), she is so impressed by the demonstration of the origin of her symptoms that this sequence of events does not recur.

(B) TREATMENT OF THE UNDERLYING CONDITION

1. Rickets (p. 487) and osteomalacia (p. 495).

2. The malabsorption syndrome (p. 939).

3. Chronic renal failure (p. 820). In this condition temporary benefit is usually the most that can be expected unless haemodialysis is being employed; symptoms should be treated as they arise with parenteral calcium.

4. When tetany follows removal of a parathyroid gland and if there is any residual parathyroid tissue, this usually undergoes compensatory hypertrophy. In the interval intravenous calcium gluconate may be required to control the tetany (p. 717). If all the parathyroid tissue has been removed, prolonged replacement

therapy with calciferol is commonly used to maintain a normal serum calcium concentration. One tablet (50,000 units or 1·25 mg.) daily is usually adequate, though 2-3 tablets daily may be required at first. The serum calcium concentration should be estimated at intervals, as persistent hypercalcaemia which might follow prolonged high doses of vitamin D would lead to widespread metastatic calcification and rapidly progressive renal failure (p. 491).

Dihydrotachysterol (AT1O), an analogue of vitamin D, is also a useful substitute in parathyroid insufficiency, but it is more expensive than calciferol and its formulation at present is unsatisfactory.

METABOLIC DISEASES OF BONE

There are a number of clinical conditions in which the bones are demineralised. This is often first recognised radiologically. The diseases concerned include the following:

1. Osteoporosis (p. 498).
2. Rickets and osteomalacia (p. 487).
3. Hyperparathyroidism with bone involvement (p. 712).
4. Metastatic malignant disease involving bone.
5. Myelomatosis (p. 657).

PAGET'S DISEASE OF BONE
(Osteitis deformans)

Although there is no reason for believing that this common condition is of endocrine origin, it is most conveniently considered here. The incidence of the condition increases with advancing years, and it is seldom seen before the age of 50 years. Both sexes may be affected. Histologically and radiologically there is evidence of increased osteoblastic and osteoclastic activity as indicated by areas of increased bone formation and density alternating with areas of rarefaction. The lesions may be found in the pelvis, skull, humerus, spine, femur, tibia or elsewhere. The distribution is characteristically irregular, so that normal bone may be found between affected areas.

Aetiology. This is unknown.

Clinical Features. Many patients have no symptoms and the disease is only recognised accidentally when radiological examination is made for some other reason. In others, pain in the bones may be severe, and the affected areas are often tender on pressure. They may be unusually warm on palpation, due to the increased vascularity of the lesions. When the skull is involved, headache may be troublesome and hearing impaired; vision is rarely affected. Deformity may follow involvement of other bones, but is unusual unless the condition is gross. Fractures may occur spontaneously or after minor trauma but usually heal normally. Osteogenic sarcoma is an uncommon late complication of the disease.

Occasionally the bone lesions are so widespread and so vascular that they form, in effect, an arteriovenous shunt. The cardiac output is therefore increased, and in some patients heart failure may ultimately appear.

Chemical Pathology. The serum calcium and phosphorus concentrations are normal, except during periods of immobilisation, when they may be considerably raised. The serum alkaline phosphatase concentration, which in these circumstances is a measure of new bone formation or osteoblastic activity, may be increased to as much as 100 (King-Armstrong) units/100 ml. or more (normal 3-12 units).

Treatment. Little can be done to alter the course of the disease. It is liable to be of long duration and is often accompanied by apparent remissions. Symptomatic treatment for pain in the bones or headache may be required, and if fractures occur they should be treated as if the bone were otherwise normal.

THE ADRENAL (SUPRARENAL) GLANDS

ANATOMY AND PHYSIOLOGY

The adrenal glands lie in relation to the upper poles of the kidneys. Each consists of an inner medulla, which secretes adrenaline and noradrenaline, and an outer cortex formed of three layers. These, from without inwards, are the *zona glomerulosa*, *fasciculata* and *reticularis*. More than 30 steroid hormones have already been isolated from the adrenal cortex, but it is probable that some of these are produced by the chemical processes used in their separation from other hormones. Two of the most important are cortisol (hydrocortisone) and aldosterone. Both have now been partially synthesised and are available for the treatment of disease, though in practice synthetic analogues are more commonly used.

The secretion of most adrenocortical hormones is controlled by the pituitary adrenocorticotrophic hormone (corticotrophin, ACTH). This in turn is dependent upon the corticotrophin releasing factor found in the hypothalamus and transmitted to the adenohypophysis through the portal system of blood vessels linking the median eminence with the anterior lobe of the pituitary gland. When ACTH is no longer being produced, as in hypopituitarism (p. 685), the secretion of adrenocortical hormones virtually ceases, with the exception of aldosterone. The mechanism controlling the production of this steroid appears to be largely independent of the pituitary and ACTH and recent evidence suggests that the dominant role is played by the renin-angiotensin system. Renin is secreted by the juxtaglomerular apparatus of the kidney, and amongst the various conditions known to stimulate the secretion of renin, sodium depletion is important.

In Addison's disease the adrenals atrophy or have been destroyed, usually by tuberculosis, so that cortical hormones, including aldosterone, cannot be formed, and no response could be expected from endogenous or administered ACTH. For this reason electrolyte abnormalities may occur in untreated Addison's disease, whereas they are most unusual in untreated hypopituitarism.

Increased secretion of adrenocortical hormones may be due to excessive production of corticotrophin by the anterior pituitary, as in Cushing's disease, or to hyperplasia or the formation of a neoplasm in the adrenals. The effects of excessive secretion may be simulated by the administration of corticotrophin or corticosteroids. Occasionally ovarian tumours secrete hormones which produce some of the effects characteristic of excessive adrenocortical activity. Thymic and pulmonary tumours may also be associated with Cushing's syndrome, possibly because they sometimes secrete material with corticotrophin-like activity.

The adrenocortical hormones may be classified into three groups according to their metabolic effects and other actions.

1. The 'glucocorticoids' or carbohydrate regulating corticosteroids. Cortisol (hydrocortisone) is responsible for these effects, which in general are antagonistic to the actions but not to the production of insulin. With large doses the blood glucose is raised, and if, as sometimes happens, the renal threshold for glucose is exceeded, glycosuria will occur. Glucose may be formed from amino acids derived from protein breakdown, and this gluconeogenesis is largely responsible for the raised blood glucose concentration. Liver glycogen stores are increased. The number of circulating blood eosinophils and lymphocytes is depressed. The 'inflammatory' response to injury and infection is suppressed, hence the glucocorticoids are sometimes referred to as 'anti-inflammatory' steroids. Alkalosis with sodium retention, and chloride and potassium depletion may occur. These changes are only evident when the adrenals are persistently overactive or excessive hormone has been administered for long periods.

2. The sodium retaining hormones ('mineralocorticoids'). This form of adrenocortical activity is normally due to aldosterone, but may be reproduced by the administration of synthetic analogues such as fludrocortisone or deoxycorticosterone acetate (DCA). Retention of sodium and increased excretion of potassium is the usual response. Water is also retained and the body weight increases. Hypertension, oedema and chloride and potassium depletion with alkalosis may follow excessive treatment with these steroids, though oedema is seldom encountered in the rare condition of primary aldosteronism (Conn's syndrome) (p. 733).

3. The 'sex hormones' formed in the adrenal cortex include androgens such as androsterone and dehydro*epi*androsterone (DHEA), the oestrogens, such as oestradiol, oestrone and oestriol, and progesterone. Depending on the predominance of one group or the other, so the effect may be virilising, e.g. hirsutism, deepening of the voice, enlargement of penis or clitoris, increased muscular development and the development of acne, or on the other hand, feminisation may be produced in the male. The nitrogen-retaining activity of the androgenic hormones is antagonistic to the 'glucocorticoid' hormones which increase protein breakdown and nitrogen excretion. Another example of antagonism between the cortical hormones is provided by the sodium retaining hormones which tend to increase the excretion of

potassium: androgens, on the other hand, by virtue of their protein anabolic effect may cause some potassium retention.

In pathological conditions such as rheumatoid arthritis cortisone may modify the activity of the disease, but there is no evidence that this disease and many others benefited by treatment with the 'glucocorticoids' and their analogues are due to a deficiency of the hormones. This 'anti-inflammatory' action bears no clear relation to the metabolic effects of these hormones, and indeed the latter may be so troublesome as to interfere with the treatment of disease (p. 723).

CORTICOSTEROIDS IN THE MANAGEMENT OF DISEASE

In the literal sense the term corticosteroid should be restricted to cortisol and the other thirty or more steroids secreted by the adrenal cortex. In practice, its meaning has been extended to include a wide variety of synthetic steroid analogues of cortisol with similar actions. These include prednisone and prednisolone, fludrocortisone, methylprednisolone, triamcinolone, dexamethasone and betamethasone. Corticotrophin (ACTH), a protein hormone secreted by the pituitary gland, increases the output of endogenous adrenocortical steroids other than aldosterone, and in this way provides an effective method of treatment with corticosteroids. For this reason it should be included in any discussion of this subject.

Cortisone and ACTH first became available for the treatment of disease in 1948. Probably no other group of drugs has received so much attention as that devoted to studies of the corticosteroids. In spite of this their fundamental mode of action remains unknown and their use is still based largely upon empirical considerations. Used with discrimination, they can be of great value in controlling many forms of disease.

Broadly speaking, these drugs are used for three main purposes. In the first instance, they are used in physiological (replacement) doses in the treatment of Addison's disease, hypopituitarism, and after bilateral adrenalectomy. Secondly, they are used occasionally to suppress and to replace adrenocortical activity, for example in congenital adrenal hyperplasia (p. 731), when the adrenal cortex is unable to synthesise cortisol, and the abnormal steroids being secreted are virilising in their action. The corticosteroids are used in pharmacological doses for the treatment of a wide variety of disorders, including the so-called collagen diseases and diseases of allergic origin. In some of these diseases the therapeutic effects of these steroids would appear to be related to their capacity to block the manifestations of an unduly vigorous and harmful antigen-antibody reaction or even the immunological reaction itself. Their lympholytic action is also of value in the management of lymphatic leukaemia and other lymphoproliferative diseases (p. 654).

The complications which may occur in patients under treatment (p. 724) may seem so formidable that the value of drugs with such potentially dangerous side-effects might be questioned. However when the indications for their use are sufficiently clear, the possible occurrence of complications need not act as a deterrent to their administration.

For the patient with adrenal insufficiency, replacement therapy with corticosteroids in physiological doses is indicated. The only serious danger is the failure of the doctor to prescribe, or the patient to take, adequate amounts of the drug to provide for his varying requirements. During any intercurrent illness, infection, injury or operation, patients with adrenal insufficiency, whether due to disease of the pituitary or adrenal glands or to treatment with corticosteroids (see below), should have their dose of corticosteroid increased three or four fold, and in some cases parenteral administration may sometimes be required as well (p. 729).

When these drugs are given to patients with intact adrenals, and particularly in pharmacological doses sometimes greatly exceeding the amount required for replacement therapy, several other considerations arise. Of these, the most important is the suppressive effect on the ability of the pituitary to secrete corticotrophin. If treatment has been in progress for periods of a few weeks or months, this inhibitory effect may persist for a long time after the corticosteroids have been withdrawn. Such patients may fail therefore to respond in the normal way to the stress of injury, infection or operation by an increased output of ACTH and corticosteroids. Thus patients who have recently been treated with steroids or indeed who are still being treated with small doses of steroids, may collapse and succumb rapidly without any satisfactory explanation emerging other than adrenal insufficiency.

Because of this danger sudden withdrawal of treatment with corticosteroids is strongly contraindicated. These patients should always be warned to inform any doctor they may consult that they are being or have been treated with corticosteroids, and it is also a valuable precaution for them to carry a card with appropriate details of their past and present treatment with corticosteroids, in the same way as diabetics are advised to do in regard to their treatment with insulin.

Many of the other dangers of corticosteroid therapy are a sequel to the use of large doses for prolonged periods which may ultimately produce the metabolic and clinical features of Cushing's syndrome (p. 731). Such a regime may also occasionally activate a peptic ulcer and even lead to perforation. Osteoporosis may develop and particularly in the elderly this may be sufficiently severe to cause collapse of vertebrae. These drugs may also modify the normal response to a major illness so that important diagnostic features such as pain, tenderness or fever may be abolished, while the response to inflammation may be poor and healing impaired. In this way treatment with these drugs may be responsible for masking the more typical and sometimes dangerous consequences of a variety of illnesses.

Mental symptoms occasionally may be troublesome: euphoria is usual in the patient on large doses and may be partly justified if the disability is responding to treatment. Depression however sometimes occurs and may be serious, especially when the dose of steroid is being reduced or the drug has been withdrawn. For all these reasons corticosteroids should always be withdrawn gradually when treatment is nearing completion.

ADRENAL INSUFFICIENCY
(ADDISON'S DISEASE)

Aetiology. This condition is due to deficiency of the adrenocortical hormones and occurs when the adrenals atrophy, are removed, or are destroyed by disease.

Since cortisone became available as substitution therapy, total bilateral adrenalectomy has been performed on many patients with Cushing's syndrome (p. 732). This operation is also employed sometimes in the management of patients with severe recurrences or metastases from mammary carcinoma, the ovaries also being removed; in some patients remarkable temporary regression of the disease occurs. For a number of reasons it is widely assumed that these operations succeed because they remove the remaining sources of sex hormones, and so control the progress of forms of cancer which are sometimes shown to be dependent on sex hormones for their growth. This induced form of adrenal insufficiency is treated in exactly the same way as Addison's disease, and if substitution therapy is omitted or is inadequate, the same dangers arise.

Adrenal insufficiency is also a most important feature of hypopituitarism, with the difference that in this condition aldosterone continues to be secreted, and electrolyte metabolism is not usually disorganised. In congenital adrenal hyperplasia the adrenal glands are incapable of synthesising cortisol, and adrenal insufficiency may be an important complication. Finally, in patients treated with corticosteroids for prolonged periods, the pituitary may become incapable of secreting corticotrophin, and acute adrenal insufficiency may follow injuries, operations or similar stresses which would normally elicit an adrenocortical response (p. 723). Acute adrenal insufficiency may also occur in severe meningococcal septicaemia associated with purpura (Waterhouse-Friderichsen syndrome).

The description which follows is primarily concerned with Addison's disease, but with obvious exceptions, the same remarks apply to patients with adrenal insufficiency for any of the other reasons mentioned.

Morbid Anatomy. The usual causes of Addison's disease are *tuberculosis* or *atrophy of the adrenals*; the latter is now regarded as a form of auto-immunisation analogous to Hashimoto's disease in the thyroid gland. Very much rarer causes are *metastatic carcinomatous deposits*, *syphilis* or *amyloidosis*. Haemorrhage occasionally occurs into both adrenals in severely ill patients (adrenal apoplexy). Both glands must be grossly affected before adrenal insufficiency becomes apparent.

Chemical Pathology (p. 727).

Clinical Features

1. *Onset*. This is usually insidious, occurring most frequently between the ages of 30 and 50 years.

2. *Asthenia.* The patient complains of weakness and tiredness. These symptoms fluctuate, but if untreated become progressively more severe. Loss of weight may be considerable, due to loss of sodium and extracellular water as well as a poor appetite. There may be a moderate degree of anaemia, which is modified, however, by haemoconcentration due to dehydration. The full extent of the anaemia is only apparent after adequate treatment has been instituted and the haemoconcentration corrected.

3. *Hypotension.* The systolic blood pressure is frequently found to be less than 100 mm. Hg. and symptoms such as unsteadiness on standing up may be caused by postural hypotension. Tachycardia is usually present.

4. *Pigmentation.* This is due to the accumulation of the brown pigment melanin, especially in exposed areas (hands and face), sites exposed to friction (belt areas) and sites normally pigmented (axillae and nipples). It may be well-marked in the creases of the hands, and is sometimes found in patches on the mucous membrane of the lips and cheeks.

5. *Gastrointestinal Symptoms.* Anorexia, nausea, vomiting, diarrhoea and constipation are common complaints.

6. *Crises.* A sudden exacerbation in symptoms may occur spontaneously or may be precipitated by even a mild infection, an attack of diarrhoea, by chilling, fasting or by drugs such as morphine, anaesthetics or potassium salts. In particular insulin administration is dangerous because the antagonistic action of the glucocorticoids is absent, and the fall of blood glucose concentration is more profound and more prolonged than would follow the injection of a larger dose of insulin in a normal individual. Induced or spontaneous hypoglycaemia may be responsible for the stupor or even coma in the adrenal insufficiency of Addison's disease or hypopituitarism. Pyrexia is common in a crisis (the temperature in Addison's disease is usually subnormal), and severe vomiting, dehydration and marked hypotension occur. Epigastric pain is a frequent early complaint, and may give warning of an impending crisis. Unless vigorous treatment is instituted, death may well ensue.

The enhanced susceptibility of these patients to stresses of all kinds must always be borne in mind, and they and their relatives should be trained to report even relatively trivial incidents which a normal person would safely ignore.

7. *Symptoms of the Primary Disease.* While tuberculosis used to be the most common cause of Addison's disease, in many countries the modern treatment of infections of this type has not only reduced the incidence of tuberculosis, but also that of Addison's disease. If the infection is obvious elsewhere, the disease in the adrenals may be overlooked; on the other hand, tuberculous adrenal disease may occur without evidence of infection in any of the more common situations. Radiological examination of the abdomen may show calcification of the adrenals when the disease is due to tuberculosis.

8. *Chemical Pathology.* In the absence of a crisis, no abnormality may be found. When changes do occur, the serum sodium is low (normally 135-150 m.Eq/*l.*) and the serum potassium is high (normally 3·6-5·3 m.Eq/*l.*). The blood urea concentration is usually raised under these circumstances. Such changes are only found in severe cases or during crises and should not be depended upon for diagnosis. There is often a tendency to spontaneous hypoglycaemia, especially following a carbohydrate meal. The abnormalities of steroid hormone secretion that occur are described below.

Diagnosis. In the past a variety of indirect tests such as dietary sodium restriction, potassium administration, the use of intravenous insulin, water loading tests, fasting and sweat electrolyte determinations, were used to demonstrate adrenal failure to secrete corticosteroids. Improvements in the reliability and simplification of assay techniques for these steroids in blood and urine have led to more precise methods of assessing adrenocortical function.

1. *Steroid excretion in urine.* The precursors of the 17-oxosteroids (ketosteroids) found in urine are normally produced by the adrenal cortex and the testis. In Addison's disease the excretion of these steroids is low in men and very low or absent in women (normal adult male excretion, 8-15 mg. per 24 hours; female, 5-12 mg.). However excretion is also low in hypothyroidism, and, as might be expected, in hypopituitarism. The measurement of 17-hydroxycorticosteroid (17-OHCS) excretion has now replaced 17-oxosteroid estimations as an index of adrenocortical function, since the 17-OHCS in urine are largely metabolites of cortisol and are derived entirely from adrenocortical

sources. A low basal excretion (<5 mg. per 24 hours) or failure to obtain an increase in output after adequate treatment with corticotrophin is strong presumptive evidence of adrenal insufficiency.

Metyrapone may be used to test the integrity of the control exercised through ACTH by the pituitary gland on the adrenal cortex. Under normal conditions administration of this drug blocks the formation of cortisol by the adrenal; a fall in the blood concentration of cortisol is followed by the release of pituitary ACTH, and this in turn by an increase in the production of adrenocortical steroids other than cortisol. This can be recognised by a rise in urinary 17-OHCS excretion. Failure to obtain this response is an indication of adrenal or pituitary disease, but if a good response is obtained to injected ACTH, then the defect can be attributed to pituitary or possibly hypothalamic failure.

2. *Fluorescence tests for 11-OHCS in blood and urine.* These are relatively simple and, although not specific for cortisol, have proved to be most valuable in the assessment of both adrenal hyperfunction and insufficiency.

3. *Kepler's water excretion test.* This test was designed to demonstrate the inability of patients with Addison's disease to excrete water rapidly. When a fasting normal subject is given one litre of water to drink, he would be expected to excrete at least 70 per cent. of this volume as urine within four hours. In adrenal insufficiency the proportion excreted is usually less than 50 per cent., but this returns to normal when cortisone is given.

If improvement does not follow with cortisone the delayed excretion of water may be due to hepatic, renal or malabsorptive disorders.

Differential Diagnosis. Other conditions associated with pigmentation may be mistaken for Addison's disease, for example cirrhosis of the liver, the malabsorption syndrome (p. 939), haemochromatosis, rheumatoid arthritis, latent uraemia, pregnancy, a negroid strain, pellagra and drugs such as arsenic or silver taken over a long period. In individuals with pediculosis there are often areas of pigmentation which have been caused by scratching itchy skin. The weakness which is so striking a feature of Addison's disease is often attributed to neuroses, especially when pigmentation is not marked and the blood electrolytes are normal. Certain of the features of adrenal insufficiency may be present in pulmonary tuberculosis, but radiological examination of the chest should eliminate this possibility. Occasionally pulmonary and adrenal tuberculosis may coexist, or amyloidosis secondary to tuberculous or other disease elsewhere may damage the adrenals.

Treatment. The remarks which follow apply equally to patients after total adrenalectomy as to those with Addison's disease. The prognosis of this condition has been vastly improved by the introduction of corticosteroids, both in duration and in the sense of well-being which these steroids confer.

In the replacement therapy of *chronic adrenal insufficiency*, two requirements must be met. In the first place cortisone, or a suitable substitute must be given. Doses of 25-50 mg. daily in divided doses are usually required. When more than 50 mg. daily is given for prolonged periods, signs of overdosage resembling Cushing's syndrome may be expected. Secondly, the loss of aldosterone secretion must be replaced. In certain patients the larger doses of cortisone sometimes used will meet a limited need for a sodium-retaining steroid, while in others, particularly when smaller doses of cortisone are being used, some more specific steroid of the sodium retaining variety will be required. Fludrocortisone (9α-fluorohydrocortisone) resembles aldosterone in promoting sodium retention and potassium excretion, and doses of 0·1-0·3 mg. daily by mouth are usually adequate, provided cortisone is also being given.

Acute adrenal insufficiency (*crisis*) may occur when replacement therapy has been inadequate or has been omitted altogether. A crisis may be precipitated by the stress of injury, an operation or anaesthetic, by infection, fever and prolonged fasting, and is a particular hazard in patients who have been treated with corticosteroids for long periods (p. 723). In addition, the patient may have been vomiting and in this way losing electrolytes as well as failing to retain any steroid taken by mouth. In such circumstances vigorous treatment with intravenous isotonic saline or glucose and saline will be urgently required. The factor responsible for the crisis, for example a pulmonary or urinary infection, should be treated appropriately. Hydrocortisone sodium succinate 100 mg. should be given as an initial intravenous injection, followed by the continuous infusion of the same steroid in doses providing approximately 100 mg. in each eight hours. Alternatively cortisone acetate may be given in similar doses by intramuscular injection, but is less satisfactory for the early treatment of such a crisis, as it may not be properly absorbed. DCA in oil should be given in single daily doses of 10 mg. intramuscularly for 1-2 days only, and the dose should then be reduced rapidly, or replaced by an oral substitute such as fludrocortisone. When the patient's blood pressure has returned to normal and the acid-base balance is regarded as satisfactory, cortisone may be given by mouth in doses which are reduced to maintenance levels as soon as the factors responsible for the crisis have been treated effectively. If pulmonary or systemic oedema is noted or even suspected, the treatment should be reviewed immediately, and a diuretic (p. 853) given if, for example, the venous pressure is found to be raised.

In the early stages of a severe crisis with profound hypotension an intravenous infusion of metaraminol (Aramine) may be required; it should be given in a concentration of 200 mg./l. of isotonic glucose and saline at such a rate as to maintain a systolic blood pressure of 100 mm. Hg., and a pulse pressure of 30 mm. Hg. at least.

Patients with Addison's disease, or others who have been treated by adrenalectomy must be suitably warned of the possibility of acute adrenal insufficiency. They should be advised to double or treble their dose of cortisone if this danger appears possible, and to seek medical advice immediately.

They should always carry a card indicating the type and dose of steroid upon which they depend.

HYPERFUNCTION OF THE ADRENAL CORTEX

The defect responsible for initiating this disorder may be in the pituitary gland, namely basophil hyperplasia or a basophil adenoma. Either is presumed to maintain excessive adrenocortical activity by increasing the secretion of corticotrophin, and this in turn is responsible for the bilateral adrenal hyperplasia found in about 70 per cent. of cases of Cushing's syndrome. In 20 per cent. a benign tumour (adenoma) and in 10 per cent. a carcinoma may be found in one of the adrenals. Other exceptional causes such as a thymoma, ovarian tumour or a bronchogenic carcinoma (p. 375) may be found. Some oat-celled bronchogenic tumours have been shown to secrete a hormone apparently identical in every way with ACTH.

Clinical Features. The clinical features of adrenal hyperfunction in the individual patient will depend on the duration of the disability, and the amount and type of steroid hormone or the group of hormones being produced.

In *children*, disorders are usually associated with *congenital adrenal hyperplasia*, due in turn to inability of the adrenals to synthesise normal steroids, particularly cortisol. Some of the abnormal steroids produced are virilising. The clinical result may include adrenal insufficiency, to which the child may succumb in infancy or early childhood. If the adrenocortical defect is incomplete and the child survives sufficiently long without treatment, precocious sexual development may occur in boys, and virilisation or pseudohermaphroditism (intersex) in girls. Growth may be abnormally advanced at first, but if the disorder is not successfully treated, retarded growth may become apparent later.

Primary aldosteronism (p. 733) follows when an aldosterone secreting tumour is present.

The *adrenogenital syndrome* is due to excessive secretion of androgens in females who develop signs of masculinisation. The clinical features may merge with those of Cushing's syndrome.

Feminisation of the male has been described in a few cases where adrenal oestrogen secretion was greatly increased.

Cushing's Syndrome. Most of the features of this condition, which is more common in females, can be reproduced by prolonged treatment with relatively large doses of corticosteroids, and it is clear that the changes noted in the condition as it occurs spontaneously are attributable to an excess of circulating cortisol. An early and striking sign consists of changes in the distribution of body fat which is increased about the face, neck and trunk, but tends to spare the limbs, so that they may appear wasted by contrast. The bloated appearance of the face and rounding of the features is sometimes referred to as 'mooning', and the changes elsewhere as 'buffalo obesity'. Purple striae (lineae distensae) may occur on the skin of the abdomen, buttocks and thighs, and a tendency to bruise unduly readily is often noted. Acne is common. Osteoporosis (p. 498) may be sufficiently severe to produce not only radiological changes in the vertebral bodies, but also complaints of backache, a kyphosis and even shortening of the vertebral column. Weakness is frequently noted, and may be due to both muscular wasting and the potassium depletion occurring as part of the metabolic alkalosis sometimes seen in these patients.

Hypertension of some degree is almost a constant finding. Impairment of carbohydrate tolerance, sometimes amounting to frank diabetes mellitus, may occur. Amenorrhoea usually develops when the disorder is active, and mental symptoms, in particular depression, may require attention. In the female, hirsutism of some degree may be accompanied by other signs of virilisation such as enlargement of the clitoris, recession of the hair line on the forehead and deepening of the voice, in addition to acne and amenorrhoea. Cases of this type may merge into the clinical group described as the *adrenogenital syndrome*, in which virilisation is the prominent feature.

The possibility that some of the clinical features might be due to metastases from an adrenal carcinoma should always be remembered.

Diagnosis. For this purpose a full clinical, biochemical and radiological investigation will be required. When the existence of abnormal steroid production has been demonstrated, the primary site of the disorder will have to be decided, for example the pituitary gland, ovary or adrenal cortex. The further diagnosis between hyperplasia, adenoma and carcinoma may not be possible until laparotomy has been undertaken. In recent years and with the improved prognosis in Cushing's syndrome, signs of a pituitary tumour have made their appearance for the first time sometimes several years after adrenalectomy. Basophil tumours of the pituitary often remain too small to be clinically apparent for long periods.

Treatment. In congenital adrenal hyperplasia treatment with cortisone or one of a number of analogues will suppress the abnormal activity of the adrenals. Ovarian and adrenal tumours when identified should, of course, be removed. Irradiation of the pituitary is still occasionally used when that gland is considered to be primarily responsible for the symptoms present.

The majority of cases of Cushing's syndrome are associated with bilateral adrenal hyperplasia, and at present the only satisfactory treatment is bilateral adrenalectomy and substitution therapy.

ALDOSTERONISM

Since aldosterone was identified in 1953 the importance of this steroid in mineral metabolism has become clearer (p. 721). In view of this it is now possible to identify patients with adrenocortical tumours secreting aldosterone. The most consistent symptom is weakness, often episodic, and attributable to potassium deficiency. Polyuria and polydipsia, also due to the effects of potassium depletion on renal tubular reabsorption of water, commonly occur. Some patients develop hypertension.

Primary aldosteronism is most likely to be confused with essential or even malignant hypertension (p. 234), with myasthenia gravis (p. 1234), or with primary renal disease associated with excessive potassium losses (p. 845). Tetany (p. 716) is also an occasional presenting symptom precipitated by the metabolic alkalosis associated with potassium depletion in this condition. Oedema occurs rarely.

Secondary aldosteronism occurs in cirrhosis of the liver with ascites, in the nephrotic syndrome (p. 805), and less consistently in congestive cardiac failure. It may also occur in patients with unilateral renal ischaemia due to renal artery stenosis, a form which can be cured by surgical correction of the arterial defect.

Treatment. The primary form should be treated by removal of the adrenocortical tumour. In the secondary form, treatment is naturally aimed at the condition responsible for the stimulus to aldosterone secretion, and the aldosterone antagonist spironolactone may be worth a trial.

TUMOUR OF THE ADRENAL MEDULLA

This rare tumour, the *phaeochromocytoma*, secretes adrenaline and noradrenaline. As a consequence hypertension is produced which is usually paroxysmal at first, but may later become persistent. Phaeochromocytoma is responsible for less than 1 in 200 of all cases of hypertension encountered clinically. Episodes of headache, vomiting, sweating, weakness and dizziness are common complaints. Transient glycosuria may occur. Estimation of the catechol amines in the urine (adrenaline and noradrenaline) or their metabolite 3-methoxy-4-hydroxymandelic acid (HMMA) is most helpful in establishing the diagnosis. *Treatment* consists of removing the tumour.

DISORDERS OF THE MENOPAUSE

The term menopause should be used to describe the cessation of the menstrual cycle, and should not be employed as a synonym for the climacteric, which includes many of the clinical features associated with the 'change of life.' The menopause, which occurs in most women between the ages of forty-five and fifty, may occur abruptly or gradually, and is the direct result of the failure of the ovaries to produce oestrogens and progesterone. As a consequence of this failure the pituitary becomes more active and produces gonadotrophic hormones in greater quantity. Biological tests for these substances, which are excreted in the urine, may occasionally be of value in distinguishing primary (ovarian) amenorrhoea from secondary amenorrhoea due to failure of the pituitary to secrete gonadotrophins. A male climacteric is sometimes described. If it produces symptoms at all, they are certainly much less clearly defined than those occurring in the female, and occur at a considerably later age.

Clinical Features. The ease with which a woman adapts herself to the change of circumstances associated with the menopause varies widely. In some women the loss of reproductive capacity leads to a loss of self respect and may be regarded with resentment; in others adjustment is readily achieved and may be unattended by any emotional reaction. In the group of patients who are troubled by symptoms, nervousness, emotional instability, irritability, insomnia, tremor and particularly hot flushes and cold sweats are common complaints. Occasionally involutional melancholia may occur with profound mental disturbance, depression and suicidal tendencies. The thyroid may be palpably enlarged and frequently it is difficult to be certain whether the symptoms present are due to a mild degree of hyperthyroidism or to the climacteric. *Obesity* may first appear, or, if previously present, may increase at this time. *Hirsutism*, especially the appearance of dark hair on the upper lip and chin, is not uncommon and may be sufficiently pronounced to require treatment for cosmetic reasons. *Arthritis*, of a type related to osteoarthritis, may be responsible for considerable disability, particularly in the obese (p. 444). *Osteoporosis*, described as post-menopausal in the female, and senile when it occurs in the male, affects the spine predominantly (p. 498).

Pruritus vulvae is a common complication which is frequently associated with atrophic changes in the mucous membranes of the genital tract. *Leukoplakia vulvae* may develop and if untreated may progress to carcinoma. *Senile vaginitis*, which not infrequently occurs, may cause considerable distress from irritation, dysuria and vaginal discharge, especially if complicated by secondary infection.

Treatment. Irrespective of the symptoms present, the essential basis of treatment is replacement of oestrogens. The synthetic oestrogens are active when given by mouth and of these the most powerful is ethinyl oestradiol. The daily dose required to suppress menopausal symptoms in different individuals varies from 0·01 to 0·1 mg. of ethinyl oestradiol, or 0·1 to 1·0 mg. of stilboestrol, and one or other should be given in courses lasting for 14 days, repeated if necessary. Local applications of drugs of this type often result in the relief of symptoms when these are due to atrophic changes in the vulva and vagina.

Other appropriate measures, such as dietary control of obesity and local treatment of arthritis, may also be required. Excessive growth of hair on the lip and chin may be removed by shaving or depilatory wax or cream, or may be made less conspicuous by bleaching with hydrogen peroxide. Involutional melancholia is a common form of depression complicating the menopause which responds well to psychiatric treatment (p. 1275).

HYPOGONADISM IN THE MALE

There are a number of conditions commonly encountered in practice which are related to diminished testicular function. The defect may only involve impaired spermatogenesis in the seminiferous tubules of the testis, or the Leydig (interstitial) cells of the testis may also be affected so that the secretion of testosterone by these cells is reduced in amount. If the interstitial cells are defective, then tubular dysfunction is inevitable.

Aetiology. Hypogonadism may be part of the syndrome of hypopituitarism, which has already been described (p. 685). In addition there are many cases in which the adenohypophysis is intact but the testes have been destroyed or damaged. Trauma, tuberculosis, gonococcal infections, syphilis, malignant disease, orchitis, as in mumps, and surgical castration are recognised causes of primary testicular failure. Maldescent or failure of descent will also lead to failure of the tubular epithelium to develop. Haemochromatosis, cirrhosis of the liver and oestrogen administration may all be associated with testicular insufficiency. A special group has recently been recognised in whom the disorder is due to abnormalities of the sex chromosomes (p. 117). Many cases remain however for which an aetiological diagnosis is still not possible, and these form the majority of patients who present with infertility as their only complaint.

Clinical Features. The results of testicular failure depend upon the age of the patient at the time of the onset of the disease. When this occurs *before puberty* the external genitalia and the secondary sex characteristics fail to develop. In these circumstances the epiphyses of the long bones do not close at the usual age and in consequence the patient may grow to an excessive height. The typical pre-pubertal eunuch develops into a tall man with a hairless face, a high-pitched voice, small genitalia and an immature emotional make-up. Some of these patients become obese and others develop gynaecomastia (enlargement of the breasts), usually in the variety known as Klinefelter's syndrome (p. 117).

When the onset of the disease is *post-pubertal* the changes are less striking. Growth is not affected and there is regression rather than disappearance of the secondary sex characteristics. The external genitalia undergo partial atrophy. Tiredness, loss of initiative and of sexual desire (libido) are common complaints. In some patients, particularly when the deprivation is sudden as in surgical castration, there may be 'menopausal symptoms' such as hot flushes and profuse sweating.

Treatment. Whatever the cause or the time of onset of hypogonadism, replacement therapy with testosterone is worthy of trial and in some cases it has dramatic and most beneficial results. The most satisfactory and economical form of therapy is the implantation of 600-1,000 mg. of testosterone in the form of 3-5 fused pellets into the subcutaneous tissue of the anterior abdominal wall. Such an implant is gradually absorbed over a period of six to eight months, after which it may be renewed.

Alternatively fluoxymesterone, a synthetic analogue of testosterone, can be given by mouth in doses of 10-20 mg. daily.

Impotence. Impotence, that is inability of the male to have sexual intercourse, is due to psychological causes in 80 per cent. of cases, and in these circumstances is not due to hypogonadism. Rarely it may be an important early symptom in organic diseases such as diabetes mellitus, disseminated sclerosis and tabes dorsalis. In hypogonadism due to anterior pituitary deficiency, a complaint of impotence is most unusual; such patients have little or no interest in sexual function, and are most unlikely to make this complaint spontaneously.

Infertility in the Male. Sterility in the husband is believed to be responsible for the infertility in approximately one-third of all childless marriages. The cause is usually defective development of the germinal epithelium in the seminiferous tubules, with oligospermia or azoospermia, but may follow hypogonadism due to any of the causes described earlier.

Cryptorchidism. Cryptorchidism (undescended testis) may occur for several reasons. In some cases the condition is due to an anomaly of the pathway of descent which occasionally may be surgically remediable; usually the descent of the testis is merely delayed and takes place normally before or at puberty. Only rarely can an endocrine cause be found to account for the disability. Carcinoma is more common in undescended than normal testes. If the glands remain in the inguinal canal they are more liable to trauma than if situated in the scrotum. The seminiferous tubules will fail to develop in undescended glands, and if the condition is bilateral sterility will follow. It is therefore important that an attempt should be made to correct failure of descent if it has not already occurred by the time that signs of puberty are appearing or might have been anticipated. Even in testes which remain undescended into adult life the interstitial cells function normally, so that the secondary sex characters develop in the usual way.

DISORDERS OF SEXUAL DETERMINATION

Recent investigations have shown the importance of chromosomal aberrations in the aetiology of disorders of sexual development and function. These matters are discussed on p. 105-122.

J. A. Strong.

Books recommended:

Williams, R. H. (1968). *Textbook of Endocrinology*, 4th ed. London: Saunders.

Loraine, J. A. & Bell, E. T. (1966). *Hormone Assays and their Clinical Application*, 2nd ed. Edinburgh: Livingstone.

* * * * * *

DIABETES MELLITUS

More than 45 years have now elapsed since the discovery of insulin, but the facts regarding the nature and cause of diabetes mellitus and its treatment have continued to increase in complexity. The incidence of the disease too is certainly much greater than earlier surveys would suggest. This increase may be due in part to a real growth in frequency, but is probably also the result of more critical methods of assessment. In some countries improvements in economic status and in opportunities for overfeeding may have aggravated the problem. Recent surveys in Great Britain suggest that more than 1 per cent. of the population, or rather more than half a million persons, are diabetics, though about half of these remain undetected.

The complications associated with the disease are common and are often most disabling, and every system in the body may be involved. Since the disease occurs in all age groups, and since there is no cure, every branch of the medical profession and many outside it are constantly involved in dealing with the problems of the life-long control and care of the diabetic patient.

Definition. Diabetes mellitus is a clinical syndrome characterised by hyperglycaemia, due to deficiency or diminished effectiveness of insulin. The disease is chronic and affects the metabolism of carbohydrate, proteins, fats, water and electrolytes, sometimes with grave consequences.

Aetiology

The precise aetiology of most cases of diabetes is uncertain. although several contributing factors are known to be involved,

PRIMARY (IDIOPATHIC) DIABETES.

(1) *Heredity*. A familial tendency to diabetes undoubtedly exists but neither the specific biochemical defect nor its mode of inheritance has yet been identified. Genetic factors are probably more important in those who develop diabetes before the age of 40, but in both young and old environmental and other factors also operate and may determine which of those with a genetic predisposition actually develop the clinical syndrome and when this occurs.

(2) *Age*. The disease may appear at any age, but 80 per cent. of cases occur after the age of 50, and the highest incidence of new cases is in the 60 to 70 age group. Diabetes is therefore principally a disease of the middle-aged and elderly.

(3) *Sex*. There are rather more young male diabetics than female; in middle age women are more often affected. Pregnancy and increasing parity may add to the likelihood of developing diabetes.

(4) *Obesity*. The association of obesity and diabetes has long been recognised, but it is still uncertain whether obesity is the result or the cause of diabetes. The majority of middle-aged diabetic patients are obese, but only a minority of obese people develop diabetes.

(5) *Infections*. These may unmask latent diabetes, especially staphylococcal infections.

(6) *Stress*. Either physical injury or emotional disturbance is sometimes suggested as the initial cause of the disease, just as in

many other diseases that arise mysteriously and unexpectedly. However, since corticosteroid administration or ACTH therapy may be associated with the development of clinical signs of the disease, and since surgical operations and severe infections appear to precipitate the disease, stress, in so far as it elicits an adrenocortical response, must be regarded as a factor of importance. A severe stress, such as a car crash, does not cause diabetes in people who would otherwise never have had it, but it may change a latent form of the disease into clinical diabetes.

Secondary Diabetes. A minority of cases of diabetes occur as a result of a recognisable pathological process.

1. In pancreatic diabetes the pathological disorder causes destruction of the pancreas and leads to impaired secretion and release of insulin. For example, pancreatitis, haemochromatosis and carcinoma of the pancreas can all cause diabetes; diabetes will also follow pancreatectomy.

2. In another group of cases, diabetes occurs because there are abnormal concentrations of hormones in the circulation which are insulin antagonists.

(*a*) Administration of *growth hormone* can produce permanent diabetes in experimental animals and about 30 per cent. of patients with acromegaly are diabetic.

(*b*) *Adrenocortical hormones*, such as cortisol, raise the concentration of glucose in the blood by increasing protein breakdown and by inhibiting utilisation of glucose by the peripheral tissues. Thus, many patients with Cushing's syndrome show impaired carbohydrate tolerance; conversely increased sensitivity to insulin is an important feature of Addison's disease and of hypopituitarism, and this can be corrected by the administration of corticosteroids.

(*c*) *Adrenaline* has a mild and transient effect on the blood glucose concentration, achieved by increasing the breakdown of liver glycogen. Patients with phaeochromocytoma frequently show a diabetic blood glucose curve on glucose tolerance testing and the incidence of these uncommon tumours is relatively high among diabetic patients.

(*d*) *Thyroid hormone* in excess will aggravate the diabetic state and some patients with hyperthyroidism show impaired glucose tolerance.

(*e*) *Gestational diabetes* refers to the hyperglycaemia which can occur temporarily during pregnancy in individuals who have an inherited liability to develop the disorder. During normal pregnancy there is an increased production of hormonal antagonists to insulin, which in turn demands an increased rate of secretion and release of insulin. A failing pancreas may be unable to meet this demand.

3. Various forms of therapy may precipitate *iatrogenic diabetes* in those genetically susceptible. For example, *steroid diabetes* can occur as a result of the therapeutic administration of corticosteroids; certain diuretics, particularly the thiazide group, can also have a diabetogenic effect.

4. Liver disease, particularly cirrhosis and hepatitis, may be associated with impaired glucose tolerance.

Chemical Pathology. The hyperglycaemia characteristic of diabetes arises from two main sources, namely a reduced rate of removal of glucose from the blood by the peripheral tissues, and an increased rate of release of glucose from the liver into the circulation.

The mode of action of insulin is still not fully understood but its physiological actions are well defined. Insulin lowers the blood glucose by facilitating the entry of glucose into the cells and by augmenting the formation of glycogen in the muscles and liver and the formation of fat in the adipose tissues. Insulin also promotes protein synthesis.

Although diabetes is a syndrome which combines several different pathological processes in a common clinical picture, it can be asserted that in every case the insulin secreted by the pancreas is either insufficient in amount or ineffective in action for one or more reasons. In either event increased gluconeogenesis will occur.

In most cases of primary diabetes, morbid histological changes can be demonstrated in the islets of Langerhans at autopsy and the majority of younger patients have little or no endogenous insulin detectable in their plasma. However, appreciable amounts of endogenous insulin can be measured in the plasma of many patients, particularly the obese, and in such cases diabetes can be presumed to be due to increased antagonism to insulin. For this purpose an insulin antagonist may be defined as any substance capable of interfering with the action of insulin. Such interference might occur in the synthesis of insulin in the pancreas or in its release into the portal circulation; an antagonist might increase the rate of degradation of insulin, modify or combine with circulating insulin so as to inhibit its biological activity, or depress the response of the target organ to the action of insulin. Several substances including hormones can act as insulin antagonists, but their role in the production of diabetes has yet to be established.

In summary the characteristic hyperglycaemia of diabetes mellitus may be caused by one or more of the following factors:

Failure to produce insulin.
The presence of insulin antagonists.
Excessive gluconeogenesis.

Consequences of Hyperglycaemia.

Glycosuria. This occurs when the glucose concentration in the blood exceeds the capacity of the renal tubules to reabsorb it from the glomerular filtrate. This 'renal threshold' is usually about 180 mg./100 ml., but may vary considerably.

Polyuria. Glucose increases the osmolality of the glomerular filtrate and prevents the reabsorption of water as the filtrate passes down the renal tubular system. In this way the volume of urine is increased in diabetes, and serious water and salt depletion may contribute considerably to the total metabolic disorder.

Fat Metabolism. Because the diabetic patient is unable to use the glucose in the circulation, fat is mobilised and at least in part is metabolised. Acetoacetic acid is one stage in the breakdown of fats. Under normal circumstances the body has no difficulty in oxidising this acid; but when the mobilisation of fat is proceeding to a disproportionate extent, acetoacetic acid and its derivatives, β-hydroxybutyric acid and acetone, begin to accumulate and appear in excessive amounts in the blood, producing *ketosis* (p. 764). The acidosis that develops is associated with dehydration and can lead to coma and death unless treated with vigour.

The increase in fat catabolism and consequent ketosis that may occur in diabetes is probably stimulated by several factors, including hormones. In some circumstances growth hormone produces ketosis.

With increased mobilisation of fat, the liver may become

enlarged and infiltrated with fat. Occasionally the serum may be milky (lipaemic) through excess of suspended neutral fat.

Protein Metabolism. A steady loss of glucose in the urine may be partly compensated by increased gluconeogenesis from the proteins of the tissues. The result is an increase in urinary nitrogen and wasting of muscles, an important clinical feature of severe diabetes.

Morbid Anatomy. Histological examination of the pancreas at autopsy shows striking abnormalities in the islets of Langerhans in many cases. In the younger age groups, that is those under the age of 40, there is usually a slight or moderate reduction in the total amount of islet tissue with a marked reduction in the number of beta cells. The remaining beta cells show evidence of overactivity; the nuclei are commonly enlarged and there is degranulation of the cytoplasm.

In the middle-aged and elderly the total mass of beta cells is usually reduced by 40-50 per cent. There is no sign of beta cell hyperactivity and the islet stroma shows marked fibrosis and hyalinisation.

In long-standing diabetes the only pathognomonic finding outwith the pancreas is a widely distributing thickening of the basement membrane in the capillary blood vessels. The main clinical and pathological impact of this microangiopathy is to be found in the retinal vessels and in the renal glomeruli (p. 769). The other pathological changes in diabetes mellitus can be related mainly to other degenerative lesions in the vascular tree, but these are not specific to the disease.

Clinical Types of Diabetes Mellitus

There are two main types.

1. The *juvenile-onset type* usually develops during the first 40 years of life in patients of normal or less than normal weight Insulin administration is required for their survival; hence the alternative name *insulin-dependent*. They develop *keto-acidosis* readily when insulin is withdrawn, and they do not respond to the oral hypoglycaemic drugs.

2. The *adult or maturity-onset type* usually appears in middle-aged or elderly patients who are often obese and in whom hyperglycaemia can be controlled by dietary means alone or, if not, by an oral hypoglycaemic compound. For this reason it is sometimes

described as the *insulin-independent type.* Patients in this category are less prone to develop ketosis and the disease is less severe than in the juvenile-onset type.

RELATED STATES. The following conditions have long been recognised; they have been precisely defined recently.

Potential diabetics are persons specially prone to develop the disease for one or more of four reasons.

(1) Having an identical twin who is diabetic.
(2) Both parents are diabetic.
(3) One parent is diabetic and the other has a definite family history of diabetes.
(4) A woman who has given birth to an abnormally large baby (weighing more than 4·5 kg.).

All these individual would be regarded as potential diabetics.

Latent diabetics are persons in whom the glucose tolerance test is normal, but who are known to have given an abnormal result during pregnancy, during infection or some other severe stress, or when overweight. Patients who have an abnormal glucose tolerance test only after treatment with cortisone would also be classified in this way.

Clinical Features. Diabetes may be discovered in one of several ways. Many patients are first noted to have glycosuria in the course of some routine examination, for example for insurance, for employment purposes or pre-operatively. Frequently they have had no symptoms, and no abnormal physical signs may be found. Secondly, the patient may present with symptoms due to one of the complications of diabetes, for example, failing vision, peripheral vascular disease, neuropathy or infection of the skin, lungs or urinary tract. Finally, some patients are first seen complaining of symptoms more directly attributable to the diabetic state. These include weakness, excessive thirst and polyuria, a dry mouth or nocturia. Loss of weight is common and may be disproportionate to any reduction in appetite or in the amount of food eaten. Pruritus vulvae is a frequent and distressing complaint in the middle-aged or elderly obese diabetic. The external genitalia are specially prone to infection by fungi (monilia), which flourish on the skin and mucous membranes contaminated by glucose.

Sometimes diabetes may first present as a fulminating illness associated with an acute infection or even without any evident precipitating cause, and epigastric pain and vomiting may be the only complaints. This is more likely to occur in the juvenile-onset type associated with keto-acidosis (p. 764). Cases of this type are emergencies of the first order; they could nearly all be saved if the medical service available is equal to the urgency of the situation.

The physical signs elicited will depend very much on the mode of presentation. There may be no abnormality other than glycosuria. Evidence of the complications of diabetes may be noted. Vulvitis may be found or, less commonly, balanitis in the male. Ophthalmoscopy may show retinal capillary microaneurysms or some other features of diabetic retinopathy (p. 771 and Plate I).

In the fulminating case the most striking features are those of dehydration, with a loose dry skin which lifts in folds, and a dry furred tongue with cracked lips causing difficulty in articulation. The intra-ocular pressure may be obviously reduced. A rapid pulse and a low blood pressure may then be anticipated. Breathing is deep and sighing in the acidotic patient and should attract the doctor's notice. The breath is usually foetid and the sickly sweet odour of acetone may be noticeable, but this of course is not specific for diabetes. Mental apathy may pass into stupor or even coma.

Diagnosis. Diabetes may be suspected because it presents with some of the clinical features or complications of the disease and the diagnosis is then virtually confirmed if glucose and perhaps ketone bodies are detected in the urine.

Many cases of mild diabetes are encountered in whom glycosuria is slight or episodic and clinical features are absent; in such cases a more critical assessment of the diagnosis, using blood glucose estimations and the glucose tolerance test will be required.

Glycosuria. Benedict's test is the traditional method for detecting reducing substances in urine. It has now been replaced by modern alternatives. (*a*) Clinistix (Ames & Co.), consists of a paper stick impregnated with an enzyme preparation which turns purple when dipped in urine containing glucose. No other urinary constituent gives this reaction: it therefore provides a rapid and specific qualitative test for glucose. (*b*) Clinitest tablets (Ames & Co.), provide an easy, semi-quantitative method of testing urine for reducing substances, including glucose.

When Benedict's reagent or Clinitest tablets only are used to detect reducing substances in the urine, it may be necessary to establish the identity of the urinary reducing agent. Glucose can easily be identified with Clinistix paper. Other reducing substances, however, occasionally occur in urine, including lactose which may be found in the later stages of pregnancy or during lactation. Pentosuria, fructosuria and galactosuria may all occur as manifestations of rare genetic disorders and special methods are required for the identification of these reducing substances when they occur in urine.

Detection of Ketone Bodies in Urine. Ketone bodies are always present in the blood and are excreted in the urine in small amounts even by healthy persons. They can be detected by the nitroprusside reaction which is conveniently carried out using Acetest tablets or Ketostix test papers (Ames & Co.). Ketonuria may be found in normal people who have been fasting for long periods, who have been vomiting repeatedly or who have been eating a diet very high in fats and low in carbohydrate. Ketonuria is therefore not pathognonomic of diabetes, but if both ketonuria and glycosuria are found, the diagnosis of diabetes is practically certain.

It is common practice to examine overnight specimens of urine for glucose. By using such a procedure the milder cases of diabetes will be overlooked and these are particularly the types that require identification. If a sample collected during the two hours following a meal is examined, then more of the milder cases will be recognised, but a higher proportion of patients with 'lag storage' or a low renal threshold will be included. In order to distinguish cases of this type from patients with mild diabetes, suitable tests of carbohydrate tolerance will be required.

The Oral Glucose Tolerance Test (Fig. 49). The patient, who should have been on an unrestricted carbohydrate intake of at least 250 g. for three days or more, fasts overnight. Outpatients should rest for at least half an hour before starting the test. A sample of blood is taken to measure the fasting blood glucose level and 50 g. glucose dissolved in about 200 ml. of water is then given by mouth. Thereafter samples of blood are collected at half-hourly intervals for two hours, and their glucose content is estimated.

The WHO Committee on Diabetes (1965) recommended that

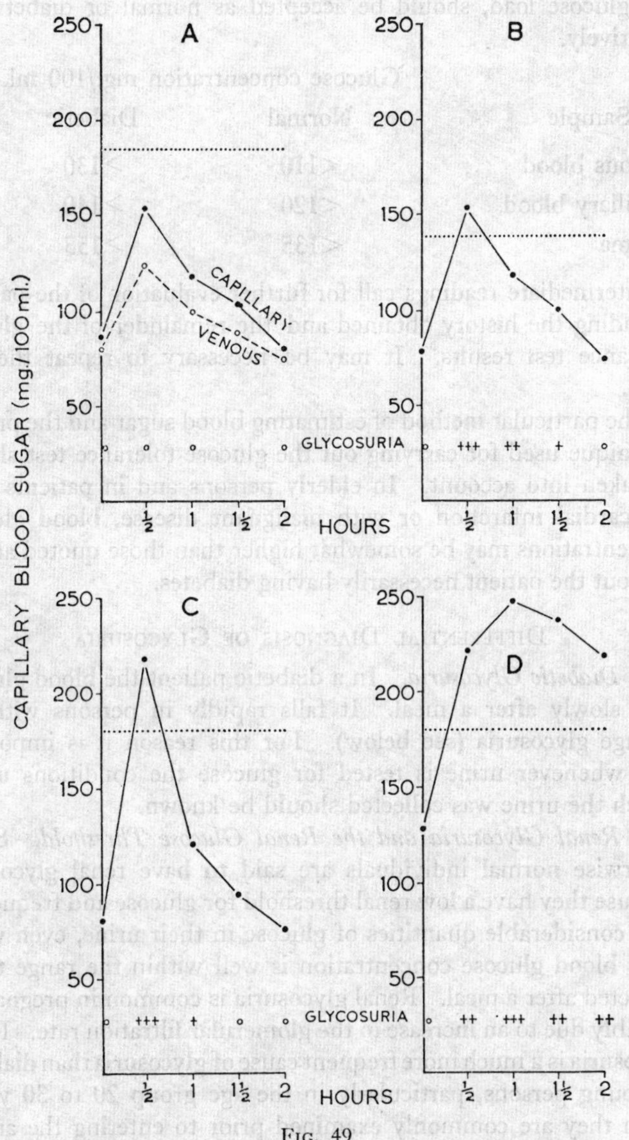

FIG. 49

The Glucose Tolerence Test: blood glucose curves after 50 g. glucose by mouth, showing (*A*) normal curve, (*B*) renal glycosuria, (*C*) alimentary (lag storage) glycosuria and (*D*) diabetes mellitus of moderate severity.

the following levels of glucose, either fasting or two hours after the glucose load, should be accepted as normal or diabetic respectively.

	Glucose concentration mg./100 ml.	
Sample	Normal	Diabetic
Venous blood	<110	>130
Capillary blood	<120	>140
Plasma	<135	>155

Intermediate readings call for further evaluation of the patient, including the history obtained and the remainder of the glucose tolerance test results. It may be necessary to repeat the test later.

The particular method of estimating blood sugar and the precise technique used for carrying out the glucose tolerance test should be taken into account. In elderly persons and in patients after myocardial infarction or with malignant disease, blood glucose concentrations may be somewhat higher than those quoted above, without the patient necessarily having diabetes.

Differential Diagnosis of Glycosuria

1. *Diabetic Glycosuria.* In a diabetic patient the blood glucose falls slowly after a meal. It falls rapidly in persons with lag storage glycosuria (see below). For this reason it is important that whenever urine is tested for glucose the conditions under which the urine was collected should be known.

2. *Renal Glycosuria and the Renal Glucose Threshold.* Some otherwise normal individuals are said to have renal glycosuria because they have a low renal threshold for glucose and frequently pass considerable quantities of glucose in their urine, even when their blood glucose concentration is well within the range to be expected after a meal. Renal glycosuria is common in pregnancy, possibly due to an increase in the glomerular filtration rate. Renal glycosuria is a much more frequent cause of glycosuria than diabetes in young persons, particularly in the age group 20 to 30 years, when they are commonly examined prior to entering the armed services, professions and industry. In the older age groups the reverse holds, and hyperglycaemia in excess of 200 mg. per 100 ml. can occur without any glycosuria. For this reason if urine tests for

glucose are used as a method of screening for diabetes, some cases will be missed, so that a glucose tolerance test or at least a single blood glucose estimation two hours after an oral dose of 50 g. of glucose should be used whenever possible.

It may be important to determine the renal threshold for glucose, and this can only be done reliably by testing samples of urine for glucose taken at intervals of half an hour in the course of a glucose tolerance test and relating the results to the blood glucose concentrations. This information may be specially important in the occasional diabetic with a low renal glucose threshold who, if attempts are made to control his diabetes on urine tests alone, is likely to be kept in a persistent state of hypoglycaemia.

Some forms of renal tubular disease may be associated with glycosuria.

3. *Alimentary* (*Lag Storage*) *Glycosuria*. In some individuals an unusually rapid but transitory rise of blood glucose follows a meal and the concentration exceeds the normal renal threshold; during this time glucose will be present in the urine. This response to a meal or to a dose of glucose is known as 'lag storage' and is not uncommon as a cause of symptomless glycosuria. It may occur in otherwise normal people or after a partial gastrectomy, when it is due to rapid absorption, or in patients with hyperthyroidism or hepatic disease. This form of diminished carbohydrate tolerance is usually regarded as benign and unrelated to diabetes; it occurs about as frequently as renal glycosuria.

4. *Other Metabolic Disorders*. As already described (p. 740), several hormones may act as insulin antagonists and impair carbohydrate tolerance, sometimes sufficiently to cause glycosuria. This may be transient or permanent. For example, adrenaline produced by emotional stress will mobilise liver glycogen and cause transient hyperglycaemia and glycosuria. Transient hyperglycaemia may occur with phaeochromocytomas which secrete adrenaline. In acromegaly and Cushing's syndrome glycosuria is common. Impaired carbohydrate tolerance can be demonstrated in hyperthyroidism; the condition of diabetic patients will deteriorate if they develop hyperthyroidism, and will improve when the hyperthyroid state has been corrected.

5. *Raised Intracranial Pressure*. A cerebral tumour, haemorrhage or injury, may be associated with glycosuria.

6. *Liver Disease*. Disease of the liver, particularly advanced

cirrhosis or severe acute necrosis, may also be associated with impaired carbohydrate tolerance.

7. *Starvation.* This, or a diet containing little carbohydrate will reduce carbohydrate tolerance. This may be demonstrated by tolerance tests, but does not usually lead to glycosuria.

THE MANAGEMENT OF DIABETES MELLITUS

Aims of Treatment

1. The abolition of symptoms of diabetes while avoiding hypoglycaemia.
2. The correction of hyperglycaemia and glycosuria.
3. The attainment and maintenance of an appropriate body weight.
4. The prevention of complications.

The patient should realise as early as possible that it is upon him that success or failure will depend. The doctor can only advise. As adherence to a dietary regimen demands from the patient self-discipline and a sense of purpose, every effort should be made to ensure that he understands the object of each aspect of his management. Accordingly, time must be spent on the education of the patient and in clinics this can be undertaken on a group basis. As soon as the diagnosis is certain the patient should be told that he has diabetes; at the same time he should be reassured, especially if a near relative has died of the disease.

There are three methods of treatment and each involves an obligation for the patient to adhere to a dietary regimen for the remainder of his life.

1. Diet alone.
2. Diet and oral hypoglycaemic drugs.
3. Diet and insulin.

When a diabetic is seen for the first time it must be decided whether or not the diabetes is severe enough to require immediate treatment with insulin; this will usually depend upon the presence of ketosis as well as other factors discussed below.

If insulin is to be given, the diet will have to be weighed at first. By adjusting the amount and type of food and the time of meals with the dose and type of insulin (or other hypoglycaemic agent) used, it is usually possible to prevent an excessive rise in the blood glucose after each meal, and at the same time prevent hypoglycaemia.

Approximately 40 per cent. of new cases of diabetes can be controlled adequately by diet alone, about 30 per cent. require insulin and another 30 per cent. will need an oral hypoglycaemic drug. A patient may pass from one group to another temporarily or permanently.

Diet

General Principles. The treatment of all diabetic patients, especially those who require insulin, involves some dietary restrictions if control is to be satisfactory. Hence it is essential to understand the general principles underlying the recommendations in a diabetic diet. If the monotony of a fixed diet is to be avoided some kind of exchange system is necessary, and this is the basis for the construction of nearly all diets in use today. Many doctors are intimidated by the number and variety of diet sheets published and feel that, since they are not trained dietitians, they cannot treat diabetes. A dietitian is certainly most helpful but is not indispensable; the basic principles of an exchange system of dietary treatment are simple, although the education of a patient in their use is time-consuming.

The first step in preparing any dietary regimen is to map out a timetable of the patient's day including a description of his usual meals. This is an essential step and one which is too often omitted. The total daily requirement of calories must next be decided. The diet must be nutritionally adequate for the patient's needs, and it must, therefore, be estimated for each individual patient after considering such factors as age, sex, actual weight in relation to desirable weight (Table 17) activity, occupation and financial resources. An approximate range for the various groups might be (1) an obese, middle-aged or elderly, patient with mild diabetes, 1,000 to 1,600 Cal. daily, (2) an elderly diabetic but not overweight, 1,600 to 2,000 Cal. daily, (3) a young, active diabetic, 2,000 to 3,000 Cal. daily. The importance of maintaining the body weight at or slightly below the ideal for the patient's height (Table 17) cannot be over-emphasised. Thus the calorie range of group 2 may have to be extended if it is not sufficient to maintain weight, and young patients in group 3 who are overweight may have to reduce their daily intake to below 2,000 Cal., perhaps temporarily only.

Next the proportion of calories derived from carbohydrate, protein and fat must be allocated. The approximate ratio in British diets is, protein 12 per cent., fat 38 per cent. and carbohydrate 50 per cent. The percentage of calories derived from carbohydrate should usually be reduced, and those from protein increased if this is practicable. In most diabetic diets therefore, the percentage of calories derived from carbohydrate should be approximately 40 per cent., from protein about 15 per cent. and the remaining 45 per cent. from fat.

The daily intake of carbohydrate to be prescribed ranges from the minimum sufficient to prevent ketonuria, that is, 100 g. daily, to a maximum of 240 to 260 g. The upper limit is imposed by the fact that it is difficult to achieve satisfactory blood glucose levels throughout 24 hours with a daily carbohydrate intake greater than this. If the daily intake of carbohydrate is 240 g., approximately 50 g. of carbohydrate will usually be provided by each of the three main meals, 20 g. by each of three snacks and 30 g. by one pint of milk (540 ml.) taken in the course of the day. Experience has shown that it is very difficult to prevent an excessive rise in the blood glucose concentration after each meal with amounts larger than this. A simple method of calculating the carbohydrate content of the diet is to allocate a figure equivalent to one-tenth of the total calories to carbohydrate, that is, if a diet of 2,000 Cal. is prescribed it should contain about 200 g. of carbohydrate, providing 800 Cal. or 40 per cent. of the total.

The consumption of *protein* is largely determined by social and economic considerations and it is not usually possible to make much change in an individual's habits. It will usually lie in the range of 60 to 110 g. daily.

The *fat* intake should be adjusted to bring the total calories to the level desired, and will usually amount to 50 to 150 g. daily.

When the patient's requirements have been assessed the figures must be translated into practical and comprehensible instructions for the patient, using one of the types of diet prescription sheets described below.

Each patient should be given a cyclostyled or printed copy of the list of exchanges (p. 1300) with instructions regarding the meals at which they may be taken. The diet sheet and exchanges must be discussed with the patient repeatedly and with a relative if necessary until the system is fully understood. No pains should be spared in teaching him how to manage his disability and a high standard of discipline should be demanded.

Weighed Diets. These are required for two groups of patients: (1) those who are not overweight and who require insulin or an oral hypoglycaemic agent, and (2) those who are overweight and require a reducing regimen.

Each patient should be provided with a simple balance for weighing his food and he should be asked to weigh all food at first. After a few weeks most patients are capable of assessing with sufficient accuracy the weight of portions by eye and regular weighing becomes less necessary. However, it is necessary to check visual assessments by weighing from time to time.

A method of constructing a sample diet of 2,000 Cal. (Diet 12) suitable for patients in group 1 is described on page 1302. The exchanges for carbohydrate, protein and fat, on which it is based, are set out on pages 1300 and 1301. It is important to realise that the exchanges or portions employed as units are arbitrary and are decided mainly in the light of the food habits of the population as a whole. It should be noted also that a carbohydrate exchange contains some protein and fat in addition to carbohydrate, while a protein exchange contains some fat. In this system the carbohydrate exchange contains 10 g. carbohydrate, as recommended in 1965 by the British Diabetic and Dietetic Associations.

Diabetics who are obese should be urged to accept a reducing regimen. The method of achieving reduction in weight is the same for obese diabetic patients as for those with simple obesity. Diet No. 3 (p. 1287) will meet the needs of many. Foods with a high carbohydrate content listed in the footnote must be avoided. If the patient is sufficiently intelligent, advice can also be given on how to avoid monotony by using the list of exchanges for diabetic diets provided on p. 1300.

Many diabetic patients need advice regarding the consumption of alcohol. There is no medical objection to taking alcoholic drinks in moderation provided the patient realises that he must take account of their calorie value and sometimes of their carbohydrate content. Beer for example may contain 10 to 30 g. of carbohydrate per half litre (one pint approximately) and with the alcohol this will provide 150 to 400 Cal., depending on the strength of the beer. Sweet wines and cider all have a high carbohydrate content, and spirits such as whisky and gin, while free of carbohydrate, contain about 70 Cal. per 30 ml.

Advice may also be asked about sweetening agents and so-called diabetic foods and drinks. Saccharin has been employed as a sweetening agent for many years. It has no calorie value. Sorbitol, a glucose derivative, and fructose are also added to 'diabetic' foods and drinks for sweetening purposes. In moderate quantities neither will interfere with the action or requirements of insulin. Sodium cyclamate is also an acceptable substitute for sugar. If a patient is having difficulty in reducing weight or in maintaining a normal weight, then the use of substitutes for sugar should be discouraged, since they may perpetuate the patient's desire to eat sweet foods and thus make it more difficult for him to tolerate dietary restrictions. Diabetic chocolate has a high fat content and this must be taken into account.

Unweighed Diets. If insulin or oral hypoglycaemic agents are not required it may not be necessary for the patient to follow such an accurate diet. Sometimes it may be impracticable to do so because of the patient's mental, visual or other physical incapacity or unwillingness to co-operate. Many patients develop the disease when they are already middle-aged or elderly and have a mild type of diabetes often associated with moderate obesity. For such patients an unweighed anti-obesity diet may be adequate, and they should be given a list of foods and instructions as described on p. 1303.

INSULIN

Unfortunately no method of giving insulin has yet been found that will control the blood glucose accurately throughout the 24 hours without some risk of hypoglycaemia. However, with one or more of the preparations of insulin available it is usually possible to keep the blood glucose within reasonable limits throughout the day and night without undue risk of hypoglycaemia.

Two main forms of insulin are available, namely soluble and depot, and there are several varieties of depot preparations. These vary in the rate of onset and duration of their effect, as shown in

Table 12. Depot insulins are made in concentrations of 40 and 80 units per ml. and soluble insulin is also available in a concentration of 20 units per ml.

Soluble Insulin. This is a clear solution in contrast to the depot insulins (PZI and IZS) which are cloudy. When injected subcutaneously, soluble insulin is rapidly effective (Table 12) but the action is relatively shortlived. A patient stabilised on soluble insulin alone would therefore need at least two injections in the day.

TABLE 12

Preparation of Insulin	Hypoglycaemic effect	*Approximate* duration of effect in hours		
		Start	Maximum	Termination
Soluble	Rapid onset and short duration	½	4–6	6–10
Globin	Intermediate	2–3	6–10	10–14
IZS amorphous				
Isophane (NPH)				12–22
PZI	Slow onset and long duration	4–6	8–14	20–30
IZS crystalline				

Most diabetic patients requiring insulin are treated with a depot preparation and many have soluble insulin as well. Soluble insulin is essential in the following circumstances:

(*a*) For new cases with severe glycosuria or ketosis.

(*b*) For emergencies associated with ketosis, such as acute infection, gastroenteritis and some surgical operations.

(*c*) For the treatment of nearly all young patients.

(*d*) For patients whose food intake or glucose tolerance fluctuates widely (and sometimes unaccountably) from day to day, particularly in diabetic children and adolescents.

Depot Insulins. These have the advantage that with their aid some patients can be controlled by a single daily injection. The most useful is protamine zinc insulin.

Protamine Zinc Insulin (*PZI*). The addition of zinc and protamine to soluble insulin delays its release from the site of injection, so that PZI exerts its maximum effort on the blood glucose later and the duration of action is longer than soluble insulin (Table 12). Despite its prolonged action PZI does not always keep the blood glucose within acceptable limits throughout the 24 hours. Glycosuria is most likely to occur before the morning injection has taken full effect, and a dose of soluble insulin is generally required in the morning and sometimes in the evening, especially in young patients. Merely to increase the morning dose of PZI may result in severe hypoglycaemia later in the day or at night. Indeed it is a good rule that the dose of PZI should not exceed 40 units at a single injection. When giving soluble insulin and PZI together, the two should not be mixed in the syringe, but may be given through the same skin puncture. If the two are mixed the excess of protamine in the PZI will convert some of the soluble insulin into PZI.

Insulin Zinc Suspensions. The rate of release of these insulins from the tissues is related to the size of the insulin particles which are suspended in acetate buffer. Three preparations are available:

(*a*) IZS amorphous (*semilente*) insulin has a duration of action which is intermediate between that of soluble and protamine zinc insulin.

(*b*) IZS crystalline (*ultralente*) insulin is slower in action than IZS (amorphous) insulin (Table 12).

(*c*) IZS (*lente*) insulin is a mixture of three parts of amorphous with seven parts of crystalline material. This usually achieves uniform reduction of the blood glucose over 24 hours. It is dispensed when IZS is prescribed unless the prescription specifically orders semilente (amorphous) or ultralente (crystalline).

Globin Insulin. This is another depot insulin, intermediate in duration of action between soluble and protamine zinc insulin.

Isophane (*NPH*) *Insulin.* This is similar in action to globin insulin, though its effect is slightly more prolonged.

In summary, while some patients requiring insulin can be controlled with a single daily injection of a depot insulin, most severe diabetics do best on PZI with one or two supporting doses of soluble insulin.

Oral Hypoglycaemic Drugs

A number of compounds are effective in reducing hyperglycaemia in patients who would otherwise require insulin. The sulphonylurea compounds, tolbutamide and chlorpropamide, and to a lesser extent the biguanides, metformin and phenformin, have a place in the management of about 30 per cent. of diabetic patients. The action of both groups appears to depend upon a supply of endogenous insulin. The sulphonylureas stimulate the secretion or release of insulin from the pancreas, and reduce the release of glucose from the liver. The action of the biguanides is less well established, but they may potentiate the action of insulin by increasing the uptake of glucose by tissues other than the liver. It is futile and dangerous to attempt to control juvenile-onset diabetics with these compounds. Their use should be restricted to adult-onset cases who are not overweight and whose glycosuria has failed to respond to a proper trial of dietary measures alone.

Chlorpropamide is excreted very slowly, and an effective concentration can be maintained in the blood by a single dose at breakfast. The usual dose is between 100 and 375 mg. daily; larger doses should not be used. Tolbutamide is metabolised and excreted more rapidly, so that it is given in two or three divided doses of 0·5 to 1 g. each.

The biguanides are less widely used in Britain than the sulphonylureas, because of the higher incidence of side-effects, though these are usually mild. On the other hand it is easier to avoid an increase of weight with the biguanides than with the sulphonylureas. The biguanides are therefore to be preferred when it is essential to treat a patient with adult-onset diabetes who is overweight. Metformin is less likely to cause gastro-intestinal side-effects that phenformin, and is given with food in two or three daily doses of 0.5 to 1.0 g. each. As the biguanides are believed to be synergistic with the sulphonylureas, there is a place for combining the two when the sulphonylureas alone have proved inadequate (primary failure), and when, as happens with 5 to 10 per cent. of patients, initial success is followed after several months or even one to two years by loss of control (secondary failure).

Patients of normal weight may be started on an oral hypoglycaemic drug as soon as it is clear that dietary measures alone are inadequate. It is usually possible to reach a decision on the success or failure of these drugs within a week, though occasionally a full response may not be apparent for considerably longer. Diabetics treated successfully in this way for prolonged periods may ultimately need an alteration of dose or a change of regime temporarily or permanently; in particular they may require insulin to meet the needs created by a severe infection, an operation or other stress.

Toxic effects are few and include a variety of skin eruptions. Diarrhoea, nausea, anorexia, vomiting and jaundice may also occur occasionally. Hypoglycaemia in an over-responsive patient, particularly the elderly, can be dangerous with chlorpropamide, and is an immediate indication for withdrawing the drug and adjusting the dose later. The side-effects of alcohol may be exaggerated in a patient using drugs of this type.

For the aged and infirm and particularly the blind, these new drugs are a great boon.

Choice of Therapeutic Regimen

It cannot be over-emphasised that the regimen eventually adopted in each case of diabetes is chosen by a process of trial, and that changes may be needed as more is learnt about the patient and the kind of diabetes which he has.

The chief indications for the main types of therapeutic regimen are:

1. Practically all young patients who develop diabetes before the age of 40 require treatment with insulin, and the majority will be best controlled by taking PZI and soluble insulin in the morning, often combined with an additional dose of soluble insulin before the evening meal.

2. Many patients over the age of 40 (adult-onset diabetics) can and should be controlled by diet alone. This applies particularly to obese patients, but others may do well on dietary therapy alone.

3. Those over the age of 40 who fail to achieve satisfactory control by dietary measures alone will usually respond well to a sulphonylurea if they are not obese, or to a biguanide if they are obese. If adequate control is not achieved by one drug, a combination of sulphonylurea and biguanide may be tried. If this fails insulin will be required.

4. Elderly patients who require insulin will often do well with a relatively small dose (20 units) of a depot insulin alone, such as PZI. A few, particularly those who would otherwise require more than 40 units of PZI a day to be adequately controlled, should be given soluble insulin in addition.

It is important that obese patients should be treated by dietary restriction and weight reduction rather than by the administration of insulin or other hypoglycaemic agent. The advent of the 'insulin era' has obscured the remarkable improvement in glucose tolerance which usually results from reduction in weight. Insulin and the sulphonylureas increase the appetite, and thus may increase weight and intensify the total disability.

Initiation of Treatment and Assessment of Control

It is usually unnecessary to admit diabetic patients to hospital for the establishment of a therapeutic regimen. The patient can learn to manage his disorder as an outpatient while leading a relatively normal existence at home and at work. However, patients being stabilised on insulin have to be seen daily at first and if this is not otherwise possible, admission to hospital will be necessary. This will also be essential for patients with keto-acidosis.

As soon as the diagnosis is made a careful search is necessary to detect early evidence of the complications to which the diabetic is prone (p. 764). These include coronary artery disease and hypertension, obliterative arterial disease, peripheral neuropathy, cataract, retinopathy, nephropathy, pulmonary tuberculosis and other infections, particularly of the skin.

The patient must be taught how to test his urine with a Clinitest set and Acetest tablets and to keep a record of the results in a notebook and to understand their significance. He must learn to measure his dose of insulin accurately with an insulin syringe (B.S. 1619), to give his own injections and to adjust his dose on the basis of urine tests and other factors such as illness, unusual exercise and insulin reactions. He must be told that any drugs may have undesirable effects on the diabetic state. He should be advised to come to the doctor or the clinic at once, without prior appointment, as soon as he is aware of any deterioration in his health or urine tests. Such instruction is time consuming and repeated practical demonstrations may also be required. However, it is only in this way that diabetic patients can safely undertake all normal activities while maintaining good control of their disease. If the patient is a child, or is blind, mentally defective or otherwise incapable of operating a syringe, instructions in these matters must be given to a parent, guardian or some other attendant.

Diabetics should be seen at regular intervals for the remainder of their lives. The object of these visits is to check the degree of control and to watch for any complications. Records should be kept so that the doctor is immediately on the alert if changes in health occur. The frequency of visits is determined by the severity of the disability and the reliability of the patient. For example:

1. An intelligent minister living in the country, who has mild diabetes not requiring insulin, can be relied upon to keep himself in health for at least six months and to come for help sooner if there is anything wrong.

2. A schoolboy living in an overcrowded slum home, requiring large doses of insulin and with a history of several previous admissions to hospital in coma, may need to be seen every day or every week until he and his parents are educated thoroughly in the control of diabetes.

For the general practitioner with diabetic patients scattered widely in his practice, this supervision may be difficult. For this reason and because of the need to develop and apply new and better techniques for the control of diabetes, many hospitals arrange Diabetic Clinics.

Urine Testing. Proper assessment of control is impossible unless in the course of his normal activity the patient tests samples of urine regularly. By selecting suitable times for the tests and tabulating the results, it is easy for the doctor or the experienced patient, to decide whether the dose of insulin or hypoglycaemic drug should be increased or reduced, or whether the carbohydrate content of the diet or the time when it is taken should be altered.

Diabetics taking insulin should test samples of urine obtained before breakfast, before the mid-day and evening meals, and at bedtime (prior to a bedtime snack if this is taken). The patient must empty his bladder and discard this urine about 30 minutes before passing a specimen for testing. Otherwise the pre-meal specimen will include urine secreted into the bladder after the previous meal and will give the impression that the blood glucose concentration before meals is higher than it really is.

Patients treated by diet alone or with oral hypoglycaemic agents should test the first morning specimen and samples passed about two to four hours after the main meals of the day; the majority of such specimens should be either free of or contain ¼ per cent. of glucose or less.

While the patient is being stabilised, tests will have to be carried out three or four times daily; when control is established the frequency can be greatly reduced. Three or four tests on a single day once or twice weekly are much more informative about the state of control than a single test carried out daily. A full series of tests should be undertaken therefore on one or more selected days each week.

Blood Glucose Estimations. At the patient's regular visits to the diabetic clinic, it is advisable to measure the blood sugar level as an additional index of the degree of control. In assessing the result it is important to consider the interval between taking the sample and the last meal and also previous physical activity. A series of estimations made over several months, or even years, provides a useful record of the patient's ability to control his disease. This is particularly important during pregnancy when the renal threshold may fall temporarily.

Insulin Reactions and Hypoglycaemia

If soluble insulin is administered to a normal person the blood glucose falls, producing symptoms that may begin to appear when the concentration is about 50 mg./100 ml. and are fully developed at about 40 mg. In diabetics who are constantly hyperglycaemic, the same symptoms may develop at much higher levels, *e.g.* 120 mg. or more.

In order of frequency the symptoms include a feeling of being weak and empty, hunger, sweating, palpitation, tremor, faintness, dizziness, headache, diplopia and mental confusion. Abnormal behaviour, leading occasionally to arrest by the police on a charge of being drunk and disorderly may also occur. Alternatively, and particularly in children, there may be lassitude and somnolence, muscular twitchings, deepening coma and convulsions.

Hypoglycaemia induces secretion of adrenaline, and this in turn causes sweating, tachycardia and tremor. Adrenaline, by mobilising liver glycogen, combats the hypoglycaemia. This homoeostatic reaction on the part of the body partly explains why patients rarely die of hypoglycaemic coma from too much soluble insulin. By contrast, coma is dangerous when it arises from a large dose of depot insulin or from an overdose of a sulphonylurea, particularly chlorpropamide. The latter condition although relatively uncommon is peculiarly resistant to treatment, since the drug reduces the hepatic release of glucose, and because the half-life of the drug is so long. Repeated profound hypoglycaemia may lead to permanent mental changes. The brain is dependent on the blood glucose for the energy necessary for its activity. For this reason, hypoglycaemia should be prevented from recurring by prompt reduction of the dose of insulin or of sulphonylurea.

Hypoglycaemia due to overdosage with soluble insulin comes on rapidly, at the time when the insulin is having its maximum effect (Table 12, p. 755), and usually passes off soon. Reactions from excessive IZS (lente) given before breakfast usually occur in the late afternoon and those from PZI at night or early next morning. These reactions begin gradually with little adrenaline response and become persistent and profound unless vigorously treated. The predominant symptoms are very variable and include headache, malaise, night sweats, nausea leading sometimes to troublesome vomiting, mental confusion and drowsiness, especially in the morning. Coma may follow.

Differential Diagnosis of Coma in a Diabetic. Confusion between coma due to hypoglycaemia and that associated with ketosis should seldom arise; the distinction is clear.

It should be noted that diabetic coma may occasionally pass undetected into hypoglycaemic coma through too enthusiastic treatment; likewise, vomiting induced by hypoglycaemia from a depot insulin may continue until diabetic coma develops.

	Hypoglycaemic Coma	*Coma with Ketosis*
History:	no food	too little or no insulin
	too much insulin	an infection
	unaccustomed exercise	digestive disturbance

Onset:	in good health immediately before	ill-health for several days before
	related to time of last injection of insulin	
Symptoms:	of hypoglycaemia (occasional vomiting from depot insulins)	of glycosuria and dehydration; abdominal pain and vomiting
Signs:	moist skin and tongue	dry skin and tongue
	full pulse	weak pulse
	normal or raised blood pressure	low blood pressure
		reduced intra-ocular tension
	shallow or normal breathing	laboured breathing ('air hunger')
	brisk reflexes	diminished reflexes
	plantar response usually extensor	plantar responses usually flexor
Urine:	no ketonuria	ketonuria
	no glycosuria, provided that the bladder has been recently emptied	glycosuria
Blood:	hypoglycaemia	hyperglycaemia
	normal plasma bicarbonate	reduced plasma bicarbonate

Treatment of Hypoglycaemic Reactions. Since hypoglycaemia can easily be corrected if recognised early, it is useful for diabetic patients to experience the condition under supervision. In this way they learn to recognise the early symptoms. They must be made to realise that the most frequent causes of the condition are unpunctual meals and unaccustomed exercise, and seek to avoid both or to make adjustments to meet these circumstances. They should always carry some tablets of glucose or a few lumps of sugar for use in an emergency. Unless an attack of hypoglycaemia is adequately accounted for, the patient should reduce the next and subsequent doses of insulin by 20 per cent., and seek medical advice.

If the patient is so stuporous that he cannot swallow, he should be given an intravenous injection of 25 g. of glucose (50 ml. of a 50 per cent solution). This may have to be repeated. If this is not available, a subcutaneous injection of 0·5 ml. of 1 in 1,000 solution of adrenaline may be tried, but it is relatively ineffective. Alternatively, the insulin-dependent patient may be given a subcutaneous or intramuscular injection of 1 mg. of glucagon, repeated if necessary after 10 minutes. This has the advantage of convenience and can be given by anybody capable of learning to use a syringe, but it is unlikely to be effective in severe and prolonged hypoglycaemia due to depot insulins. Glucagon stimulates the secretion of insulin and it should not be used to treat hypoglycaemia induced by an oral hypoglycaemic agent, since this may simply aggravate the disability by provoking further insulin secretion.

As soon as the patient is able to swallow, he should be given 30 g. of sugar by mouth. Full recovery may not occur immediately, especially if the patient has been in coma for some time. Further, when hypoglycaemia has occurred in a diabetic using a depot preparation of insulin or a sulphonylurea, particularly chlorpropamide, the possibility of relapse within a day or more should be anticipated.

Repeated episodes of hypoglycaemia may lead to permanent intellectual deterioration; accordingly, adjustments to prevent recurrences are essential.

THE COMPLICATIONS OF DIABETES MELLITUS

Diabetic Keto-acidosis

Prior to the discovery of insulin more than 50 per cent. of diabetic patients ultimately died of keto-acidosis. Today this complication is preventable and accounts for less than 2 per cent. of diabetic deaths. However, the mortality rate is still regrettably high. A clear understanding of the biochemical disorders involved is essential for its efficient treatment which should aim at having the patient out of danger within 24 hours.

Water and Mineral Depletion. The osmotic diuresis arising from an increase in the osmolar concentration of the urine due to glycosuria depletes the body of water, sodium and potassium. As the concentration of glucose in the blood rises the extracellular fluid becomes hypertonic and water leaves the cells. In the early stages, before the volume of the extracellular fluid is grossly reduced, the patient will have relatively few clinical features, but as the loss of water and electrolytes continues evidence of salt and water depletion becomes apparent (p. 841). In the later stages of keto-acidosis, vomiting contributes to the fluid and electrolyte loss.

The deficit of total body water in a severe case may be about 6 litres. About half of this is derived from the intracellular compartment and occurs relatively early in the development of acidosis; the remainder represents loss of extracellular fluid sustained largely in the later stages. It is at this time that marked contraction of the size of the extracellular space occurs, with haemoconcentration, a decrease in plasma volume, and finally a fall in blood pressure with associated renal ischaemia and oliguria.

The concentration of sodium and potassium in the serum gives very little indication of body losses, and they may even be raised due to disproportionate losses of water. Sodium loss, mainly from the extracellular space, may amount to as much as 500 mEq.

Glycogen and protein are present in the cells in association with water and intracellular electrolytes. As the glycogen and protein are catabolised, glucose, nitrogen, water and electrolytes, particularly potassium, are released into the extracellular space. An increased excretion of potassium, magnesium and phosphate occurs early in keto-acidosis. Potassium loss from the cell may be 400 mEq. or more. The concentration of potassium in the plasma in these circumstances is dependent on the balance between catabolism of protein and glycogen and haemoconcentration on the one hand, and urinary excretion on the other. Since the former generally exceeds the latter a high level of plasma potassium is likely to be present initially, in spite of a total body deficit. However, within a few hours of beginning treatment with insulin, there is likely to be a precipitous fall in the plasma concentration of potassium. At least three mechanisms are responsible for this: dilution of extracellular potassium by the administration of potassium-free fluids, the movement of potassium into the cells as the result of insulin therapy, and the continued renal loss of potassium.

Keto-acidosis. Ketone bodies raise the osmolality of the plasma and so also lead to withdrawal of water from the cells. They are strong acids which dissociate readily and release hydrogen ions into the body fluids. The fall in *p*H is reduced by the buffers of the blood, the most important being bicarbonate. The fall in plasma *p*H stimulates pulmonary ventilation. Clinically hyperpnoea or 'air hunger' is observed and measurement of plasma bicarbonate will show a lower value than normal.

Clinical Features. Any form of stress, particularly an acute infection, can precipitate severe keto-acidosis in even the mildest diabetic. A common cause is neglect of treatment due to carelessness, misunderstanding or illness, and failure to adjust the therapeutic regimen in the event of an acute infection.

The *symptoms* of diabetic keto-acidosis invariably include intense thirst and polyuria. Constipation, muscle cramps and altered vision are common. Sometimes, especially in children, there is abdominal pain, with or without vomiting. Hence diabetic keto-acidosis is important in the differential diagnosis of the acute abdomen. Weakness and drowsiness are commonly present, but it should be remembered that the state of consciousness is very variable and a patient with dangerous ketosis requiring urgent treatment may walk into hospital. For this reason the term diabetic keto-acidosis is to be preferred to the traditional 'diabetic coma', which suggests that there is no urgency until unconsciousness occurs. In fact it is imperative that energetic treatment is started at the earliest possible stage.

The *signs* include a dry tongue and soft eyeballs due to dehydration: 'air hunger' indicated by long, deep, sighing respirations; a rapid, weak pulse, and low blood pressure; sometimes abdominal rigidity and tenderness; the smell of acetone in the breath; ultimately coma supervenes.

Laboratory tests show (1) ketonuria and heavy glycosuria; (2) blood glucose usually between 400 and 800 mg./100 ml., but it may be much higher; (3) low plasma bicarbonate and blood *p*H; (4) normal or raised serum sodium and potassium; (5) leucocytosis.

Treatment. This condition should be treated with the utmost urgency in hospital. Intravenous therapy is required since even when the patient is able to swallow, fluids given by mouth may be poorly absorbed. Treatment must also be checked against the blood concentration of glucose, potassium and bicarbonate estimated at intervals of not longer than two hours. Only in this way can the metabolic disorder be corrected accurately and rapidly. The aim should be to overcome with all speed:

1. Ketosis, by means of insulin to permit glucose utilisation.
2. Circulatory collapse, acidosis, and water and electrolyte depletion, by means of appropriate intravenous fluids.
3. Infection, if present, by means of antibiotics.

Figure 50 (p. 768), shows an example of a moderately severe case of diabetic ketosis treated on these lines.

Ketosis and dehydration render the comatose patient very resistant to insulin. Only soluble insulin should be used and 100 units should be given immediately the diagnosis is made, half intravenously and half intramuscularly. The total amount of insulin required varies widely and must be assessed in the light of changes in the blood glucose level; severe cases will usually need at least 500 units in the first 24 hours and may require considerably more. As long as there is evidence of circulatory collapse some of the insulin should be given intravenously.

The deficit of extracellular fluid, which is likely to be of the order of 3 litres, should be made good by saline which is isotonic in respect of sodium. In cases which are also severely acidotic (bicarbonate < 12 mEq./*l.*), one-third to one-half of the isotonic saline should be replaced by either isotonic sodium bicarbonate or, if this is not available, by isotonic sodium lactate solution (p. 863). The intracellular deficit of water, usually amounting to 2 to 3 litres, must be replaced by giving 5 per cent. glucose and not by more saline. It is best given when the blood glucose is approaching normal. It is important to continue the intravenous glucose together with appropriate doses of soluble insulin subcutaneously until the ketonuria has disappeared and the water deficit has been made good.

If the patient is admitted in profound circulatory failure, or the blood pressure remains low after the administration of saline and bicarbonate, it may be necessary to give blood or plasma. Vasopressor drugs as used for the treatment of shock may also be required.

Every patient in diabetic keto-acidosis is potassium depleted

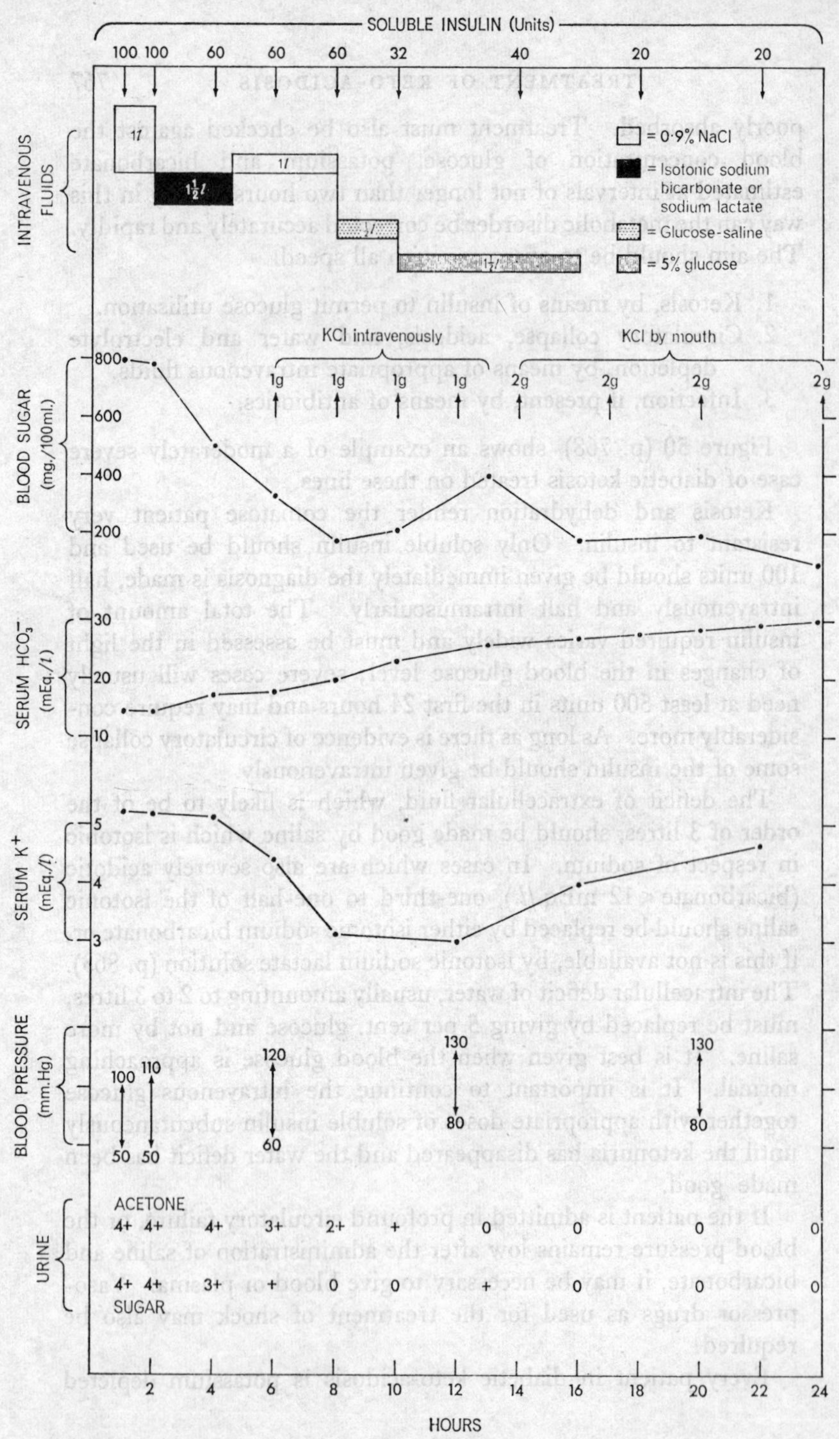

FIG. 50

Chemical pathology and response to treatment of a moderately severe case of diabetic ketosis during the first 24 hours in hospital.

and many will require intravenous potassium to prevent the development of dangerously low levels of potassium (p. 845) during the course of treatment. As the serum potassium is often high at the time of diagnosis it is important not to start potassium therapy until the level in the serum has fallen to normal, the peripheral circulation has been restored, and the urinary output is adequate. Approximately 80 mEq. of potassium may safely be given by vein in the first 16 hours but much more than this may be required. It is important to realise that sufficient potassium must be given to maintain a normal serum concentration, and this can only be confirmed by frequent estimations. It is customary to add 1 g. potassium chloride (13·4 mEq. potassium) to each 500 ml. of glucose and water given intravenously. Once oral feeding has started 2 g. potassium chloride should be given 4-hourly for two to three days to restore the total body deficit.

In a stuporous or comatose patient, gastric aspiration should be undertaken to avoid the risk of inhalation of vomitus.

Infections must be carefully sought and vigorously treated since it may not be possible to abolish ketosis until they are controlled. Once ketosis has been overcome, and the water and salt deficit made good (usually in about 24 hours), feeding by mouth can be started with frequent small fluid feeds each containing about 25 g. of carbohydrate. Five examples of such feeds are (1) 100 ml. (3½ oz.) fruit juice plus 15 g. (½ oz.) of cane sugar or glucose. (2) 200 ml. (7 oz.) milk plus 180 g. (6 oz.) of porridge. (3) 200 ml. (7 oz.) milk plus 20 g. (¾ oz.) Ovaltine, Horlicks or similar preparation. (4) 200 ml. (7 oz.) milk plus 10 g. (⅓ oz.) cereal plus 7 g. (¼ oz.) sugar. (5) 200 ml. (7 oz.) milk plus 20 g. (⅔ oz.) Benger's food. Enough insulin should be given to prevent any further ketonuria or glycosuria. Only soluble insulin should be used for several days until the patient has been stabilised.

Vascular Disorders

Diabetes mellitus is associated with changes in blood vessels of all sizes, but the thickening of the basement membrane of the capillaries is probably the earliest and possibly the only vascular abnormality that can be regarded as specific to diabetes. These changes are almost certainly secondary to the metabolic abnormalities occurring in diabetes since they are found in both primary and secondary diabetes and can be produced experimentally in animals rendered diabetic by various methods. Strict control probably offers the best chance of delaying the onset and progress of the vascular complications of diabetes. Unfortunately, however, they may develop despite every effort by both patient and doctor to maintain precise control of the diabetic state.

Thickening of the basement membrane develops, probably due to disordered metabolism of the glycoprotein of which the membrane is composed. These changes in the capillary walls lead eventually to serious disorders of vision and renal function (p. 771).

Atherosclerosis occurs commonly and extensively in diabetics. An integral part of the pathology of atherosclerosis is the deposition of cholesterol in the intima of the arteries; hyperlipaemia in diabetes perhaps contributes to this. Atherosclerosis in diabetics affects particularly the arteries of the legs, heart and kidneys, rendering them more prone at an earlier age than other people to intermittent claudication, gangrene of the toes and feet, myocardial infarction and nephropathy. Seventy-five per cent. of diabetics ultimately die from the effects of one or other of these vascular disorders.

In the absence of sufficient knowledge of the cause of atherosclerosis (p. 278), it cannot be prevented in diabetics any more than in other patients. It seems logical, however, to assume that the special prevalence of atherosclerosis in diabetes may be associated with the hyperglycaemia and lipaemia which are commonly present, and to treat the total disorder assiduously.

Diabetic Gangrene. Defective circulation in the legs resulting in poorly nourished tissues predisposes to the dangerous complication of gangrene. If a painless peripheral neuropathy (p. 772) is present, this may also be of aetiological importance, since the patient will tend to ignore or neglect injuries and other damage to the tissues. Diabetic gangrene usually starts in one foot, following a trivial injury—the cutting of a corn or a burn from a hot water bottle. Toxic absorption from necrosis of tissue and secondary infection may kill the patient unless the limb is amputated. Amputation of a toe, a foot, or even a whole leg is sometimes necessary to save life.

A great deal can be done to prevent this serious complication by instructing diabetics with a poor circulation to wear properly fitting shoes, to use bed-socks rather than hot water bottles, never to cut their own corns and to 'keep their feet as clean as their face'. The services of a skilled chiropodist are invaluable.

Diabetic Nephropathy. A specific type of renal lesion may occur as a result of the changes in the basement membrane of the glomerular capillaries. This is known as *diabetic glomerulosclerosis*, and there are two types, diffuse and nodular: the former is the more common and consists of a generalised thickening of glomerular capillary walls. The nodular type is a development of this, and in these cases rounded masses of acellular, hyaline material are superimposed upon the diffuse lesion in the glomeruli. These nodules are sometimes called Kimmelstiel-Wilson bodies. Diabetic glomerulosclerosis can be seen by light microscopy in about 70 per cent. of diabetic patients at autopsy. In the early stages of diabetes there may be little or no clinical evidence of renal involvement, and even with well-established diabetic glomerulosclerosis the patient may exhibit only slight to moderate proteinuria. In some cases, however, the patient develops marked proteinuria and the nephrotic syndrome with increasing renal failure and uraemia.

Diabetic Retinopathy. This has a specific appearance (Plates I and II) which sometimes enables the physician to make the initial diagnosis of diabetes. On examination with an ophthalmoscope, microaneurysms on the capillaries and circular haemorrhages and waxy exudates may be seen. These are the consequences of the changes in the capillaries previously mentioned. Changes in the veins and formation of new blood vessels (retinitis proliferans), both of which lead to pre-retinal or vitreous haemorrhages are extremely dangerous, inasmuch as fibrosis secondary to the haemorrhage can and often does cause blindness. In the latter type of lesion, before it has advanced too far, hypophysectomy may occasionally be effective in arresting progress of the disorder.

Other Ocular Disorders

Blurring of vision may occur in a severe diabetic before treatment, and may be especially troublesome after starting treatment with insulin. It is due to transitory osmotic abnormalities in the eye, especially in the lens, and may persist even for several weeks after initiating treatment.

Very rarely a specific type of opacity of the lens (cataract) occurs in diabetic children whose disease has not been adequately controlled. Cataract also occurs in elderly diabetics, but is said to be no more common than in other elderly people.

Infections

Any type of infection is of importance in diabetes, particularly if the disease is inadequately controlled. The following forms are especially important.

Carbuncle. Staphylococcal infections often cause a large increase in insulin requirements. The development of a carbuncle may unmask latent diabetes; it may even precipitate ketosis and coma. The diabetic state brought on by a carbuncle is not invariably permanent; glucose tolerance may return to normal (at least temporarily) when the infection subsides.

Cleanliness is a special virtue in the prevention of skin infection in diabetes. Once infection has occurred a suitable antibiotic must be used.

Pulmonary Tuberculosis. If a diabetic under treatment shows unexplained loss of weight, increase in insulin requirements or symptoms of pulmonary disease, clinical and radiological examination of the lungs should be undertaken. Pulmonary tuberculosis may be arrested in its early stages by prompt recognition and specific treatment, and every newly recognised diabetic should have a radiological examination of his chest.

Urinary Tract Infections. The presence of glucose in the urine provides a favourable medium for the growth of bacteria. Intractable infections of the urinary tract frequently occur, and for this reason catheterisation should be avoided if possible. Once infection has occurred treatment consists in controlling the glycosuria and the administration of suitable antibiotics as for any other case of urinary tract infection (p. 812).

Diabetic Neuropathy

Peripheral neuropathy is a frequent and troublesome complication. Motor, sensory or autonomic nerves may be involved, usually in a symmetrical manner. The most common types are:

1. Acute peripheral neuropathy which occurs usually in poorly controlled severe diabetics and which attacks one or many nerves.

The clinical features are those of peripheral neuropathy (p. 1217). Pain, felt particularly in the anterior aspect of the legs at night, is prominent. It is thought to be a metabolic neuropathy since it often improves rapidly when the diabetes is controlled.

2. Chronic peripheral neuropathy, which may be due to ischaemic damage to the sensory portions of peripheral nerves consequent upon diabetic angiopathy, and is therefore more common in older diabetics with long-standing disease. The clinical features are those of a painless neuropathy affecting the legs, including sometimes the appearance of a Charcot joint, and closely resembling those of tabes dorsalis (p. 1167).

3. Involvement of the autonomic nervous system may cause diarrhoea, overflow incontinence of urine, impotence or postural hypotension.

4. Diabetic amyotrophy consists of bilateral symmetrical wasting and weakness of the pelvic girdle musculature with concomitant pain.

Disorders of the Skin

The major changes found are those related to acute infections such as boils and carbuncles. Fungal infection of the feet and elsewhere may occur. Pruritus vulvae associated with a fungal infection is so typical as to be almost pathognomonic of diabetes. Abnormal lipid deposits in the skin (xanthoma) are sometimes found, but are not confined to diabetic patients.

SPECIAL PROBLEMS IN THE MANAGEMENT OF DIABETES

Diabetes in Children

Fortunately diabetes is not common in childhood, but when it occurs it is relatively severe and always requires treatment with insulin. The therapeutic problem of matching the dose of insulin to the food intake raises practical difficulties.

Food. The nutritional needs of diabetic children are essentially no different from those of other children. Since they should be growing, their caloric requirements are large in proportion to their size, by comparison with adult standards. Difficulties may be experienced in finding the best means of providing the requisite calories. In children, likes and dislikes for particular foods are often fickle and unpredictable. It is important to make sure that the child does not become too fat; hypoglycaemia due to too much insulin can lead to excessive appetite and hence to obesity. A dietitian can do much to help a diabetic child and his parents with proper advice. A diabetic child must not have sugar or sweets, but the essential composition of his diet need differ little from that of his friends. It is important that everything possible should be done to avoid distinguishing him from his contemporaries. Once properly trained, he may go with them to a summer holiday camp if he so desires, provided that the camp organiser understands his disease. The British Diabetic Association runs special camps for diabetic children.

Insulin. Day-to-day requirements for insulin are often very variable. Children must not be expected to lead the steady life of a business man or housewife; their emotions and activities fluctuate unexpectedly—sometimes wildly active and sometimes sulking. This may have an important effect on their daily needs for insulin; excessive activity may result in hypoglycaemia, whilst lethargy may lead to hyperglycaemia. The latter may also be caused by any one of the numerous infectious diseases to which all children are prone. A combination of one of the depot insulins and soluble insulin before breakfast and usually a second dose of soluble insulin before supper is a suitable arrangement for most diabetic children.

Pregnancy in Diabetes

One of the important consequences of the discovery and use of insulin is that diabetic women can now have children, whereas in the pre-insulin era they were almost always amenorrhoeic and infertile. If a diabetic woman wishes to have a child there is no reason why she should avoid pregnancy, provided that she suffers from none of the more serious complications of diabetes and provided she remains constantly under expert medical care.

Nevertheless pregnancy in a diabetic woman carries certain definite risks; in the later stages of pregnancy she may develop an excessive accumulation of amniotic fluid (hydramnios); in addition the foetus is sometimes unusually large leading to difficulty in labour. Small babies are liable to die, either shortly before delivery or soon after birth. The chances that a diabetic mother may lose her baby either from a stillbirth or in the early neonatal period are greater than those of a non-diabetic mother, even with the most careful supervision.

The proper treatment of a pregnant diabetic patient requires the close and co-ordinated supervision of a team, consisting of physician, obstetrician, anaesthetist, nurse and dietitian. The sooner the pregnancy is diagnosed the better. Some non-pregnant diabetic women often miss one or more menstrual periods especially if their disease is poorly controlled. For this reason a Hogben pregnancy test is often helpful. There are grounds for suggesting that oral hypoglycaemic agents might be teratogenic, and any diabetic patient who is taking these drugs and becomes pregnant should change to a preparation of insulin as soon as the pregnancy is diagnosed.

It is desirable that the expectant mother should spend a week as an ambulant in-patient in hospital towards the end of the third month of pregnancy. This will enable the patient and the team to get to know each other. Every effort must be made at this time to see that her diabetes is under the best possible control; further education of the patient may be needed in the proper management of her diet and insulin while at home. The diet, at first at least, need differ in no important respect from the diabetic diet (Diet No. 12, p. 1302) to which she has been accustomed, but may need adjustment later, particularly with additional milk. Practical problems may be created for the physician and dietitian by bouts of vomiting that commonly occur in the early stages of any pregnancy, and by the peculiar food fads which many pregnant women develop.

After the diagnosis of pregnancy has been made the patient should be seen at first at fortnightly and later at weekly intervals. Continued full control of the diabetes may be complicated by other factors. First, the renal threshold for glucose often falls as pregnancy advances. This is a normal phenomenon, but in the diabetic it means that the tests for glycosuria which she carries out at home may cease to be a reliable index of diabetic control. Further, in the later stages of pregnancy lactosuria may occasionally occur and may lead to confusion. If excessive amounts of glucose are lost in the urine because of the lowered renal threshold, it may be necessary to give additional carbohydrate feeds between meals and sometimes at night, covered by suitable amounts of soluble insulin. Then, too, the requirements for insulin often increase as pregnancy advances. Frequent estimations of blood glucose are needed to ensure that an increase in insulin dosage, based on misleading urine tests, is not producing hypoglycaemia; or alternatively, that hyperglycaemia is not insidiously building up through failure to give enough insulin to meet an increase in insulin requirements.

Pregnancy in a diabetic woman should seldom if ever be allowed to proceed to term. The chances of survival for the infant are greatly enhanced if it is delivered between the thirty-sixth and thirty-eighth weeks by induction of labour or if necessary by Caesarean section. Following delivery the insulin requirements of the mother fall considerably. Frequent blood glucose estimations and co-operation between the physician and dietitian are needed to ensure an uneventful return to the former diet and insulin dosage.

A final word of warning is necessary. It has already been indicated that glycosuria is not unusual during normal pregnancy, either because of a fall in the renal threshold for glucose or through lactose appearing in the urine. The finding, however, of reducing substances in the urine of a pregnant woman should never be lightly dismissed as a normal phenomenon. Full clinical investigation to exclude diabetes is essential; otherwise a preventable catastrophe may follow.

Surgery and Diabetes

Any surgical operation, however minor, and the accompanying anaesthetic cause a metabolic stress which the diabetic is less well able to meet than the normal person. The stress is temporary and will not be aggravated by a mild hyperglycaemia, but an accompanying acidosis will prejudice normal recovery. The position is worse if there is tissue wasting with much breakdown of fat and protein and the excretion of large amounts of potassium, phosphate and other intracellular electrolytes.

Two points must be kept in mind: first, the need to provide an adequate supply of energy for the tissues, and secondly, the need to be constantly on the alert for acidosis.

In practice there are two separate problems. The first is the management of a stabilised diabetic who has to undergo an operation at a time which can be chosen by the surgeon and physician. The second is that of a diabetic whose disease may not be well controlled and who suddenly has to be operated upon because of trauma, acute sepsis or a major abdominal or other catastrophe, or one who is first discovered to be diabetic immediately before operation.

As both the severity of the diabetes and the extent of the operation will vary greatly, it is not possible to set out details of management. Each patient is an individual problem.

Elective Surgery in a Stabilised Diabetic. All diabetics must be admitted to hospital about three days before an operation, even a minor one. During this period the control of the diabetes can be checked thoroughly. Provided a diabetic goes to the theatre in good condition, there is unlikely to be any significant change in the blood glucose, plasma bicarbonate or ketone levels during the time he is undergoing surgery. In fact, hypoglycaemia is more likely to occur than acidosis. For this reason it is generally advisable to give no insulin immediately before operation. During the day preceding the operation the patient's usual diet and doses of insulin should be given though doses of depot insulin of more than 20 units should be reduced by half and a supplementary dose of soluble insulin given later that day instead. It will usually be possible to arrange for the operation to take place in the morning. The patient should receive no breakfast and nothing by mouth before operation. Before being transferred to the theatre the fasting blood glucose level should be determined. If this lies between 120 and 200 mg./100 ml. then no glucose or insulin need be given. If the level is below 120 then about 25 to 40 g. of glucose should be given intravenously, preferably in hypertonic solution, in order to prevent possible hypoglycaemia during the operation. No insulin is necessary. If the fasting blood sugar is over 200, which is infrequent, then some insulin will be required. About one-third of his usual total daily dose is indicated, in the form of soluble insulin, but its administration can usually be postponed until after operation.

Recovery from the anaesthetic must be carefully supervised. The sooner the patient returns to his usual diet the better. This interval may be a few hours or several days, depending on the nature and severity of the operation. Within a few hours of recovery from the anaesthetic many patients are able to take a fluid or semi-fluid feed containing 25 g. of carbohydrate (p. 769) at three- to four-hourly intervals, covered by suitable doses of soluble insulin. Some insulin-dependent diabetics after a major operation may need to have most of their energy requirements supplied as glucose, either intravenously or by mouth. If all has gone well, a single determination of the fasting blood glucose each morning will suffice. If recovery is stormy, measurements may be necessary at four-hourly intervals or even more frequently. Determination of the plasma bicarbonate or CO_2 combining power and electrolytes in the blood will also be helpful. The insulin dosage will depend on these findings, and until stability has been regained only soluble insulin should be used.

Each specimen of urine must be tested for sugar and ketone bodies. If ketosis develops it is essential to take immediate steps to increase the metabolism of glucose by adjusting the dose of insulin.

Diabetes and Surgical Emergencies. Circumstances vary so much that it is impossible to consider them except in the most general way. The essentials are to maintain the oxidation of glucose by the tissues at a sufficient rate and to combat acidosis and electrolyte disturbances when they occur. This can only be done effectively if the state of the diabetic control is assessed continuously and accurately. A laboratory service that can provide rapid results is thus essential. As long as the surgical condition remains untreated and the 'metabolic stress' continues, the diabetic condition is likely to get worse. Once the patient's surgical condition is under control he may be expected to respond promptly to the appropriate therapy for his diabetes.

Prognosis

The prognosis in diabetes has improved steadily since the introduction of insulin; but even with its use the average expectation of life is still rather less than that of a non-diabetic. It may be difficult to estimate the prognosis of an individual patient because so many variable factors have to be considered. Thus the child of parents poor in means and education, who is first seen in coma, obviously has a very different future compared with the middle-aged lady in easy circumstances who complains of nothing but a little thirst and pruritus, and can afford the time and the means to follow precisely the diet prescribed for her. The incidence of the complications of diabetes is mainly related to the duration of the disease but probably also to the precision with which it has been controlled.

General Prevention

Diabetes is a disease of the prosperous, and in wealthy countries it is one of the major health problems. The hardships of the Second World War were associated with a marked decline in the incidence of diabetes in European countries; rationing of both food and petrol was probably responsible. The importance for health of sufficient exercise (p. 454) and of avoiding dietary excess has been stated repeatedly (p. 459). Diabetes, like obesity and atherosclerosis, is likely to arise in predisposed persons who eat too much and exercise too little. Excess of dietary carbohydrate may strain the limited capacity of the pancreas to produce insulin, especially if it is in the form of sugar or other refined carbohydrate; excess of dietary fat may accelerate the complications of diabetes; atherosclerosis is a common cause of death in diabetics. In any event the public should be warned primarily against an overall excess of calories.

Screening. It is much easier to control the disease and to maintain the health of the patient in a state which allows him to lead a normal life, if the diagnosis is made early in the course of the disease. In many patients, the biochemical changes can be detected before the symptoms are sufficiently severe to make them seek medical advice. Any screening technique is expensive and should only be used if it is likely that a significant number of new diabetics will be recognised. High-risk groups, for example the first degree relatives of known diabetics, the obese and the mothers of babies weighing more than 10 lb. at birth, will give a particularly high yield. The prevalence of diabetes in different communities varies from 0·5 to 5 per cent. About half of these may be unaware that they have the disease. These figures vary widely according to the social and economic state of the people and the educational and medical services available.

Urine testing has been widely used as a screening procedure. As up to 3 per cent. of people may have renal glycosuria and so will have to be recalled for blood tests, this is a wasteful procedure. Whenever practicable, blood glucose examination is recommended as the screening procedure. Auto-analysers enable large numbers of samples to be tested daily (p. 748).

Nearly 50 surveys in various countries have been described. Their value is now established and regular surveys will probably be incorporated in many public health programmes in the future.

Genetic Counselling. Diabetic patients will often consult their doctor about the advisability of having children and sometimes it is his duty to warn them of the dangers. They can be told that the risks of pregnancy and delivery are little greater for a diabetic mother than for a normal woman, provided she submits to the strict discipline required (p. 774). The chances that she will produce a healthy baby are also good, but not quite so good as for a normal mother. The chances that her child will subsequently develop diabetes are considerable. If both parents have diabetes, the probability is that about half their children will develop the disease at some stage in life. The risk is about half this if only one parent is affected but the other has a family history of the disease. Many diabetics have healthy children, and how strongly a doctor should word these necessary warnings is a matter for judgment in each case. The family history, the severity of the disease in the parents and their educational and economic background, must all be considered. Should a diabetic decide to have a child, both parents must be told of their responsibility for keeping a careful watch for early symptoms of the disease in their offspring, whose future may depend on its prompt recognition.

Conclusion. It is a wise precaution for diabetic patients who are taking insulin or oral hypoglycaemic drugs to carry a card with them at all times stating their name and address, the fact that they are diabetic, the nature and dose of any insulin or other drugs they may be taking, and, in addition, giving the name, address and telephone number of their family doctor and any special diabetic clinic they may be attending. Suitable cards are provided by the British Diabetic Association for the use of members.

Finally, the prevention of the *complications* of diabetes offers a great opportunity for good medical practice; there are few other chronic diseases in which the practice of preventive medicine can make so much difference to a patient's life.

J. A. STRONG.
JOYCE D. BAIRD.

Books recommended:

Dunlop, Sir Derrick Alstead, S., & Macgregor, A. G. (1968). *Textbook of Medical Treatment*, 11th ed. Edinburgh: Livingstone.

Williams, R. H. (1960). *Diabetes*. New York: Hoeber.

DISEASES OF THE KIDNEY AND URINARY SYSTEM

STRUCTURE AND MODE OF ACTION OF THE KIDNEYS

THE kidneys are each composed of approximately one million similar functional units called nephrons. Each nephron consists of a small tube, the upper end of which is dilated to form an epithelial sac (Bowman's capsule). Freely communicating loops of capillaries which arise from afferent arterioles lie within the sac and with it form the glomerulus. The glomeruli lie in the cortex of the kidney and are surrounded by convolutions of the proximal and distal tubules. From most glomeruli the proximal convoluted tubule leads to a thin segment which enters the medulla and which ultimately forms the loop of Henle. Each loop consists of thin descending and ascending limbs which are arranged in parallel, some of which penetrate as far as the renal papillae. The ascending limb of the loop then returns towards the renal cortex and enlarges there to form the distal convoluted tubule. These ultimately end in collecting ducts which once more descend into the medullary region, lying between the loops of Henle, and drain the urine into the renal pelvis at the renal papillae. For a short distance the afferent arterioles and distal convoluted tubules are in contact, and at this point the tubular cells become tall and columnar in character, forming the macula densa. The wall of the arteriole is thickened by cells which contain large secretory granules. These structures together constitute the juxtaglomerular complex which is believed to be the source of renin and to be intimately concerned in the regulation of the volume of the extracellular fluids and blood pressure.

The blood supply of the kidney is relatively large and amounts to about one-quarter of the cardiac output at rest, i.e. 1,300 ml. per minute. The afferent arterioles which give rise to the glomerular capillaries arise from branches of the renal artery. Emerging from the glomeruli the capillaries unite to form the efferent arterioles which then supply blood to the convoluted tubules. The medullary region of the kidney is supplied by arterioles which arise from those glomeruli situated in the deeper regions of the cortex (juxtamedullary glomeruli).

The hydrostatic pressure within the glomerular capillaries of about 70 mm. Hg. results in the filtration of fluid from the plasma into Bowman's capsule. This fluid is identical in its composition with plasma except that it normally contains no fat and very little protein. The filtrate thus formed, then flows through the various parts of the tubule and is modified according to the needs of the body by tubular secretion and by the selective reabsorption of its constituents.

The Functions of the Kidneys

In health the volume and composition of the body fluids vary within narrow limits. The kidneys are largely responsible for maintaining this constancy and the excretion of the waste products of metabolism represents merely one aspect of this task. The various renal functions are conveniently considered under the following headings and some are shown diagrammatically in Figure 51.

1. **Regulation of the water content of the body.** About seven-eighths of the water filtered by the glomerulus is reabsorbed by the proximal tubules. The remaining water passes through the distal tubules and collecting ducts where its reabsorption is regulated chiefly by vasopressin, the antidiuretic hormone of the posterior pituitary. In the presence of vasopressin the collecting ducts become permeable to water which is then passively reabsorbed in response to the high concentration of sodium chloride and urea which exists in the medullary interstitium. The urine then becomes concentrated. In the absence of vasopressin the collecting ducts are impermeable to water. In these circumstances a dilute urine is formed by the tubular reabsorption of sodium without water. Disorders of the water-regulating mechanism which result in oliguria or polyuria are described on p. 787.

2. **Regulation of the electrolyte content of the body.** The electrolyte content of the body is kept remarkably constant as a

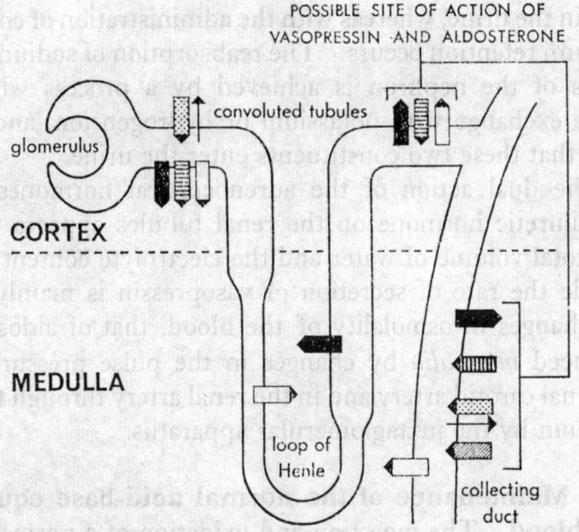

Functions of the Nephron

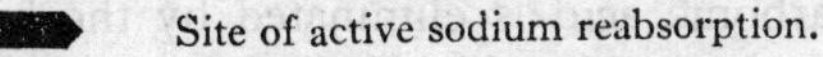

Site of active sodium reabsorption.

Site of active potassium reabsorption or secretion.

Site of passive water movement.

Site of hydrogen ion secretion, and bicarbonate ion generation and reabsorption.

Site of ammonia secretion.

Fig. 51

Arrangement of some of the events concerned in urine formation. In the proximal tubule about seven-eighths of the filtered sodium, potassium and water are reabsorbed. The greater part of the filtered bicarbonate is also reabsorbed here by a process which involves the secretion of hydrogen ions in exchange for sodium. The sodium reabsorbed in the ascending limb of the loop of Henle is largely responsible for the hyperosmolarity of the medullary interstitium. In the distal tubule and collecting duct potassium and hydrogen ions are exchanged for sodium ions, ammonia is secreted and water is passively reabsorbed in the presence of vasopressin.

result of selective reabsorption by the renal tubules. A large part of the filtered sodium and probably all the potassium are reabsorbed in the proximal convoluted tubules. The intrinsic mechanisms by which these functions are performed are unknown. The remainder of the sodium passes into the distal tubule and collecting ducts where its reabsorption appears to be under the influence of hormones of the adrenal cortex especially aldosterone. With reduced secretion of these hormones, excessive quantities of sodium and chloride ions are lost in the urine, whereas with the administration of corticosteroids, sodium retention occurs. The reabsorption of sodium in the distal parts of the nephron is achieved by a process which involves ionic exchange with potassium or hydrogen ion, and it is in this way that these two constituents enter the urine.

The dual action of the adrenocortical hormones and of the antidiuretic hormone on the renal tubules appears to determine the total volume of water and the electrolyte content of the body. While the rate of secretion of vasopressin is mainly determined by changes in osmolality of the blood, that of aldosterone is influenced *inter alia* by changes in the pulse pressure within the internal carotid artery and in the renal artery through the liberation of renin by the juxtaglomerular apparatus.

3. **Maintenance of the normal acid-base equilibrium of the blood.** The ingestion and oxidation of a normal diet results in the formation of substances which yield hydrogen ions in aqueous solution. Carbonic acid is eliminated by the lungs as carbon dioxide but the other acids which include acetoacetic acid and the oxidative products of sulphur containing foods require the collaboration of an elaborate mechanism within the kidney for their disposal. These inorganic and organic acids are in the first instance partly neutralised by the blood and other buffer systems as described on p. 860. By itself this process leaves the blood abnormal in three respects, i.e. the hydrogen ion concentration remains increased above normal, the concentration of bicarbonate is reduced and the anions of the acids still require to be excreted. These abnormalities are corrected as follows:

1. Carbonic acid is generated within the renal tubular cells from CO_2 and H_2O under the influence of carbonic anhydrase.
2. The hydrogen ions of this acid are secreted into the tubular lumen in exchange for filtered sodium which is then reabsorbed into the blood.
3. Some of the hydrogen ions are buffered in the urine by disodium hydrogen phosphate to form dihydrogen sodium phosphate and by ammonia to form ammonium ions. The anions of the inorganic and organic acids are then excreted in the urine largely as ammonium salts.
4. The bicarbonate ions liberated from the carbonic acid made

locally in the renal tubular cells are reabsorbed into the blood and restore the concentration of plasma bicarbonate to normal values and also regenerate other buffers in the body which have been titrated by the invading acids.

The degree to which these mechanisms operate is adjusted in accordance with the nature of the food ingested and the amount of endogenous acid production. In health, on a normal diet, 40-80 m.Eq of acid are excreted daily into the urine. When alkali or an alkali-ash diet is taken (i.e. a diet consisting mainly of fruit and vegetables) alkaline sodium phosphate and bicarbonate are excreted in the urine and tubular secretion of hydrogen and ammonium ions is suppressed.

In disease states in which abnormally large amounts of organic acids are being formed (e.g. β-hydroxybutyric acid and acetoacetic acid in diabetic acidosis), these processes are fully active and may be overwhelmed. Excess acid is retained in the blood and acidosis occurs. When renal tubular activity itself is severely affected by kidney disease these regulatory mechanisms fail and acidosis of renal origin develops.

4. Retention of other substances vital to body economy, e.g. glucose, amino acids, phosphate, bicarbonate, proteins. Glucose is normally reabsorbed so completely by the proximal tubules that none can be detected in the urine by clinical tests. *Renal glycosuria* (p. 748) is a genetically determined benign defect of tubular reabsorption in which glucose appears in the urine in the presence of normal blood levels. More rarely other congenital or acquired abnormalities of tubular transport result in abnormal loss in the urine of amino acids, phosphate, sodium, potassium, calcium and water. These defects may occur singly or in combination. Examples of these disorders are *cystinuria, essential hypophosphatasia, nephrogenic diabetes insipidus* and the *Fanconi syndrome*, a disease chiefly of infancy and childhood. In health the great bulk of the bicarbonate filtered by the glomeruli is removed from the urine by tubular reabsorption, and this becomes complete when the urine is acid. *Idiopathic renal tubular acidosis* is a rare congenital disease in which there is a defect in the power to acidify the urine which usually contains significant amounts of bicarbonate in the face of systemic acidosis. A similar tubular defect may be acquired as a result of renal disease such as pyelonephritis. Both types are apt to lead to osteomalacia and ectopic calcification, especially in the kidneys, and to hypokalaemia.

In health it seems likely that only a small amount of protein (10 mg. per cent.) reaches the fluid in Bowman's capsule. The volume of glomerular filtrate, however, is so great that if this small amount were not reabsorbed over 15 g. of protein would be excreted in the urine in 24 hours. The relative extent to which increased permeability of the glomerular membrane and failure in tubular reabsorption of protein contribute to the proteinuria in such diseases as acute glomerulonephritis, membranous glomerulonephritis or in other causes of the nephrotic syndrome is unknown. Evidence from electron microscope studies however suggests that abnormalities in glomerular permeability are responsible for proteinuria in the great majority of instances.

5. **Excretion of waste metabolic products, toxic substances and drugs.** The end-products of metabolism, especially those of protein, include urea, uric acid, creatinine, phosphates, sulphates.

6. **Hormonal functions.** The juxtaglomerular complexes within the kidneys are believed to secrete renin, which is converted in the blood to angiotensin. This substance increases the rate of aldosterone secretion by the adrenal cortex. This may be the sequence of events by which renal ischaemia produces hypertension. The kidney is the main source of erythropoietin necessary for normal erythropoiesis (p. 605).

THE DIAGNOSIS OF RENAL DISEASE

In the majority of patients suffering from renal disease, symptoms and signs are not usually referred to the anatomical site of the kidneys. This is due to the fact that clinical features of renal disease most frequently arise from abnormalities in the chemical composition of the body or from hypertension. Their true origin therefore may be suspected only after the detection of urinary abnormalities, and the importance of a routine examination of the urine in clinical practice cannot be over-emphasised. The examinations which may be of value include the determination of the volume of urine passed in 24 hours, the presence of abnormal urinary constituents and bacteriological examination. Under certain standardised conditions the determination of the specific gravity and the hydrogen ion concentration (pH) of urine is of value. In addition it may be necessary to obtain further information by some or all of the following investigations.

1. Chemical analysis of the blood and urine.
2. Tests of glomerular and tubular function.
3. Radiological examination of the abdomen, intravenous pyelography, cystoscopy, ureteric catheterisation with collection of urine samples from each kidney, retrograde pyelography, renal angiography, isotope renography and renal biopsy.

URINARY VOLUME

In health and in temperate climates the volume of urine excreted usually lies within the range of 800-2,500 ml. per 24 hours. There is a limit to the power of the kidneys to concentrate urine and on a normal diet a minimum volume of 800 ml. is required to excrete the solid urinary constituents which consist mainly of urea and electrolytes. Less solute has to be excreted when a diet rich in carbohydrate and fat and low in protein and salt is eaten, and as little as 250 ml. of urine per 24 hours is sufficient in these circumstances.

Oliguria is the production of insufficient urine to enable solute to be excreted in adequate amounts and the *milieu intérieur* of the body to be preserved. If the concentrating power of the kidneys is seriously reduced or if the solute to be excreted in the urine is increased above the normal, as occurs, for example, in severe infections, a daily output of as much as 2-3 litres of urine may even be insufficient. Oliguria develops in conditions associated with a reduction in renal blood flow and rate of glomerular filtration, e.g. diseases giving rise to water and salt depletion, hypotension, cardiac failure, acute glomerulonephritis, and other parenchymal diseases of the kidneys. In these circumstances urine flow sometimes ceases completely and anuria develops. Anuria from this cause should be distinguished from urinary retention. In the latter case distension of the bladder will be found on examination of the abdomen, confirmed if necessary by catheterisation.

Polyuria. This term denotes a persistent increase in urinary output. It must be distinguished from frequency of micturition, which may be defined as the frequent passage of small quantities of urine without an increase in the total volume.

There are several mechanisms which give rise to polyuria. It may be due either to the excretion of an abnormally large amount of solute so that elimination of increased volume of water is required, or to a limitation in the ability of the kidney to concentrate urine and conserve water. The latter defect may arise because of lack of circulating vasopressin or insensitivity of the concentrating mechanism within the kidney to its action. Polyuria occurs in the following clinical circumstances:

(*a*) Diabetes mellitus in which an osmotic diuresis occurs because of glycosuria due to hyperglycaemia.

(*b*) Chronic parenchymal renal disease with uraemia or the recovery phase of some cases of acute renal failure in which the elevated concentration of urea in the blood acts as the osmotic diuretic.

(*c*) Conditions in which there is decreased responsiveness of the collecting ducts to vasopressin, e.g. in some cases of chronic renal disease, hyperparathyroidism and potassium depletion, and in familial nephrogenic diabetes insipidus.

(*d*) Diabetes insipidus of neurohypophyseal origin in which there is diminished secretion of vasopressin.

(*e*) Inhibition of vasopressin secretion due to excessive drinking of fluid either from choice or from psychiatric causes.

(*f*) The elimination of oedema, e.g. in recovery from congestive heart failure or the nephrotic syndrome.

SPECIFIC GRAVITY OF URINE

The specific gravity of urine is defined as the ratio between the weight of a given volume of urine and the weight of an equal volume of distilled water. It is therefore a measure of the quantity of solids in solution and is an approximate measure of osmolality. For clinical purposes measurement of the specific gravity is made by a hydrometer (urinometer) which is calibrated to read 1·000 at 16° C. (60° F.) in water. In health, urea and sodium chloride are the main solutes contributing to the specific gravity of urine. In diabetes mellitus, on the other hand, the quantity of glucose in the urine may far outweigh the total of all the other solutes present;

water containing 1 per cent. glucose has a specific gravity of 1·004. Sometimes the urine from a patient with diabetic polyuria appears to be dilute because it is pale in colour, but it may in fact have a high specific gravity due to the presence of as much as 10 per cent. glucose. Protein has almost the same effect in increasing the specific gravity as a similar quantity of urea. Urea, however, is present in a concentration of 2 per cent. in normal urine, while protein, even in the most severe cases of the nephrotic syndrome, is seldom present in such large quantities. Thus 4 g. protein per litre, which gives a strong reaction with Albustix, raises the specific gravity by only 0·001. The specific gravity of urine varies with the nature and quantity of food eaten as well as with the amount of water or other fluid taken. When determination of the specific gravity of urine is used to assess renal function, these factors should be controlled.

Maximal concentration of urine. The maximal capacity of the kidneys to concentrate urine may be determined either after depriving the patient of fluid for a standard time or by the injection of pitressin. In health, fluid deprivation results in a rise in serum osmolality which acts as a stimulus for production of endogenous antidiuretic hormone. The urine becomes progressively more concentrated as fluid deprivation is continued, and in experimental subjects increasing values for urine osmolality are found up to three days. This is far too long a period of time for clinical application but deprivation of fluid for at least 20 hours is necessary for consistently accurate results to be obtained in temperate climates. With this procedure urinary concentrations corresponding to specific gravity of from 1·022 to 1·040 are obtained in healthy individuals. Restriction of fluid to this extent is nearly always unpleasant and in the case of diabetes insipidus may actually be dangerous. As an alternative to fluid restriction the patient may be given 5 units of pitressin in oil by intramuscular injection, the specific gravity of all specimens of urine passed in the next 24 hours being measured. During the test the patient may eat and drink normally. The results obtained with this method are slightly lower than those found after fluid restriction but, in health, values of 1·020 or above are achieved. If a random or pre-breakfast sample of urine is found to have a specific gravity of 1·020 or more there is clearly no need to carry out the tests described above.

Minimal concentration of urine. The minimal concentration of urine that can be attained is determined after the ingestion of 1 litre of water or the intravenous infusion of 1 litre of 5 per cent. dextrose in water to the fasting subject. The ingestion or the infusion of the fluid should not take longer than 20 minutes and the urine should be collected hourly thereafter for four hours. During this time a normal subject excretes at least 70 per cent. of the water load and the concentration of at least one specimen should be below 1·004.

The following precautions should be taken in measuring the specific gravity of urine.

(*a*) The urinometer should be tested periodically in order to confirm that the reading in distilled water is 1·000.

(*b*) When the specific gravity is being taken the urinometer should not touch the side of the vessel containing the urine.

(*c*) The reading on the urinometer should be made at the level of the bottom of the meniscus.

(*d*) The urine should be allowed to cool to room temperature (16° C.) before the reading is made. Erroneously low values will be obtained unless this precaution is taken.

Diminution in the power to concentrate urine may be due to an inability to produce vasopressin, to a failure of the concentrating mechanism to respond to endogenous or exogenous vasopressin or to an osmotic diuresis in which there is an increase in the amount of solute excreted per nephron. Although defects in urinary concentrating power are usually accompanied by restriction in urinary diluting power, this is not invariable, and the latter may persist long after concentrating power is lost.

REACTION OF THE URINE AND ACID EXCRETION

In health and on a normal diet 40-80 m.Eq of acid are excreted daily in the urine. The greater part of this acid is excreted in buffered form partly as dihydrogen phosphate, which constitutes the bulk of the titratable acidity of the urine, and partly as ammonium ions. A very small amount of free hydrogen ion is also excreted and it is this which is measured when the pH of the urine is determined. Little information is gained from the routine determination of urinary pH in random samples of urine. In certain circumstances the ability of the renal tubules to excrete hydrogen ions is depressed and the demonstration of this is of clinical significance. It is important to examine fresh specimens of urine since urea may decompose to form ammonia and give a false result if urine is left to stand. Infections of the urinary tract with organisms other than *Esch. coli* or tubercle bacilli also cause the urine to be alkaline owing to the breakdown of urea.

Procedure used to estimate the tubular capacity to secrete acid. The administration of ammonium chloride by mouth to the normal subject rapidly leads to a fall in the urinary pH and to a progressive rise in titratable acidity and in the amount of ammonium ions in the urine. This is due to the conversion of the NH_3 in the ingested salt to urea, leaving HCl to be buffered in the body and subsequently excreted in the urine. For most clinical purposes this function is tested by the oral administration of 7 g. of NH_4Cl in gelatin-covered capsules taken over a period of 60 minutes in the fasting state with 1 litre of water. Urine is collected without catheterisation at one *or* two-hourly intervals for seven hours and the pH of each specimen is determined. Normally the pH of the urine is found to have fallen to less than 5·0 and this value is also reached in most patients with chronic renal disease. Failure to acidify the urine following the administration of ammonium chloride is characteristic of *renal tubular acidosis* occurring either as an inherited or acquired defect, and may also occur in potassium deficiency and in some patients with hypercalciuria and nephrocalcinosis. Additional information can be obtained by determining the titratable acidity and the rate of excretion of ammonium. These measurements give a value of the power of the renal tubules to secrete hydrogen ions in buffer form as monosodium dihydrogen phosphate and the ammonium ion. Titratable acidity and ammonia excretion are reduced in chronic renal insufficiency and in some patients with nephrocalcinosis. While titratable acidity is also reduced in potassium depletion and renal tubular acidosis, the power to excrete ammonia appears to be normal.

THE MEASUREMENT OF RENAL CLEARANCE

The ability of the glomeruli to perform their function in health and disease may be estimated by the measurement of 'clearance.'

The term 'clearance' does not imply the complete removal of a substance from the plasma. It is an arbitrary, but quantitatively valid measurement which relates the amount of a substance present in the urine, produced over a unit of time, to its concentration in the plasma. It is measured from the following equation

$C=\frac{UV}{P}$ in which:

C is the clearance.
U is the concentration of the substance in the urine.
P is the concentration of the substance in the plasma.
V is the volume of urine in ml. secreted per minute.

If a substance in the plasma passes freely through the glomerular filter, and is neither absorbed nor excreted by the tubules, the quantity excreted in the urine, UV, is identical with the quantity filtered by the glomeruli. The clearance of such a substance is therefore equal to the rate of glomerular filtration. Endogenous creatinine and the polysaccharide, inulin, appear to be excreted in this way and their clearances are used to estimate the rate of glomerular filtration, which for the average adult is about 120 ml. per minute. Since urea is partly reabsorbed by the tubules its clearance is less than that of the creatinine or inulin. The clearance of creatinine is determined by collecting urine over a 24-hour period and withdrawing one sample of blood during the day. It is advisable to check the accuracy of an abnormal result by repeating the test on several occasions.

ABNORMAL CONSTITUENTS OF URINE

1. **Protein.** The presence of protein in the urine is always of clinical significance. Proteinuria detectable by the use of Albustix or salicylsulphonic acid does not usually occur in disease of the lower urinary tract, though a small amount can be detected in severe urinary infection or obvious haematuria. Proteinuria almost invariably indicates the presence of parenchymal disease of the kidneys but its magnitude bears little relation to the degree of renal failure. In the absence of inflammation in the urinary tract, the protein is derived from plasma proteins which have been filtered by the glomeruli. Because of its smaller molecular size, albumin predominates over the globulins.

Small amounts of protein are usually found in the urine in severe chronic renal disease, in the course of febrile illnesses and in congestive heart failure. Larger amounts of protein (e.g. 3 g./day or more) are found in the nephrotic syndrome (p. 805). Bence Jones proteins may be found in myelomatosis and in other diseases of the reticulo-endothelial system. Postural proteinuria is discussed on p. 796.

2. **Blood.** Blood is found in the urine in a wide variety of clinical conditions, and haematuria usually indicates serious disease of the urinary tract and the cause must always be sought. If an episode of haematuria is neglected and time is allowed for the symptom to recur in order to confirm the patient's observation, many potentially curable cases will advance to an incurable stage. The appearance of the urine varies with the amount of blood and is normal to the naked eye when traces only are present. When larger amounts of blood are present the urine may be smoky in appearance, bright red or reddish-brown. The brown discolouration is due to the formation of acid haematin from haemoglobin.

Red blood cells are found in varying numbers in the urine in acute glomerulonephritis, embolic nephritis, malignant hypertension, polyarteritis nodosa, renal lupus erythematosus, renal tuberculosis, congenital polycystic disease, haemorrhagic diseases, renal infarction and trauma to the kidneys. Red cells occur in the urine also in inflammation and tumour of the kidney and of the urinary tract, in senile hyperplasia and carcinoma of the prostate, and in the presence of urinary calculi. They are absent or very scanty in nephrosclerosis, in chronic, minimal lesion and membranous glomerulonephritis and most other causes of the nephrotic syndrome.

Many of these conditions can be diagnosed by the presence of characteristic symptoms and signs in addition to haematuria. On the other hand when haematuria is the sole or presenting symptom the cause is likely to be one of the following conditions:

Renal	*Bladder*	*Prostate*
tumour	papilloma	senile hyperplasia
calculus	carcinoma	carcinoma
tuberculosis		

When blood appears only at the beginning of micturition, the rest of the urine voided being clear, the source of bleeding is distal to the bladder. When blood is uniformly mixed with the urine, it may have come from any part of the urinary tract other than the urethra. Renal colic accompanying haematuria indicates that the bleeding is renal or ureteric in origin.

To establish the presence of small quantities of blood in the urine it is essential to examine microscopically the centrifuged deposit of a fresh specimen. If the specimen is not fresh, the hypotonicity of a dilute urine or the hypertonicity of a concentrated urine may destroy or deform the red cells. Even if the urine is obviously red it is necessary to demonstrate the presence of red cells microscopically, in order to distinguish haematuria from other rarer causes of discolouration of the urine with which there may be confusion. These are:

(*a*) Haemoglobinuria, which accompanies various rare intravascular haemolytic crises. The urine gives the chemical and spectroscopic tests for haemoglobin, but no red cells are present.

(*b*) Phenolphthalein in an alkaline urine. Phenolphthalein is an ingredient of many proprietary purgatives, and self-medication with alkalis and purgatives is common. As urine tends to become alkaline on standing it may turn pink if phenolphthalein is present. The addition of acid dispels the colour.

(*c*) Beetroot, senna, medicinal rhubarb, dyes used to colour sweets and a few other substances taken by mouth may redden the urine.

(*d*) **Congenital and intermittent porphyria.** These are rare diseases in which large amounts of porphyrins are excreted in the urine. Fresh urine from such cases may appear normal, but on standing for some hours a dark red colour may develop. In some cases the presence of porphobilinogen may be suspected from the red colour produced by the addition of Ehrlich's aldehyde reagent. In contrast to that produced by urobilinogen, this colour is not extracted by chloroform. The identification of such porphyrins, however, is too complicated for sideroom analysis, and urine should be sent to the laboratory for examination. The diagnosis should be suspected in the presence of one or more of the following clinical features: unexplained abdominal colic, polyneuritis and mental disturbance.

3. **Pus Cells and Bacteria.** Pus cells may be found in the urine in inflammation of any part of the urinary tract. Microscopical examination of the urine is the only method that can be recommended for their recognition. The urine should always be cultured when urinary tract infection is suspected. In obtaining the specimen for culture it is best to avoid catheterisation. A midstream specimen should be obtained from both male and female patients, and a culture should be made of this immediately. When this is not possible, the specimen should be refrigerated and sent to the laboratory within 24 hours.

4. **Urinary Casts.** Casts are cylindrical structures of microscopic size which are found in the urinary deposit. They are formed in the renal tubules by the coagulation of protein. Red blood corpuscles or epithelial cells may be impressed upon this matrix, producing blood and epithelial casts respectively; such casts are found in the early stages of acute glomerulonephritis and other diseases in which there is glomerular inflammation. Granular casts are formed by degeneration of the impressed cells. Epithelial and granular casts are indicative of inflammation and degeneration of the renal tubules. Hyaline casts, found in chronic glomerulonephritis and occasionally in very small numbers in normal urine, are formed by coagulated protein without the addition of cellular elements.

Although the number of cells and hyaline casts passed in the urine in the course of the day by the healthy adult is considerable, in practice microscopic examination of the centrifuged deposit reveals only an occasional cell or hyaline cast in each low power field.

5. **Bile and Urobilinogen.** These may also occur in the urine in abnormal amounts (p. 1003).

CHEMICAL ANALYSIS OF THE BLOOD

With progressive impairment of renal function the composition of the body fluids becomes abnormal. These abnormalities may be detected by blood analyses. The products of metabolism which in health are excreted in the urine are retained in the blood, and the concentration of urea, creatinine and the anions such as phosphate and sulphate increases. Determination of the concentration of blood urea gives a useful indication of the degree of renal failure, but it should be remembered that this does not rise above the accepted normal maximum until renal function is reduced by at least 50 per cent. The diminishing capacity of the kidneys to secrete hydrogen ions results in their accumulation in the blood, and the severity of the consequent metabolic acidosis may be estimated by measurement of the concentration of bicarbonate in the blood. Estimation of serum sodium, potassium, calcium and protein concentrations is of value in certain circumstances. A table of normal values for some blood constituents is given under 'Useful Data' (see end-paper).

POSTURAL PROTEINURIA

(Syn.: Benign Proteinuria; Orthostatic Albuminuria)

In a number of apparently healthy children and adolescents, and less commonly in adults, protein is excreted in the urine in variable but usually small amounts without associated disease of the kidneys. The urine formed while these individuals are recumbent is free from protein so that examination of the first specimen voided immediately on rising in the morning is normal. On the other hand urine formed while the individual is in the erect position or following exercise is found to contain protein. Tests of renal function show no abnormality.

There is evidence that the proteinuria in some cases is due to a rise in pressure in the renal veins produced by a kinking of the inferior vena cava as it passes through the diaphragm. It has been suggested that this kinking depends upon the forward rotation of the liver and the degree of fixation of the inferior vena cava to the posterior surface of the liver. Extreme lordosis while upright or recumbent produces proteinuria in the majority of young subjects. In others a reduction in blood flow known to occur on assuming the erect position may be an important factor. Hyaline casts, red cells, epithelial cells and leucocytes increase in proportion to the degree of proteinuria. Proteinuria of the orthostatic type is sometimes seen in the presence of renal disease. It should be regarded as a benign condition only if careful investigations fail to reveal any other abnormality.

GLOMERULONEPHRITIS

The term 'glomerulonephritis' is used to describe a bilateral disease of the kidneys which predominantly affects the glomeruli. In practice, cases can usually be placed in one of three clearly defined categories which are described below under the headings of acute proliferative, minimal lesion and membranous glomerulonephritis. In the past there has been difficulty in correlating the morbid histology with the clinical findings. The development of the technique of renal biopsy now permits a degree of clinico-pathological correlation hitherto unattainable. In the early stages of all three disorders the histological pictures are distinct. In cases of acute proliferative glomerulonephritis which fail to recover completely, and in the later stages of membranous glomerulonephritis which is a chronic disease, the morbid histological features become less clearly distinguishable. The fact that hypertension may accompany some stage of these two diseases complicates the pathology still further by the changes due to arteriolosclerosis. There is no evidence that the three types of glomerulonephritis are related aetiologically.

ACUTE PROLIFERATIVE GLOMERULONEPHRITIS

(Syn.: Ellis Type I Nephritis; Acute Nephritis; Acute Glomerulonephritis)

This condition is characterised by a diffuse inflammation of the glomeruli of both kidneys.

Aetiology. The great majority of cases of acute proliferative glomerulonephritis follow infection with haemolytic streptococci. This may occur as acute tonsillitis, scarlet fever or upper respiratory infection. The streptococcus responsible in the majority of cases has been shown to be Type 12 (Group A). A latent period is usual, the features of glomerulonephritis developing one to three weeks after the infection has subsided. A previous history of an acute infection is more commonly obtained in children than in adults. The infection may be slight and even pass unnoticed, and there is no relationship between its severity and the probability of the development of the disease.

The disease occurs most commonly in childhood and adolescence but can occur at any age. As in the case of acute rheumatic fever and scarlet fever, the condition has become less common in recent years.

Pathology. The earliest lesion is a diffuse inflammation of the glomerular capillaries with swelling and proliferation of the endothelial cells and accumulation of polymorphonuclear leucocytes in the tuft and the glomerular space. There may be proliferation of the outer layer of Bowman's capsule to form epithelial crescents. In the majority of cases these changes disappear with clinical recovery and the kidney returns to normal. In *progressive cases* the epithelial crescents which are believed to arise as a result of the presence of red blood cells and inflammatory exudate in Bowman's space, increase in size. Progressive fibrosis of crescents and glomeruli occurs and the glomerular capillaries gradually become obstructed, resulting in secondary degeneration in the tubules. Ultimately many nephrons may be replaced by fibrous tissue, leading to small contracted kidneys.

Pathogenesis. The time interval between infection and the onset of acute nephritis is reminiscent of that between the injection of therapeutic serum and the onset of serum sickness. This interval, and the absence of bacteria in the renal lesions and the urine, suggest that the disease has an immunological basis. This view is supported by recent developments in immunological techniques which have shown a diminution in the titre of serum complement and have demonstrated that antigen antibody complexes are deposited on the basement membrane.

Clinical Features. The onset may be insidious, but is usually abrupt, the most constant features being puffiness of the face, low urinary output and blood-stained urine. In addition there may be the general symptoms and signs of an acute infection, malaise, fever, anorexia, vomiting and headache. Breathlessness due to pulmonary oedema may be present and epistaxis may occur. Discomfort in the renal angles occasionally occurs. Subclinical cases may be discovered by routine examination of urine.

The pale puffy face gives an appearance which is almost pathognomonic. Oedema around the ankles may be detected if the patient is ambulant. In severe cases there may be extensive pitting oedema and effusions into the serous sacs.

The distribution of the retained fluid is probably determined by gravity and the striking oedema around the eyes is explained by the laxity of the tissues in this region.

The early appearance of generalised oedema, especially in the face, has given rise to a popular theory that there is generalised capillary damage throughout the body. The evidence suggesting this explanation has never been satisfactory, and it is now believed that the oedema is caused by fluid retention consequent on reduced filtration due to glomerular damage and to increased reabsorption of water and salt by the tubules. Congestive heart failure may sometimes be a contributory factor.

The cardiovascular system may be affected as indicated by hypertension, a rise in the jugular venous pressure, a slight outward displacement of the apex beat, a soft apical systolic murmur, reversed splitting of the second sound and bilateral basal crepitations.

In the *urine* the following changes are found at the onset:

1. Oliguria. The daily output is usually between 300 and 700 ml., due to reduction in the rate of glomerular filtration and increased tubular reabsorption. Anuria may occur in very severe cases.

2. Haematuria. The urine may appear red or smoky owing to the presence of blood.

3. Specific gravity. The urine is concentrated at least in the earlier stages, as tubular function is preserved and the specific gravity is high.

4. Proteinuria. This is of moderate degree, seldom exceeding 4 g. per day, but the amount of protein present is out of proportion to the haematuria.

5. Urinary deposit. Microscopic examination of the deposit reveals erythrocytes, some leucocytes, and red blood cell, epithelial and granular casts.

Retention of nitrogenous substances in the blood is common except in mild attacks. In a few cases hypertensive encephalopathy due to cerebral arteriospasm and oedema occurs. These attacks are characterised by headache, restlessness, transient blindness or paresis, vomiting and generalised convulsions. There is no correlation between the occurrence of the seizures and the degree of nitrogen retention in the blood. Retinal examination may reveal papilloedema, haemorrhages and exudates.

Course and Prognosis. *Complete recovery* occurs in over 90 per cent. of children who suffer from the disease. The prognosis is worse in adults and after middle age when complete recovery occurs in only about 50 per cent. of cases. In most instances the acute manifestations lessen in the course of three to four days, the temperature, pulse rate and blood pressure falling to normal. Diuresis occurs, and the oedema, haematuria and number of casts in the urine diminish. Small amounts of blood may be present in the urine for 10 to 14 days, while proteinuria may persist for several weeks or months.

In the rare very severe case, with marked hypertension, extreme oliguria and recurrent convulsions, death may occur within a few days from acute cardiac failure and pulmonary oedema or in two or three weeks from uraemia. Treatment by dialysis has improved the mortality in this group but it still remains high.

In a small number of cases the symptoms and signs persist for months or years. In some of these cases the proteinuria becomes massive and gross generalised oedema develops. Some authors call this stage subacute glomerulonephritis. Uraemia and acidosis slowly increase and the patient may die while oedema persists.

Latent Stage of Glomerulonephritis. In about 10 per cent. of cases the hypertension and haematuria subside and the patient apparently regains normal health. Proteinuria however persists, and after many years chronic glomerulonephritis with hypertension and renal failure develops.

Renal Function Tests. In the early stages renal concentrating power is usually unimpaired, and the specific gravity of the urine is high. The rate of glomerular filtration is reduced and the concentration of urea in the blood is raised. A moderate degree of acidosis is usual. When recovery occurs the filtration rate rises and the blood urea concentration falls to normal.

Diagnosis. Acute glomerulonephritis should be distinguished from:

1. Angioneurotic oedema, in which swelling of the eyelids is a frequent feature. This condition is usually associated with swelling of the lips or tongue, and urinary abnormalities are absent. In addition, the patient may be known to be an allergic subject, similar attacks may have occurred previously, and eosinophilia is often present.

2. Henoch-Schönlein purpura (p. 670) in which the hypersensitivity reaction often involves the glomeruli with resulting haematuria.

3. Polyarteritis nodosa and lupus erythematosus are both conditions which may involve the glomeruli with consequent haematuria and proteinuria. Red blood cells casts may also be found in the urine. Other organs of the body are usually involved in the pathological process, and the diagnosis of these two diseases is suspected on this basis. Polyarteritis nodosa and lupus erythematosus are occasionally confined to the kidney and renal biopsy is necessary to establish the nature of the condition.

4. Acute pyelonephritis, in which oedema is absent while pain and tenderness in the renal region and frequency of micturition are prominent. The urine contains micro-organisms, more pus cells than red blood cells and casts are absent or scanty.

5. Haematuria due to tuberculosis or tumours of the kidney or urinary tract. In these conditions oedema does not occur and there are no cellular casts in the urine.

6. Embolic nephritis due to subacute bacterial endocarditis, in which microscopic haematuria is a valuable diagnostic sign, and uraemia may develop.

7. Acute recurrent focal nephritis. This is a condition of unknown, but probably multiple aetiology in which recurrent episodes of haematuria occur over a period of months or years. There are no other symptoms or signs of acute proliferative glomerulonephritis or Henoch-Schönlein's purpura. The diagnosis is made by renal biopsy in which endothelial cell proliferation is found affecting only a proportion of glomeruli. Repeated episodes may lead to progressive glomerular destruction with renal failure and hypertension.

Treatment. There are three chief principles in the treatment of acute proliferative glomerulonephritis:

1. Rest and warmth. 2. Dietary regulation. 3. Antibiotic therapy.

Rest and Warmth. The patient should be kept warm in bed and protected from cold and draughts; rest in bed should be maintained until haematuria, hypertension, oedema and proteinuria have disappeared, and this may occur in from two to four weeks. Opinions vary as to how long rest in bed should be enforced in those cases which show persistent abnormalities in the urine beyond this time. When the patient feels well, but protein and red cells in the urine fail to show any diminution over a period of several weeks, it is doubtful whether further rest in bed is of benefit and the patient should be allowed up and encouraged to resume normal activities gradually.

Diet. There is no evidence that modifications of the diet make any significant difference to the *healing* process in nephritis, but protein restriction controls the degree of uraemia. Complete restriction of protein with an adequate caloric intake from carbohydrate and fat ensures minimum protein breakdown. For most cases, however, reduction of the protein intake to 20-40 g./day appears to be satisfactory.

In addition to protein restriction, treatment should be directed to maintaining fluid and electrolyte balance.

In cases of *mild to moderate* severity:

1. *Fluid* should be restricted while oedema is present to ½ litre per day plus the volume of the previous day's urinary output. If there is evidence of pulmonary oedema, fluid should be withheld entirely.

2. *Food* should be given in such quantities as the patient desires, but consisting mainly of carbohydrate and fat, e.g. bread, biscuits, cereals, jam, syrup, sugar and vegetables. Not more than half a pint of milk per day may also be taken. Sufficient protein is present in such foods to reduce the breakdown of body protein for essential needs to a low level (Diet 9, p. 1295).

3. *Salt* should not be used in cooking nor added to food. If the oedema is severe a low salt diet should be given.

In the occasional rare case of *severe* nephritis with anuria or extreme oliguria which shows no improvement on the measures mentioned above within three or four days, the regimen described on p. 825 should be adopted.

When hypertension and haematuria have subsided and diuresis has occurred, a light diet with a moderate restriction of protein (an egg at one meal and a small helping of fish, poultry or meat at another meal) is given for a few days before the resumption of a normal diet (Diet 10, p. 1296).

Antibiotic Therapy. Benzylpenicillin in doses of 500,000 units 12-hourly should be injected intramuscularly daily for five days. Residual streptococcal infection may thus be eliminated.

Treatment of Hypertension and Convulsions. This is similar to that of hypertension and hypertensive encephalopathy from non-renal causes and is discussed on p. 231.

Focal Sepsis. Removal of infected tonsils or other septic foci should be delayed until convalescence is advanced, as tonsillectomy may be followed by an exacerbation, especially if carried out during the acute stage. However, in a few cases of nephritis with persistence or repeated recurrence of symptoms and signs, these features may disappear only after the removal of a focus of chronic infection, e.g. apical teeth abscesses. It is important to search for these and other possible foci of infection. In the event of operative treatment being needed, penicillin should be given on the day of operation and for three days after it.

MINIMAL LESION GLOMERULONEPHRITIS AND MEMBRANOUS GLOMERULONEPHRITIS

(Syn.: Ellis Type II Nephritis)

Minimal lesion and membranous glomerulonephritis are conditions associated with an increase in the permeability of the glomerular basement membrane. This leads to proteinuria which is often so severe that hypoproteinaemia and oedema develop. They are described together because clinically they are usually indistinguishable.

Aetiology. The aetiology of both types of glomerulonephritis is unknown. Unlike acute glomerulonephritis neither disease is preceded by any recognisable infection. The possibility that an immune process plays a part is supported by some evidence but there is no proof that such a mechanism is primarily responsible for initiating the disease processes.

Pathology. Renal tissue obtained by biopsy shows two easily distinguishable lesions. In membranous glomerulonephritis the histological appearances consists of a diffuse hyaline thickening of the glomerular capillary walls with little or no evidence of inflammation. As the disease progresses the thickening becomes more severe and the glomerular tufts are converted into structureless hyaline tissue. In minimal lesion glomerulonephritis, the glomeruli show no lesion when examined by light microscopy. However, abnormalities of glomerular structure involving especially the epithelial cells are revealed by the electron microscope. The evidence suggests that this condition does not progress to glomerular destruction as is the case with membranous glomerulonephritis.

Clinical Features. The diseases are insidious in onset. If the proteinuria is slight they may persist without symptoms and remain undetected for months or years. When proteinuria increases in severity oedema occurs and it is in this way that attention may be drawn to their existence. The oedema is generalised, involving first the subcutaneous tissue and later the serous sacs and lungs. The face presents a pale and puffy appearance. The general health may remain good for some considerable time but eventually becomes progressively impaired, with increased liability to infection of the oedematous tissues or the serous cavities.

The urine contains protein in moderate amounts though as much as 30 g. may be excreted per day in occasional patients. Granular and hyaline casts are seen on microscopic examination, red cells being scanty or absent.

At first chemical examination of the blood shows little or no increase in nitrogenous end-products. Plasma cholesterol is raised commonly to 300-500 mg. per 100 ml. and the serum and ascitic fluid may look milky due to a coincidental increase in fat and β-lipoproteins. Total serum proteins are greatly reduced, e.g. to 3-4 g. per 100 ml. There are quantitative changes in the various globulin fractions, but the chief reduction affects the serum albumin. Proteins of larger molecular weight, especially α_2 globulin, are retained in the blood and hence are increased relatively to the other plasma proteins. The resulting fall in colloid osmotic pressure of the serum is mainly responsible for the massive oedema which is the prominent clinical feature. The ensuing oligaemia stimulates the secretion of aldosterone which promotes further electrolyte and water retention.

In the early stage of the diseases renal function tests reveal no impairment of glomerular filtration rate or of the ability to concentrate urine.

Course and Prognosis. In the majority of cases the oedema persists for months or years, with occasional spontaneous but temporary remissions. Prior to the use of effective diuretics, antibiotics and corticosteroids, recovery rarely occurred. The majority of patients died either from intercurrent infection in the oedematous phase or from renal failure. There is growing evidence that in patients with minimal lesion glomerulonephritis corticosteroid treatment causes the proteinuria to subside and the condition to resolve. In membranous glomerulonephritis, however, the prognosis is much less favourable. Arterial hypertension and hypertensive retinopathy develop and progressive renal destruction ultimately reduces the rate of glomerular filtration. Proteinuria diminishes, and consequently the serum proteins rise and oedema becomes less. There is gradual impairment of renal function as the disease progresses to chronic glomerulonephritis (p. 807) with uraemia.

Differential Diagnosis of the Nephrotic Syndrome. The term 'nephrotic syndrome' is sometimes used to describe the clinical state of hypoproteinaemic oedema associated with marked proteinuria irrespective of its aetiology. Minimal lesion glomerulonephritis is the most common cause of the nephrotic syndrome in children and is responsible for about 20 per cent. of cases in the adult. Membranous glomerulonephritis is more common in adults and both must therefore be distinguished from other renal disorders which give rise to a similar clinical picture. Sometimes the aetiology of the nephrotic syndrome is obvious from the presence of other clinical features of the causative disease. In many patients it is necessary to carry out a renal biopsy in order to make the diagnosis. Causes of the nephrotic syndrome other than these two types of glomerulonephritis are as follows:

(*a*) Acute glomerulonephritis is occasionally associated with heavy proteinuria and massive oedema. In many patients the clinical history and the course of the disease are sufficient to make this diagnosis clear, but in others the true nature of the syndrome is only detected after renal biopsy.

(*b*) The nephrotic syndrome associated with diabetic nephropathy is discussed on p. 771.

(*c*) Amyloid disease is usually secondary to rheumatoid arthritis, multiple myeloma, tuberculosis or chronic suppuration anywhere in the body. It gives rise to proteinuria as a result of the deposition of amyloid material in the glomerular capillaries. Renal biopsy is usually necessary to provide histological evidence of amyloid infiltration.

(*d*) Poisoning due to drugs, e.g. mercury, gold and troxidone.

(*e*) Renal vein thrombosis is a rare cause of the nephrotic syndrome. It should be suspected when proteinuria occurs in a patient with evidence of deep venous thrombosis in the lower limbs or if an illness is complicated by pain in the loins and the subsequent development of the nephrotic syndrome.

(*f*) Rarely the syndrome develops as the presenting feature in the course of disseminated lupus erythematosus. It also may occur in polyarteritis nodosa.

(*g*) Quartan malaria is an important cause of the syndrome in children in parts of Africa.

The nephrotic syndrome must also be distinguished from:

(*a*) *Congestive cardiac failure* with severe oedema, in which dyspnoea is prominent, the venous pressure is increased, signs of underlying cardiac disease are present, oedema is usually absent from the face, and proteinuria is less severe.

(*b*) *Chronic glomerulonephritis and nephrosclerosis*, in which oedema is due to congestive cardiac failure, resulting from hypertension, and there is impairment of renal concentrating power.

(*c*) *Hypoproteinaemic oedema*, due to causes other than loss of protein in the urine, namely failure of intake, digestion, absorption or synthesis of protein and in protein losing enteropathy.

In hepatic oedema in which ascites is usually out of proportion to the oedema elsewhere and proteinuria is slight or absent.

Treatment is directed toward the relief of oedema and the control of proteinuria.

1. *Relief of Oedema.* (*a*) Dietary protein. So long as the blood urea is not elevated, a liberal intake of protein is desirable in an attempt to make good the urinary loss of protein. At least 90-100 g. protein per day should be given. This may be supplemented with Casilan or Lonolac which are salt-free protein concentrates (Diets 7 and 8, pp. 1292 and 1293).

(*b*) Salt intake should be restricted by prohibiting extra table salt, avoiding salty foods and reducing the amount used in cooking. Although drastic salt restriction occasionally produces dramatic results, 'salt-free' diets are so unappetising that patients will not tolerate them for more than a few weeks.

(*c*) Diuretics are of great value in controlling the oedema. One of the thiazide group of diuretics, chlorthalidone or frusemide or ethacrynic acid given orally or mersalyl by injection may be equally effective (p. 191).

(*d*) If oedema is resistant to these measures relief is often obtained by giving plasma, salt-free albumin or dextran intravenously.

2. *Control of Proteinuria*. Corticosteroids (p. 547) provide the main chance of cure in the treatment of minimal lesion glomerulonephritis. In the great majority of cases this treatment abolishes proteinuria. Prednisone should be given in doses of 60-80 mg./day for about three weeks and then reduced to 20 mg./day and continued for at least six months. Corticosteroids are ineffective in membranous glomerulonephritis.

CHRONIC GLOMERULONEPHRITIS

Aetiology. Chronic glomerulonephritis is the terminal stage of progressive acute proliferative or membranous glomerulonephritis. In many cases, however, no history of either disease is obtained and in these, post-mortem studies of the kidney suggest that the pathological change has been developing insidiously over many years.

Pathology. The kidneys are small; the capsules strip with difficulty, leaving a granular surface; the peripelvic fat is increased and there is great reduction of parenchyma. The normal distinction between cortex and medulla is obscured. On *microscopical* examination there is fibrosis or hyalinisation of most of the glomeruli with fibrous replacement of many tubules. Remaining nephrons may show hypertrophy and arteriolosclerosis is usually present.

Pathogenesis. The clinical features of chronic glomerulonephritis are attributable to the effects of chronic renal failure combined usually with an arterial hypertension. As renal failure develops, the composition of the body fluid becomes abnormal, particularly with regard to its water and salt content, its acid-base equilibrium, and the concentration of nitrogenous compounds which are normally excreted by the kidney. These alterations ultimately combine to produce the clinical picture of severe uraemia which is the terminal stage of renal failure.

Clinical Features. A history of acute glomerulonephritis or of the nephrotic syndrome is obtained in some cases. The earlier stages of the disease may be unattended by symptoms but may come to light only by discovery of proteinuria or hypertension during the course of a routine examination. Later, because of the widespread consequences of renal failure, the symptoms and signs are referable to almost every system in the body and patients suffering from the disease present with complaints which at first sight may not suggest their renal origin. The patient may seek medical advice because of polyuria, nocturia, thirst, loss of energy, weakness, nausea, vomiting, or diarrhoea. Polyuria develops both because of diminished power for tubular reabsorption of water and because the elevated blood urea produces an osmotic diuresis. Anaemia is the main cause of the loss of energy and it is usually normocytic. The high blood pressure may have been detected in the course of a general examination or the patient may have sought advice for headache, loss of vision or breathlessness or because of the occurrence of cerebrovascular insufficiency.

As the disease progresses, renal function deteriorates and uraemia increases. The blood concentration of urea and other nitrogenous compounds steadily rises. The patient looks more ill and the complexion is sallow, often accompanied by a yellow-brown discolouration attributed to the retention of urinary pigment. With the exception of those who develop cardiac failure from hypertension and those in whom the chronic stage of membranous glomerulonephritis has followed rapidly upon the initial oedematous stage, the patients are not only free from oedema but usually exhibit signs of water and salt depletion. The skin and tongue are dry and the blood pressure may fall from its previous high level. Acidosis contributes to the dyspnoea and the respirations are deep (Kussmaul's respirations). Hiccough, muscular twitchings, fits, drowsiness and coma may occur. A tendency to bleed may develop in the terminal phase, as evidenced by epistaxis, bleeding gums, bruises, purpura, haematemesis and melaena. Hypertensive retinopathy of any degree may be present and visual impairment may result from numerous hard exudates arranged in star shape around the macula. Some patients complain of vague muscle or bone pain and in a few cases this becomes severe. Radiological examination occasionally reveals the appearances of osteomalacia, osteitis fibrosa (p. 712) and areas of osteosclerosis. Renal failure is associated with the development of resistance to the action of vitamin D and there is impaired absorption of calcium from the intestine. In young individuals this interferes with normal growth and the condition has been called renal rickets. Peripheral neuritis due to uraemia also occurs.

Laboratory Data. During the early stages of the disease, and before nitrogen retention in the blood is detectable, the urine is found to contain protein, usually in small amounts; red blood cells and granular and hyaline casts are present in small numbers. Glomerular filtration may be reduced to less than 10 per cent. of normal and there is a gradual rise in the concentration of plasma urea, creatinine and phosphates. The ability of the kidneys to form concentrated or dilute urine is impaired. Ultimately this power is lost completely and the urine is of a fixed specific gravity (1·010). The plasma concentration of bicarbonate diminishes as acidosis occurs. The serum concentration of sodium and calcium is frequently lowered. Potassium occasionally accumulates in the blood and is one of the factors causing death by its effect on the heart.

Course and Prognosis. The disease progresses steadily over months or years to a fatal termination. The course may be punctuated by exacerbations of acute proliferative glomerulonephritis which hasten the progress of the disease. When nitrogen retention and acidosis are severe, the outlook is grave and most patients die in a few months or a year. Papilloedema is a bad prognostic sign and unless treatment with hypotensive drugs is instituted before uraemia becomes severe, most patients who show it die within a few months. The cause of death is generally uraemia frequently complicated by infection to which such patients are extremely susceptible; in other cases the patient dies from a cerebral haemorrhage, congestive cardiac failure or myocardial infarction. A terminal non-bacterial pericarditis is common. Haemorrhage from any site or enterocolitis is also an ominous feature.

Diagnosis. The distinction between chronic glomerulonephritis and other causes of chronic renal failure with hypertension is difficult and may be impossible. A similar clinical picture may also arise in the following diseases.

1. Other conditions which primarily affect the glomeruli with their eventual destruction include polyarteritis nodosa, lupus erythematosus, amyloid disease and diabetes mellitus. Patients suffering from these conditions may die ultimately of renal failure and uraemia.

2. Essential hypertension may occasionally lead to nephrosclerosis and uraemia. This should be suspected if there is a clear family history of high blood pressure; also in the malignant phase of hypertension from any cause evidence of renal disease is invariably present and renal failure is rapidly progressive.

3. Congenital polycystic disease of the kidneys, which may be diagnosed by the family history, by palpation of the enlarged, firm and irregular kidneys and by pyelography.

4. Chronic pyelonephritis, which is more common in women, and hypertension may be absent. There may be a history of acute pyelonephritis and organisms can sometimes be cultured from the urine.

5. Bilateral hydronephrosis, in which diagnosis may be confirmed by retrograde pyelography.

6. Congenital renal hypoplasia with bilateral small kidneys is occasionally the cause of death from uraemia in children.

Treatment. Although the natural history of the disease cannot be altered and there is progressive deterioration in renal function, the patient's health and feeling of well-being may be considerably improved with suitable treatment.

Food. When there is nitrogen retention the onset of severe uraemia may be delayed by restricting protein intake to 40 g. per day and by ensuring an adequate caloric intake from carbohydrate and fat (Diet 9 p. 1295). In the later stages when the blood urea concentration rises to 200 mg./100 ml. further protein restriction to 20 g./day is indicated. It is best to provide this as first class protein in the form of meat, milk and eggs and to avoid protein of lesser biological value in vegetables and cereals.

Fluid. Fluid restriction is contraindicated since, in view of the impaired concentrating power, a large volume of urine is needed to excrete end-products of metabolism. Except in the presence of congestive cardiac failure a fluid intake sufficient to produce at least 2½ litres of urine per day should be advised.

Salt. In the absence of oedema, congestive cardiac failure or arterial hypertension, salt restriction is contraindicated. In a few cases of chronic nephritis there is an excessive loss of salt in the urine due to a failure of tubular reabsorption, and this may be aggravated by an enforced high fluid intake. Water and salt depletion occur and this aggravates the uraemia (p. 842). Clinical improvement will result in such cases from the addition of 5-10 g. salt per day. The limit to the additional salt is set by the occurrence of systemic or pulmonary oedema, or by an aggravation of the hypertension. Sodium bicarbonate should be substituted in part for sodium chloride when acidosis is severe and giving rise to symptoms.

When nausea, vomiting or coma make it impossible to control water and salt depletion and acidosis by oral administration, fluid and electrolytes should be given by intravenous infusion. The volume of fluid required depends upon the severity of the salt and water depletion and the degree of acidosis (p. 843). An average amount for a case of moderate severity is 5 litres given in 24 hours, one part of isotonic sodium bicarbonate, two parts of normal saline and two parts 5 per cent. dextrose. The infusion should be continued until the bicarbonate concentration of the blood has been increased, if possible to within the normal range and until the patient is adequately hydrated.

Miscellaneous. Obvious foci of infection, e.g. tonsils, infected sinuses or root abscesses should be removed in order to reduce the likelihood of an exacerbation of acute glomerulonephritis. Anaemia should be treated by slow blood transfusions though it is probably not desirable to increase the concentration of haemoglobin above 60 per cent., as a rapid rise in blood viscosity is apt to cause a fall in renal plasma flow and a temporary aggravation of the uraemia; oral or parenteral iron therapy is ineffective unless there is evidence of a complicating iron deficiency. Intractable nausea, hiccoughing or vomiting may be relieved with chlorpromazine (25 mg. intramuscularly). Treatment of cardiac failure or cerebrovascular accidents may be required in the late stages. If bone pain is severe and if the dominant radiological picture is that of osteomalacia vitamin D should be given orally in doses of up to 300,000 units daily for some weeks. The treatment should be controlled by chemical estimations of serum calcium and alkaline phosphatase, for there is a significant risk of producing hypercalcaemia and calcification of the tissues. The presence of uraemia is no contraindication to the treatment of co-existing hypertension provided that care is taken to see that hypotensive treatment does not cause a rise in the concentration of blood urea. The choice and use of drugs should be made according to the recommendations given on p. 239.

If the patient's health continues to deteriorate in spite of all these measures, it is doubtful whether one should insist on withholding a more liberal diet.

Within the last two years it has been possible to preserve the life of some patients with chronic renal failure who are virtually devoid of all renal function by repeated intermittent haemodialysis. Facilities for this form of treatment are likely to increase in the future. The practicability of transplantation of a normal kidney from a healthy donor or a cadaver to patients with chronic irreversible renal failure is also under active investigation at the present time. Discrete enquiries should be made concerning the existence of an identical twin. If the healthy twin is willing to act as a donor the prospects of renal transplantation being successful are good and very much better than renal transplants from other sources.

URINARY TRACT INFECTION

Infection of the urinary tract is an extremely common clinical problem. The infection may be considered to involve the urethra, the bladder, the ureters and the kidneys themselves. In any individual case it is difficult on clinical grounds to be certain of the extent of the invasion of the various parts of the urinary tract. In recent years the tendency has been to assume that the kidneys and the upper urinary tract are involved in every case, even when the symptoms of the infection are those solely of cystitis or urethritis. However, many patients develop recurrent symptoms of lower urinary tract infection without apparently suffering deterioration of renal function in later life.

ACUTE PYELONEPHRITIS (ACUTE PYELITIS)

This is characterised by an acute inflammation of the parenchyma and pelvis of the kidney. The term 'pyelitis' is still frequently used, but the inflammation involves the renal tissue as well as the pelvis. The disease may be unilateral or bilateral.

Pathology. The renal pelvis is acutely inflamed and there is often a coincident inflammation of the bladder. In those cases with macroscopic involvement of the renal parenchyma, groups of small abscesses may be seen on the surface of the kidney when the capsule has been stripped. On section, small cortical abscesses and linear streaks of pus in the medulla are often evident. On histological examination a focal infiltration of the renal parenchyma by polymorphonuclear cells is evident.

Aetiology. Acute pyelonephritis is an infection commonly associated with some obstruction in the urinary tract. In view of the importance of preventing chronic pyelonephritis, the existence of a predisposing lesion should be suspected in every case. In men this is commonly due to prostatic enlargement, in pregnant women to obstruction by the uterus and atonia of the ureters due to the action of progesterone, and in children to congenital malformation of the urinary tract. Calculi, foreign bodies or tumours may also be responsible. Pyelonephritis may occur in infancy and in adult women, however, without evidence of an obstructive lesion. The infection ascends in most cases via the ureter and in some it is blood borne. About 75 per cent. of the infections are due to *Esch. coli*, the remainder being mostly due to streptococci, staphylococci or the Proteus group of organisms.

The predominance of urinary infections in the female suggests that the anatomical relation of the short urethra to the rectum is a predisposing factor. Catheterisation of the bladder is particularly liable to introduce organisms into the urinary tract, and this procedure may be responsible for the later development of acute or chronic pyelonephritis in some patients. Catheterisation should be reduced to the minimum and when indicated should be carried out with strict antiseptic precautions.

Clinical Features. In many cases there is a sudden onset of pain in one or both loins, radiating to the iliac fossae and suprapubic area. There may be dysuria (difficult or painful micturition) and strangury (a painful desire to pass urine though the bladder is empty), with the frequent passage of small amounts of scalding, usually cloudy urine, due to an associated cystitis. The temperature rises rapidly to 38°C.-40°C., with the general manifestations of fever. A rigor may occur, and there may be vomiting. Tenderness and muscular guarding may be present in the renal angle and the lumbar region. There is a leucocytosis. The urine in *Esch. coli* infections is nearly always acid; in other infections it may be acid or alkaline. On microscopic examination there are numerous pus cells and organisms, some red cells and epithelial cells. When the organisms are motile gram-negative bacilli and the urine is acid in reaction, the infection may be assumed to be due to *Esch. coli*.

Acute pyelonephritis may occur with few or no symptoms referable to the urinary tract. This is particularly the case during pregnancy. Routine culture of a midstream specimen of urine has revealed the presence of asymptomatic bacteriuria in about 7 per cent. of all pregnancies during the early months. If no antibiotics are given progression to acute pyelonephritis occurs in about 40 per cent. of such cases, and this is rare in those in whom the urine was sterile at the original examination. Investigation by intravenous pyelography after the termination of pregnancy shows a high incidence of abnormalities of the urinary tract in those women with bacteriuria. Suppressive chemotherapy at the asymptomatic stage has been found to prevent the development of acute symptoms and progressive renal damage.

Pyelitis in children, like infections of the throat and middle ear, often presents as a fever without any localising symptoms. The initial feature may be a convulsion. In the feverish child, particular attention should be paid to these sites and the urine should be examined routinely for pus cells and organisms.

Diagnosis. Acute pyelonephritis should be distinguished from:

1. Acute appendicitis, salpingitis, cholecystitis and diverticulitis, especially by the absence of pus and organisms in the urine.
2. Diaphragmatic pleurisy, with or without pneumonia. Pain

is usually made worse by coughing or a deep breath. Tenderness with guarding similar to that occurring in pyelonephritis may be present, but there are no abnormalities in the urine and abnormal physical signs may be detected in the chest.

3. Perinephric abscess due to infection by *Staph. aureus*. The illness is severe and the characteristic clinical features are pain and tenderness in the renal region, high remittent fever and polymorphonuclear leucocytosis. Urinary symptoms are absent and there are usually no pus cells or organisms in the urine. Oedema may obliterate the normal hollow in the loin, and an abscess may eventually point in the loin or groin, or it may rupture into the peritoneal or pleural cavity. Careful enquiry frequently elicits the history of a recent boil.

Course and Prognosis. With adequate treatment the disease subsides rapidly in the great majority of cases. Fever, pain, frequency and dysuria disappear in a day or two. The urine usually becomes sterile within a few days.

In some cases, although the acute symptoms subside, a low-grade infection may persist, and the disease may pass into the chronic stage. More rarely the disease may be severe and cause necrosis of the papillae (acute necrotising papillitis). Fragments of renal tissue are then excreted in the urine and can be identified histologically. This complication, which may lead to renal failure, is particularly liable to occur in diabetic patients and in those addicted to phenacetin. In view of the frequency of acute pyelonephritis, the curable nature of the condition, and the fact that chronic pyelonephritis is a common cause of renal failure and hypertension, the importance of adequate treatment of the acute stage cannot be overstressed.

Treatment. The patient should be confined to bed and the general measures for the treatment of fever applied (p. 18). The precise treatment will depend upon the infecting organism and its sensitivity, and a midstream specimen of urine should be sent to the laboratory before treatment is begun. Since infection is usually due to *Esch. coli* it has been customary for many years to start treatment with sulphadimidine in doses of 1 g. three times a day after a loading dose of 2 g. before the results of urine culture are available. Although this therapy was justified prior to the introduction of antibiotics which were bactericidal to infection of the urinary tract, the prescription of sulphonamides, especially for such a potentially dangerous disorder as pyelonephritis, is debatable. It is true that the majority of cases of urinary tract infection due to *Esch. coli* respond excellently to sulphadimidine and that the drug is much cheaper than cycloserine. On the other hand the sulphonamides are bacteriostatic drugs to which an increasing number of strains of *Esch. coli* are becoming resistant. Undesirable toxic effects are infrequent with both sulphadimidine and cycloserine but even less so with the latter. For these reasons many authorities believe that cycloserine is the drug of choice for the treatment of pyelonephritis and that it should be given in doses of 250 mg. twice daily for 14 days for initial treatment, while awaiting the report of the sensitivity of the infecting organism to various antibiotics. A second midstream specimen of urine should be sent to the laboratory from four to six weeks after the completion of the initial course of treatment to make sure that the infection has been eradicated. If this has not been accomplished further treatment with the appropriate antibiotic must be given, depending on the bacteriological findings. The midstream specimen must reach the laboratory within two hours of voiding or be refrigerated at 4° C. for a period not exceeding 24 hours. Cycloserine should not be given in the presence of renal failure as it accumulates in the body and may cause convulsions. In the very severe case and if septicaemia occurs kanamycin is the drug of choice. Ampicillin is of value in proteus infections and carbenicillin (p. 74) in infections with *Ps. pyocyanea*.

In every case the possibility of calculus, renal tuberculosis or an obstructive lesion of the urinary tract must be considered and treated if found.

CHRONIC PYELONEPHRITIS

Aetiology. The disease may follow an attack of acute pyelonephritis which has been inadequately treated. It may be caused also by infection above an obstruction to the urinary tract e.g. calculus, stricture or prostatic disease. Other cases may follow cystitis due to stasis as a result of cystocele or interference with the innervation of the bladder, e.g. in paraplegia or disseminated sclerosis. *Esch. coli* is the organism responsible for most cases. Other infecting agents are proteus, *Pseudomonas pyocyaneus*, staphylococci, etc. In conditions in which the outflow tract of the bladder is deranged, reflux of urine into the ureters may occur during micturition. The question as to whether vesico-ureteric reflux occurs in the absence of such pathological lesions is unknown but if it does it is not clear to what extent it contributes to the development of pyelonephritis. Chronic pyelonephritis also occurs in conditions leading to nephrocalcinosis (p. 829).

Pathology. The changes may be unilateral or bilateral, and of any grade of severity. The fully developed case usually shows gross scarring of the kidneys, which may be much reduced in size with narrowing of the cortex and medulla. Microscopically there is patchy fibrosis with chronic inflammatory cell infiltration, tubular atrophy, periglomerular fibrosis and eventual disappearance of nephrons. The arteries and arterioles may show sclerosis and narrowing.

Clinical Features. In many cases no symptoms arise directly from the renal lesions, and the patient may consult the doctor because of lassitude, tiredness and vague ill-health or for symptoms of uraemia or arterial hypertension. The discovery of hypertension or proteinuria on routine examination may be the first indication of the presence of the disease. Symptoms arising from the urinary tract, however, may also be present and include frequency of micturition, dysuria and occasionally aching lumbar pain. The urine may contain pus cells, a small amount of protein and many epithelial cells, though in some cases it may be normal.

Diagnosis. In all cases of chronic pyuria, investigations such as rectal or vaginal examination, cystoscopy and pyelography must be carried out to discover the nature of any underlying mechanical factor causing obstruction to the flow of urine and to determine the extent of the infection. Chronic pyelonephritis should be distinguished from renal tuberculosis by cystoscopy, pyelography and bacteriological examination of the urine. In the later stages, when hypertension and uraemia have developed, the condition may be difficult to distinguish from chronic glomerulonephritis and nephrosclerosis. The presence of pus and organisms in the urine and a past history of frequency and dysuria support the diagnosis of chronic pyelonephritis. Full investigation may be required, as listed on p. 786.

Course and Prognosis. The course is usually a long one and may be punctuated by acute exacerbations. The infection is difficult to eradicate, even when underlying mechanical obstructions are found and relieved. Some cases progress to chronic uraemia, which may be alleviated for a year or two by treatment. In elderly people, in diabetic patients and in cases of tabes dorsalis or paraplegia, the infection may become fulminating and be the immediate cause of death.

Complications. Hypertension and uraemia have been discussed above. Pyonephrosis may occur, especially in the presence of renal calculi. It is characterised by persistent lumbar pain, intermittent pyrexia, often with rigors, emaciation, pyuria, and, if both kidneys are involved, uraemia. One or both kidneys may become palpable.

Treatment. Medical treatment of chronic pyelonephritis is similar to that described for the acute disease. The chronic infection is usually more difficult to eradicate. Attempts should be made to remove obstructive lesions or renal calculi by appropriate surgical procedures. A bactericidal antibiotic to which the organism is sensitive should be given for 14 days (p. 816). If the infection is not eradicated suppressive antibiotic treatment may be required for many months, the antibiotic used being indicated by the changing pattern and sensitivity of the organisms in the urine. Ampicillin and cycloserine are of the greatest value for this purpose. A moderate degree of uraemia may be present which progresses little for months or years. This is especially so when hypertension is absent or minimal; in such cases salt and water depletion is often present due to failure of tubular reabsorption, and this aggravates the uraemia (p. 842). Considerable benefit may result from an additional intake of salt as described under chronic glomerulonephritis (p. 811). When the renal infection is unilateral or if pyonephrosis has developed, nephrectomy may be indicated; rarely, high blood pressure may be cured by the removal of the diseased kidney.

CYSTITIS, URETHRITIS AND THE URETHRAL SYNDROME

Reference has already been made to the possibility that some infections of the urinary tract may be confined to the urethra or bladder. In these the features of systemic illness are slight and the symptoms are those of frequency and dysuria. Intense scalding pain is felt in the urethra during micturition. Suprapubic pain of cystitis is felt before, during and a few moments after voiding urine. Although the bladder is empty there may be an intense desire to pass more urine (strangury), due to spasm of its inflamed wall. Tenderness is often present in the suprapubic region, and the urine may have an unpleasant odour and appear cloudy. Pus cells, red cells and organisms may be seen on microscopical examination of the urine. Sometimes the urine is grossly bloodstained. Cystitis is particularly common in women and young girls, and the infection is usually due to *Esch. coli*.

Investigation for a possible predisposing cause is essential though this is found in only a minority of cases. This may entail digital examination of the prostate and bladder and gynaecological examination. Cystoscopy, must be postponed until the acute condition has subsided. If there is reason to suppose that the kidneys are also involved, the examination should proceed with ureteric catheterisation with the collection of samples of urine from each kidney, and retrograde pyelography.

Therapy is similar to that of acute pyelonephritis. In the majority of instances this is effective and there is no recurrence of the symptoms. In some patients, however, the clinical features of infection persist or recur.

The possible causes of failure to respond to treatment, or of relapse, are:

1. Infection with organisms resistant to the chemotherapeutic agent employed.

2 Tuberculosis, with or without secondary infection.

3. Continued infection from above, e.g. pyelonephritis associated with calculi.

4. Obstruction below the base of the bladder by:

(*a*) prostatic hyperplasia, carcinoma of the prostate, or urethral stricture in the male;

(*b*) chronic urethritis or stricture in the female.

5. Involvement of the bladder by:

(*a*) malignant tumour arising in the bladder or in adjacent organs;

(*b*) vesical calculus; foreign bodies may have been inserted into the bladder;

(*c*) inflammation from adjacent structures, e.g. diverticulitis of the colon.

6. The presence of urethral caruncle, cystocele, urethrocele or cervicitis in the female or a meatal fissure in the male. The latter may be noted as a tender induration on examination of the meatus.

7. Paraplegia, in which urinary infection is frequent, persistent and often the ultimate cause of death.

In some patients with symptoms suggestive of urethritis and cystitis, no organism can be cultured from the urine. The term 'urethral syndrome' has been applied to this category of patients who are predominantly female. The cause of the symptoms is unknown although a variety of explanations, which include allergy, congestion of the urethra possibly related to sexual activity and infection of the urethral glands, have been put forward. In Reiter's syndrome an unexplained urethritis may be associated with arthritis, conjunctivitis and sometimes diarrhoea (p. 543).

RENAL FAILURE AND URAEMIA

Introduction. The term 'uraemia' has been used for more than a century to describe the clinical state which arises from renal failure. The retention of abnormal amounts of urea in the blood in renal disorders was amongst the early discoveries resulting from the application of biochemical methods to the elucidation of disease and the symptoms of chronic renal failure were long attributed to it. The newer knowledge of renal physiology has shown that as renal function becomes impaired other complex biochemical changes occur and that these are probably more responsible for the clinical features of uraemia than the elevation of blood urea. These changes include disturbances in hydrogen ion concentration and abnormalities in water and electrolyte balance. In addition, renal failure is accompanied in the majority of cases by arterial hypertension, and this fact complicates still further the clinical picture and renders difficult any attempt to ascribe symptoms and signs to their basic cause.

Classification. Uraemia is invariably the consequence of impairment of renal function. This commonly results from disease affecting the renal parenchyma and this form of uraemia is called *renal uraemia.* The renal failure may be acute or chronic. A wide variety of conditions give rise to acute renal failure *with structural renal damage* and these include acute proliferative glomerulonephritis, acute severe bilateral pyelonephritis, malignant hypertension, polyarteritis nodosa, renal involvement in lupus erythematosus and eclampsia. Chronic renal failure arises as a result of diseases which destroy tissue more slowly, e.g. progressive proliferative glomerulonephritis, the late stages of membranous glomerulonephritis, chronic glomerulonephritis and chronic pyelonephritis, bilateral hydronephrosis, polycystic disease, hypertension, diabetic nephropathy, amyloid infiltration, tuberculosis and conditions causing hypercalcaemia.

Acute uraemia occurs also in patients in whom initially there is no primary parenchymal renal disease but in whom acute circulatory failure leads to sudden reduction in renal blood flow: this reduces the capacity of the kidneys to perform their functions normally. This occurs in states associated with water and salt depletion, shock, haemorrhage, etc. (p. 822). Since the origin of the uraemia is not directly related to renal disease, the terms *prerenal* or *extrarenal uraemia* have been applied to it. With appropriate treatment this type of uraemia is reversible and the prognosis is generally good. In a proportion of cases of prerenal uraemia due to acute renal circulatory failure, renal ischaemia may be so severe and prolonged as to produce necrosis of the renal parenchyma. When the necrosis affects only the tubules the condition is called *acute tubular necrosis.* More rarely the whole of the renal cortex is involved, the glomeruli as well as the tubules becoming necrotic. This has been called *renal cortical necrosis.*

Impairment of renal function arises also in conditions in which there is obstruction to the renal tract, e.g. senile hyperplasia of the prostate. This type of uraemia is called *post-renal uraemia* and is described on p. 827.

CHRONIC RENAL FAILURE AND URAEMIA

The clinical features and treatment of renal uraemia occurring as a result of chronic glomerulonephritis have been described on pp. 808 and 810. The clinical features of renal uraemia occurring in the course of other chronic kidney diseases are similar.

PRERENAL URAEMIA

The performance of normal renal function is dependent upon the maintenance of an adequate renal circulation. The renal share of the cardiac output is normally about 25 per cent. at rest. If the cardiac output falls the renal blood flow is disproportionately reduced. In this event, the glomerular filtration rate is reduced and oliguria results. While systemic hypotension often precedes prerenal uraemia, it appears that renal ischaemia may occur in its absence. Regional vasoconstriction is a means by which the blood pressure may be maintained in the face of oligaemia, and the success of this mechanism may deprive the kidneys of a large part of their blood supply. The urine that is formed is small in volume and the concentration of urea in the blood gradually rises. The more common causes of prerenal failure include:

1. *Loss of blood* from any cause including complications of pregnancy, trauma or gastrointestinal bleeding. This should be treated by blood transfusion.

2. *Loss of plasma* as in burns and crushing injuries. This should be treated by intravenous infusions of plasma or dextran.

3. *Loss of fluid*—

(*a*) *From the gut* in severe vomiting, diarrhoea, acute intestinal obstruction, paralytic ileus and fistulous drainage.

(*b*) *In the urine* in diabetic coma and Addison's disease.

(*c*) *From the skin* in excessive sweating (heat stroke).

4. General anaesthetics and surgical operations reduce renal blood flow and may precipitate renal failure in those whose blood volume is precariously balanced.

5. Serious infections, especially septicaemia from *Esch. coli*, may produce shock, and reduce renal blood flow.

All these conditions should be treated by appropriate fluids given intravenously and by specific measures as indicated in the treatment of diabetic ketosis, Addison's disease, infection, etc. Prompt and effective replacement of blood, water and salt is essential. In many cases vigorous treatment in the early stages prevents the occurrence of significant degrees of renal failure. If oliguria or anuria persists in spite of the return of the blood pressure to normal, acute tubular necrosis must be assumed to have occurred and should be treated accordingly.

ACUTE RENAL FAILURE AND URAEMIA DUE TO ACUTE TUBULAR NECROSIS

Acute renal failure with tubular necrosis is a disease affecting both kidneys, characterised by anuria or oliguria with low specific gravity urine and rapidly developing uraemia.

Much of the earlier information about acute renal failure was obtained from studies of the 'crush' syndrome which occurred during the air raids of the Second World War.

Aetiology. Acute tubular necrosis occurs as a complication of various conditions which are associated with marked hypotension, arteriolar constriction and severe dehydration, and which are listed as causes of prerenal uraemia on p. 822.

In other cases acute tubular necrosis develops unattended by any general circulatory disturbance. It occurs in some instances for example following incompatible blood transfusion or during acute haemolytic crises; it is also occasionally seen in patients with obstructive or hepatocellular jaundice, severe infection and septicaemia. Certain drugs are also capable of producing acute renal failure. These include sulphonamides and mercury given as organic mercurial diuretics. Poisoning by substances, such as sodium chlorate, which produce renal parenchymal necrosis, may also be responsible.

Pathogenesis. Severe shock and water and salt depletion are accompanied by generalised vasoconstriction. Renal ischaemia results from the hypotension and afferent arteriolar vasoconstriction. If the ischaemia is severe and of sufficiently long duration, focal necrosis of the renal tubules occurs. The pathogenesis of renal tubular necrosis in cases unassociated with severe circulatory disturbances is not fully understood though it is believed that renal ischaemia may result from regional restriction in the renal blood flow with maintenance of the systemic blood pressure. In other cases, e.g. following mercurial diuretics, sulphonamides or sodium chlorate, direct damage to the renal parenchyma from toxic or allergic reactions is responsible.

Clinical Features and Course. The clinical features of acute renal failure are those of the causal condition together with oliguria or anuria. Any urine that is formed contains protein, casts and red and white blood cells. The specific gravity is usually about 1·010 early in the course of the disease, and this persists for several days or weeks. At first the patient may feel well, but after some days the features of uraemia appear. Initially these are anorexia, nausea and vomiting; apathy is followed by mental confusion and later muscular twitching, fits, drowsiness, coma, and bleeding episodes occur. At this stage the main dangers to life are pulmonary oedema due to the injudicious administration of excessive amounts of fluid, potassium intoxication due to the rise in the concentration of serum potassium which is especially likely if there is haemolysis or massive soft tissue damage, the occurrence of severe systemic infection to which such patients are highly susceptible, and uraemia itself.

The anuric or oliguric phase of the disease usually lasts for one to three weeks. If the patient does not succumb the daily volume of urine increases and may rapidly reach several litres. This is called the diuretic phase and coincides either with healing of the renal tubules or reduction in intrarenal tension. During this phase there is uncontrolled water and mineral loss, and sometimes flaccid paralysis due to loss of potassium occurs in the absence of treatment. The concentration of blood urea ceases to rise and then gradually falls. Virtually complete recovery of renal function then takes place slowly over a period of three to six months.

Treatment

1. *Causal Condition.* With a view to preventing or minimising the renal lesion, the underlying cause should be treated urgently and the appropriate repair solutions administered.

2. *Oliguria or Anuria.* The treatment of oliguria or anuria due to tubular necrosis has undergone many changes, and it is of some interest to review these alterations and the reasons for them. Formerly treatment was based upon the crude assumption that the kidneys could be forced to secrete urine by giving large amounts of fluids intravenously or by the use of osmotic diuretics such as sodium sulphate. There seems little doubt that the high mortality which varied from 60-90 per cent. was largely due to these procedures.

It is now evident from clinical and pathological studies that during the oliguric phase, filtration at the glomerulus is much reduced and necrotic lesions are present in the tubules. Both defects are usually reversible provided the patient can be kept alive for this period of time. Treatment is designed to minimise the need for renal function until healing occurs. In the anuric and oliguric phase uraemia is delayed by providing calories largely in the form of sugar, thus reducing protein metabolism to a minimum. Water balance is maintained by replacing the obligatory loss through the skin and lungs, estimated at 600 ml. per day, and no electrolytes are given, since none are being lost from the body.

Use is made of the knowledge that an intake of 100 g. of sugar per day has a maximum protein sparing effect and enables the body to utilise its own fat stores. If more sugar can conveniently be given, some of the weight loss will be prevented but endogenous protein metabolism will not be further depressed. The recommended treatment for an adult therefore consists of giving 100-300 g. lactose in 500 ml. of water daily by mouth or stomach tube. Lactose is preferable to glucose because it is less sweet and less nauseating. If dependent oedema or pulmonary crepitations are present or appear during treatment, the quantity of water should be reduced. In the event of vomiting, oral treatment should be replaced by 50 g. of fructose in 500 ml. of water infused through polythene tubing introduced through a peripheral vein. Instead of glucose, 10 per cent. fructose is recommended because it is less liable to produce venous thrombosis.

Water and salt depletion due to vomiting or diarrhoea should be treated by isotonic saline and by the appropriate amount of isotonic sodium bicarbonate (p. 863). The latter is indicated only if the concentration of bicarbonate in the blood is greatly reduced. In febrile patients an extra allowance of water is required to replace fluid lost through visible perspiration and a further small supplement equal to the volume of urine passed each day should be added. No salt is given during the oliguric phase.

In many patients in whom the acute renal failure is mild in degree and relatively short in duration this treatment prevents the blood urea from rising more than 20 mg. per 100 ml. per day, and the accumulation of potassium from protein catabolism is usually not sufficient to have serious consequences. When the oliguria is more prolonged this regimen is tiresome for the patient and unsatisfactory since it does not prevent continuing loss of weight. For this reason it is now customary to add 20 g. of first class protein to the diet with the object of relieving its monotony and helping to preserve the composition of the body (p. 462). In suitable cases this does not significantly increase the uraemia. If considerable elevation of serum potassium level occurs attempts should be made to reduce it, employing cation exchange resin. A sodium or calcium charged resin which removes potassium from the body should be given orally in doses of 30 g. three or four times per day. If the patient becomes nauseated and vomits, the resin may be given by retention enema. Treatment should be controlled by repeated serum electrolyte determinations. If a suitable resin is not available a temporary fall in serum potassium concentration can be achieved by giving 20 units of soluble insulin subcutaneously and an intravenous infusion of 50 g. of glucose.

In some patients, however, and especially in those suffering from severe infection or massive tissue damage, or in whom blood has become loculated in one of the tissue spaces, the rate of rise of blood urea and potassium is much more rapid and life is threatened from uraemia within a few days. The conservative measures already described are then insufficient and the patient should be transferred to a centre equipped with the means for extracorporeal dialysis (artificial kidney). Multiple haemodialyses may be required over a period of several weeks before renal function returns. Peritoneal dialysis has recently been advocated as an alternative to haemodialysis. While this method has a place in the treatment of a moderately severe case or in small children, it is a prolonged, uncomfortable and sometimes painful procedure.

Diuresis. When diuresis commences, a light diet, containing not more than 45 g. protein per day and ample fruit, should be provided (Diet 9, p. 1295). Sufficient fluid must be given to replace the uncontrolled loss of water in the urine. The fluid intake must be increased by the volume of the previous day's urinary output. Salt supplements are usually needed during the diuretic phase to compensate for increased urinary loss. On average about 3 g. of sodium chloride and 2 g. of sodium bicarbonate are needed for each litre of urine passed. The fruit usually compensates for the potassium loss, though in many cases a supplement of potassium chloride by oral administration may also be required.

As the blood urea concentration returns to normal values and renal function improves a normal diet may be taken.

Patients with severe acute renal failure are seriously ill and require skilled nursing, preferably in single rooms designed to prevent aerial or contact infection. Great care must be exercised in the use of drugs which are normally excreted by the kidneys.

Prognosis. The high mortality accompanying acute renal failure with tubular necrosis has been greatly reduced by the measures described above. Prognosis depends upon the speed and efficiency with which the therapeutic measures are put into operation, the prompt recognition and effective treatment of complicating infection, and the nature and the severity of the condition precipitating the syndrome.

POST-RENAL URAEMIA

Uraemia may result from obstruction at any point in the urinary tract. This obstruction may occur:

(1) *In the ureters*, due to calculi, peri-ureteral fibrosis or congenital ureteral achalasia, malignancy, severe urinary tract infection with blockage due to pus, blood clot or the precipitation of crystals, e.g. sulphonamide, or to accidental ligation at operation.

(2) *At or below the outlet of the bladder*. This is commonly due to benign enlargement or carcinoma of the prostate gland, and less often to other obstructions such as urethral stricture or congenital abnormalities.

When the obstruction is distal to the bladder the following effects are liable to arise:

1. Because of the failure to empty the bladder completely, there occur (*a*) progressive enlargement and hypertrophy of the bladder with diverticulum and calculus formation; (*b*) hydro-ureter and hydronephrosis; and (*c*) atrophy of kidney parenchyma with progressive uraemia if the obstruction is not relieved.

2. Obstruction is sooner or later followed by infection behind the block. Hence cystitis, ascending pyelonephritis and pyonephrosis develop.

Diagnosis. The diagnosis may be suggested by a history of previous urinary symptoms such as pain in the loins, haematuria, renal colic, nocturia or difficulty in micturition. In the event of obstruction distal to the bladder, clinical signs include:

1. Enlargement of the bladder, evidence of which can usually be seen or felt on examination of the abdomen.
2. Alteration in the size or consistency of the prostate, which may be assessed by digital examination through the rectum.
3. The presence of residual urine in the bladder after the patient has voided, as detected by radiography after intravenous pyelography or by catheterisation.

If these features are not present and the obstruction is within the ureters, cystoscopy and ureteral catheterisation will be required to establish the diagnosis.

Treatment. Surgical treatment is required for all cases of post-renal obstruction. Uraemia may be severe, yet relief of the obstruction followed by a high fluid intake results in recovery of adequate renal function in many patients, provided that this treatment has not been delayed too long.

RENAL HYPERTENSION AND UNILATERAL RENAL DISEASE

The frequent occurrence of hypertension in patients with bilateral parenchymal renal disease has been recognised for many years. As has been described above its occurrence influences adversely both the course and the prognosis of renal disease and is reflected in the pathological appearances of the kidneys themselves. Unilateral renal disease, though a rare cause of hypertension, is also recognised as being capable of producing severe elevation of the blood pressure which may be remedied by nephrectomy. It is now recognised that surgical treatment is likely to be of value only when the renal lesion causes under-perfusion of the kidney (renal ischaemia). Renal artery stenosis commonly due to atheromatous plaques in the main renal artery in the elderly and to fibromuscular dysplasia in the young or chronic pyelonephritis with endarteritis in the intrarenal arteries are the most frequent causes of unilateral renal ischaemia. The presence of these lesions should be suspected if there is a history suggestive of pyelonephritis or renal trauma, in malignant hypertension, or if a systolic murmur is heard over the upper rectus abdominis or over the low thoracic regions posteriorly. Intravenous pyelography may show features of chronic pyelonephritis or renal ischaemia with reduction in kidney size, contraction of the calyces, delayed appearance of dye and increased concentration of the contrast medium within the pelvis. In both conditions the radiohippuran renogram shows evidence of disparity in function. Nephrectomy or surgical reconstruction of the renal artery should be considered in young hypertensive patients in whom these investigations and the estimation of function in each kidney have demonstrated unilateral ischaemic disease. Over the age of 40 years renal artery stenosis may be a secondary feature of the hypertension rather than its primary cause, and treatment with hypotensive drugs is the therapy of choice in the majority of patients.

RENAL AND VESICAL CALCULI AND NEPHROCALCINOSIS

Aetiology. Urinary calculi have long presented fascinating aetiological problems which are still largely unsolved. Two or three centuries ago vesical calculus was so common in Britain that a respectable living could be made as a lithotomist, but the incidence is much lower at the present time for reasons that are not known. It is indeed surprising that renal and vesical calculi or nephrocalcinosis do not occur more frequently since some of the constituents of urine are present in a concentration in excess of their maximum solubility in water. It seems likely that urine contains certain substances, e.g. mucoproteins, hyaluronic acid and citric acid, which, by forming complexes, keep otherwise insoluble salts in solution in the urine. Other authorities believe that the primary cause of urinary calculi is a pre-existing renal or vesical lesion which acts as a nidus on which urinary constituents precipitate. The following conditions are frequently associated with stone formation: (*a*) climate or occupation which necessitates living or working under conditions where excessive loss of water from sweating occurs, thus causing constituents to be precipitated because of their high concentration in the diminished volume of urine excreted ; (*b*) urinary infection and stagnation; (*c*) conditions leading to hypercalciuria which increases the liability to the formation of stones consisting mainly of calcium phosphate and calcium oxalate. These include idiopathic hypercalciuria, prolonged immobilisation, hyperparathyroidism, Cushing's syndrome, sarcoidosis, multiple myeloma and vitamin D intoxication. Calcium phosphate stones tend to occur in alkaline urines and this may be an important factor determining their occurrence in idiopathic renal acidosis and in some patients with chronic pyelonephritis; (*d*) certain rare congenital abnormalities, e.g. cystinuria and primary hyperoxaluria, which may lead to the production of cystine or oxalate stones respectively; (*e*) conditions causing increased excretion of uric acid, e.g. gout and leukaemia; (*f*) dietary factors such as an excessive intake of milk or absorbable alkali.

Since the constituents of renal and vesical calculi are present in numerous articles of food it is not surprising that physicians have long believed that diet must be of aetiological importance. In support of this view are many experimental investigations in animals which have shown that by increasing the calcium content of the diet and reducing the intake of vitamin A, renal and vesical calculi can be produced regularly. Likewise, the remarkable fall in the incidence of vesical calculi in children and young adults, which occurred in Britain in the nineteenth century, coincided with a marked improvement in the nutrition of the nation. Against this view is the undoubted fact that in Britain and other prosperous countries renal calculi occur frequently in well nourished, healthy young men in whom the most careful clinical and laboratory investigations frequently reveal no cause for stone formation.

Pathology. Urinary concretions vary in size from particles like sand to large round stones and staghorn calculi which fill the whole renal pelvis and branch into the calyces. Such stones are usually associated with hydronephrosis and chronic pyelonephritis. Deposits of calcium may also be present throughout the renal parenchyma, giving rise to nephrocalcinosis. This is especially liable to occur in cases of hyperparathyroidism, renal tubular acidosis, vitamin D intoxication, and in healed renal tuberculosis.

Clinical Features. These vary according to the size, shape and position of the stone, and the presence and nature of the underlying condition. Renal calculi or nephrocalcinosis may be present for many years and yet themselves give rise to no symptoms. While nephrocalcinosis never gives rise to pain, the most common complaint arising from renal calculi is an intermittent dull pain in the loin or back, increased by movement or a sudden jolt. Some abnormal constituents of the urine, e.g. red cells, protein or pus cells, can be found at one time or another in most cases. When a stone is small enough to enter the ureter and large enough to obstruct it, an attack of renal colic develops. The patient is suddenly aware of pain in the loin, which soon radiates round the flank to the groin and often into the testis or labia in the sensory distribution of the 1st lumbar root. The pain steadily increases in intensity to reach a maximum in a few minutes. The patient is restless, and generally tries, unsuccessfully, to obtain relief by assuming various positions, both lying and sitting, and by pacing about the room. There is pallor, sweating, and often vomiting, and the patient may groan in agony. Frequency and haematuria may occur. Without treatment the intense pain usually subsides within two hours but may continue unabated for several hours or some days. In many cases the pain is constant during the attack, though slight fluctuations in severity may occur. Contrary to what is often believed, it is rare for attacks to consist of intermittent severe pains, coming and going every few minutes for some hours.

Diagnosis. When renal colic occurs the diagnosis is usually easily made as it can be established by the history and by the finding of red cells in the urine. All patients suspected of having renal calculus, including those with renal colic, should have a radiological examination of the urinary tract, including retrograde pyelography in some instances. If there is doubt about the cause of the abdominal pain, an intravenous pyelogram during the attack may be helpful. When the pain is due to a stone in the ureter, the radiograph shows a dense renal shadow with delay in the appearance of the dye in the renal pelvis. Appropriate investigations should be undertaken to discover the presence of any underlying condition which might be responsible for the development of renal calcification or lithiasis.

Prognosis. This varies greatly depending on the underlying cause and on whether the patient passes the stone in the urine or whether it continues to obstruct the ureter. In the latter case, if the stone is not removed surgically, hydronephrosis and pyelonephritis are likely to develop in time.

Treatment and Prevention. The immediate treatment of renal pain or renal colic is rest in bed, the application of warmth to the seat of pain, and the administration of analgesic drugs, e.g. pethidine (100 mg.) or morphine (15-30 mg.), and antispasmodic drugs, e.g. atropine sulphate (0·8 or 1·2 mg.). These should be injected subcutaneously and may be repeated within two hours. Attempts to dissolve calculi in the kidneys have not been successful. Stones in the renal pelvis and urinary bladder must be removed surgically. Stones in the ureter usually pass naturally if left alone and surgical removal is apt to be followed by stricture and its complications. When, however, pain persists or frequent bouts of pain become intolerable, the insertion of a ureteric catheter is often followed by the passage of the stone. Urgent surgical intervention is necessary in the event of anuria. It is also required if the stone has not moved for some months and hydronephrosis is developing or there is continuing infection in the urinary tract. A stone larger than 1 cm. in diameter generally requires surgical removal. Suitable medical or surgical measures should be instituted for the correction of any primary cause of renal lithiasis that may have been discovered.

With regard to dietary restrictions prescribed with the object of preventing the formation of further stones, opinion is now in favour of the view that with certain exceptions mentioned below these are not likely to achieve any worthwhile results. In addition dietary restrictions cause considerable inconvenience and possible harm to the patient. This view is based first on the fact that it is now known that the urinary output of calcium and of oxalates and urates, which are common constituents of stones, depends more on endogenous metabolism than on exogenous sources. Secondly, since stones seldom consist of a single substance, the dietary treatment of mixed stones presents grave practical difficulties. Two possible exceptions must be mentioned: first, the elimination of rhubarb and spinach from the diet, articles which have a very high content of oxalate, may be worthy of trial in patients with recurrent oxalate stones; the other exception is the avoidance of liver, kidney, sweetbreads, fish roe, sardines and sprats, articles with a very high purine content, by persons who have passed several uric acid or urate stones, as occurs sometimes in gouty persons or in patients with leukaemia. Even if the above dietary restrictions fail to alter the course of the disease, they at least cause little or no inconvenience or hardship. Since the distribution of phosphorus occurs so widely in foodstuffs, dietary restriction for the treatment of phosphatic calculi is unlikely to be of any value. Phosphatic calculi are found only in alkaline urine, hence acidifying the urine by administering ammonium chloride daily may be effective. In contrast, cystine and urate stones may be prevented or sometimes dissolved by making the urine persistently alkaline, especially if combined with a high output of urine.

Lastly, the most important therapeutic and prophylactic measure for all forms of stones is the provision of an adequate fluid intake as this helps to flush out from the urinary passages particles of gravel which in time may develop into calculi. A daily output of urine of at least 3 *l.* is advisable; hence the intake of fluid should be approximately 4 *l.* daily. If the climate or the patient's occupation causes much sweating the fluid intake requires to be greatly increased.

POLYCYSTIC DISEASE OF THE KIDNEYS

Polycystic kidney disease is a genetically determined abnormality of renal structure and is often associated with other congenital abnormalities, e.g. cystic liver.

The condition may be found during infancy, but symptoms often do not develop until adult life. Both kidneys are affected, are several times the normal size, and consist of masses of cysts with a variable amount of renal parenchyma which often shows extensive fibrosis and arteriolosclerosis.

The clinical features include pain in the renal angles, haematuria, uraemia and usually a slowly developing arterial hypertension. Often one or both of the kidneys can be palpated and the surface may be nodular. When renal failure is present polyuria occurs, with urine of fixed specific gravity. Marked retardation of growth and bone changes simulating rickets are found in children. In course, prognosis and treatment, the disease resembles chronic glomerulonephritis, and death occurs in middle age from uraemia, cerebrovascular accident or cardiac failure.

RENAL CARCINOMA

Renal carcinoma is the most common tumour of the kidney. This was formerly called a hypernephroma on the mistaken view that it arose from adrenal rest tissue within the kidney. Haematuria is the most frequent presenting feature and blood clots may give rise to renal colic. Sometimes the tumour causes vague abdominal pain and it may also be responsible for long continued fever. Occasionally patients present first with symptoms arising from metastatic foci in the lungs, liver or bones. On rare occasions polycythaemia occurs, and this is believed to be due to excessive production of erythropoietin (p. 605). The diagnosis may be suspected from the history or the tumour may be palpable. Radiological investigation is usually essential, and aortography may distinguish the filling defect from that due to a simple cyst. Early surgical treatment affords the only prospect of cure.

HYDRONEPHROSIS AND PYONEPHROSIS

In hydronephrosis, the pelvis of the kidney dilates as a result of obstruction of the urinary tract. An aching pain may be felt in the back, flank or occasionally in the hypochondrium, and haematuria may occur. Some cases are symptomless and the renal swelling is detected on routine examination of the abdomen. Surgical treatment is necessary to remove the obstruction, and in many cases nephrectomy is required.

Pyonephrosis is an infected hydronephrosis. The clinical features are similar to those of acute pyelonephritis, but in addition the kidney may be palpable. Chemotherapy and surgical relief of the obstruction or nephrectomy are required.

In addition to hydronephrosis and less frequently pyonephrosis, other diseases in which the kidneys may be palpable are polycystic disease, solitary cyst, renal carcinoma and other tumours. It should be remembered however that in some normal people all of the right kidney, and occasionally the lower pole of the left kidney may be felt on clinical examination. This is particularly true in women. On the other hand, pathologically enlarged kidneys are not always palpable. When a kidney can be felt, however, it may be possible to appreciate departures from the normal size, smooth surface and firm consistency.

RENAL TUBERCULOSIS

Tuberculosis of the kidney is invariably secondary to tuberculosis elsewhere in the body and occurs as a result of blood-borne infection. It is rarely encountered at the present time. The initial lesion develops in the renal cortex and if untreated may ulcerate into the pelvis with consequent involvement of the bladder, epididymes, seminal vesicles and prostate. The disease tends to occur in young people and may manifest itself with recurrent haematuria and dysuria due to secondary involvement of the bladder. In addition the general features of tuberculosis, i.e. malaise, fever, lassitude and weight loss, may be present. Culture of the urine by ordinary methods may be sterile in spite of pyuria. The extent of the infection should be ascertained by cystoscopic examination, by retrograde pyelography, and by culture of the urine from both ureters. Combinations of streptomycin, para-aminosalicylic acid and isoniazid should be given as for tuberculosis elsewhere in the body (p. 425). Partial or complete nephrectomy may be necessary in those in whom the disease has advanced to the stage of producing serious destruction of renal tissue with cavitation.

CERTAIN PRESENTING CLINICAL FEATURES ARISING FROM DISEASES OF THE URINARY TRACT

Pain. Renal pain is experienced only when the disease process involves the pelvis or stretches the renal capsule; there is no pain associated with the nephrotic syndrome, chronic glomerulonephritis, nephrosclerosis or malignant hypertension, in all of which there may be gross disease and destruction of kidney substance. Occlusion of a renal artery or one of its main branches is sometimes painful, though most infarcts of the kidney are painless. Pain sometimes occurs in acute glomerulonephritis and is probably due to acute distension of the renal capsule. Pain is commonly present in perinephric abscess, acute pyelonephritis and pyonephrosis, and it may occur with chronic hydronephrosis or stone in the renal pelvis. It is sometimes a symptom of polycystic disease, tumour or tuberculosis of the kidney. The pain in all these conditions is felt mainly in the back, between the 12th rib and the iliac crest. When a calculus or other material such as blood clot or caseous matter obstructs the ureter, renal colic may occur. This is one of the most painful conditions encountered in medical practice (p. 830).

Frequency of Micturition. The most common cause of frequency of micturition occurring in the absence of dysuria and as a sole complaint is anxiety. The desire to urinate occurs especially at times which are most inconvenient, such as at social functions. The symptom may fluctuate in severity from time to time, and there may be great variability in the quantity of urine that can be retained. The absence of nocturia or of nocturnal enuresis (bed-wetting) is evidence that bladder capacity is normal and that there is no organic disease to account for the frequency. In these cases there are no chemical or microscopic abnormalities of the urine. It should be noted, however, that when, as commonly occurs, insomnia is associated with anxiety, frequency may persist during the night.

Two important organic causes of frequency occurring as a sole complaint are:

1. Pregnancy, especially during the first 12 weeks and near full term.
2. Any condition causing partial obstruction distal to the bladder, e.g. pressure on the urethra from fibroids or retroverted gravid uterus, urethral stricture, hyperplasia or carcinoma of the prostate.

Blood in the Urine. The passage of red or dark urine subsequently found to be due to the presence of blood usually indicates serious disease of the urinary tract and a cause must always be sought. Any of the conditions given on p. 793 may be the cause of macroscopic haematuria. In practice, however, the majority of cases presenting with haematuria as the sole or major symptom are due to a small number of diseases of the urinary tract whose diagnosis can be readily established.

Unpleasant or foul-smelling urine. Patients sometimes report that their urine smells unpleasantly. There are two main causes.

1. Infected urine without other symptoms. This is diagnosed by microscopic and bacteriological examination of the urine, and the case is investigated and treated along the lines already indicated. *Esch. coli* imparts a fishy odour to the urine, whereas in most other infections there is an ammoniacal smell.

2. Concentrated urine. The smell may be noticed, for instance, by the mother of a feverish child. If the urine is normal on examination the cause may be explained to the patient or mother.

It is worth while noting that when asparagus has been eaten the urine may have the unpleasant smell of methyl mercaptan.

PREVENTION OF DISEASES OF THE KIDNEY AND THE URINARY TRACT

In recent years the incidence of acute proliferative glomerulonephritis has considerably diminished. This is probably due to a combination of factors which include the wider use of antibiotics in the treatment of streptococcal infections in the respiratory tract, and improved social conditions. However, since acute glomerulonephritis may follow a slight throat infection for which the patient does not attend a doctor, prophylactic chemotherapy is not always practicable. In any case neither chemotherapy for tonsillitis nor tonsillectomy necessarily prevents the subsequent development of acute nephritis. Accordingly there is little hope of preventing these attacks until more is known of the unusual reaction of the body to infection which occurs in this condition and of the factors which determine the prevalence and spread of haemolytic streptococci. However, in the event of an epidemic of streptococcal infection with a nephritogenic strain occurring in a closed community, the prophylactic administration of penicillin should be given to all contacts and to streptococcal carriers.

There is no known method of preventing minimal lesion or membranous glomerulonephritis. The liability to develop diabetic nephropathy may be reduced by careful control of the diabetes. When the nephrotic syndrome is due to amyloid infiltration of the kidneys secondary to tuberculosis or other infection, adequate treatment of the latter may reverse the process of amyloid infiltration to some extent with great improvement in the clinical state.

With regard to prevention of infections of the urinary tract, the early diagnosis of the cause and the complete elimination of the infection are very important factors in preventing the development of chronic pyelonephritis. This is of particular importance in the asymptomatic urinary tract infection in pregnancy. All pregnant women should be screened with routine culture of mid-stream specimens of urine. Suppressive chemotherapy should be given to those in whom organisms are found in the urine. Reference to the section on Renal Calculi and Nephrocalcinosis will indicate various prophylactic measures of value in this condition. Acute renal failure may be prevented in some cases by prompt action to restore the blood pressure in hypotension. The incidence of polycystic disease might be reduced by appropriate genetic advice. The frequency of carcinoma of the urinary bladder could be reduced by precautions in the gas, dye and rubber industries, and possibly by giving up cigarette smoking.

A large consumption of phenacetin has been held responsible for the development of chronic renal failure in some patients, particularly in Scandinavia and the United States of America. Until more information is available it is wise to avoid giving phenacetin to patients with chronic renal disease or pyelonephritis and to endeavour to withdraw the drug from those who have become habituated to it.

Finally, the adequate and early investigation of a symptom such as haematuria frequently leads to the discovery of the causal condition at a stage amenable to radical cure.

J. S. ROBSON.
E. B. FRENCH.

Books recommended:

Black D. A. K. (1967). *Renal Disease*, 2nd ed. Oxford: Blackwell.
de Wardener, H. E. (1967). *The Kidney*, 3rd ed. London: Churchill.

DISTURBANCES IN WATER AND ELECTROLYTE BALANCE AND IN HYDROGEN ION CONCENTRATION

WATER AND ELECTROLYTE BALANCE

THE chemical events, collectively called metabolism, require the concentration of hydrogen ions and electrolytes to remain within narrow limits within the tissue cells and in the fluid which bathes them. Derangement of water and electrolyte balance and disturbances in hydrogen ion concentration occur in a wide variety of clinical conditions which are separately described in the appropriate chapters of this book. It is convenient, however, to summarise here the relevant physiological facts and to describe briefly the more common abnormalities.

THE NORMAL DISTRIBUTION OF WATER AND ELECTROLYTES

Water. The body of a normal man of 65 kg. contains approximately 40 litres of water. About 28 litres of this is intracellular, and 12 litres extracellular. The latter is composed of 9-10 litres of interstitial fluid and 2-3 litres of plasma. Using tritiated water, it has been shown in human subjects, that water readily passes through all membranes of the body and permeates easily into all fluid compartments. Its final distribution between the compartments is determined by osmotic and hydrostatic pressures and under normal conditions the total amount of water in the body is kept remarkably constant in a dynamic equilibrium.

Electrolytes. The inorganic ions dissolved in the body water include sodium, potassium, calcium, magnesium, chloride, phosphate, bicarbonate and sulphate. These are not dispersed in the same concentrations throughout the various body fluid compartments. Sodium and chloride are confined mainly to the extracellular fluids where they are present in average concentrations of 142 m.Eq/*l.* and 100 m.Eq/*l.* respectively. These ions contribute the major part of the total osmolar concentration of the plasma and extracellular fluids. Potassium, magnesium, phosphate, and sulphate are present in highest concentration inside the cells where they maintain the osmolar concentration analogous to that of sodium and chloride in the extracellular fluids. Potassium is present in extracellular fluid in a mean concentration of only 4·5 m.Eq/*l.* and magnesium in a concentration of about 2 m.Eq/*l.* Bicarbonate is found in the fluid outside the cells and in the tissue cells themselves in concentrations of 25 m.Eq/*l.* and 10 m.Eq/*l.* respectively. Hydrogen ions are present in a concentration of only 40 nanoEq/*l.* They are present within cells at a higher concentration than in the extra-cellular fluids.

Because of the permeability of the capillaries, the concentration of electrolytes in the plasma and in the extracellular fluids in the tissue spaces is very similar. Interchange between these extracellular compartments is limited, however, in respect of protein molecules, the concentration of the latter being many times greater in the plasma than in the interstitial fluid. The volume of the plasma is largely the resultant of hydrostatic pressure which tends to force water outwards, and the osmotic pressure of the plasma proteins which draws water back into the vascular bed. In spite of the differences in the ionic pattern inside the cells as compared with that of the fluid which bathes them, under normal conditions the osmotic pressure is believed to be identical in extracellular and intracellular fluids. The differences in composition are established and maintained by the activity of ionic pumps within or near the cell membrane and are essential to life.

DISTURBANCES IN WATER AND ELECTROLYTE BALANCE

The complexity of the composition of body fluids is reflected in the variety of disturbances that may occur in them either as a result of disease processes or as a consequence of therapeutic endeavour and drug administration. Such disturbances not only contribute to the clinical picture of many diseases, but are themselves a hindrance to recovery. As a result, much of modern therapy is directed towards maintaining the chemical composition of the body fluids and correcting as far as possible any derangements that may arise. It is important that these disturbances are recognised and adequately treated. The labelling of many such abnormalities simply as 'dehydration' and the indiscriminate use of intravenous 'normal' saline in an attempt to correct them is to be deprecated. The more common disturbances in water and electrolyte balance are as follows:

1. Salt depletion.
2. Water depletion.
3. Potassium depletion.
4. Potassium intoxication.
5. Magnesium deficiency and intoxication.
6. Water intoxication.
7. Sodium and water accumulation.

1. Salt (sodium) Depletion

Normal salt balance depends upon an equality between the amount of sodium excreted and the amount ingested. In health and in temperate climates negligible amounts of sodium are lost in the stools and from the skin. In the absence of renal disease the power of the kidneys to conserve sodium in the face of reduced intake is considerable and normal salt balance may be maintained with a very small daily intake. For these reasons salt depletion generally occurs because of excessive loss of salt from the body rather than because of inadequate intake.

Because of the intimate relations of salt and water balance, loss of sodium is usually accompanied by a corresponding reduction in the water content of the body. *Pure* salt depletion unattended by significant water loss is rare and probably occurs only as a result of abnormal loss of salt and water when an unrestricted intake of water has been permitted or encouraged. This may arise, for example, from excessive sweating in unfavourable environments when fluid loss is replenished by salt free liquids. In these circumstances the change in total body water may be negligible in spite of a considerable deficit of body salt. More commonly, however, conditions giving rise to sodium depletion are attended by proportionate water loss and unless large amounts of salt-free fluids have been given, the depletion is really a *mixed* one, though the salt loss usually predominates over the water loss.

Causes of salt depletion. In temperate regions predominant salt depletion arises as a result of excessive loss of salt in the urine or because of increased loss of sodium-containing fluids from the gastrointestinal tract. These are as follows:

1. Failure of the kidney to conserve salt may develop because of intrinsic renal disease or inadequate hormonal control. Examples are found in some patients with pyelonephritis (i.e. 'salt-losing nephritis'), the diuretic phase of acute renal failure of ischaemic origin, Addison's disease and to a lesser extent in hypopituitarism. Excessive loss of salt in the urine together with water loss occurs in the osmotic diuresis of uncontrolled diabetes mellitus. If diabetic ketosis and acidosis develop, urinary sodium loss is further increased as the mechanism for hydrogen/sodium ion exchange is unable to cope with the severer degrees of acidosis (p. 784). Salt depletion may also be induced by the excessive or prolonged use of diuretic drugs.

2. Gastrointestinal causes of salt depletion include all conditions involving external loss of salt-containing fluids, i.e. acute or chronic diarrhoea, intestinal fistulae, aspiration of gastrointestinal contents and vomiting.

Consequences of predominant salt depletion. Because sodium is predominantly extracellular, salt depletion quickly reduces the volume of the extracellular fluids. Any disproportionate loss of salt to that of water tends to render the extracellular fluids hypotonic. This tendency however is mitigated by two events. (1) The volume of water excreted in the urine is initially increased in order to restore the normal total osmolar concentration. (2) Some extracellular water migrates into the cells so that the threatened extracellular dilution is minimised. As a result, there is a further diminution in the volume of extracellular fluid, including plasma, while the water content of the cells may even increase. The fact that predominant salt depletion chiefly affects the volume of the extracellular fluid is responsible for many of the clinical features such as loss of elasticity of the skin, diminution of intra-ocular pressure and dryness of the tongue. Thirst is not a prominent complaint, and its absence may be due to the hypotonicity of the body fluids. The decrease in blood volume leads to a fall in blood pressure and in the rate of glomerular filtration; oliguria then occurs. The capacity of the body to rid itself of urea diminishes and prerenal uraemia develops (p. 822). The pulse rate rises. Selective vasoconstriction diminishes the circulation through the skin so that the skin and the limbs become cold. Vomiting and anorexia are common and these add to the difficulties of oral treatment. Although the serum sodium concentration may be within normal limits, in severe cases it may be reduced to 120 m.Eq/*l*. or less.

Treatment. The administration of water or of glucose in water in conditions associated with salt depletion is fraught with danger because the hypotonicity may be further aggravated. As more salt-free fluid is given, the kidneys respond by the excretion of large volumes of dilute urine in an attempt to restore the normal osmolar concentrations. The ill-effects of such treatment, moreover, are all too easily obscured by the conventional fluid balance chart which records only water intake and urine output, without reference to sodium balance. Adequate treatment consists of giving salt and water by mouth or isotonic saline intravenously. The latter is required in all but very mild cases with normal blood pressure. Two to three litres of normal saline given intravenously in two hours represents average adult requirements. In the more severe cases with marked circulatory impairment deficits equivalent to 4-8 litres of normal saline occur. Such deficits should be repaired largely by normal saline (0·9 g. per cent. NaCl). The first 2-3 litres should be given rapidly within the first two to three hours, the remainder being given within 24 to 48 hours. The best guides to the amount required are the disappearance of the clinical signs of salt depletion and the restoration of blood pressure and pulse rate and pressure. Serum sodium determinations are useful in controlling the treatment of severe cases, especially when the causative disease is likely to lead to continued salt loss (e.g. severe and persisting diarrhoea). Excessive administration of saline is to be avoided; the bases of the lungs should be frequently examined in order to detect crepitations, and the neck veins should be inspected carefully in order to detect an increase in venous pressure.

Severe salt depletion is almost invariably associated with water depletion and disturbance in acid-base balance. Frequently potassium balance and occasionally magnesium metabolism are also disturbed (p. 850). When accompanied by these disturbances the treatment of salt depletion requires to be modified accordingly.

2. Primary Water Depletion

Pure or predominant water depletion is one of the simplest of chemical disorders. The water content of the body is reduced both absolutely and relatively to the salt content, and the osmolar concentration of the extracellular fluids tends to rise. Between 600 and 1,000 ml. of water is lost daily from the body in the expired air and by evaporation from the skin. This daily loss continues irrespective of the water intake. The urine is the other main channel of excretion of water but its volume can be reduced if necessary by increasing its concentration up to a limit determined by renal concentrating ability and the amount of solute to be excreted.

Causes of water depletion. Primary water depletion occurs less commonly in clinical practice than salt depletion. In contrast to salt depletion it usually arises because water intake is reduced below an amount necessary to maintain balance. This is liable to occur in patients who suffer from dysphagia or have obstructive lesions of the oesophagus or more simply in those who are comatose, depressed or apathetic, as is common, for example, in the aged. Water deficit then occurs because the intake falls below the amount being lost from the lungs and the skin. This obligatory daily loss of water from the lungs and skin is increased by hyperpnoea or pyrexia. Excessive loss of water in the urine is a rare cause of water depletion but occurs in patients in whom the renal power of concentration is restricted, as for example in diabetes insipidus, hyperparathyroidism and other diseases associated with hypercalcaemia and potassium depletion, and in water-losing nephritis.

Consequences of water depletion. As water is lost from the body the extracellular fluid becomes hypertonic. Water then migrates from the cells in accordance with this increase in osmotic pressure and intracellular dehydration occurs. The overall body water loss is thus shared by the extracellular and intracellular fluids. For this reason the symptoms and signs of dehydration are not so obvious as those of salt depletion. Thirst is usual unless the patient is senile or confused. The migration of water from the cells to the extracellular fluids helps to maintain the volume of the extracellular fluid within normal limits for a time, so that the blood pressure, packed cell volume and serum and blood concentrations remain unaltered until considerable depletion has occurred. The patient, however, may exhibit mental confusion or complain of vertigo and difficulty in swallowing. In severe cases the skin and tissues acquire a curious 'doughy' consistency. Ultimately renal blood flow is reduced and the blood urea concentration rises. The serum sodium concentration and the packed cell volume become elevated.

Treatment. Water depletion should be treated by giving salt-free fluids. The use of 'normal saline', which is isotonic with the blood but which contains sodium and chloride in greater concentrations than those occurring in plasma is contraindicated. If the patient is conscious and is not vomiting, water should be given by mouth until thirst is quenched and thereafter in amounts of between 1,500 ml. and 2,500 ml. per day are usually sufficient. If the patient is unable to swallow fluids in sufficient amounts, 5 per cent. glucose in water should be given by intravenous infusion. The amount required varies with the degree of depletion. In moderately severe cases 2-4 litres of 5 per cent. glucose in the course of 24 hours is usually sufficient. In severe water depletion 5-10 litres may be needed. The best guides to the amount of fluid required are the clinical improvement of the patient and the increase in the volume of urine, which should rise to about 1,500 ml. per 24 hours. If water depletion is due to water losing renal diseases, it may be necessary to continue administering large daily amounts of water.

It must be remembered that when water depletion is associated with salt loss, isotonic saline and water are both required and should be given together in relative amounts determined by clinical assessment of the degrees of the two deficiencies.

3. Potassium Depletion

The extent to which potassium depletion is responsible for various clinical features in a wide variety of diseases has only been fully appreciated in recent years. Depending upon the daily intake, the healthy individual in potassium balance excretes about one-third of his daily potassium intake in the stools and two-thirds in the urine. The bulk of urinary potassium is secreted by the cells lining the distal renal tubules into the tubular lumen. These cells exchange potassium or hydrogen ions for sodium filtered by the glomerulus.

Causes of potassium depletion. Potassium depletion occurs as a result of excessive loss of potassium from the gastrointestinal tract or in the urine.

(*a*) Alimentary loss occurs as a result of acute severe or chronic diarrhoea due to infection, malabsorption, neoplasm of the small or large bowel or excessive use of cathartics, and loss of intestinal fluid from vomiting, fistulous drainage or aspiration.

(*b*) Renal wastage of potassium is more complex in its development and occurs in circumstances which lead to an increase in the rate of sodium/potassium exchange in the renal tubules. These disorders include Cushing's syndrome and primary or secondary aldosteronism; the administration of large amounts of sodium-containing fluids, the use of mercurial or other diuretics and corticosteroids also lead to excessive loss of potassium in the urine. Since hydrogen ions compete with potassium for exchange with sodium, drugs or diseases which suppress tubular secretion of hydrogen ions result in excessive potassium loss. These include acetazolamide, chlorothiazide and its derivatives and diseases such as renal tubular acidosis of idiopathic or acquired origin and metabolic alkalosis. Since almost all of the potassium in the body lies within the cells, factors which lower the gradients between the cells and the extracellular fluids are also capable of leading to potassium depletion and increased urinary loss. These conditions include anoxaemia, impaired oxidation of carbohydrate and acidosis of metabolic or respiratory origin.

Consequences and clinical features of potassium depletion. Significant depletion of potassium may occur without alteration in the serum potassium concentration and the diagnosis of intracellular potassium deficit is made difficult by the inaccessibility of the intracellular fluid to analysis. Biochemical evidence of potassium lack may be suggested by an elevation in plasma bicarbonate concentration or a diminution in plasma sodium concentration. These effects are believed to be due to the migration of hydrogen and sodium ions from the extracellular fluids into the cells respectively. Symptoms attributable to potassium deficiency include apathy, muscular weakness, mental confusion and abdominal distension. It is clear that such features arise in the course of many diseases. Nevertheless, their occurrence in circumstances which are known to lead to potassium deficiency, and their relief after potassium administration justify the diagnosis. In recent years the effect of potassium deficiency upon renal, function has been defined more precisely and it is now known that potassium depletion reduces the ability of the kidney to concentrate. Polyuria and resultant thirst commonly occur. Potassium depletion also gives rise to increased susceptibility to intoxication with digitalis glycosides. Severe potassium depletion lowers the cardiac output and this may give rise to oedema.

Potassium deficiency sufficiently severe to be associated with reduction of the serum concentration is more easily recognised, but is less common than simple intracellular depletion. It may occur in any of the conditions mentioned above if the deficiency is severe enough and is particularly liable to develop in cases of diabetic ketosis which have been vigorously treated with saline or glucose saline and insulin; this therapy causes a migration of potassium from the extracellular to the intracellular space with resulting hypokalaemia. The clinical picture of extracellular potassium deficit is characterised by generalised muscular weakness with paresis or flaccid paralysis and ileus. Paraesthaesiae are also commonly present. The electrocardiogram commonly shows a small T wave, prolongation of the Q-T interval and S-T depression. If untreated death may occur.

Treatment. Potassium depletion should be treated by giving a potassium salt orally or intravenously. The former route is more commonly used and is less dangerous than parenteral administration. The normal daily intake of potassium is about 2-3 g. Established deficiencies of moderate severity (about 400 m.Eq) can be remedied by giving 10-15 g. of potassium chloride per day orally in divided doses for some days in addition to a diet rich in potassium i.e. containing fruit and fruit juices. Potassium chloride tablets, even when enteric coated, are sometimes irritating to the gastrointestinal tracts. 'Slow release' tablets of potassium chloride are less troublesome in this respect, each tablet containing 600 mg. of KCl. Some patients tolerate effervescent potassium tablets more readily and these appear to be less nauseating. Some effervescent tablets contain chloride which is useful in correcting the metabolic alkalosis associated with potassium depletion and which is frequently due to concurrent chloride depletion (p. 866). Each tablet contains 0·25 g. of potassium. Intravenous infusions of potassium chloride are needed for patients who are unable to take potassium by mouth, but should be given only when the existence of hypokalaemia is established by chemical analysis. Such infusions should rarely be given in the presence of anuria or oliguria and only when facilities for repeated chemical analysis are available. If oliguria is due to associated water and salt depletion these should be treated first. For intravenous administration, potassium chloride (2 g. in sterile ampoules) can be conveniently added to 500 ml. of normal saline or 5 per cent. glucose solution. This solution then contains 52 m.Eq/*l.* respectively and should be given slowly over two to three hours. Repeated determinations of the serum potassium are necessary to determine whether further infusions are required. Administration of potassium by mouth should be started as soon as possible, as the major portion of the deficit can be corrected only by this means. When the depletion of potassium has arisen because of persistent vomiting and is associated with alkalosis due to loss of gastric hydrochloric acid, potassium is conveniently given with sodium and ammonium chloride as described on p. 866. Prophylactic administration of potassium chloride (3-4 g. daily) or effervescent potassium tablets should be given to patients who are being treated by drugs known to increase urinary loss of potassium. These include corticosteroids, chlorothiazide and its derivatives and other diuretics (p. 853).

4. Potassium Excess and Intoxication

Causes. Abnormal accumulation of potassium in the blood and extracellular fluid usually occurs in association with severe oliguria or anuria. It is commonly found in conditions leading to acute renal failure, e.g. circulatory failure from blood loss or injury and severe cases of Addison's disease and Addisonian crisis; it may occur in diabetic coma prior to adequate treatment with insulin and intravenous saline. Some patients in the terminal stages of chronic renal failure develop hyperkalaemia. Hyperkalaemia is readily induced if potassium supplements are given to patients with severe renal impairment or those who are being given a spironolactone.

Consequences of potassium excess. Patients with hyperkalaemia are dull and lethargic and gradually become confused. Asthenia develops and progresses to flaccid paralysis. These features are indistinguishable from those of hypokalaemia. The pulse becomes irregular and bradycardia develops from heart block of variable degree. Hyperkalaemia is of considerable clinical importance because of the danger of cardiac arrest with levels of serum potassium above 7·5 m.Eq/*l.* The diagnosis is made more frequently by knowing the circumstances in which intoxication is likely to arise and confirming the suspicion by serum potassium analysis than from any specific clinical feature. Typical electrocardiographic changes occur; these include increase in the amplitude of the T wave, atrioventricular and intraventricular conduction defects and ultimately ventricular standstill.

Treatment. It is important to prevent the occurrence of potassium intoxication in conditions associated with oliguria and anuria. The recommendations made with regard to the diet in acute renal failure (p. 825) are designed with this aim in view. When dealing with an established case of hyperkalaemia, the following measures are advised:

(*a*) Immediate restriction of foods rich in potassium, i.e. fruit and fruit juices and foods rich in protein.

(*b*) The repair of any associated depletion of water or salt with the aim of re-establishing a normal circulation as early as possible and the correction of acidosis of metabolic or respiratory origin by appropriate methods (p. 864).

(*c*) The sodium or calcium loaded ionic exchange resin (Resonium A and Zeocarb) absorbs potassium in the intestine from the blood and intestinal secretions and contents. A suspension of 30 g. in a small volume of water should be given by mouth three or four times per day or as required. In the event of vomiting the resin may be administered as a retention enema.

(*d*) The administration of glucose and insulin in order to encourage migration of potassium from the extracellular fluids into the cells. Twenty units of soluble insulin subcutaneously and 50 g. glucose by mouth should be given and may be repeated every two to four hours. The beneficial effect of this treatment is increased if ½ to 1 litre isotonic sodium bicarbonate is given simultaneously by intravenous injection.

(*e*) Calcium gluconate (10 per cent.), 10 ml. given intravenously and repeated in two to three hours, has been shown to reduce the cardiotoxic effect of potassium.

(*f*) If these methods fail or if the rise of concentration of potassium is rapid, removal of potassium by peritoneal or haemodialysis (artificial kidney) is indicated.

5. Magnesium Deficiency and Intoxication

Until recently disorders of magnesium metabolism have been difficult to recognise. Rapid methods for determination of magnesium in body fluids have recently become available and their application to human diseases has shown that disorders of magnesium metabolism are occasionally responsible for otherwise puzzling clinical features and are susceptible to therapeutic control. The most frequent cause of magnesium deficiency is prolonged diarrhoea or vomiting, in which parenteral fluid and electrolyte therapy without magnesium supplements are given. It occasionally follows long continuous diuretic therapy, and is associated with chronic diarrhoea and severe undernutrition, such as occurs in kwashiorkor and the malabsorption syndrome. Aldosteronism and hyperparathyroidism also lead to magnesium deficiency. Clinical features of magnesium deficiency are predominantly neuromuscular with tremor, choreiform movements and aimless plucking of the bedclothes. Mental depression, confusion, agitation, epileptiform convulsions and hallucinations also occur. The diagnosis should be confirmed by finding the concentration of magnesium in the plasma to be less than 1·5 m.Eq/*l*.

Magnesium deficiency may be treated orally by giving about 150 m.Eq/day of magnesium chloride or hydroxide for several days. This is approximately equivalent to 7 and 4 g. respectively per day. When parenteral treatment is necessary 100 m.Eq of magnesium chloride may be added to 1 litre of 5 per cent. glucose solution or isotonic saline and given over a period of several hours. The infusion should be repeated daily until the serum concentration remains within the normal range.

Magnesium intoxication mainly occurs in acute and chronic renal disease, and contibutes to the central nervous features associated with uraemia (p. 808). Its treatment is that of the primary disorder and is discussed on page 810.

6. Water Intoxication

Healthy individuals can safely drink very large volumes of water and respond to this by a vigorous water diuresis. The capacity of the body to excrete water when given without electrolytes is dependent upon many factors which include the rate of glomerular filtration and the power of the distal tubules of the kidney to produce a dilute urine. Many patients who are ill for a variety of reasons have a restricted ability to dilute the urine when given large amounts of water. These include patients suffering from acute and chronic renal disease, severe congestive heart failure, adrenocortical insufficiency and hepatic cirrhosis. Occasionally tumours of the bronchus or ovaries secrete a polypeptide with antidiuretic properties, like antidiuretic hormone, which leads to water intoxication. Post-operative subjects are also incapable of diluting the urine because of the liberation of vasopressin by the stress of the operation. In all these circumstances even a modest water intake reduces the serum osmolality and the concentration of sodium and produces symptoms which are primarily those of disordered cerebral function; these include dizziness, headache, nausea and mental confusion. Severe water intoxication can produce convulsions, coma and death. Diagnosis depends upon being aware of the circumstances in which water intoxication is likely to occur, and the demonstration of a serum sodium concentration below 130 m.Eq/*l*. Symptomatic treatment consists of restricting water intake for a few days. In severe cases 100 ml. 5 per cent. saline should be given intravenously and repeated in a few hours if there is little or no response. The use of fludrocortisone is beneficial in cases of hyponatraemia due to tumours and is also indicated in Addison's disease (p. 724).

7. Sodium and Water Accumulation

In health, the total amount of sodium in the body is kept within narrow limits in spite of great day-to-day variations in the amount ingested. Positive sodium balance with consequent accumulation of sodium in the body results from a renal excretion that is inadequate in relation to the amount ingested. The accumulation is generally accompanied by the retention of water so that the concentration of sodium in the extracellular space is usually not materially altered. When the distribution of the retained fluid is generalised, the expansion in the volume of the extracellular space does not become clinically detectable until the increase is of the order of 15 per cent.

The primary mechanisms responsible for the accumulation of water and salt which accompanies all types of oedema vary with the nature of the disease and they are discussed in the appropriate sections of this book. They include reduction in the osmotic pressure from hypoproteinaemia as occurs in the nephrotic syndrome (p. 805), and increase in venous hydrostatic pressure with migration of fluid from the vascular space to the tissue spaces, an important factor in congestive heart failure (p. 169), primary renal retention of salt and water as in acute proliferative glomerulonephritis and in low output cardiac states. In addition several compensatory reactions occur which promote further retention of water and salt. These include increased secretion of aldosterone and a rise in the levels of circulating vasopressin (p. 1026). The therapeutic use of cortisone, corticotrophin, DCA and testosterone may also give rise to water and sodium retention by virtue of their action on the kidney. Some oedema is not uncommon in normal women during the premenstrual stage of the menstrual cycle, but the mechanism of this is unknown. Oedema may be present in pregnancy and this may be due either to renal disease or merely to the increase in adrenocortical hormones in this condition. Other disorders associated with generalised oedema include nutritional oedema (p. 442), vitamin B deficiency and potassium deficiency. In some diseases several mechanisms appear to be operating simultaneously. This is exemplified particularly in the oedema and ascites of hepatic cirrhosis in which portal hypertension, hypoproteinaemia and possibly salt-retaining and antidiuretic agents all contribute to the abnormal retention of water and salt. It has to be admitted, however, that the knowledge of the cause of oedema in the above-mentioned diseases is far from complete. The clinical features of water and salt excess depend to some extent upon the distribution of the retained fluid. These are described under the various diseases in their respective sections.

Principles of Treatment. The principles guiding therapy are as follows:

(*a*) The use of measures designed to remedy specific factors leading to the oedema. These include digitalis in congestive heart failure, corticosteroids in some forms of glomerulonephritis, the intravenous administration of plasma salt-poor albumin in conditions associated with hypoproteinaemia, and a high protein diet in oedema of nutritional origin, hepatic cirrhosis and the nephrotic syndrome

(*b*) The depletion of the body of salt and water by the use of effective diuretics.

(*c*) The restriction by dietary means of the raw materials necessary for the formation of extracellular fluid, i.e. water and salt. The necessity for these restrictions has been greatly modified with the introduction of modern diuretics.

Diuretic Therapy. Before the discovery of modern diuretics oedema was a persisting and serious complication of several diseases, e.g. cardiac (p. 174), hepatic (p. 1025), renal (p. 804) and nutritional diseases (p. 442). Nowadays it is rare for oedema to be resistant to modern treatment and the vast majority of patients who suffer from it can be totally relieved. The greatest advance has been the discovery of drugs which specifically block renal tubular reabsorption of sodium. As a result of this effect these agents induce negative sodium balance and by increasing the amount of solute particles in the tubular fluid a large volume of water is eliminated. The treatment of oedema by these diuretics is generally successful even when the pathological processes leading to water and salt retention are beyond therapeutic control. The most important diuretics are as follows.

ORGANIC MERCURIAL DIURETICS. For reasons discussed on page 191 the use of mersalyl has greatly diminished in recent years. Mersalyl should only be prescribed when undesirable reactions or insensitivity to other diuretics develop. It exerts an effect on sodium reabsorption throughout the nephron but predominantly reduces the sodium reabsorbed by the distal tubule. Responsiveness to organic mercurials varies with the reaction of the body fluids, sensitivity being reduced as these become more alkaline. This is one reason why resistance to mersalyl may develop following repeated administration and has led to the coincident administration of the acidifying salt ammonium chloride (p. 191).

CARBONIC ANHYDRASE INHIBITORS. Acetazolamide is the best known example of this group of drugs which exert a mild diuretic effect by blocking the tubular reabsorption of sodium bicarbonate. This rapidly results in acidosis and the diuretic effect is self limited. For this reason and because profound potassium depletion occurs with its use, acetazolamide is no longer recommended as a diuretic. Its interest lies in the fact that its discovery led to the most important group of oral diuretics so far discovered, namely the benzothiadiazine drugs.

BENZOTHIADIAZINE DIURETICS. Diuretics belonging to this group exert two separate effects on renal function. Like mercurial diuretics they depress distal tubular reabsorption of sodium but they also inhibit carbonic anhydrase and sodium bicarbonate reabsorption in the proximal convoluted tubules. This double effect promotes sodium chloride and sodium bicarbonate loss in the urine. Potassium depletion occurs because of the delivery of increased amounts of sodium to the site of sodium/potassium exchange in the distal tubule. In addition, however, potassium depletion is further aggravated by the reduction of secretion of hydrogen ions consequent upon carbonic anhydrase inhibition. The first compound of this group of diuretics was chlorothiazide. Since then a series of thiazide diuretics have been produced by various modifications to the molecule which have altered their relative solubilities and stability within the body (p. 189). These characteristics are mainly responsible for differences in potency which is the only way in which drugs in this group differ from each other. The benzothiadiazine diuretics in common use are chlorothiazide (1-2 g.), flumethiazide (1-2 g.), hydrochlorothiazide (100 mg.) and bendrofluazide (10 mg.).

One of the thiazide diuretics should be the first choice in the treatment of congestive heart failure and in the nephrotic syndrome. Because of their tendency to produce potassium depletion and the neurological features of hepatic insufficiency they are sometimes less valuable than other diuretics for the treatment of oedema of hepatic cirrhosis (p. 1033). Toxic reactions are rare but hyperglycaemia and diabetes are occasionally produced in susceptible patients in whom there is a family history of the disease. A rise in uric acid also occurs and for this reason the drugs should not be given in gout or when the blood concentration of uric acid is elevated. The occurrence of agranulocytosis and thrombocytopenic purpura has occasionally been observed.

Other Diuretics. *Chlorthalidone* (100-200 mg. by mouth) is a sulphonamide derivative similar in its action to benzothiadiazine drugs (p. 854). It produces a slower and more prolonged diuresis extending over 48 hours.

Frusemide is one of the most recently introduced diuretics. It is chemically unrelated to the diuretics discussed above. This substance may be given orally (40-80 mg.) or intravenously (10-20 mg.). The onset of the diuresis is extremely rapid and is generally complete within six hours. Contrary to original claims frusemide also causes potassium loss. It appears to eliminate a greater volume of water than can be accounted for solely by the osmotic effect of sodium within the renal tubules. It may therefore have an important role in severe congestive heart failure with hyponatraemia.

Ethacrynic acid is another new diuretic of considerable potency and represents a new class of diuretics. It is given orally in doses of 50-200 mg. per day. As in the case of frusemide it appears to eliminate a greater volume of water than can be accounted for by the osmotic effect of sodium. Indications for its use are probably similar to those for frusemide.

Triamterene (200 mg.) is a much less potent diuretic than any of the thiazides or the mercurial compounds and does not lead to potassium deficiency. This may be due to the fact that part of its natruretic effect is due to inhibition of sodium reabsorption at the site of sodium/potassium exchange. Triamterene is not a diuretic of first choice and is generally used in conjunction with other diuretics.

In severe cases, however, when the measures discussed above are only partially or temporarily successful their combination with a *diet very low in salt* is necessary (Diet 8, p. 1793). With this multiple therapy the possibility of producing serious derangements in the chemical composition of the body fluids is considerable, and such a combination should not be used where facilities for blood analyses may not be available. Occasionally oedema resistant to these measures will respond to the administration of the aldosterone antagonist, *spironolactone* (Aldactone A). This drug is ineffective when given alone.

Abnormalities in electrolyte balance and in hydrogen ion concentration which may occur following intensive diuretic therapy include potassium depletion, metabolic alkalosis and, more rarely, sodium depletion. Chlorothiazide and its derivatives, frusemide and ethacrynic acid produce *potassium depletion* more rapidly than mersalyl, though both groups of drugs are capable of doing so, especially when given repeatedly over long periods of time and when combined with diets low in sodium. In these circumstances, symptoms of potassium deficit may arise before satisfactory loss of oedema has been achieved and are then superimposed upon the clinical features of water and salt accumulation. This state of affairs is especially prone to develop in the treatment of the more severe grades of congestive cardiac failure. This complication is particularly unfortunate since it can give rise directly to increased sensitivity to digitalis, with the development of toxic manifestations to this drug before adequate digitalisation and control of the congestive heart failure has been attained. Pulsus bigeminus and other cardiac arrythmias may develop. In hepatic disease with oedema and ascites the potassium depletion may seriously aggravate or precipitate the neurological features of hepatic insufficiency. Once severe potassium deficiency has occurred in these conditions, restoration of the normal body content may be extremely difficult and even impossible. It is for this reason that prophylactic administration of potassium chloride or effervescent potassium tablets (p. 847) is essential when diuretics are being given for long periods. *Metabolic alkalosis* as a result of diuretic therapy is only seen following continued use of mersalyl or other mercurial preparations.

Excessive administration of diuretics is capable of giving rise to *severe salt depletion.* This low salt syndrome is only likely to occur when treatment is long continued and when additional mechanical methods such as repeated abdominal paracenteses are being used. These patients exhibit some of the features of sodium depletion although they are still oedematous. They become apathetic and suffer from anorexia and vomiting. The circulatory characteristic of sodium depletion is present, namely hypotension with an increase in the pulse rate. Chemical analysis shows that the blood urea concentration is increased (prerenal uraemia) and that the serum sodium concentration is reduced to 130 m.Eq/*l.* or less. Such patients are usually seriously ill and may be in the last stage of their disease. Persistent attempts to reduce the oedema by any of the measures described above leads to further deterioration in their condition. These remedies should be withheld and a diet unrestricted in its salt content permitted. In a few instances the intravenous administration of hypertonic saline may be dramatically successful in relieving the symptoms of the low salt syndrome. Two hundred ml. of 5 per cent. saline should be given slowly by intravenous infusion, and may be repeated after 24 hours.

SUMMARY

It is apparent from this summary of the consequences of body depletion of sodium, water and potassium and of potassium intoxication that these disturbances present considerable diagnostic difficulty and are not characterised by pathognomonic signs or symptoms. The apathy of potassium depletion is indistinguishable from that of hyperkalaemia; severe sodium depletion is attended in the majority of instances by considerable water deficit so that these cases do not exhibit a clearly defined clinical picture. Furthermore, it is not uncommon for dual electrolytic deficits to develop simultaneously. For example, in diabetic ketosis potassium depletion may occur in conjunction with predominant salt depletion. In addition the symptoms of lethargy, apathy and mental confusion are common accompaniments of many diseases in which no significant body fluid distortion exists.

It has to be admitted also that the results obtained from biochemical analyses of blood by routine procedures are of only limited diagnostic value. Potassium or magnesium deficit may occur without significant alteration in serum potassium concentration, and serious sodium depletion may develop with serum sodium concentrations within the recognised limits of normality. A low serum sodium may not even indicate salt depletion, and hyponatraemia is frequently seen in the late stages of malignant disease, generalised tuberculosis and more rarely in association with vasopressin secreting tumours or other causes of water intoxication. The suggestion that diagnosis may be based upon easily detected abnormalities in the urine is unfortunately not supported by experience. A simple side-room test for urinary chloride using silver nitrate has been advocated as an easy method for detecting salt depletion. It is true that in certain conditions, e.g. excessive sweating, the urine is virtually free of sodium or chloride. However, in the majority of cases of salt depletion met with in clinical practice the depletion has arisen as a result of abnormal urinary loss; the test becomes valueless in these circumstances, and differentiation from simple water depletion is not possible by its use.

Accurate diagnosis largely depends upon a knowledge of the conditions and diseases which may give rise to abnormalities in water and electrolyte balance. In the presence of such diseases, the suspicion that these abnormalities may exist is strengthened by the presence of the clinical features known to occur with them and possibly by the results of appropriate biochemical and electrocardiographic examinations.

By understanding the mechanism by which the economy of the fluids of the body becomes disturbed and by the intelligent use of the reparative fluids which have been described, much can be done to restore the distortions of body fluid balance wrought by disease. Table 13. (p. 859) provides a list of the conditions associated with the disturbances in water and electrolyte balance discussed.

HYDROGEN ION CONCENTRATION

Life is possible only if the blood is kept within a range of alkalinity, and in health a physiological hydrogen ion concentration corresponding to a pH of between 7·35 and 7·45 is maintained by two widely different mechanisms which are closely integrated. A proper understanding of these mechanisms is necessary for a full appreciation of the clinical implications of acidosis and alkalosis.

The blood is alkaline because it contains bicarbonate, phosphate and proteins which are quite strong bases. It also contains carbonic acid and the pH of the blood depends principally upon the ratio of the main acid component, carbonic acid and the main base bicarbonate. The concentration of carbonic acid in the plasma is determined by the partial pressure of carbon dioxide (P_{CO_2}) in the alveoli. The latter is normally about 40 mm. Hg. and this gives rise to little over 1 m.Eq/*l.* of carbonic acid in physical solution in the plasma. The alveolar partial pressure of carbon dioxide is itself maintained steady by the equality between its rate of production by the tissues and the rate at which ventilation eliminates it from the body. On the other hand, the concentration of

TABLE 13. CAUSES OF WATER AND ELECTROLYTE IMBALANCE

Predominant Salt Depletion	Primary Water Depletion	Potassium Depletion	Potassium Excess and Intoxication	Magnesium Depletion	Sodium and Water Excess (generalised oedema)
Acute severe diarrhoea	Apathy due to illness, senility, psychosis	Acute severe diarrhoea	Diabetic coma (before treatment)	Malabsorption syndrome	Congestive cardiac failure
Chronic diarrhoea	Diseases causing dysphagia	Chronic diarrhoea	Peripheral circulatory failure from burns and blood loss	Diarrhoea	Hepatic cirrhosis
Intestinal fistulae	Coma	Vomiting	Acute renal failure (oliguric phase)	Vomiting	The nephrotic syndrome
Gastrointestinal aspiration	Diabetes insipidus and other renal water-losing conditions, e.g. hyperparathyroidism	Aspiration of gastro-intestinal contents	Addison's disease	Aldosteronism	Acute glomerulonephritis
Vomiting	**Water Intoxication**	Malabsorption syndrome	Chronic renal disease	Hyperparathyroidism	Excessive use of corticotrophin, corticosteroids and testosterone
Diabetes mellitus and diabetic ketosis	Post-operative period	Chronic starvation and anorexia		Long continued diuretic therapy	Premenstrual phase of cycle
Chronic nephritis and pyelonephritis (salt-losing)	Acute and chronic renal disease	Diabetes mellitus and diabetic ketosis (after treatment)		Diuretic phase of acute ischaemic renal failure	Toxaemia of pregnancy
Diuretic phase of acute renal failure	Adrenocortical insufficiency	During and after treatment with corticosteroids and corticotrophin		**Magnesium Intoxication**	Malnutrition
Addison's disease	Severe congestive heart failure and hepatic cirrhosis	Excessive use of mercurial diuretics, acetazolamide thiazide diuretics, frusemide, ethacrynic acid		Acute and chronic renal failure	
Hypopituitarism		Cushing's syndrome and aldosteronism			
Excessive sweating (with unrestricted water intake)		Post-operative period			
Excessive use of diuretics		Acidosis and alkalosis			
		Dehydration			
		Chronic tissue hypoxia (e.g. congestive heart failure)			

bicarbonate is regulated by the tubular epithelium of the kidneys and in health is kept at about 22 to 24 m.Eq/*l* by the mechanism described on p. 784. A great many metabolic processes result in the production of acids and these must be eliminated from the body if the reaction of the tissue and the blood is to remain within the normal range. The route of disposal of these acids depends upon whether or not they are capable of being oxidised completely to carbon dioxide and water. Carbon dioxide forms carbonic acid within the body and is eliminated as carbon dioxide by ventilation. Other acids such as acetoacetic acid or sulphuric acid which is derived from the oxidation of sulphur-containing proteins are excreted by the kidneys. At the site of their production in the tissues and during their carriage in the blood all acids increase the hydrogen ion concentration. The extent of this increase is minimised by the stabilising power of the blood and tissues which in turn depends on the presence of the physiologically important buffers.

Carbonic acid is produced by metabolic reactions in far greater amounts than any other acid. A small part of the carbon dioxide is transported in the blood reversibly bound to haemoglobin as a carbamino compound. A greater part is converted to carbonic acid in the red blood cells under the influence of carbonic anhydrase and is then buffered by haemoglobin as it gives its oxygen to the tissues and is converted to reduced haemoglobin The hydrogen ions of the carbonic acid are taken up by the haemoglobin in the red cells while the bicarbonate ion moves out from the red cells to the plasma in exchange for chloride ions (chloride shift, Fig. 52).

Most of the carbonic acid added to the blood therefore appears not as acid but as bicarbonate ion. As the blood passes through

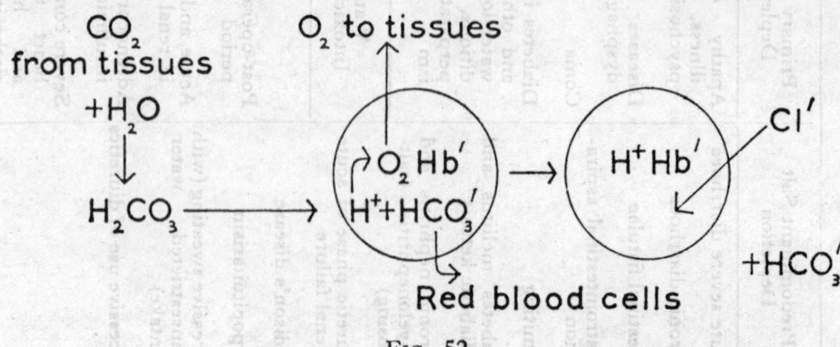

FIG. 52

the lungs and the haemoglobin is re-oxygenated this process is reversed and the carbon dioxide formed is expelled by ventilation.

In health a small amount of inorganic acid is produced each day and being non-volatile requires to be excreted by the kidney. No significant amount of organic acid is produced in normal conditions but in diabetic ketosis for example a large amount of acetoacetic acid is formed. The tissue and blood are buffered against these acids by a different mechanism which involves in particular the sodium bicarbonate and carbonic acid buffer system in the plasma. The addition of acid to the plasma for example, results in a movement of the reactions given in the direction indicated by the broad arrow (Fig. 53).

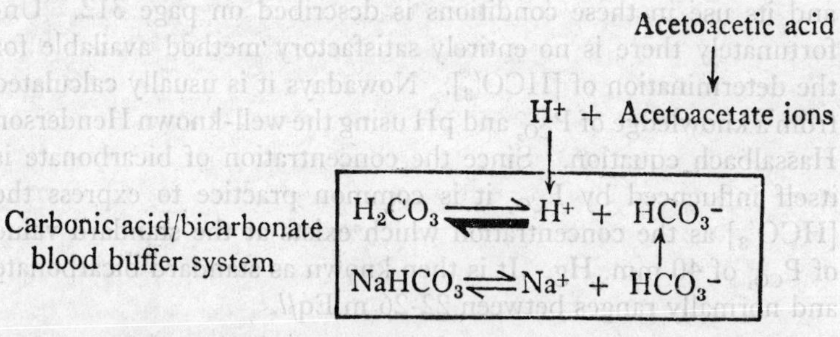

FIG. 53

As a result of this and of a similar reaction on the part of the other buffer systems, many of the hydrogen ions which would otherwise increase the acidity of the plasma are removed to form increased amounts of carbonic acid. There is a corresponding diminution in the concentration of bicarbonate ions. By this means the pH of the plasma falls far less than it would do if the buffers were not present. The fall in pH stimulates ventilation and the excess carbonic acid is removed from the body as carbon dioxide. The anion of the acid (i.e. acetoacetate) and the depleted body bicarbonate are dealt with simultaneously by the kidney. The renal tubules form carbonic acid, much of the hydrogen ion of which is used to form ammonium ions which are then excreted in the urine with the acid anion. The bicarbonate ion generated in this process is returned to the blood and reconstitutes the depleted blood buffer (p. 784).

These buffering and excreting mechanisms are continually in operation in response to the normal production of acids derived from the food and its metabolism. It is clear from this simplified description that the important limiting factor in the buffering power of blood is the available haemoglobin and bicarbonate. The limiting factor in the body's ability to rid itself of anion derived from inorganic and excess organic acid is the excretory power of the kidneys.

DISTURBANCES IN HYDROGEN ION CONCENTRATION

Abnormalities in the reaction of the body may be caused by changes in the concentration of carbonic acid (i.e. P_{CO_2}) and by alterations in body base, notably that of bicarbonate. The estimation of P_{CO_2} is of particular value in respiratory disorders and its use in these conditions is described on page 312. Unfortunately there is no entirely satisfactory method available for the determination of $[HCO'_3]$. Nowadays it is usually calculated from a knowledge of P_{CO_2} and pH using the well-known Henderson Hassalbach equation. Since the concentration of bicarbonate is itself influenced by P_{CO_2} it is common practice to express the $[HCO'_3]$ as the concentration which exists at the standard value of P_{CO_2} of 40 mm. Hg. It is then known as standard bicarbonate and normally ranges between 22-26 m.Eq/*l*.

Metabolic Acidosis

Metabolic acidosis arises as a result of the production or ingestion of acids other than carbonic acid, or as a consequence of body depletion of the base bicarbonate. The condition is characteristic by a fall in pH, a marked reduction in the concentration of bicarbonate in the plasma. The P_{CO_2} is reduced secondarily by the hyperventilation produced by respiration stimulation and this mitigates to some extent the reduction in pH due to the fall in $[HCO'_3]$.

The production of large amounts of lactic acid in vigorous exercise is probably the most common cause of acidosis and is to be regarded as physiological. Shock causes metabolic acidosis because of hypoxia of the tissues and the accumulation of organic acids, particularly lactic acid. Other important causes of acidosis are diabetes mellitus and ketosis, and renal failure. In the former condition, β-hydroxybutyric acid and acetoacetic acid are produced in abnormally large amounts, and at a rate which is greater than the capacity of the body for their oxidation. In patients with renal failure, the power of the kidneys to generate bicarbonate ions and to produce and secrete hydrogen and ammonium ions is impaired and their excretion is diminished. This is seen particularly in chronic glomerulonephritis and chronic pyelonephritis.

Diminution in blood bicarbonate occurs from direct loss of sodium bicarbonate in the stools in chronic or acute severe diarrhoea or from loss of intestinal contents from fistulae or by intestinal aspiration. The therapeutic administration of acetazolamide (Diamox) for glaucoma or ammonium chloride may also give rise to acidosis. In the latter case the ammonium radical is converted to urea, and the hydrochloric acid remaining reduces the available bicarbonate in the blood. Acetazolamide depresses the power of the kidneys to generate bicarbonate and secrete hydrogen ions which accumulate in the blood.

Consequences of metabolic acidosis. The most obvious consequence of acidosis is the stimulation of the respiratory centre by the abnormally high blood concentration of hydrogen ions. In severe cases the respirations become deep and rapid (Kussmaul's respiration). It is clear, however, from the list of causes given above that the clinical picture in the individual case is largely determined by the underlying condition and by the presence of other concomitant disturbances in water and salt balance. By the time acidosis is severe in diabetic coma, considerable water and salt depletion has usually occurred. The acidosis of chronic diarrhoea is similarly associated with salt loss and especially with potassium deficit. The failure of ammonium and hydrogen ion production by the kidney in chronic nephritis, which leads to acidosis, is necessarily accompanied by abnormal loss of cation in the urine giving rise to salt depletion. As in the case of disturbances in water and electrolyte balance, the diagnosis of metabolic acidosis is facilitated by an awareness of those pathological conditions in which it is likely to arise. The diagnosis should be confirmed by the determination of the concentration of bicarbonate in the blood. In acidosis of moderate degree this value is reduced to 15 m.Eq/*l.*, while levels below 10 m.Eq/*l.* represent severe degrees of acidosis.

Treatment. Since metabolic acidosis is commonly associated with some degree of salt depletion and water deficiency, it would seem reasonable to correct these disturbances, in the first instance, by the administration of suitable amounts of isotonic saline, as already described. Isotonic saline is a neutral solution and by itself might be expected to have only a little influence on the reaction of the blood and tissues. In point of fact, however, provided the kidneys are not primarily diseased and provided the degree of salt and water depletion is not so severe as to impair renal function seriously, the intravenous administration of normal saline is usually effective in correcting metabolic acidosis of moderate severity. The success of this is dependent upon the capacity of the kidneys to generate bicarbonate from carbon dioxide and water and to retain this with the infused sodium, rejecting the chloride in the urine.

In the presence of renal disease or with severe acidosis and salt depletion giving rise to prerenal uraemia, it is unwise to depend upon the collaboration of the kidney for the alkalising effect of sodium chloride. In these circumstances, isotonic sodium bicarbonate should be given by intravenous infusion in addition to isotonic saline. The two solutions should be given in a ratio of 1 to 2 and need not be mixed. The total volume of the combined solutions required varies with the severity of the salt depletion and with the degree of acidosis. A moderately severe case of diabetic coma, for example, may require as much as 4-6 litres in the first 24 hours, of which 1 to 2 litres should be the isotonic sodium bicarbonate solution. The latter infusion should be given for as long as there is evidence of acidosis, as determined by the estimation of the bicarbonate concentration in the blood. When this has returned to normal levels, it may be necessary to continue the intravenous infusion of normal saline alone. This is indicated if there is still evidence of predominant salt depletion.

In severe shock or cardiac arrest due, for example, to myocardial infarction, acidosis develops without salt depletion. In these circumstances it is best to give sodium bicarbonate in a small volume of hypertonic concentration, i.e. 200-300 ml. 5 per cent. solution intravenously in the course of 10 to 15 minutes.

Metabolic Alkalosis

Metabolic alkalosis arises most commonly as a result of the abnormal loss from the body of hydrochloric acid in the course of prolonged or severe vomiting. It is also now known that chloride deficiency itself leads to alkalosis by stimulating the renal tubular reabsorption of bicarbonate. More rarely alkalosis may arise from the ingestion of large amounts of sodium bicarbonate given, for example, in the treatment of peptic ulcer. This is especially likely to occur if there is associated pyloric spasm or stenosis, with vomiting. Potassium depletion also gives rise to alkalosis by the mechanism described on p. 847.

Consequences of Alkalosis. The sequence of events which occurs when hydrochloric acid is lost from the body as a result of vomiting, is shown in Figure 54.

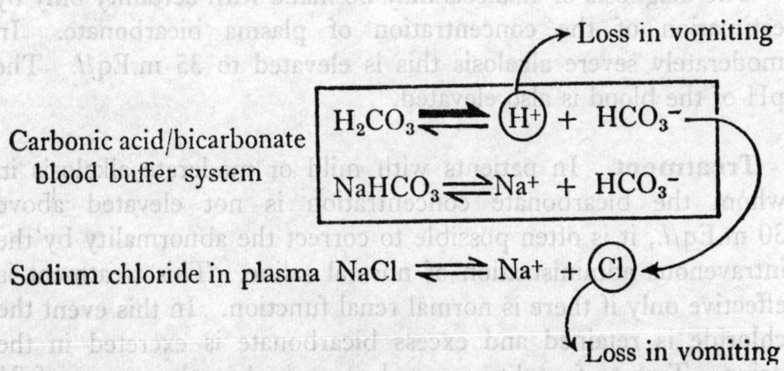

FIG. 54

The loss of hydrogen ions in severe and continuous vomiting lowers the hydrogen ion concentration of the blood and leads to alkalosis. This effect is mitigated by an increase in the ionisation of blood carbonic acid to hydrogen and bicarbonate ions, as indicated in the diagram by the board arrow. The former tends to restore the hydrogen ion concentration towards normal, and the latter replaces the chloride in the blood which has also been lost in the gastric contents. For as long as the chloride deficiency persists increased tubular conservation of bicarbonate sustains the alkalosis.

Alkalosis of some duration is often associated with significant depression of renal function with uraemia. Protein and casts are found in the urine, and the diagnostic error of attributing vomiting due to pyloric stenosis to primary renal disease must be avoided. In spite of the existence of metabolic alkalosis, the urine may remain acid. There are two causes for this paradoxical aciduria. The alkalosis is frequently associated with chloride depletion, and under these circumstances a very alkaline urine cannot be elaborated. Secondly, respiratory compensation for the alkalosis results in a rise in P_{CO_2} which is also known to increase renal tubular reabsorption of bicarbonate. Apathy, personality changes, delirium, and stupor occur; since the patient usually suffers from associated water and potassium depletion, it is probably wrong to attribute these features solely to the effect of alkalosis. Tetany may occur spontaneously or be induced by the Trousseau manœuvre.

The diagnosis of alkalosis may be made with certainty only by estimation of the concentration of plasma bicarbonate. In moderately severe alkalosis this is elevated to 35 m.Eq/*l.* The pH of the blood is also elevated.

Treatment. In patients with mild or moderate alkalosis in whom the bicarbonate concentration is not elevated above 30 m.Eq/*l.*, it is often possible to correct the abnormality by the intravenous administration of normal saline. This treatment is effective only if there is normal renal function. In this event the chloride is retained and excess bicarbonate is excreted in the urine. Two to four litres may be required in the course of 24 hours. In severe cases the administration of ammonium chloride by intravenous infusion has been found effective and is conveniently prepared in a solution which is designed also to repair the commonly associated potassium deficit. This is called the 'gastric solution'. One litre of a solution containing 63 m.Eq/*l.* of sodium chloride, 17 m.Eq/*l.* of potassium chloride and 70 m.Eq/*l.* of ammonium chloride may be given in four to six hours and repeated as indicated by blood analysis. The use of this solution is of particular benefit in these patients who are being prepared for operation for relief of pyloric obstruction and in whom repeated daily gastric lavage is needed to prevent vomiting and reduce the size of a dilated stomach.

Ketosis

The excessive production of β-hydroxybutyric acid and acetoacetic acid in diabetes mellitus and coma has already been described as a cause of acidosis. Abnormal amounts of acetoacetic acid also arise in the body when the carbohydrate in the food is inadequate and increased amounts of fat are being utilised for energy. This is commonly found in cases of cyclical or severe vomiting in children, hyperemesis gravidarum, starvation, and in post-operative vomiting. Two opposing tendencies are obviously in operation, the ketosis tending to increase, and vomiting tending to decrease the concentration of hydrogen ions in the blood. In these cases it is not uncommon, therefore, to find that metabolic alkalosis coexists with ketosis. The student should be aware of the fact that the presence of acetoacetic acid in the urine does not necessarily imply the existence of acidosis, and that the existence of the latter is established only by the determination of the blood pH or bicarbonate concentration.

Apart from the possible need to treat concomitant acidosis or electrolyte disturbances, ketosis is best remedied by restoring the consumption of carbohydrate to normal. In cases of diabetes mellitus the administration of insulin is essential. In the other forms of ketosis this need not be given. Ample supplies of glucose should be provided: if this cannot be taken by mouth an intravenous infusion of 5 per cent. glucose in water may be given. Two to four litres of this solution may be needed in the course of the day.

Respiratory Acidosis and Alkalosis

Respiratory acidosis arises when the effective alveolar ventilation does not keep pace with the rate of CO_2 production (p. 308). As a result the P_{CO_2} and carbonic acid concentration of the blood increase, and the pH falls. The distinction between respiratory acidosis and metabolic alkalosis is usually easily made from a knowledge of the cause of the disturbance. The reaction of the arterial blood is decisive; in both the P_{CO_2} is increased, but in respiratory acidosis pH is reduced, whereas in metabolic alkalosis the pH is increased. The kidney responds to an increase in P_{CO_2} by excreting an acid urine and conserving sodium bicarbonate. The causes and consequences of respiratory acidosis are given on p. 312.

Respiratory alkalosis occurs when there is excessive loss of carbonic acid by over-ventilation of the lungs. Most commonly this occurs in hysterical over-breathing, though it may arise also in the course of meningitis, encephalitis and with salicylate administration. Tetany may ensue.

Electrolyte repair solutions play no part in the treatment of respiratory acidosis or alkalosis, and therapy should be directed to the underlying disorder. The treatment of hypercapnia is described on p. 321.

Respiratory alkalosis is best treated by the administration of 5 per cent. carbon dioxide and oxygen, or more simply by asking the patient to re-breath his own carbon dioxide by breathing into a paper bag. Tetany may be treated by an intravenous injection of 10 ml. of 10 per cent. calcium gluconate if necessary. The underlying causative factors should receive appropriate attention.

J. S. Robson.

Books recommended:

Black, D. A. K. (1967). *Essentials of Fluid Balance*, 4th ed. Oxford: Blackwell.
Robinson, J. R. (1967). *Fundamentals of Acid-Base Regulation* 3rd ed. Oxford: Blackwell.

DISEASES OF THE DIGESTIVE SYSTEM

THE SYMPTOMATOLOGY OF GASTROINTESTINAL DISEASE

It is generally agreed that history taking is the most important part of the examination of the patient. In gastrointestinal disease we are particularly dependent on an accurate history, but this is of little value unless the significance of symptoms and physical signs can be properly interpreted. Unfortunately this may prove difficult. Symptoms should be regarded as the patient's expression of a disorder of function, but the same disorder of function can be due to different disease processes.

This may be illustrated by an example such as vomiting. This symptom may result from diseases of the stomach such as peptic ulcer, carcinoma of the stomach or acute gastritis. On the other hand vomiting frequently accompanies extragastric conditions such as intestinal obstruction, biliary or renal colic, hepatic or renal disease, pregnancy, increased intracranial pressure, migraine or emotional disturbances. The value of vomiting as a diagnostic symptom is discussed on p. 874. Accordingly it is helpful to consider some of the symptoms of the digestive system and what is known of the underlying disorder of function.

Pain

Pain is the most common symptom of any patient with gastrointestinal disease. In the past, visceral pain arising in the gastrointestinal tract was considered to be distinct from pain of somatic origin. Any distinction observed is more likely to be due to differences in richness of innervation or in the adequacy of stimuli, rather than to an essential dissimilarity in the mechanisms of visceral and somatic pain.

Pain nerve endings are free nerve endings whose cell stations lie in the posterior root ganglia. Afferent impulses reach the cord by the splanchnic nerves and then pass up the anterolateral tracts. From certain viscera, impulses may travel up both sides of the cord and this may explain why some pains, such as intestinal colic, are felt in the midline of the body.

Though the distribution of pain nerve endings in different parts of the gastrointestinal tract is not accurately known, it seems likely that certain regions are less well supplied than others. This might explain the existence of so-called 'silent areas' of the gut, such as the cardiac end of the stomach and the caecum, where lesions tend to be symptomless.

Equally important as the richness of innervation in the production of pain is the adequacy of the stimulus. The type of stimulus that is painful on the surface of the body is not necessarily painful inside the abdomen.

Adequate stimuli which commonly give rise to pain in the abdomen are:

1. Strong contractions of smooth muscle as in intestinal, biliary, ureteric or uterine colic, particularly if inflammation is present.
2. Inflammation of the parietal peritoneum as in perforation of a peptic ulcer or in appendicitis.
3. Stretching of the capsule of a viscus, e.g. the liver, as in cardiac failure, or the spleen, as in splenic venous thrombosis.

Tissues which appear to be relatively insensitive, are:

1. Gastric and intestinal mucosa. Thus intense gastritis or enteritis gives rise to no more than slight discomfort, if there is no associated muscular contraction of the gut.
2. Parenchyma of liver, spleen, kidney, etc. Thus large secondary growths in the liver may be completely painless.

Quality of Pain. Patients use different and often dramatic expressions to describe their sensations. The one quality of pain they can all determine is whether it is superficial or deep. Though the description of the quality of the pain may not be helpful, its time relations, intensity, its site and its reference are of the greatest value.

Reference of Pain. Some process must take place in the sensorium to localise the site of origin of a pain and this process may be called reference. This process can only take place if there is some kind of map of the body in consciousness, or 'body image' as it is called, to which reference can be made. All of us have some kind of mental image of our bodies, which includes particularly the limbs and face, the front of our bodies more vividly than the back and which does not extend deeper than the superficial layers. When part of the actual body is lost as after the amputation of a limb, this amputated part does not disappear from the 'body image'. Sensations from the same segments of the spinal cord which supplied the amputated limb are now 'referred' back to that part of the body image and the patient is said to have a 'phantom limb'. The patient can then feel a leg which is no longer there or even experience angina down the inner side of a non-existent arm. The gastrointestinal tract, however, appears to occupy little place in the normal body image except as something vaguely deep to the abdominal wall. It is therefore not surprising that resection of the stomach or colon produces no phantom viscus. On this basis it is possible to explain the 'reference' to the surface of the body of pain coming from the viscera, since the sensorium cannot project back sensations to parts of the body it does not recognise. It will however always refer them to the same segments of the spinal cord from which the original sensations were transmitted.

Pain Threshold. The pain threshold is the level of the intensity of a stimulus necessary to produce pain. It seems likely that changes of pain threshold in the gastrointestinal tract can occur so that stimuli which are usually painless become painful. These alterations of threshold might be produced by inflammatory change as on the surface of the body. If the sensitivity of the stomach to stimuli is largely dependent on the degree of inflammation present, this alteration in threshold might explain changes of ulcer pain which occur without changes in the size of the ulcer niche, or in the amount or quality of gastric secretion.

Reactivity. Not only do we experience pain, but we react to it. It seems that the thresholds to sensation on the surface of the body do not vary greatly in different patients, but that these patients have widely different levels of reactivity. In other words, the patient who appears to 'feel' pain easily has probably the same pain threshold as the 'normal' but reacts to it at a much lower level of intensity. It is possible that these conclusions are also true of visceral pain.

Associated Phenomena

Reflex rigidity and 'referred tenderness'. Of the phenomena we associate with pain in the abdomen, the most striking is muscular rigidity. This sign is sometimes considered peculiar to inflammations in the abdomen but is in fact associated with deep pain everywhere in the body. For example, pain from sinusitis produces corresponding muscular rigidity in the face. Sometimes this reflex rigidity in the abdomen is spoken of as guarding, implying that it is protective. It is in fact a reflex spasm occurring in a muscle supplied from the same spinal segment which innervates the inflamed viscus, but the muscle concerned does not necessarily lie directly over the diseased organ. Rigidity in the abdomen usually results from peritoneal inflammation and may be present even if the original pain has disappeared. It should be sought for most carefully.

'Referred tenderness'. There is no good phrase to describe the tenderness which may be elicited at a distance from the diseased organ. In certain diseases, as in inflammation of the gall-bladder, not only may pain be felt in a situation distant from the gall-bladder but there may also be tenderness on pressure over the right lower ribs posteriorly which can persist after the original pain has subsided. The mechanism of this phenomenon is not clear.

Hunger, Appetite and Food Habit

Over a long period animals, including man, take in and give out equal amounts of energy and thereby maintain their weight with but little variation. The host of complex factors which control this homeostatic mechanism are imperfectly understood, but its efficiency is proved by the difficulty many patients have, of either increasing or decreasing their weight. In animals there is evidence for the existence of certain stimuli which signal the need for more food to a regulatory centre in the hypothalamus, while regulation of the volume of food ingested is mediated in part through oropharyngeal receptors and receptors in the upper alimentary tract which respond to distension and produce the sensation of satiety. Energy requirements influence these mechanisms. In dealing with a patient the physician is concerned with his symptoms, and these can be divided into hunger and appetite sensations which roughly correspond to the stimulation of gastric and oral afferents.

Though the terms 'hunger' and 'appetite' are used synonymously by most patients to describe any desire for food, they are in fact distinct sensations. The lack of a general desire for food is termed anorexia.

Hunger is usually described as an unpleasant sensation, part of which is localised to the epigastrium. In addition to this localised sensation, the subject may experience certain general sensations, e.g. weakness, irritability, occasionally headache or even nausea. If carefully observed the epigastric sensation of hunger is intermittent, and this sensation is thought to arise from active movements of the stomach and duodenum, so-called 'hunger contractions'. These contractions occur for a period and then die away as the stomach passes into a resting phase. In certain diseases of the stomach, as in an infiltrating carcinoma, these movements are diminished or disappear and coincidentally the patient may complain of anorexia. It is clear, however, that the urge to eat is not conditioned by these sensations alone, as patients continue to eat after a complete gastrectomy.

Appetite is described by most people as a pleasant sensation and though less easily localised than hunger, is usually felt in the mouth or palate. It appears to depend more on the odours and memory of pleasant foods and is clearly distinct from hunger. It is possibly related to olfactory acuity. Anorexic drugs such as amphetamine which reduce appetite have no action on the movements of the stomach. If the sense of smell is completely destroyed, as may occur in a fracture of the base of the skull, the patient loses interest in food, though eating continues from habit. Food habits are not closely related to the physiological suitability of any particular diet and are notoriously rigid and difficult to alter.

Apart from these factors of hunger, appetite and food habit, all of which affect the urge to eat, it is obvious that food has certain associations, so that the intake of food may be affected by psychological factors and both obesity from overeating and leanness due to anorexia, may be caused in this way. The persistent refusal of food from psychological causes is termed anorexia nervosa (p. 983) and may even be of such severity as to cause death.

Nausea

Nausea is an unpleasant sensation easily recognised though with difficulty described. It is felt in the epigastrium and may precede vomiting. It is not a continuous sensation but may be recognised as coming in waves and may be accompanied by salivation, pallor and sweating. Its physiological basis is probably a change of motility pattern in the upper alimentary tract, with loss of tone in the stomach. Fat causes increased tone in the duodenum and inhibits movements of the stomach, and this may explain why some people feel nauseated when large amounts of fatty food are eaten. If the feelings of nausea are slight and not due to serious abdominal disease, they may be abolished by measures which encourage peristaltic movements down the gut. Such measures include food and aperients, and this is possibly the explanation of the well-being ascribed to a morning dose of Epsom salts.

Vomiting

The act of vomiting is a movement caused by the active contraction of the abdominal wall against a fixed diaphragm, with the cardiac sphincter relaxed. Vomiting is often preceded by nausea and salivation. Reflex salivation is called waterbrash, and the fluid either runs directly out of the mouth or is swallowed and then regurgitated from the oesophagus. Vomiting is a reflex act, which may be elicited by a variety of stimuli and over a wide area. Therefore for this reason vomiting is not a useful localising symptom. In the abdomen, the most common causes of vomiting are diseases of the stomach or small intestine, peritonitis, appendicitis or cholecystitis. Diseases of the large bowel cause vomiting less frequently. Outside the abdomen there are numerous conditions which may be responsible, e.g. migraine, meningitis, uraemia etc.

When vomiting has an abdominal cause, it is usually preceded by nausea; when the vomiting is due to direct stimulation of the vomiting centre in the medulla, it may occur suddenly without any warning. Vomiting in the morning occurs in pregnancy and alcoholic gastritis or may be psychogenic in origin. If the size of the vomitus is unaccountably large, there must be dilatation of the stomach, most probably due to obstruction of part of the pyloroduodenal canal. Vomiting that produces relief of pain is likely to be due to an obstructive cause. If there is a history of repeated vomiting unattended by any loss of weight, the vomiting is probably psychogenic in origin. In assessing the significance of vomiting as a symptom, it is helpful to find out if the patient vomits readily and has frequently vomited in the past with but little cause. The significance of vomiting in such a patient is unlikely to be great.

Flatulence

Many patients complain of a symptom which they call 'wind' or 'flatulence'. This may mean they believe that their abdominal discomfort is due to increased gas in some part of their gastro-intestinal tract or the term is used to describe the passage of an excessive quantity of gas either from the stomach or the colon, or the borborygmi which accompany the movement of gas in the gut. There is no doubt of course that gas exists in the gastro-intestinal tract and that it may give rise to symptoms, but the patient frequently interprets his sensations incorrectly.

The physiological problem of gas in the alimentary tract is basically simple. If we believe that no secretion of gas occurs into the gut, as it does in the swim bladder of fishes, then the passage of gases across the gut wall must proceed according to the laws of diffusion. If this is so, the ways in which gas can enter or leave the gut are:

1. (*a*) *Swallowing of air.*
   (*b*) *Expulsion of gas from the stomach or colon.*

Everybody swallows some air with his meals. When the stomach contracts, this swallowed air is easily expelled up the oesophagus particularly if there is a fluid trap preventing its passage through the pylorus. If the stomach is empty of fluid when it contracts, as during hunger contractions, the air tends to pass through the pylorus rather than up the oesophagus, and the sounds of its passage into the intestine are called borborygmi and sometimes worry an introspective patient. Gas in the stomach is eructated without difficulty when the stomach contracts, provided the subject is in an upright position. If, on the other hand, the patient is lying horizontally as after an operation, the gas cannot be completely eructated and some must pass into the intestine. Gas in the lower colon or rectum can be readily evacuated but it is possible it may get trapped in a loop of bowel such as the splenic flexure.

2. *Diffusion of gas.* Movement of gas across the gut wall takes place in either direction according to the laws governing diffusion, that is, gas passes from a region of high partial pressure to one of lower pressure. This means that any mixture of gases in the bowel will tend to reach equilibrium with the gases in the blood.

3. *The formation and absorption of gas.* Carbon dioxide is formed to the amount of 3-4 litres a day in the small intestine from the interaction of acid gastric juice and alkaline pancreatic secretion. Gas can also form by fermentation of carbohydrates and by putrefaction of proteins. Neither of these reactions normally takes place in the stomach, except in pyloro-duodenal obstruction when foul inflammable gas may be formed and eructated. Both however occur particularly in the large bowel and the gas is either expelled from the bowel or is absorbed, and passing by the portal blood stream, may be detoxicated in the liver before being excreted through the lungs. The greater part of the gas formed in the gut is removed in this way.

A few gases, such as hydrogen sulphide, may be removed by chemical combination in the intestine. Therapeutically, charcoal has been used to absorb unwanted gases. Though, with certain gases, charcoal may do this very effectively when in a finely divided dry state, there is no evidence that it is of any value under the moist conditions in the intestine.

Symptomatology

Gastric Flatulence. It is difficult to understand how swallowed air in the stomach can ever give rise to any but the most temporary symptoms. Directly gas is introduced into the stomach experimentally, the intragastric pressure rises, and it requires great determination on the part of the subject to resist belching. The complaint therefore of gas in the stomach that cannot be eructated must be due to a misinterpretation of sensation; either gas is not the cause of the symptoms at all, or the sensation is really derived from gas elsewhere in the alimentary tract. Some people in an attempt to rid themselves of imaginary gas in the stomach swallow more and develop the habit of aerophagy. This trick has been shown to be due to the entry of gas into the oesophagus and not into the stomach from where it is expelled. Unpleasant gas can of course be eructated in pyloro-duodenal obstruction, especially when achlorhydria is present.

INTESTINAL FLATULENCE. The small intestine is normally completely empty of all gas as judged radiologically, but we must assume that gas is passing through the gut and it only becomes visible either when in excessive amounts or when the gut is paralysed and the gas is able to separate itself from the fluid contents. In intestinal obstruction distension with gas is one of the main clinical features. The existence of gas does not by itself produce symptoms unless the gut is able to contract, hence post-operative 'gas pains' are not felt till the gut recovers its tone about the third post-operative day.

COLONIC FLATULENCE. Sometimes the passage of excessive quantities of gas is a complaint. If the gas is odourless it may be either nitrogen that is derived from increased amounts of air that have been swallowed, or carbon dioxide that has been produced by carbohydrate fermentation. If the gas is foul smelling, it must mean putrefaction of proteins and this may be due to intestinal hurry or to defective pancreatic secretion so that excessive quantities of undigested protein are brought into the large bowel. The gas must also have been produced too fast for absorption into the blood stream and consequent detoxication in the liver.

Absorption of gas depends mainly on an adequate mucosal blood flow.

HEARTBURN

Heartburn is a feeling of burning behind the lower end of the sternum and is often accompanied by regurgitation of fluid into the pharynx. The sensation strongly suggests the burning effect of acid, but drinking decinormal hydrochloric acid does not immediately produce heartburn in a normal oesophagus though it will do so if the gullet is inflamed. The symptoms have been produced by stretching the lower end of the oesophagus or by producing oesophageal spasm. Hence it seems possible that heartburn is a muscular sensation. It is common in pregnancy. Heartburn may be experienced following meals, or following change of posture, such as lying down or after heavy lifting. The heartburn following meals is frequently associated with a duodenal ulcer, while that associated with a rise of intra-abdominal pressure is due to incompetence of the oesophageogastric sphincter, and is found most frequently in association with a hiatus hernia.

Sense of Fullness

Certain patients complain that as soon as they eat they feel 'full up'. The stomach, like other hollow viscera, relaxes to receive an increasing quantity of food, so that the resulting intraluminal pressure does not rise; this may be termed receptive relaxation. The stomach fails to do this in two types of patient, in those with an anxiety state and in those with organic disease of the stomach such as a carcinoma. The first type is by far the more common.

DISEASES OF THE MOUTH

The mouth acts as a receptacle in which food can be broken down into small particles during mastication. Into the mouth flows the saliva which is secreted in response to the sight, taste and smell of food, and also by the act of chewing. Saliva has several functions. It is essential for speech and it moistens the food and lubricates the process of swallowing. By its solvent action on the foodstuffs, it enables tasting to take place. It also contains an enzyme ptyalin which is concerned in the digestion of polysaccharides to disaccharides.

The Teeth

The reduction of foodstuffs to a soft pulp by efficient mastication is an important prerequisite to good digestion. It is essential therefore to determine whether the patient has an adequate number of teeth in his mouth, and whether those which are present are directly in apposition in the lower and upper jaw. If dentures are used, they must be comfortable, otherwise they may be worn for social functions only, but removed at mealtimes. At one time it was widely believed that focal sepsis located in the teeth and jaws was an important factor in the production of diseases of the digestive system. The lesions held to be responsible were of two types; the first is pyorrhoea alveolaris in which pus can be expressed from the pockets lying between the teeth and the margin of the gum. The second is apical infection, from which an abscess at the root of a tooth may develop. In pyorrhoea alveolaris the septic material is swallowed and hence might theoretically produce an inflammation of the gastric mucosa, particularly in an achlorhydric stomach. In root abscess the bacteria or their toxins may be absorbed into the general circulation. The importance of focal sepsis as a cause of disease is not as widely accepted today as it was thirty years ago. However, it seems only hygienic to consult a dentist at regular intervals with the object of preventing and treating foci of infection in the teeth. Where possible teeth should be preserved and extraction should be undertaken only after the most careful consideration. When such a decision has been reached it is a wise precaution to give the patient a prophylactic injection of penicillin both before and after the operation of extraction, if valvular disease of the heart is present (p. 75).

Stomatitis

Stomatitis, or inflammation of the mouth, is of several varieties.

1. *Simple catarrhal stomatitis* occurs in poorly nourished children during the eruption of the first teeth, in adults after excessive smoking or drinking, during the course of febrile disease, in association with severe dental sepsis, and in seriously ill people whose mouths are not regularly cleaned. The lack of normal salivary flow from mastication and dehydration is a contributory cause. The gums and mouth are painful and, except in the teething infant, usually dry. The mucous membrane is reddened, the tongue swollen and covered with a dry brown fur, and in severe cases the breath is foetid. Simple catarrhal stomatitis may be prevented, and when present, treated by careful oral hygiene, especially during illness, when the mouth should be washed repeatedly with hydrogen peroxide solution and swabbed with glycerine of boric acid (B.P.) or glycerine and lemon.

2. *Stomatitis due to deficiency of nutritional factors.* Stomatitis is frequently seen in patients suffering from a deficiency of nutritional factors. Such a deficiency may arise directly from an insufficient intake of essential food factors (p. 441) or indirectly as a result of impaired absorption (pp. 939 and 943). The food factors responsible for the prevention of stomatitis belong to the B group of vitamins, especially nicotinic acid, riboflavine, folic acid and cyanocobalamin. Stomatitis is a characteristic feature of pellagra, sprue and pernicious anaemia. It also occurs in anaemia due to iron deficiency, especially when the condition is severe and chronic. When the nutritional deficiency is acute and severe the tongue is raw, red and painful; when the deficiency is chronic and

less severe the tongue appears smooth, moist and unduly clean because of papillary atrophy. All these types of stomatitis respond to replacement therapy.

3. *Stomatitis* occurs in a large number of blood dyscrasias, such as purpura, agranulocytosis, the leukaemias, etc. (p. 663).

4. *Stomatitis* may be due to infection with the specific micro-organisms causing diseases such as scarlet fever, diphtheria or syphilis. In Britain and in many other countries stomatitis, from such infections, is now rarely encountered. Ulcerative stomatitis (Vincent's angina) is also a disease which is now rarely seen but used to occur, mainly in adults, in conditions associated with malnutrition and overcrowding. Ulcers with ragged necrotic margins are seen on the gums, lips, palate, fauces or inner sides of the cheeks and the breath has a foul odour. Vincent's spirochaetes and fusiform bacilli are found in these ulcers in large numbers and are believed to be the primary cause of the disease. The condition responds rapidly to penicillin lozenges (500 units per lozenge) sucked every two hours for three to four days. To prevent spread of infection the patient's cups, plates and cutlery must be sterilised.

Parasitic stomatitis (*Thrush*). This form of stomatitis is due to an infection with the fungus *Candida albicans*. It is found in the advanced stages of debilitating diseases such as cancer, but it is also associated with the prolonged use of antibacterial substances and after treatment with corticosteroids. White sloughs covering areas of superficial ulceration appear on the gums, palate and cheeks, and they may enlarge and coalesce to form an easily detached membrane. In infants, thrush should be prevented by keeping the mouth clean and by sterilising feeding bottles and teats, and in debilitated adults by oral hygiene. The disease is treated by gently swabbing off the membrane and painting the areas with 1 per cent. aqueous solution of gentian violet twice a day for four days. If this is not successful a fungal antibiotic such as nystatin (p. 84) should be used orally. Every attempt must be made to improve the nutrition of the patient.

5. *Stomatitis* is also a feature of certain virus infections, e.g. those of herpes simplex, herpes zoster, measles, smallpox, etc.

6. *Stomatitis* can also result from a local allergic reaction to certain chemicals as in toothpastes, dentures or mint sweets, or

to antibiotics, particularly if they have been used locally. It may also be a feature of angioneurotic oedema.

7. *Stomatitis* may be caused by metals, e.g. bismuth, mercury, gold, lead or arsenic, but this is now very rarely seen. Treatment of the stomatitis consists in removing the patient from contact with the metallic poisons or stopping their administration. In severe cases dimercaprol (p. 551) should be given.

8. *Stomatitis* may be caused by phenytoin, an anticonvulsant drug used in the treatment of epilepsy, which produces a considerable overgrowth of the gums.

9. *Aphthous stomatitis* occurs both in children and in adults, in the course of various gastrointestinal disorders, or sometimes for no obvious reason in perfectly healthy persons. The lesion is extremely painful; it appears as a small vesicle which then forms an ulcer which may remain shallow or may become deep. The ulcers are often multiple. They tend to occur in patients with emotional problems, and if these can be resolved a reduction in the number of attacks may follow. The ulcers are best treated by coating them with a dental paste containing triamcinolone acetonide 0·1 per cent. after meals. The pain may be relieved by analgesic lozenges containing amethocaine.

10. Finally, there are a number of skin diseases, such as lichen planus, with oral manifestations.

The Tongue

In health the tongue is moist with only a slight white fur on the dorsum. The papillae are readily seen. Mouth breathing causes a dry tongue, but otherwise dryness of the tongue is an indication of dehydration.

The tongue may be coated with a whitish-yellow fur in persons who smoke excessively. The tongue is dry and covered with a dirty brownish fur in febrile diseases. In general, the presence of fur on the tongue has little clinical significance.

Glossitis, acute or more usually chronic, may be a prominent feature of stomatitis resulting from nutritional deficiency (p. 532).

Simple ulceration of the tongue may occur in association with various forms of stomatitis, or as a result of trauma from the sharp edges of damaged teeth, badly fitting dentures, or epileptic fits.

Chronic ulceration of the tongue. In all cases of chronic ulceration of the tongue it is essential to exclude a carcinoma and if any doubt exists biopsy should be carried out.

Syphilis of the tongue may occur as a primary chancre, in the secondary stage as 'mucous patches,' or in the tertiary stage as painless gummatous ulcers. All of these manifestations are now rare in Britain, but are common in many underdeveloped countries.

Leukoplakia of the tongue is a chronic affection characterised by the presence of white, firm, smooth patches beginning at the edges and later spreading over the dorsum. In the early stages the tongue is not painful but later the patches are split by fissures with resultant pain and tenderness. Leukoplakia is thought to be a chronic infective process not infrequently associated with syphilis and is considered by many to be a pre-cancerous state.

Treatment is that of the causal condition.

Hereditary telangiectasia may manifest itself by the occurrence of small red or purplish papules on the tongue.

The Salivary Glands

Ptyalism

Ptyalism, or excessive salivary secretion, may be a response to irritation or inflammation in the mouth, e.g. oral sepsis, or it may develop reflexly as in trigeminal neuralgia; it is an important symptom in oesophageal obstruction. An increased amount of saliva may be secreted in post-encephalitic Parkinsonism. Certain drugs such as potassium iodide and the heavy metals, especially mercury, are excreted in the saliva and this may cause an increased secretion. Reflex salivation as the cause of waterbrash has already has already been mentioned (p. 874).

Treatment. Treatment depends on removal of the underlying cause. Symptomatic treatment consists of the administration of parasympathetic paralysants such as atropine.

Xerostomia (dry mouth)

Xerostomia is usually defined as a deficient secretion of saliva though a dry mouth may be seen in mouth breathers and in persons who sleep with their mouth open. The condition is most commonly found to be associated with acute febrile conditions' and in other states of marked dehydration, such as diabetes mellitus, or when severe diarrhoea is present. Xerostomia, due to degeneration of the parotid gland associated with defective lacrimation is one of the features of a condition called Sjögren's syndrome (p. 553). As already noted, parasympathetic paralysants will depress salivary secretion.

Treatment. This consists of measures to treat the fever and cure the dehydration. Symptomatic treatment consists of the use of acidulated sweets, chewing gum, bitter tonics before meals, and very exceptionally the use of cholinergic drugs such as pilocarpine which may be required to stimulate salivary secretion when all other methods have failed. In the treatment of patients with early Sjögren's syndrome corticosteroids have been shown to cause the return of normal salivary secretion.

Parotitis

Inflammation of the parotid glands may be due to the virus of mumps (specific parotitis), the clinical features and treatment of which are described on p. 55, or to bacterial infection of the glands which tends to develop during severe febrile illnesses and after major surgical operations if adequate attention is not given to careful oral hygiene and to the prevention of dehydration and toxaemia. Septic parotitis is much more rarely encountered today than formerly. Its treatment consists in the parenteral administration of penicillin and surgical drainage if abscess formation has occurred.

* * * * * *

THE OESOPHAGUS

Anatomy. The oesophagus is a muscular tube extending from the pharynx to the cardiac end of the stomach. It has two functional sphincters, one at its junction with the pharynx, the other at its junction with the stomach. There is in addition a narrowing of the lumen where the aorta passes across the oesophagus. The oesophagus is lined with squamous epithelium and contains mucus secreting glands.

Swallowing in its first stage is a voluntary act, but once the bolus of food is on its way, it is carried on by involuntary peristalsis. The musculature of the upper part of the oesophagus is striated, but lower down it becomes smooth muscle. Though gravity helps the passage of food through the cardia, swallowing can be successfully carried out with the subject standing on his head. The exact mechanism of the lower sphincter is not clearly understood. Anatomically there is no intrinsic sphincter, but recent work has demonstrated a physiological sphincter just above the cardia. Part at least of the sphincteric action appears to depend on the angle at which the oesophagus enters the stomach. Once the attachment of the oesophagus to the diaphragm is loosened, and herniation of the stomach into the thorax occurs, regurgitation of gastric contents readily takes place as this sphincteric action is lost. If regurgitation continues to take place over any lengthy period, oesophagitis may follow. Sphincteric incompetence can take place in the absence of a hiatus hernia.

Methods of Examination. Of some value in the diagnosis of dysphagia is the ability of the patient to localise roughly the site of the obstruction.

Radiology. It is preferable for the patient to fast before the examination. In all cases the thorax should be screened and this screening may show the dilated oesophagus of achalasia, or fluid levels in hernias or diverticula. The patient is then asked to swallow a barium emulsion, which should be thicker than is usually used for stomach examinations, and he is screened erect in various oblique positions. Subsequently he should be examined in the prone position. To outline oesophageal varices a special technique is used.

Endoscopy. The whole of the gullet can be directly examined through the oesophagoscope, either through a rigid instrument under general anaesthesia or a flexible instrument under local anaesthesia. In the hands of a skilled examiner the method is almost without danger. Not only may a lesion be inspected but if necessary a biopsy specimen can be obtained.

Manometry. Manometry of the oesophagus is carried out by getting the patient to swallow tubes with small balloons at their tips arranged 5 cm. apart. These are connected through transducers to equipment which records the pressure changes. A 'swallow' is recorded and the tubes are then withdrawn and another 'swallow' is recorded. In this way it is possible to localise the boundary between thorax and abdomen, and the rhythm and the intensity of oesophageal contractions. It is a useful method when the diagnosis is obscure.

DYSPHAGIA

Dysphagia is defined as a difficulty in swallowing. Since the only function of the oesophagus is the transmission of food from mouth to stomach, most diseases of the oesophagus cause dysphagia.

Causes of Dysphagia

1. Painful diseases of the mouth and pharynx, e.g. stomatitis, tonsillitis, quinsy, tuberculous laryngitis, tumours, pharyngo-oesophageal pouch. These disorders produce dysphagia, but they do not usually cause confusion with extrinsic or intrinsic disease of the oesophagus as the site of the lesion is so readily localised. Pharyngo-oesophageal diverticulum at first only produces slight discomfort in the pharynx, but later there is more definite dysphagia. If symptoms are severe, the pouch may require excision.

2. Nervous disturbance of deglutition, e.g. diphtheritic neuritis, myasthenia gravis, bulbar paralysis, globus hystericus, achalasia and spasm of the oesophagus. These are not uncommon causes of dysphagia but are usually associated with other symptoms and signs referable to the central nervous system.

3. Extrinsic compression of the oesophagus, e.g. enlargement of thyroid, mediastinal glands, or aorta; pericardial effusion, neoplasms of bronchus. Compression may be caused by a large variety of tumours in the neck and mediastinum with resulting dysphagia. Such dysphagia, however, is rarely a presenting symptom nor is it commonly the major complaint of the patient.

4. Intrinsic disease of the oesophagus.

(*a*) Congenital abnormalities, e.g. short oesophagus.

(*b*) Inflammatory and degenerative processes, e.g. peptic oesophagitis and peptic ulcer, corrosive oesophagitis and stenosis, traction diverticulum, sideropenic dysphagia.

(*c*) Neoplasms. Carcinoma of oesophagus; carcinoma of stomach. Sarçoma and benign tumours of the oesophagus are very rare.

INTRINSIC DISEASE OF THE OESOPHAGUS

(*a*) *Congenital abnormalities.* A short oesophagus can probably occur as a congenital abnormality though it is now thought that most of the cases described as such in the past are in fact acquired, secondary to inflammation.

(*b*) *Inflammatory and degenerative processes.*

(i) Inflammation due to stagnation of food, mucus, etc. in oesophageal obstruction as occurs in achalasia and carcinoma.

(ii) Inflammation due to acid-pepsin regurgitation as occurs with incompetence of the lower sphincter in certain cases of hiatus hernia. This type of reflux oesophagitis may finally lead to oesophageal stenosis.

(iii) Oesophageal stenosis can occur from the swallowing of corrosives such as caustic soda.

(iv) Other causes of dysphagia are sideropenic dysphagia and the collagen disease, scleroderma (p. 559).

For patients with difficulty in chewing or swallowing a semi-fluid low-roughage diet (Diet 1 or 2, pp. 1284, 1285) may be indicated.

Sideropenic Dysphagia (Plummer-Vinson Syndrome)

This name is given to a condition of dysphagia, localised to the upper sphincter, which occurs mainly in women of middle age and is usually associated with an iron deficiency anaemia, diminished gastric secretion, glossitis and perhaps with koilonychia; it is believed to be due to a deficiency of the vitamin B complex, or iron, or a combination of both resulting in a degeneration and atrophy of the epithelium on the tongue, pharynx, oesophagus and stomach. In Europe and North America the syndrome is much milder and much less frequently encountered than formerly. Pathologically there is a pharyngo-oesophagitis which may be sufficiently severe to produce anatomical changes.

Treatment. The anaemia should be treated with iron (p. 616) and the deficiency of the vitamin B complex corrected by a preparation of yeast and a well-balanced diet. Dilatation is occasionally necessary.

Complications. There is an undoubted predisposition for carcinoma to develop in the hypopharynx in later years.

OESOPHAGEAL HIATUS HERNIA

The diaphragm has several openings through which herniation of abdominal viscera into the thorax can occur. Of these openings the most important is the oesophageal hiatus. In middle-aged and elderly people particularly, the oesophageal attachment weakens so that herniation of the intra-abdominal oesophagus and stomach readily occurs.

The three types of hiatus hernia usually described are:

1. *Congenital short oesophagus.* The stomach is drawn up into the thorax due to congenital shortening of the oesophagus but it is now probable that this is usually acquired.

2. *Para-oesophageal hiatus hernia.* In this condition a knuckle of stomach herniates alongside the oesophagus through the hiatus, while sometimes the entire stomach may lie above the diaphragm.

3. *Oesophagogastric or 'sliding' hernia.* In this variety both the lower part of the oesophagus and part of the fundus of the stomach herniate into the thorax and gastric reflux readily occurs. It is by far the most common form.

Aetiology. Type 2 and type 3 hernias usually develop in middle life and are probably associated with some weakness of the connective tissue holding the oesophagus to its hiatus. They are more common in women than in men, and in the flabby rather than in the lean and muscular subject. The actual herniation may be precipitated by any condition that increases intra-abdominal pressure, the most common causes being pregnancy and obesity.

Clinical Features. Many of these hernias are symptomless and are discovered accidentally by the radiologist, if he makes a practice of examining all his patients not only standing up but also lying down. Hiatus hernia usually only gives rise to symptoms in so far as the sphincteric action at the cardia is lost and free regurgitation of acid peptic juice occurs. This produces the condition of reflux oesophagitis. The patient may present with unexplained iron deficiency anaemia. Type 2 hernias are less commonly associated with oesophagitis as the sphincteric mechanism at the cardia tends to be maintained. The patient may complain of a substernal feeling of discomfort following food, due to distension of the hernial sac.

Treatment. Symptomless hernias require no treatment. If reflux oesophagitis is present medical or surgical treatment will be required.

REFLUX OESOPHAGITIS

Definition. An inflammation of the oesophagus that may lead to ulceration or stenosis produced by regurgitation of the acid peptic juice from the stomach.

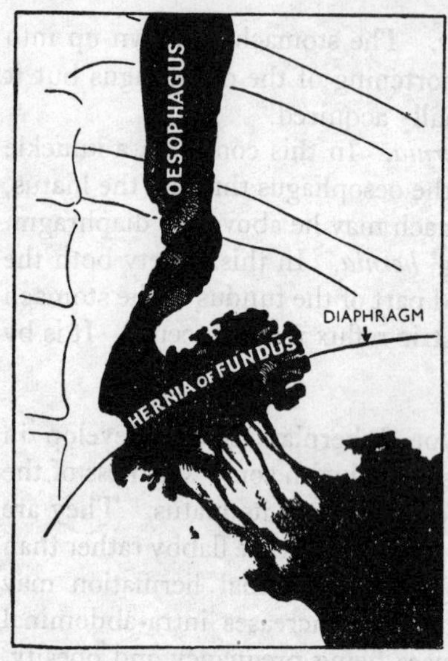

FIG. 55

Lower part of oesophagus and upper part of stomach following barium meal, showing oesophagus and part of fundus of stomach above diaphragm—chronic oesophagitis and hiatus hernia (sliding type or type 3).

Aetiology. Reflux oesophagitis may occur after repeated vomiting but usually clears up quickly when the vomiting subsides. The most common cause is the repeated regurgitation of gastric juice which occurs due to the lack of sphincteric action in patients with hiatus hernia. How the cardiac sphincter precisely acts is still disputed, but there is no doubt that much of its efficacy is lost when herniation of the stomach into the thorax occurs.

Clinical Features. The cardinal symptom of reflux oesophagitis is heartburn, which is felt substernally and may be accompanied by regurgitation of fluid into the mouth. This heartburn may occur after meals but is more typically associated with a change of posture, e.g. bending down at housework, or lifting or straining, which produces a rise of intra-abdominal pressure. It may even occur on lying down at night and may waken the patient, who obtains relief from sitting up. This nocturnal pain, which occurs within an hour of retiring, should not be confused with the nocturnal pain of duodenal ulcer, which usually comes on between 2 and 3 a.m. There is no other pain produced in the alimentary tract which is so closely linked to change of posture.

The patient may also complain of more severe pain or the sensation of food sticking which may amount to dysphagia. Such substernal pains may be confused with angina pectoris, with which they may be identical in site, character and radiation, but the absence of any relation of the pain to effort, its relation to posture, and its relief by antacids usually makes the diagnosis clear.

Bleeding not infrequently occurs in patients with hiatus hernia, and may be suspected as the cause of an obscure iron deficiency anaemia. Severe haematemesis from peptic oesophagitis is rare but when it occurs it usually comes from a small ulcer in the hernial sac.

Diagnosis. If a clear description of postural heartburn is obtained, the diagnosis may be made with considerable confidence on this alone. The diagnosis is confirmed by the radiologist, who demonstrates a hernia with oesophageal reflux. The endoscopic appearances of sliding hernias are striking and characteristic. In normal persons the oesophagus is dry save for a little swallowed saliva which can be rapidly sucked away. When, however, the sphincteric action of the cardia is lost, free regurgitation of the stomach contents occurs and with each breath the fluid wells backwards and forwards. On inspection inflammatory change or actual ulceration may be seen in acute oesophagitis, while leucoplakia of the oesophagus is commonly present when the condition is chronic.

Treatment. The majority of patients with reflux oesophagitis are in the fourth or fifth decade and can usually be maintained free from symptoms by medical treatment. The patient should take a bland diet, and if there is obesity the weight must be reduced. This is the most important item of treatment (p. 449). Patients who are particularly distressed with pain at night should be taught to sleep in a semi-upright position, with the head of the bed raised on to blocks, to diminish regurgitation of gastric juice. If the pain is at all severe, the regimen should be of the ulcer type with hourly antacids continued until the oesophagitis subsides. Anaemia which is due to bleeding should be treated with oral iron or in severe cases with blood transfusion. Oesophagitis which persists despite efficient medical treatment may require surgical treatment for its relief. Such pain is likely to be associated with ulceration and some degree of stricture formation. A stricture remaining after the oesophagitis has subsided is frequently amenable to dilatation with a mercury bougie. The patient is taught to pass this daily or sufficiently frequently to maintain a clear passage.

Traction Diverticulum

The most common site for traction diverticula is in the middle of the oesophagus near the bifurcation of the trachea. This is due to symptomless adherence of the diverticulum to inflamed lymph glands. The diverticulum is most often found accidentally during a routine radiological examination; it is usually wiser not to disclose the finding to the patient. Surgical treatment is rarely necessary.

Spasm of the Oesophagus

Spasm can occur anywhere in the oesophagus. At the upper sphincter in the oesophagus it produces the sensation of a 'lump in the throat'. A synonym for this spasm is 'globus hystericus' and the condition is not a true dysphagia as there is no difficulty in swallowing. It is usually the expression of some emotional disturbance and the symptom can be treated by explanation and reassurance and, if possible, the removal of the underlying psychological causes. Spasm can also occur in the lower part of the oesophagus in an otherwise normal organ, or in association with oesophagitis. Such spasm is painful and tends to be precipitated by nervous tension and may cause a complete blockage which persists for some minutes. The organ normally relaxes spontaneously but the sufferer may discover some helpful device to relieve it, such as forcing down a mouthful of water. Tab. trinitrin is sometimes of value in relieving spasm.

ACHALASIA

The cardinal feature of achalasia is deranged motility of the oesophagus associated with abnormal post-ganglionic cholinergic innervation. These changes affect both propulsive movements and sphincteric action so that a complete motor incoordination results.

Persistalsis in the lower oesophagus is weak and the sphincter fails to relax normally. The cause of this change is unknown and pathological examination has not always revealed changes in the ganglion cells of the narrowed segment. In certain parts of the world nutritional deficiencies are thought to be responsible.

The dysphagia, whose site is usually localised behind the sternum, is at first intermittent. Later the difficulty in swallowing becomes persistent and may be so severe that it prevents the patient from living an ordinary social life or feeding in public. If the retained contents of the oesophagus spill over into the bronchial tree, the patient may give a history of recurrent pulmonary infections.

Radiology. The radiological appearances are usually diagnostic unless the case is seen at an early stage when the achalasia is intermittent; the oesophagus may then appear normal. At a later stage, however, the barium swallow shows an absence of propulsive waves with some dilatation and elongation of the oesophagus. When the column of barium reaches a height of some inches it is seen to run through into the stomach. The outline of the oesophagus is usually smooth and has a pointed termination. The smooth outline may be broken, however, if oesophagitis is present. Carcinoma in this site has usually a much more ragged edge, and the resultant dilatation is not so marked as it is in achalasia.

Manometry. Manometric investigations show that cholinergic drugs such as Mecholyl, when given in doses of 1-5 mg. intramuscularly, will produce violent and sometimes painful contractions of the denervated section of the oesophagus. This response is characteristic and may be used to differentiate achalasia from other lesions of the oeosphagus.

Oesophagoscopy. Oesophagoscopy should always be carried out to exclude an obstructive lesion. It will usually be necessary to wash out the oesophagus first, and the changes seen will be those of inflammation occurring in a dilated oesophagus.

Diagnosis. From the history, the radiological, endoscopic and, if necessary, manometric examinations the diagnosis is usually obvious.

Treatment. Instrumental dilatation is recommended. A bougie is passed into the oesophagus with a bag tied on its lower end and is so arranged that the bag lies in the last part of the oesophagus at the level of the cardiac sphincter. Using water pressure the bag is then dilated with sufficient force to rupture some of the circular fibres of the oesophagus. A single dilatation may cure the patient permanently. If the patient remains unrelieved after two such dilatations, operation should be considered. Heller's operation, consisting of an anterior incision through the narrowed segment of the oesophagus and the cardia is the procedure generally recommended.

CARCINOMA OF THE OESOPHAGUS

Carcinoma of the oesophagus is mainly a disease of the male sex and tends to occur at a later age than other cancers. It has some association with smoking. The most frequent site is in the lower third of the oesophagus. It is less common in the middle third and least common in the upper third. As in cancer elsewhere the morphological appearance may vary and the growth may be described as polypoid, ulcerative or scirrhous, resulting in the formation of a stricture. Histologically, the growth is squamous-celled. Where an adenocarcinoma is found, it has probably arisen from a gastric carcinoma that has invaded the oesophagus.

Clinical Features. The most common complaint is that of dysphagia, noticed first with solid foods, and which, starting as the mildest of symptoms, develops progressively in severity. The early and occasional discomfort grows into more constant pain, and with increasing stenosis regurgitation of food develops. By the time the patient is first seen by a doctor, which is usually some months after the initial symptoms have appeared, there is considerable loss of weight.

On questioning, the patient will frequently localise the site of obstruction accurately. Apart from wasting, which may be extreme, and possibly the enlargement of lymphatic nodes and liver from metastases, there may be no obvious abnormal physical signs.

Radiology. In the great majority of cases radiological examina-ion reveals the lesion as an irregularity of outline of the wall of the oesophagus with perhaps some stenosis and dilatation above (Fig. 56). There may be difficulty in distinguishing a carcinoma of the oesophagus from an extension of a carcinoma of the cardia. Also a carcinomatous stricture may simulate a benign stricture or an ulcerating carcinoma may be confused with a benign peptic ulcer of the oesophagus. In most cases, however, the radiological diagnosis is not difficult.

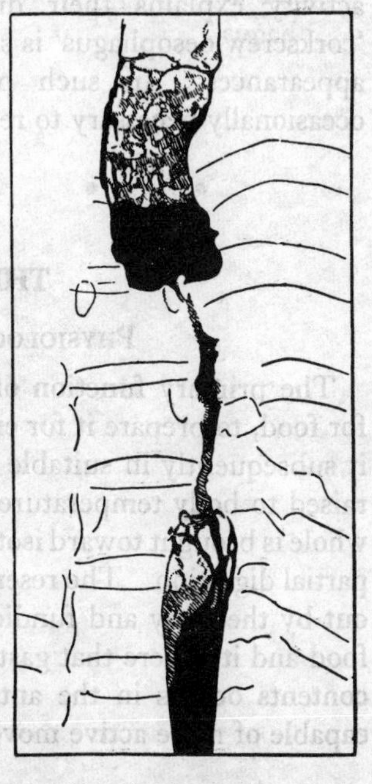

Fig. 56

Oesophagus following barium swallow showing long irregular stricture with barium and food residue above it—carcinoma of oesophagus. Only slight dilatation of oesophagus above the carcinoma.

Oesophagoscopy. Endoscopy should always be carried out and provides the opportunity of removing tissue for microscopy. In malignant disease, a high proportion of positive results may be obtained by passing a small brush into the stricture and examining microscopically a stained smear of the cells thus obtained.

Treatment. The choice of treatment lies between surgery and radiotherapy and conflicting claims in their support have been made from different centres. It is probable however, that radiotherapy is the treatment of choice. Whichever treatment is adopted, a small percentage of three-year and five-year 'cures' can be achieved. If radical measures have failed, dilatation of a stenosing carcinoma may help the patient and sometimes an artificial dilator may be permanently inserted into the growth. Gastrostomy as a palliative procedure provides little prolongation of life and adds further discomfort to a weary patient.

OESOPHAGEAL DYSKINESIA

The introduction of manometry into the investigation of dysphagia has revealed in some patients with oesophageal spasm, a series of strong contractions which are non-propulsive. In other patients, usually elderly, a bizarre pattern of incoordinated motor activity explains their difficulty in swallowing. The name 'corkscrew oesophagus' is sometimes applied to these radiological appearances. In such patients a longitudinal myotomy is occasionally necessary to relieve their symptoms.

* * * * * *

THE STOMACH

Physiology of the Stomach

The primary function of the stomach is to act as a reservoir for food, to prepare it for entry into the duodenum and to deliver it subsequently in suitable amounts. In this process the food is raised to body temperature, is reduced to a semiliquid state, the whole is brought toward isotonicity, while some foodstuffs undergo partial digestion. The reservoir function of the stomach is carried out by the body and fundic portion which relaxes to receive the food and it is here that gastric secretion is added. Mixing of the contents occurs in the antral portion, the part of the stomach capable of more active movements.

Movements of the Stomach. Changes in intragastric pressure can be recorded from a tube which has been swallowed. The end of the tube may be open or have a small balloon attached. In the fasting subject, the tracing indicates that the stomach goes into phases of activity—'hunger periods'—lasting usually some 30 to 40 minutes with intermediate periods of quiescence. These hunger periods, with their strong contractions, underlie the sensation of pangs of hunger in the normal subject, and the sensation of 'hunger pains' in some cases of peptic ulcer. Though the movements occur spontaneously, they may be prolonged by cholinergic drugs.

The above type of study, though useful in research, is less convenient clinically than the radiological examination of a subject following a barium meal. The stomach, which cannot be visualised when empty, is seen when filled with barium sulphate, and the motility and rate of emptying can then be directly observed. Waves may be seen to form in the body of the stomach, deepening as they move down the lesser curvature, until, in the antrum, they form deep constrictions. The rate of emptying of a barium meal may also be observed, the stomach being re-examined at certain intervals after ingestion. Normally, the stomach is empty in four hours, but should always be completely empty of barium in six hours.

Emptying of the Stomach. Gastric evacuation depends on various factors. Basically the rate of emptying of the stomach varies with the volume of contents, i.e. the greater the volume the faster the rate of emptying. Various factors affect this rate; both an increase in acid and an increase or decrease in osmolality act as 'brakes' on the rate of emptying through a reflex mechanism, while a buffered iso-osmolar fluid meal empties extremely rapidly. A fatty meal delays emptying through the release of a local hormone in the upper small intestine. In the pathological stomach it is clear that the rate of emptying and degree of motility are not synonymous. A stomach with vigorous contractions is typical of early pyloric stenosis, and this empties slowly; while the 'leather-bottle' stomach, with absent contractions, empties very rapidly. Therapeutically, when it is desired to increase gastric motility, drugs of the cholinergic group, such as Mechothane (urethane β-methyl choline chloride) may be employed and are particularly useful in the atonic stomach following vagotomy. Drugs which inhibit movement include the parasympathetic paralysants, such as atropine, and ganglionic paralysants—such as the hexamethonium salts.

Gastric Secretion. Another important function of the stomach is to secrete a digestive juice. This juice contains hydrochloric acid, pepsin, mucus, and the intrinsic factor of Castle, essential for normal haemopoiesis. There are specific cells for the secretion of acid (parietal cells), for pepsin and for mucus. In man the site of production of intrinsic factor is the body and fundus of the stomach and its source may be the parietal cells.

The secretion of both hydrochloric acid and pepsin is under the control of a nervous and hormonal mechanism, and stimulation of the vagus by hypoglycaemia, or of the vagal nerve endings by cholinergic drugs produces a secretion of pepsin.

The secretion of mucus is enhanced by the mechanical rubbing action of food, but it is uncertain if its secretion is also under nervous control.

The nervous mechanism is actuated through the vagus, and acid secretion can be stimulated following the sight or smell of food; this appetite juice has been shown to disappear in man after cutting the vagus. This secretion may also be abolished or reduced by atropine. The injection of insulin, 15 units intravenously, into a fasting patient, by producing a hypoglycaemia, causes the stomach to secrete an acid juice. This test has been used after vagotomy as a measure of the completeness of section of the nerve.

Acid can also be secreted in response to the presence of food in the stomach, and a hormone, gastrin, is responsible for this action. The secretory action of the vagus is largely through the release of gastrin from the pyloric antrum. Gastrin has now been isolated in pure form, its structure characterised and its synthesis achieved. It is an extremely powerful compound. Histamine is also an effective stimulant of acid secretion and there is evidence that gastrin stimulates acid secretion through the release of histamine.

According to one theory it is believed that the primary secretion of the parietal cell is roughly isotonic with the blood, and by stimulation of the human stomach with pure gastrin or with large doses of histamine, it is possible to obtain hydrochloric acid of about 150 m.Eq/*l*., that is, very near the theoretical maximum. This primary acidity, as secreted directly by the parietal cells, is then diluted and partly neutralised by secretion from non-parietal sources; it may of course be further diluted with stomach contents. The output of acid represents the product of a number of parietal cells termed the 'parietal cell mass', and it is more accurate to refer to 'output of acid' rather than to 'acid concentration.

Secretory tests. Any test of the acid secretory capacity of the stomach can only yield information about:

(*a*) The number of parietal functioning cells. An estimate of the 'parietal cell mass' may be made by measuring the output of acid from the stomach in a given time following maximal stimulation. The details of the test are given below.

(*b*) The response of these parietal cells to certain stimuli, nervous and hormonal. There is no satisfactory method of measuring the stimuli to which a given stomach is being subjected, or the responsiveness of the parietal cells. It may be that in certain patients, there is an increased vagal tone so that the parietal cells are being subjected to an abnormally intense or a more prolonged stimulation. It may also be that in other patients increased amounts of gastrin are being released. For the moment these hypotheses remain unproven.

(*c*) The effectiveness of the inhibitory mechanism. Of the precise nature of the inhibitory mechanisms little is known, but at present it does not seem likely that they are of much clinical importance.

The most useful test, therefore, within the limitations of our present knowledge, is one which measures the 'parietal cell mass'. This estimate is made by measuring the output of acid from the stomach obtained under conditions of strong stimulation over a fixed period since the amount secreted is probably directly related to the number of parietal cells in the gastric mucosa. The ideal stimulant would be the pure hormone gastrin but this is unobtainable commercially. Histamine is widely used together with an antihistamine drug to prevent some of the side-effects and is extremely effective. Histamine acid phosphate in a dose of 0·04 mg./kg. body weight is given subcutaneously preceded by an intramuscular injection of mepyramine maleate 50-100 mg. half an hour before the injection of histamine. Antihistamine drugs have no effect in blocking the action of histamine on the parietal cells. As an alternative stimulant there is now available a small polypeptide, structurally related to gastrin, pentagastrin (Peptavlon), which gives closely similar results to histamine in a dose of 6 μg./kg. body weight subcutaneously.

The practical procedure is to pass a soft rubber tube into the stomach, through the nose, which is anaesthetised by amethocaine. The tube should be radio-opaque and the terminal holes must be of adequate size, as in the Levin type. The position of the tube in the stomach must be checked by fluoroscopy and it is then attached to a suction pump, with the patient lying on his left side. Continuous aspiration is then begun, and samples collected. After an hour's resting secretion has been obtained, the appropriate stimulant is given and the juice collected for a further hour. The volumes are measured, the juice titrated, and the output calculated.

Intrepretation. The mean output of a group of patients with duodenal ulcer is higher than the mean output of a group of normals, and the mean output of the normal group is higher than the mean output of a group of patients with gastric ulcer. There is, however, an overlap between the groups so that the diagnostic value of the test is limited. The measurement of acid output is of value in deciding whether operation is indicated. Surgical results are likely to be more satisfactory if operation for duodenal ulcer is only undertaken when acid secretion falls within the duodenal ulcer range. The surgeon may also use this value to guide him in determining the extent of the operation which is necessary to reduce gastric secretion.

Achlorhydria. Achlorhydria may be defined as the absence of any hydrochloric acid in the gastric juice; such a finding is obviously related to the effectiveness of the stimulant employed and the sensitivity of the method used to detect the presence of the acid. In this sense the definition is arbitrary. If the most potent stimulus to gastric secretion is applied, such as maximal doses of histamine or gastrin, and achlorhydria is defined as a failure to lower the pH of the neutral resting juice by more than one unit, then it is extremely uncommon to find achlorhydria except in patients who have pernicious anaemia or who are going to develop it.

Interpretation. If the output of acid from the stomach is directly related to the number of parietal cells present, the anatomical basis for achlorhydria would be an absence of such cells, and in general this is true. Decreased output of acid is often related to the presence of gastritis, and may be found in gastric ulcer, gastric carcinoma and idiopathic gastritis. If the gastritis improves, as with healing of a gastric ulcer, acid secretion may return towards normal.

Gastric Investigation

In clinical practice the human stomach can be examined by various methods:

1. Physical examination.
2. Radiology.

3. Endoscopy.
4. Laboratory tests, particularly those assessing secretion (p. 896).
5. Biopsy.

Physical methods. There are three physical signs of great value in gastric disease.

1. *Pointing sign.* The patient with a history suggestive of ulcer dyspepsia is asked to indicate, with one hand, where he gets his pain. The sign is positive if the patient localises the pain accurately with a finger, or group of fingers. A positive sign strongly suggests, but is not pathognomonic of, peptic ulcer. This is the best physical sign of ulcer we possess.

2. *Muscular rigidity.* Muscular rigidity is well recognised in cases of generalised peritonitis, but it should be carefully sought for in all cases of dyspepsia, when it may be demonstrated in a much milder form, by careful palpation first of one rectus and then of the other. If one rectus is persistently firmer and more resistant than the other, there is unilateral rigidity, and this reflex is most likely to have arisen from peritoneal inflammation, due to an ulcer.

3. *Visible peristalsis.* To elicit this sign, the examiner should kneel down by the side of the bed, so that the light strikes across the abdomen. The epigastrium should then be carefully watched for waves passing from left to right. A carbonated drink is a useful stimulus or the waves may be started by flicking the skin over the epigastrium with the finger. Unless the abdominal wall is extremely thin, a positive sign always means some degree of pyloric obstruction, most commonly due to a stenosing duodenal ulcer.

Though the normal stomach is not palpable, tumours of the body or antrum may be felt in patients with advanced carcinoma.

Radiology. Next to taking a careful history, the radiological examination is the most important diagnostic method; this method (using a barium meal), gives some idea of the motor activity of the stomach and its rate of emptying. It is also possible to outline ulcer craters, and to show filling defects from carcinomatous infiltration, and herniation through the diaphragm. The mucous membrane pattern may be delineated by using small quantities of barium, and, with a tilting table, the stomach may be examined in various positions. By such manipulations the accuracy of ulcer diagnosis in certain sites of the stomach can be extraordinarily high. In the cardia and the antrum mistakes are more readily made, while the radiology of an artificial stoma is perhaps most difficult of all. The distinction between a benign and a carcinomatous ulcer may baffle the most experienced.

Endoscopy. It is possible with a flexible gastroscope to inspect most of the interior of the stomach. The operation, in experienced hands, is reasonably safe, and with a co-operative patient occasions little distress. A recently developed instrument called the fiberscope, consisting of a bundle of fine, coated, quartz fibres, is particularly successful for inspection of the antrum. Gastroscopy may be looked on as a useful diagnostic method, accessory to radiology. It is also possible to photograph the interior of the stomach. These endoscopic methods are particularly valuable in giving a practitioner a vivid insight into a living pathology.

Biopsy. It is now possible, using a flexible tube, to obtain specimens of gastric mucosa. The manœuvre is comparatively safe and causes little distress.

PEPTIC ULCER

Aetiology. The term 'peptic ulcer' refers to an ulcer found either in the lower end of the oesophagus, the stomach, the duodenum, the small intestine anastomosed to the stomach, or rarely, at the junction of a Meckel's diverticulum with the small intestine, and is caused by the acid-pepsin digestion of the mucosa. Since normal stomachs secreting acid and pepsin do not develop ulcers, we must postulate the existence of some protective mechanism. The central equation of ulcer aetiology may be written:

Acid-pepsin versus *Mucosal Resistance*

The evidence that ulcers can only occur in the presence of acid and pepsin is very strong. Peptic ulceration has never been found in patients with pernicious anaemia, and if rigid criteria are used (p. 898) it is doubtful if an active ulcer has ever been shown to occur in association with achlorhydria.

In the past, most attention has been paid to the left-hand side of the equation, and investigators have sought for abnormalities in secretion which might explain ulcer formation. These abnormalities might be (1) qualitative, but there is no evidence that the parietal cell in a case of duodenal ulcer secretes acid of higher concentration than does a similar cell in the stomach of a normal person; or (2) quantitative, that is, an excessive response to a meal, or a prolonged secretion during the interdigestive period. In the case of chronic duodenal ulcers, both these factors may operate.

Such abnormalities, however, are not found in all ulcer patients, and indeed in patients with gastric ulcer secretion is usually lower than normal, hence it is necessary to look for factors affecting the mucosal resistance to acid peptic digestion. The nature of these factors is unknown, but four possibilities should be considered:

1. *Mucus.* Alkaline mucus is the first line of defence for the gastric mucosa, and probably acts simply as a protective antacid barrier against the acid fluid. Of great importance is the ability of the superficial layer of mucous cells to renew itself every two or three days.

2. *The nutrition* of the stomach mucosa must be of importance in maintaining its health. However it is doubtful if malnutrition plays any significant part in the aetiology of peptic ulceration in Britain, except possibly in some patients with gastric ulcer.

3. *Blood supply.* One of the classical theories of ulcer formation is that which ascribes the lowering of mucosal resistance to poor blood supply and it is possible that some of the gastric ulcers occurring in the elderly are due to thrombosis, venous or arterial. The possibility of a 'shunt' circulation in the mucosa may provide a possible anatomical mechanism.

4. *Hormonal factors.* There is a striking sex difference in the incidence of duodenal ulcer which may indicate a greater immunity of women to ulceration. This immunity seems to increase in pregnancy, so that active ulceration producing bleeding or perforation is then almost unknown. When pregnancy has ended, reactivation of the ulcer may occur quite rapidly. These observations have led to a search for humoral substances which might hasten ulcer healing.

Constitutional Factors.

Heredity. There seems no doubt that in peptic ulcer there is a definite hereditary factor and a certain tendency for the disposition to ulcer formation to run true to type, that is, for patients with duodenal ulcer to beget children who develop duodenal ulcer, and likewise for gastric ulcer. A strong family history is frequently found in patients who develop ulcers in childhood or soon after puberty.

ABO blood groups. There is a striking association of peptic ulcer with blood group O, an association which has been confirmed in a large number of countries. There is no satisfactory explanation of this association.

Seasonal Factor. There is a strong seasonal factor which can be shown in the seasonal variations in mortality rate and in the recurrence of symptoms of ulcer. In Britain ulcer mortality is at its lowest in August and September, and begins to rise in October. Symptoms also tend to recur at this time, and there is a further exacerbation of symptoms in the spring. The cause of this seasonal variation is unknown.

Stress. The occurrence of acute ulcers following physical or mental trauma or a surgical operation, is undoubted. Such episodes may be accompanied by the excretion of increased amounts of cortical steroids in the urine. It is therefore tempting to postulate a causative stress mechanism which acts through the adrenal cortex.

Pathology. Ulcers occurring in the stomach and duodenum may be acute or chronic, the acute being frequently multiple, and occurring less regularly in those well-defined sites which chronic ulcers tend to occupy, i.e. either on or near the lesser curve above the angulus, or, less frequently, near the pylorus. Both types are found less commonly near the cardia, and only rarely on the greater curvature or on the anterior wall. In the duodenum they are usually on the anterior or posterior walls.

Clinical Features. While there are grounds for thinking that gastric and duodenal ulcer are separate aetiological diseases, it is convenient to give the general features of 'peptic ulcer' as inclusive of both, noting differences where they occur.

Peptic ulcer may manifest itself in various ways. The most common history is of a chronic dyspepsia, extending over months or years. The ulcer may, however, come to notice as an acute episode with bleeding or perforation with little or no previous history. Rarely the patient may present with pyloric obstruction, having had negligible previous dyspepsia.

Dyspepsia. In the early stages it is typically intermittent, with intervals of relief in which the patient can do and eat anything;

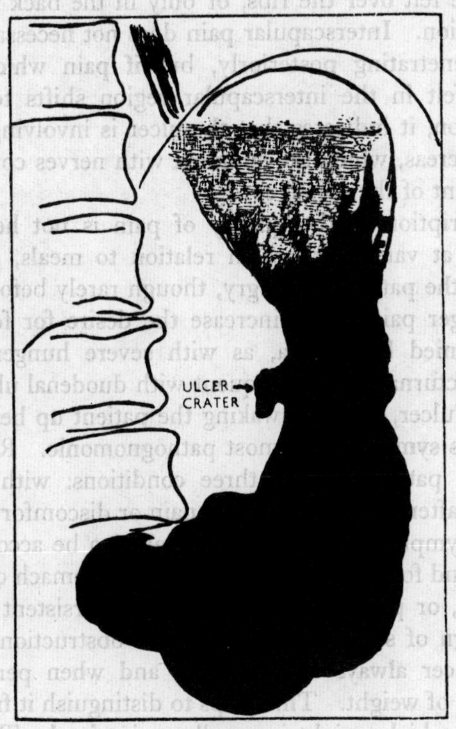

Fig. 57
Stomach following barium meal showing large projection from lesser curvature—gastric ulcer.

but later these intervals lessen, and the discomfort becomes persistent. The cause for these relapses can only rarely be found. Seasonal factors are responsible in a small percentage of cases, the dyspepsia returning with the colder weather in October and November, with possibly a further exacerbation in the spring. Sometimes a psychological stress is blamed, sometimes some article of diet and sometimes alcoholic overindulgence. Infection seems to be an occasional cause. Most commonly, no reason can be found for the relapse.

Pain. This symptom may vary in severity, and it is often useful to get the patient to qualify it as 'pain', or as 'discomfort', to get an idea of its intensity. It is felt in the epigastrium, the lower chest or the back, in the segments supplied by Th. 5-8. The pain may only be felt over the ribs, or only in the back in the interscapular region. Interscapular pain does not necessarily indicate an ulcer penetrating posteriorly, but if pain which has been previously felt in the interscapular region shifts to the upper lumbar region, it indicates that the ulcer is involving structures, e.g. the pancreas, which are supplied with nerves coming from a lower segment of the spinal cord.

The description of the quality of pain is not helpful. The pain is felt at varying times in relation to meals, often before food, when the patient is hungry, though rarely before breakfast. These 'hunger pains' may increase the desire for food, or may be accompanied by nausea, as with severe hunger in normal people. Nocturnal pain is frequent with duodenal ulcer and rare with gastric ulcer, the pain waking the patient up between 2 and 3 a.m. This symptom is almost pathognomonic. Relief of pain is noted by patients under three conditions: with food, after antacids, or after vomiting. While pain or discomfort is the most prominent symptom, the dyspepsia may also be accompanied by heartburn, and followed by regurgitation of stomach contents into the pharynx, or possibly by waterbrash. Persistent vomiting is usually a sign of some degree of pyloric obstruction. Vomiting in peptic ulcer always relieves pain and when persistent may result in loss of weight. This helps to distinguish it from nervous vomiting, in which weight is usually maintained. Though there is no constant change of bowel rhythm during an ulcer relapse, some patients experience the symptoms of 'spastic colon' when the ulcer dyspepsia reappears.

Physical Signs. Of all the physical signs, the 'pointing sign', as already described, is the most valuable. The accurate localisation of pain, localised tenderness and rigidity over one rectus muscle, when present together, are practically diagnostic of ulcer.

Radiology. While an acute ulcer (p. 909) is frequently invisible radiologically, practically all chronic ulcers are detectable by a good radiologist. The characteristic sign is the niche, either seen in profile (Fig. 57) or seen *en face* with radiating mucosal folds. In the case of a deeply penetrating ulcer, the niche may show a fluid level. An experienced radiologist will miss very few ulcers on the lesser curvature or posterior wall, but may miss them in the antrum or near the cardia. In the duodenum it requires careful technique to demonstrate the niche, which is most usually shown *en face* with radiating folds (Fig. 58). The cap will be distorted by spasm, and if scarring occurs it will produce permanent deformity.

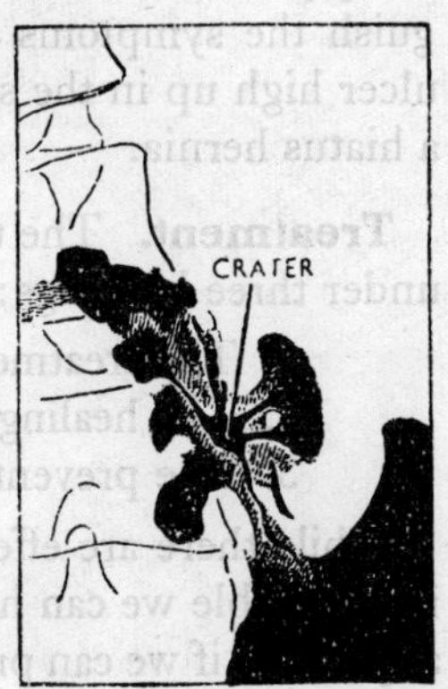

Fig. 58

Oblique view of duodenal cap showing ulcer crater with typical general deformity and radiating folds from the ulcer.

Endoscopy. Endoscopic examination of the stomach will confirm the presence of an ulcer if it is situated in an accessible site, that is, on the lesser curvature or posterior wall of the stomach. It may be difficult to find an ulcer high up on the posterior wall, and ulcers near the pylorus are seen less easily. Gastroscopy may help to decide whether an ulcer is benign or malignant, and it is possible to watch the healing of an ulcer by examination at intervals. It is justifiable, and occasionally useful to employ gastroscopy to determine the source of bleeding in a severe haematemesis.

Laboratory Procedures. *Secretion test* (p. 896). This test is of limited diagnostic value but gives some indication of the intractability of the ulcer and may suggest a need for surgery.

Occult blood. In all disorders of the gastrointestinal tract a useful test is that for the presence of occult blood in the stool. The O-tolidine tablet test (Haematest, Ames & Co.) is simple, accurate and convenient.

Diagnosis. The diagnosis of peptic ulcer is suggested by the history and confirmed by radiological examination. The history of ulcer pain is typical, but if ulcer pain is ultimately related to the sensitisation of nerve endings by inflammation, then the same symptoms might occur in a patient with gastritis or duodenitis alone or with some other lesion such as a carcinoma of the stomach.

Nervous dyspepsia may give rise to difficulty, but the history is rarely as clear cut, the pain cannot be localised, and there is no sharply defined tender area. It is sometimes difficult to distinguish the symptoms of pain and heartburn caused by a gastric ulcer high up in the stomach, from reflux oesophagitis caused by a hiatus hernia.

Treatment. The treatment of peptic ulcer may be considered under three headings:

1. The treatment of symptoms,
2. The healing of an individual ulcer,
3. The prevention of recurrence.

While there are effective methods of removing symptoms, and it is possible we can hasten the healing of an ulcer, it is doubtful, at present, if we can prevent its recurrence, or can alter the natural tendency to remit and relapse. It must never be forgotten that the relief of symptoms, which is naturally the main concern of the patient, does not mean the healing of the ulcer. Relief of symptoms can occur in a few days; healing of an ulcer may take six weeks or longer. Once the patient is in this painless phase, the ulcer may persist for many months without any further recurrence of pain, and without any change in its size. The more chronic an ulcer the less chance there is of obtaining healing, and such ulcers may require surgical treatment. It should, therefore, be our aim to heal an ulcer in the early stages in the hope of preventing this irreversible development. Unfortunately, this ideal is difficult to attain for economic reasons, as the patient is frequently unable to afford the time off work. Hospitalisation is usually reserved for those patients with complications, such as stenosis, bleeding or intractable pain, and for those with large gastric or duodenal ulcers—or where any question of malignancy arises.

1. Rest. For the relief of ulcer pain and the promotion of healing, rest is the single most effective measure. This may be undertaken at home under the supervision of the family doctor or in hospital, where more complete freedom from domestic and business cares may be obtained. Rest implies bed rest, though visits to the toilet and bathing are allowed. With this régime pain frequently disappears in a few days.

2. Diet. It has been said that a suitable diet should be mechanically and chemically non-irritating, and should consist of small

frequent meals. Much of this advice has little experimental evidence to support it. It has been shown, for example, that hourly feedings of milk provoke more acid secretion in the stomach than does the ordinary routine of four meals a day: nor is there any evidence that the rate of healing of an ulcer is increased by taking the traditional bland ulcer diet. However, the patient often appreciates frequent feedings, and gets relief from a glass of milk in between his meals. For a suitable diet see Diet 2 (p. 1285) and the instructions for a patient with dyspepsia (p. 1286).

3. SMOKING. There is good evidence for believing that smoking delays healing. There are therefore grounds for prohibiting smoking, at any rate for a trial period. If patients find from experience that relapses are prevented, they should naturally be encouraged to abstain permanently from smoking.

4. DRUGS. *Antacids.* The common antacids used are sodium bicarbonate, magnesium oxide, hydroxide and carbonate, calcium carbonate, bismuth carbonate, aluminium hydroxide and magnesium trisilicate. The disadvantage of the absorbable alkalis, such as sodium bicarbonate, is that they may produce alkalosis. This however rarely occurs except with excessive dosage, vomiting or when renal disease is present. For this reason, aluminium hydroxide and magnesium trisilicate are often prescribed, though patients do not get such rapid relief from them due to their slower neutralising action. It is possible, by giving antacids frequently, to reduce the level of acidity in the stomach sufficiently low to prevent peptic digestion, i.e. above pH 5, and to do this it is theoretically necessary to relate the dose of antacid to the secretory capacity of the stomach. It has not, however, been shown that such intensive alkali therapy is essential to the healing of an ulcer, or indeed hastens it; antacids are usually given in less heroic dosage to relieve pain. If pain is severe, however, antacids should be given frequently and there need be no hesitation in giving 1-2 g. hourly of Pulv. Mag. Trisil. Co. B.P.C. Antacids are also available in tablet form which can be conveniently carried in the pocket (Gelusil, Nulacin). The composition of a mixture of antacids can be altered so that by increasing the amount of magnesium salt, a laxative effect will be produced, while increasing the amount of calcium salts or aluminium hydroxide tends to cause constipation.

Vagal paralysants. Belladonna and atropine have been used for many years for their action in inhibiting vagal stimulation and thus reducing gastric motility and secretion. Innumerable substitutes have been synthesised with the object of increasing the desired effect on the stomach, and of reducing the undesirable side-effects e.g. on salivary secretion. There is no conclusive evidence that this goal has yet been reached and atropine and belladonna appear to be as cheap and convenient as any of the synthetic substitutes while with tincture of belladonna the dose can be easily regulated. Anticholinergic drugs seem most valuable in relieving nocturnal pain and for this purpose should be pushed to the limit of tolerance so that the patient wakes up with a dry mouth or blurred vision. The dose is then somewhat reduced. A suitable starting dose is 3 ml. of the tincture of belladonna. Such large doses cannot of course be given by day to ambulant patients and they are ill tolerated by the elderly. Of the synthetic substitutes propantheline 15 mg. and poldine methy sulphate (2-6 mg.) are perhaps best. These drugs are contraindicated in glaucoma, prostatism and gastric retention.

Many practitioners find sedative drugs most useful in the treatment of ulcer patients, particularly those who are often described as 'highly strung'. For these patients phenobarbitone is a reliable sedative in relieving some of their tension. Tranquillisers such as chlorpromazine may be helpful, starting with a dose of 25 mg. t.d.s. There is evidence from clinical trials that a derivative of liquorice, carbenoxolone sodium (Biogastrone) expedites the healing of gastric ulcers in ambulant patients. It should be given in a dosage of 50-100 mg. three times a day but it causes sodium and water retention and this may prove risky to elderly subjects. No beneficial effect on duodenal ulcers has yet been demonstrated.

Surgical Treatment. Operative treatment must be *considered* for the following conditions:

1. An ulcer which has failed to heal under efficient medical treatment, and when symptoms persist or recur.
2. An ulcer which has produced pyloric or duodenal stenosis or hour-glass stomach.
3. An ulcer which is thought to be malignant.
4. A jejunal ulcer following gastrojejunostomy.
5. Perforation of a peptic ulcer.
6. Haemorrhage, severe or recurrent.

There is as yet no single, ideal surgical operation. For gastric ulcer the operation of choice is that of partial gastrectomy in which the ulcer itself and the ulcer-bearing area of the stomach is resected. Anastomosis of the gastric stump to the duodenum may be possible. For duodenal ulcer various procedures are available, including partial gastrectomy, the object being to remove sufficient of the acid-secreting area to allow the ulcer to heal. An alternative operation is that of vagotomy, which aims at reducing the nervous stimulation of gastric secretion. This operation, which also interferes with gastric emptying, must always be combined with some form of drainage procedure such as pyloroplasty or gastro-enterostomy. The choice of operation is to some extent guided by measurements of the secretory capacity of the stomach. When this is very high, some surgeons prefer to combine partial gastrectomy with vagotomy in order to ensure that the secretion is sufficiently reduced. The anastomosis of a highly secreting stomach to the jejunum may result in a jejunal ulcer so that a simple gastrojejunostomy should only be carried out for duodenal stenosis when the measured secretory capacity of the stomach is low. For a jejunal ulcer following a previous anastomosis, either vagotomy alone or a further resection of the stomach should be considered (p. 917). No matter which type of elective operation is advised it is important that the patient should not be over-persuaded to accept it.

Complications. The common complications of peptic ulcer are haemorrhage, perforation, and pyloric obstruction. Ulcer-cancer is discussed under *Carcinoma.*

Gastro-duodenal Haemorrhage

Bleeding, in the sense of a positive test for occult blood in the stools, can be detected at some time or another in the great majority of cases of peptic ulcer. Gastro-duodenal haemorrhage, as a complication, is taken to mean bleeding of sufficient severity as to cause symptoms on its own account.

Aetiology. The common causes in Britain are:

1. Acute gastric ulcer.
2. Chronic gastric ulcer.
3. Chronic duodenal ulcer.

4. Carcinoma of the stomach.
5. Portal hypertension.

The first three cover 90 per cent. of all cases. Acute ulcers range from minute erosions to shallow ulcers an inch or two in diameter and involving only the mucosa. They may be related to infection, stress, intracerebral lesions and to the taking of aspirin. Their presence is only manifested by bleeding or perforation and there may be no previous history of dyspepsia. They are difficult to demonstrate on radiological examination, and heal rapidly. Bleeding from oesophageal varices secondary to portal hypertension can be extremely severe and may demand special measures for its management (p. 1034). Bleeding from an area of oesophagitis is usually of a much milder degree (p. 889).

Haemorrhage shows itself by the vomiting of blood (i.e. haematemesis), or by the passage of altered blood in the stools (i.e. melaena). If the blood has been in the stomach for any length of time, it appears brown and granular in the vomit—so-called 'coffee grounds.' The blood passed per rectum makes the stool black and sticky, but if bleeding is rapid, there is little time for this change to take place. Since rapid bleeding is more likely to produce vomiting, the prognosis is worse with a haematemesis than with a melaena. Apart from the rate of bleeding, the whole outlook in gastro-duodenal haemorrhage naturally depends on whether the bleeding will stop spontaneously, and this in turn depends on the type of vessel involved. If the bleeding is coming from a sclerotic vessel, which cannot retract, the outlook for spontaneous cessation is poor. If bleeding is capillary, and the vessels can retract, natural cessation of haemorrhage will follow. It therefore follows that the main prognostic factor in haemorrhage is the extent and type of vascular disease, which is usually related to the age of the patient.

Bleeding from oesophageal varices secondary to portal hypertension is at present rarer in Britain than in the United States, but is increasing in frequency.

Clinical Features. The patient complains of a feeling of weakness, often specifically mentioned as being in the legs, nausea, sweating, faintness, and this is followed by the actual vomiting, or passage of blood. Frank blood can traverse the gut, and appear from the rectum within minutes of the onset of symptoms.

On examination, the patient is pale, faint, sweating and anxious. The pulse rate is always raised, and the blood pressure may show a fall. The pulse rate is the most sensitive objective measurement of the extent of the bleeding. The ordinary laboratory tests are of limited value. Until haemodilution occurs, the haemoglobin level will not alter, and this may not take place for some hours, nor be complete for some days. There is, in fact, no simple laboratory procedure which will give any estimate of the amount of blood loss until the haemodilution is complete, and this, therefore, throws great responsibility on clinical judgment.

Management. The patient should be put to bed, and given morphine 15 mg. to allay anxiety. Thereafter a sedative such as phenobarbitone should be given. Blood should be taken for haemoglobin estimation, and for blood grouping. An hourly record should be kept of the patient's pulse and blood pressure. The immediate decision to be made, on clinical grounds, is whether to give blood transfusion. If the patient is elderly, and has obviously lost a good deal of blood, there is no doubt that blood is not only necessary but needs to be given rapidly in large amounts. If the patient is young, and has bled slightly, it should be quite safe to wait. The main indications for blood transfusions are the severity and persistence of bleeding. If there is doubt about whether bleeding is continuing, a soft rubber tube can be introduced into the stomach and samples removed at hourly intervals for inspection.

After haemorrhage food should be given as soon as the patient asks for it and he should be encouraged to eat an ordinary ulcer diet. Iron should also be given to aid in the restoration of a normal blood count (p. 616).

It is possible to examine the patient radiologically during the acute episode and identify the causative lesion in the majority of instances. For this purpose it is safer to use Gastrografin (Schering, Ltd.), instead of the usual barium sulphate suspension. Some physicians prefer to defer radiological examination until bleeding has ceased, but examinations at this time will frequently be negative owing to healing of an acute ulcer.

The persistence or recurrence of bleeding causes the physician much anxiety. The first 48 hours is the most critical period. In such cases it may be necessary to repeat the transfusion. Not only may massive transfusion be necessary, but an emergency operation will have to be considered. Surgeons differ in their management of such patients, but good results are claimed for resection of the stomach in patients with a palpable chronic ulcer at laparotomy. Where no ulcer is obvious gastrotomy should be done, and if an acute ulcer is found, bleeding can be stopped by underrunning it with a suture.

Prognosis. The prognosis in gastro-duodenal bleeding is related largely to age. Before transfusion was employed, it was rare for death to occur under 35; with massive transfusion, the mortality is slight till after 55; while above this age bleeding becomes a dangerous hazard. A patient with a chronic ulcer, who has had a previous haemorrhage, should therefore be offered elective surgery.

Acute Perforation

When free perforation occurs, the contents of the stomach escape into the peritoneal cavity. If perforation of the stomach occurs without loss of contents, as in the accidental perforation of the empty stomach at gastroscopy, few symptoms are produced, and the accident may even pass unnoticed. It follows that the symptoms of perforation are those of peritonitis, and are in proportion to the extent of peritoneal soiling. It may occasionally happen that the symptoms of perforation appear and rapidly subside; this occurs when the perforation closes spontaneously. The appearances of the stomach at operation for gastrectomy not infrequently suggest that some ulcers have perforated locally, but have escaped recognition. Perforation occurs more commonly in duodenal than in gastric ulcers, and usually in ulcers on the anterior wall.

Clinical Features. Though perforation may occur as the first sign of an ulcer, there is much more commonly a history of dyspepsia. The most striking symptom of an acute perforation is pain. Its onset may be so incisive that the patient can time it to a minute. It may be very severe, and its general distribution follows the spread of the gastric contents over the peritoneum. If these reach the diaphragm, shoulder-tip pain will be produced, but this is often disregarded by the patient as unconnected in position and eclipsed in severity by his chief agony. The pain is accompanied by pallor, sweating and shallow respiration; vomiting is common. The abdomen is held immobile, and there is rigidity which becomes generalised. Intestinal sounds are absent. The liver dullness to percussion may disappear due to the presence of gas under the diaphragm, and this is shown by a radiograph taken in the vertical position. In this context, this sign is pathognomonic of perforated ulcer. After some hours the symptoms improve, though the abdominal rigidity remains. This period of improvement may deceive the physician seeing the patient for the first time. After this temporary improvement, the symptoms of general peritonitis appear, and the patient's condition gradually deteriorates.

Differential Diagnosis. The all-important point is to decide whether the patient requires laparotomy. All the causes of the 'acute abdomen,' or those which simulate it, must be considered (p. 946).

Treatment. The orthodox view is that acute perforation should be treated surgically, an exception being made if the symptoms spontaneously subside due to natural sealing of the perforation. Conservative measures consisting of continuous suction of the stomach contents, chemotherapy and parenteral maintenance of water and electrolyte balance have been recommended. Although there is evidence to support these views, the great majority of surgeons believe that surgical treatment is indicated in all cases of perforation, either by simple closure or, in the case of perforation of a chronic ulcer, by partial gastrectomy.

Prognosis. The condition carries a considerable mortality of from 10 per cent. to 25 per cent. in various series. The outlook depends on the degree of peritoneal soiling, and therefore on the size of the perforation and the amount of stomach contents at the time of perforation. Of great prognostic importance is the interval elapsing between the onset of perforation and the time of operation.

'Pyloric Obstruction'

A complication of ulcer in the region of the pylorus, whether on the gastric or duodenal side, is that of gastric retention due to constriction from benign ulcer—most commonly a chronic duodenal ulcer. A pyloric carcinoma is a rarer cause. The obstruction may be due to actual organic narrowing from scar tissue, or to oedema and spasm produced by the ulcer; frequently it is a combination of all three. It should also be noted that gastric ulcers may arise in a stomach which is the subject of pyloric obstruction due to duodenal ulcer and that in such patients the ulcer is aetiologically related to the retention.

In infants congenital hypertrophic pyloric stenosis occurs which manifests itself within the first few weeks of life. It is best treated surgically. A type of hypertrophic pyloric stenosis, whose aetiology is unknown, occurs in adults.

Obstruction is loosely described as 'pyloric' stenosis, even where the actual site is distal to the pylorus in the duodenum. There thus arises in the 'pyloric' obstruction of duodenal stenosis the paradoxical situation in which the pylorus itself is seen radiologically to be abnormally dilated.

Clinical Features. All these types of obstruction have many features in common. In the majority of patients there is a preceding history of ulcer, though sometimes the ulcer is unsuspected, and obstructive vomiting is the first sign. When there has been a history of dyspepsia the symptoms change and vomiting becomes the prominent feature and nausea replaces a normal appetite. Vomiting produces such striking relief that a patient may even start to eat or prepare food immediately after the stomach has been emptied. If the obstruction progresses, further dilation of the stomach occurs so that ultimately surprisingly large amounts may be brought up. Articles of food which have been taken 24 hours previously may be recognised in the vomit. The loss of gastric contents results in water and electrolyte depletion. If large amounts of hydrochloric acid are lost, as occurs particularly in pyloric obstruction due to duodenal ulcer, alkalosis develops (p. 864). Physical examination may show some wasting and dehydration, and the changes of alkalosis. Splashing may be elicited in the stomach four hours or more after the last meal or drink and sometimes the patient notices it. In normal persons it only occurs for a short time after a meal since gastric emptying is normally rapid. The sign of greatest value in pyloric obstruction is visible gastric peristalsis, and this should be searched for carefully and can be elicited in the majority of cases. Another test for obstruction of the pylorus is the demonstration of food residue aspirated, before breakfast, through a stomach tube.

If the patient takes a fluid diet with large amounts of milk the signs of obstruction may be masked and nutrition may be maintained, even resulting in obesity.

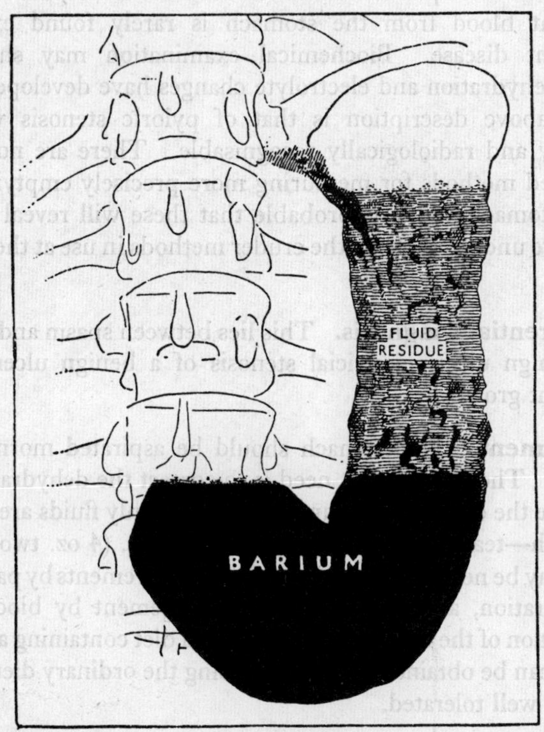

FIG. 59

Stomach following barium meal showing dilated stomach with fluid residue—obstruction in pyloric region.

Radiological Examination. The condition is confirmed by radiological examination (Fig. 59). The radiological signs are (1) an increase in fasting residue of the stomach; (2) the presence of dilatation of the stomach, with or without excessive peristalsis; (3) a lesion near the pylorus; and, (4) a delay in emptying of the stomach. If pyloric obstruction is suspected, it may be advisable to aspirate the gastric residue and wash out the stomach before the radiological examination is made. The distinction between spasm and true organic narrowing may be made by following the course of the disease over a period.

Laboratory Tests. The absence of acid in the stomach contents after histamine stimulation rules out a peptic ulcer. Apart from those patients with active haematemesis, the aspiration of bright blood from the stomach is rarely found except in malignant disease. Biochemical examination may show that severe dehydration and electrolyte changes have developed.

The above description is that of pyloric stenosis which is clinically and radiologically recognisable. There are now being developed methods for measuring more precisely emptying rates of the stomach and it is probable that these will reveal changes which are undetectable by the cruder methods in use at the present time.

Differential Diagnosis. This lies between spasm and oedema of a benign ulcer, cicatricial stenosis of a benign ulcer, and a malignant growth.

Treatment. The stomach should be aspirated morning and evening. The most urgent need is to correct the dehydration and to restore the electrolyte balance. Initially, only fluids are allowed by mouth—tea, broth, fruit drinks, milk, etc. (4 oz. two-hourly) and it may be necessary to make up fluid requirements by parenteral administration, and to control the management by biochemical examination of the blood (p. 853). A fluid diet containing adequate calories can be obtained by homogenising the ordinary diet. Such diets are well tolerated.

Course. The majority of patients seen with gastric retention and visible peristalsis can be greatly improved by these measures, and the stomach returns to normal emptying. It is then necessary to decide whether an operation, such as a gastroenterostomy with or without a vagotomy, or partial gastrectomy, should be advised.

The Zollinger-Ellison Syndrome

This is a rare but important syndrome in which intractable ulceration of the duodenum or even jejunum may occur (p. 1065).

COMPLICATIONS FOLLOWING OPERATIONS ON THE STOMACH

Though the great majority of operations on the stomach can be regarded as highly successful, over 90 per cent. in certain centres, there are certain complications, both local and systemic, which may follow. The physician is only concerned with the late post-operative complications.

Jejunal Ulcer

When the jejunum is anastomosed to the stomach in a patient who has had a duodenal ulcer, a second ulcer may develop at the junction of the stomach and the small intestine. The cause of such an ulcer is thought to be the continued action of the acid and pepsin of the stomach eroding the mucosa of the small intestine which is particularly vulnerable to peptic digestion. Because of this complication, simple gastroenterostomy in cases of chronic duodenal ulcer has fallen into disrepute.

Clinical Features. For some months or years after the operation, the patient obtains complete relief from his previous ulcer pains; then they return. The pains are similar to the original ulcer pains in quality and in time relationship to food though they may occur sooner after a meal. They are accompanied by localised tenderness which may be felt somewhat near the midline. Vomiting is not infrequent. Melaena may be the complaint that brings the patient to the doctor. Excessive indulgence in alcohol is sometimes a factor in recurrence of haemorrhage.

Physical examination often shows localised tenderness with possibly some rigidity.

Radiographic examination of the anastomotic area is a difficult task and the most skilled radiologist may miss an ulcer. At gastroscopy, the stoma can usually be seen, and often in addition the mucosa of one or both loops of small bowel at its junction with the stomach. Since the ulcer is on the intestinal side it is normally hidden from view. The test for occult blood may be positive.

Management. In some patients recurrent ulcers may heal spontaneously and in others it is possible to relieve symptoms temporarily by medical management on the lines already discussed. Many patients, however, will need surgery, the nature of which will depend on the original operation. Vagotomy, a comparatively simple operation, by diminishing a high gastric secretion, results in healing in a large number of cases. In others, partial gastrectomy may be the operation of choice.

Complication. A rare complication of a jejunal ulcer is a gastro-jejuno-colic fistula, in which a communication develops between the jejunum and the colon. The fistula is most easily demonstrated radiologically by a barium enema. The clinical features of the malabsorption syndrome in its most severe form rapidly develop (p. 942).

Ulcer of the Gastric Remnant

The jejunal ulcer which may follow partial gastrectomy must be distinguished from an ulcer which appears on the gastric side of the anastomosis in the remnant of the stomach. This ulcer is usually near the anastomosis and is sometimes due to ischaemia produced by sutures; at gastroscopy a suture thread may sometimes be seen sticking up from the ulcer crater. Such ulcers of the gastric remnant are associated with low acid outputs as opposed to the finding in jejunal ulcers where high outputs are almost invariable. Ulcers of the gastric remnant should be treated medically and do not usually need resection.

Post-cibal Syndromes

In a considerable number of patients after gastrectomy, symptoms may appear following the taking of food. Two separate syndromes can be distinguished, which may be classified as 'early' or 'late', according to the time of onset in relation to the meal. These syndromes occur in normal people and also in those with peptic ulceration, but are more common and more severe in those who have had some form of gastric operation. They should therefore be looked on as an exaggeration of a normal response to food.

'Early' Syndrome. The symptoms consist of a feeling of intense drowsiness coupled with muscular weakness, and this sensation of asthenia may be described as 'tiredness' or 'fatigue'. The patient may even find it necessary to lie down. There may also be associated symptoms of tachycardia with awareness of the heart's action. They usually develop immediately after a meal but may be delayed for half to one hour.

The pathogenesis of these early symptoms is still uncertain, but it is probable that they are reflexly produced by the stimulation of the small intestine by gastric contents which have left the stomach too rapidly. This stimulation may be mechanical, e.g. from distension with gastric contents; thermal, as by drinking hot fluids; or osmotic, e.g. hypertonic solutions of sugar. Clinical experience shows that this train of symptoms disappears in time in the majority of patients, as they become adapted to these stimuli.

Treatment. The patient should be given an explanation of the symptoms, reassured, and encouraged to anticipate that the attacks will diminish and disappear. Avoidance of hot fluids like soup or strong sweet tea may prevent attacks. Meals should be taken dry and fluids taken in between meal times. If it is found that a bulky meal is the chief offender, it may be eaten at the end of the day when the patient has the opportunity of resting thereafter. Of the drugs that may be tried, hexamethonium salts (125-250 mg. by mouth with each meal) are perhaps the most useful.

'LATE' SYNDROME. This syndrome is due to hypoglycaemia and comes on usually one to one and a half hours after a meal; it is almost always associated with exertion. The symptoms are those of weakness, tremor, a hungry or empty sensation in the epigastrium, and faintness with occasionally loss of consciousness, particularly in elderly patients. The hypoglycaemia may be due to an excessive secretion of insulin following the rapid absorption of sugar. If the attacks can be reproduced by giving insulin intravenously, the diagnosis is confirmed, and their disappearance can be demonstrated to the patient by giving glucose. Attacks can then be prevented by taking glucose at the appropriate time, or better still, by taking ample amounts of meat or fat at the two main meals. This reduces the emptying rate of the stomach and hence reduces the tendency to hypoglycaemia. Elderly patients who are subject to these attacks may have to be warned of the dangers of driving a car.

POST-OPERATIVE DIARRHOEA

Vagotomy which is undertaken to depress gastric secretion, also affects movements of the stomach and intestine and is nowadays always associated with some additional operation for drainage, such as pyloroplasty or gastroenterostomy. There is frequently some looseness of the bowels following this operation which rarely inconveniences the patient and in fact is sometimes welcomed. Occasionally it is disabling and it is worth trying cholinergic drugs for relief such as Mechothane 25-50 mg. sublingually. If it is associated with steatorrhoea, it may be due to a failure to achieve proper mixing of the duodenal contents with the pancreatic juice, and may be helped by treatment with a pancreatic substitute (p. 1061). If vagotomy has produced a marked depression of the acid secretion the diarrhoea is sometimes associated with an unusual growth of bacteria in the small intestine. It is then worth trying a short course of chemotherapy with neomycin 0·5 g. four times a day to alter the bacterial flora.

Anaemia. Anaemia is a common late sequel of operations on the stomach particularly after a partial gastrectomy. The anaemia is usually due to inadequate absorption of iron (p. 616). Megaloblastic anaemia is much rarer but may occur as there is a tendency for the remainder of the stomach to atrophy following gastric operations and the serum level of vitamin B_{12} has been observed to fall slowly over the years.

Ultimately a megaloblastic anaemia may develop which responds excellently to vitamin B_{12} (p. 623). Some practitioners would advise giving this vitamin routinely as a prophylactic following gastric operations.

In a proportion of patients there is some nutritional impairment following gastric surgery, a danger which increases with the extent of the resection.

CARCINOMA

Carcinoma of the stomach is a common form of cancer but it is certainly decreasing in the U.S.A. and also in Britain. It tends to occur in the age groups over 45, and in males more often than females. Nothing is known of its aetiology, though there is a striking hereditary influence in certain families. There also appears to be a clear association between blood group A and carcinoma of the stomach. Attempts have been made to discover a pre-cancerous lesion of the stomach, and there is evidence that chronic atrophic change precedes gastric carcinoma.

Pathology. Macroscopically, the lesions seen are of several types. Most common is a lesion at the pylorus, which is sharply limited to the stomach and does not spread across to the duodenum. A growth in this site may produce symptoms of pyloric obstruction. Next in frequency is a lesion of the body of the stomach, often involving the greater curvature, producing a

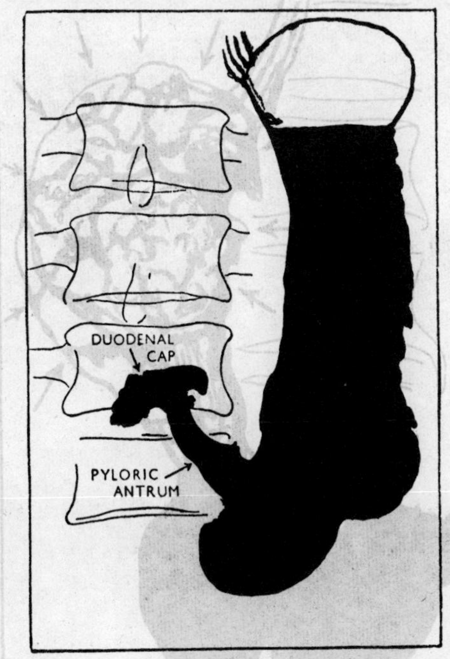

FIG. 60
Stomach following barium meal showing persistent narrowing of pyloric antrum—Gastric Carcinoma.

fungating, ulcerated mass. Least common is a diffuse, infiltrative lesion, with much fibrosis, producing the so-called 'leather-bottle' stomach. The carcinomatous growth spreads directly, by lymphatic permeation, and by embolism via the portal blood stream and the systemic blood stream.

ULCER-CANCER. Much discussion has taken place in the past as to how often a benign ulcer of the stomach becomes cancerous, and how often cancer may be attributable to an original benign ulceration. While different views are still held, most authorities believe that chronic peptic ulcer and carcinoma of the stomach are separate diseases, and that the possession of the first carries no special danger of the second. It is still a very important problem for the clinician to decide, whether a given ulcerating lesion seen radiologically is, in fact, simple or malignant.

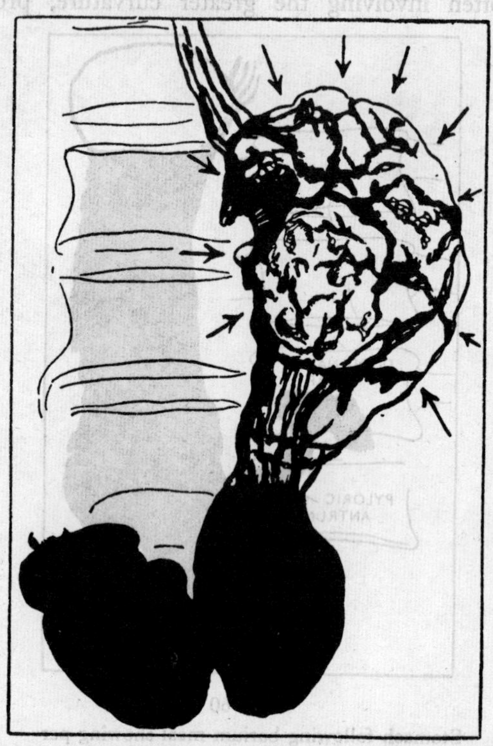

FIG. 61
Stomach following barium meal showing large irregular filling defect involving its fundus and proximal part of body—gastric carcinoma. The surface of the tumour is outlined by a thin film of barium.

Clinical Features. The classical picture of carcinoma of the stomach usually given in the textbooks of medicine is that of a patient complaining of dyspepsia for about a year or less with worsening of symptoms during the preceding few months, and with increasing anorexia, nausea, discomfort or pain, vomiting and loss of weight. On examination there is much wasting, and a mass is visible and palpable. This is a picture of hopeless, inoperable cancer, and a diagnosis made at this stage is too late. With this haunting picture in mind, clinicians have assiduously sought for the early symptoms of cancer. Unfortunately, many cancers metastasise before they give arise to symptoms at all, and there are therefore no symptoms which can be called 'early', though some appear sooner than others. Loss of appetite, slight nausea, and discomfort occurring for the first time, may be the first heralds of a carcinoma of the stomach, but they are in no way characteristic. Cancer should be suspected in anyone over 45 who has dyspepsia for the first time, and whose dyspepsia fails to clear up completely in two or three weeks with simple treatment. There are other modes of presentation. Carcinoma as the cause of haematemesis or melaena should always be remembered—or of an unexplained iron deficiency anaemia. In a growth near the cardia, dysphagia may be the earliest symptom. Reflex diarrhoea associated with a rapidly emptying stomach may be a confusing feature. Rarely, a perforated ulcer may prove to be malignant, and sometimes it is the presence of metastases elsewhere which first brings the patient to the physician.

Diagnosis. Physical examination in the early case may reveal nothing. In the more advanced case, a mass may be palpable or visible peristalsis may be present in the abdomen. There may be pallor and cachexia, or evidence of metastases in the liver or lymphatic glands, supraclavicular and left axillary, or above the prostate on rectal examination.

Radiology. The radiographic appearances vary. The most common appearance is a filling defect in the antrum or body of the stomach (Figs. 60 and 61). There may be a niche in the pyloric antrum or elsewhere. The initial radiological picture may be that of pyloric obstruction, and until the examination is repeated after washing out the stomach, it may not be possible to determine whether the lesion is benign or malignant. In the rare form of diffuse scirrhous carcinoma of the stomach, the picture is that of a rigid tube through which barium pours rapidly into the intestine (Fig. 62). If dysphagia is the presenting symptom, a lesion at the cardia will probably be found, but symptomless lesions in this area can very easily be missed.

Special investigations. *Secretory studies* usually show diminished secretion of acid. Blood in the aspirated juice is highly suggestive of carcinoma.

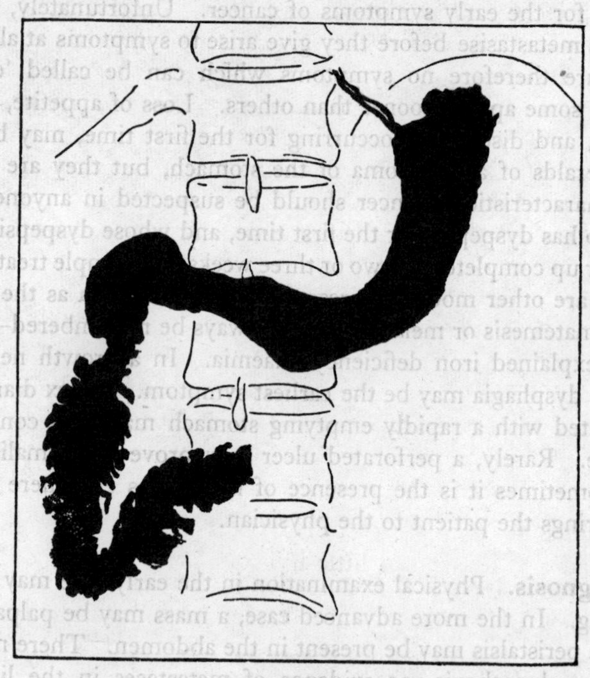

FIG. 62
Stomach following barium meal showing uniform narrowing with mucosal destruction and absence of peristalsis—diffuse infiltrating carcinoma ('leather-bottle' stomach).

Gastroscopy may help to decide if a doubtful lesion is malignant, but is unnecessary for obvious cancers of the body. The newer instruments enable the observer to inspect the antrum more exactly, and endoscopy is probably the best method of deciding if an antral lesion is malignant. The operability of a growth cannot be decided from endoscopic inspection.

Examination of the blood may show a hypochromic anaemia and the sedimentation rate may be raised.

Exfoliative cytology will confirm the diagnosis of cancer of the stomach if cells which can be obtained from stomach washings are unequivocally malignant. In collecting and staining of the exfoliated cells, it is essential to adhere to a rigid technique. This diagnostic method offers little promise of improving the early diagnosis of carcinoma of the stomach since it is hardly practicable to carry it out routinely on the population generally. By the time the patient has symptoms, the diagnosis can usually be made by other methods.

Treatment. The only curative treatment is gastrectomy, partial or total. Partial gastrectomy may be curative or palliative, and a palliative operation is worth while if pyloric obstruction is present, even if there are secondary deposits; such an operation may produce surprisingly little disturbance, gives the patient some extra life, and relieves the obstruction. Careful pre-operative treatment is most essential. It consists of the restoration of fluid and electrolyte balance, the correction of any anaemia present, and the improvement of the nutrition of the patient. After total gastrectomy, however, the patient may have difficulty in regaining his normal weight and returning to a manual occupation.

Prognosis. The prognosis in carcinoma of the stomach is very bad and has shown little improvement during the past 40 years. Of all patients with cancer of the stomach, only a percentage find their way to hospital: of these, only a proportion are fit for operation; in only a few of those operated on is radical removal possible, and of those who survive only a small fraction live for five years. Experience only reinforces the conviction that there is little hope for patients with this disease until some entirely new approach to the problem can be devised.

GASTRITIS

Gastritis signifies an acute or chronic inflammation of the stomach.

Our knowledge of these changes in the gastric mucosa has been obtained in three ways:

1. By direct observation of the gastric mucosa in a patient with gastrostomy, as in the case of Alexis St. Martin observed by Beaumont over a century ago, and in the more recently studied Tom.
2. By gastroscopic observation of the mucosa.

3. By histological examination of specimens removed at operation, or of specimens obtained post-mortem from a stomach which had been fixed in formalin immediately after death, or from biopsy in the living subject (pp. 900, 943).

Classification. If histological specimens obtained in this way are examined, it is very rare to find a normal stomach, free from any signs of inflammation. In this sense, 'gastritis' is a universal finding in adults. There are, however, gross departures from this 'normal', even if, as Beaumont originally observed, they do not give rise to symptoms.

The classification of gastritis has occasioned much difficulty, but most authors would agree that there exist acute inflammatory changes (acute gastritis, either exogenous or endogenous) and chronic atrophic changes (chronic atrophic gastritis). It is doubtful if a condition called simple gastric atrophy in which no evidence of preceding inflammation can be found, can be separated as a distinct entity rather than as the final stage of an atrophic process. The term 'hypertrophic gastritis' has sometimes been given by endoscopists to the appearance of the stomach in which the rugae are enlarged and which show a granular or nodular character. Histological examination from biopsy specimens has failed to support the existence of this variety.

Acute gastritis

Macroscopically, there is engorgement of the mucosa, with swelling, patches of adherent mucus, and sometimes small erosions. Microscopically, there is hyperaemia, infiltration with many inflammatory cells, and desquamation of the superficial layer. An exogenous gastritis can occur from an external irritant, such as alcohol or some unsuitable food; an endogenous gastritis can arise from an infection such as influenza.

Clinical Features. In his original observations on Alexis St. Martin, Beaumont noticed the considerable degree of inflammation that might exist in the stomach without symptoms. This finding has been repeatedly confirmed and the gastric mucosa seems a relatively insensitive tissue.

Symptoms associated with acute inflammation of the stomach from an external irritant such as alcohol or a haematogenous infection are anorexia, nausea, vague discomfort, heartburn and giddiness. Severe irritants produce vomiting, and diarrhoea if there is an associated enteritis. It is possible that the symptoms of a duodenal ulcer can be simulated by acute antral gastritis, and that this accounts for some of the cases where there is a typical ulcer history but no radiological evidence of an ulcer.

Radiology. Gastritis cannot be diagnosed with certainty from radiological examination, though such studies can show the size and form of the mucosal folds.

Gastroscopic Examination. The visible changes of acute inflammation are swelling and hyperaemia. The mucosa is easily damaged, and erosions may occur.

Secretory Studies. Any inflammatory process is likely to decrease the acid output by depressing the parietal cells and also by increasing the secretion of the alkaline non-parietal component. Acid secretion will tend to recover after the inflammation has subsided.

Diagnosis. The clinical diagnosis of acute gastritis in a patient who has taken excessive alcohol, irritant foods, or drugs, is easy. The symptoms will disappear spontaneously in a few days, though it may be much longer before the mucosa returns to normal. Similarly, the gastritis associated with specific fevers (such as influenza) disappears as the infection subsides. There remains a group of patients who spontaneously, or from some slight error of diet, get periods of discomfort and nausea. Radiological examination shows no organic change. Such patients are often called neurotic, but it is possible that a chronic gastritis is responsible for their symptoms.

Treatment. Treatment of the gastritis associated with peptic ulcer or carcinoma is that of the parent cause. There is also a group of patients, possibly with recurrent antral gastritis, who get bouts of dyspepsia of ulcer type; these cases may be helped by an ulcer diet, antacids and belladonna. No method is known for preventing gastric atrophy, or for stimulating the mucosa to regenerate.

Atrophic gastritis

Macroscopically there is little to be seen. Microscopically, there is considerable atrophy of glandular tissue, with the presence of plasma cells, lymphocytes, eosinophils and fibrosis in varying amounts; leucocytes are scanty. This condition has been thought to occur as the result of repeated attacks of acute gastritis, but usually no history of such attacks is obtained. It may also be found in association with gastric ulcer or carcinoma. These appearances can also be seen in patients with hypopituitarism and Addison's disease. It is possible that the atrophic changes are due to an auto-immune process. Evidence in support of this hypothesis is the presence of lymphocytic and plasma cell infiltration histologically, the detection of gastric antibodies in the circulating bloodstream, and an association with circulating antibodies to other tissues such as the thyroid.

Radiology. With atrophic change the folds may be thinned or even, as in advanced cases of pernicious anaemia, completely absent.

Gastroscopic Examination. If the mucosa is atrophic, folds tend to be absent, and it is possible at gastroscopy to see the submucous plexus of veins through the thinned mucosa. From an erosion in such an atrophic mucosa bleeding from the stomach readily occurs and this is a not uncommon cause of bleeding from the stomach. This atrophic appearance is constantly present in pernicious anaemia, and is often seen in localised patches with gastric ulcer and gastric carcinoma, only rarely is it seen with duodenal ulcer.

Diagnosis. Atrophic changes in the stomach produce no gastro-intestinal symptoms and its existence can only be suspected from an associated anaemia or the finding of diminished or absent secretion of acid or intrinsic factor and can only be confirmed by biopsy examination.

Treatment. Except in those patients with hypopituitarism or Addison's disease where replacement therapy is possible, no method is at present known for stimulating the mucosa to regenerate.

DISEASES OF THE SMALL INTESTINE

The small intestine is a muscular tube, lined with a secretory mucous membrane, whose function is to complete the digestion of foodstuffs and to absorb water, mineral salts, vitamins and the products of digestion. It is about four times as long as the large intestine. The process of absorption is enhanced by the presence of villi which increase enormously the effective surface area. Examination by the electron microscope has shown microvilli of the epithelial cells (the 'brush border') which further increase the surface area of these cells by a factor of 24.

Methods of Examination

Physical Examination. Inspection of the abdomen may show the distended gut of intestinal obstruction running transversely, and its peristaltic movements may be seen. Palpation may reveal masses of thickened and inflamed bowel affected by regional ileitis, while auscultation may be extremely valuable in the diagnosis of the 'acute abdomen.' The loud sounds of the actively contracting gut in intestinal obstruction contrast strikingly with the silence present in paralytic ileus.

Radiology. A radiograph of the abdomen in both the upright and the lying positions without any barium is of the greatest value in suspected intestinal obstruction. Normally gas is seen in the stomach and colon, but not in the small intestine. Directly obstruction or paralysis of the small intestine occurs, gas shadows, often with fluid levels can be easily demonstrated by radiological examination and the site of the obstruction can frequently be localised. Paralysis of the intestine occurs readily as a temporary phenomenon, lasting 12-48 hours, in abdominal diseases associated with severe pain such as obstruction of the biliary tract or a twisted ovarian cyst. Paralysis from peritonitis may be much more protracted.

Radiological examination with a barium meal reveals the mucosal pattern, the rate of transit through the bowel, and any abnormal appearances of the gut such as narrowing, filling defects or dilatation. The mucosal outline shows a coarse herring-bone appearance in the jejunum and upper ileum, which may be absent in the lower ileum. In certain states associated with the 'mal-absorption syndrome' (q.v.) this appearance is changed.

In addition to the mucosal appearance, radiological examination gives information about the rate of passage of barium through the bowel. The barium passes rapidly through the upper part of the intestine, but slows up in the lower part of the ileum, which is not usually empty until five to eight hours after ingestion of the meal.

Lesions in the small intestine will be discovered only if the radiologist watches the head of the barium meal in its passage through the gut, an examination that takes considerable time. The difficulties caused by the overlapping of the stomach shadow with the jejunal loop and its intermittent filling from the stomach may sometimes be overcome by introducing barium directly into the small intestine by intubation.

The last part of the ileum can not only be filled by a barium meal but may also be examined by a barium enema.

Laboratory Procedures (p. 943).

Biopsy (p. 943).

Motility Studies. There are techniques for recording the changes in the intraluminal pressure in the intestine, either by the swallowing of a tube or by the use of a small swallowed capsule, which radiates a signal of the pressure changes to a recording instrument. It is likely that the development of such techniques will provide useful information about a part of the gut which has hitherto been somewhat inaccessible.

Food Poisoning

Definition. The most common disease affecting the small intestine is acute enteritis due to food poisoning. Food poisoning is a difficult term to define, but through common usage it is accepted as meaning an acute gastroenteritis developing some hours (up to 48) after the consumption of unwholesome food or drink. It is customary not to include under this term (*a*) such specific infectious diseases as enteric fever, dysentery or cholera which are also spread by infected drinking water and food, because their incubation period is longer and gastritis is not an essential feature, (*b*) food idiosyncrasy or food allergy, since the food ingested is wholesome (e.g. shellfish), but the patient's reaction to it is abnormal, (*c*) digestive upsets resulting from the eating of food which is too rich (e.g. fat), or mechanically irritating (e.g. unripe fruit). Children are particularly prone to such upsets.

Aetiology. In contrast to enteric fever which is relatively uncommon in Britain at the present time, an increase in the reported incidence of food poisoning has occurred during the last few years.

Food poisoning may be due to the ingestion of inherently poisonous foods or to the consumption of food contaminated with chemicals or pathogenic bacteria and their products.

Poisonous foods. Inherently poisonous foods include fungi, especially the 'death cap' fungus, which may be mistaken for the harmless edible mushroom, and certain tropical fishes.

Chemical food poisoning. Poisoning may also be due to injurious chemical substances in the food, but, fortunately, nowadays, such cases are rare. The poison may contaminate food which has been placed in a container previously used for holding a chemical poison, or the food may be contaminated as a result of placing acid liquids such as lemonade or stewed fruits in cheap enamel or zinc vessels with the consequent liberation of antimony or zinc.

Food poisoning due to viral infections. (p. 982).

Bacterial food poisoning. Food poisoning of bacterial origin is by far the most common type and is usually divided into two main groups:

1. The 'toxin' type.
2. The 'infection' type.

'*Toxin*' *type*. Food poisoning due to bacterial toxins is most commonly caused by the exotoxin produced by the *Staph. pyogenes* which, in the great majority of instances, is transferred by a food handler who has a septic lesion of the hands or arms, or who is a carrier of the organism in his nose or throat. The exotoxin is very resistant to heat and is not destroyed by cooking or even by boiling for a short time. The 'toxin' type of food poisoning is much less commonly due to haemolytic and non-haemolytic streptococci and very rarely to the anaerobic organism *C. botulinum*, which causes a very serious and usually fatal disease of the central nervous system with minimal gastrointestinal disturbance.

'Infection' type. The organisms mainly responsible belong to the *Salmonella* group which has its natural reservoir in certain birds, mammals and reptiles. *Salmonella typhimurium* has been found to be the organism causing at least three-quarters of the cases of food poisoning of the 'infection' type in Britain. Food may be contaminated with infected excreta of mice or rats, etc., or infection may be transferred by flies or by human carriers employed in the handling of food. The possibility that the infection is due to a virus should be remembered (p. 982).

It is important to note that the size of the infecting dose of bacteria bears a close relationship to the speed of onset of symptoms and to the severity of the illness. This indicates clearly the dangers of bacterial multiplication which may take place when food is exposed to infection and thereafter remains at a warm temperature, as in a kitchen, for many hours or even days. The types of food which are particularly likely to be infected are twice cooked meat dishes, stews, gravies, soups, custards, milk and synthetic cream; also tinned foods which, though usually initially sterile, may become infected if not immediately consumed after the tin has been opened. While hens' eggs are very rarely infected, ducks' eggs are quite commonly infected because the duck is a carrier of *Salmonella* organisms in its oviduct and alimentary tract. Hence ducks' eggs are not suitable for the preparation of lightly cooked foods such as custards, milk puddings etc., because it has been shown that boiling for 10-15 minutes is necessary if sterilisation is to be secured.

Experience has shown that outbreaks of food poisoning are especially liable to occur whenever large amounts of food are prepared and when the remaining food not consumed is kept for future meals. The danger of infection is greatly increased if such food is kept at a warm temperature instead of being stored in a refrigerator. It is not surprising therefore that food poisoning is reported far more frequently from canteens, restaurants, hospitals and other institutions than from private houses.

Pathology. In all types of food poisoning the mucosa of the stomach and small intestine shows varying degrees of inflammation and even ulceration. In severe cases, the lesions may extend into the large intestine and there may be an accompanying septicaemia.

Clinical Features. In food poisoning it is common to find other members of the household or institution affected simultaneously and when this feature is present it makes diagnosis easier. The incubation period of the different types is a useful pointer to their aetiology. If vomiting starts within half an hour of the ingestion of a poisonous food, it is likely to be due to a chemical poison; if it occurs within six hours, it is probably due to a bacterial toxin; whereas, if it arises 12-48 hours later, it is probably due to a *Salmonella* infection, as multiplication of the organisms must occur before toxaemia results.

The symptoms in any single outbreak vary widely in severity depending on the type and amount of the poisonous substance ingested. The principal symptoms are nausea, vomiting, diarrhoea and abdominal pain, the latter being due to small intestinal colic. In severe cases there may be prostration, collapse and signs of dehydration. In the 'chemical' and 'toxin' types of food poisoning the onset tends to be sudden and severe and the patient rapidly passes into a state of collapse and frequently has a subnormal temperature. Recovery however usually occurs within 24 hours. In the 'infection' type, symptoms develop more slowly and there may be a rise in temperature. The patient may be ill for several days. The stools are watery and offensive, and there may be a little blood and some mucus, in contrast to bacillary dysentery where there is in addition much pus.

The most important point to decide, especially in children, is whether a surgical condition of the abdomen is present. It should be remembered that acute abdominal pain, vomiting and diarrhoea may occur in acute appendicitis, intestinal obstruction, intussusception and volvulus.

Investigation of a Suspected Case. A specimen of the patient's vomit and faeces collected during the acute stage of the disease should be sent immediately to the nearest central laboratory. Suspected articles of food, if available, should also be sent. Organisms of the *Salmonella* group can usually be readily isolated. Notification of suspected cases to the appropriate Medical Officer of Health is compulsory in Britain, but isolation in an infectious diseases hospital is not mandatory.

Treatment. Most cases are mild and can be treated at home with rest in bed, warmth and plenty of bland fluid drinks. Patients who are moderately or severely ill and show signs of collapse and dehydration should be admitted to hospital since skilled nursing is essential and fluid and electrolyte loss may require intravenous replacement. Hospitalisation is also indicated when home nursing is difficult or impossible because of overcrowding or inadequate toilet facilities. If the poisoning is believed to be due to a chemical or a poisonous food such as the 'death cap' fungus, the patient's stomach should be washed out with warm normal saline and the appropriate antidote given. In all cases the patient should be encouraged to drink warm saline as this helps to counteract dehydration. If this becomes unduly severe intravenous glucose saline should be administered. Symptoms normally pass off spontaneously in a day or two if food is withheld, and only fluids, such as fruit drinks, tea or broth are allowed. As the condition improves, the patient may take a light diet containing bread and butter, eggs, pounded fish, soft puddings and jellies (Diet 1, p. 1284). To control the diarrhoea, kaolin may be given in 15 g. doses, two-hourly, suspended in a little water. Codeine, 30-60 mg. doses, is also useful. Of the chemotherapeutic agents, neomycin is of most value in doses of 0·5 g. six-hourly orally for five days. If the organisms are resistant to neomycin, Colomycin should be given orally in doses of 3 million units t.d.s. for five days. If, as occasionally happens, it is suspected that a septicaemic state has developed, ampicillin 1·5 g. six-hourly should be given orally for 21-28 days.

Prevention. In *Salmonella* food poisoning the excreta should be treated by the addition of disinfectants such as 1:20 carbolic acid and the patient should not be allowed to handle food until laboratory tests have shown that the organism is no longer being excreted in his stools. The carrier state persists on the average for about 14 days after infection but may be much longer.

A reduction in the high incidence of food poisoning can best be achieved by improving the standards of personal hygiene, especially in those handling food, and by giving advice on the disinfection of toilets and the importance of washing the hands after using the lavatory. Increasing the facilities for low temperature storage of food which has to be kept for some hours or days before being consumed is of the greatest importance. Steam disinfection of bedding and fomites, as is undertaken in enteric fever, is not required.

ACUTE APPENDICITIS

Though this condition is rightly regarded as surgical, it is of such importance as the most common cause of the 'acute abdomen' (p. 946) that it should be discussed in a textbook of medicine.

Aetiology. The disease occurs in both sexes, and though it may occur at any age it is more common in young people. There is no satisfactory theory to account for the causation of appendicitis but it seems likely that obstruction of the appendicular lumen with faecoliths is frequently followed by distension and infection of that organ. Inflammation and swelling of the lymphoid tissue by viral infection is possibly a precipitating cause.

Clinical Features. The classical history is that of a central abdominal pain accompanied by nausea and vomiting in the great majority of cases. This is followed by a shift of the pain to the right lower quadrant with the development of localised tenderness and rigidity as the peritoneum becomes inflamed. The pulse rate is increased. The temperature is raised, though seldom above 38° C. (100° F.). Accordingly a high fever makes the diagnosis of appendicitis unlikely. Of the laboratory examinations, only a leucocyte count is of much value and this is usually raised to about 15,000 per c.mm.

Though a case with this classical history and course offers no difficulty in diagnosis, the inflamed appendix may lie in abnormal positions and so can simulate many other diseases of the abdomen. For this reason rectal examination is helpful. In the retrocaecal position renal disease may be simulated; lying on the psoas muscle, pain may be caused by outward rotation of the hip thus suggesting arthritis; an inflamed appendix lying under the liver may suggest cholecystitis or a perforated peptic ulcer. In a woman, salpingitis must be remembered.

Another condition which may easily be mistaken for appendicitis is non-specific mesenteric lymphadenitis, an inflammatory lymphadenopathy, probably due to a virus. It occurs in children and is characterised by pain in the right iliac fossa, accompanied by nausea and vomiting and some alteration of bowel rhythm; there is a slight fever. Examination reveals some tenderness and perhaps rigidity in the right lower quadrant. The distinction from appendicitis is difficult, and if in doubt, it is safer to operate. If the diagnosis of lymphadenitis can be made with confidence, only symptomatic treatment is necessary.

Treatment. While there is no doubt that removal of the diseased appendix is the only proper procedure, there is some difference of opinion as to the optimal time of removal if abscess formation or peritonitis is present at the time the diagnosis is made.

CHRONIC APPENDICITIS

While no one would question that recurrent attacks of acute appendicitis can occur in the same person, there is considerable doubt whether chronic inflammatory appendicitis is a pathological entity. It is generally acknowledged that many patients operated on for 'chronic appendicitis' derive only temporary relief from their symptoms and later return with further digestive complaints. There is little doubt that most of such patients are suffering from an overactive state of the bowel in the ileo-caecal region unassociated with organic disease but often associated with an anxiety neurosis.

REGIONAL ENTERITIS

(Crohn's disease; Regional ileitis)

This disease is characterised by localised areas of non-specific chronic inflammation of the small, or more rarely, of the large bowel. It is a disease mainly of young people, and typically shows remissions and relapses over many years. Crohn's disease and regional ileitis are other names for the condition which possibly includes several disease entities.

Aetiology. The cause of this disease is still unknown, no specific organism having been identified from the bowel content, the bowel wall or the regional lymphatic glands. The condition has been distinguished from chronic tuberculosis of the bowel, which it somewhat resembles both clinically and histologically. When the disease affects the large bowel, it may be difficult or even impossible to distinguish it from ulcerative colitis. It has been suggested that the disease is a manifestation of sarcoidosis (p. 433). but though there is almost identical histology, the clinical courses of the two diseases are dissimilar. The current concept of auto-immunity has aroused speculation that Crohn's disease may be an example of this mechanism but the hypothesis awaits proof.

Pathology. Though the disease may occur throughout the small and the large intestine, in the great majority of cases it is the terminal ileum which is mainly involved. Macroscopically, the bowel is engorged and oedematous in all layers, producing narrowing of the lumen. The mucosa is ulcerated and the change from normal mucosa to the affected part is quite abrupt. Microscopically, all grades of inflammation may be seen with giant cell formation but without caseation.

Clinical Features. There is usually a history suggesting colic of the small intestine, and pain localised to the lower rightquadrant of the abdomen. Diarrhoea, which tends to follow a bout of pain, is frequent, but is not usually so severe as in ulcerative colitis. Stools may be formed or loose and rarely contain frank blood, mucus or pus unless the diarrhoea is severe. Most cases have a low-grade fever, and moderate anaemia. Loss of weight is common. The condition may be discovered when the abdomen is opened after an erroneous diagnosis of acute appendicitis has been made.

The cardinal physical sign is a tender mass in the right lower quadrant, palpable by abdominal and frequently by rectal examination. The mass consists of inflamed loops of bowel bound together and may be of any size. Fistulae are a feature of this disease; they may open on to the surface of the abdomen, may communicate internally, or may appear in the perianal region. Clubbing of the fingers is often found.

Radiological Examination. This is most helpful. A barium meal should be given and the small intestine carefully examined. The bowel may show alteration of mucosal pattern, evidence of narrowing, as in the almost pathognomonic 'string sign', or areas of dilatation above the lesion with irritability and difficulty in filling the gut. The caecum is usually unaffected. Segments of the bowel may be involved with normal tissue intervening. Such segments are sometimes called 'skip' lesions, and these may easily be missed at radiological examination, as barium passes through them so quickly and they may only be found at subsequent laparotomy.

Laboratory Examinations. These are of limited value. Pus cells and red blood corpuscles may be found on microscopic examination of the faeces. Bacteriological examination yields nothing specific. Some patients show evidence of malabsorption, most commonly of cyanocobalamin, if the appropriate tests are carried out.

Differential Diagnosis. The symptoms, signs and radiological findings are usually sufficient to point to a lesion in the lower part of the small bowel. The other common diseases in this part of the intestinal tract are appendicitis or an appendix abscess, carcinoma of the caecum, ulcerative colitis extending into the ileum, and, but rarely in Britain, tuberculosis of the ileocaecal region and caecal amoebiasis. Even when the bowel is inspected at operation, the diagnosis may remain uncertain. Although tuberculosis of the ileocaecal region is becoming rare, it must always be borne in mind if only for its satisfactory response to specific treatment with streptomycin and PAS. It is not likely to be missed if the primary lesion in the lung is obvious and gross, but it can occasionally occur in patients in whom the primary infection is minimal and has been completely overlooked. The Mantoux test should always be done.

Treatment. Treatment of regional enteritis is unsatisfactory. Resection or short circuiting of the affected area of the gut was carried out formerly with considerable optimism, but careful observations of patients followed over a period of years have shown a depressingly high recurrence rate. Modern opinion veers towards the view that management should be primarily conservative unless there are clear indications, such as obstruction, for surgical treatment.

Medical management will be necessary to steer a patient through a mild relapse, when the disease is insufficiently severe to warrant operation. Bed rest may be required for many months by those patients with more severe lesions. The diet should be low in residue but otherwise adequate (Diet 2, p. 1285). Treatment with corticosteroids is worth a prolonged trial in the same dosage as in ulcerative colitis (p. 963). In the acute inflammatory stage of the disease it may prove very successful. Alternatively, sulphasalizine may be given as in ulcerative colitis during the acute phase, 4-6 g. daily. For the prevention of relapse some physicians believe that corticosteroids given over a long period and in low dosage, e.g. prednisolone 10 mg. daily, are of value. In the same way sulphasalazine has been tried in doses of 2 g. daily. A short course of phthalylsulphathiazole or a suitable antibiotic may be given in the hope of reducing secondary infection of the ulcerative bowel, and subacute attacks of obstruction may be treated with gastric intubation (p. 951) and parenteral feeding. Patients can often prevent these attacks by paying meticulous care to their diet.

There is no unanimity of opinion as to the best surgical procedure to adopt. In some cases a simple short-circuiting operation will be sufficient, while in others anastomosis combined with resection of the affected part may be indicated.

THE MALABSORPTION SYNDROME

Definition. A number of disorders are encountered in clinical practice in which the primary defect is malabsorption of one or more of the necessary foodstuffs, mineral salts or vitamins. These disorders are associated with some or all of the following features: diarrhoea, loss of weight, anaemia, mineral and vitamin deficiency, tetany and abdominal distension. In the past some of these conditions have been called the steatorrhoeas, since the difficulty in absorbing fat was the most evident single feature. It is essential to think of the defect of absorption in more general terms. Hence the general title of 'the malabsorption syndrome.'

Aetiology. The process of absorption can occur in two main ways: (1), by diffusion, whereby substances move from a higher to a lower concentration, and (2), by a process of active transport necessitating the expenditure of energy, whereby a substance can move against the concentration gradient. While the products of protein and carbohydrate digestion are water soluble, fat and fatty acids are insoluble in water and it is usually with these substances that difficulties in absorption first arise. While the small intestine is the chief site for absorption, it is not the only one; for example water is absorbed from the colon and it may also be sparingly absorbed from the stomach.

The causes of malabsorption may be classified as follows:

1. *Inadequate preparation of foodstuffs for absorption.* This may be due to a lack of digestive enzymes consequent on deficiency of pancreatic secretion. A lack of enzymes produced by the small intestine has also been demonstrated and this deficiency may be congenital or possibly acquired. The absence of bile, as in complete biliary obstruction, will also result in steatorrhoea. When the mixing of food and enzymes is inadequate, even a partial deficiency of pancreatic enzymes may lead to a failure in digestion. Such a situation may develop after operations on the stomach when the jejunum is anastomosed to the stomach and food enters the intestine without the intermingling with bile and pancreatic enzymes that inevitably occurs in its ordinary passage through the duodenum. Loss of weight and signs of mineral deficiency may develop after partial gastrectomy.

2. *Diversion of foodstuffs by intestinal organisms.* It has been known for a long time that intestinal organisms can synthesize certain vitamins, especially those belonging to the B group. More recently it has been shown that under certain circumstances an abnormal intestinal flora can divert to its own use substances (e.g. cyanocobalamin) which are essential for the health of the body and which are only needed in minute amounts. Infection of the small intestine with the fish tapeworm can produce a similar result.

A clinical example of this phenomenon is the so-called 'blind loop' syndrome (pp. 620, 627). A severe state of nutritional deficiency may develop as a consequence of a gastro-jejuno-colic fistula. The resulting malabsorption may be due to the invasion of the small intestine by colonic bacteria which act in the way described above, as well as to intestinal hurry consequent upon the mechanical short-circuiting of the intestine.

3. *Reduction in the amount of surface of the bowel.* Clearly, the extent of the surface available for absorbtion is of great importance (pp. 620, 626). Evidence of severe clinical malabsorption does not appear until more than 50 per cent. of the gut has been resected, as for example following an extensive mesenteric thrombosis. Intestinal fistulae which short-circuit areas of the small intestine may produce similar results.

It is doubtful if intestinal hurry in the normal gut is ever responsible for malabsorption.

Intrinsic movements of the villi, by their pumping action, continually change the intestinal milieu and the cessation of this action might result in a diminished rate of absorption.

4. *Damage of the intestinal mucosa.* Examination of a piece of the intestinal mucosa obtained by biopsy has revealed the association of histological change with certain types of malabsorption. Whether this change precedes or follows the malabsorptive state is still uncertain. In coeliac disease of children and its counterpart in adults, malabsorption is due to an idiosyncrasy to gluten, a protein in wheat and certain other cereals. In the tropics the intestinal mucosa may become damaged for reasons that are not known, and the malabsorptive condition which may follow is known as tropical sprue. Some other causes of damage to the intestinal wall are infiltration by malignant tissue, e.g. the reticuloses, and chronic inflammation as occurs in regional enteritis and tuberculosis. Finally, there are cases of the malabsorption syndrome in which the histology of the intestinal mucosa is similar to that found in patients with gluten induced enteropathy but for which no cause can be found. Such cases are classified as idiopathic steatorrhoea.

5. *Insufficient lymph or blood flow.* Even though substances are adequately prepared for passage through the intestinal epithelium, absorption may be defective on account of insufficient flow of lymph or blood. Thus, steatorrhoea may result from interference with the flow of lymph consequent on obstruction of lymph channels by tuberculous or malignant disease of the small intestine. Changes in blood flow are less easily recognised, but there is evidence in intestinal obstruction that they play a part in the failure of the gut to absorb gases.

Clinical Features. The patient with malabsorption can present in various ways. There may be general malnutrition, with loss of weight and energy and a slow deterioration in health or, in a child, a failure to grow and thrive. Abdominal distension is often a striking feature. Steatorrhoea may be the presenting symptom. The patient complains of diarrhoea, with the passage of loose, pale, bulky and offensive stools which float on water, so that to cleanse the toilet-pan may require several flushes from the cistern. This difficulty is almost pathognomonic of steatorrhoea. The patient may have an anaemia which is the direct consequence of a deficiency of iron, cyanocobalamin or folic acid (p. 626). Apart from changes in the blood picture, haemorrhagic phenomena due to a deficiency of vitamin K, a fat soluble vitamin, may be an occasional presenting feature. Tetany may occur as a result of hypocalcaemia, because in the presence of excessive fatty acids in the gut, calcium absorption may be impaired. The features of rickets or osteomalacia and various other disorders due to deficiency of vitamins may be noted, such as sore tongue, angular stomatitis, dry and atrophic skin, or hair which undergoes early greying or fails to grow. There is frequently clubbing of the fingers; pigmentation and hypotension may be present so that Addison's disease is mimicked.

Diagnosis. Though the syndrome may be suspected from the history, physical examination and appearance of the stools, various ancillary methods of investigation, including tests for absorption, may be required if the diagnosis of the underlying mechanism is to be established.

Radiology. Radiological examination of the alimentary tract may reveal various causes of malabsorption. In certain types of intestinal disease there is an alteration of mucosal pattern due to the outpouring of mucus which produces some flocculation of the barium. Though this may occur in certain malabsorptive states, it is not pathognomonic as it may be seen, for example, in patients with pyloric stenosis, where large amounts of gastric mucus pass into the intestine. Intestinal diverticulosis may be visible though the extent of its involvement is rarely appreciated from the film, since many diverticula remain unfilled. In the small intestine the features of regional enteritis or the changes of tuberculosis or malignant disease may be evident. In the large bowel there may be changes of a 'regional colitis' which point to a regional ileitis that has escaped previous radiological observation. A barium enema may also reveal a gastro-jejuno-colic fistula.

Biopsy of small intestine. This can be carried out by using a biopsy capsule which the patient swallows and which is carried into the small intestine by peristalsis. A fragment of mucosa is obtained by applying suction to the attached polythene tubing which activates a sliding knife within the capsule. The biopsy specimen should be examined by means of a low power microscope. The macroscopic appearances are most instructive and may show changes which may be missed on histological examination alone. Microscopically, changes may range from normality to complete disappearance of the villi.

Tests of absorption. Various tests are available but all depend on one of three principles.

(*a*) It is possible to give a known amount of a substance by mouth and then to measure the amount that appears in the stool. This is one method commonly used for testing fat absorption. The simplest technique is to put the patient on an ordinary ward diet containing 50-100 g. fat and 70-100 g. protein, and collect the stools over a period of three days or longer; the fat in the stools can be estimated by hydrolysis and titration of the fatty acid thus produced, the biochemical estimation being simple and rapid. Normally not more than 5-6 g. of fat are excreted in the stools per day. The amount of nitrogen in the stools can be easily estimated by the Kjeldahl method. Normal persons excrete up to 2·5 g. N. per day (1 g. N. = 6·5 g. Prot.) and this figure will rise in various malabsorptive states, in particular those associated with pancreatic disease.

In recent years it has been shown that various nutrients can be labelled with radioactive isotopes. By this means it is possible to study their absorption through the intestinal wall and their ultimate metabolism. This type of test has been of particular value in clinical practice for the study of the absorption of iron and cyanocobalamin.

(*b*) The rise and fall of the concentration in the venous blood of substances taken orally can be measured. In the case of glucose such changes are the result of two simultaneous processes, that of absorption and that of utilisation. Theoretically, a flat glucose curve could indicate that no absorption was taking place, but in practice it usually indicates that utilisation is occurring at the same rate as absorption. The rise and fall of the serum iron, as estimated by chemical analysis, can also be followed after an oral dose of iron, but this test also is subject to the same difficulties of interpretation.

(*c*) The amount of a substance administered orally which is excreted in the urine over a period of time can be estimated. The urinary excretion of xylose, a pentose sugar which is not metabolised in the body, has been used as a test of sugar absorption. The absorption of folic acid has been studied in a similar way.

In addition, malabsorption of certain vitamins and minerals may be suspected by indirect methods, e.g. vitamin K from prolongation of the prothrombin time, and calcium from hypocalcaemia, elevation of the alkaline phosphatase level in the serum and radiographic evidence of demineralisation of the skeleton.

All these tests show that there are many nutrients whose absorption is impaired in the malabsorption syndrome. As the severity of the disorder progresses, even the simplest substances, such as electrolytes and water, may only be absorbed with difficulty.

In investigating a case of the malabsorption syndrome, a test for steatorrhoea should be carried out first because the absorption of fat is so frequently impaired. This is usually followed by a glucose absorption test since it distinguishes very clearly between the steatorrhoea of pancreatic disease and the steatorrhoea of intestinal malabsorption. In the former, there will be either a diabetic or pre-diabetic type of curve (p. 746), while in the latter, the curve is flat.

Chronic pancreatitis as a cause of steatorrhoea can usually be diagnosed by the glucose tolerance test alone, but other tests of pancreatic function may be necessary, namely, estimations of the output of pancreatic digestive enzymes obtained by duodenal intubation (p. 1055). If, in addition to the features of malabsorption, there is a history of intestinal pain, this suggests organic disease of the small intestine, such as regional enteritis, neoplastic infiltration, the presence of adhesions causing obstruction, or tuberculous enteritis. The history of a previous operation, with an abdominal scar, may suggest resection or short-circuiting of the small intestine, and also the possibility of a 'blind loop' or intestinal fistula. If a gastroenterostomy has been performed, a gastro-jejunal ulcer, with a gastro-jejuno-colic fistula, is a possibility. In the case of a child, gluten sensitive enteropathy is the most probable diagnosis, and this is also true of the majority of cases occurring in adults if malabsorption appears spontaneously and insidiously.

Treatment. From the foregoing discussion, it is clear that some patients with malabsorptive states, such as those with fistulae, are curable, while in others the disorder can only be treated symptomatically. The treatment of diseases of the pancreas is discussed on p. 1061. It is not always possible to demonstrate by radiological examination intestinal abnormalities such as multiple jejunal diverticulosis or a cul-de-sac, and it may therefore be necessary to advise abdominal exploration. In fact it is wise to advise laparotomy in all patients with the malabsorptive state which is undiagnosed and certainly in all those in whom pain is a feature. Improvement following oral chemotherapy is consistent with a malabsorptive state induced by abnormal bacterial growth. Where no cause is found a gluten sensitive enteropathy must be considered, and it may be necessary to give a gluten-free diet a thorough trial, even for several months. If improvement is obtained, further confirmation can be gained by deliberately giving gluten and thus provoking a relapse. Where no remediable cause can be found the malabsorptive state can only be treated symptomatically. For this purpose a low-fat/high-protein diet (Diet 6, p. 1290) should be prescribed, and the deficiencies of minerals and vitamins, as indicated by clinical and laboratory investigation, should be corrected.

If there has been persistent steatorrhoea for some time, calcium salts such as calcium gluconate or lactate should be given by mouth, supplemented by vitamin D. Intravenous calcium salts, such as 10 ml. of 10 per cent. calcium gluconate given slowly, will relieve tetany. Vitamin K should be given if there is any haemorrhagic tendency. Glossitis, cheilosis and 'crazy paving' skin are indications for the administration of the vitamin B complex. Anaemia should be treated with iron orally if there is evidence of iron deficiency. Parenteral iron therapy is of particular value in cases resistant to oral therapy (p. 617). Folic acid in particular (5-20 mg. orally) or cyanocobalamin (parenterally) should be given if a megaloblastic anaemia is present (p. 623). In some cases of idiopathic malabsorption cortisone or prednisolone has been shown to have a striking though temporary effect in ameliorating the condition.

Tumours

Tumours, simple or malignant, rarely develop in the small intestine though there is some evidence that reticuloses are more likely to develop in patients who have had chronic malabsorption. Of special interest is the carcinoid tumour whose symptomatic effects are related to the over-production of 5-hydroxytryptamine, a very important and highly potent pharmacological substance.

THE ACUTE ABDOMEN

Definition. A group of abdominal emergencies exist which require an immediate and accurate diagnosis to decide whether surgical operation should be performed or withheld. These abdominal emergencies, which are usually accompanied by severe pain, are collectively referred to as 'the acute abdomen,' a piece of jargon now hallowed by long usage. Their differential diagnosis is naturally the particular concern of the surgeon, but since certain medical diseases may simulate the acute abdomen, and since surgical emergencies such as perforation of a peptic ulcer or intestinal obstruction may readily occur in family practice and in medical wards, it is necessary for all doctors to be keenly aware of these conditions. In no other branch of medicine has the diagnostician the power to save or destroy life so dramatically.

Classification. No classification of the causes of the acute abdomen is entirely satisfactory. They may be roughly divided into three groups: (1) inflammations of the abdominal viscera, (2) the colics and (3) vascular lesions.

(1) Inflammations of the Abdominal Viscera. Since the perforation *per se* of a viscus such as stomach or colon is painless, the symptoms of perforation must be regarded as entirely due to the resulting peritonitis. Chemical irritation of the peritoneum

from the stomach contents in a perforated ulcer, produces an immediate reaction, but the contents of the large bowel, though far more highly infected, produce no immediate reaction from the peritoneum, and symptoms and signs of peritonitis are therefore delayed.

Acute inflammation of the gall-bladder, pancreas and appendix usually follows an initial period of obstruction.

(2) THE COLICS. Colic is a difficult term to define but denotes a severe pain, most frequently muscular in origin, arising in a tube or passage, usually from an obstruction. Renal, biliary and intestinal colic are the most common forms.

Intestinal colic can occur simply from acute inflammation as in acute enteritis when it is accompanied by diarrhoea. When associated with constipation and distension it is due to obstruction. Intestinal colic without diarrhoea or distension occurs in lead poisoning.

(3) VASCULAR LESIONS. The principal vascular lesions are acute mesenteric thrombosis, dissecting abdominal aneurysm (p. 283) and ruptured ectopic gestation. Acute mesenteric thrombosis usually occurs in elderly patients with arterial disease and is accompanied by severe abdominal pain. It is probable that some of the less severe attacks of abdominal pain in the elderly are really due to a localised mesenteric thrombosis which never reaches the stage of requiring surgical treatment. Blood may be passed rectally.

Ruptured ectopic gestation will usually present as a very severe internal haemorrhage, the intraperitoneal collection of blood forming a swelling palpable on vaginal or rectal examination. Irritation of the diaphragm by blood will produce shoulder tip pain.

Of the causes listed above, the more commonly encountered are acute peritonitis from perforated ulcer, acute cholecystitis, acute appendicitis, biliary and renal colic, and intestinal obstruction. The most important medical conditions which may simulate the acute abdomen, and which should always be borne in mind, are lobar pneumonia, acute pyelonephritis, diabetic coma and coronary thrombosis.

Examination of the Acute Abdomen. The history is the most important part of the clinical examination. Particular attention must be paid to the description of the onset of the pain, its site and radiation, its severity and its course, and whether it is accompanied by restlessness as in most colics, or whether the patient keeps still as in peritonitis. A general examination of all systems of the body must be carried out, though naturally particular attention will be paid to the abdomen. The abdomen should be carefully inspected; in intestinal obstruction the outline of distended coils may be visible while the abdominal wall may be withdrawn in severe peritonitis. The abdomen is palpated gently to elicit tenderness, to detect swellings, and to estimate rigidity. Light percussion may be employed and may reveal absent liver dullness, as occurs when a peptic ulcer perforates. Auscultation should always be practised. The combination of a wave of abdominal pain with a rush of bowel sounds is pathognomonic of intestinal obstruction, while if the gut is paralysed as may occur with peritonitis or with severe pain, sounds are absent. Palpation of the hernial orifices and examination of the rectum should never be omitted. Urinary examination may show blood in a case of renal colic, pus in an acute pyelonephritis, bile following a biliary colic, sugar in pancreatitis, and sugar and ketone bodies in a diabetic coma and porphyrins in porphyria. The urinary amylase may also be measured in a suspected pancreatitis. Other useful laboratory examinations include a white cell count, and estimation of serum amylase. If facilities are available radiological examination of the abdomen should always be carried out, with the patient in the horizontal and the vertical position. If an obstruction is present an experienced radiologist will diagnose its site with some certainty, while the presence of air under the diaphragm always indicates a perforation, usually from a peptic ulcer. An electrocardiogram should be taken if a coronary thrombosis is suspected. In all cases of the acute abdomen, the opinion of a surgical colleague must be sought. If in any doubt, it is always safer to explore the abdomen. The old aphorism is still true: it is better to look and see than to wait and see.

INTESTINAL OBSTRUCTION

Definition. Intestinal obstruction may be defined as any condition which delays or prevents the onward passage of the contents of the gut. Alternatively the term 'ileus' is sometimes used. An important distinction must be drawn between those conditions in which the obstruction is mechanical and those in which the defect is due to paralysis of the intestinal muscle. Intestinal obstruction is not, of course, a disease entity, but is symptomatic of many different conditions.

Classification. Many attempts have been made at classifying intestinal obstruction, but the important questions the physician should ask himself are:

Is the obstruction mechanical or paralytic?

Is the obstruction high (jejunum and upper ileum) or low in the intestinal tract (lower ileum and colon)?

Is strangulation present? Strangulation is a condition which results from obliteration of the arterial or venous components or of both components of the mesenteric circulation.

Is an obstructed *closed* loop of bowel present?

Causes. A. *Mechanical obstruction.* In Britain the common causes in adults are:

External and internal hernias.

Bands and adhesions from previous operations, or inflammatory disease.

Carcinoma of the large bowel.

Volvulus.

Intussusception. This is the most frequent cause of obstruction in children.

B. *Paralytic ileus.* This is commonly due to the development of peritonitis after an operation, or consequent on perforation of a peptic ulcer or of a colonic diverticulum. It may also occur temporarily following any severe abdominal pain.

Pathology. Despite a large amount of clinical and experimental observation, the underlying pathology of intestinal obstruction is far from understood. Many of the symptoms of obstruction, particularly if high up in the intestine, are due to the loss of fluid and of electrolytes. The loss may occur in two ways, firstly, by vomiting, and secondly, by stagnation in dilated intestinal loops whereby the secretions are lost to the circulation. It has been calculated that the total amount of all digestive secretions entering the gut is of the order of 8 litres in the 24 hours. Not only these secretions but also any additional fluid which may be ingested, may be lost in the ways already described. The fluid vomited or lost is nearly neutral in reaction, so that there is no special tendency to acidosis or alkalosis.

Though loss of water and electrolytes may explain many of the symptoms of high intestinal obstruction, it does not explain the symptoms of obstruction in the colon where distension from retained gas and fluid seems to play a very important part. This distension is thought to cause reflexly circulatory changes which may lead to peripheral circulatory failure. With a rise in intraluminal pressure secondary changes take place in the intestinal wall which may reduce the circulation of the blood, alter permeability, and interfere with absorption. If strangulation occurs, the wall of the gut is even less capable of dealing with absorption of gases and fluids. There is evidence that some toxic substance is elaborated in the obstructed bowel which, when absorbed into the circulation, can cause death.

Clinical Features. In mechanical obstruction, the cardinal symptom is pain which comes in waves, and these episodes are accompanied by loud borborygmi. After some hours the pain may become more constant; in strangulation it is usually severe and persistent.

In a paralytic ileus the bowel is paralysed and there is no pain. Constipation in all types of ileus is ultimately complete, but in the earliest stages of mechanical obstruction it may be preceded by diarrhoea. Vomiting is a sign of both types of obstruction but is present only when the site of the obstruction is high in the intestine. Colonic obstruction will not produce vomiting for some days.

Physical Examination. The hernial orifices must be examined as a routine, and the presence of any scars indicating a previous abdominal operation noted. Distension is a characteristic sign, occurring more readily with obstructions in the lower ileum or colon. Dilated loops may sometimes be seen lying transversely. Palpation may reveal a mass producing the obstruction, more commonly on the left side. Rectal examination usually reveals an empty rectum. An intussusception may be palpable per rectum, and blood and mucus may then be found on the examining finger. Auscultation of the abdomen should never be omitted. The sounds of peristaltic activity are very marked with mechanical obstruction and occur synchronously with colicky pain; in paralytic ileus no sound except an occasional tinkle is heard.

Radiology is the most important diagnostic method, and it can also help to localise the site of the obstruction. In any suspected case a straight radiograph should be taken of the abdomen in the vertical position in order to detect distended loops with fluid levels. This sign may become positive within a few hours of the onset. A radiograph taken of the abdomen with the patient in the horizontal position gives the best chance of identifying the site of the obstruction. If intestinal obstruction is evident, or even if it is only suspected, a barium meal should not be ordered as it may easily convert a partial into a complete obstruction. It is, however, possible to give a radio-opaque fluid which is absorbable and therefore innocuous.

Management. Once obstruction of the intestine is suspected, the patient should be moved immediately to hospital, or if in hospital, the advice of a surgeon should be sought, even if non-operative measures are to be used initially.

While most cases of mechanical obstruction will require surgical intervention, most cases of paralytic ileus can be relieved by non-operative measures. Even if surgery is indicated, the patient may require medical treatment to bring him into better condition for operation.

In all cases water and electrolyte loss should be corrected by the parenteral administration of the appropriate solution. A record should be kept of the intake and output of fluids and in this way a balance sheet may be drawn up of gains and losses. The control of electrolyte equilibrium is not easy, except in a hospital with full laboratory facilities, which make it possible to follow the levels of the electrolyte concentrations in the plasma. Potassium loss may contribute to the paralysis of the intestinal muscle. Potassium salts may be given safely by slow infusion, but it is unwise to do so unless there are facilities for the estimation of potassium in the serum (p. 847).

Gastric or intestinal intubation can be a lifesaving measure. If it is used in strangulation of the bowel or in closed bowel obstruction to the exclusion of surgical operation, it can prove a lethal mistake. In such cases immediate operation is required.

Decompression of the obstructed gut by intestinal intubation using the Miller-Abbott tube is infrequently carried out because it is an exacting and time consuming procedure. Continuous evacuation of gastric contents by suction through a Levin tube (gauge 10) passed through the nose into the stomach is nearly as effective and much easier to undertake.

Intubation should be used in all cases of paralytic ileus and by this means operation is usually avoided. It may be usefully employed as a temporary measure when bands or adhesions cause mechanical obstruction of the small intestine and may even render operation unnecessary if the obstruction relieves itself.

Distension is a prominent feature of intestinal obstruction and is mainly due to swallowed air which cannot pass on. Of the swallowed air, oxygen is partly absorbed, leaving the relatively insoluble nitrogen behind. This is only absorbed slowly and tends to remain in the bowel. Its natural removal by diffusion may be hastened by the patient breathing oxygen in high concentration, which reduces the nitrogen tension in the blood and thus aids the diffusion of the nitrogen from the bowel into the blood. If intubation has been carried out successfully the remainder of the gas can be removed by suction.

In paralytic ileus various drugs such as prostigmine, pitressin, and cholinergic drugs have been tried but with no striking success.

DISEASES OF THE LARGE INTESTINE

Anatomy and Physiology

The colon and rectum constitute the large bowel; this is the terminal portion of the gut and its main fuctions are the absorption of water from the chyme, the storage of faeces and their excretion at convenient intervals. The large bowel begins at the ileo-caecal junction and removal of this 'valve' can promote hurry and malabsorption under certain conditions. The large bowel ends in the anal canal and the external anal sphincter.

The motor and secretory functions of the large bowel are controlled through the sympathetic and parasympathetic nerves as elsewhere in the alimentary tract. The wall of the bowel is insensitive to touch and to painful stimuli so that injections of sclerosing agents can be given quite painlessly as in the treatment of piles. Pain arises only when the bowel is stretched or stimulated to contract strongly.

The motor activity of the colon, which is very sluggish compared to the small bowel, has been studied by radiological methods and by the introduction of balloons and other pressure recording devices into the lumen. In general, parasympathomimetic drugs stimulate colonic motility and autonomic blocking agents tend to reduce it though therapeutically their effect is disappointing.

Absorption of water, sodium and chloride, occurs in the right side of the colon, while faeces are stored on the left side. The rectum is normally empty and the stimulus to defaecation occurs when faeces enter it. The mucosa of the colon is flat and histologically can be seen to contain a layer of columnar epithelial cells with many goblet cells secreting mucus. The colon contains large numbers of micro-organisms whose role has long been disputed. In health they may play some part in the synthesis of the vitamins of the B complex, but under conditions of disease it is possible that they may become harmful.

Physical Examination. The large intestine is accessible to palpation over part of its course. The normal bowel is palpable only in the right and left iliac fossae, where, respectively, the caecum and the sigmoid colon can be rolled under the finger. If a tumour is present in the sigmoid colon, part of the mass palpated is usually faecal. If the colon is inflamed as in dysenteric colitis, ulcerative colitis, or diverticulitis, it will be tender on palpation. When these conditions have become chronic the bowel may also be obviously thickened, especially in diverticulitis. In the functional disorder called 'irritable colon,' the bowel is spastic and may be rolled as a hard cord in the left iliac fossa though it is not usually tender. The colon is not normally visible, but if it is obstructed by a neoplasm or stricture, it may become very distended and is then easily seen on inspection of the abdomen.

Rectal examination should never be omitted. Routinely it is best done in the left lateral position with the knees drawn up. The anal sphincter should always be stretched very gently; the more resistance encountered, the less hurried should be the dilatation. In the left lateral position the index finger may reach 10 cm. up the rectum, but in order to palpate the area of the rectosigmoid junction which is about 16 cm. from the anus, it is necessary to examine the patient in the squatting position and ask him to bear down gently. A tumour at the rectosigmoid junction may sometimes be palpated in this way.

Stool Examination. The consistency of the stool varies with the amount of food ingested, the type of food—a vegetarian diet producing a soft stool—and the activity of the colon. In a spastic colon, the faecal mass may be hard, dry and indented or in the form of a collection of compressed pellets. In disease of the lower bowel the stools may be ribbon-like in appearance. The colour of the stool should be noted. It is light on a milk diet and darker on a meat diet; it is greyish-white in obstructive jaundice, creamy in the sprue syndrome, shiny black and sticky in consistency when melaena has occurred, dull black with iron and green with bile. The colour of the stools may also be altered by various drugs.

The odour of the normal stool is not unduly offensive but if there is excessive protein present due to intestinal hurry, putrefaction occurs in the large bowel and the odour can become very unpleasant. Mucus may be a sign of inflammation or of new growth and occurs with blood in the loose watery stools of dysentery and ulcerative colitis; or it may be present in large amounts in functional disorders of the colon (p. 986).

Endoscopy. Proctoscopy or sigmoidoscopy may be of diagnostic value in any case of rectal or colonic disease and is a preliminary to radiological examination by barium enema. The examination is safe and produces only slight physical discomfort if the anal canal is first dilated with the finger and the instrument is warmed and well lubricated. The unpleasantness of the examination is psychological and this should be overcome by discussion with the patient. For the examiner, the best posture of the patient is the knee-chest position. This attitude is somewhat tiring to a patient, and in a debilitated subject it will be necessary for him to adopt the left lateral position. The rectum may be seen in every patient while in the majority the instrument will pass the rectosigmoid junction, at about 16 cm. distance, and the lower sigmoid colon can be inspected. The normal mucosa is orange-red with the submucosal vessels plainly visible. Inflammation is indicated by engorgement of the mucosa with disappearance of the submucosal vessels; an inflamed mucosa is easily traumatised and bleeds spontaneously. There may be mucus or mucopus on the surface of the bowel. Tumours may also be observed endoscopically and a biopsy specimen may be removed for section. Normally the bowel motility is slight and only occasional contractions are seen in the sigmoid, but in inflammatory states or in patients showing functional spasm, the bowel may be seen to contract actively.

Radiology. The colon may be examined radiologically in two ways: (1) by giving a barium meal and following it through into the large bowel, or (2) by giving a barium enema. The latter is preferable. Barium is run in gently and the tone of the bowel, its distensibility and the rapidity of filling is visualised on the screen at fluoroscopy and a search made for filling defects. As in the stomach, various techniques have been tried for depicting the mucosal relief pattern, such as inflation of air after the barium has been evacuated; their success depends on getting the colon absolutely clean prior to examination. Lesions in the rectum, or in the sigmoid colon if there are many loops, may be missed by the radiologist. Fortunately, it is this part of the bowel that is so readily accessible to palpation and endoscopic inspection.

Microscopic examination of the stools is valuable but is insufficiently practised.

The cellular elements commonly seen in diseases of the colon are polymorphonuclear neutrophils, red blood corpuscles and macrophages. Polymorphonuclear leucocytes are present in large numbers in diffuse inflammatory lesions such as ulcerative colitis or bacillary dysentery. The cytological examination may be of great value in distinguishing bacillary from amoebic dysentery.

The remnants of foodstuffs may be distinguished in the faeces; microscopic examination may show fat globules which stain well with Sudan III, starch granules which stain with iodine, and meat fibres, which if undigested, retain some of their normal striated appearance. All of these may be present in the normal stool and it requires considerable experience to decide whether they are present in excess.

In addition to cellular elements and the remains of foodstuffs, there are normally found numerous bacteria which are considered to be harmless saprophytes. To identify the pathogens, stool culture is necessary, the only exception being the tubercle bacillus, which is detected by microscopic examination of stained films made from the stool which may require previous concentration. The most valuable chemical examination of the stool is that for occult blood. Recording the motility of the colon is a procedure requiring special apparatus, but it is likely to become more widely used in the future and will help in the diagnosis of disorders of the large bowel.

DYSENTERY

Dysentery is an inflammation of the colon and rectum characterised by tenesmus and the passage of frequent stools, containing blood and mucus. Its causes are bacterial, protozoal, e.g. from *E. histolytica*, and helminthic, e.g. from *S. mansoni*.

BACILLARY DYSENTERY

The bacilli belong to the genus *Shigella* of which there are three main pathogenic groups, often known as *Shiga*, *Flexner* and *Sonne*, the last two having numerous strains. The *Shigellae* are Gram-negative bacilli, non-sporing, non-motile and are easy to grow on ordinary culture media. In Britain over 95 per cent. of cases of bacillary dysentery in recent years have been caused by *Sh. sonnei*.

Epidemiology. Bacillary dysentery in an endemic form is an extremely widespread disease all over the world. It occurs in epidemic form wherever there is a crowded population with poor sanitation, and in this way it has been a constant accompaniment of wars. In the tropics it is spread by flies, but in Great Britain, though it may be spread by contaminated food, it seems that personal contact is the most important factor. Outbreaks are not uncommon in institutions. The disease is notifiable.

Pathology. There is a generalised inflammation of the large bowel, which sometimes involves the lower part of the small intestine. The mucosa is red and swollen with a layer of mucopus and there are patchy haemorrhagic areas. Ulcers may form and the adjacent lymph glands are enlarged.

Clinical Features. There is great variation in severity. The disease, particularly from infection with *Sh. sonnei*, may be so mild as to escape detection and the patient remains ambulant with a few loose stools and perhaps a little colic, or it may be sufficiently severe to cause death within 48 hours.

In a moderately severe illness, the patient will complain of diarrhoea, colicky pain and, if the rectum is inflamed, tenesmus. The stools will be small, and after the first few evacuations, will contain blood and purulent exudate and little faecal material. There will be fever, with dehydration and weakness if the diarrhoea persists. On physical examination, there will be tenderness over the whole colon more easily elicited over the sigmoid part in the left iliac fossa. In *Sonne* infection the illness often takes the form of a fever and diarrhoea may be mild or even absent; there is usually some headache and muscular aching, with bronchitis. It is possible to overlook a mild attack of dysentery unless other more severe cases appear, when suspicion will be aroused, and the stools cultured.

In a minority of cases of dysentery the diarrhoea becomes chronic and the picture then becomes indistinguishable from chronic ulcerative colitis.

Diagnosis. Diagnosis depends essentially on microscopic and bacteriological examination of the faeces. Microscopic examination of the stool shows the presence of numerous pus cells while culture of dysentery bacilli is pathognomonic. Radiography is hardly possible in the acute stage, nor is it necessary.

Treatment. The patient inevitably takes to bed with bacillary dysentery of any severity. Mild cases, however, who may remain ambulant, should preferably be confined to prevent spread of infection. If diarrhoea has been severe it will be necessary to repair the water and electrolyte deficit incurred, and parenteral administration may be necessary. A semi-fluid low roughage diet (Diet 1 or 2, pp. 1284, 1285) should be given, depending on the severity of the diarrhoea. Weakness may be due to potassium loss, which may be remedied by giving potassium salts (p. 847) orally. For the relief of pain tincture of opium may be necessary.

When Shigella organisms are sensitive to sulphonamide drugs, phthalylsulphathiazole can be recommended. Phthalylsulphathiazole is given to an adult in a dose of 3 g. initially followed by 1-2 g. four-hourly. The dose may be reduced when the stools become faeculent.

In Britain many strains of the Shigella group are now insensitive to sulphonamides, in which case 500 mg. of neomycin or ampicillin should be given six-hourly for approximately five days, the duration of treatment depending on the severity of the infection.

Prophylaxis. Prevention of faecal contamination of food, milk and drinking water, the isolation of proved cases, and the discovery and treatment of carriers, are obvious methods which are excellent in theory, but may be very difficult to apply unless one is dealing with a limited outbreak.

Amoebic Dysentery (p. 591)

NON-SPECIFIC ULCERATIVE COLITIS

Apart from the bacillary dysenteries, amoebic colitis, and tuberculous enterocolitis, which all produce colonic ulceration, there is a group of cases in which no specific organisms can be isolated, but which are characterised by inflammation and ulceration of the colon. To this group the name 'non-specific ulcerative colitis' is applied.

Aetiology. The aetiology of ulcerative colitis is unknown. It is possible that some unknown primary agent produces a change in the colon wall and that subsequent bacterial invasion then occurs. Some authorities believe that a psychological factor is, if not causative, at any rate, contributory. There is no doubt that many patients with ulcerative colitis for some months, with loss of weight and with frequent bowel motions, show considerable psychological changes. It seems probable, however, that such changes are largely due to the disease, since they greatly improve or disappear during a remission or following a successful colectomy. Psychological features are not peculiar to ulcerative colitis, since they may also occur in any patient with a comparable loss of weight and a similar severity of diarrhoea. Nevertheless, there is little doubt that psychological trauma such as a bereavement or an unhappy love affair can act as a trigger in initiating an attack or in provoking a relapse.

Present interest in the concept of so-called 'auto-immune' disease has raised the question whether ulcerative colitis may not be an example of this disease process. The occurrence of ulcerative colitis with disease in other viscera, such as the joints, the liver, the skin and even the parotid gland, together with auto-immune reactions, such as the presence of antinuclear factor or L.E. cells in the blood, provides evidence to support this hypothesis.

Pathology. Ulcerative colitis usually appears first in the rectum, and involving the colon, may spread towards the caecum. From the caecum it may spread to the last part of the small intestine. In the early stage the mucous membrane of the rectum is slightly swollen and roughened in appearance and earns the name of 'granular proctitis'. There is congestion of the mucosa, which bleeds easily with slight trauma and small ulcers may be seen with some inflammatory exudate. In the more chronic stages, the mucous membrane of the colon may become hyperplastic so that a polypoid appearance results.

Clinical Features. The disease occurs with equal frequency in men and women between the ages of 20-40. It is rare after 60. At present there is no completely satisfactory classification. The course is essentially chronic and relapsing. The onset is usually insidious and is characterised by periodic attacks of diarrhoea with blood and mucus. The patient may complain of pain or discomfort in the abdomen preceding the passage of a motion, and tenesmus if there is much proctitis. Tenderness may be present over the colon and particularly in the left iliac fossa, where the colon may be palpated under the finger. There is no colonic distension unless there is an associated stricture or the patient is severely ill. There may be generalised wasting and the skin may show changes of vitamin deficiency, such as follicular hyperkeratosis, and 'crazy paving.' The disease is attended by variable fever, loss of weight and anaemia, and signs of vitamin deficiencies, such as glossitis, are common. This is a description of a case of moderately severe colitis. The condition may, however, be much milder with looseness of the stools unaccompanied by macroscopic blood or mucus. The condition is then recognised only from the proctoscopic appearances and the microscopical appearance of pus cells and red cells in the stools. Some writers regard the type of disease which remains confined to the rectum as a separate entity from ulcerative colitis proper. A very severe variety is also seen, with many motions every day, severe anaemia and toxaemia, exhaustion from frequent bowel actions and with considerable tachycardia and hectic temperature. There is also a chronic stage, when the disease has apparently gone into continued remission. The colon in such cases is a rigid tube, incapable of absorbing fluid properly or acting as a faecal reservoir. Such a patient though not robust, suffers little from toxaemia but may remain subject to persistent diarrhoea.

The cause of relapse, as in peptic ulcer, cannot usually be identified by the patient. Infections can undoubtedly be responsible; some patients blame a particular foodstuff; emotional stress is probably a cause, while the effect of pregnancy is inconstant. A relapse following pregnancy, however, is nearly always severe.

Complications. INTESTINAL. These include stricture, perforation, massive haemorrhage, and polypoid and carcinomatous change in the colon.

Polypoid change is a common complication and represents the remains of islands of mucosa; stricture occurs most commonly in the anal canal. Perforation is usually an end result and often passes undiagnosed owing to the small reaction immediately produced. Carcinomatous change is particularly liable to occur in young patients or in those who have had the disease for many years. The risk of carcinoma of the large bowel in such patients is probably at least 30 times greater than in a comparable normal group.

SYSTEMIC. These include arthropathy, lesions of the skin and damage to the liver. Septicaemia may occur in severely ill patients.

Diagnosis. Proctoscopy or sigmoidoscopy should be undertaken in every case except in those too ill to be examined. The pathological appearances have already been described. It is also possible to see polypi which may not have been found by the radiologist. The examination is made, not only for diagnostic purposes but so that the progress of the disease can be judged at subsequent examinations.

Radiology. While endoscopy determines the existence of ulcerative colitis, radiological examination demonstrates its extent. If the rectum only is affected, as in an early case, the radiologist may see nothing abnormal on examination. If the disease has spread higher into the colon various changes of the mucosal pattern may appear. There is also frequently loss of haustration though this is not pathognomonic of ulcerative colitis. In the final stage of ulcerative colitis the colon will be narrowed and shortened (Fig. 63). Radiological examination by barium enema is dangerous in the acutely ill patient, as it may produce perforation. If the diagnosis is in doubt in such patients, a radiograph of the abdomen will show sufficient outline of the gas-filled colon to enable a diagnosis to be made.

Laboratory Procedures. The stools should be examined microscopically for blood, pus and amoebae. Culture reveals a mixed group of organisms and is not helpful except to exclude the *Shigella* group. Blood examination may show an anaemia and a mild leucocytosis; the sedimentation rate is raised and repeated estimations may be used as an index of progress. Of chemical changes in the blood, the most frequent and important is hypoproteinaemia due to the loss of protein in the stool, to inadequate intake and to a deterioration in the ability of the liver to make plasma albumin (p. 1000).

A biopsy of rectum can be obtained and is of some value in assessing progress of the disease.

Treatment. The management of patients with ulcerative colitis differs according to the grade or stage of the disease.

For patients whose general health is not affected and their only symptoms are those of passing stools more frequently, with the passage of blood from time to time, treatment of the local lesions by prednisolone enemata is indicated and this may be combined with corticosteroids given orally.

Hospitalisation is indicated for those patients with more severe bowel symptoms and general systemic disturbance.

Though no specific therapy exists for ulcerative colitis a very great deal can be done by intense supportive treatment to maintain

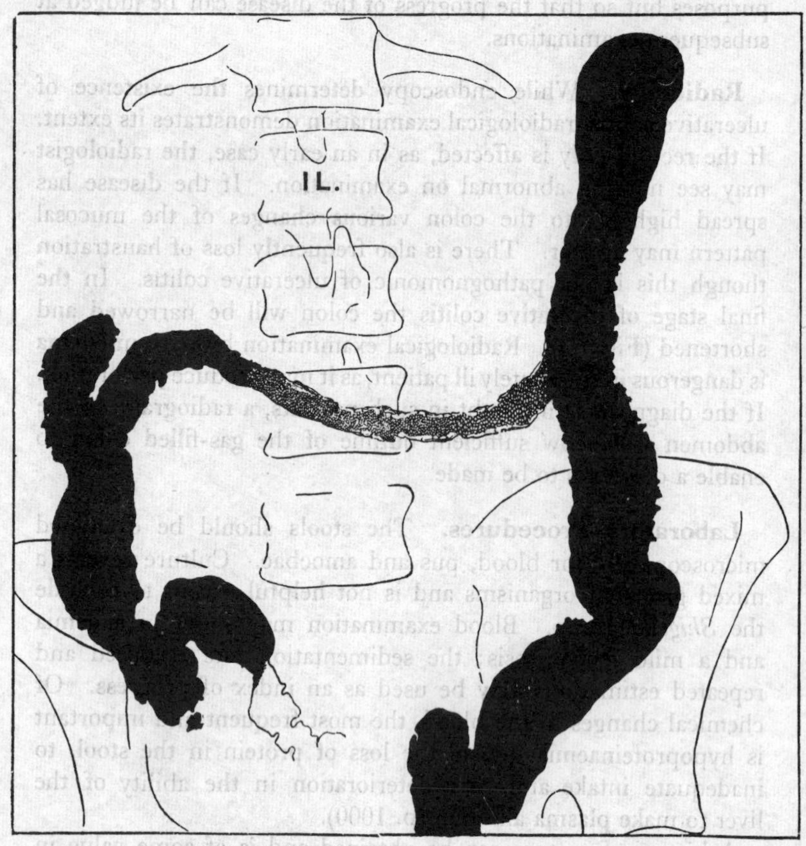

FIG. 63

Barium enema showing shortening and narrowing of colon with lack of haustrations and presence of numerous small ulcer craters giving a shaggy outline—generalised ulcerative colitis.

the patient, either through the relapse to a natural remission or as a preparation for surgery. No immediate results can be expected from such methods of treatment, which may have to be continued persistently for many weeks, or even months. During this time the patient may be miserable, as are many patients with a chronic bowel disorder, and he will need firm and optimistic management. In few other diseases can medical and nursing care be rewarded by the recovery of such apparently hopeless cases.

Though the patient must be encouraged to eat a full diet, low in residue and with ample protein (Diet 2, p. 1285), he is unfortunately often unable to tolerate it, and with a continual loss of protein in the stool, may pass into a state of negative nitrogen balance. This state is exceedingly difficult to treat, but plasma infusions may supply some of the needed protein. Diet 1 (p. 1284) which is semi-fluid and low in roughage may be indicated.

Of electrolyte losses, the one likely to be overlooked is potassium loss. If there is hypokalaemia, potassium salts (p. 847), should be given by mouth until normal electrolyte figures are obtained. If there is anaemia, iron should be given. Blood transfusions may also be required, and they seem to produce beneficial results out of proportion to the improvement in the haemoglobin level.

The sulphonamides have proved disappointing. Salicylazosulphapyridine has been widely used but it may be accompanied by toxic symptoms. There is evidence that it will produce a remission, though it is less effective than the corticosteriods, but should be prescribed if they have failed. Given in small doses of 2 g. daily it may help to prevent a relapse. Broad spectrum antibiotics are best reserved for the treatment of complications or as a pre-operative measure. Their prolonged use is contraindicated because of the danger of producing 'superinfection' with resistant organisms (p. 80). There is no satisfactory drug for controlling diarrhoea. Small doses of tincture of opium 0·3-1·3 ml. (5-20 min.) may be necessary to relieve severe diarrhoea or pain. Codeine phosphate, 15-30 mg. t.d.s. is of some value but may produce nausea.

The introduction of corticosteroids and corticotrophin has proved a definite advance in the management of this condition though it is not yet clear which is the most valuable drug. Of the various corticosteroids available, prednisone or prednisolone is recommended. These are given in doses of 30 mg. daily and this may be increased to 50 or 60 mg. a day if necessary, accompanied by supplements of potassium salts. The usual contraindications to the use of these drugs must be observed (p. 722). The corticosteroids tend to produce an optimistic outlook and sense of well-being. In addition they may produce such an increase in appetite that the problem of getting the patient to take sufficient food is often solved. There is also some indication that in cases with profuse diarrhoea the loss of protein in the stools is decreased. The good effects of corticosteroid therapy have been well established by careful trial and they seem to be more effective in the first attack of ulcerative colitis than in subsequent relapses. The corticosteriods in no sense provide a cure, but they greatly increase the chance of a remission. They are valuable as a means of improving the state of gravely ill patients so as to fit them for major surgical procedures. Corticotrophin seems to be the more valuable drug in the treatment of a relapse, though its use is likely to be attended by more complications than are usually produced by corticosteriods. It is given in doses of 40-120 units daily.

The principles of management of the more severely ill patient do not differ from those already outlined, but greater difficulties are encountered in putting them into practice. The problem of maintaining life and promoting a remission may tax all the resources of the physician and nurse. Since the faecal losses of fluid, electrolytes and blood will be much greater, an accurate record of them must be kept, and scrupulous care taken to replace them. The most difficult problem is that of maintaining nitrogen balance. Frequent transfusion of blood and of plasma should be given, and the anabolic steroids, such as nandrolone phenylpropionate (Durabolin) 25 mg. intramuscularly weekly may be of some help. Psychologically the patient will need constant support, reassurance and encouragement. The use of corticosteroid drugs has undoubtedly improved the prognosis and they should be prescribed as already indicated. If all these measures are assiduously carried out, the great majority of patients in this grade will eventually pass into remission.

When all acute activity of the disease has subsided and the patient is in a continued remission, he has usually adapted his mode of life to meet the demands of a permanently damaged colon. The danger of a severe relapse is now less. The main danger is that of polypoid change with bleeding or malignant degeneration. This latter danger is very real and the advisability of having a total proctocolectomy has to be carefully considered. It is not always easy, however, for a patient, who is managing to live reasonably well with his condition, to accept such an extensive prophylactic operation as colectomy. If operation is not considered, or has been refused, then an annual examination by barium enema should be advised.

Surgical Treatment. Surgical treatment has become increasingly practised for this condition. It may be indicated in cases of perforation, for the complication of stricture, and for cases of polyposis in young people where the risk of colectomy is less than the risks of a carcinoma developing. There remains a group of cases in which the indications are less certain. Clearly the mild case with only rectal involvement does not require an operation. At the other extreme, the acute fulminating case presents a very difficult problem and the mortality will be high whatever treatment is undertaken. Since, however, nearly all such patients will need colectomy if they recover, it is probably wisest to advise operation if the patient fails to improve significantly within a few days. The cases for which surgery is most clearly indicated are the chronic relapsing and remittent types, where there are bouts of diarrhoea with fever and general ill-health. In the period of remission, such patients never return completely to normal, and the colon passes into an irreversible pathological state. The operation of ileostomy and colectomy produces a very dramatic improvement in the majority of patients belonging to this group. The diseased rectum is either removed at the same time as the colon or at a later stage. Now that it is possible to seal an ileostomy bag to the skin around the ileostomy opening, much of the unpleasantness previously associated with this operation has gone and such patients can expect to take part in any kind of physical activity.

Prognosis. It is extremely difficult to give a prognosis in ulcerative colitis. The extent of involvement of the colon is important, the outlook being much better for example if the rectum only is involved. The prognosis is very grave in patients with fulminating disease however they are treated. The outlook is also poor in the elderly in a second attack. Broadly speaking, the overall mortality is probably somewhere about 10 per cent., but this figure can be very greatly reduced when the patient is treated by those with special medical and surgical experience of the disease. The mortality of a total proctocolectomy done during a remission by an experienced surgeon is approximately 1 to 2 per cent.

DIVERTICULOSIS AND DIVERTICULITIS

Though diverticula occur throughout the gastrointestinal tract, they are most common in the large bowel. The presence of diverticula is known as diverticulosis; when they are inflamed the condition is known as diverticulitis. Such inflammation commonly occurs only in diverticulosis of the colon.

Aetiology. The aetiology of diverticulosis is unknown. The formation of diverticula in the colon could be explained by weakening of the bowel wall or by increased intracolonic pressure. Males and females are equally affected. The condition occurs especially in middle age or in the elderly. Radiological examinations have shown that approximately 5-10 per cent. of all colons examined by barium enema show this change. What proportion of the population with diverticulosis develops diverticulitis is uncertain, but it may be somewhere about 10 per cent.

Pathology. The sigmoid colon is the part most commonly involved. The diverticula are pouchings of the mucosa and serosa with little of the muscular coat. They usually occur near the entrance of blood vessels from the mesentery, where the wall may be weaker; they tend to increase in size with age. It is not clear how they become inflamed. Radiological examination frequently shows the presence of a faecolith in a diverticulum, and it may be that infection only results when it is closed off, as occurs in appendicitis. Such inflammation may resolve, or end in suppuration which in turn may lead to perforation and peritonitis. Repeated attacks of diverticulitis result in a chronically inflamed bowel, with narrowing of the lumen and pericolic adhesions.

Clinical Features. By definition, only diverticulitis and not diverticulosis gives rise to symptoms. Pain or discomfort felt in the left iliac fossa is a frequent complaint and this is associated with localised tenderness. A common symptom is alteration of bowel habit, either of increasing constipation or constipation interspersed with diarrhoea. This is the most important symptom of colonic disease and can occur with any lesion. By middle age, bowel habits are firmly established and a definite alteration always betokens organic change in the colon such as carcinoma or diverticulitis. Acute diverticulitis can give rise to a clinical picture similar to appendicitis, but the pain is on the left side of the abdomen. A severe rectal haemorrhage may be the first sign of diverticulitis. If the lesion narrows the bowel there may be symptoms of subacute obstruction, with increasing distension of the abdomen and pain of a colicky type. Urinary symptoms of frequency or discomfort on distension of the bladder may be present.

On examination of the sigmoid colon in the left iliac fossa, it may be found to be palpable, thickened and tender. Rectal examination is negative. Sigmoidoscopy is of no value in detecting the diverticula as only very rarely can the opening into a sac be observed. The associated inflammation, however, may produce an irritable condition of the gut which may be visible on endoscopic examination.

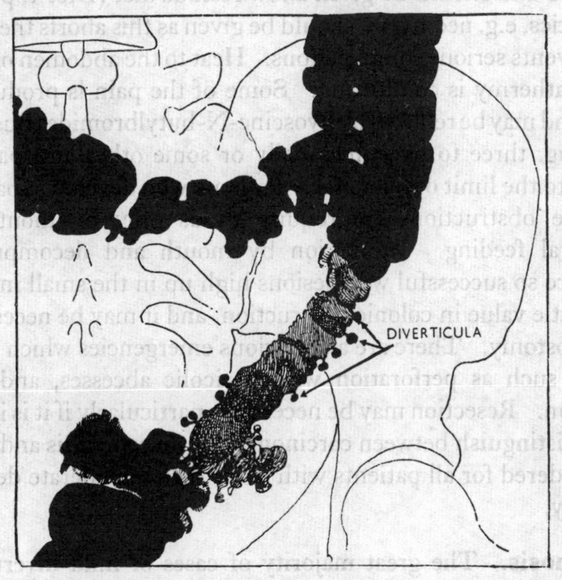

FIG. 64

Barium enema showing numerous diverticula with general narrowing and irregularity in descending and pelvic colon—diverticulitis.

Radiology. Radiological examination is the most valuable diagnostic procedure. Diverticulosis produces a characteristic radiological picture in which the sacs are outlined as pouchings from the main contour of the gut (Fig. 64). If a faecolith is present in the diverticulum, the barium partially surrounds it in a crescentic fashion. When a barium enema is evacuated, barium is frequently left behind in the diverticula which are clearly visualised. If diverticulitis is present, there will be in addition narrowing, rigidity and lack of normal haustration of a segment of colon. The main diagnostic difficulty is to distinguish this appearance from a carcinoma and the distinction may be impossible. A further difficulty may be that with an obstructing carcinoma of the sigmoid colon, the obstruction itself may render visible diverticula above the carcinoma.

Treatment. Diverticulosis requires no treatment. If diverticulitis is present with pain, fever and leucocytosis, the patient should be in bed and should be given a low residue diet (Diet 1, p. 1284). Antibiotics, e.g. neomycin, should be given as this aborts the attacks and prevents serious complications. Heat to the abdomen or short-wave diathermy is comforting. Some of the pain is produced by spasm and may be relieved by hyoscine-N-butylbromide (Buscopan) 10-20 mg. three to five times daily or some other antispasmodic pushed to the limit of tolerance. Patients who develop subacute or complete obstruction will require fluids only by mouth, and parenteral feeding. Intubation by mouth and decompression, which are so successful with lesions high up in the small intestine, are of little value in colonic obstruction, and it may be necessary to do a colostomy. There are also various emergencies which require surgery such as perforation with pericolic abcesses, and fistula formation. Resection may be necessary, particularly if it is impossible to distinguish between carcinoma and diverticulitis and should be considered for all patients with more than a moderate degree of disability.

Prognosis. The great majority of cases of mild diverticulitis settle down and remain well on simple measures. Patients with obstructive symptoms may require a partial colectomy or permanent colostomy.

CARCINOMA OF THE COLON AND RECTUM

While carcinomas are rare in the small intestine in Britain they occur in the large intestine more frequently than anywhere else in the gut.

Aetiology. As elsewhere in the body, search has been made for a pre-cancerous condition. The only diseases known to be clearly associated with cancer are ulcerative colitis, when it has been present for many years, and familial multiple polyposis.

There is no established association between carcinoma and diverticulitis.

Pathology. The most common site for cancer of the large bowel is the rectum, with the sigmoid, caecum and ascending colon next in order of frequency. Macroscopically, several types are recognised according to the amount of cellular and fibrous tissue present; there may be fungating growths or ring-like strictures. Microscopically, nearly all tumours are adenocarcinomas, except the epitheliomas around the anus. In general, these tumours are slow growing. Metastases spread through direct extension, lymphatic permeation and embolism, and by the blood stream in the portal and general circulations. The liver is the organ where secondary deposits are most commonly found.

Clinical Features. Carcinoma of the large bowel affects the older age groups and men and women in about equal frequency. There is a difference in the symptomatology of carcinoma in the descending and ascending colon. Carcinomas of the descending colon tend to produce obstruction, while cancer of the ascending colon is usually associated with symptoms of toxaemia from absorption through the ulcerated growth. Very important is the symptom of altered bowel habit already mentioned, in the form of increasing constipation or diarrhoea, or an alternation of both. If the lesion is a stricture and occurs on the left side of the abdomen the earliest symptoms will be obstructive. The patient may complain of attacks of pain, and constipation will become more persistent and severe. Discomfort is not necessarily felt at the site of the lesion, but may be felt as far round as the caecum even with an obstructive lesion in the descending colon. Sometimes the patient notices the presence of excessive borborygmi; later there may be an associated distension. If the lesion ulcerates, pus and frank blood may be seen in the stools or they may pass unnoticed until the development of the symptoms and signs of anaemia draws attention to the need for microscopical and chemical examination of the faeces. A large ulcerated lesion, particularly on the right side, will produce symptoms of loss of weight, anaemia and general ill-health. In the rectum, bleeding is the most important sign. There is often discomfort in the rectum and usually a change in bowel habit. Piles may form as the result of obstruction of the porto-systemic anastomosis at the junction of the inferior mesenteric and superior haemorrhoidal veins, and the finding of piles in the elderly should always lead to the search for an underlying cancer.

The physical appearance of the patient ranges from the normal to the cachectic. The abdomen may be distended and palpation may reveal a tumour. Even if the tumour is small, there is often a retained mass of faeces above a stricture which makes its detection easier. Rectal examination must always be done (p. 953).

Sigmoidoscopy. Nearly three-quarters of the malignant tumours of the large bowel occur in a part accessible to direct inspection, i.e. the rectum and lower sigmoid. Endoscopic examination must never be omitted. The whole or part of the growth may be seen and a biopsy specimen can be removed, though sometimes the lesion is invisible because the field is obscured by blood and mucus. A negative pathological report based on examination of a piece of tissue removed from outside the malignant area should not mislead the practitioner if other evidence is in favour of carcinoma.

Radiology. The barium enema is a more useful method of examination for diseases of the colon than the 'follow-through' of a barium meal, though the latter may be satisfactory for examination of the ascending colon. The rectum and the lower sigmoid are difficult to examine radiologically, and at any rate in the rectum, large growths may be missed. For diagnosis in this region, reliance should be placed on endoscopy. The usual radiological appearances of a carcinoma are either those of a stricture or a filling defect in the barium outline (Fig. 65).

Laboratory methods are not helpful. If there is an ulcerating lesion, examination of the blood may show an iron deficiency anaemia and occult blood and pus may be present in the faeces. Though the sedimentation rate will probably be raised in an ulcerating lesion, it may be perfectly normal in a carcinomatous stricture.

Diagnosis. There are no pathognomonic signs of carcinoma of the bowel. It is only possible to emphasise the need for perpetual vigilance and always to remember the possibility of carcinoma when anyone of middle age has bleeding from the rectum, or a change of bowel habit. There is on the average an interval of approximately six to nine months from the onset of symptoms to the diagnosis of the condition. The doctor who omits a rectal examination must accept responsibility for delay in diagnosis.

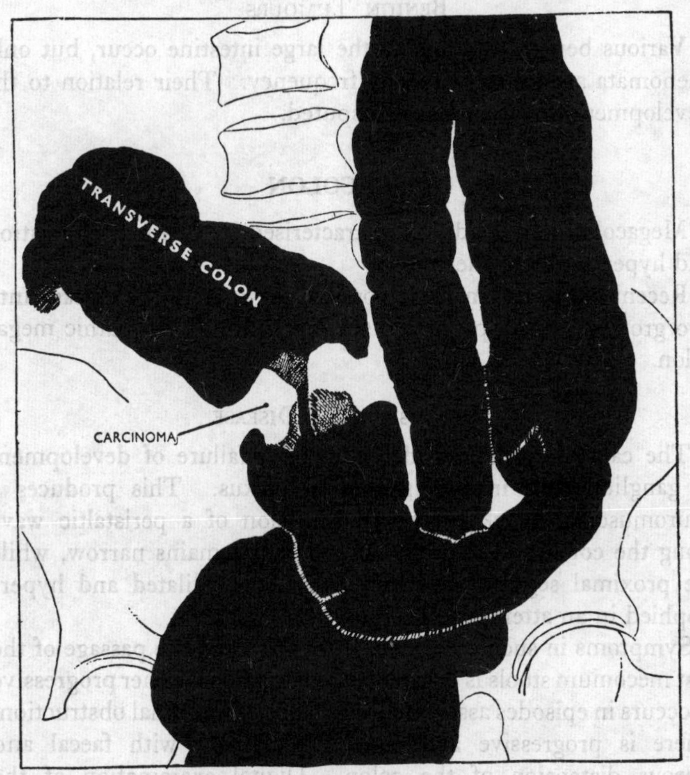

Fig. 65
Barium enema showing localised narrowing in transverse colon due to a carcinoma.

Treatment. The treatment of choice is resection of the tumour, preceded if necessary by colostomy for the immediate relief of colonic obstruction. If there is no colonic obstruction, time should be spent in getting the patient into the best possible condition for operation by correcting any dehydration, electrolyte imbalance and blood loss. The general outlook in carcinoma of the colon is considerably less gloomy than in carcinoma of the stomach, and in the most experienced hands, 80 per cent. of tumours are resectable and of these patients half are alive five years later. A bland diet low in roughage (Diet 2, p. 1285) may be indicated.

Benign Tumours

Various benign tumours of the large intestine occur, but only adenomata are found with any frequency. Their relation to the development of carcinoma is disputed.

MEGACOLON

Megacolon is a condition characterised by dilation, elongation and hypertrophy of the colon.

Recent study has made it possible to separate the disease into two groups, Hirschsprung's disease proper and idiopathic megacolon.

Hirschsprung's Disease

The cause is now considered to be a failure of development of ganglion cells in the intramural plexus. This produces a neuromuscular block to the transmission of a peristaltic wave along the colon and the affected segment remains narrow, while the proximal segment becomes enormously dilated and hypertrophied in an attempt to overcome the block.

Symptoms in such cases date from birth and the passage of the first meconium stools is delayed. Constipation is either progressive or occurs in episodes associated with signs of intestinal obstruction. There is progressive abdominal enlargement with faecal and gaseous distension of the colon. Digital examination of the rectum reveals no abnormality and the passage is empty. Radiographic examination demonstrates the lower, narrowed segment of rectum and colon, while above it there is enormous dilatation. The diagnosis can be confirmed by establishing the absence of ganglion cells in a biopsy specimen removed through a sigmoidoscope.

Treatment is surgical and the abnormal segment is excised. This allows normal movement of the propulsive wave to occur and the colon can be emptied. If the symptoms of obstruction develop at birth, it may be necessary to do a colostomy. The prognosis is excellent.

Idiopathic Megacolon

In this group of cases there is no such definite aetiology as in Hirschsprung's disease proper and both colon and rectum show general dilatation. Constipation is present sometimes from birth but is much milder in degree. Radiographic examination fails to demonstrate the sharp demarcation between dilated proximal colon and the narrowed distal segment.

Reasonably good health can be maintained by a diet containing ample roughage, and by giving lubricants or laxatives. It may be necessary to irrigate the colon with saline 'washouts.' In more severe cases sympathetic denervation of the colon may be done and this has been of value in many cases.

CONSTIPATION

Acute constipation is associated with intestinal obstruction, whether mechanical or paralytic in origin, of which it forms one of the cardinal symptoms. The chronic form is by far the more common and is the type usually denoted by the term 'constipation.' It may be defined as an infrequent evacuation of the faeces. What constitutes 'infrequency' differs in different persons, some have a bowel movement after each meal, while others only open their bowels every two or three days. Each of these rhythms is compatible with normal health. Chronic constipation is generally considered to be of two main types.

1. Colonic constipation. 2. Dyschezia.

Colonic Constipation

Colonic constipation denotes delay through the colon as a whole due to insufficient propulsive movements, although segmental movements may actually be increased. Colonic constipation may also be due to mechanical interference with the passage of faeces. Deficient movement may result from inadequate stimulation of the colon from insufficient faecal bulk due to diminished intake of food. Some nurses, and even some doctors, regard any patient as constipated who does not have his bowels open daily, even if he has been taking no food by mouth. A starved patient obviously cannot have a daily bowel action and movements will not return until two or three days after he has started eating again. Inadequate stimulus to colonic movements is also a sequel to a previous purgation which leaves the bowel empty. Many people have irrational ideas of the value of cleansing the colon and a horror of retaining faeces for longer than a day. Such patients may take purgatives daily or have what is known as a 'clean out' once a week as part of a purification ritual. Their colon is never allowed the chance of normal stimulation from the faecal mass and of acquiring a natural rhythm.

Severe dehydration from any cause may be followed by constipation. A spastic colon which abstracts an undue amount of water from the faecal mass may also be a cause.

Defective movement also occurs from hypothyroidism which is often associated with constipation, sometimes as the first symptom. Such constipation is soon relieved by giving thyroxine. Chronic constipation can also occur from a stricture of the bowel which is usually carcinomatous, but may be due to diverticulitis. Constipation is also a symptom of a depressive state.

Dyschezia

The most common cause of simple non-organic constipation is a habitual failure to empty the rectum. This type of constipation has been named 'dyschezia.' Various factors have been suggested to account for this condition.

Aetiology. 1. Improper training in childhood, insufficiency of lavatory accommodation and a persistent neglect to answer the call to defaecate.

2. Lack of roughage or fibre content in the diet.

3. Weakness of the abdominal muscles and the muscles of the pelvic floor. This may be a causative factor in the constipation of the aged.

4. Posture at defaecation. Some races defaecate in the squatting position with the thighs flexed on the abdomen and this seems to hold certain anatomical advantages, which are lost if the more usual sitting position of western civilisation is adopted.

Symptomatology. Apart from a little discomfort due to retained faeces which seems to be mainly mechanical, and possibly also slight headache, it is doubtful if constipation produces any symptoms.

Physical Examination. The finding of a rectum distended with faeces coupled with an absence of any desire to defaecate is pathognomonic of dyschezia. Faeces may also be palpated in the sigmoid colon. Radiological examination may be necessary to exclude an organic cause for the constipation. The typical finding in dyschezia is the enormous distensibility of the rectum.

Diagnosis. It is important in the first place to be certain that constipation actually exists. Some people have acquired the habit of taking laxatives to rid themselves of some condition such as headache, or eczema, and only need to discontinue these aperients to cure themselves. If simple constipation exists, it is usually due to persistent disregard of the normal signal to empty the bowel.

Treatment. The patient should first be educated in the physiology of defaecation and the importance emphasised of attending to the call to stool and thus re-educating his bowel. All strong laxatives should be forbidden and enemas should be discontinued. As a substitute for purgatives, while the bowel is being re-educated, liquid paraffin alone, or with one of the hydrophilic colloids such as agar, is very suitable. A diet with increased fibre content, that is containing fruits, green vegetables, and whole-meal bread, is helpful (Diet 11, p. 1297). These articles of diet have presumably the same action as the hydrophilic colloids like agar or tragacanth, but the patient may prefer them as being more 'natural' than the use of 'drugs'. In the elderly or wasted, it may be necessary to improve the tone of the abdominal and pelvic muscles by means of exercises. Many cases of long-continued constipation will require a mild laxative, e.g. senna or cascara, in addition to the measures discussed above.

Complications. The only important complication of constipation is faecal impaction. In the aged, who suffer from constipation from any cause, faeces may accumulate in the rectum forming a mass which finally produces the symptoms of a partial intestinal obstruction. The patient usually takes laxatives in an attempt to relieve the condition and liquid faeces may be passed without the original faecal mass being expelled, so-called spurious diarrhoea. This condition must be kept in mind if chronic or subacute intestinal obstruction is seen in an elderly or bedridden patient. The condition is treated by manual removal of the faecal mass, an operation which may require an anaesthetic.

CHRONIC DIARRHOEA

Chronic diarrhoea is not a disease *sui generis* but a symptom of many diseases and disorders. Acute diarrhoea, which is usually due to dietetic indiscretions, or to alimentary infections and food poisoning, is discussed on p. 930.

Aetiology. It is possible to list the diseases which are most commonly responsible for chronic diarrhoea. Such a list, however, is only applicable to a particular clinic at a particular time. Probably in hospital outpatient practice in Britain, combining both medical and surgical cases, the most common causes are nervous diarrhoea, carcinoma of the colon, diverticulitis, ulcerative colitis and diarrhoea following gastric surgery.

The differential diagnosis can usually be made from:

(*a*) The history and physical examination.
(*b*) Examination of the faeces; macroscopic, microscopic, bacteriological and biochemical.
(*c*) Endoscopic examination.
(*d*) Radiographic examination.

Diarrhoea which closely follows the eating of food suggests the expression of a sensitive gastro-colic reflex, due either to rapid emptying of the stomach, as for example in a carcinoma of the stomach or as the result of a gastric operation, or to inflammation in the colon, as in ulcerative colitis. Diarrhoea associated with pain usually indicates infective or ulcerative disease of the intestine or a neoplasm producing obstruction or a spastic colon. It may be possible to localise the site of the inflammation in the small intestine from a history of small intestinal colic, or in the rectum in there is definite tenesmus. Painless diarrhoea occurs with gastrogenous diarrhoea, nervous diarrhoea, the malabsorption syndrome, and the diarrhoea of pancreatic insufficiency. The alternation of constipation and diarrhoea can occur with almost any affection of the colon and is in no way pathognomonic of neoplasm. If the colon is sufficiently stimulated to empty itself completely, a day or two is bound to elapse before it fills up again, and during this time constipation is present. Diarrhoea occurring in the elderly is most likely to be due to neoplasm of the colon, diverticulitis or the misuse of purgatives. Diarrhoea associated with a palpable, tender mass in the right iliac fossa is probably due to neoplasm of the caecum or colon, or to Crohn's disease. Tuberculous enterocolitis and amoebic colitis are other possibilities uncommonly encountered in Britain. Diarrhoea associated with a mass in the left iliac fossa is likely to be due to a carcinoma of the sigmoid colon or a diverticulitis. Diarrhoea associated with some emotional situation may be purely a nervous diarrhoea, but it may also be due to some organic cause such as ulcerative colitis in which emotion acts as the trigger. Hyperthyroidism as a cause of diarrhoea is liable to be overlooked if overt signs of thyrotoxicosis are absent. Nocturnal diarrhoea which may waken the patient and is almost explosive in character, sometimes occurs as a complication of severe diabetes mellitus or multiple jejunal diverticulosis. It is possibly an expression of an autonomic neuropathy. The diarrhoea associated with the latter will sometimes respond to cyanocobalamin in the doses used in the treatment of pernicious anaemia (p. 623).

Examination of the Faeces. Visible red blood in the faeces from a patient with chronic diarrhoea is most frequently due to a lesion of the colon such as dysentery, ulcerative colitis, or a neoplasm of the colon or rectum. It occurs less commonly with regional enteritis. Mucus may be found in association with blood in any inflammation of the large bowel, or from a tumour, but it may also be passed by itself or with a normal motion from a patient with the syndrome of 'irritable colon.' Pus can best be detected by microscopical examination of the faeces and occurs in large amounts in ulcerative colitis and bacillary dysentery. Search should also be made for amoebae or amoebic cysts. Parasites may also be detected by microscopical examination. In the malabsorption syndrome, the stools may be bulky, frothy or greasy in appearance. The stool should also be examined on repeated occasions for occult blood.

Endoscopy. Practically all cases of bacillary dysentery and ulcerative colitis show lesions in the rectum on endoscopic examination. Malignant growths of the rectum or rectosigmoid colon can usually be inspected and a biopsy taken. Amoebic inflammation frequently shows localised ulcers in the rectum but the intervening mucosa is normal. Active motility of the sigmoid colon in diverticulitis and in the functional disorder of the 'irritable colon' can also be seen.

Radiology. Radiological examination is very valuable in the investigation of any patient with diarrhoea. Examination of the stomach with a barium meal will show the rate of gastric emptying. In the small intestine, cases of the malabsorption syndrome may show a 'deficiency pattern' (p. 942). Slight lesions of the small intestine such as occur in the early stages of Crohn's disease may be missed. Most lesions of the small intestine causing diarrhoea, however, occur in the lower ileum where the movement of barium is slower and observation is therefore easier. Radiological examination of the colon is essential to show disease which is outside the range of endoscopic examination. Even if ulcerative colitis has been diagnosed by proctoscopy, radiography is of value in determining the extent of the disease. Diverticulitis and neoplasms above the rectosigmoid junction of the colon may be detected by radiography. Not only may the colon be examined by a barium enema but the fluid passes through the ileo-caecal valve, and lesions in the last part of the ileum may thus be visualised.

PROTEIN-LOSING ENTEROPATHY

It has been recognised for many years that ulcerative colitis could be associated with a considerable loss of protein in the stools and that this constituted one of the main problems in the management of a severely ill patient. The concept of increased loss of protein through disease of the alimentary tract has been extended to include a number of other conditions. The loss of protein may be from intestinal juices, from desquamated cells or from albumin transudation. In some of these conditions the faecal nitrogen is normal as the excessive loss of protein into the gut is digested and reabsorbed. Provided the liver can make good the loss by protein synthesis, no hypoproteinaemia results; but if synthesis does not balance the loss, hypoalbuminaemia may be found. The investigation of albumin metabolism requires highly sophisticated techniques. A cause for unexplained hypoalbuminaemia should always be sought in the alimentary tract.

The diseases in which this condition has been reported include a type of hypertrophic gastritis, gastric carcinoma, idiopathic steatorrhoea, regional enteritis, 'blind loop' syndrome and ulcerative colitis.

DISEASES OF THE PERITONEUM

The peritoneum lines the abdomen and consists of two parts, the parietal peritoneum lining the inside of the abdominal wall and the visceral peritoneum covering the abdominal organs. Between these two layers is a potential space, the peritoneal cavity, divided into two sacs, the greater and the lesser. The peritoneum is a membrane across which water, electrolytes, and gases can pass.

Acute Peritonitis. Inflammation of the peritoneum can result from either chemical irritation or bacterial infection. Hence peritonitis is commonly due to rupture of an appendix, perforation of a peptic ulcer or an inflamed diverticulum, or it may follow surgical operations.

Clinical features are abdominal pain, tenderness, muscular rigidity and paralytic ileus. Abdominal pain is generalised and severe, and the sufferer lies immobile. This immobility contrasts with the restlessness of a patient with biliary or renal colic. Tenderness may be elicited by abdominal palpation and by rectal examination when pelvic peritonitis is present. The muscular rigidity is related to the area of peritoneum involved. Paralytic ileus is commonly present and is shown by distension of the abdomen and absent bowel sounds on auscultation.

The treatment is that of the causative condition and may be surgical, e.g. the removal of an appendix, or the suture of a perforated peptic ulcer. In addition if the patient's condition deteriorates a suitable antibiotic should be given. Kanamycin sulphate can be given in a dose of 1 g. intramuscularly for five days, while the drug should also be given intraperitoneally 0·25 g. in 500 ml. of saline twice daily for three days. Paralytic ileus is treated by intestinal decompression and maintenance of electrolyte balance.

Primary Peritonitis. This is an uncommon condition usually occurring in children, especially girls, which may be due to a pneumococcus which invades the peritoneum through the genital tract.

Tuberculous Peritonitis is mainly a disease of childhood and although it has now become extremely rare in Britain, it is still a common condition in the Middle East, Asia and Africa. The condition usually arises from a tuberculous focus in the abdomen, e.g. a mesenteric gland. There is an outpouring of fluid rich in protein into the peritoneal cavity and the mesentery becomes thickened and palpable. The patient is ill with some pyrexia, tachycardia and lassitude, and the general wasting contrasts strikingly with the enlarged abdomen. Tubercle bacilli may be isolated from the peritoneal fluid.

Treatment of the condition consists of nursing the patient under sanatorium conditions while streptomycin together with PAS and isoniazid is undoubtedly a most effective combination.

Malignant Peritonitis. The dissemination of malignant growths in the peritoneal cavity produces a reaction with an exudation of fluid which is usually rich in protein and of high specific gravity, similar to that occurring in bacterial peritonitis. These findings help to distinguish the fluid of malignant peritonitis from ascites due to chronic liver disease. The diagnosis may sometimes be confirmed by the detection of malignant cells in sediment obtained from the fluid. The growths responsible may arise anywhere in the abdomen, but the stomach and ovary are common primary sites. The symptoms, excluding those due to ascites, are those of the parent tumour. Paracentesis as required gives symptomatic relief, and antimitotic drugs are sometimes given into the peritoneal cavity.

ALLERGY OF THE INTESTINAL TRACT

Manifestations of allergy of the skin and respiratory tract are usually well defined, but allergic reactions occurring in the alimentary tract are more difficult to identify, so that there is even doubt of their very existence. When however episodes of vomiting and abdominal pain are associated with reactions in the skin such as urticaria and angioneurotic oedema, the most sceptical observer must be convinced that manifestations of intestinal allergy can occur.

Allergens are thought to be protein in nature, and manifestations in the skin subsequent to the oral ingestion of the allergen implies passage of protein molecules through the gut wall. It is known that this can occur normally in animals for a short period after birth, and it is assumed that this may also occur under pathological conditions. There is no doubt that food allergy is more common in the human infant than in the adult. In some cases the offending allergen may be obvious, e.g. if the ingestion of oysters produces a skin disturbance with abdominal symptoms. Frequently the specific allergen is unknown, and is difficult to identify since there is no simple means of testing for it. Skin testing is unreliable. Sometimes the patient appears to be multisensitive, and the allergic state may then depend more on the reactivity of the patient than on a particular allergen.

The main symptoms of an acute attack of intestinal allergy are abdominal pain of a colicky nature, vomiting and diarrhoea. They may be sufficiently severe to suggest the 'acute abdomen' Melaena may be present with or without purpura in Henoch Schönlein disease (p. 671). Radiographic examination of the small intestine with either barium or gastrografin during an attack reveals a bizarre picture of irregular mucosal folds, and re-examination some 24 hours later usually shows a dramatic return to normal. The pathology of the condition has not been studied since there is normally no indication to explore the abdomen. The attacks respond dramatically to injections of adrenalin, and the symptoms usually subside in a few hours. The use of corticosteroids as in status asthmaticus is rarely necessary.

The undoubted existence of acute allergic manifestations in the gut has suggested the possibility of chronic allergic states. Evidence has been produced that some patients with ulcerative colitis are sensitive to milk protein. It is not certain however whether reactions of this kind indicate the cause of the condition or whether the inflammatory process has allowed the passage of a foreign protein into the blood stream. The existence of chronic allergic states as a cause of alimentary disease must be regarded as still unproven.

The nature of allergic reactions and the clinical features and treatment of allergic diseases are discussed on pages 20-26.

VIRAL DISEASES OF THE INTESTINAL TRACT

The study of viruses as a cause of disease has lagged behind bacteriology owing to the much greater technical difficulties involved. There are however a number of diseases of the alimentary tract in which a viral origin is either certain or highly probable.

Diarrhoeal disease in which no causative bacteria can be identified may be due to viruses, and in some outbreaks infection has been transmitted to volunteers by oral administration of bacterial-free faecal filtrates. It is not always possible to identify the virus responsible for an epidemic of diarrhoea since viral infection is so common, particularly in children. Proof of a causal relationship is therefore difficult while some viruses have not yet been cultivated in the laboratory.

The problem of chronic diarrhoeal disease like ulcerative colitis and tropical sprue is even harder, and it is difficult to prove the existence of a viral aetiology and almost impossible to disprove it.

Some viruses affect the skin and mucous membranes, producing vesicles. In the moist conditions of the mouth these readily break down, producing ulceration, and a number of such ulcerative conditions have been identified as due to viruses. No virus has yet been isolated as responsible for simple aphthous ulcers of the mouth.

A number of adenoviruses have a predilection for lymphoid tissue and may be responsible for some instances of mesenteric adenitis in children. It is also possible that the association between acute appendicitis and oropharyngeal infection which occurs in some patients, and which has long been recognised, is due to a common viral origin.

Glands associated with the alimentary tract may be affected. Parotitis can be produced by the virus of mumps, and this virus can also infect the pancreas. It is possible that some enteroviruses may be responsible for infection of the pancreas. The liver may be involved in a number of virus infections apart from the virus of infectious hepatitis.

Further research is likely to identify a number of alimentary diseases as of viral origin and may ultimately make available antiviral compounds which are therapeutically effective.

FUNCTIONAL DISORDERS OF THE GASTROINTESTINAL TRACT

The general problems related to the causation and treatment of functional disorders are the same whether the clinical features are referred to the gastrointestinal, respiratory, cardiac or central nervous system (p. 1248). A discussion of some of the more important specific syndromes of the gastrointestinal tract follows.

SPECIFIC SYNDROMES

Anorexia Nervosa

Anorexia may be defined as a loss of the general desire to eat without dividing this desire into its component factors of hunger, appetite and food habit. Sucking concerns the infant within a few hours of birth, and the importance of food continues throughout life. Food, quite apart from its nutritive value, acquires psychological connotations and the giving of food is symbolic of friendship and love in all countries of the world. It is not therefore surprising that an alteration of appetite can be an expression of a psychological disorder. The attitude of people to food differs widely; some express an entire indifference and derive no enjoyment from it; others get much satisfaction from the pleasures of the table. Anorexia of mild degree is a common symptom of anxiety neuroses and is not infrequently encountered in psychotic states. The term 'anorexia nervosa' should be restricted to the syndrome in which the loss of appetite is severe in degree and is conditioned by a hysterical reaction. The type of patient to develop such a hysterical reaction is one who is emotionally immature and unstable and usually highly suggestible. The psychological disturbance is often repressed into the subconscious mind and is replaced by a physical symptom.

The patient is usually a young unmarried woman. In some cases the exciting cause may be easily discovered, e.g. a desire to slim, or a childish method of attracting attention. Occasionally there seems to be a mental association between the idea of getting fat and that of becoming pregnant. In many cases the underlying cause, being deeply repressed, is difficult to elicit. The distaste for all foods is complete, and if the patient is forced to take food it may be vomited. The patient may go to extreme lengths to conceal food which she is supposed to have eaten at table, and which is afterwards thrown away. Following the anorexia there is loss of weight which may be extreme, but it should be noted as of considerable diagnostic importance that there is little change in physical or mental activity until very late in the disease. Other clinical features are an associated amenorrhoea and a downy growth of hair on the body.

Treatment is best carried out in a hospital. Psychological treatment should be undertaken with the object of persuading the patient to eat. In many cases this can be carried out by the physician, but if he fails, the opinion of a psychiatrist should be sought. It should be emphasised to the patient that she has lost the eating habit, and that the desire for food will not return until she forces herself to eat. The appetite in fact grows by what it feeds on. It may be necessary for the doctor or nurse to be present at meals to see that the patient does in fact eat the food, and not hide it away. Meals should be small in size, appetising, well-cooked, and daintily served.

Entirely opposite to anorexia nervosa with its attendant wasting is obesity induced by psychological causes. The taking of food can serve to relieve tension, and some people acquire the habit of eating excessively for this reason. Obesity and anorexia nervosa can even alternate in the same patient.

Glossodynia

Occasionally a patient will complain of a persistent unpleasant taste in the mouth or a painful tongue. No change in appearance is visible on examination, nor has the pain any relation to particular foodstuffs, such as rusks, salted foods, vinegar, or hot liquids, as occurs with a true glossitis. The psychological origin of the symptom is always deep seated, and the complaint may virtually amount to a delusion. The symptom cannot easily be removed. If the patient cannot accept any psychological explanation for its cause he should be encouraged to accept the disability as one that does not interfere with eating and that is due to a hyperacute sense of taste, or an unduly sensitive tongue.

Globus Hystericus (p. 890)

Nervous Dyspepsia

This term is used to describe a condition in which complaints of vague dyspeptic symptoms, such as a feeling of satiety, abdominal discomfort, nausea, anorexia or vomiting are associated with certain psychoneurotic features such as anxiety, irritability, insomnia, loss of weight, attacks of sweating, weakness, tachycardia, or a feeling of tension. The precise mechanism by which psychological disturbances produce gastric symptoms is uncertain. There is no doubt that emotion can alter gastric secretion, motility, and blood flow, and it is likely that some altered pattern of gastric behaviour is the underlying basis of functional disease of the stomach.

Clinical Features. There is no constant group of complaints in nervous dyspepsia. The symptoms may have been present for a long time, altering from day to day, and having no constant relationships either to time or to food. The discomfort is usually referred diffusely across the abdomen and is rarely sharply localised. These features contrast strongly with those found in a subject with peptic ulcer, who typically describes an unvarying train of events and accurately localises the site of his pain. The appetite is usually capricious or impaired and there is often nausea. Constipation is often present. Aerophagy may have developed as a habit following a feeling of discomfort ascribed to excessive 'wind' in the stomach, which the patient attempts to eructate. Physical and radiological examination yield negative results and no occult blood can be detected in the stools.

Treatment. Once organic disease has been excluded, the patient should be told that while he may have an irritable stomach, there is no organic disease. The nervous origin of his symptoms should be explained to him, and he should be treated on the general lines discussed on p. 1248. Frequently such patients recognise that they have a 'weak stomach' which bears the brunt of recurrent stress, but they come to a doctor for fresh reassurance from time to time. Often they have some private ritual or magic diet to which they attach great importance. Provided such a diet is harmless and does not exclude essential foodstuffs it can be left unaltered.

Psychogenic Vomiting

This is not uncommon and usually occurs on getting up or after breakfast; only rarely does it appear later in the day. It is often unattended by any loss of weight despite its occurrence over long periods, and this is of value in distinguishing it from vomiting due to organic disease. If psychogenic vomiting is a symptom of a functional anxiety state it will disappear if the causes leading to the emotional tension can be resolved. In some cases, as in the famous instance of Charles Darwin, the patient may have to accept the disability. If the vomiting occurs in the morning only, the disability may be circumvented by arranging to eat later in the day. Anti-emetic drugs such as chlorpromazine, 25-75 mg. or promethazine, 25 mg. are sometimes effective in severe cases.

IRRITABLE BOWEL

Functional disorders of the small and large intestines are probably the most common gastrointestinal conditions which a doctor encounters. A disorder of intestinal function takes the form either of a motor dysfunction resulting in painful spasm or diarrhoea, or much more rarely a secretory dysfunction resulting in the passage of large amounts of mucus. Both may be present in the same patient.

In the past various names have been given to designate these different types such as spastic colon, 'mucous colitis,' nervous diarrhoea, but it is probably better to admit their unity of origin and call all such manifestations examples of the syndrome of the 'irritable bowel.' The term 'mucous colitis' is particularly unfortunate, as the condition is emphatically not an inflammation of the colon. The behaviour of the colon is only part of a general picture of autonomic disturbance which may affect the whole gastrointestinal tract, and indeed, the whole body.

Aetiology. The aetiological factors underlying functional disease have already been discussed. The provoking cause for the appearance of symptoms may sometimes, though not invariably, be traced to a particular stress. Allergy has been suggested as the trigger, which initiates the attacks, but with little real evidence to support it. The symptoms may be associated with menstruation or may be troublesome during the menopause. Mental and physical fatigue are precipitating factors, as also is the taking of irritating purgatives.

Clinical Features. Both sexes are affected. There seems some tendency for the condition to run in families. Either this tendency is actually inherited or the disorder is suggested to the child from the preoccupation with bowel symptoms of an introspective parent. The patient complains of recurring attacks of abdominal pain lasting some hours, which are not usually severe. The pain may be dull, aching or cramp-like. The lower left quadrant is a common site. These attacks of pain are associated with an alteration of bowel rhythm but may be interspersed with attacks of diarrhoea often brought on by the taking of purgatives. Constipation is common. Scybalous stools are passed during the attacks, sometimes together with large amounts of mucus; hence the name 'mucous colitis' used to describe this syndrome. Between the episodes the bowel rhythm may be normal. There may be associated irritability of the pyloro-duodenal region with symptoms suggesting an ulcer. Vomiting is uncommon.

On physical examination, palpation may reveal a hard pencil of gut in the left iliac fossa which is contracted but not tender. There is no associated abdominal rigidity and fever is absent. The abdominal scar of an appendicectomy for 'chronic appendicitis' is a common stigma. Rectal examination is normal and the rectum is usually empty. Sigmoidoscopy helps to distinguish the condition from certain organic diseases such as ulcerative colitis. The sigmoid colon frequently appears to be extremely motile, showing contraction and relaxation, quite unlike the inert state of the normal colon. A record of movements of the colon confirms this striking activity. On radiological examination by barium enema the outline of the colon shows considerable variation and may show spasm and narrowing in various areas, the sigmoid colon being most frequently affected. Haustration may disappear temporarily, giving the appearance often associated with ulcerative colitis. If the progress of a barium meal be watched through the gut, the small intestine may also show abnormal patterns.

Treatment. If there are obvious causes of underlying tension they should be relieved: the common fear of cancer is one that proper examination should remove. Treatment of insomnia is important, and phenobarbitone is of value in relieving emotional tension, as is methylpentynol, 250-500 mg. For the spastic constipation, one of the hydrophilic colloids such as agar should be prescribed. For the treatment of spasm, atropine sulphate or tincture of belladonna may be given. Should these fail, the following antispasmodic preparations may be tried: hyoscine-N-butylbromide (Buscopan) 10-20 mg. t.d.s. or tricyclamol (Lergine) 50-100 mg. t.d.s.

Nervous Diarrhoea

This condition occurs in the highly strung individual and is characterised by the passage of loose stools after meals or as a result of some situation producing emotional strain. The sufferer may become so conscious of, and so obsessed with, his condition that visits to a theatre or travel in a train without access to a toilet become impossible. There are no abnormal physical signs beyond those of general reactivity such as tachycardia and brisk reflexes. Examination by barium enema and sigmoidoscopy are normal.

After organic disease has been excluded, the doctor should discuss the condition with the patient and reassure him. Phenobarbitone may help him to avoid some of the effects of an emotive situation, and codeine in doses of 15 mg. is a most helpful drug in aiding the patient to regain control of his bowel activity. At first it is taken one to three times a day as required until the motions are formed. Tablets should be carried by the patient. Soon the patient will regain his confidence and can reduce the frequency of administration. Finally he may only require to take a tablet on occasions known to be associated with particularly severe emotional stress. This treatment very rarely fails.

PREVENTION

Diseases and disorders of the digestive system are responsible for a considerable proportion of the work of general practitioners and physicians in hospitals. It is, therefore, all the more unfortunate that such is our ignorance of the aetiology of many of the most common diseases of the digestive system that little scope for their prevention is possible at the present time. An adequate diet, good mastication, sufficient time for meals and relaxation, and the avoidance of excessive smoking and drinking are measures that all contribute towards health without preventing any particular disease. The disorders of the alimentary tract which are commonly encountered in practice are:

(1) **Functional Disorders.** The mechanisms underlying the production of various functional disorders and the general

measures for their prevention and treatment are fully discussed in the appropriate sections on pp. 983-988. A reduction in functional disease in general and of the alimentary tract in particular presents an intricate and highly important medical problem. The great frequency of functional disease makes it all the more desirable to investigate the best methods for its prevention. Consideration must be given to measures for improving the nation's mental health which include the breeding of a psychologically more robust population, the rearing and education of children in the best way to fit them for making adequate adjustments to life, and the guidance of adults, and especially of parents, in their attitude towards work, play and family responsibilities. The solution of these problems requires the co-ordinated efforts of the geneticist, the educationalist, the psychologist, the industrialist, the priest and particularly the family doctor.

(2) **Peptic Ulcer.** The vexed question of aetiology of peptic ulcer has been fully discussed on p. 900. Suffice it to say that the cause of peptic ulceration is not known. If it is a disease of modern life, there seems no immediate prospect of changing the pattern of modern life. There is, however, some scope for preventing some of its complications. Deaths from ulcer occur from perforation, haemorrhage, and from operations on the stomach. While some perforations occur with no warning, others follow an acute exacerbation of dyspepsia associated with pain and rigidity. If at this stage the patient is treated in bed, subsequent perforation may be prevented. We may also be able to forestall haemorrhage by operating during a quiescent period in an ulcer patient who is known to have a chronic ulcer that is unlikely to heal.

(3) **Infections.** Infections of the alimentary tract may be bacterial, protozoal or helminthic. These are extremely common in tropical countries and theoretically all are preventable. In temperate climates and in civilised countries their incidence has been greatly reduced by the provision of a pure water supply and a water carriage system of sewage disposal. There are still, however, in Britain many cases of food poisoning and there is much scope for improvement in the preparation and handling of food in our shops and restaurants and for the provision of proper washing facilities in all lavatories, public or private.

(4) **Malignant Disease.** Since little is known about the factors which are responsible for the development of malignant disease, little can be done to prevent its occurrence. It would, however, be possible to mitigate its effects if early diagnosis were possible. The fact that malignant disease of the stomach and intestine is not visible to direct inspection except sometimes with the aid of special instruments, and that symptoms may be absent or indefinite for a considerable period of time, makes early diagnosis especially difficult. There is little evidence to suggest that pre-cancerous states commonly occur in the alimentary tract.

W. I. CARD.

Books recommended:

Avery Jones, F. & Gummer, J. W. P. (1968). *Clinical Gastro-enterology*, 2nd ed. London: Butterworth.

Bockus, Henry L. (1963). *Gastroenterology*, 2nd ed. Philadelphia: Saunders.

DISEASES OF THE LIVER AND BILIARY TRACT

DISEASES OF THE LIVER

ANATOMICAL CONSIDERATIONS

On histological examination the liver appears to be composed of radial columns of cells arranged in lobules around a central efferent vein. At the periphery of the lobules lie portal tracts, each containing a small branch of the hepatic artery and of the portal vein and a small bile duct. Between the columns of liver cells are sinusoids lined with cells of the reticulo-endothelial system known as Kupffer cells. Small bile canaliculi lie between the liver cells, forming a network which opens eventually into the interlobular ducts situated in the portal tracts.

From the portal vein and from the hepatic artery in the portal tract, blood passes into the sinusoids and reaches the central vein, which drains into the hepatic veins. Mixing of portal venous and hepatic arterial blood appears to occur in the sinusoids. When the normal architecture of the liver including pre-sinusoidal sphincters on the arterioles is damaged by disease, direct transmission of the high arterial pressure to the portal system may be partly responsible for the portal venous hypertension found in such conditions.

Bile, secreted by the liver cells, passes, in reverse direction to the blood flow, through canaliculi to the periphery of the lobule. There, the bile ducts are lined with cuboidal epithelium and gradually become larger as they progress to the porta hepatis. Ultimately the common hepatic duct is formed by the union of the ducts from the right and left lobes of the liver, and this, with the cystic duct from the gall-bladder, forms the common bile duct. This usually traverses the substance of the head of the pancreas, where it is joined, in the majority of cases, by the pancreatic duct. The united ducts then open into the second part of the duodenum through the ampulla of Vater, the opening being controlled by the sphincter of Oddi.

Blood Supply. The liver is unique in that the greater part of the blood flowing to it is venous and comes via the portal vein which drains the large and small intestine, stomach, pancreas and spleen. The total blood flow through the adult human liver averages 1500 ml./minute. This frequently becomes considerably reduced in chronic hepatic disease. Though the hepatic artery supplies only about 20 per cent. of the blood to the liver, it carries up to 50 per cent. of the oxygen utilised by the organ. The large supply of venous blood results in an oxygen supply that is probably always precarious, so that the liver is vulnerable to chronic anoxia. In chronic passive congestion, for example, there is degeneration and sometimes necrosis of the cells furthest from the entry of well-aerated blood, i.e. in the centre of the lobule. Centrilobular necrosis is found also in thyrotoxicosis, in which the oxygen demand by the liver cells is increased. In addition, in the majority of acute toxic or infective liver diseases, in which there is neither anoxia nor excessive oxygen utilisation, necrosis in this zone is commonly found. Damage to the parenchymal cells in these conditions may be aggravated by the relative oxygen deficiency in the centre of the lobule.

The blood supply to the liver through the portal vein is believed to follow two main streams, one from the stomach, spleen and descending colon to the left lobe, and one from the small intestine and ascending colon to the right lobe. This distribution of blood does not correspond strictly to the anatomical lobes of the liver. Acute massive necrosis, which may in part, at least, be due to dietary inadequacy (p. 1009), may show damage predominantly in the left lobe, presumably because essential dietary constituents are especially deficient in blood draining the stomach, spleen, and descending colon. Likewise, abscesses from an infected appendix occur mainly in the right lobe.

METABOLIC ACTIVITIES OF THE LIVER

The manner in which blood gains intimate contact with hepatic cells facilitates the rapid transfer of metabolites. Apart from the Kupffer cells of the reticulo-endothelial system, all the cells of the liver are undifferentiated and appear capable of performing the many functions of the liver.

(1) **Carbohydrate Metabolism.** The liver is the most important organ in the body for the maintenance of a normal concentration of blood glucose. It is able to convert glucose, fructose, galactose, glycerol, certain amino acid residues, and 2- and 3-carbon compounds (e.g. lactate, pyruvate and oxalo-acetate) to glycogen. In hypoglycaemia it hydrolyses stored glycogen to glucose. These mechanisms are intrinsic functions of the organ but they are influenced by many extrahepatic factors, e.g. insulin, adrenaline, thyroxine, cortisol and glucagon.

(2) **Protein Metabolism.** The liver is the most important site of deamination of amino acids, as a preliminary step in their interconversion and oxidation. Urea synthesis from the amino groups made available by this process occurs solely in the organ. Plasma albumin, prothrombin, fibrinogen and the other clotting factors V, VII, IX and X are synthesised perhaps exclusively in the parenchymal cells of the liver. α and β globulins are mainly formed in the liver, while γ globulin is formed by cells of the reticulo-endothelial system. As a result of these syntheses, the protein pattern of the plasma is to a large extent determined by liver function.

(3) **Lipid Metabolism.** The liver plays an important part in fat metabolism. Fats are oxidised in the liver as far as the four carbon chain stage (ketone bodies). The amount of this oxidation depends, *inter alia*, upon the availability of carbohydrate and is greatly increased when sugar is absent (e.g. in fasting) or when there is difficulty in its use (e.g. in diabetes mellitus). The ketone bodies themselves do not appear to be oxidised in the liver and are liberated into the blood stream for peripheral oxidation. Triglycerides are formed in the liver and synthesis of phospholipid from fatty acid, glycerol, phosphate and a nitrogenous base, e.g. choline, also occurs largely in the liver. Cholesterol is synthesised in the liver and is also esterified there. Cholesterol and triglycerides circulate in the blood as lipoproteins; not only is the liver an important source of these complexes which maintain lipid in colloidal solution, but also it contains an enzyme which can break the lipid-protein bond.

(4) **Vitamin Metabolism.** The liver is directly or indirectly concerned with the metabolism of many of the vitamins. Fat-soluble vitamins depend to some extent for their absorption upon

a normal biliary secretion. Vitamins A, D, E, K, B_{12} and folic acid particularly are stored in the liver. Vitamin K is required by the hepatic cells for the production of prothrombin and factor VII. The liver contains enzymes which can convert tryptophane to nicotinic acid and synthesise many coenzymes and prosthetic groups. The phosphorylation of thiamine (aneurin), which is a necessary preliminary to its function as a co-enzyme, and the methylation of nicotinic acid also occur in the liver.

(5) **Inactivation of Hormones.** Oestrogens, corticosteroids and other steroid hormones are conjugated in the liver with glucuronic acid and excreted in the urine, though other modes of inactivation also occur. Thyroxine and vasopressin of the posterior pituitary gland are probably inactivated in the liver, but the mechanisms are unknown.

(6) **Detoxication of Drugs.** Many drugs are either conjugated or oxidised in the liver, and the purpose of this is generally considered to be detoxication. Alkaloids such as morphine or atropine are partly destroyed in the liver, ammonia is converted to urea, barbiturates undergo oxidation of their side chain and are rendered pharmacologically inert. Conjugation with glucuronic acid occurs with salicylates, tribromethanol (Avertin), morphine and chloral hydrate, and these conjugates are less active than their precursors. Acetylation of sulphonamides also occurs, though this process makes these drugs less soluble and relatively more toxic.

(7) **Biliary Excretion.** Bile is produced by the liver and passes through the intrahepatic biliary channels to the common hepatic duct and thence to the gall-bladder. The main constituents, apart from water and inorganic salts, are bilirubin, bile acids, cholesterol, alkaline phosphatase and mucin.

(*a*) *Bilirubin.* Haemoglobin is broken down by reticulo-endothelial cells mainly in the spleen, liver and bone marrow. The bile pigment, unconjugated bilirubin (prehepatic bilirubin) is derived from the non-iron-containing residue after the separation from globin. In the blood it is maintained in solution through binding with plasma albumin and as a consequence it does not pass readily through the glomerulus of the kidney into the urine. Unconjugated bilirubin is actively transported from the blood to the bile by the liver cells and during its passage it is separated from its protein and is conjugated with glucuronic acid. This conjugation, into mono- and di-glucuronides which occurs in the microsomes of the liver cells by the activity of glucuronyl transferase, renders the pigment water soluble so that it becomes capable of being more freely excreted in the urine. This compound is called conjugated bilirubin (post-hepatic bilirubin).

In the small intestine conjugated bilirubin is metabolised by bacteria to a series of isomers of stercobilinogen which on oxidation forms the main faecal pigment stercobilin. The bulk of these pigments is excreted in the stool (250 mg./day) but some is reabsorbed from the gut. Most of this is excreted by the liver cells into the intestine and a small part is excreted in the urine (2-4 mg./day) where it is called urobilinogen. Urobilinogen and its oxidation product urobilin are chemically identical with stercobilinogen and stercobilin, respectively.

(*b*) *Excretion of Bile Acids and Cholesterol.* Bile acids are formed from cholesterol solely in the liver. They are secreted by the hepatic cells into the biliary canaliculi along with considerable amounts of cholesterol and enter the intestine where they facilitate emulsification of water insoluble lipids.

(*c*) *Excretion of Enzymes.* The serum alkaline phosphatase is derived mainly from hepatic cells in the adult and is normally excreted in the bile. An isoenzyme produced by the osteoblasts accounts for a variable proportion of alkaline phosphatase activity in children and in diseases of bone. In pregnancy another isoenzyme is produced by the placenta.

JAUNDICE

Jaundice or icterus is a condition characterised by increase in the bilirubin content of the blood above the normal range of 0·2-0·8 mg./100 ml. serum. When the increase is slight (serum bilirubin $<$2 mg. per 100 ml.) its presence can often be detected only by serum analysis, and latent jaundice is then said to exist. When the increase is greater, there is visible yellow colouration of the skin, sclerae and mucous membranes, and clinical jaundice is present. Internal tissues are also stained. Bilirubin does not pass the blood-brain barrier except in the immediate neo-natal period. Pathological mechanisms giving rise to jaundice fall into three well-defined groups.

1. Obstructive Jaundice

Obstructive jaundice occurs when there is a block to the pathway between the site of conjugation of bile in the liver cells and the entry of bilirubin into the duodenum. Stasis occurs within the dilated bile ducts and canaliculi, and conjugated bilirubin and other constituents of bile are retained and enter the blood stream.

Causes. Obstructive jaundice may be broadly divided into two categories: (a) extrahepatic cholestasis where there is obstruction to the main bile ducts, and (b) intrahepatic cholestasis where the lesions responsible lie within the liver between the cells and the main bile ducts. The most common extrahepatic causes of obstructive jaundice are impaction of gall-stones in the common bile duct and carcinoma of the head of the pancreas or ampulla of Vater. Other causes include carcinoma of the gall-bladder and metastatic carcinoma of lymph nodes in the porta hepatis. Intrahepatic obstructive jaundice occurs in the presence of patent main bile ducts and is of multiple aetiology. Certain drugs commonly employed in clinical practice occasionally produce jaundice of this type which is believed to be due to a drug sensitivity as a result of which inflammation develops around the intrahepatic biliary canaliculi. These include chlorpromazine and other phenothiazine derivatives, para-aminosalicylic acid, arsenical compounds, thiouracil, chlorpropamide and nitrofurantoin. Other drugs which may cause cholestatic jaundice are methyl testosterone, anabolic steroids such as norethandrolone and sulphadiazine. The resultant jaundice in this latter group is not due to drug sensitivity but appears to be a genuine intoxication. The steroids that have been implicated in this way are all C17 α-alkyl substituted testosterones. This is important since oral contraceptives contain such compounds; reactions from their use have been rare in Britain but comparatively common in Scandinavia and Chile.

Intrinsic disease of the liver itself is often associated with intrahepatic cholestasis, and complicates the jaundice which occurs in diseases which damage hepatic cells, e.g. infective hepatitis (p. 1007).

Clinical Features, apart from those of the causative disease, include yellow colouration of sclerae and skin, pale or clay-colouted bulky stools containing an excessive amount of fat and a deficiency of stercobilinogen, and the presence in the urine of bilirubin, which renders it dark. Pruritus, anorexia and a metallic taste in the mouth may occur. Bradycardia is sometimes found in the early stages and may be produced by an increase in vagal inhibitory tone due to circulating bile salts. Owing to the impairment in fat absorption in the intestine as a result of the absence of bile salts, vitamin K absorption is diminished, with consequent increase in coagulation time and in the one-stage prothrombin time from prothrombin and factor VII deficiency, and a tendency to haemorrhage. Tests of liver function which are dependent upon the metabolic activities or integrity of the parenchymal cells, e.g. flocculation tests, tend to be normal in the initial stages. There is usually, however, slight elevation of the serum enzyme levels (p. 1004). In long-standing obstructive jaundice, parenchymal liver cell damage occurs, with consequent impairment of metabolic function, and ultimately a drowsy, semi-stuporous state may ensue prior to death (hepatic encephalopathy).

2. Haemolytic Jaundice (p. 629)

Excessive destruction of red blood cells results in increased bilirubin formation. The liver excretes conjugated bilirubin into the intestine to the maximum of its capacity, and a healthy liver can handle a bilirubin load six times greater than normal before unconjugated bilirubin accumulates in the plasma. This accounts for the fact that except in the newborn, jaundice due to haemolysis is usually mild.

Causes. The rate of destruction of red blood cells is increased either because of a congenital defect in the red cells which renders them unduly fragile (congenital spherocytosis, sickle cell anaemia, thalassaemia) or because various extracorpuscular factors act on the red cells and cause excessive haemolysis. These factors include infections, poisons and circulating red-cell antibodies as in idiopathic acquired haemolytic anaemia, incompatible blood transfusion and erythroblastosis foetalis.

Clinical Features. The following features are common to all types of haemolytic jaundice and are independent of its cause. The jaundice may be latent or overt but is rarely severe, the total serum bilirubin being less than 4 mg./100 ml. Enlargement of the spleen is found in the majority of the cases and is due to excessive activity of the reticulo-endothelial system. Reticulocytosis is almost invariably present, but the degree of anaemia varies with the severity of the haemolytic process and the power of the bone marrow to increase its productive activity (p. 629). The stools are brown or orange in colour and contain large amounts of stercobilinogen and stercobilin. Part of the stercobilinogen in the intestine is reabsorbed and appears in the urine (urobilinogen). Freshly voided urine is therefore of normal colour, since no bilirubin is present, but oxidation of excess urobilinogen to urobilin quickly renders the urine dark. Pruritus which is believed to be due to retention of bile salts does not occur. Tests of liver function which are dependent upon parenchymal cell metabolic activities are normal.

3. Hepatocellular Jaundice

This type of jaundice is usually associated with damage to the parenchymal cells of the liver by toxic or infective agents, the power to transfer bilirubin from the blood to the biliary canaliculi being, in consequence, diminished. The cellular degeneration and necrosis permit diffusion into the blood of bilirubin that has reached the canaliculi; swelling of the cells and oedema add an intrahepatic obstructive element which causes regurgitation of bilirubin from the canaliculi into the blood (intrahepatic cholestasis).

Causes

1. Infection with the virus of infective hepatitis is by far the most important cause of hepatocellular jaundice (p. 1007).
2. Other infections, e.g. leptospirosis, yellow fever, septicaemia.
3. Poisonous substances (p. 1006).
4. Deficiencies of specific food factors, e.g. methionine, choline and cystine. Deficiencies in these substances produce liver damage in experimental animals. The extent to which they produce acute massive necrosis and hepatic infiltration with fat in man is not known.
5. As a consequence of a primary defect in bilirubin transport or conjugation within the liver. The best example and one which is particularly common in premature infants

was originally called 'physiological jaundice of the newborn'. The condition is now known to be due to immaturity of the enzymic mechanisms responsible for conjugation of bilirubin.

A few otherwise apparently normal subjects show episodic or permanent elevation of serum bilirubin above 1 mg. per 100 ml. This disorder is often called congenital non-haemolytic hyperbilirubinaemia. A number of syndromes have been described; they fall into two groups, in one of which the mild jaundice is due to increase of circulating unconjugated bilirubin, and in the other of conjugated pigment.

There are two main conditions. In the first (Gilbert's disease) the fault lies in the mechanism for transport of bilirubin to its site of conjugation in the liver cell. The defect in the second less common disorder (Dubin-Johnson syndrome) is in the transport of conjugated bilirubin from the liver cells into the bile canaliculi; one diagnostic feature of this condition is that the liver cells contain black pigment.

Clinical Features. The clinical features of hepatocellular jaundice vary according to the aetiology. Icterus may be mild or very severe. For further details of the clinical picture and laboratory data of a typical example of hepatocellular disease see p. 1008.

LIVER FUNCTION TESTS

Liver function tests are performed for three main reasons:

1. To assist in the differential diagnosis of jaundice, with the chief aim of distinguishing between jaundice requiring surgical treatment and jaundice requiring medical treatment.
2. To obtain confirmation of suspected liver disease.
3. To estimate hepatic function as a guide to progress and an aid to prognosis.

The various hepatic functions are not impaired to the same degree in any one case of liver disease, irrespective of its aetiology. As a direct consequence of this differential depression of function, a series of tests covering different functions is best applied. As a corollary, a single negative result of a test indicates neither that the liver is normal nor, if the liver is known to be diseased, that the test is necessarily insensitive.

'Surgical' or extrahepatic obstructive jaundice is not associated with marked parenchymal lesions in the liver, at least in the initial stages. As a result, metabolic functions carried out by the parenchymal cells are not affected, while those activities which involve biliary excretion are impaired. To some extent the reverse situation obtains in 'medical' jaundice (hepatocellular jaundice), which usually results from parenchymal damage. Thus the tests of metabolic functions are impaired, and the tests of excretory functions are depressed only in so far as they are a part of hepatic cell metabolism.

Tests of Metabolic Functions

This group of tests provides estimates of parenchymal cell liver function. The particular functions concerned are not directly dependent upon the patency of the bile ducts and are therefore performed normally in the early stages of biliary obstruction. Prolonged biliary obstruction naturally causes parenchymal cell damage, and such functions do in time become impaired as a consequence of this. In the past the power of the liver to convert laevulose or galactose to glycogen was tested by serial blood sugar determinations following the oral or intravenous administration of one or other of the above sugars. While this test is used in the detection of galactosaemia—a rare inborn error of metabolism in infants—it has been superseded by other methods which are more sensitive tests of liver function and which are discussed below.

Protein Metabolism. The power to synthesise plasma proteins, particularly albumin, is evaluated by determination of plasma albumin and globulin concentrations. In diffuse parenchymal liver disease albumin concentration falls, while there is a rise, for reasons unknown, in the globulin fractions. A quantitative change in the fractions of serum globulin also occurs, affecting mainly α or γ globulin fractions, particularly the latter, and these may be demonstrated by paper electrophoresis of serum proteins. These distortions, with the lowered serum albumin, provide the physico-chemical basis of *flocculation tests*, which include cephalin-cholesterol flocculation, zinc sulphate turbidity and thymol turbidity and flocculation. These tests are influenced to a varying extent by the different plasma protein components. Since many disorders disturb the plasma protein pattern, e.g. multiple myeloma, the flocculation tests are not specific for liver disease and must always be interpreted in relation to the clinical picture and other laboratory findings.

The distortion of the plasma protein pattern, particularly a fall in fibrinogen concentration, is also responsible for the fact that a low erythrocyte sedimentation rate is sometimes found in the presence of active liver disease.

In the early stages of the large majority of cases of jaundice due to extrahepatic obstruction, these flocculation tests are negative or only slightly positive.

Diminution in the blood content of prothrombin and factors VII and IX (Christmas factor), as detected by the one-stage prothrombin time (prothrombin and factor VII) and Thrombotest (all three clotting factors), occurs either as a result of diffuse parenchymal liver disease or in states of vitamin K deficiency. In the case of the former, parenteral administration of vitamin K has little effect upon the prothrombin time. When, however, the prolonged prothrombin time is the result of failure of absorption of vitamin K, the intramuscular injection of 5-10 mg. of menaphthone brings the time back to normal in 6-12 hours (p. 667). This effect is seen, for example, in cases of obstructive jaundice in which the absence of bile salts in the intestine prevents the absorption of vitamin K. The distinction, however, is not so clear as to be of value in the assessment of hepatic function or in the differentiation between obstructive and hepatocellular jaundice.

Tests which, though Primarily of Metabolic Function, are Dependent upon the Patency of the Bile Ducts

These tests provide estimates of parenchymal cell hepatic functions which are directly dependent upon the patency of the biliary tree. As a result, they will detect alterations in function due either to parenchymal cell damage or to obstruction to the bile ducts.

1. **Serum Alkaline Phosphatase Activity.** This enzyme is excreted by the hepatic parenchymal cells into the biliary canaliculi and eventually into the intestine. Normal serum values in adults range from 3-12 King-Armstrong units per 100 ml.

serum, though levels up to 25 units are found in growing children. In acute or chronic parenchymal liver disease a moderate elevation up to 30 units can occur, while in obstructive jaundice concentrations between 30 and 100 units are found in the great majority of cases. Values above 50 units are also found in many cases of diffuse metastases within the liver. It is to be remembered that high concentrations of serum alkaline phosphatase occur also in conditions in which osteoblastic activity is a feature, e.g. rickets, Paget's disease, hyperparathyroidism, benign and malignant tumours of bone, and metastatic tumours in bone. Multiple myeloma on the other hand, a malignant disease which affects bone extensively is not associated with much bone repair and seldom shows a raised serum alkaline phosphatase.

2. **Bromsulphthalein Excretion (BSP).** This dye, after intravenous injection, is removed from the blood by the parenchymal cells and the Kupffer cells of the liver and excreted in the bile. This capacity may be estimated by determining the concentration of BSP in the blood 45 minutes after the injection when less than 5 per cent. is found in the blood of healthy individuals. The test is sensitive and is positive in about 80 per cent. of cases of infective hepatitis in the pre-icteric phase, and in a very large number of patients with chronic liver disease without jaundice. The test is not useful in the presence of jaundice, both by virtue of difficulty in estimation of the dye in the blood in the presence of increased amounts of bilirubin, and because, as a test of parenchymal cell function, the result is vitiated by the presence of biliary obstruction.

Tests of Biliary Excretion

These tests, though affected to some extent by parenchymal cell damage, are directly dependent upon the patency of the biliary channels. They are used primarily, therefore, in deciding questions regarding the patency of the biliary tree and in estimations of variations in the degree of obstruction present.

1. **Total Serum Bilirubin.** The serum bilirubin normally ranges from 0·2 to 0·8 mg. per 100 ml. serum. It is elevated in all forms of jaundice and provides an accurate measure of the depth of the jaundice, and a useful indication of the trend of the disease. Values above 2·0 mg. per 100 ml. coincide with visible

jaundice. In the majority of parenchymal liver diseases the serum bilirubin rises to a maximum then gradually subsides as the disease process recedes. Fixed high levels of serum bilirubin in combination with acholic stools imply complete biliary obstruction, and this occurs most commonly in malignant obstruction of the bile ducts. Fluctuating levels are found in 'surgical' jaundice due to obstruction by gall-stones.

Methods of estimating conjugated and unconjugated bilirubin separately are too complex for routine use. In practice their chemical distinction is of clinical value only in jaundice of the newborn in which the level of unconjugated bilirubin is the important factor in deciding on the need for exchange blood transfusion.

2. **Urinary Bilirubin.** In recent years a test has been devised using a tablet containing a stable diazo dye (Ictotest). This test is sensitive and is simple to perform. Bilirubin is present in the urine in cases of obstructive and hepatocellular jaundice, though in the latter it tends to vary inversely with urobilinogen. It is absent from the urine in haemolytic jaundice.

3. **Urinary Urobilinogen.** The simple qualitative test for urobilinogen in urine using Ehrlich's aldehyde reagent is an important procedure in all cases of liver disease and jaundice. In complete obstructive jaundice bilirubin does not enter the intestine, and therefore urobilinogen disappears from the urine. When there is no obstruction to the biliary channels, an increase in urobilinogen may occur (a) because a damaged liver is unable to excrete the normal amounts of urobilinogen presented to it (parenchymal liver disease), or (b) because a normal liver is unable to re-excrete adequately the excessive quantity of urobilinogen presented, as occurs when there is excessive haemolysis (e.g. congenital or acquired haemolytic anaemia). Accordingly, in the non-jaundiced patient the presence of an abnormal amount of urobilinogen in a single specimen of freshly voided urine is one of the most sensitive indications of liver damage, provided haemolytic disease (including pernicious anaemia) can be excluded. It occurs in the congestion of the liver associated with congestive heart failure. Serial tests in typical cases of hepatocellular jaundice reveal the presence of increased amounts of urobilinogen

in the early stages, and the absence of bile. As intrahepatic biliary obstruction becomes more severe and jaundice deepens, bilirubin increases in the urine and urobilinogen gradually disappears. Recovery is associated with relief of the obstruction to the canaliculi in the liver so that bile once more enters the intestine. As a result, bilirubin decreases in the urine and urobilinogen reappears.

Tests of Liver Cell Damage

The parenchymal cells of the liver contain certain enzymes in relatively large amounts. These may be released into the plasma when the cell is damaged and their measurement in the serum may be used as an estimate of liver cell damage. Of these the most important for clinical purposes are alanine aminotransferase (glutamic pyruvic transaminase GPT), and aspartate aminotransferase (glutamic oxalacetic transaminase GOT), only small amounts of which are present in normal plasma or serum. In patients suffering from acute parenchymal disease of the liver with or without jaundice, the activity of the enzymes rises in the blood above the upper limit of normal (35 units/ml.) and usually reaches values of several hundred units within the first few days. In patients with obstructive jaundice the activities of the enzymes are often slightly increased but seldom reach values of over 100 units. The determinations of serum GPT and GOT are of real value in helping to distinguish hepatocellular jaundice from obstructive jaundice and they are specially helpful in the early diagnosis of infective hepatitis. It should be noted that serum GOT but not serum GPT is elevated in cases of myocardial infarction. Lactate dehydrogenase (LD5) and isocitrate dehydrogenase (ICD) are other enzymes which are released into the plasma when liver cells are damaged. The two tests most commonly undertaken in Britain are for GPT and ICD and their estimation produces comparable information.

SUMMARY

These tests for the different types of hepatic disease provide an insight into hepatic function but they can be performed only when adequate laboratory and hospital facilities are available. In general practice, however, much information can be obtained from tests for urobilinogen and bile in the urine, and observations of the colour of the stools. In the non-jaundiced patient, urobilinogen is present in abnormal amounts in the urine of a high proportion of cases with diffuse parenchymal hepatic disease. Urobilinogen is absent from the urine if there is complete biliary obstruction, irrespective of its cause. It is present in abnormally large amounts in the urine in haemolytic jaundice, in which disease the stools are well coloured.

It is difficult to distinguish, by the use of these procedures, the jaundice due to extrahepatic obstruction from hepatocellular jaundice which is associated with severe intrahepatic cholestasis. It may sometimes be necessary in these cases to perform a laparotomy, in order to establish the cause of the jaundice.

The flocculation tests, performed in combination with serum alkaline phosphatase and transaminase determinations, are most useful in differentiating obstructive jaundice due to extrahepatic block and jaundice of hepatocellular origin. This is particularly true if the tests are performed early in the course of the disease.

In the absence of jaundice, the other tests of metabolic function are refinements for hospital practice, to be used in detecting or in following hepatic impairment.

PARENCHYMAL DISEASE OF THE LIVER

Parenchymal disease of the liver may be acute, subacute or chronic. In some cases, chronic parenchymal liver disease may be attributable to a previous episode of acute hepatic disease; in others the condition is insidious in onset and no frank history of acute liver disease can be elicited.

ACUTE PARENCHYMAL DISEASE OF THE LIVER

Acute parenchymal liver disease is the result of hepatic cell degeneration or necrosis. This is brought about largely by the action of infective or toxic agents. Idiosyncrasy, allergy and nutritional factors may also play a part.

Infections. Virus of acute infective hepatitis, of serum hepatitis and of yellow fever; leptospirosis; severe septicaemia, e.g. due to *Esch. coli* or pneumococci; severe cases of infectious mononucleosis; infection with *Entamoeba histolytica.*

Toxic substances. Carbon tetrachloride; ethylene glycol; methyl chloride; phosphorus; chloroform; halothane; dinitrophenol; tetrachlorethane; cinchophen; mepacrine; arsenic and antimony compounds; gold-containing compounds; ferrous sulphate; poisonous fungi (*Amanita phalloides*); sulphonamides; isoniazid; para-aminosalicylic acid; phenylbutazone; thiouracil; mono-amine oxidase inhibitors (e.g. iproniazid) pheniprazine, phenelzine and nialamide.

Of the infective and toxic agents mentioned above, infection with the virus of infective hepatitis and poisoning with carbon tetrachloride are the most common.

In addition, hepatic cell degeneration and necrosis may accompany hyperemesis gravidarum and eclampsia. The respective parts played by infective, toxic and nutritional factors in the aetiology of these two conditions are not known.

The severity of the illness following hepatic injury from any cause varies with a number of factors which include the nature and virulence of the infecting organism or the size of the dose of the toxic agent, and the resistance of the patient. The latter represents the reaction of the patient to hepatic insult and is determined by the existing nutritional state, the occurrence of previous liver damage and the resulting degree of hepatic reserve, individual idiosyncrasy, the age of the patient, heredity and perhaps other factors. In general, the susceptibility of the liver to toxic agents is increased when it is depleted of glycogen as a result of partial starvation. In addition, an adequate supply of protein has been shown to be necessary for the maintenance of the resistance of the liver to injury, and this seems to be related to the intake of the sulphur-containing amino acids, methionine and cystine.

Pathologically, the damage to the liver falls into two more or less clearly defined forms:

1. Acute zonal necrosis, in which necrosis occurs in the same zone of all the lobules of the liver, the central zone being most commonly affected.

2. Acute massive necrosis in which widespread necrosis affects entire hepatic lobules throughout large expanses of the liver, sometimes leaving other areas relatively unharmed.

Although these types of necrosis are to some extent determined by the severity of the disease, irrespective of the aetiological agent, certain agents typically tend to produce one or other of the patterns of necrosis. Acute infective hepatitis is, for example, a common cause of centrilobular necrosis. The other agents which tend to produce zonal necrosis include carbon tetrachloride, phosphorus, chloroform, arsenic and gold, and it occurs in hyperemesis gravidarum and eclampsia. Serum hepatitis which is caused by a virus similar to that of infective hepatitis, also produces zonal necrosis; this type of necrosis is found in some cases of yellow fever and leptospirosis (Weil's disease).

Massive necrosis of the liver is associated with a very much more severe clinical picture than is zonal necrosis and may occur as an exaggerated reaction to agents which usually produce zonal necrosis. Acute massive necrosis can be produced in animals by a diet deficient in selenium. The relatively high incidence of massive hepatic necrosis in tropical countries with poor standards of nutrition, and during pregnancy and lactation in Britain suggests that the human disease may also be due to direct or conditioned deficiency of animal protein or amino acids. Occurring in the course of infective hepatitis, it may be regarded as a complication of this nature. It has to be admitted, however, that apart from the few cases which are due to intoxication with such agents as cinchophen, mepacrine, tetrachlorethane and dinitrophenol, no satisfactory explanation can be found for the majority of cases of massive necrosis occurring in Britain.

The distinction between these types of necrosis, although not always clinically possible, is of importance because of the different clinical and pathological courses which they subsequently follow, i.e. zonal necrosis (p. 1008), massive necrosis (p. 1013); and post-necrotic scarring (p. 1028).

ACUTE INFECTIVE HEPATITIS

In its clinically recognisable form this common infectious disease is characterised by febrile jaundice, a long incubation period and a low mortality rate. It is due to a virus which may be spread by human faeces and which usually enters the body by the oral route. In some instances entry via the respiratory tract has been suggested, but limited experimental attempts to demonstrate this have failed to confirm this portal of entry. On rare occasions it may enter the body through infected blood as in the case of serum hepatitis.

Infective hepatitis may be contracted by direct personal contact either with cases incubating or suffering from the disease, or with apparently healthy carriers of the virus. In some epidemics water, milk and shell fish have been incriminated as vehicles of infection. The incubation period is 15-35 days. In peace-time children are most commonly affected, while in war-time the majority of the cases are young adults, and the disease is frequently epidemic.

Pathology. While the disease is systemic in distribution with some involvement of the gastrointestinal tract, heart, pancreas, spleen, etc., the main lesion is in the liver and consists of a zonal necrosis affecting the centrilobular cells; in the typical case the reticulum framework of the liver is not involved and the hepatic architecture is correspondingly not deranged. This permits, in the vast majority of cases, complete regeneration of liver lobules without distortion or fibrosis when recovery occurs. Swelling of the parenchymal cells, with associated inflammatory cell infiltration, results in compression of the small intrahepatic biliary ducts with dilatation of the intralobular canaliculi. Intrahepatic obstructive jaundice is thus superimposed upon hepatocellular jaundice. In some outbreaks hepatic cell necrosis may be slight and the main lesion consist of inflammation around the biliary canaliculi, giving rise to intrahepatic cholestasis.

Clinical Features. In the case of average severity, prodromal symptoms precede the development of jaundice by a period of from a few days to two weeks. They are the usual manifestations of an acute infectious disease, and include chills, headache and malaise. Gastrointestinal symptoms may be prominent: anorexia is a common and early complaint, and nausea, vomiting and diarrhoea may follow. A severe, non-colicky upper abdominal pain occurs as a result of stretching of the peritoneum over the liver as the organ enlarges. Physical signs are scanty in the initial stages; the liver is usually tender, though not readily palpable. Tender enlarged cervical lymph nodes are commonly found and splenomegaly may occur, particularly in children. Signs and symptoms of acute infection in the upper respiratory tract develop in some epidemics.

The appearance of bile in the urine and a yellow tint to the sclera heralds the onset of jaundice. As the element of obstruction to the biliary canaliculi develops, the jaundice deepens, the stools become paler and the urine darker, while the liver becomes more easily palpable. At this time the appetite often improves and gastrointestinal symptoms diminish in intensity. After a variable period of time, usually of weeks, the great majority of cases gradually recover, jaundice subsides and the liver enlargement regresses.

It is now recognised that in many patients the disease may run a milder non-icteric course. The condition may be asymptomatic and be suspected only because of biochemical evidence of hepatic dysfunction. In others there are short-lived vague gastrointestinal complaints associated with malaise.

Course and Prognosis. The vast majority of cases proceed to complete recovery within 3 to 6 weeks, the mortality in children and young adults being 0·2 per cent. A small number tend to relapse in late convalescence; this can sometimes be attributed to too early resumption of activity or neglect of advice about abstinence from alcohol. In these cases the symptoms and signs return and subsequently subside, with complete recovery. Occasionally a moderately severe attack of infective hepatitis may not be followed by subsidence of activity and healing of the liver. Serial biopsy studies may show a continuation of focal hepatic cell degeneration and inflammatory cell infiltration, with increasing fibrosis, over many months or years. There may be no symptoms until chronic hepatic insufficiency develops; occasionally recurrent symptoms and signs such as abdominal discomfort, intolerance to fat, bouts of jaundice and diarrhoea, pruritus, and persistent elevation of serum bilirubin, may persist to the stage at which hepatic cirrhosis is fully established. It is not known whether the development of chronic hepatitis is due to the persistence of the virus infection or the result of an auto-immune mechanism. Rarely the disease is fulminant and death ensues in the acute phase, often associated with renal failure. Such cases are commonly those in whom a superimposed nutritional factor increases the susceptibility of the liver cells to necrosis, e.g. as a conditioned deficiency in pregnant women, elderly patients, and alcoholics in Britain, or as a direct deficiency in persons taking a poor diet lacking in animal protein, as occurs commonly in Asia and Africa. Hormonal imbalance appears to affect the course of the disease and girls at menarche and women at the menopause are apparently more susceptible to hepatitis. The mortality in these groups may be as high as 50 per cent. Clinically, jaundice increases, and the features of acute massive liver necrosis may develop (p. 1013). Occasionally, in such cases, the patient survives the acute phase, only to develop at a later date the symptoms and signs of chronic hepatic insufficiency, due to post-necrotic scarring (p. 1028).

Laboratory Data. The urine contains excess urobilinogen in the initial stages of infective hepatitis before the appearance of visible jaundice. Urobilinogen increases in the urine as jaundice develops. If complete intrahepatic biliary obstruction occurs, urobilinogen temporarily disappears from the urine and bilirubin becomes detectable. A mild degree of proteinuria is usual. Serum bilirubin is elevated in most cases. Serum flocculation tests (p. 1000) are positive in over 90 per cent. of cases and are of great value in doubtful cases in which differential diagnosis from extrahepatic obstructive jaundice is difficult. Other tests of parenchymal function may show corresponding depression. Serum alkaline phosphatase rarely exceeds 30 King-Armstrong units/100 ml., but SGPT is elevated in the early stages of the disease to 100-2000 units/ml.; indeed estimation of SGPT is the best diagnostic test in the pre-icteric phase of the disease and is particularly helpful in screening contacts. The total white count is either normal or less than normal in the uncomplicated case, and there may be a relative lymphocytosis. This finding is of considerable diagnostic value and helps to distinguish the condition from Weil's disease (p. 1011).

Treatment. There is no specific therapy for acute infective hepatitis. Chemotherapeutic agents and antibiotics have been shown not to be effective. Infectivity is greatest in the early stages of the disease before jaundice has developed. Isolation is unnecessary, but the ordinary precautions for preventing spread of enteric infections should be adopted. Supportive therapy including suitable modifications to the diet, which should be applied to all types of acute parenchymal liver disease is discussed on p. 1017.

Differential Diagnosis is discussed on p. 1016.

SERUM HEPATITIS

A form of viral hepatitis has been shown to occur in a small proportion of patients receiving injections of human plasma, serum and blood, especially after transfusion with pooled dried human plasma, and measles, mumps or yellow fever inoculations. It has been noted also after intradermal, subcutaneous, intramuscular or intravenous injections or following venepuncture for the withdrawal of blood. Under these circumstances contamination of syringe or needle with the virus is responsible. The virus exists in the blood stream of certain individuals without producing frank disease, and is closely allied to the virus of infective hepatitis. The two diseases are indistinguishable pathologically, and the clinical courses are similar, though the incubation period of serum hepatitis is longer and ranges from 40-100 days and the mortality rate is higher.

An analysis of the records of about 1,500 patients with viral hepatitis admitted to hospitals in Boston, U.S.A., showed that the mortality rate for those with post-transfusion hepatitis was 12·5 per cent., in contrast to a mortality rate of 0·5 per cent. for patients with classical infective hepatitis. The majority of the post-transfusion cases of hepatitis belonged to an older age group than the patient with infective hepatitis and many had serious underlying illness which made blood transfusion necessary. In view of these differences between the two groups it does not follow that the virus causing serum hepatitis is necessarily more virulent than the virus causing infective hepatitis.

Treatment. There is no specific treatment for serum hepatitis at the present time. Supportive therapy is described on p. 1017. Precautions which may be taken to prevent the occurrence of the disease are discussed on p. 1051.

SPIROCHAETAL JAUNDICE (WEIL'S DISEASE)

This disease is caused by infection with *Leptospira icterohaemorrhagiae*. The spirochaete, harboured in rats and excreted in their urine, enters the human body through skin abrasions or the mucous membrane of the nasopharynx or the alimentary tract. The disease is mainly occupational, and is found in sewage and abattoir workers, miners, workers in rice and sugar-cane fields and fish workers; it may be contracted by bathing in canals.

Pathology. In some cases, foci of degeneration, including fatty change, are found in the liver. Separation of liver cells by oedema and inflammatory exudate leads to intralobular biliary stasis. In severe cases, centrilobular zonal degeneration may proceed to necrosis, and in fatal cases this becomes massive. Lesions in other organs also occur and may predominate; a combination of direct invasion of the kidney and hypotension from myocardial involvement may lead to acute renal failure.

Clinical Features. The incubation period is from 7-13 days. In cases of moderate severity, the disease begins abruptly with rise in temperature, muscular pain, anorexia, vomiting and prostration. Haemorrhage into the skin, from the nose, or fram the alimentary tract may be present: hae morrhagic herpes labilis is common. Hyperaemia of the conjunctivae is a striking feature. This febrile stage lasts for about five days. During the second stage (toxic or icteric stage) jaundice appears and prostration becomes more severe. The liver becomes palpable: generalised lymph node enlargement is unusual and splenic enlargement is rare. The cardiovascular system is affected and hypotension may develop; bradycardia, ectopic beats and other arrhythmias are common. Oliguria or anuria, uraemia, and the other features of acute renal failure are found in severe cases (p. 823). Direct infection of the meninges occurs in about 10 per cent. of cases and produces symptoms and signs of meningitis. During recovery the temperature falls by lysis; in some patients it rises again temporarily in association with recurrence of muscle pains. Relapses may occur. It should be noted that in mild cases clinical jaundice may never be present. The mortality varies from 5-20 per cent. in different countries.

Laboratory Data. The jaundice is hepatocellular in origin, with an obstructive element (intrahepatic) superimposed. Bilirubin and urobilinogen are present in the urine, and albumin, red blood cells, and cellular and granular casts are also found. The blood urea is elevated in severe cases. There is a polymorphonuclear leucocytosis. Tests of liver function give results which reveal parenchymal damage.

The diagnosis can be made by inoculating a guinea-pig with blood in the first week or with urine in the second and third weeks. Specific antibodies can be demonstrated in the serum from the second week of the disease and show a rising titre.

Specific Treatment. The giving of specific antileptospiral serum (20-40 ml. intravenously) during the first week of the illness is effective, but is rarely practicable because diagnosis is difficult before the onset of jaundice. *Leptospira icterohaemorrhagiae* is sensitive to benzylpenicillin *in vitro*, and in the guinea-pig, and on this account its use in doses of 500,000 units twice daily is advised in human cases of this infection. Its effect in reducing the mortality has been disappointing and this is probably due to the fact that the organisms being mainly intracellular, are only partially accessible to its action. In the event of acute renal failure with oliguria, the treatment described on p. 824 should be initiated. The protection of food from contamination by rats is important, and exposure of skin to water suspected of being the source of infection should be avoided.

Differential Diagnosis (p. 1016).

Canicola Fever

Infection with *Leptospira canicola* produces a disease similar to a mild form of Weil's disease, except that jaundice is much less common. *L. canicola* is harboured in dogs and very rarely in pigs, so that the disease tends to be a domestic rather than an occupational hazard. Infectivity is low and the disease usually affects one member of the household. Headache, stiffness of the neck, muscle tenderness and fever are common. Meningitis occurs in about 80 per cent. of cases, with a pleomorphic cell picture in the cerebrospinal fluid. Recovery is usually complete in one or two weeks. Diagnosis may be confirmed by guinea-pig inoculation with blood in the first week, or by a positive leptospiral agglutination test from the second week onwards. Antibiotic treatment is similar to that employed in Weil's disease.

ACUTE MASSIVE LIVER NECROSIS

(Acute Yellow Atrophy)

This rare condition, which is more common in women, is characterised by the acute onset of massive cell necrosis, shrinkage of the liver, deep jaundice, mental confusion, aminoaciduria, coma and usually death. It occurs rarely in the course of acute infective hepatitis and Weil's disease and is seen occasionally in pregnancy complicated by eclampsia. A few cases are due to intoxication with cinchophen, mepacrine, tetrachlorethane, phosphorus and dinitrophenol. In other cases no satisfactory explanation can be found for its occurrence.

Pathology. Histologically, the liver shows extensive parenchymal cell necrosis. Large expanses of liver tissue are affected, leaving other areas relatively unharmed: in the most severe cases, the whole hepatic parenchyma may become necrotic. The organ is enlarged in the initial phase; as the necrotic tissue is absorbed, the organ becomes correspondingly small. If recovery occurs, the normal architecture of the organ is destroyed: massive strands of fibrosis replace dead tissue, and this, with irregular regeneration of liver cells in other areas, eventually leaves the organ shrunken and coarsely nodular (post-necrotic scarring).

Clinical Features. General weakness, nausea, vomiting and complete anorexia occur at the outset. Pyrexia invariably develops later, even in the absence of infection. Pain in the right hypochondrium is common. Jaundice, hepatocellular in type, occurs rapidly, becomes very intense, and may fluctuate. The breath often has a characteristic and pungent odour, known as foetor hepaticus. This is probably due to the presence of methyl mercaptan, which has been shown to be excreted in the urine of such subjects. A generalised haemorrhagic tendency is common. Petechiae, ecchymoses, haematemesis, melaena and menorrhagia occur as a result of deficiency of coagulation factors and perhaps also abnormal fibrinolysis. On physical examination, the liver is enlarged in the first instance, but subsequent shrinkage of the organ is common and can be noted from day to day. The spleen is usually only slightly enlarged. Generalised oedema and ascites occur in some cases, as a result of a disturbance in water metabolism and of an alteration in plasma protein concentration.

Course and Prognosis. The majority of patients with acute massive necrosis enter a state of increasing mental confusion and mania which is followed by stupor and coma. Yawning and hiccoughing may be severe. There is evidence of central nervous system involvement, with extensor plantar reflexes, muscle spasticity and choreiform movements. A flapping tremor of the hands demonstrated by extending the patient's arms is characteristic but not specific to severe hepatic failure. Oliguria and a pronounced rise in temperature occur. Death takes place usually within a week, without convulsions. The mechanism of production of these symptoms and signs is not fully understood. They result from gross hepatic insufficiency and may be due to the entry into the systemic circulation of toxic nitrogenous substances absorbed from the intestine. An abnormally high concentration of ammonia in the arterial blood and cerebrospinal fluid is found in most cases but, although the level of arterial ammonia tends to parallel the severity of clinical illness, ammonia is not considered to be the cerebral intoxicant.

A few cases survive the acute attack only to die from further repeated episodes of acute necrosis. Others recover and eventually become symptom-free for a period. A nodular liver, frequently enlarged and palpable from extensive regenerative hyperplasia, remains as evidence of the previous attack. In the end, these patients develop the symptoms and signs of chronic parenchymal disease of the liver (p. 1024).

Laboratory Data. The severity of the jaundice is reflected in a serum bilirubin concentration usually higher than in jaundice from any other cause. The tests for hepatocellular damage are positive (pp. 999-1004). Cholesterol ester disappears from the blood. The derangement of protein metabolism is so severe that many amino acids accumulate in the blood and can be found in the urine by chromatographic methods. Abnormal amounts of tyrosine and leucine in the urine have been recognised as a feature of severe liver damage for many years; they tend to crystallise in the urine when present in high concentrations and can be recognised on microscopic examination of a centrifuged deposit of urine. The stools may contain occult or macroscopic blood. The volume of the urine is reduced and it contains bilirubin and urobilinogen; proteinuria is common. White blood cell counts vary from leucopenia to leucocytosis. Blood cultures, which should be undertaken frequently may reveal the existence of septicaemia.

Treatment. There is no specific therapy. Supportive treatment is discussed on p. 1017.

DIFFERENTIAL DIAGNOSIS OF ACUTE PARENCHYMAL DISEASE OF THE LIVER

The differential diagnosis of the various types of acute parenchymal disease is not difficult in the majority of cases. When a young person develops jaundice, preceded by gastrointestinal upset, and associated with pale stools and dark urine, it is presumptive evidence of infective hepatitis. A history of recent contact with a case of jaundice makes this diagnosis more certain. The preicteric phase of acute infective hepatitis may be confused with other acute infective diseases and in particular with infectious mononucleosis. In the latter condition there is enlargement of the lymph nodes and a typical blood picture. Later the Paul-Bunnell reaction becomes positive in high dilutions. There is increasing recognition that hepatitis and hepatic cell necrosis may accompany septicaemia, particularly with organisms such as *Esch. coli.* When this occurs the patient is profoundly ill and febrile and the diagnosis is confirmed by blood cultures. The hepatocellular jaundice of acute massive necrosis should be suspected if there is a history of exposure to a known hepatotoxic agent. In the absence of such a history, the severity of the illness, the depth of the jaundice, and the development of lethargy and coma suggest that massive necrosis has occurred.

Infective hepatitis must also be differentiated from Weil's disease. In a typical case of leptospirosis of moderate severity, the onset is abrupt and haemorrhages, e.g. epistaxes and petechiae, are common: these are rare in infective hepatitis. Weil's disease is associated with leucocytosis, and blood and casts are found in the urine, whereas in infective hepatitis leucopenia is common, and these abnormal urinary constituents are absent, in the uncomplicated case. The patient with Weil's disease is likely to give a history of occupational exposure to infection, and the diagnosis can be confirmed by appropriate bacteriological methods. Infective hepatitis is clinically indistinguishable from serum hepatitis. The history of receiving plasma or serum or having been subjected to subcutaneous or intramuscular injection or to venepuncture one to three months previously suggests the latter condition.

The most difficult problem in diagnosis is the differentiation between the jaundice of infective hepatitis and extrahepatic obstructive jaundice due to a 'silent' stone in the common bile duct or to obstruction of this duct by neoplasm, especially if the jaundice in infective hepatitis persists without marked improvement for more than three weeks. The distinction is made more difficult by the knowledge that in many patients with viral hepatitis the effect on the liver is predominantly due to intrahepatic stasis in bile ducts rather than to parenchymal cell necrosis. Fever may be present in both types of jaundice, in the one as a result of virus infection, and in the other as a result of ascending cholangitis (p. 1029). It is particularly important to make a correct diagnosis. since the operative interference which is indicated in extrahepatic obstructive jaundice may have serious effects in cases of infective hepatitis and other types of hepatocellular jaundice. Radiographs of the abdomen should be taken in every case. They are helpful when radio-opaque stones are seen in the gall-bladder or common bile duct and more rarely in showing calcification of the pancreas following pancreatitis. In the absence of these findings, repeated liver function tests (p. 999) become of great value. The initial determinations should be performed as early in the course of the jaundice as possible and the decision to operate should be determined largely by them when the clinical picture is equivocal. In obstructive jaundice the serum alkaline phosphatase is rarely less than 30 units and SGPT rarely more than 100 units/ml., while in jaundice due to hepatocellular disease alkaline phosphatase values tend to be less than 30 units, while SGPT values often reach several hundreds of units per millilitre. In those cases in which both the results of liver function tests and the clinical picture are indeterminate, liver biopsy, carried out by liver puncture under local anaesthesia or intravenous cholangiography often provide evidence upon which an accurate diagnosis may be based.

TREATMENT OF ACUTE PARENCHYMAL DISEASE OF THE LIVER

Apart from the specific therapy of Weil's disease to which reference has already been made, the treatment recommended is as follows:

1. *Bed Rest*. This is best imposed until evidence of activity has subsided. The appetite should have improved, enlarge-

ment and tenderness of the liver on palpation should have disappeared and normal colour should have returned to the stools before the patient is allowed up. For the average case of infective hepatitis this usually involves two to three weeks bed rest. Slight persistent jaundice (serum bilirubin $<1{\cdot}5$ mg. per 100 ml.) is not by itself an indication for continued confinement to bed. It will be impossible to adhere to these criteria in the few cases in whom activity of the disease process continues for months or years.

2. *Drugs.* Those which are known to be inactivated by the liver are best avoided, as are also potential hepatotoxic agents. The former include morphine and some barbiturates. Abstinence from alcohol should be advised for at least six months.

3. *Dietary Regime.*

(a) *In mild and moderately severe cases.* Recent work suggests that the best results are obtained by giving a diet of 3,000 calories from the onset of the disease and for several weeks after the acute symptoms have subsided. A similar diet is recommended for cirrhosis of the liver and the basis of its construction is given in Diet 7 (p. 1292). Owing to nausea and malaise many patients are unable to tolerate such a high calorie diet in the first few days of acute parenchymal disease. In these circumstances a light diet supplemented with carbohydrate in the form of fruit drinks and glucose will be found to be acceptable; the actual content of the diet should however be largely dictated by the patient's desires. The high calorie diet, rich in protein, however, should be given as soon as possible. In the great majority of cases complete recovery occurs within a few weeks and the patient may be allowed a normal diet. In the small proportion in whom the activity of the disease persists for months or years the diet should be continued.

(b) *In severe cases.* In a few cases of acute infective hepatitis and Weil's disease and in almost all cases of massive liver necrosis, the patient is seriously ill and is unable to ingest an adequate amount of food because of nausea or vomiting. The mentality is clouded or the patient may be in coma, and the neurological manifestations of severe parenchymal failure may be present (p. 1027). Hitherto such patients were often given methionine or choline orally or by injection or casein hydrolysate by stomach tube or intravenous infusion. These measures were adopted in an attempt to maintain a reasonable intake of essential amino acids and because of the beneficial effects of such dietary supplements observed in experimental liver disease in animals.

It is now established that such patients may be harmed by these supplements, which are capable of precipitating or aggravating mental confusion and hepatic coma (p. 1027). In the presence of such features nitrogen-containing foods and supplements, i.e. all proteins, should be prohibited. The best results are obtained by giving lactose or glucose by stomach tube or glucose or fructose by intravenous infusion. Recently there has been a tendency to replace glucose for intravenous infusion by fructose because this carbohydrate is believed to be more easily oxidised by the liver and is less prone to cause local venous thrombosis. A 10-20 per cent. solution of glucose or fructose may be delivered into a large peripheral vein through a polythene tube and up to 300 g. of sugar may be given in the course of the day. The amount of saline used as carrier for the glucose should be evaluated from day to day, taking into account the urinary output and the state of electrolyte balance. Parentrovite Forte, which is a high-potency mixture of B vitamins and ascorbic acid, is added to the fluid prior to its administration, or can be given by separate intravenous or intramuscular injection. Thiamine (20 mg./day) should be added to the fluid prior to its administration, and potassium salts (pot. chloride, 2 g. q.i.d.) may be given orally. Even in the absence of protein feeding the bacterial flora in the gut appear to contribute to the clinical picture, probably by producing toxic nitrogenous compounds. Because of this, oral neomycin, 1·0 g. six-hourly, is recommended, and evacuation of the colon by daily enema is advised initially. Excitement and restlessness during episodes of confusion are best controlled by intramuscular injections of sodium phenobarbitone or paraldehyde.

The value of corticosteroids and corticotrophin is still uncertain, but when a *severe* case of hepatitis shows deterioration despite the above measures, administration of large doses of either prednisone (60 mg.) or corticotrophin (120 units) is worthwhile. These measures may transform a case of severe hepatic failure into one who can tolerate food by mouth, and may dramatically improve the level of consciousness. Protein should then once more be included in the diet. It is advisable to start with no more than 25 g. per day, the amount being slowly increased to about 40 or 50 g. per day. It is generally found that patients who survive hepatic coma or who have had the neurological signs attributable to nitrogenous intoxication are unable to tolerate much more than 50 g. of protein in the day.

CHRONIC PARENCHYMAL DISEASE OF THE LIVER (CIRRHOSIS OF THE LIVER)

Cirrhosis of the liver is a generic term applied to chronic diffuse liver disease of multiple aetiology, characterised by destruction of parenchymal cells, distortion of the normal lobular architecture with nodular regeneration of the parenchymal cells and overgrowth of fibrous tissue. There are three basic pathological types of cirrhosis:

1. **Diffuse Hepatic Fibrosis** (Portal or Laennec's Cirrhosis). Diffuse hepatic fibrosis appears to occur as a sequel to two kinds of lesion: (a) infiltrative disease of the liver without previous necrosis, the most common example of which is fatty infiltration of the liver, and (b) zonal necrosis, following which fibrosis may rarely occur if complete restoration of tissue is prevented either by repeated episodes of necrosis, e.g. repeated attacks of infective hepatitis, or by chronic interference with cell nutrition or oxygenation, e.g. in malnutrition or chronic congestive heart failure. Every lobule is involved in the fibrosis, which begins around the central veins and the portal tracts. As a result of the diffuse regenerative hyperplasia, the organ becomes finely granular. Depending on the stage of the process and the degree of infiltration, the organ is increased, normal or diminished in size.

2. **Post-necrotic Scarring.** Post-necrotic scarring occurs in livers which have been the seat of massive hepatic necrosis. The collapse of the reticulum framework of the liver lobules which follows the removal of the dead cells in massive necrosis permits extensive development of fibrous tissue in wide bands throughout the liver. Areas of relatively normal hepatic tissue remain as islets, and from these grow new hepatic cells which do not assume the normal lobular arrangement, producing an organ which is grossly and irregularly nodular.

3. **Biliary Cirrhosis.** In the great majority of cases biliary cirrhosis occurs as a result of biliary obstruction and superimposed infection, i.e. cholangitis and cholangio-hepatitis. *Esch.*

coli and *Strep. viridans* are the most common infecting organisms. Distension of the bile canaliculi, proliferation of the bile ducts in the portal tracts and degeneration and inflammatory infiltration of the parenchyma around the portal tracts result in a diffuse fibrosis which is predominantly portal and periportal. Parenchymal cell regeneration is usually marked. The fibrosis spreads and classically surrounds single lobules or groups of lobules. Fibrosis around the central vein is less marked than in portal (Laennec's) cirrhosis. The term 'primary biliary cirrhosis' is used to describe a similar condition associated with chronic intrahepatic cholestasis of unknown origin which is seen predominantly in middle-aged women.

AETIOLOGICAL FACTORS IN THE PRODUCTION OF CHRONIC PARENCHYMAL DISEASE OF THE LIVER

1. **Diet.** There is much evidence to suggest that hepatic cirrhosis may result from dietetic deficiency. Experimental work on animals has clearly shown that cystine deficiency can lead to acute massive necrosis: dietetic deficiency may thus be implicated in the aetiology of post-necrotic scarring in human subjects. Diffuse fatty infiltration of the liver can be produced experimentally in animals by diets deficient in certain food constituents, which, by value of their power to remove neutral fat, are termed lipotropic substances. Part of the fat in the liver is phosphatide, and the formation of phosphatide from neutral fat, phosphoric acid and choline probably occurs solely in this organ. Choline is therefore essential, and its deficiency leads to an accumulation of neutral fat in the liver. Methionine is also a lipotropic agent and probably acts by virtue of possessing a labile methyl group needed in the synthesis of choline. Infiltration of the liver with fat may thus be regarded as a result of a deficiency of labile methyl groups. Whether directly as a result of fatty infiltration, or because of an associated metabolic defect, diffuse fibrosis occurs around both the central veins and portal tracts (portal or Laennec's cirrhosis).

2. **Alcohol.** Although acute alcoholic intoxication can produce parenchymal cell degeneration, it is doubtful if alcohol by itself produces cirrhosis of the liver. Many chronic alcoholics eat a diet deficient in protein and lipotropic food factors, and since their

caloric intake derived from alcohol is usually large, there results a disparity between the intake of calories and of essential food factors. This may result in fatty infiltration, which appears to be a precursor of diffuse hepatic fibrosis. A contributory factor to fibrosis in some cases may be the iron which is laid down in the parenchymal cells of the liver due to the increased absorption of iron from the alimentary tract which occurs in the presence of alcohol and to the high iron content of many alcoholic beverages. A history of chronic alcoholism was formerly almost invariably present in cases of diffuse hepatic fibrosis occurring in Britain. While this association is still frequently encountered in the United States of America, it is now a less common feature of the disease in this country.

3. **Hepatic Infection and Auto-immunity.** Acute infective hepatitis and serum hepatitis are the most common infective diseases of the liver in Great Britain, and are usually followed by complete recovery. About one-third of the cases of cirrhosis, however, give a history of previous episodes of jaundice which was apparently neither obstructive nor haemolytic. In severe cases of infective hepatitis characterised by massive necrosis in which death does not occur, post-necrotic scarring is inevitable. Diffuse hepatic fibrosis (portal or Laennec's cirrhosis) appears also to follow infective hepatitis; it is possible that repeated attacks of zonal necrosis are necessary for this development to take place. The demonstration that a small number of patients with chronic relapsing hepatitis who develop hepatic fibrosis possess some of the features associated with auto-immune disease has led to the suggestion that immune mechanisms may play a part in sustaining the hepatic damage in chronic liver disease. Such patients exhibit liver infiltration with lymphocytes and plasma cells, hyper globulinaemia, occasionally positive L.E. tests and other immunological disturbances such as positive tests for rheumatoid factor, positive Coombs' test and false positive Wassermann reaction. They sometimes show a dramatic response to corticosteroid therapy. Although this is an attractive theory the concept that auto-immunity plays any part in the pathogenesis of chronic hepatitis and hepatic cirrhosis requires more proof before it is accepted.

4. **Obstruction of the Bile Ducts.** Long-standing obstruction of the bile ducts, associated with an ascending cholangitis, usually

leads to biliary cirrhosis. In most cases obstruction is extrahepatic in situation, e.g. stone in the common bile duct. This is followed by an ascending infection of the biliary tree which results in a variable degree of intrahepatic inflammatory biliary obstruction. Such cholangio-hepatitis may lead to the development of biliary cirrhosis even if the extrahepatic obstruction is removed. Rarely biliary cirrhosis may develop from cholangio-hepatitis which has arisen in the absence of extrahepatic biliary obstruction. In some of these cases the infection may start *de novo*, while in others it may be initiated by obstruction to the intrahepatic biliary tree, e.g. by stones, duct tumours or xanthomatous deposits.

5. **Chronic Congestive Cardiac Failure.** Diffuse hepatic fibrosis following centrilobular degeneration and necrosis occurs occasionally as a result of long-standing congestive heart failure. It is most frequently associated with mitral stenosis, tricuspid incompetence or chronic constrictive pericarditis.

6. **Hepatic Infiltrations.** Substances infiltrating the hepatic parenchymal or connective tissue have been shown to be associated with diffuse hepatic fibrosis. Fatty infiltration has already been discussed in relation to dietary deficiency of labile methyl groups (e.g. methionine). Fatty infiltration is found commonly also in diabetic subjects, and the liver may be palpably enlarged as a result. Excessive glycogen infiltration occurring in children from birth in von Gierke's disease leads to diffuse fibrosis. Gaucher's disease, Niemann-Pick disease and xanthomatosis also produce hepatomegaly, due to infiltration of the reticulo-endothelial cells in the liver by kerasin, sphingomyelin and cholesterol respectively: diffuse fibrosis occurs as a result. Amyloid disease, which involves the walls of the sinusoids, occasionally results in diffuse hepatic fibrosis. Wilson's disease (p. 1191), in which there is an abnormal accumulation of copper in the liver, is associated with hepatic fibrosis. Haemochromatosis is a condition in which iron is absorbed in large amounts from the alimentary tract and deposited in excessive amounts, both in the liver parenchyma and in the cells of the reticulo-endothelial system. In the liver, cell degeneration and diffuse fibrosis develop (p. 1035).

Finally, it should be stated that in many cases of cirrhosis of the liver all investigations fail to reveal any aetiological factor.

CLINICAL FEATURES OF DIFFUSE HEPATIC FIBROSIS (PORTAL OR LAENNEC'S CIRRHOSIS)

Cirrhosis of the liver is more common in men than in women. It may be entirely latent during life and discovered only at post-mortem examination. In some cases, the incidental finding of a firm palpable liver may be the first indication of the disease. The hepatomegaly which is common in the early stages of cirrhosis, results from fatty infiltration or parenchymal hyperplasia. The organ has a smooth edge, and is not tender. Later, with increased fibrosis and parenchymal destruction, the liver shrinks and becomes smaller than normal. The main clinical features of the condition are attributable to portal hypertension, hepatic insufficiency, or a combination of both.

Portal Hypertension. Elevation of hydrostatic pressure in the portal system occurs as a result of partial obstruction to the flow of portal venous blood through the liver, and this is probably due to fibrosis, which decreases the vascular bed and distorts the vascular tree, and to transmission of hepatic arterial pressure to the portal venous system. As a consequence of portal hypertension, there develop features related to the gastrointestinal tract, haemopoietic system, spleen, portal vascular tree and abdominal cavity.

Vague digestive complaints are frequent in the initial stages of the disease and result from congestion of the gastrointestinal tract. They include flatulence, nausea, anorexia and vomiting, especially in the morning. Later, pain in the right hypochondrium occurs, usually after meals. Abdominal distension is common and is due to impaired intestinal gaseous absorption and to ascites. Anorexia aggravates the poor nutritional state usually already present. In those with an alcoholic history, polyneuritis, rough skin and smooth tongue are not infrequently present.

Splenomegaly is a primary result of portal hypertension. In addition to the factor of congestion, hyperplasia of the reticulo-endothelial cells of the spleen occurs as a direct consequence of hepatic damage. The mechanism of this is uncertain. The organ is usually hard, but only moderately enlarged except in children in whom it may be considerably increased in size.

Evidence of the presence of *collateral circulation* appears wherever there is communication between portal and systemic veins. These sites are at the lower end of the oesophagus and the upper end of the stomach, the anus and lower rectum, at the normally obliterated embryological circulation through the falciform ligament, and between colon, omentum and spleen and the retroperitoneal veins. Oesophageal and gastric varices are common and their rupture, producing haematemesis, may be fatal. A haematemesis may be the first sign in a hitherto unsuspected case of hepatic cirrhosis. The demonstration of the presence of oesophageal varices from the mucosal pattern following a barium swallow or by carefully performed oesophagoscopy is a valuable means of substantiating the diagnosis of hepatic cirrhosis or detecting the cause of unexplained melaena, occult blood in the stools, frank haematemesis or splenomegaly. Haemorrhoids developing in a middle-aged person for no obvious reason, or the appearance of large veins in the abdominal wall and around the umbilicus, should arouse suspicion that cirrhosis of the liver is present.

The injection of a radio-opaque substance into the spleen (transcutaneous splenovenography) may be used in selected patients to demonstrate the extent of collateral venous channels and to determine the patency of the splenic and portal veins.

Anaemia, hypochromic and microcytic, or, more rarely, normochromic and macrocytic, occurs. The former is usually due to blood loss. The latter is very rarely associated with a megaloblastic reaction in the marrow, which may be due to associated nutritional folic acid deficiency or to lack of intrinsic factor from gastritis and consequent malabsorption of vitamin B_{12}. An associated moderate thrombocytopenia and leucopenia may be present, and these are generally attributed to concomitant hypersplenism (p. 659).

Ascites is commonly, though not invariably present, in cases of hepatic cirrhosis. It is usually associated with, but is out of proportion to ankle and lower limb oedema. There are probably several factors responsible for water and salt retention and ascites in hepatic disease. Possible mechanisms which have been suggested include (1) a lowering of the osmotic pressure of the plasma as a result of failure of the liver to synthesise albumin; (2) portal hypertension and lymphatic obstruction produced by the fibrosis in the liver substance which may be responsible for the localisation of most of the retained fluid in the peritoneal cavity; (3) failure on the part of the liver to inactivate aldosterone and vasopressin. These lead to excessive reabsorption of salt and water in the tubules of the kidney; and (4) a lowering of the glomerular filtration rate, which is probably responsible for excessive tubular reabsorption of salt and other electrolytes.

Hepatic Insufficiency. The principal clinical features of hepatic insufficiency are the following:

Clinical Jaundice. This is rarely severe and is present in only a minority of cases, usually in the terminal stages of the disease. It occurs as a result of parenchymal cell damage (hepatocellular jaundice) and intrahepatic obstruction to bile canaliculi. In cirrhosis associated with alcoholism recurrent bouts of superimposed acute toxic hepatitis cause phases of jaundice mainly as a result of interference with bilirubin transport and conjugation in the liver.

Oedema. This is probably the result of a fall in plasma osmotic pressure and of the hormonal factors discussed above, and is to be regarded as evidence of hepatic failure.

Spider angiomata, capillary dilatations in the skin (telangiectases) flushing of the palms and *gynaecomastia.* These features are frequently seen, and are believed to be produced by an excess of circulating oestrogens, which probably results from the failure of the damaged liver to inactivate them. The spider angiomata occur predominantly on the forehead, neck, forearms and hands. In the male these compounds may occasionally produce hypogonadism, i.e. female distribution of hair, gynaecomastia and testicular atrophy.

Cyanosis, hyperdynamic circulation and finger clubbing. These features are seen in a few patients. The most likely explanation is veno-arterial shunting of blood in multiple pleural and intrapulmonary telangiectases.

A generalised haemorrhagic tendency. This occurs only in advanced cirrhosis of the liver and is largely due to prothrombin, factor VII and factor IX deficiency. Thrombocytopenia due to hypersplenism, if marked, is a contributory factor. Epistaxis, purpura, menorrhagia or melaena may develop.

Generalised pigmentation of the skin. This is due mainly to increased deposition of melanin in the skin, and occurs in a minority of cases. It may be related to a disturbance of amino acid (tyrosine) metabolism.

Hepatic encephalopathy (*portal-systemic encephalopathy*). The severe mental changes progressing to coma and the neurological features which have been described in relation to acute massive necrosis (p. 1013) occur also in patients suffering from hepatic cirrhosis. However, these features usually tend to be more chronic and intermittent. In addition to the factor of severe parenchymal cell failure, it seems likely that the presence of collateral venous circulation by-passing the liver permits certain nitrogenous compounds absorbed from the intestine to enter the systemic circulation directly and so produce the abnormal behaviour and the neurological features. The condition is easily precipitated in a susceptible patient by the giving of nitrogen-containing food and drugs; it tends to improve if the bowel is emptied or sterilised. Neuropsychiatric complications may overshadow the associated liver disease. This may lead to the patient's being admitted to a mental institution because of the incorrect diagnosis of primary mental disorder. If the anastomotic channels are extensive these features may occur even in the presence of relatively good hepatic cell function and in the absence of jaundice. This is a particularly unfortunate but not uncommon sequel to the operation of portacaval anastomosis.

Apart from the role of nitrogen in the production of encephalopathy, it may also follow gastrointestinal bleeding, infection or hypokalaemia. After bleeding the resultant anaemia and hypotension may cause further liver damage, and the blood reaching the colon provides a protein substrate for bacterial action.

Dupuytren's contracture of the hand is occasionally seen in hepatic cirrhosis in which alcoholism is a prominent feature of the history. The cause is unknown.

Course and Prognosis. In the absence of haematemesis or melaena the prognosis of cirrhosis of the liver depends upon the degree of hepatic damage and upon the intensity with which modern treatment is applied (p. 1032). Some patients may realise their full life expectancy and it is no longer correct to accept a relentless downhill course as inevitable. Bad prognostic signs are those of gross hepatic insufficiency and severe portal hypertension, leading to repeated haematemeses. Death occurs from bleeding varices in about 20 per cent. of cases. Intercurrent infection (lobar pneumonia, bronchopneumonia, peritonitis, septicaemia) is a common terminal event, and death in hepatic coma from severe hepatic insufficiency accounts for a further group of fatal cases. There is also an increased incidence of hepatoma in subjects with cirrhosis.

Laboratory Data. The concentration of plasma albumin is reduced, though it may return to normal values in some cases, following treatment. A rise occurs in plasma globulin concentration, so that the total protein concentration may be little altered. Tests for impaired parenchymal cell functions (p. 999) are positive in the majority of cases. The tendency to bleed is little affected by vitamin K administration. SGPT is commonly slightly elevated to 100 units/ml. Serum alkaline phosphatase concentration is usually increased to 20 or 30 units per 100 ml. In those patients who show no disturbance of liver function in routine tests, estimation of bromsuphthalein excretion is valuable since this is usually impaired.

In contradistinction to these positive findings of abnormal parenchymal cell metabolism, tests of bile pigment excretion are minimally affected. Serum bilirubin is usually only slightly increased and, except in advanced cases, there is no bilirubin in the urine, though urobilinogen is almost invariably present. The stools are not pale and contain normal amounts of stercobilinogen.

The ascitic fluid is usually clear, with a protein content characteristic of a transudate, i.e. about 1 g. per 100 ml.

Differential Diagnosis and Treatment. See pp. 1030 and 1032 respectively.

CLINICAL FEATURES OF POST-NECROTIC SCARRING

Post-necrotic scarring is less common than diffuse hepatic fibrosis. In the vast majority of cases it is a sequel to a previous recognisable attack of acute massive necrosis of the liver. In these cases, a history of jaundice is invariable, and one of repeated episodes of jaundice over the preceding years is frequent. In a minority of cases of post-necrotic scarring, there is no history of a previous attack of acute liver damage with jaundice. It is possible that in these cases the necrosis is less acute, and takes place over a longer period of time than in the more common type of case. The liver is enlarged early in the disease, and in some cases the edge is grossly irregular and feels similar to that in metastatic hepatic neoplasm. The clinical features and laboratory evidence of hepatic insufficiency are similar to those found in diffuse hepatic fibrosis (portal cirrhosis), but they occur earlier in the course of the disease. Accordingly the differential diagnosis from portal cirrhosis may be difficult and from a therapeutic point of view is of little importance. The disease is, however, more common in women and a history of alcoholism is usually not present. The tendency to early development of liver insufficiency makes the prognosis of post-necrotic scarring poorer than that of portal cirrhosis.

CLINICAL FEATURES OF CHOLANGIO-HEPATITIS AND BILIARY CIRRHOSIS

Biliary cirrhosis, which is more common in women than in men, usually begins with a phase of extra- or intrahepatic obstructive jaundice, which may or may not be associated with pain, depending on the nature of the obstruction (p. 996). The obstruction may be partial or complete and this accordingly determines the degree of jaundice, which may even be absent. Usually the stools are pale, and the urine dark from the presence of bilirubin. The liver is uniformly enlarged and smooth, and the spleen is not usually palpable. Flatulence and nausea may be present, and pruritus may be severe. The concomitant infection, in the form of cholangitis and cholangiohepatitis, manifests itself by the presence of the following features. Fever is usual but not invariable. It may be recurrent over many weeks or months. Hepatic enlargement may increase with febrile episodes, and be associated with upper abdominal pain. Jaundice fluctuates and becomes more intense as fever increases. With these febrile episodes and deepening jaundice, anorexia, flatulence and vomiting increase. In severe cases, rigors, prostration and a hectic temperature, similar to that of septicaemia, occur. Indeed in a few patients positive blood cultures can be obtained. A polymorphonuclear leucocytosis is frequently present, but severe infection can occur with leucopenia. Finger clubbing is common and xanthomata may eventually appear in the skin. Bone pain develops due to infiltration by fat-laden macrophages.

Biliary cirrhosis becomes established after months or years of such chronic infection and obstruction. Ascites and the signs and symptoms of portal hypertension are much less common than in either portal cirrhosis or post-necrotic scarring and, in fact, may be absent throughout the whole course of the disease. In the early stages, the clinical picture of obstructive biliary cirrhosis may be similar to that of post-necrotic scarring with jaundice. In the later stages due to the absence of bile salts from the small bowel features of malabsorption and steatorrhoea dominate the clinical picture.

Laboratory Data. In keeping with the pathogenesis of the disease, laboratory investigations usually reveal the features of obstructive jaundice in the early stages (p. 1001). This is true even when the obstruction is not found in the extrahepatic passages, but is intrahepatic in situation. Later in the course of the disease, especially if the obstruction is not relieved, or if chronic infection persists in the liver, tests of parenchymal function are abnormal (p. 1000). Total blood cholesterol is increased.

Course and Prognosis. Biliary cirrhosis may be prevented in patients in whom prompt surgical removal of the obstruction to the biliary passages is possible. If this is not done, or if the obstruction is intrahepatic, continuing liver damage is inevitable and the patient will probably survive for not more than four or five years. Jaundice is a prominent feature over this period and death usually occurs from hepatic insufficiency or more rarely from the bleeding of varices due to secondary portal hypertension.

DIFFERENTIAL DIAGNOSIS OF CIRRHOSIS OF THE LIVER

(Diffuse Hepatic Fibrosis, Post-Necrotic Scarring and Biliary Cirrhosis)

The differential diagnosis includes consideration of other causes of chronic dyspepsia (p. 903) and haematemesis (p. 909). When enlargement of the liver is present, the following should be considered:

1. Congestive heart failure (p. 169). The liver is large and smooth, frequently tender, and less hard than the cirrhotic liver. Other symptoms and signs of heart failure are present. Oedema of the lower limbs is usually in proportion to the degree of ascites

and as in cirrhosis of the liver the ascitic fluid protein concentration is that of a transudate. Cardiac cirrhosis may be suspected if congestive heart failure has been of long standing and the liver is hard on palpation or exhibits pulsation as in tricuspid incompetence.

2. Secondary carcinoma of the liver (p. 1038). The spleen is not enlarged and a few large nodules may be felt along the edge of the liver. The primary tumour, e.g. carcinoma of bronchus, may give rise to symptoms and its discovery indicates the cause of the hepatomegaly. Peritoneal involvement produces ascites in which the ascitic fluid contains a relatively high concentration of protein, i.e. 3-5 g. per 100 ml., and may be haemorrhagic. Tumour cells may be seen in the fluid.

3. Rarer causes of enlargement of the liver in Britain are Hodgkin's disease, leukaemia, amyloid disease, sarcoidosis, amoebic abscess and hydatid cysts. In tropical countries hepatic enlargement is frequently associated with kala azar, malaria and schistosomiasis.

4. Primary carcinoma of the liver (p. 1037). Its incidence varies greatly in different parts of the world; it is a rare tumour in Britain but it is one of the most common forms of malignant disease in the South African Bantu. It usually occurs in association with hepatic cirrhosis. Under these circumstances the diagnosis is difficult but should be suspected if the liver rapidly enlarges and if there is a sudden deterioration in the patient's condition which is otherwise unexplained. Jaundice is more frequent than in uncomplicated portal cirrhosis and fever is common.

Differentiation of portal cirrhosis and post-necrotic scarring from other types of cirrhosis of the liver is generally not difficult. Biliary cirrhosis is usually associated with the features of obstructive jaundice or there is a history of such an episode. Fever may be present in the initial phases, and a history of intermittent jaundice, cholecystitis or biliary colic is common. The enlargement of the liver is progressive, while ascites and haematemeses are uncommon until the disease is far advanced. The cirrhosis of haemochromatosis, of other infiltrations of the liver and of hepato-lenticular degeneration is characterised by the other features of these diseases. Other causes of hepatomegaly, e.g. blood diseases, reticuloses and infections, must be excluded by appropriate methods.

If a consideration of the clinical features and laboratory tests fails to establish the diagnosis in a case of hepatomegaly, it may be necessary to obtain a biopsy specimen either at laparotomy or by liver puncture. In selected cases the latter procedure has proved itself to be of great value.

TREATMENT OF CIRRHOSIS OF THE LIVER

Diffuse Hepatic Fibrosis and Post-necrotic Scarring. There is no doubt that adequate medical treatment can influence the prognosis of cirrhosis of the liver by favouring hyperplasia of the parenchymal cells, by preventing further progression of the fibrosis, by increasing the hepatic reserve and by inhibiting the development of fluid retention and encephalopathy. This is especially so in cases of diffuse hepatic fibrosis. Medical measures do not influence established portal hypertension, so that resultant haematemesis cannot be prevented by such means.

Bed rest is not necessary in the average case, but is indicated in the presence of gross hepatic insufficiency or of massive ascites, and following a haematemesis.

Diet. It is generally agreed that dietary deficiency plays a part in the genesis of some cases of hepatic cirrhosis. As a result, a high calorie diet (approximately 3,000 calories per day) which is rich in protein (120 g.), and which contains approximately 400 g. carbohydrate, is recommended (Diet 7, p. 1292). If jaundice is absent a fat intake of 100 g. per day can be given to most cases of cirrhosis of the liver, provided the fat is obtained mainly from milk, butter and cheese. Such patients usually have little difficulty in digesting milk fats in moderate quantities. Positive nitrogen balance may be obtained by these diets and improvement in hepatic function may be shown over periods of months, by an increasing albumin concentration in the blood and by other liver function tests. When oedema or ascites is present it may be desirable to replace 20-40 g. of protein in the diet by Casilan, given in water or milk. This preparation of milk protein is particularly useful because it is nearly salt-free and facilitates the provision of a high protein diet low in salt, (Diet 8, p. 1293). The danger of a high protein diet precipitating hepatic encephalopathy is discussed on page 1015. Alcoholic drinks should be forbidden.

Other dietary supplements which have been used, and for which there is theoretical justification, include yeast, thiamine (aneurin), nicotinamide, riboflavin, choline and the sulphur-containing amino acids, methionine and cystine. A moderate intake of thiamine (aneurin), nicotinamide and riboflavin is ensured by the protein-rich diet recommended above. Nevertheless additional daily supplements should be given orally, yeast ¼-½ oz., thiamine 5 mg., nicotinamide 50 mg. and riboflavin 5 mg. per day representing adequate amounts. Theoretically, methionine and choline are most likely to be effective in the stage of fat infiltration, prior to the development of marked diffuse fibrosis. This is especially so if there is a definite history of prolonged dietary insufficiency due to poverty, ignorance or a large intake of calories in the form of alcohol. In practice, methionine and choline are rarely prescribed in this condition because of their expense and because there is reason to believe that the body can be supplied with adequate amounts of these substances if a high protein diet containing ample quantities of milk is taken.

Ascites and oedema may respond to the improvement in hepatic function brought about by the above measures. As a first step the patient may be allowed salt in cooking but be forbidden soups, ham, bacon and salt at the table. This will reduce his intake to about 2 g. of sodium per day. If further salt restriction is necessary a special 0·5 g. sodium diet should be prescribed (Diet 8, p. 1293). Frusemide, ethacrynic acid and thiodiazine diuretics are all effective but should be used with care, since they frequently aggravate or precipitate hepatic encephalopathy. It is particularly important to prevent the development of hypokalaemia by using potassium supplements (p. 847). A specific aldosterone antagonist, spironolactone (Aldactone-A), may be given in addition in a dose of 25 mg. four times per day. A small number of patients with ascites and oedema are found to be resistant to all the therapeutic measures discussed above. For such cases the intravenous administration of salt-poor albumin preparations (25 g.) given in 5 per cent. dextrose solution and repeated daily for some days is often helpful. Abdominal paracentesis is nowadays rarely necessary. Occasionally diuresis may be promoted by osmolar loading with an intravenous infusion of mannitol.

In the small proportion of cases in which the mentality becomes clouded and abnormal neurological features develop, the treatment recommended on page 1019 should be given.

Blood transfusion is necessary when haematemesis or melaena is sufficiently severe to produce a state of clinical shock or significant anaemia. If bleeding continues the patient should receive 20 units of vasopressin in 100 ml. dextrose over a period of 10 minutes; this acts by reducing portal venous pressure consequent on mesenteric vasoconstriction. The procedure may be repeated every two hours. Should haematemesis still persist then bleeding may be controlled by using a Sengstaken tube. This tube possesses two balloons which when inflated exert pressure both in the fundus of the stomach and in the lower part of the oesophagus.

Surgical treatment offers the only hope of reducing portal hypertension. As the block is in the liver, splenectomy alone will fail to relieve the hypertension. For this purpose the blood must be shunted from the portal to the systemic circulation by anastomosing the splenic vein after splenectomy to the left renal vein, or the portal vein to the inferior vena cava. The latter procedure is more effective. It has also been suggested that haemorrhage may be prevented by resecting the area of varices at the lower end of the oesophagus and the upper end of the stomach. Such surgical procedures are difficult to perform and carry a considerable risk to life. These major operations are indicated when the risk of death from haemorrhage is greater than the risk of death from liver failure. In such cases encouraging results have been reported. They should not be undertaken if hepatic cell function is very severely diminished or if ascites cannot be controlled by medical measures.

Biliary Cirrhosis and Cholangio-hepatitis. Biliary cirrhosis can be prevented in a proportion of cases by prompt surgical treatment of obstructive jaundice. Laparotomy should be carried out in all cases with features of obstructive jaundice if the jaundice does not subside within a few weeks, unless there is good reason to believe that the patient has acute parenchymal disease of the liver with superimposed intrahepatic obstruction. The exclusion of the latter is frequently difficult and is discussed on p. 1016. When no obstruction to the extrahepatic bile ducts is found at operation, treatment is unsatisfactory and largely symptomatic. Cholangio-hepatitis is an infection which is difficult to control; antibiotics should be reserved for acute exacerbations of fever. Sometimes the organisms responsible may be isolated by blood culture, in which case sensitivity tests will indicate the appropriate antibiotic. If it is not possible to isolate the causative organism the recommendations given on p. 1043 should be followed. Recurrent attacks of fever may be prevented by long term use of a suppressive dose of ampicillin. Jaundice is usually severe, and antihistamine drugs (e.g. mepyramine maleate and promethazine hydrochloride) may help to alleviate the pruritus. Alternatively methyltestosterone (25 mg. sublingually) or norethandrolone (10 mg. t.i.d.) can be used. A new approach to this serious problem is the use of an oral ion exchange resin, cholestyramine, which adsorbs bile salts. The principles of dietetic therapy recommended for portal cirrhosis should be followed, with the qualification that fat is usually less well tolerated (Diet 6, p. 1290). If jaundice persists for months or years, fat soluble vitamins should be given parenterally, as they may not be absorbed from the intestine. Monthly intramuscular injections of 10 mg. vitamin K (Synkavit), and 300,000 units of vitamin D given every three months are usually adequate. A water soluble form of vitamin A should be given by mouth. Sodium glycocholate and taurocholate (0·1-0·5 g.) or dehydrocholic acid (Dehydrocholin, 0·25 g. tabs.) may be given three times a day to relieve dyspepsia associated with steatorrhoea. Calcium supplements are also essential and may be given in the form of skimmed milk and calcium effervescent tablets, 4 tablets three times a day.

OTHER MISCELLANEOUS DISEASES INVOLVING HEPATIC FIBROSIS

1. **Haemochromatosis.** (Pigment Cirrhosis: Bronzed Diabetes.) This is an uncommon disease which usually affects males over 45 years of age. There is dispute about its aetiology. In some families the condition appears to be inherited as an autosomal dominant with impaired penetrance (p. 112). When no genetic predisposition is evident there is often a history of excessive alcohol intake. For unknown reasons excessive absorption of iron in the intestinal tract occurs over many years. The deposition of this iron in the tissues appears to be responsible for most of the features of the condition. Pathologically, the findings include the distribution of iron-containing pigment (haemosiderin) throughout many organs in the body, but particularly the liver, heart and pancreas. Possibly as a result of direct mechanical destruction of

parenchymal cells, diffuse hepatic fibrosis occurs. The clinical features include those of hepatic cirrhosis, and the symptoms and signs of diabetes mellitus are also present as a result of pancreatic fibrosis, and frequently constitute the presenting complaint. A leaden-grey colour of the skin is characteristic, and is due to deposition of iron pigment and excess melanin. The diagnosis may be confirmed by a liver biopsy, in which iron can be demonstrated histochemically and by the finding of an elevated serum iron level and complete or nearly complete saturation of the serum iron binding capacity. Haemochromatosis must be distinguished from haemosiderosis which may result from repeated blood transfusions or from excessive administration of iron parenterally; tissue siderosis induced in this way is seldom accompanied by cell damage or fibrosis. Treatment involves a combination of therapies for hepatic cirrhosis (p. 1032) and for diabetes mellitus (p. 750). The body stores of iron should be reduced by repeated withdrawal of blood. Approximately 500 ml. (which contains about 225 mg. of iron) should be removed once weekly until the serum iron level falls to 100-150 μg./100 ml. and thereafter venesection should be done at suitable intervals in order to keep the serum iron in this range.

2. **Hepato-lenticular Degeneration (Wilson's Disease).** This is a very rare familial disease transmitted by autosomal recessive inheritance (p. 112) in which hepatic fibrosis appears to be secondary to the deposition of large amounts of copper in the liver parenchyma. The copper-containing protein (caeruloplasmin) normally present in the blood is reduced in amount and there is an associated excessive absorption of copper from the intestine. The condition develops mainly in young adults and children. While in most cases neurological symptoms consisting of tremor, rigidity, dysarthria and a facies similar to that found in Parkinsonism (p. 1188) dominate the picture, a few show features which are hepatic in origin, including ascites, evidence of abnormal collateral circulations, jaundice, and hepatomegaly. Diagnosis is made from the familial nature of the disease, the presence of Kayser-Fleischer rings, which consist of greenish deposits at the margin of the cornea seen best on slit lamp illumination, and the associated neurological features. It is confirmed by the demonstration of reduced amounts of serum caeruloplasmin and by the

presence of increased urinary copper. The excretion of copper in the urine can be increased by the administration of chelating agents, particularly penicillamine, a compound related to penicillin. Penicillamine is the drug of choice because it is the most powerful agent for this purpose and can be given by mouth. In some cases of hepatolenticular degeneration striking clinical improvement follows its use (p. 1193).

3. **Syphilitic Cirrhosis.** Congenital and acquired syphilis are rare causes of fibrosis of the liver. The former is associated with other stigmata of congenital syphilis, and the liver is enlarged as a result of intralobular and interlobular fibrosis. In acquired syphilis hepatic involvement is rare, but when it occurs the lesions present are usually gummata, which undergo fibrosis and scarring; the liver may be considerably enlarged.

4. **Schistosomiasis (Bilharziasis).** Infection with *Schistosoma mansoni* or *japonicum* is an important factor in causing hepatic fibrosis in countries where bilharziasis is endemic. Malnutrition is usually present in these areas and probably contributes to the development of the cirrhosis. The liver and spleen may be greatly enlarged.

5. **Congenital Hepatic Fibrosis.** This rare disorder is probably part of the visceral manifestations of polycystic disease. The principal features are a large hard liver, splenomegaly, portal hypertension and abnormalities of the kidneys. Liver function is usually normal.

NEW GROWTHS OF THE LIVER

Primary Carcinoma of the Liver (p. 1031). This condition occurs mainly in males over middle age. The tumour may be of liver cell or bile-duct type, and develops either as a large carcinomatous nodule, sometimes almost completely occupying one lobe of the liver, or as a more diffuse form, with several nodules throughout the organ.

Symptoms and signs include vague gastrointestinal complaints, weakness, ascites, loss of weight, right upper quadrant pain and occasionally symptoms referable to metastatic foci. Unexplained fever is a common feature, and if this occurs in a known case of hepatic cirrhosis and is associated with rapid development of ascites or marked loss of weight, hepatic carcinoma should be suspected. It is now possible, using various radioactive isotopes, to obtain a map of the liver by scanning the organ using a scintillation counter. The demonstration of a filling defect in the liver profile may be of considerable diagnostic aid.

Secondary Neoplasms of the Liver. These are relatively common, and are often secondary to primary carcinoma in the bronchus, breast, abdomen or pelvis. The metastatic foci may be multiple or single. Dissemination throughout the peritoneum frequently results in ascites.

Symptoms of the primary neoplasm are absent in about half the cases and the presence of cirrhosis of the liver may be suspected from the hepatomegaly. The spleen, however, is rarely enlarged. There is usually a rapid enlargement of the liver, fever, weight loss and jaundice. Tests of liver function may show no impairment until late in the course of the disease. Diagnosis may be made by needle biopsy of an enlarged area of the liver, laparotomy or radio-isotope scanning.

DISEASES OF THE GALL-BLADDER AND BILE DUCTS

ANATOMY AND PHYSIOLOGY

The normal gall-bladder concentrates 5 to 10 times the bile secreted by the liver, and this is accomplished by the absorption of water and salt by the mucous membrane. Thus it acts as a reservoir for the discharge of bile into the duodenum. About 1000 ml. of bile are secreted by the liver continuously throughout the 24 hours, and the greater part of this enters the gall-bladder through the cystic duct, the sphincter of Oddi being closed. After the ingestion of food the sphincter of Oddi relaxes, the gall-bladder contracts, and its contents are expelled through the cystic duct into the common bile duct and duodenum. The stimulus for this activity is the presence of food in the upper part of the small intestine. Fats and foods rich in fat are especially effective in causing bile to be discharged by the gall-bladder. It is believed that, as a result of this stimulus, a hormone, cholecystokinin, is secreted into the blood by the mucosa of the duodenum and jejunum, and that this compound acts directly on the wall of the gall-bladder causing it to contract. In addition, the gall-bladder and sphincter of Oddi appear to be reciprocally innervated: vagal stimulation results in contraction of the gall-bladder with relaxation of the sphincter, while stimulation of the sympathetic nerves produces the reverse effects. Over-activity of the sympathetic or parasympathetic systems or disturbance of the hormonal mechanism responsible for the simultaneous contraction of the gall-bladder and relaxation of the sphincter of Oddi may be the cause of functional disorders of the biliary tract. These include biliary dyskinesia (p. 1049) and the bilious vomiting associated with such conditions as migraine.

The sympathetic nerves to the gall-bladder are connected, through the coeliac plexus, with the lower six thoracic segments in the spinal cord. This fact probably explains the referred pain, tenderness and hyperaesthesia over the area of somatic distribution of the lower thoracic nerves posteriorly which is frequently found in gall-bladder disease. The pain in the shoulder which is more rarely present in biliary disease is probably due to direct irritation of a branch of the phrenic nerve below the diaphragm.

EVALUATION OF GALL-BLADDER STRUCTURE AND FUNCTION

Available methods permit the estimation of the concentrating power of the gall-bladder and its ability to contract, and an assessment of the patency and configuration of the bile ducts. These procedures have become an essential part of the investigation of patients suspected of having gall-bladder disease, and accuracy in diagnosis has been greatly increased by their use.

1. **Radiography of the Abdomen.** A plain film of the abdomen may demonstrate the presence of stones in the gall-bladder or ducts, gas in the biliary tract or calcification in the pancreas.

2. **Cholecystography** is the most useful single procedure in the diagnosis of gall-bladder disease. An organic iodine-containing compound (e.g. Telepaque) is taken by mouth on the evening

before the examination, following a light, fat-free supper. The compound is absorbed, secreted by the liver in the bile and concentrated in the normal gall-bladder. Under these circumstances, a shadow is seen in the area of the gall-bladder on radiological examination the following morning, about 14 hours later. The patient is then given a meal containing fat (e.g. $\frac{1}{2}$-1 oz. of butter on toast with milk or egg) and a final film taken after one hour, when partial evacuation of the normal gall-bladder should have occurred. Interpretations of results in terms of gall-bladder activity can be made only in the absence of vomiting, diarrhoea, severe hepatic insufficiency, and obstructive and hepatocellular jaundice. When these conditions are not present and provided the patient has taken the iodine-containing compound as instructed, failure to visualise the gall-bladder indicates gall-bladder disease or obstruction in the cystic duct (non-functioning gall-bladder). If the gall-bladder is functioning sufficiently to produce a shadow, any non-opaque stones will probably be demonstrated. This is of great importance, since only a minority of stones, namely those containing a sufficiently high calcium content, are seen as definite shadows in the gall-bladder area on radiological examination of the abdomen. Tumours of the gall-bladder may also be seen.

3. **Cholangiography.** Biligrafin (iodipamide methylglucamine) is a substance which is given intravenously and is concentrated and excreted by the liver. In subjects with reasonably normal liver function and with the serum bilirubin concentration less than 2 mg. per cent., the dye permits visualisation of the main biliary ducts. In the cholecystectomised patient it is the only method of demonstrating the bile ducts and the presence of a stone, and it is valuable in showing the existence of intrahepatic stones or other pathology.

In operations on the biliary tract the patency of the ducts may be demonstrated by the injection of the non-irritant radio-opaque substance, diodone, into the extrahepatic ducts. A similar procedure should be used post-operatively before withdrawing a drainage tube which has been inserted into the common bile duct.

ACUTE CHOLECYSTITIS

Aetiology and Pathogenesis. Acute cholecystitis is rarely due primarily to infection of the gall-bladder, but almost always occurs in association with obstruction to the cystic duct or neck of the gall-bladder, upon which infection is usually superimposed. By far the most common cause of obstruction is gall-stones but inspissated bile, oedema of the duct, or more rarely enlarged lymph nodes or tumour may produce the same effects. The gall-bladder swells as a result of the obstruction, which prevents evacuation of bile, and from the accumulation of inflammatory exudate and mucin. In consequence, its vascular supply is compressed and necrosis and perforation may follow. The most common infecting organisms are *Strep. faecalis* and *Strep. viridans*, and *Esch. coli*. Whether the infecting organisms reach the gall-bladder via the bile ducts, the lymphatics or the blood stream is uncertain. It is possible that cholecystitis may sometimes be initiated by the chemical irritation of bile salts, when the latter reach abnormally high concentration in the gall-bladder; this could occur either when the outlet to the organ is obstructed and absorption of water and inorganic salts continues, or from an increase in the concentration of the bile acids secreted by the liver.

Acute bacterial cholecystitis can occur without obstruction in the course of typhoid or paratyphoid fever. It may also rarely develop in the septicaemic stage of other infective processes, without obstruction to the cystic duct.

Pathology. The organ may show any degree of change from slight congestion to gross inflammation, swelling and tenseness. In the latter case, ulceration of the wall may be present. Occasionally, the gall-bladder may be full of pus (empyema) and this is usually associated with complete blockage of the cystic duct by a stone.

Clinical Features. Although the disease can occur at any age, patients are most commonly women who have borne children and are aged between 40 and 60 years. Obesity is often present.

When there is no obstruction in the cystic or common bile duct, the patient is nauseated, complains of discomfort in the upper abdomen and is febrile. On examination tenderness is maximal in the right hypochondrium when the patient takes a deep breath. When obstruction occurs, as it does in the majority, the patient develops a sudden severe pain due to biliary colic, and becomes restless. The full clinical features are described on p. 1044.

Jaundice is in most cases absent or slight, and if present suggests obstruction (stone or oedema) in the common bile duct, or ascending cholangitis and cholangiohepatitis. A history of attacks of abdominal pain is commonly obtained.

Laboratory Data. Polymorphonuclear leucocytosis is usual. In some clinically non-jaundiced cases serum bilirubin is found to be elevated, and tests for bile in the urine may also be transiently positive. Cholecystography is contraindicated in the acute phase, but a plain radiograph of the upper abdomen may be helpful by showing radio-opaque stones.

Course and Prognosis. In the majority of cases of acute cholecystitis, the symptoms subside in a few days with conservative therapy, though a recurrence of the attack after weeks, months or years is common. In a few cases, however, serious complications occur, which, if left untreated, can be fatal. In severe infections with complete obstruction, the gall-bladder becomes acutely tender, and muscular rigidity spreads. Empyema of the gall-bladder may develop in a few hours, and perforation with localised or rarely generalised peritonitis can follow. Subphrenic abscess, acute pancreatitis (p. 1056), or ascending cholangitis and cholangiohepatitis (p. 1045) may also result. When such complications develop the patient is clearly seriously ill, with high fever and rapid pulse.

Differential Diagnosis must be made from other causes of severe upper abdominal pain. These include appendicitis, perforation of a peptic ulcer, myocardial infarction, renal colic, acute pyelonephritis, intestinal colic, herpes zoster, pleurisy, acute pancreatitis, epidemic myalgia (Bornholm disease) and acute porphyria.

Treatment. There is a difference of opinion with regard to treatment of cases of acute cholecystitis. The increased operative mortality in the complicated case leads some authorities to advise surgical intervention in all cases of acute cholecystitis at the outset of the disease (cf. appendicitis). The great frequency, however, with which clinical features subside on conservative therapy is a strong argument in favour of advising surgical intervention in the acute stage only when signs and symptoms which suggest the development of empyema occur; these are persisting pyrexia, increasing tenderness, appearance of a mass or the least suspicion of peritonitis. Each case must therefore be evaluated on its own merits, and should be carefully watched for evidence of complications. In the acute stages, medical therapy consists of maintaining salt and water balance, and the relief of pain by the measures described for the treatment of biliary colic (p. 1047). Opinions vary as to the appropriate antibiotic to be used. Formerly penicillin and streptomycin were almost uniformly successful, but with alterations in sensitivity patterns to these agents this is no longer true. If, as is usual, the bacteria responsible for the infection cannot be isolated ampicillin is the drug of first choice. If infection is severe or septicaemia is present kanamycin should be tried. Surgical removal of the gall-bladder should be advised after the acute symptoms have subsided, especially if gall-stones are proved to be present and if there have been previous attacks. If surgical interference is contraindicated, dietetic and other measures described in the treatment of chronic cholecystitis should be applied (p. 1048).

CHRONIC CHOLECYSTITIS

The term 'chronic cholecystitis' is used to denote chronic disease of the gall-bladder whether due to calculi, to infection or to the deposition of cholesterol.

CHOLELITHIASIS (GALL-STONES) AND CHRONIC CALCULOUS CHOLECYSTITIS

Gall-stones (cholelithiasis) occur in 5-10 per cent. of the population and are found about five times more commonly in females than males. In a few cases no evidence of cholecystitis is found, but in the majority the cholelithiasis is associated with chronic inflammation of the gall-bladder of varying degree. The wall may be greatly thickened and fibrosed, and the organ is frequently shrunken. The destruction of mucosa leads to impairment in concentrating power.

Aetiology of Gall-stones. The detailed mechanism of gall-stone formation is unknown. The increased incidence of gall-stones containing cholesterol which is stated to occur in pregnancy and diabetes mellitus, in which conditions a slight but significant increase in plasma cholestorol is present, suggests that a change in the metabolism of cholesterol may be partly responsible. The cholesterol/bile salt ratio is important in maintaining the former in solution, and it may be significant that the chronically diseased gall-bladder can usually absorb bile salts more rapidly than normal, thus producing a fall in their concentration, so that cholesterol may be precipitated. Other factors, which include alterations in pH of the bile, the presence of infection, diminution in the hepatic formation of bile acids, increase in the excretion of bile pigment, the occurrence of biliary stasis and sedentary habits, may play a part in what is clearly a complex biochemical event.

Classification of Gall-stones. There are three main types of gall-stones:

(1) *Cholesterol stones.* These are composed almost entirely of cholesterol and are frequently called 'metabolic stones'. They occur singly or in pairs in most cases, and are very probably formed as a result of alteration in cholesterol/bile salt ratio. Infection is believed to play no part in their production.

(2) *Pigment stones.* These stones, which are always numerous, are composed almost entirely of bile pigment. They occur in association with haemolytic diseases (e.g. congenital or acquired haemolytic anaemia) and presumably result from the excessive excretion of bilirubin by the liver. They are rare.

(3) *Mixed stones.* These are the most common type of stone; they are usually present in large numbers and consist of lamellated layers of cholesterol, calcium and bilirubin.

Clinical Features. Patients are most commonly obese women of middle age. The nature and severity of their complaints depend upon the position of the stones in the biliary tract and upon the degree of associated infection. If the stones remain in the gall-bladder, there may be no symptoms.

Biliary colic is the cardinal symptom of chronic calculous cholecystitis. It occurs when a stone lodges in the cystic or common bile duct, and it is frequently the first and only clinical evidence of the presence of gall-stones. The attack may be precipitated by dietary indiscretion or undue physical effort, or it may occur without apparent reason. A sudden pain is felt in the epigastrium, and this gradually increases with slight wave-like exacerbations, and usually moves to the right hypochondrium. The pain, which is frequently agonising, may then be referred, as in acute cholecystitis, to the right side and back, or to the right shoulder. Vomiting and nausea frequently occur. The pain lasts several hours, and then subsides, often suddenly, leaving a feeling of soreness which persists for some days. During the attack tenderness and muscle spasm in the right upper quadrant of the abdomen are found and, if the stone remains in the cystic duct, acute cholecystitis may develop. Jaundice appears in a little over half of the patients in whom the stone lodges in the common bile duct, and its occurrence is dependent upon the degree of blockage of the duct. The jaundice may be slight or latent and revealed only by serum bilirubin determination. Commonly in such cases, however, bile may appear transiently in the urine, or the patient may give a history of having noted a temporary darkening of the urine. In other cases frank obstructive jaundice develops simultaneously with episodes of biliary colic. The obstruction is not usually complete, and often lasts for little more than one to two weeks. In some of these cases the symptoms and signs of cholangitis and cholangio-hepatitis develop: fever and rigors occur, and the liver may enlarge.

A proportion of patients with chronic calculous cholecystitis complain of chronic flatulent dyspepsia definitely related to meals and frequently precipitated by fatty or fried foods. Most patients describe this as discomfort in the epigastrium and a feeling of fullness and nausea. Constipation with transient attacks of diarrhoea may be present. This symptom complex has been called 'gall-bladder dyspepsia', and organic disease of the gall-bladder or the presence of gall-stones has been held responsible for its production. Since, however, many patients with organic disease of the gall-bladder never complain of dyspepsia, and since similar clinical features occur in association with other organic and functional conditions of the gastrointestinal tract, such dyspepsia should be attributed to gall-bladder disease only when other causes have been carefully excluded.

Laboratory and Radiological Data. The urine may or may not contain bilirubin, depending upon the presence of obstruction to the common bile duct. It may be present in the urine, however, in the absence of clinical jaundice, perhaps for only a few hours. Urobilinogen is found also in the urine if previous episodes of gall-bladder disease have resulted in hepatic parenchymal damage. After the subsidence of an acute attack of colic, radiological examination of the abdomen should be carried out and cholecystography should be performed. By these means stones and/or a poorly functioning gall-bladder will usually be demonstrated.

Differential Diagnosis. In the absence of biliary colic and obstructive jaundice, the diagnosis of chronic calculous cholecystitis presents considerable difficulty. Other conditions associated with dyspepsia, e.g. cardiospasm, hiatus hernia, peptic ulcer, carcinoma of the stomach, chronic gastritis, biliary dyskinesia and chronic pancreatitis, have to be excluded by appropriate methods. It is a sound rule not to diagnose organic disease of the gall-bladder from the presence of dyspepsia alone without the radiological demonstration of gall-stones or an abnormal cholecystogram. In the differentiation of biliary pain due to cholelithiasis from other conditions producing acute abdominal pain (p. 1042) it is helpful to note that it occurs in discrete episodes of usually less than a day and separated by symptom-free periods of weeks or months. Cholecystography is again necessary to confirm the origin of the symptoms and signs. It should also be appreciated that patients with organic disease of the biliary tract not infrequently have disorders elsewhere in the alimentary tract, in particular hiatus hernia and diverticulosis of the colon. Symptoms arising from these conditions must be carefully assessed before advising cholecystectomy.

When obstructive jaundice is present differential diagnosis between stone in the common bile duct and carcinoma of the head of the pancreas or of the biliary tract should be attempted. Loss of weight may be marked in the latter condition and biliary colic is absent, while the jaundice is usually progressive and without fluctuation. The palpation of a smooth, tender, distended gall-bladder favours obstruction of the common bile duct by neoplasm rather than stone, since a gall-bladder which is the seat of chronic inflammation and gall-stones is usually incapable of distension. The differential diagnosis between obstruction of the common bile duct by a neoplasm and obstruction due to a 'silent' stone, i.e. a stone impacted in the duct which does not produce the symptoms of biliary colic, is especially difficult. Such 'silent' common duct stones may be found at operation in patients in whom neoplasm was suspected pre-operatively.

Treatment. There is no satisfactory treatment for chronic calculous cholecystitis other than surgical removal of the gall-bladder and any stones that may be in the blliary tract. Operation, however, should not be undertaken for the presence of stones *per se*, but advised for patients who have suffered one or more attacks of biliary colic or episodes of acute cholecystitis, or in whom jaundice and evidence of cholangitis are present and have persisted for a period of some weeks. Operation is strongly contraindicated for symptoms of 'gall-bladder dyspepsia' in the absence of additional evidence of organic gall-bladder disease. It should be avoided if possible in patients who are poor surgical risks (e.g. those with severe cardiovascular, pulmonary or renal disease or with marked obesity), and elderly patients who prefer to retain their gall-stones should be allowed to do so.

Medical management of chronic calculous cholecystitis includes the treatment of the acute attack of biliary colic, the treatment of infection in the gall-bladder and biliary tract, the treatment of dyspepsia and obesity and non-surgical biliary drainage, which is applicable to the minority of patients for whom conservative therapy has been recommended.

Biliary colic. Although morphine sulphate is known to cause contraction of the sphincter of Oddi, it remains one of the most effective drugs for the relief of biliary colic, provided it is given in large enough doses, i.e. 15-20 mg. subcutaneously and repeated in one hour if relief is not obtained. Concomitantly, a tablet of glyceryl trinitrate 0·5 mg. sublingually every 30 to 60 minutes, or an intramuscular injection of propantheline bromide (30 mg.) should be given to relieve spasm. In less severe cases pethidine, 100 mg., by intramuscular injection, may be satisfactory, and may be repeated in two hours. Local application of heat is indicated in all cases.

Infection in the biliary tract. Antibiotics and chemotherapeutic agents should be used when fever is present, i.e. either in acute cholecystitis or in acute cholangitis and cholangio-hepatitis developing in the course of chronic calculous cholecystitis. Their use in these conditions is described on p. 1043.

Dyspepsia and obesity. Dietetic treatment is of value in patients in whom surgical removal of the gall-bladder is not to be undertaken. Foods which precipitate or aggravate symptoms should be avoided. These include cooked fats and fried foods. Eggs may be allowed in moderation if they do not produce symptoms. Since biliary stasis is believed to predispose to the formation of gallstones, a moderate intake of uncooked fats is permitted in the form of milk, butter and cream cheese. This promotes drainage of the gall-bladder and bile ducts. Otherwise the diet should be bland, and should contain adequate quantities of protein (60-80 g./day) and of carbohydrate (300-400 g./day). However, if obesity is present a low calorie diet should be prescribed.

Chronic Non-calculous Cholecystitis

This is a relatively rare cause of symptoms referable to the gall-bladder. Infection of the gall-bladder is probably secondary to mechanical or chemical factors. Partial obstruction of the cystic duct by inflammatory swelling can result in a chronic inflammation of the wall of the gall-bladder.

Clinical Features are the same as those associated with calculous cholecystitis but are usually milder. Biliary colic and mild jaundice can also occur, the latter being due to ascending cholangitis.

Diagnosis of chronic cholecystitis without stones depends upon the clinical features and the objective findings of gall-bladder disease as revealed by cholecystography, namely the presence of a gall-bladder which fails to function normally and in which gallstones cannot be demonstrated.

Treatment of the confirmed case of non-calculous cholecystitis is similar to that described under calculous cholecystitis (p. 1047), except that medical treatment may be given a longer trial before resorting to surgery. In those cases in which operation is not advisable, medical therapy directed to eliminate biliary stasis and increase bile flow can be more vigorous than in calculous cholecystitis, since the danger of a stone becoming impacted in the common bile duct is absent. Magnesium sulphate taken before breakfast and olive oil before lunch and the oral administration of bile salts have a more important place in treatment.

Cholesterolosis of the Gall-bladder

This condition may occasionally be found at operation in patients diagnosed as suffering from chronic calculous cholecystitis. The mucosa of the gall-bladder is red and studded with deposits of cholesterol and other lipid material; cholesterol calculi may be present. The mechanism of the cholesterol deposition is unknown, though infection is not believed to play a part. Autopsy studies show that cholesterolosis can exist without symptoms. The patients are predominantly obese females; symptoms, when present, are due to associated cholelithiasis or calcification of the gall-bladder wall (porcelain gall-bladder). The presence of cholesterolosis is not usually suspected, and is revealed only at operation. Cholecystography usually shows impairment of gall-bladder concentrating power, and cholesterol crystals may be seen in large numbers in the fluid obtained by duodenal aspiration. Treatment is similar to that for chronic calculous cholecystitis (p. 1047).

FUNCTIONAL DISORDERS OF THE GALL-BLADDER AND BILIARY TRACT

(Biliary Dyskinesia)

Biliary dyskinesia has been defined as an obstruction to bile flow into the duodenum due to a neuromuscular disturbance of the sphincter of Oddi, as a result of which symptoms suggestive of organic disease of the gall-bladder are present. Its existence is disputed by many authorities. It is however extremely rare to find a patient with vague fat-intolerant dyspepsia and mild biliary colic attributed to the disorder, in whom there are not present other more tangible mechanisms such as hiatus hernia, pancreatitis, ulceration of the second part of the duodenum or psychoneurosis. The failure of sphincterotomy to give relief to all but a few substantiates this impression. In suspect cases a trial of antispasmodic drugs, e.g. propantheline bromide 15 mg. given every four hours or glyceryl trinitrate 0·5 mg. as required is justified.

TUMOURS OF THE GALL-BLADDER AND BILE DUCTS

Primary Carcinoma of the Gall-bladder

This disease is not common and occurs in females more frequently than in males. Chronic calculous cholecystitis predisposes to the development of malignant disease.

Clinical Features. Most patients are elderly women who give a history of calculous cholecystitis for many years. Frequently the symptoms do not differ from those of chronic cholecystitis, diagnosis being made at operation. Pain in the epigastrium and right upper quadrant of the abdomen gradually becomes constant and severe. A palpable mass can be felt in the gall-bladder area in about 50 per cent. of cases. Complete obstructive jaundice, from compression or invasion of the common bile duct, is common and persists without remission. Fever, loss of weight and vomiting are usual in the late stages. The occult blood test of the faeces is frequently negative.

Diagnosis is usually made at operation undertaken for obstructive jaundice, suspected to be due to stone in the common bile duct or carcinoma of the head of the pancreas.

Treatment. Removal of the gall-bladder in the early stage is the only successful therapy.

Primary Malignant Tumours of the Extrahepatic Biliary Ducts

Tumours of these ducts are rare. An insidious onset of jaundice is almost invariable, and eventually the features are those of complete obstructive jaundice (p. 996). Pain is common and may be similar to that of biliary colic; the features of superimposed cholangio-hepatitis often develop. The occult blood test of the faeces is usually positive.

Treatment. Operative removal of the tumour is rarely possible.

Benign Tumours (Papilloma)

Benign tumours of the gall-bladder or bile ducts are rare and in the latter situation may give rise to obstructive jaundice.

PREVENTION OF DISEASES OF THE LIVER AND BILIARY TRACT

The specific measures adopted for the prevention of diseases of the liver and biliary tract vary with the cause.

Acute Parenchymal Disease of the Liver

The hazards from exposure to toxic agents used in industry, e.g. carbon tetrachloride, tetrachlorethane, phosphorus and others, have been greatly reduced in recent years by appropriate measures enforced by Acts of Parliament. Acute parenchymal liver disease following chloroform poisoning is now relatively rare as this compound has been largely replaced by newer anaesthetics. Acute hepatic disease may result from the therapeutic use of gold, antimony, arsenic and cinchophen. Such toxic reactions are, however, rare and are often a manifestation of idiosyncrasy. During treatment by these drugs careful watch should be kept for signs which suggest liver damage, e.g. jaundice and the presence of urobilinogen in the urine; if these appear the administration of hepatotoxic drugs should be stopped immediately. It is obvious that they should not be used in patients already suffering from chronic parenchymal liver disease. A number of organic chemicals may cause damage to the liver, including such drugs as chlorpromazine and oral contraceptive agents which are widely prescribed. The Dunlop Committee on Drug Safety has been set up to safeguard patients as much as possible from this form of iatrogenic disease and to encourage surveillance and care in the use of all new drugs.

Acute infective hepatitis is the most important acute parenchymal liver disease of infective origin. The difficulty in diagnosing the sporadic case before the onset of jaundice renders preventive measures virtually impossible. The problem is further aggravated by the doubt which exists with regard to the mode of transmission and the fact that infectivity is greatest during the pre-icteric phase. In epidemics specific measures of prevention include those applicable to all infectious diseases and in selected epidemics the administration of γ-globulin to those whose exposure to infection is great. The occurrence of serum hepatitis can be prevented to a large extent by screening blood donors and eliminating all those giving a history of jaundice. The use of liquid plasma, stored for three to six months, appears to result in the smallest incidence of serum hepatitis. The highest incidence (5-10 per cent.) follows the use of large pools of dried plasma. If, however, pooling of dried plasma cannot be avoided for practical reasons, the pool size should be no greater than 10 donors. Adequate sterilisation of syringes and needles is essential. Ideally, this is accomplished by autoclaving syringes and needles for 20 minutes at 120° C. Alternatively disposable needles and tubing should be used. In the absence of these facilities, syringes and needles should be washed in 2 per cent. lysol, then boiled in water for 20 minutes. These precautions are especially necessary when venepuncture is to be undertaken.

The control and prevention of Weil's disease depends upon adequate destruction of rats in mines, farms and sewers, and attention to rat-proofing in premises in which rat infestation is likely to occur, e.g. food stores, granaries and fish-curing establishments. These methods are more likely to be successful than the wearing of rubber boots or other protective clothing, or the use of vaccines.

The nutritional state of the individual is important in determining the occurrence and degree of liver damage which results from any of the above causes. Death from acute infective hepatitis is much more common in the native populations of countries in which there is a poor standard of nutrition than it is in Britain.

Chronic Parenchymal Disease of the Liver and Disease of the Biliary Tract

Prevention of chronic disease of the liver consists partly of preventing the occurrence of acute hepatic disease. This is particularly true in the case of post-necrotic scarring and post-infective cirrhosis. The high incidence of cirrhosis of the liver in tropical countries in which the dietary intake of first-class protein and essential food factors is deficient could undoubtedly be reduced by the provision of a more satisfactory diet. Such a diet can be made available only if there develops greater co-operation on the part of economists, agriculturalists and statesmen of many countries than exists today. Diffuse hepatic fibrosis occurring as a sequel to fat infiltration may occur where there is a large disparity between the intake of calories and of essential food factors. This was formerly seen commonly among chronic alcoholics. The reduction in the consumption of alcohol, advances in education and improved living standards have all contributed to a decline in the number of cases of alcoholic cirrhosis. Alcohol is still considered to be a cause of relapse in patients convalescing from hepatitis and should be forbidden for at least six months after the acute illness. Likewise, known hepatotoxic drugs should not be given in the presence of established liver disease or in patients recovering from hepatitis; until more information is available it would be wise to include the contraceptive pill in this category.

Biliary cirrhosis, which most commonly results from unrelieved obstruction to the common bile duct, with associated infection, can usually be prevented by prompt surgical relief of the biliary obstruction and treatment of the underlying infection. Biliary obstruction itself is most commonly the result of cholelithiasis and impaction of a stone in the common bile duct. The restriction of foods containing large amounts of cholesterol is of doubtful value in preventing calculus formation. A moderate intake of neutral fat, with the avoidance of sedentary habits, helps to prevent biliary stasis, which is a potent factor in stone formation. The association of gall-bladder disease and cholelithiasis with obesity provides additional justification if any more is needed for the prescription of an anti-obesity diet as a preventive measure in persons who are overweight.

There is no known method of preventing the hepatic fibrosis which results from infiltration of the liver with glycogen, kerasin, sphingomyelin or cholesterol. Progressive deterioration of liver function can be prevented in haemochromatosis by regular venesection in the early stages and in hepatolenticular degeneration by penicillamine; moreover the genetic nature of these two rare diseases makes it possible to anticipate their development and to take the necessary prophylactic measures.

J. S. Robson.
John Richmond.

Books recommended:

Popper, H. & Schaffner, F. (1961). *Progress in Liver Diseases*, vol. 1. New York: Grune & Stratton.

Popper, H. & Schaffner, F. (1965). *Progress in Liver Diseases*, vol. 2. New York: Grune & Stratton.

Read, A. E. (1967). *The Liver*. *Colston Papers No.* 19. London: Butterworth.

Sherlock, S. (1968). *Diseases of the Liver and Biliary System*, 4th ed. Oxford: Blackwell.

DISEASES OF THE PANCREAS

ANATOMY AND PHYSIOLOGY

MOST of the pancreatic tissue consists of acini of serous cells which are the site of the most active protein synthesis in the body. Their secretion plays an important part in digestion and is discharged into the duodenum through the pancreatic duct. The latter enters the duodenum along with the common bile duct at the sphincter of Oddi, but in about 10 per cent. of individuals the main outflow of pancreatic juice reaches the duodenum by a separate duct. The pancreas also contains isolated areas of specialised cells (the islets of Langerhans), which quite independently produce an internal secretion, insulin, which is intimately concerned with carbohydrate metabolism. Diabetes mellitus (p. 739) is associated with insufficiency or diminished effectiveness of insulin which is secreted by the beta cells of the islets. The alpha cells of the islets produce a hormone (glucagon) which influences blood sugar levels by promoting breakdown of glycogen to glucose.

Pancreatic juice is an alkaline secretion containing sodium bicarbonate and about a litre is secreted daily. In addition to various salts it contains three main enzymes: amylase (diastase) is a starch-splitting enzyme; lipase splits fats that have been acted on by bile; and a group of proteolytic ferments attack selected proteins and peptides. Trypsin is an important enzyme of this group and is secreted in both active and inactive forms. These enzymes are elaborated by the same serous cells and are secreted in parallel concentrations. Pancreatic juice reaches a maximum flow between two and three hours after a meal. Its secretion is stimulated partly by nervous mechanisms acting through the vagus nerves which prime the acinar cells to respond to the hormones secretin and pancreozymin formed when acid chyme comes into contact with the mucosal cells of the duodenum.

TESTS OF PANCREATIC FUNCTION

The study of variations in blood sugar levels which are related to the internal secretory function of the pancreas is described in connection with diabetes mellitus (p. 712).

Pancreatic lipase, aided by the emulsifying action of the bile salts, is responsible for the hydrolysis of fat prior to its absorption through the intestinal wall. Malabsorption of fat occurs if the supply of lipase or of bile is subnormal. When pancreatic secretion is defective the fat content of the stools is raised above the normal limit of 6 g. in 24 hours on a diet containing up to 150 g. The diagnosis of steatorrhoea depends however on chemical estimations of stools collected over a sequence of several days.

The trypsin secreted by the pancreas is the principal enzyme concerned in protein digestion, and if it is deficient in quantity the faeces will contain a marked increase in the number of undigested meat fibres; i.e. creatorrhoea. However, both meat fibres and fat globules may be found in the stools on microscopy in any patient with intestinal hurry. An increase in the normal maximum 24 hours output of 2·5 g. of nitrogen in the stools may also indicate inadequate proteolysis in pancreatic insufficiency. Amylase is partly absorbed into the blood and thereafter excreted by the healthy kidney. The amount of serum amylase can be measured by its property of starch digestion and the normal range is expressed as from 3 to 10 Wohlgemuth units per ml. of serum. In acute pancreatitis the amount of amylase in the blood and urine rises greatly to levels of 100 units or more. This test is therefore of great value in the early diagnosis of this acute disorder but it should be remembered that high levels can sometimes occur in other acute abdominal emergencies. The test is, however, of little use in the more chronic disorders of the pancreas.

A valuable test of pancreatic function can be performed by the passage of tubes into the stomach and duodenum under radiological control. The gastric and duodenal contents can then be aspirated until the latter are obtained in an uncontaminated state. The hormone secretin is then injected intravenously and the duodenal juice is collected for an hour. An intravenous injection of pancreozymin is next given and a further collection of duodenal juice is made. A full quantitative and qualitative study of the external pancreatic secretion can then be made in respect of its rate of production and bicarbonate and enzyme content. The main application of this test is the determination of chronic pancreatic disease such as chronic pancreatitis and carcinoma of the pancreas and in the exclusion of the pancreas as a cause of malabsorptive disorder, but its value is limited in that it rarely detects early disease of the pancreas. A serial rise in serum amylase levels in blood withdrawn half, one and two hours after the injection of secretin is helpful in the diagnosis of obstructive lesions of pancreatic ducts.

As yet no ideal radiological method is available for the demonstration of pancreatic disease. Photo-scanning following intravenous ^{75}selenium-methionine is used, but the pancreas may be overlapped by the scan of an enlarged liver. Other techniques include study of mucosal folds in the duodenum and selective arteriography of the mesentric and coeliac axis.

INFLAMMATORY CONDITIONS OF THE PANCREAS

ACUTE PANCREATITIS OR ACUTE PANCREATIC NECROSIS

This is a serious disorder which may proceed to a haemorrhagic necrosis of pancreatic tissue with the formation of a local or generalised peritonitis. The disease is most common between the fourth and seventh decades with an equal sex incidence.

The exact mechanism which initiates the destruction of the pancreatic tissue has not been established. A frequent association between biliary tract disease and acute pancreatitis has given rise to the widely accepted theory that an obstruction at the sphincter of Oddi due to a gall-stone, oedema or spasm, allows a reflux of bile along the pancreatic duct. This causes an activation of the enzymes, trypsin and lipase which start an auto-digestion of the pancreatic blood vessels and parenchyma. Although in only a small proportion of cases can a stone be found at operation or post-mortem, a bile-stained pancreas is seen in many cases of acute pancreatitis and a common terminal channel for both the bile and pancreatic ducts is usually present in fatal cases. It seems unlikely that infection plays an initial role as cultures made in early cases are usually sterile. Once, however, the process has started, oedema, haemorrhage and fat necrosis may continue, with destruction of much of the pancreas, the liberation of a serosanguinous exudate into the peritoneal cavity, including the lesser sac, and with chemical splitting of fat deposits in the omentum and mesentery. In Britain about 60 per cent. of cases appear to be associated with underlying biliary disease and about 20 per cent.

with a history of alcoholic excess. In some countries there seems to be a more dominant association with excessive drinking. Occasionally acute pancreatitis may occur as a complication of disseminated lupus erythematosus, pregnancy, carcinoma of the head of the pancreas, ascariasis, hyperparathyroidism and abdominal trauma.

Clinical Features. There is usually a history of preceding attacks of dyspepsia associated with pain in the back, and often of episodes of gallstone colic. There may be a known history of alcoholism or recent contact with a case of mumps. The onset is sudden with agonising pain in the epigastrium or right hypochondrium. It often occurs within 12-24 hours following the taking of alcohol or a heavy meal. The pain is usually persistent and radiates most frequently through to the back, to either shoulder, or to one of the iliac fossae before spreading to involve the whole abdomen. Nausea and vomiting are frequent and constipation is almost always present. The patient looks ill and in severe cases profound shock soon supervenes with cyanosis, clammy skin, rapid thready pulse and a subnormal temperature. In milder cases moderate fever occurs, and slight jaundice may develop, especially in cases with gall-stones.

The abdomen is soft at first, but becomes tender and rigid, especially in the upper half, as peritoneal irritation increases and the initial shock passes off. There is often general distension of the abdomen and on auscultation peristalsis may be inaudible from the outset of the attack.

Diagnosis. A most important point in the diagnosis of acute pancreatitis is for the practitioner to remember it as one of the causes of severe upper abdominal pain. Many cases are diagnosed for the first time at laparotomy, having been admitted to hospital for perforated peptic ulcer, acute intestinal obstruction or acute appendicitis. The condition may also simulate acute cholecystitis (with which it may co-exist), and myocardial infarction. In the early stage of an acute case the determination of the serum amylase is of great diagnostic importance. Within the first few hours levels in excess of 100 Wohlgemuth units per ml. of serum will be found (normal 3 to 10 units). Such amylase estimations are only useful in the early stages of the acute disease since the concentration may be normal in mild and subsiding cases. Serial estimations of amylase in serum which show rising levels during the first 48 hours are of diagnostic value. Amylase may also be found in fluid aspirated on diagnostic abdominal paracentesis. Other laboratory investigations are of less help, but hyperglycaemia may occur and the blood calcium may be lowered in the later stages. In cases with associated biliary obstruction the serum bilirubin may be raised. There is usually a moderate polymorph leucocytosis. Radiological examination of the abdomen is essential. A 'plain film' may show a 'sentinel' loop of transverse colon or jejunum distended by ileus, calcified gallstones or calcification in the pancreas, and ileus and oedema of the duodenum may be demonstrated by gastrografin studies.

Treatment. When the diagnosis of acute pancreatitis has been established pre-operatively, the present tendency is to favour conservative treatment as giving a lower mortality. Medical management consists of measures to combat shock, to relieve pain, to suppress pancreatic secretion and to prevent infection. In the stage of shock plasma transfusions are indicated and intravenous infusions may be required for several days to relieve dehydration and to restore electrolyte balance. Intravenous calcium gluconate may be required as the serum calcium level may fall due to the formation of soaps from ionised calcium and fatty acids in the areas of fat necrosis. Continuous gastrointestinal suction (p. 952) is essential to reduce vomiting and distension and to rest the pancreas by preventing the initiation of the secretin mechanism by acid chyme. Atropine by injection will reduce the acid gastric secretion entering the duodenum. For the relief of the pain repeated intramuscular injections of methadone 10 mg., or pethidine 100 mg. should be given. Hypodermic injection of morphine 10-20 mg. may be required in the pain is very severe, but this drug, and to a lesser degree pethidine, cause spasm of the sphincter of Oddi, which is not a desirable effect. This spasm is not affected by the administration of atropine but may be reduced or abolished by glyceryl trinitrate given in the form of tablets dissolved sublingually. The dose is 2 tablets, each of 0·5 mg. and this may be repeated at intervals of 30 to 60 minutes. Atropine is of value in resting the secretory function of the pancreas because of its paralysant action on the vagus nerves. It may therefore be given in an initial dose of 1 mg. and repeated in half this amount at four-hourly intervals. However, propantheline bromide (Pro-Banthine) is the more effective agent for relaxing the sphincter of Oddi and should be given in a dose of 15 to 30 mg. at six-hourly intervals. Antibiotics should be administered with the object of preventing secondary bacterial infection of the damaged tissues. Steroids are widely used in the treatment of acute pancreatitis but there is little evidence of their value in this condition. Mortality in acute pancreatitis is often aggravated by the release of an amine, kallikrinin, into the circulation with resulting hypotension and shock. Trasylol, a kallikrinin inhibitor manufactured from cat submandibular glands is now widely used by intravenous infusion but its therapeutic value is not yet established.

Prognosis. It is probable that where recovery occurs from an attack of acute pancreatitis, it is usually complete, and only a small minority of such cases experience recurrent episodes or pass insidiously into a state of chronic pancreatitis.

SUBACUTE PANCREATITIS

Inflammatory involvement of the pancreas, presumably blood-borne in origin, may occur as a complication of mumps, influenza, infective hepatitis and smallpox. This condition, often referred to as subacute pancreatitis, is not a serious one and suppuration never occurs. It is recognised by the occurrence of mild pyrexia, epigastric pain and abdominal discomfort. Rapid and complete recovery is the rule.

CHRONIC PANCREATITIS

This condition is due either to the laying down of excessive fibrous tissue in the pancreas as the result of recurrent inflammatory changes or to atrophy of acinar tissue subsequent to main duct obstruction. It may follow repeated attacks of acute or subacute pancreatitis or be associated with chronic inflammation of the biliary tract or with the penetration of a chronic duodenal ulcer into the pancreas. In many cases some cause of obstruction of the main pancreatic duct is found, including valerian stenosis, traumatic stricture, ampullary papilloma and lithiasis. In these conditions when fibrosis is present, it is most marked between the lobules of epithelial cells, and whereas the acinar tissue is destroyed, the internal secretory islet cells are spared for a long time. Pancreatic fibrosis of an intralobular type may occur in haemochromatosis with replacement of the parenchyma and early atrophy of the islet tissue. A congenital form is associated with cystic dilatation of the acini and with congenital cystic disease of the lungs and some of these patients survive to adult age. Chronic pancreatitis most commonly occurs in males in the fifth and sixth decades and many of these are alcoholics. Diffuse calcification of the sclerosed pancreas is usual in this group.

Clinical Features. These depend on the nature of the associated primary disease, the amount of destruction of the acinar and islet tissue and the degree of obstruction of the common bile duct caused by the fibrotic and sometimes enlarged head of the pancreas. Recurrent episodes of midabdominal and lumbar pain are common, often relieved by a crouching posture, lasting for three or four days, and accompanied by nausea, vomiting and pyrexia in many cases; but in some cases there may be no obvious clinical features and the condition is discovered only at autopsy or operation. Cases with haemochromatosis may show skin pigmentation (p. 1035). In others marked loss of weight occurs because of faulty digestion and absorption of foodstuffs and there is chronic diarrhoea with an excess of fat and undigested muscle fibres in the stools. Again the condition may manifest itself first by the development of painless, slowly progressive obstructive jaundice with enlargement of the liver. There may be a previous history of symptoms of chronic cholecystitis and gallstones. Ultimately the full picture of diabetes and malabsorption may supervene as both the acinar and islet tissues atrophy or are destroyed.

Diagnosis. A history of previous gall-bladder disease, especially cholilithiasis, or of excessive intake of alcohol, and succeeded by recurrent episodes of upper abdominal pain will usually be elicited. Characteristically the episodes of pain occur on the *day after* an occasion of dietary or alcoholic excess. If examination of the stools reveals an excess of fat and creatorrhoea and an increased output of faecal nitrogen, this provides strong evidence of pancreatic insufficiency in the absence of diarrhoea of intestinal origin. The association of these findings with glycosuria and a diabetic type of glucose tolerance curve is virtually diagnostic, especially when the excretion of an oral load of xylose remains normal (p. 943). Serum amylase estimations are of little value in the diagnosis of chronic pancreatitis. The pancreatic function test (p. 1056) often demonstrates low volume of secretion and reduced concentration of amylase and bicarbonate. When jaundice is present the condition must be distinguished from: (1) stone in the common bile duct, in which there is usually intermittent pain and fever and fluctuating jaundice, (2) carcinoma of the head of the pancreas or of the bile duct, in which the features are so similar that laparotomy is usually necessary to establish the diagnosis; and (3) chronic hepatitis with jaundice, in which there is some bile and an excess of fat in the stools. The finding of calcareous shadows in the region of the pancreas on radiological examination may suggest chronic pancreatitis. The uptake of ^{75}selenium-methionine in an isotope scan is poor and patchy or, in advanced disease absent. Tests for electrolyte content of sweat will be required if cystic fibrosis is suspected.

Treatment. When obstructive jaundice is present it should be relieved by surgical means. Otherwise the patient should be treated conservatively. The diet should be bland and low in roughage with small meals taken frequently. Alcohol should be prohibited. If steatorrhoea is present the fat intake should be restricted to about 45 g. daily as in Diet 6 (p. 1290). Fried, greasy and fat-rich foods must be excluded. To make up for the loss of calories from fat restriction, the diet must contain as much carbohydrate and protein as the patient can tolerate. A sufficiency of minerals and fat-soluble vitamins should be assured, the latter being given parenterally if necessary. Substitution therapy with adequate amounts of active pancreatic extracts is essential once steatorrhoea is present. These must be taken either sprinkled on the food or sipped in a liquid vehicle throughout each of the three main meals of the day. Their action is improved by the simultaneous administration of alkalis. Insulin injections are required when diabetes mellitus supervenes.

When more acute exacerbations of the chronic pancreatitis cause attacks of pain, the measures described for the relief of pain in acute pancreatitis should be employed. The surgical measures adopted in the treatment of chronic pancreatitis with episodes of pain, are the removal of gall-stones with cholecystectomy, sphincterotomy of the common bile duct, various procedures for anastomosing the pancreatic duct in the body and tail to a loop of jejunum, and splanchnic sympathectomy. Pancreatography by injecting the main duct (in the operating theatre) is the best guide to the procedure to be followed.

PANCREATIC CALCULI

Calcification occurs in about a third of cases of chronic pancreatitis and is especially common in the alcohol induced variety. Concretions of calcium carbonate in the ducts are usual, but a diffuse calcinosis in areas of fat necrosis in the parenchyma is found less often.

The condition may produce no special clinical features other than those that may be associated with chronic pancreatitis. In some cases attacks of severe, recurrent, colicky pain closely resembling gall-stone colic, may occur, though the pain may be more to the left side of the abdomen. Surgical removal of the calculi is possible in some cases where the calculi are in the main ducts. Symptomatic relief of pain by medical measures as described under acute pancreatitis is indicated where colic is severe. Retrograde drainage of the main pancreatic duct can relieve the underlying stasis and cause regression of calcification. Sympathectomy may be required in cases with persistent pain where drainage is unsuccessful or not possible.

PANCREATIC CYSTS

These are very rare and are broadly of three kinds: true acinous retention cysts of the ducts, proliferative cysts, which are tumours, and the so-called pseudo-pancreatic cysts which result from the liberation of blood and pancreatic secretions into the lesser peritoneal sac. The latter may occur after acute pancreatitis or follow traumatic rupture of the pancreas in injuries of the upper abdomen by impact or crushing. Some cysts of the pancreas give rise to very few clinical features while others may cause mechanical effects, and pseudocysts may result in persistent pain. Such cysts present usually as a tense rounded swelling in the epigastrium, and diagnosis is facilitated by a barium meal, isotope scanning or selective arteriography. Their treatment is operative and involves internal drainage into the alimentary tract, usually by anastomosis to the stomach.

TUMOURS OF THE PANCREAS

The two important tumours of the pancreas are carcinoma arising from the acinar epithelium and adenoma derived from the islets of Langerhans. Other much rarer primary pancreatic tumours occur, and secondary deposits from primary neoplasms elsewhere are not uncommon. Carcinoma arising from the ampulla of the bile duct is another important tumour occurring in this region.

CARCINOMA OF THE PANCREAS

This is an adenocarcinoma of scirrhous nature and in two-thirds of cases it is involvement of the head of the gland which causes symptoms and signs. It tends to metastasise early to neighbouring structures and to the liver. The condition is more common in males than in females, and occurs most frequently between the ages of 55 and 70.

Clinical Features. These depend very largely on the site of the growth. Epigastric pain which is one of the earliest and most significant symptoms may occasionally be absent throughout the course of the disease. The pain is variable in type but is characteristically dull and boring and radiates through to the back. It is often intensified by food and by lying supine and is especially noticed at night. It may be relieved by crouching forward. Vague dyspeptic symptoms are common and include anorexia, nausea, flatulent discomfort and sometimes vomiting. These symptoms may be the only manifestations until metastasis occurs. General emaciation occurs rapidly. In some cases jaundice is the presenting feature and may be painless and progressive. Jaundice may not appear at all in cases where the lesion affects mainly the body and tail of the pancreas, but in the majority with involvement of the head, deep obstructive jaundice with a large, firm liver eventually develops. In such cases a dilated gallbladder can frequently be palpated (p. 1046). The symptoms of diabetes mellitus (p. 744) may occasionally present in this disease.

Carcinoma of the pancreas is a rapidly progressive disease especially in cases in which the head is involved, when death usually occurs within six months of the onset of obstructive jaundice.

Diagnosis. The condition has to be distinguished from: (1) chronic pancreatitis, (2) chronic hepatitis, (3) stone in the common bile duct, and (4) other causes of obstruction to the biliary passages, especially ampullary carcinoma. Radiological examination by barium meal often shows distortion of the duodenal wall in carcinoma arising from the head of the pancreas and a pushing forward of the stomach in lesions of the body. Intravenous cholangiography in the absence of jaundice may reveal distortion of the common bile duct. In ampullary carcinoma fluctuating jaundice is common, often precedes pain, and blood may be aspirated from the duodenum and be detected on testing the stool. Pancreatic function tests should be carried out and where facilities for exfoliative cytology are available the duodenal aspirate should be examined for malignant cells. In all cases where the symptoms are suggestive or where the cause of obstructive jaundice cannot be firmly established, exploratory laparotomy should be advised. Unless this is done, those cases of stone in the common bile duct in which pain is not a prominent feature may be erroneously diagnosed as carcinoma. Isotope scanning with ^{75}selenium and selective arteriography are now established methods of delineating the tumours.

Treatment. This is by surgical means. In carcinoma of the pancreas radical surgery is rarely possible, but a by-pass may be fashioned to relieve the obstructive jaundice. Such patients, however, rarely live more than one year. In early cases of ampullary carcinoma pancreatico-duodenectomy may achieve a cure.

ISLET-CELL TUMOURS

Benign adenomas may arise rarely from the beta cells of the islets. They are usually very small and in 10 per cent. of cases are multiple. They produce hyperinsulinism and the syndrome of attacks of spontaneous hypoglycaemia (p. 764). Even more rare

are tumours, usually malignant, from non-specific islet cells which elaborate polypeptides, the secretion of which into the blood causes a variety of syndromes. The most common is the Zollinger-Ellison syndrome in which gastric hypersecretion and severe persistent peptic ulceration are present. A profound electrolyte and water-losing diarrhoea occurs in others. The treatment of these conditions is by the surgical removal of the adenomas, where possible, or by total gastrectomy in the gastric hypersecretion syndrome.

PREVENTION OF DISEASES OF THE PANCREAS

In view of the present lack of knowledge regarding the causation of most diseases of the pancreas, little can be done for their prevention. If, however, it is accepted that coincidental infective processes in the biliary tract are of aetiological importance in a proportion of cases of pancreatic conditions, measures for the prevention and early treatment of biliary infections may be considered of value in the prophylaxis of disease of the pancreas. Caution regarding the excessive intake of alcohol should be advocated for those who have had attacks of pancreatitis.

JAMES INNES.
WILFRED SIRCUS.

Book recommended:

Bockus, H. L. (1965). *Gastroenterology*, vol 3. p. 121. London: Saunders.

DISEASES OF THE NERVOUS SYSTEM

FACED with a neurological problem, the student is usually bemused by the multiplicity of symptoms and signs. A fundamental error is the belief in the 'diagnostic sign'. Charcot's triad (intention tremor, nystagmus, scanning speech) does not indicate that the patient has disseminated sclerosis but only that there is a lesion in certain cerebellar pathways, that is, it has localising value but does not indicate the nature of the pathology. The physician gets his clues from the manner in which it develops. This principle applies in every branch of medicine, but in neurology it is particularly important. The history of the illness must be considered chronologically in broad outline for this purpose. Attention to the symptoms and signs which indicate loss of function of particular parts of the nervous system then follows for purposes of localisation.

Sudden onset of symptoms which reach their maximum almost immediately, remain maximal for a short time if the patient survives, and then recover completely or with a residual deficit, indicate that the lesion is traumatic or due to a vascular catastrophe.

Inflammatory lesions such as infections develop rapidly but less acutely than traumatic or vascular catastrophies and the recovery phase is, generally, also more rapid and complete.

The paroxysmal disorders of function recover after each attack. A history of this type is always suggestive of epilepsy (p. 1116) but migraine and transient vascular attacks should be borne in mind.

Disease which progresses from an ill-defined onset and shows no tendency to improve is likely to be degenerative or neoplastic. Rapid progressive deterioration is more likely to be neoplastic, though the converse is not true since some encapsulated tumours may cause symptoms extending over many years. As a general rule, degenerative diseases affect specific cell systems and occur bilaterally (cf. paralysis agitans, Friedreich's ataxia, subacute combined degeneration of the cord, muscular dystrophy). Neoplasm, on the other hand, is no respecter of functional or anatomical boundaries and the clinical features indicate progressive involvement of anatomically adjacent nerve fibres. With neoplasm too, the pace of development accelerates and mechanical effects may be produced which cause abrupt new symptoms due to obstruction of venous or cerebrospinal fluid drainage, and physical occupation of space in a non-expansile cavity such as the skull or spinal canal.

A stair-case progression suggests a degenerative disease due to the cumulative effect of minor vascular lesions—e.g. cerebral atherosclerosis (p. 1136). A relapsing and remitting curve of inflammatory episodes with early complete remission but later cumulative loss of function, is characteristic of disseminated sclerosis (and perhaps of immunological disorders in general).

APPLIED ANATOMY AND PHYSIOLOGY

The Divisions of the Nervous System

The Motor System

Movements, whether voluntary or involuntary, are the result of the contraction or controlled relaxation of groups of muscles and never of a single muscle only. This is effected by contraction of muscles which act as prime movers and reciprocal relaxation of their antagonists. The action of the prime movers is provided with a firm base by contraction of synergists which stabilise the joints, and by appropriate adjustments of posture. The postural adjustments are largely under the control of the extrapyramidal motor system and the vestibular and spinal reflexes. Voluntary movements require the participation of the pre-central gyrus of the cerebral cortex ('motor area') and the timing and degree of contraction or relaxation of the muscles of the synergy are co-ordinated by the cerebellum, especially when a movement involves more than one segment of a limb. The action of the upper motor neurones from the motor area of the cortex, the extrapyramidal motor system and the cerebellum are brought directly or indirectly to the cells of the anterior horn of spinal grey matter or motor cranial nuclei from which the lower motor neurone runs to a group of muscle fibres ('motor unit'). Thus the lower motor neurone is the 'final common path' for all efferent impulses directed at the muscle and the groups of anterior horn cells may be considered to 'represent a muscle' in the same sense as the cells of the motor cortex 'represent a movement'. This distinction is vital to an understanding of the signs and disorders of the motor system.

Upper Motor Neurone. The fibres arise from cells in the precentral gyrus ('motor area'). These initiate movements of different parts of the opposite side of the body, the parts being represented in the following order from below upwards—tongue, face, hand, forearm, arm, trunk, thigh, leg, foot and perineal areas with considerable overlap. The cortical area representing movements of each of these parts is proportional to its functional importance rather than to its anatomical size. The projections of the upper motor neurones to the contralateral motor nuclei of the brain stem and anterior horn of the spinal cord are shown in Figure 66.

A destructive lesion of the indirect corticospinal tract above its decussation causes a loss of some voluntary movements of part of the opposite side of the body, according to the fibres involved, but automatic associated movements, such as the stretching of a paralysed arm when yawning, may persist and other voluntary or reflex movements using the same lower motor neurones and muscles may be preserved. This is the essential difference between paralysis of upper motor neurone type and that due to a lower motor neurone lesion. For the same reason stretch reflexes are retained but these are usually of heightened activity. This indicates that the pyramidal tract normally carries fibres which are inhibitory to the stretch reflex. The pattern of cutaneous protective reflexes also changes, causing the emergence of the Babinski reflex. There are thus two types of disturbance, a negative one due to loss of a particular activity, and a positive one due to the release of lower levels from control. Hughlings Jackson considered that this is a principle of general application in the nervous system and the concept is important in understanding the signs of extrapyramidal disease. Another type of positive symptom results from irritative lesions (usually incomplete damage to a nerve cell or its fibre) which cause spontaneous activity of the affected neurones. Paraesthesia is a good example of a symptom due to spontaneous activity in sensory fibres. Spontaneous activity in upper motor neurones causes involuntary movements as in focal epilepsy (p. 1120).

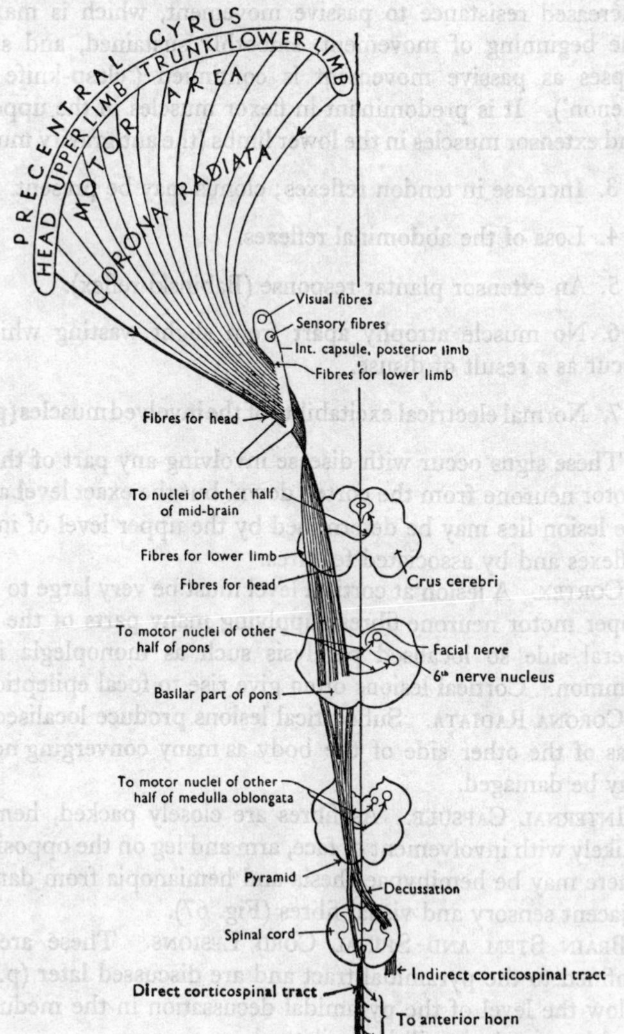

FIG. 66

THE MOTOR PATHWAYS

Disorders of the upper motor neurone cause:

1. Weakness or paralysis of movements of part of one side of the

body. (Other movements using the same muscles may be spared.)

2. Increase of tone of spastic type. This is characterised by an increased resistance to passive movement, which is maximal at the beginning of movement, smoothly sustained, and suddenly lapses as passive movement is continued ('clasp-knife phenomenon'). It is predominant in flexor muscles in the upper limbs and extensor muscles in the lower limbs (the antigravity muscles).

3. Increase in tendon reflexes; clonus may be present.

4. Loss of the abdominal reflexes.

5. An extensor plantar response (Babinski reflex).

6. No muscle atrophy apart from slight wasting which may occur as a result of disuse.

7. Normal electrical excitability of the involved muscles (p. 1073).

These signs occur with disease involving any part of the upper motor neurone from the cortex down, but the exact level at which the lesion lies may be determined by the upper level of increased reflexes and by associated features.

CORTEX. A lesion at cortical level must be very large to damage upper motor neurone fibres supplying many parts of the contralateral side so localised paralysis such as monoplegia is more common. Cortical lesions often give rise to focal epileptic fits.

CORONA RADIATA. Subcortical lesions produce localised weakness of the other side of the body as many converging neurones may be damaged.

INTERNAL CAPSULE. As fibres are closely packed, hemiplegia is likely with involvement of face, arm and leg on the opposite side. There may be hemihypaesthesia and hemianopia from damage to adjacent sensory and visual fibres (Fig. 67).

BRAIN STEM AND SPINAL CORD LESIONS. These are rarely confined to the pyramidal tract and are discussed later (p. 1083). Below the level of the pyramidal decussation in the medulla, the resulting paralysis will be ipsilateral.

Lower Motor Neurone. From the cells of the anterior horn of the spinal cord and the motor cranial nerve nuclei emerge axons which pass through the anterior nerve root to enter a mixed peripheral nerve in which they run to the muscles or glands which they supply. There are two types, a large fibred (alpha) efferent neurone and a small fibred (gamma) efferent neurone (Fig. 68). The term 'lower motor neurone' is usually confined to the large fibred system. Each lower motor neurone has a terminal branching so that it is distributed to the motor end-plates of a group of

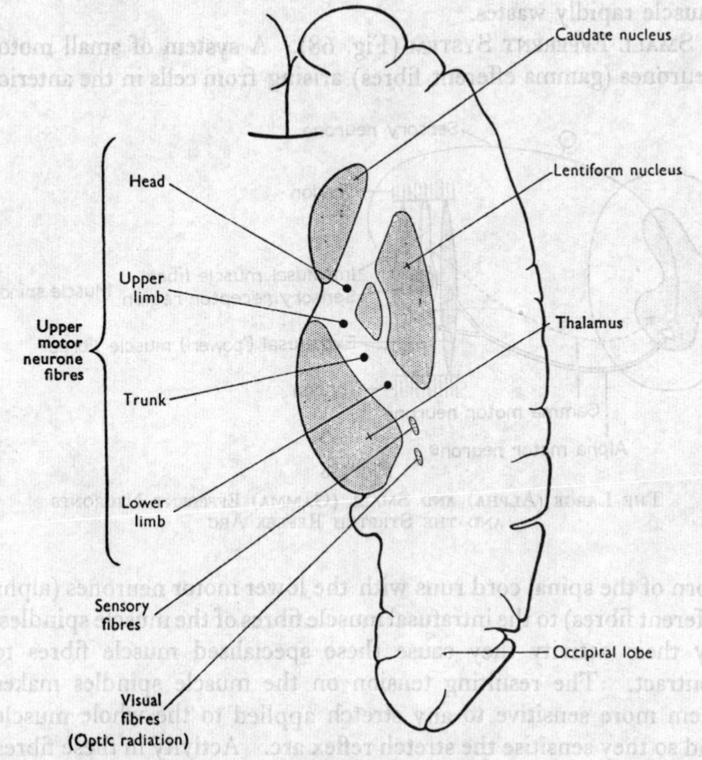

FIG. 67
SCHEMATIC HORIZONTAL SECTION THROUGH THE RIGHT CEREBRAL HEMISPHERE SHOWING POSITION OF SOME OF THE FIBRES IN THE INTERNAL CAPSULE

muscle fibres or to a gland. The anterior horn cell body, axon and a group of muscle fibres is the motor-unit and each muscle is composed of a large number of such units. The anterior horn cell is activated by impulses from the corticospinal tracts, from the extrapyramidal tracts, and from some of the posterior nerve root afferent fibres responsible for spinal reflexes. The lower motor neurone (alpha efferent fibre) is thus an integral part of the spinal reflex arc and is the final common pathway for all motor impulses, involuntary or voluntary, directed to a muscle. Normal nutrition of a muscle appears to depend on its contact with the spinal cord through the lower motor neurone since if it is interrupted the muscle rapidly wastes.

Small Efferent System (Fig. 68). A system of small motor neurones (gamma efferent fibres) arising from cells in the anterior

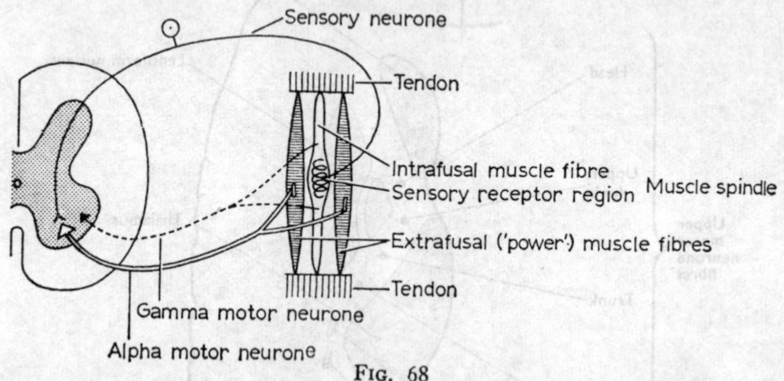

Fig. 68

The Large (Alpha) and Small (Gamma) Efferent Neurones and the Stretch Reflex Arc

horn of the spinal cord runs with the lower motor neurones (alpha efferent fibres) to the intrafusal muscle fibres of the muscle spindles. By their activity they cause these specialised muscle fibres to contract. The resulting tension on the muscle spindles makes them more sensitive to any stretch applied to the whole muscle and so they sensitise the stretch reflex arc. Activity in these fibres is regulated by supraspinal influences from the anterior lobe of the cerebellum and the reticulospinal system and will be affected in disorders of the cerebellum and extrapyramidal motor system. The small efferent system is important in the regulation of muscle tone. It may be utilised for controlled voluntary movements, the corticospinal activity first passing to the intrafusal muscle fibres of the spindles. The latter respond to the tension induced and in turn activate the alpha motor neurones which cause the main muscle fibres to contract.

Disease of the lower motor neurone results in the following signs which will be present only in those muscles supplied by the particular neurones affected:

1. Weakness or paralysis of muscles. This affects all movements in which they take part whether as prime movers or synergists, voluntary or involuntary, or in reflex contractions.

2. Loss of tone on passive movement (flaccidity).

3. Wasting of the affected muscles which appears within two or three weeks of an acute lesion (atrophy).

4. Absence of reflexes subserved by the affected neurones. Abdominal and plantar reflexes remain normal unless the neurones to the appropriate muscles are damaged when they cannot be elicited.

5. Fibrillation in a denervated muscle may be detected by electromyography. This is spontaneous contraction of single muscle fibres which appears when they are no longer influenced by the lower motor neurone. If the latter is damaged but still capable of conducting impulses it may initiate spontaneous discharges which are distributed to bundles of muscle fibres. The resulting contraction ('fasciculation') is visible under the skin but fibrillation is not. Fibrillation is always pathological but fasciculation may be physiological in overtired and anxious people.

6. Contractures of muscles due to replacement by fibrous tissue and 'trophic' changes such as dryness and cyanosis of the skin, and brittleness of the nails, partly due to impaired circulation.

7. The electrical excitability of the peripheral nerves and muscles is altered as can be shown by special tests. They may usefully be combined with electromyography to confirm that a weak and wasted muscle is denervated. Lesions of peripheral nerves short of complete interruption may cause slowing of conduction which can be measured by special techniques.

If lower motor neurones are damaged in the cord or nerve roots the muscles and reflexes affected in the ways described above will be those supplied by one or more segments of the spinal cord. If the neurones are damaged more peripherally after they have been redistributed in the nerve plexuses, the paralysis will occur in the territory supplied by the appropriate peripheral nerve and it is probable that there will be similar damage to the sensory fibres with which they are associated in the mixed nerve.

Extrapyramidal System. This consists of all descending neurones other than the corticospinal and its full complexity is not yet determined. There are three main levels which doubtless

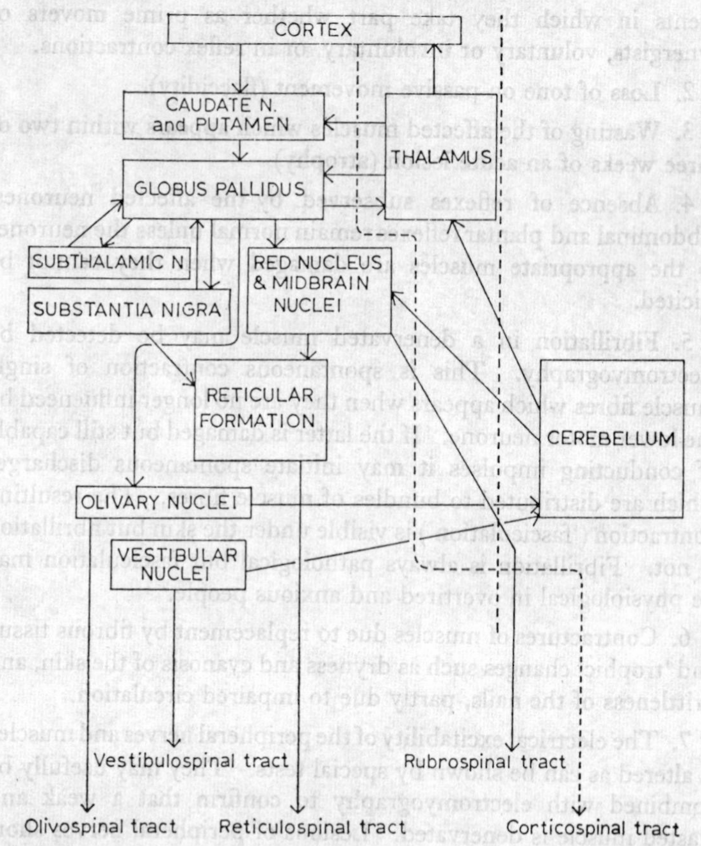

FIG. 69

DIAGRAM OF THE EXTRAPYRAMIDAL MOTOR SYSTEM

interact, the higher levels tending to control the lower by inhibition, and so the signs of disease are partly due to 'release phenomena' (p. 1068). These are (*a*) the caudate nucleus and putamen, (*b*) the globus pallidus (pallidum), and (*c*) the red nucleus, reticular formation and other lower centres (Fig. 69). It is not certain whether the main outflow from the globus pallidus is to the reticular formation of the medulla or to the cortex via the ventrolateral nucleus of the thalamus. Efferent impulses from the thalamus and cortex enter the caudate-putamen-pallidum complex (jointly called the corpus striatum). The activity of the globus pallidus is further modified by to and fro connections with the substantia nigra and the subthalamic nucleus. Some efferent fibres from the globus pallidus pass to the tegmentum and possibly to the red nucleus.

The extrapyramidal system regulates the activity of the lower motor neurones mainly through the reticulo-spinal, olivo-spinal and vestibulo-spinal tracts by a balance of facilitatory and inhibitory impulses. This regulation may be through a direct influence on the anterior horn cells, or these may be excited or depressed by regulation of the discharge of small efferent motor nerves to the spindles (p. 1072 and Fig. 68).

The functional role of the extrapyramidal system in health is not known but it is believed to control the 'set' of the muscles from which voluntary activity originates and the involuntary movements required to adjust the parts of the body for maintenance of posture. Disease of this system is characterised by: disturbance of voluntary movement; disturbance of tone; involuntary movement.

Disturbance of Voluntary Movement. There is no true paralysis in extrapyramidal disease, but rather slowness of movement and poverty of movement in that spontaneous gestures, changes in facial expression, and associated movements for postural adjustment such as swinging the arm when walking are lost on the side opposite to the lesion.

Disturbance of Tone. Tone may be increased as in Parkinsonism or decreased as in chorea. Increase in tone, of extrapyramidal type, has characteristic features. It is present throughout the whole range of passive movement; it affects opposing muscle groups equally; it may be smooth and plastic ('lead-pipe rigidity') or intermittent ('cog-wheel rigidity') which is more common.

Involuntary Movement. There are many varieties but four important types may be described. Some involuntary movements such as focal epilepsy, tics and fasciculation are not extrapyramidal in origin and are excluded from this list.

1. *Tremor*. This consists of rhythmic movements caused by alternate contraction of opposing groups of muscle. Tremor at rest is typical of Parkinsonism. Other causes

are thyrotoxicosis and anxiety neurosis but these are more rapid and finer than extrapyramidal tremor.

2. *Choreiform movements.* These are quasi-purposive, non-repetitive jerky movements of face, tongue or limbs. They give the impression that some action is about to be undertaken, but is suddenly broken off by interposition of another purposive movement.
3. *Athetosis.* Athetoid movements are slow, sinuous writhing movements of the face and limbs, being most marked peripherally.
4. *Dystonia.* Movements resembling athetosis but much slower affect the proximal parts of the limbs and the trunk which tends to rotate ('torsion spasm'). The movements are so slow that they may cause prolonged abnormal postures.

Cerebellum. The cerebellum is the most important part of the nervous system for the co-ordination of movement and the muscular contractions required to maintain posture. The cerebellum receives impulses from many sources, principally the proprioceptive end-organs, the skin, the vestibular nuclei and the cerebral cortex. The pontine nuclei and the inferior olive relay fibres from the cerebral motor cortex and basal ganglia respectively to the cerebellar cortex of the opposite side. The cerebellar cortex integrates this information about body posture, limb position and motor intention and sends efferent fibres via the cerebellar nuclei to the reticular formation, red nucleus and vestibular nucleus of the opposite side, whence fibres descend to influence both types of motor cells in the anterior horns of the spinal cord; as these descending fibres cross again each cerebellar hemisphere controls the ipsilateral side of the body. Efferent fibres from the cerebellum also ascend to the contralateral thalamus through which it influences the cerebral cortex. The cerebellum is therefore a great co-ordinating centre controlling the synergic action of muscles during voluntary and automatic movements and adjusting posture. It determines whether a movement will be carried out by the lower motor neurones directly or by the slightly slower but more controlled indirect route through the small efferent system and the peripheral reflex arc (p. 1072). Disturbance of the latter route lowers the excitability of tendon reflexes.

The effects of disease of the cerebellum are best seen in acute lesions, for in chronic lesions considerable compensation occurs so that the deficit is less than might be expected. A lesion of the cerebellar hemisphere produces all its effects on the same side of the body. The principal effects are:

MUSCULAR HYPOTONIA. The muscles are flaccid on palpation, show diminished resistance to passive movement and, when an outstretched limb is suddenly displaced, it makes a greater excursion than usual and oscillates before resuming its posture.

DISTURBANCE OF TENDON REFLEXES. The reflexes are either diminished or pendular as when the knee jerk is followed by a series of diminishing oscillations.

DISTURBANCE OF POSTURE AND OF GAIT. The head may be tilted towards the side of the lesion and the patient leans or may even fall towards that side. His gait is reeling and he tends to stagger to the side of the lesion.

DISORDERS OF MOVEMENT. Incoordination, hypotonia and the fact that muscular contraction is unregulated by the muscle spindles cause ataxia which manifests itself in different ways:

Dysmetria. Movements are not accurately adjusted to their object, so that the finger may overshoot or fall short of the object it is required to touch. If a movement is attempted with the eyes closed the finger overshoots towards the side of the cerebellar lesion ('past-pointing').

Dyssynergia. Movements involving more than one joint are broken up into their component parts.

Intention Tremor. A combination of dyssynergia and dysmetria causes faulty correction of the badly directed limb movement so that it approaches the target in a zig-zag manner. The coarse irregular tremor increases as the target is approached. It is not increased when the eyes are closed. The contraction of muscles necessary to maintain a posture may be similarly affected so that tremor at rest occasionally occurs in cerebellar disorders.

Dysdiadochokinesis. The arrest of one movement and its immediate replacement with the opposite movement requires accurate co-ordination of the various muscles of the synergy. Rapidly alternating movements are therefore disturbed and carried out in a clumsy, irregular, jerky fashion.

Rebound phenomenon. For the same reason a strong contraction cannot be arrested when resistance is suddenly removed, whereupon the limb shoots beyond the normal range.

Disorders of Articulation and Phonation. Articulation is irregular, slurred and explosive as the volume of sound is poorly controlled. A rarer form of dysarthria is scanning-speech in which the syllables tend to be separated from each other.

Disturbance of Eye Movements. Jerking nystagmus in the horizontal plane is commonly seen. It is a defect of postural fixation involving conjugate gaze (p. 1099). In a unilateral cerebellar lesion the movements are greater in amplitude and slower in rate when the eyes are deviated to the side of the lesion.

The Sensory System

Superficial sensation, which arises from the skin has four primary components, touch, pain, warmth and cold. *Deep sensations* arising from subcutaneous structures are deep pain, pressure and proprioception which enables the recognition of movements of joints and the position of the parts of the body relative to one another. Vibration is a sensation due to rhythmical stimulation of groups of deep or superficial touch receptors. Some of the afferent impulses carried in 'sensory' nerve fibres do not reach consciousness but convey impulses directly or indirectly to motor neurones for reflex functions or to the cerebellum for purposes of co-ordination e.g. impulses arising in muscle and tendon receptors. All sensory impulses arise in the sensory receptors or end-organs which are widely distributed throughout the body. It is probable, though debatable, that specialised receptors respond to specific types of stimuli. Stimulation of an end-organ causes impulses to pass along the first sensory neurone to the spinal cord. This neurone has its cell body in a dorsal root ganglion but does not synapse until it reaches a second order neurone in the spinal cord or brain stem. On entering the cord by the posterior nerve root, fibres subserving proprioception, vibration and a proportion of touch sensation turn medially and ascend in the posterior column of the same side to the lower part of the medulla oblongata to synapse with cells in the gracile and cuneate nuclei. From there, the second order neurone crosses to the other side of the medulla and ascends in the medial lemniscus to the main sensory nucleus of the thalamus.

Fibres subserving pain, warmth, cold and the remainder of touch sensation synapse in the posterior horn of the spinal cord soon after entering it. Most of the second order neurones cross at the

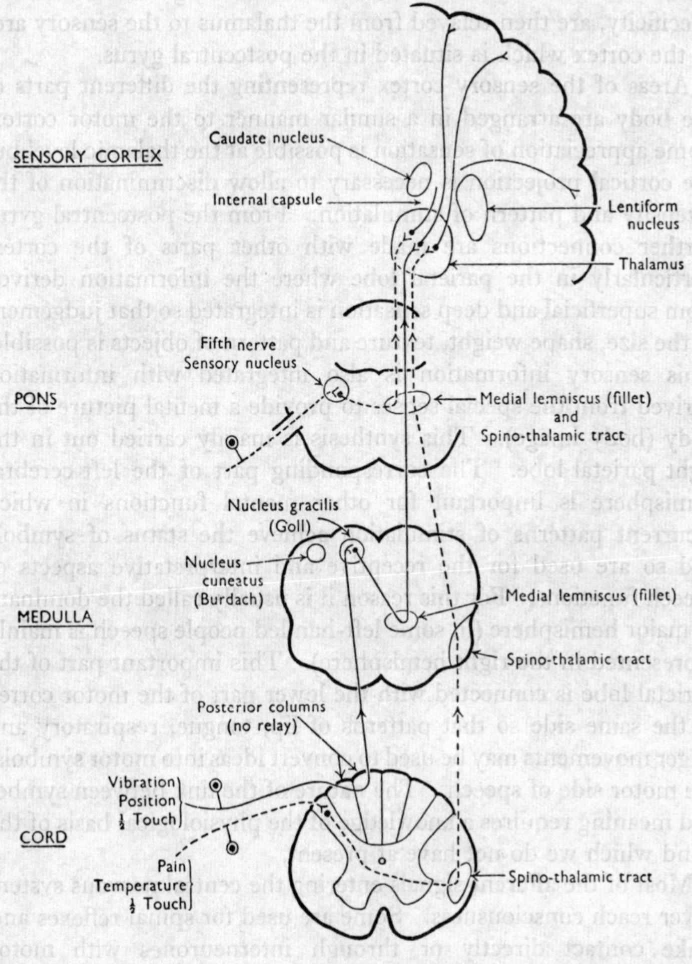

FIG. 70
DIAGRAM OF THE MAIN SENSORY PATHWAYS

same level, or one or two segments higher, to reach the antero-lateral column where they ascend to the thalamus as the spino-thalamic tract. Some of these fibres do not cross but enter the ipsilateral spinothalamic tract. As it ascends through the brain stem the tract gradually intermingles with the medial lemniscus and terminates along with it in the main sensory nucleus of the thalamus. Third order neurones, maintaining their functional specificity, are then relayed from the thalamus to the sensory area of the cortex which is situated in the postcentral gyrus.

Areas of the sensory cortex representing the different parts of the body are arranged in a similar manner to the motor cortex. Some appreciation of sensation is possible at the thalamic level but the cortical projection is necessary to allow discrimination of the intensity and pattern of stimulation. From the postcentral gyrus further connections are made with other parts of the cortex, particularly in the parietal lobe where the information derived from superficial and deep sensation is integrated so that judgement of the size, shape weight, texture and pattern of objects is possible. This sensory information is also integrated with information derived from the special senses to provide a mental picture of the body (body image). This synthesis is mainly carried out in the right parietal lobe. The corresponding part of the left cerebral hemisphere is important for other mental functions in which recurrent patterns of stimulation achieve the status of symbols and so are used for the receptive and interpretative aspects of speech functions. For this reason it is usually called the dominant or major hemisphere (in some left-handed people speech is mainly represented in the right hemisphere). This important part of the parietal lobe is connected with the lower part of the motor cortex of the same side so that patterns of lip, tongue, respiratory and finger movements may be used to convert ideas into motor symbols, the motor side of speech. The nature of the link between symbol and meaning requires a knowledge of the physiological basis of the mind which we do not have at present.

Most of the afferent signals entering the central nervous system never reach consciousness. Some are used for spinal reflexes and make contact directly or through interneurones with motor neurones. Other fibres which also originate in muscle receptors end at the base of the posterior horn in contact with second order neurones. These neurones turn laterally to the periphery of the cord to ascend in the anterior and posterior spino-cerebellar tracts to the cerebellar cortex. Most of these ascend without crossing but some second order neurones cross to the opposite anterior spino-cerebellar tract. These fibres carry some of the proprioceptive information required to enable the cerebellum to co-ordinate limb movements. Still other sensory fibres, which do not carry 'sensation' in the ordinary sense, are extremely important for the maintenance of consciousness. These are collateral branches of the main spinothalamic pathways and of the special sensory tracts which turn medially into the upper part of the reticular formation in the mid-brain. Here there is a chain of short neurones with intimate inter-connections which also receives neurones from most parts of the cerebral cortex. It is therefore an important integrating centre. At its upper end it communicates with the non-specific nuclei of the thalamus which relay impulses to all areas of the cortex. Activity in this system is considered to be essential for the conscious state and may be important in some mental functions in collaboration with the cerebral cortex.

Disease of the sensory system may be accompanied by positive phenomena such as pain or paraesthesiae due to spontaneous activity or irritation of sensory neurones, or by negative phenomena in which there is loss of the ability to appreciate some modality of sensation (anaesthesia and analgesia). These symptoms occur only with disorders of the first or second order neurones, i.e. from the end-organs to the thalamus. Suprathalamic lesions show certain differences. Paraesthesia may occur with irritative lesions of the sensory cortex but anaesthesia does not. Instead there is a loss of sensory discrimination and of the spatial and quantitative aspects of sensation.

Peripheral Nerve. With a complete lesion all forms of sensation are lost in the area supplied by the affected nerve, but the zone of anaesthesia may be limited by the fact that neighbouring nerves overlap into its territory, the extent varying from person to person. The resistance of different types of fibres to disease need not be the same so that it is common for one type of cutaneous or deep sensation to be more affected than another and indeed some may be spared. If the afferent fibres of a reflex arc are affected, as the sciatic nerve in the ankle jerk, the reflex concerned is lost. Some neuropathies (p. 1217) do not affect individual nerves but rather damage fibres selectively. As a general rule the longest fibres are most susceptible and so the sensory and motor disturbance is first noticed at the tips of all the toes and fingers, irrespective of nerve supply, and spreads proximally as the advancing disease involves progressively shorter fibres. This produces a 'glove and stocking' distribution of sensory loss.

Posterior Root. The different forms of sensation are affected by a posterior root lesion in the same way as for a peripheral nerve but the distribution of the loss follows a dermatome pattern or motor deficit. The overlap from adjacent roots may be so great that no anaesthesia can be detected. When the root is irritated pain and paraesthesia are experienced in the full dermatomal distribution of the root and pain may also be experienced in the deep structures such as muscles and ligaments which are supplied by the root. (These structures do not necessarily underlie the dermatome.) Any reflex subserved by the involved root is also lost, for example, the ankle jerk when the S1 posterior root is damaged by a prolapsed intervertebral disc.

Posterior Column. A lesion confined to the posterior column of the spinal cord will cause loss of position and vibration sense on the same side, but the sensations of pain, touch, warmth and cold will be preserved (Fig. 71). The loss of the sense of position causes sensory ataxia since the patient is unable to control his movements by awareness of the position achieved at each instant. Sensory ataxia differs from cerebellar ataxia in that it is more marked when the eyes are closed, because vision can compensate to a certain extent for loss of proprioceptive information. Thus there is unsteadiness in the finger-nose test which is greater when the eyes are closed but without the marked tremor of cerebellar ataxia. The gait is ataxic and the patient walks with a broad base to give himself a firmer foundation and steps high to make sure that his feet clear the ground which he is unable to feel with certainty. If his eyes are closed he is unable to stand with feet close together without swaying (Romberg's test). Vibration sense is abolished below the level of the lesion ipsilaterally. The same symptoms will be found if the first order neurones of the proprioceptive nerve fibres are damaged peripherally but they will then be associated with other signs of peripheral nerve disease.

Spinothalamic Tract. Lesions of the anterior and lateral spinothalamic tracts in the anterolateral columns of the cord or their continuation through the brain stem cause impairment of the ability to appreciate pain, warmth and cold on the contralateral side of the body below the level of the lesion. Touch is usually modified (it feels 'different') but not abolished because of its alternative pathway in the posterior columns. This is the situation produced by the operation of anterolateral cordotomy for the relief of intractable pain.

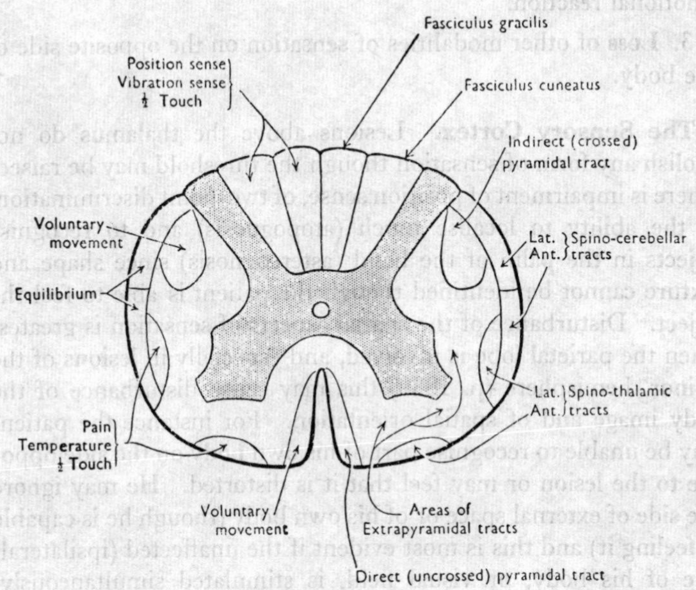

FIG. 71

CROSS-SECTION OF SPINAL CORD

Brain Stem. Since the spinothalamic tract and medial lemniscus run close together and eventually intermingle, lesions of the upper brain stem usually affect all forms of sensation on the contralateral side of the body. With mid-brain lesions the hemihypaesthesia will extend to the face, but with ponto-medullary lesions the second order neurones from the trigeminal sensory nucleus or the nucleus and descending tract of the fifth nerve may be damaged so that sensory loss will be on the same side of the face as the lesion but on the contralateral side of the rest of the body (p. 1140 and Fig. 74).

Thalamus. Lesions of the main sensory nucleus in the lateral part of the thalamus may cause:

1. Spontaneous pain of most unpleasant quality in the opposite side of the body.
2. The threshold for pain is raised on the opposite side of the body but when it is exceeded the resulting pain is exquisite and has the same unpleasant quality which often causes considerable emotional reaction.
3. Loss of other modalities of sensation on the opposite side of the body.

The Sensory Cortex. Lesions above the thalamus do not abolish any form of sensation though the threshold may be raised. There is impairment of position sense, of two-point discrimination, of the ability to localise touch (atopognosis) and to recognise objects in the palm of the hand (astereognosis) since shape and texture cannot be identified though the patient is able to feel the object. Disturbance of the spatial aspects of sensation is greatest when the parietal lobe is involved, and especially in lesions of the 'minor' hemisphere (p. 1080) this may cause disturbance of the body image and of spatial orientation. For instance the patient may be unable to recognise part of his own body on the side opposite to the lesion or may feel that it is distorted. He may ignore one side of external space or of his own body (though he is capable of feeling it) and this is most evident if the unaffected (ipsilateral) side of his body, or visual field, is stimulated simultaneously. When presented with this 'perceptual rivalry' his brain 'ignores' the stimulus on the side contralateral to the affected parietal lobe though a stimulus applied to that part alone would be recognised immediately. Lesions of the dominant hemisphere (p. 1080) in the region where parietal, temporal and occipital lobes meet (angular and supramarginal gyri) are associated with receptive dysphasia (p. 1091). This is a special case of the failure to analyse the temporal and spatial aspects of sensory stimuli.

The Reflexes

Certain functions are economically catered for by the nervous system by means of reflexes, which are short chains of neurones (the reflex arc) connecting a receptor to an effector organ such as muscle or gland, so that an appropriate stimulus invariably leads to a specific response. The quantity but not the nature of the response may be modified by other stimuli or by supraspinal influences from the cortex (p. 1070), extrapyramidal system (p. 1075) or the cerebellum (p. 1076). There are two main categories of reflex (1) postural and (2) protective. The appropriate stimuli for postural reflexes are (*a*) muscle stretch and (*b*) vestibular impulses from the inner ear. Protective reflexes are evoked by stimuli to pain receptors. They are usually superficial (cutaneous or corneal) but the protective 'spasm' of muscles around a painful lesion is similar in nature.

Stretch Reflexes (Tendon Jerks). A basic postural reflex depends on the stimulation of muscle spindles when a skeletal muscle is stretched. The afferent fibre enters the cord by a posterior nerve root and communicates directly or via a chain of interneurones with the anterior horn cells which control the stretched muscle, thus causing it to contract and so resist the displacement. A sudden tap to a tendon activates only the monosynaptic arc (in which the afferent fibre terminates at the anterior horn cell without interneurones) and this results in a sharp but brief contraction of the muscle. For the contraction to be sufficient to cause a visible movement the sensitivity of the stretch receptor must be potentiated by contraction of its intrafusal muscle fibres by the activity of the small efferent motor neurones (p. 1072). This activity may be increased by certain manoeuvres such as clenching the teeth or pulling the interlocked hands apart. This is termed reinforcement of the reflex and a tendon jerk should not be declared absent until reinforcement has failed to make it visible. The stretch reflex is inhibited by receptors in the tendon (and accessory receptors on the muscle spindles) if muscle tension rises too high, thus risking the integrity of its fibres. This may happen when the reflex is exaggerated by withdrawal of a normal inhibitory effect of the corticospinal tract (p. 1070), so that the contraction is abruptly stopped. This is the mechanism of the 'clasp-knife' response. There are also supraspinal facilitatory and inhibitory influences from the extrapyramidal system and cerebellum so lesions of these systems may abolish the reflexes.

An example of a monosynaptic stretch reflex is a knee jerk. A tap on the patellar tendon activates stretch receptors in the quadriceps muscle giving rise to impulses in first order sensory neurones which pass directly to the lower motor neurones to the quadriceps muscle making it contract. A lesion anywhere along this path will cause loss of the reflex, hence it is important in the localisation of disease to know through which spinal segment each reflex passes. The common tendon reflexes are the brachioradialis or supinator (C 5-6), the biceps (C 5-6), the triceps (C 7), the knee (L 3-4) and the ankle (S 1).

Superficial Reflexes. These are polysynaptic reflexes originating from stimuli to superficial structures. The interneurones may connect with motor neurones at several segmental levels and so the response may be a co-ordinated movement, usually designed to withdraw the stimulated part from a potentially dangerous stimulus. There are very many of these reflexes, some of which are conflicting. For example, stimulation of the sole of the foot evokes both flexion and extension reflexes. Which reflex will predominate is determined by higher influences. The nature of this influence is unknown but is believed to require the corticospinal (pyramidal) tract and damage to this tract will cause a change in the predominant reflex pattern.

The Plantar Reflex. When the outer border of the sole of the foot is stroked in normal people after infancy, there is plantar flexion of the great toe. In 1896 Babinski pointed out that when the upper motor neurone was damaged the same stimulus caused dorsiflexion of the toe. (Anatomically this is described as an extensor plantar response though physiologically it is part of the flexion withdrawal reflex.) When the reflex is well developed it can be elicited from the medial side of the sole of the foot or even from the lower part of the leg and the hallux response is accompanied by dorsiflexion and abduction or fanning of the other toes and even withdrawal of the limb. The fundamental importance of the extensor plantar or Babinski response as a sign of loss of function of the upper motor neurone is widely accepted but it may occur in transient form during temporary states such as coma or after an epileptic fit and need not indicate permanent damage. It is often extensor in normal infants during the first year of life.

The Abdominal Reflexes. When the skin on one side of the abdominal wall is stroked with a pin, there is a reflex contraction of the underlying muscles, a reflex for protection of the viscera. This may be lost on the affected side in disease of the upper motor neurone though the sign is less reliable than the plantar reflex. For instance the abdominal reflexes may be lost early in disseminated sclerosis yet retained despite severe pyramidal tract damage in motor neurone disease. The abdominal reflexes may not be obtainable on either side in elderly, obese or multiparous patients, and may be lost where operative incisions have severed the nerves concerned. The abdominal reflexes are served in their peripheral course by the intercostal nerves and segments Th. 8 to 12.

THE CORNEAL REFLEX. A light touch on the cornea provokes a blink of the eyelids on both sides. The afferent path for this reflex is the first division of the trigeminal nerve and the efferent path is the facial nerve. Loss of both corneal reflexes is a valuable indication of a deepening level of unconsciousness from any cause but should be elicited with discretion in case of accidental damage to the cornea.

Nervous Control of the Bladder and Rectum

Bladder. The nerve supply to the bladder is derived from three sources:

1. Sympathetic, from the first and second lumbar segment via the inferior hypogastric plexus and hypogastric nerves, which relax the bladder wall and contract the sphincters. (This mechanism, present in many animals, is disputed in man.)

2. Parasympathetic, from segments S. 2, 3, 4 via the pelvic nerves (nervi erigentes) which contract the bladder wall and relax the internal sphincter.

3. Somatic, from segments S. 2, 3, 4 via the pudendal nerves, which contract the external sphincter of the urethra.

Afferent impulses from the bladder wall travel via the pelvic nerves and from the sphincters via the pudendal nerves. Distension of the bladder activates stretch receptors in the bladder wall and stimulates the parasympathetic fibres by means of a reflex arc through the upper sacral segments of the spinal cord, for example in the infant when the bladder empties automatically when distension reaches a certain degree. Subsequently two descending pathways from higher levels assume control, one which inhibits the automatic reflex emptying, and the other which relaxes the inhibition when appropriate. The expression of urine is then promoted by contracting the abdominal and relaxing the pelvic muscles.

Interruption of the sacral reflex arc leads to retention of urine. This is accompanied by loss of bladder sensation if the lesion is on the afferent side of the arc, as in tabes dorsalis. Damage of the anterior sacral nerve roots causes an atonic bladder without loss of sensation ('lower motor neurone paralysis'). Lesions in the spinal cord above the sacral segments may damage the inhibitory fibres, causing urgency, precipitancy or incontinence of urine, or damage to the facilitatory fibres may cause hesitancy or retention. If the higher control is completely lost there is a period of retention with overflow from a passively dilating atonic bladder until the sacral reflex begins to function as in infancy, restoring automatic bladder emptying. The bladder is hypertonic ('upper motor neurone paralysis') and may shrink if this is not prevented. Cerebral lesions at the vertex near the motor or sensory area may also give rise to incontinence or retention, and with frontal lobe lesions the intellectual disturbance may be associated with failure to inhibit reflex emptying.

Rectum. The rectum has a dual nerve supply from the sympathetic (inhibitory) and the parasympathetic (facilitatory) systems. Disturbances of function similar to those in the bladder occur, but are less severe and more transient.

THE LOCALISING SIGNS OF DISEASE OF THE BRAIN

The Pre-frontal Lobe. This comprises the frontal lobe anterior to the precentral gyrus. It is concerned with some aspects of psychological reactions, notably the ability to make intelligent anticipations of the future, and the emotional correlations of thought. Disturbances of these functions cause vague psychiatric disorders which are difficult to diagnose in the early stages. The patient loses appreciation of the consequences of his actions, fails to take forethought and becomes apathetic or morbidly facetious. With progressing dementia his memory and intellect become impaired. His social sense is also affected; he becomes careless about his dress and appearance and may micturate in public or become incontinent without seeming to care about it. Physical signs are few but there may be generalised convulsions and a grasp reflex may be found in the contralateral hand. With this reflex, the patient involuntarily clutches at an object which is drawn lightly over the skin of the palm between the index finger and the thumb. The contralateral arm may be ataxic if the fronto-pontine fibres connecting with the cerebellum are interrupted. Expanding lesions of a frontal lobe may compress the underlying olfactory nerve causing unilateral loss of the sense of smell (anosmia). These signs may be missed in a routine examination. It is important, therefore, to search for them when confronted with a patient with early mental changes.

The Precentral Gyrus. Lesions in this region give rise to unequivocal signs. Jacksonian epilepsy (p. 1120) is common and monoplegia (p. 1070) readily develops. A lesion such as a meningioma arising from the falx cerebri involving the superior ends of both 'motor areas' may give rise to signs of an upper motor neurone lesion in both lower limbs, the upper limbs being spared. When a lesion in the dominant hemisphere extends forwards from the inferior end of the precentral gyrus it gives rise to dysphasia of expressive type (p. 1091).

The Parietal Lobe. Lesions of this area may also present with Jacksonian epilepsy, but of sensory type, and in addition there is disturbance of the quantitative and localising aspects of sensation on the opposite side of the body (p. 1080). Lesions situated more posteriorly in the parietal lobe may cause:

1. Spatial disorientation—lack of the patient's ability to find his way about.
2. Apraxia—loss of the ability to perform a pattern of movements though the patient understands its purpose and has no motor or sensory deficit.
3. Agnosia—loss of the ability to recognise a previously familiar object though the patient has good vision and sensation.

4. 'Sensory inattention' or 'perceptual rivalry'—the patient tends to ignore a cutaneous or visual stimulus on the contralateral side if it is presented simultaneously with one on the same side as the lesion though it is perceived if presented alone. This is most prominent in disease of the non-dominant hemisphere (p. 1084).

5. Receptive dysphasia—lesions of the angular and marginal gyri or the posterior temporal-parietal junction cause receptive dysphasia which may be predominantly for written or spoken speech. There may be specialised types of dysphasia such as the loss of ability to count or to recognise parts of the body such as a particular finger.

6. Homonymous hemianopia—Deep lesions in the parietal lobe may involve the optic radiation and so cause a contralateral homonymous hemianopia (p. 1095).

The Occipital Lobe. Irritative lesions cause crude visual hallucinations such as flashing lights, while destructive lesions cause a contralateral homonymous hemianopia (p. 1090).

The Temporal Lobe. Irritative lesions in the posterior temporal lobe may cause visual sensations which are more elaborate than with occipital lobe irritation. Patterns of moving colours or hallucinatory pictures may be experienced by the patient. A similar lesion of the anterior part of the temporal lobe may cause auditory hallucinations (superior temporal gyrus), gustatory and olfactory hallucinations (uncus) or misinterpretations (illusions) of auditory and visual sensations. These are often associated with altered states of consciousness such as dreamy states, automatic behaviour, temporary upsets of memory (*déjà vu*) or brief amnesia. In affections of the dominant hemisphere there may be dysphasia of receptive type (p. 1091). An important sign easily overlooked is a homonymous upper quadrantanopia due to destruction of the lower fibres of the optic radiation which sweep down into the temporal lobe (p. 1093).

Speech

Speech is the symbolic expression of thoughts in words, that is to say, in patterns of sound formed by the vocal apparatus or characters formed by the hands. It requires the learning of certain conventions which differ from one culture and nation to another. When the ability to interpret the meaning of conventional sound or visual symbols is lost, though they can be heard or seen, there is receptive dysphasia. When the ability to express ideas in sound, written or drawn patterns is absent, though there is no paralysis, there is expressive dysphasia. Failure of the symbolical aspect of speech must be distinguished from failure to pronounce or articulate correctly which is dysarthria (p. 1092). The types of dysphasia may therefore be looked on as special cases of agnosia and apraxia respectively (p. 1089). Complete loss of either aspect of speech is termed aphasia. This classification is satisfactory for routine clinical use though the expert will recognise variants from these major patterns. It should, however, be stressed that frequently mixed forms of disturbance occur. The neural mechanisms underlying speech are usually situated in the left hemisphere.

Expressive Dysphasia (Motor). Though he can articulate correctly, the patient is unable to put his thoughts into symbolic form as spoken or written words. The defect may be of varying degrees of severity from complete loss of the power of speech to occasional misplacement or misuse of words. Emotional speech is less affected than propositional speech. There is a marked tendency for the patient to continue to use one word or phrase though he is attempting to express different ideas ('perseveration'). The defect can usually be recognised readily during ordinary conversation with the patient, but in very mild cases it may be necessary to try such tests as showing him a large series of objects and asking him to name them. Though he fails to do so, he will immediately recognise the correct name when it is suggested to him. This type of defect occurs with a lesion at the posterior end of the inferior frontal gyrus (Broca's area) and the lower part of the precentral gyrus.

Receptive Dysphasia (Sensory). In this condition the patient who is neither deaf nor blind is unable to understand the meaning of words, whether spoken or written. It may be the sole defect of speech, but more commonly there is an associated defect of expression. Receptive dysphasia is detected by testing the ability to carry out simple instructions presented orally and in writing.

In mild cases, though simple instructions may be well performed, more complex instructions involving two or three movements or possible alternatives will defeat the patient.

Receptive dysphasia occurs with lesions of the dominant hemisphere situated in the posterior part of the superior temporal gyrus and the angular gyrus of the adjacent parietal lobe. Pure aphasia occurs without intellectual impairment, but the mechanisms of speech are intimately linked with symbolic thought and it is not surprising that some severe states of aphasia are associated with gross disorder of thought and expression. The diagnosis from pure mental disease may then be extremely difficult, calling for specialised examination by a skilled clinical psychologist.

Dysarthria. Dysarthria should be distinguished from dysphasia for in this condition there is no defect in the comprehension of words nor their use to express ideas, but rather a failure of the articulatory mechanism. That is, the idea is given its correct symbol but the pattern of muscle contraction is distorted in the vocal apparatus; the words are correct but they are mispronounced. Writing is not affected, in contrast to the condition in expressive aphasia where there is usually also impairment of ability to express oneself by means of written symbols.

The Visual Pathway

The optic nerve carries third order neurones, the first order neurones being very short fibres within the retina For much of its length it is surrounded by a protrusion of the meningeal membranes into which cerebrospinal fluid can pass, especially if intracranial pressure is raised. For these reasons the optic nerve is liable to suffer from different pathological states than other peripheral nerves. The visual pathway is illustrated in Figure 72. Sensory impulses from the retinae pass along the optic nerves to the optic chiasma where the fibres from the temporal halves of the retinae continue posteriorly in the lateral angle of the chiasma into the optic tracts on the same side. Fibres from the nasal halves of the retinae decussate so that the optic tract carries fibres from that part of each retina which receives light from the contralateral half of the visual field of each eye (the light rays crossing in the refractory media of the eyes). In the same way the light rays from the upper part of the visual field stimulate the lower part of each retina and the fibres arising there remain inferior throughout their further path to the cortex. The optic tracts continue to the lateral geniculate bodies where the fibres concerned with vision

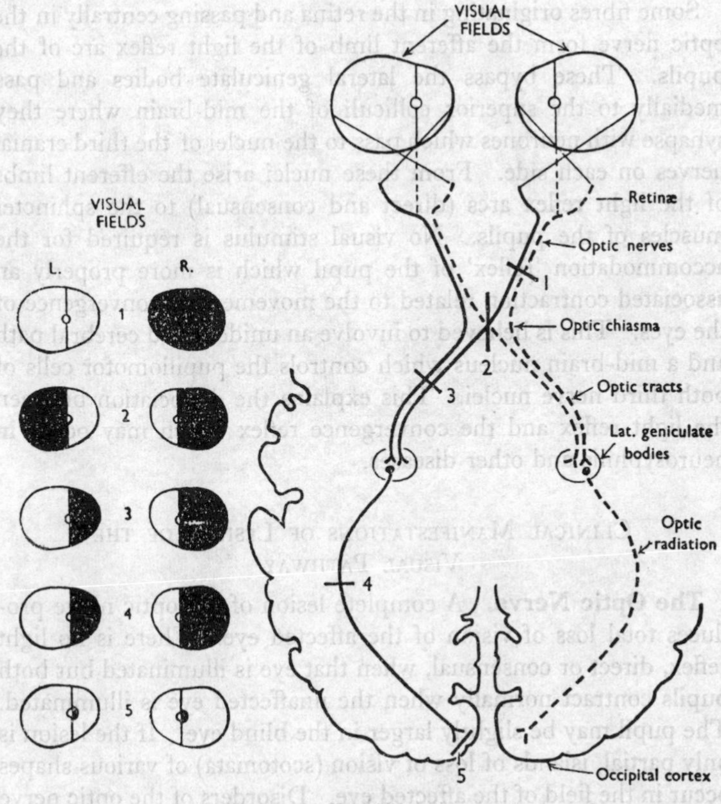

Fig. 72

Visual Pathways and Field Defects resulting from Different Lesions

synapse and the impulses are relayed along the optic radiations to the calcarine area of the occipital cortex. The uppermost fibres which carry impulses derived from the superior quadrants of each retina (lower quadrants of visual fields) pass directly through the parietal lobe, whereas the lowermost fibres which relay impulses from the lower quadrants of the retinae (upper quadrants of visual fields) sweep downwards and forwards round the temporal horn of the lateral ventricle in the temporal lobe before passing to the occipital cortex. Throughout the whole of the visual pathway fibres from the various parts of each retina maintain approximately the same relationship with each other.

Some fibres originating in the retina and passing centrally in the optic nerve form the afferent limb of the light reflex arc of the pupils. These bypass the lateral geniculate bodies and pass medially to the superior colliculi of the mid-brain where they synapse with neurones which pass to the nuclei of the third cranial nerves on each side. From these nuclei arise the efferent limbs of the light reflex arcs (direct and consensual) to the sphincter muscles of the pupils. No visual stimulus is required for the accommodation 'reflex' of the pupil which is more properly an associated contraction related to the movement of convergence of the eyes. This is believed to involve an unidentified cerebral path and a mid-brain nucleus which controls the pupillomotor cells of both third nerve nuclei. This explains the dissociation between the light reflex and the convergence reflex which may occur in neurosyphilis and other diseases.

Clinical Manifestations of Lesions of the Visual Pathway

The Optic Nerve. A complete lesion of the optic nerve produces total loss of vision of the affected eye. There is no light reflex, direct or consensual, when that eye is illuminated but both pupils contract normally when the unaffected eye is illuminated. The pupil may be slightly larger in the blind eye. If the lesion is only partial, islands of loss of vision (scotomata) of various shapes occur in the field of the affected eye. Disorders of the optic nerve are described on p. 1096

The Optic Chiasma. A lesion of the central portion of the chiasma involves the decussating fibres from the nasal halves of both retinae and so gives rise to bitemporal heminanopia. In practice such lesions are rarely symmetrical and hence the degree of involvement of the visual fields of each eye is often unequal. A pituitary tumour first compresses the lower fibres and so the bitemporal hemianopia begins in the superior quadrants, whereas a suprasellar cyst compresses the chiasma from above so that field loss starts in the lower quadrants.

The Optic Tracts. A lesion of an optic tract gives rise to a homonymous hemianopia, the lost half of the field of vision of each eye being on the side opposite to the lesion. The involvement of the two fields is often unequal ('incongruous'), being slightly greater in the field of the eye on the side of the lesion.

The Optic Radiation. The effects of a lesion of the optic radiation depend on its exact site. A lesion of the temporal lobe involves the lower fibres only and gives rise to a homonymous defect affecting mainly the upper quadrants of the visual fields. A lesion in the anterior part of the parietal lobe causes a homonymous hemianopia mainly affecting the lower quadrants as it affects fibres from the upper parts of the retinae. A lesion at the posterior part of the parietal lobe, where both groups of fibres are again adjacent, gives rise to a total homonymous hemianopia.

The Occipital Cortex. A destructive lesion of one occipital cortex gives rise to a complete (and congruous) homonymous hemianopia if it is extensive, or to a scotoma which is present in the fields of both eyes. Irritative lesions, as in the ischaemia caused by migraine, cause hallucinations of flashing lights which are referred to the contralateral fields of both eyes.

DISORDERS OF THE CRANIAL NERVES

The cranial nerves are frequently involved in generalised disease of the nervous system. In addition, there are specific conditions affecting a single cranial nerve. It is convenient for descriptive purposes to study consecutively the manifestations of lesions of the cranial nerves and their nuclei.

The First Cranial Nerve

The olfactory nerve arises from olfactory receptors in the nasal mucosae. The fine first order fibres pass through the cribriform plate in the floor of the anterior fossa of the skull. They synapse in the olfactory bulb and second order neurones run to the olfactory area of the brain (the antero-medial part of the temporal lobe) and higher autonomic centres by the olfactory tract which lies under the orbital surface of the frontal lobe. Thus tumours of the frontal lobe may compress it and cause loss of the sense of smell (anosmia) on one side of the nose. The fragile fibres passing through the cribriform plate are readily damaged by head injuries.

The Second Cranial Nerve

The anatomy and central connections of the optic nerve are described on p. 1092 and the visual field changes caused by a lesion of the nerve are discussed on p. 1094. When the fibres originating in the macular area are damaged there is a loss of visual acuity (amblyopia) which cannot be corrected by lenses. Direct and consensual light reflexes are depressed or absent when the amblyopic eye is stimulated but the convergence pupil response is unaffected.

Papilloedema. This term is applied to oedema of the optic disc or papilla from any cause. The swelling may be inflammatory (papillitis) or due to passive venous congestion. The venous drainage from the retina may be obstructed if the meningeal sheath surrounding the optic nerve is distended by cerebrospinal fluid under increased pressure. Papilloedema may arise from:

1. Increased intracranial pressure, as in some cases of cerebral tumour, abscess and meningitis.
2. Optic neuritis due to inflammatory lesions of the optic nerve (p. 1097).
3. Disease of the retinal arteries, as in malignant hypertension.
4. Obstruction of venous drainage from the orbit due to an orbital neoplasm, thrombosis of the central vein of the retina or cavernous sinus thrombosis.

The appearances of papilloedema, commencing with the earliest, are (*a*) congestion of the retinal veins; (*b*) increased pinkness of the optic disc; (*c*) blurring of the disc margin starting on the nasal side; (*d*) filling of the physiological cup; (*e*) elevation of the optic disc; (*f*) haemorrhage in and around the disc; (*g*) pallor of the disc due to optic atrophy which is the terminal stage of prolonged papilloedema.

The visual changes associated with papilloedema depend on the cause. The most important distinction is that visual acuity is relatively well preserved when papilloedema is due to pressure, though the visual fields may show peripheral constriction and enlargement of the 'blind spot'. Optic neuritis, on the other hand, causes severe loss of visual acuity for an equal degree of disc swelling and the visual fields usually show large central scotomata. These points are valuable in differentiating between two important neurological diseases, i.e. cerebral tumour and disseminated sclerosis presenting with visual failure and papilloedema.

Optic Neuritis. The most common cause of inflammation of the optic nerve is disseminated sclerosis. Syphilis is now a rare cause. The optic nerve may suffer damage (more properly called an optic neuropathy) from toxic factors such as the excessive consumption of pipe tobacco and some chemical substances, or from deficiency of the vitamin B complex. The ophthalmoscopic appearances of optic neuritis depend on the situation of the lesion in the nerve. When it is immediately behind the disc ('papillitis'), the inflammatory oedema is manifest as a papilloedema (p. 1096). Lesions further back are called retrobulbar neuritis and do not cause abnormal ophthalmoscopic appearances during the acute stage.

Retrobulbar Neuritis. The patient complains of fairly sudden onset of blurring of the vision of one eye which may progress to almost complete loss of sight in 24 to 48 hours. There may be slight discomfort on movement of the eye and tenderness on pressure over the eyeball but pain is not a marked feature. The ophthalmoscopic appearances are normal at this stage but the visual field shows a large central scotoma since the macular fibres are most readily damaged. Visual acuity begins to return rapidly in two or three weeks and has usually recovered within four to six weeks. The only residual sign may be temporal pallor of the disc due to permanent damage to the macular fibres. Retrobulbar neuritis is commonly caused by disseminated sclerosis so other manifestations of the disease should be looked for. It is often the first symptom and further relapses may not appear until months or years later and it may remain the only feature. Syphilis is a much rarer cause but vision is less likely to recover. The Wassermann reaction should be tested and treatment with penicillin started immediately if syphilis is proved to be the cause (p. 62).

Optic Atrophy. This is a terminal stage of several conditions: the more important causes are (*a*) optic neuritis (p. 1097); (*b*) long-standing papilloedema; (*c*) certain poisons, e.g. tobacco, methyl alcohol, quinine, lead; (*d*) localised pressure on the optic nerve, e.g. glaucoma and cerebral aneurysm; (*e*) thrombosis of the central retinal artery; (*f*) trauma; (*g*) primary syphilitic optic atrophy. This differs from syphilitic neuritis which is due to an endarteritis and which causes sudden visual failure. Primary atrophy is a progressive degenerative lesion of the optic neurones which usually advances to complete blindness. The optic disc is small and uniformly pale, and the visual fields initially show peripheral constriction; (*h*) familial degenerative disorders. These are sometimes associated with hereditary ataxia; (*i*) diabetes mellitus. This is a rare cause.

The ophthalmoscopic appearance of optic atrophy is an intensely white disc with a clearly defined margin and few capillaries. The visual fields show variable defects according to the cause of the atrophy. No direct or consensual light reflex is obtained from illumination of the affected eye but pupil responses are otherwise normal.

The Third Cranial Nerve

The oculomotor nerve supplies all the external ocular muscles except the lateral rectus and the superior oblique. It also supplies the levator palpebrae superioris, the constrictor of the pupil, and the ciliary muscle. It may be involved in disseminated sclerosis, meningovascular syphilis, diabetes mellitus, and cerebral aneurysms which may compress the nerve at several sites. The manifestations of a third nerve palsy are ptosis, diplopia, external deviation of the eye (divergent strabismus) due to the action of the unopposed lateral rectus muscle and defective ocular movement in the direction in which the muscles supplied by the third nerve move the eye. The patient complains of double vision but in a long standing lesion one of the images is suppressed. Complete paralysis of the third nerve also paralyses the constrictor of the pupil so it is large and fails to react to light (by the direct or consensual path) or on convergence.

The Fourth Cranial Nerve

The trochlear nerve supplies the superior oblique muscle. A lesion of the nerve gives rise to defective movement and diplopia which is maximal when the patient attempts to look down with the eye turned inwards. The pupils are not affected. An isolated lesion of the nerve is rarely encountered, as usually there is also involvement of either the third or sixth nerve.

Diagnosis of Squint. Squint (strabismus) may be paralytic or non-paralytic.

Paralytic squint is due to weakness of one or more of the extra-ocular muscles. Defective movement of the eye can be seen when the patient attempts to move the eye by the weak muscle and this usually causes diplopia. The rules for identifying the paretic muscles causing diplopia or squint are:

1. The separation of the images is greater when the patient attempts to look in the direction to which the paretic muscle should move the eye.
2. In this position, the most peripheral image is the 'false image' from the affected eye. It is identified by covering one eye with a green glass and the other with a red one.

Concomitant squint ('lazy eye') is due to failure to maintain the correct posture of an eye which is so defective in vision that its image is suppressed by the brain. There is no muscle paresis and both eyes are capable of full movements in all directions. The most common cause is an error of refraction during childhood. If recognised and properly treated with suitable spectacles the squint can be prevented though a 'latent squint' often remains.

Conjugate Paralysis of Gaze. The cerebral hemispheres control the direction of gaze by co-ordinated movements of both eyes. A supranuclear lesion therefore affects movements of both eyes together in a particular direction. Each eye when tested separately, however, shows a full range of movement. (This is an excellent example of the aphorism that 'the cortex controls movements, and the lower motor neurones control individual muscles'.)

Nystagmus

The eyes are not normally moved independently but are mutually adjusted so that corresponding areas of the retina of each eye receive light rays from the same part of the visual field. Conjugate movements of the eyes may be carried out voluntarily by pathways involving the frontal lobes (conjugate gaze to the contralateral side) or they may be initiated reflexly. One of the most important of these reflexes is the fixation reflex. It involves the cortex of the occipital and adjacent part of the parietal lobe and causes gaze to be adjusted so that the object of main interest is viewed by the macular areas of each eye and the eyes will move to keep it there if the object is moving. This following movement continues until the eyes are fully deviated to one side, then the eyes jerk back and the gaze fixes on a new object. This sequence may be repeated rhythmically (optokinetic nystagmus). Ocular fixation is disturbed by lesions of the eye or of the visual pathway including fibres which pass to the superior colliculi of the brain stem.

It is also necessary for the retinal images to be stabilised even if the head is moving in space or relative to the rest of the body. This is achieved by reflexes originating in the vestibular labyrinth and in proprioceptive receptors in the neck (Fig. 73). All these

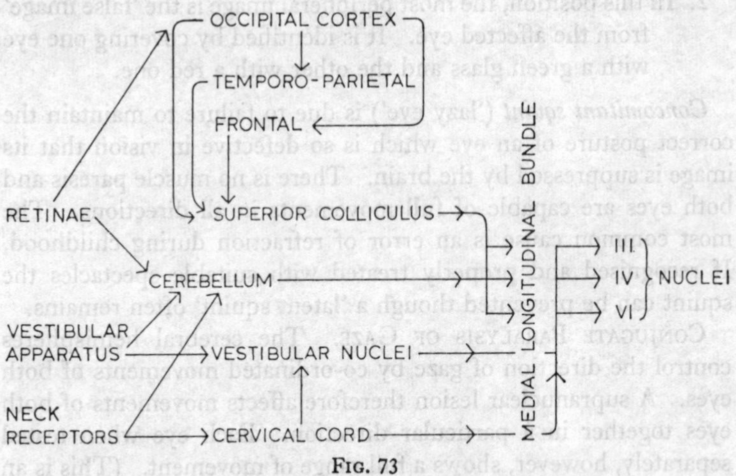

FIG. 73

DIAGRAM OF PERIPHERAL, CORTICAL, AND BRAIN STEM CONTROL OF CONJUGATE GAZE. THE EXTRA-OCULAR MUSCLES ARE CONTROLLED BILATERALLY.

influences, cortical, ocular, vestibular and cervical, are relayed by the medial longitudinal bundle to the nuclei of the third, fourth and sixth nerves on both sides, producing the reciprocal contractions and relaxation of extraocular muscles which are necessary to move the eyes conjugately. Part of the cerebellum also participates in the co-ordination of postural movements of the eyes, as it does with posture of the limbs (p. 1078).

Nystagmus is a series of rhythmic oscillations of the eyes. It may be spontaneous or induced by visual or vestibular stimulation which causes the posture of the eyes to be maintained badly. The oscillations may be equal in speed and amplitude in both directions (pendular nystagmus) or unequal (jerking nystagmus), or they may occur as a series of rotations about a central axis (rotatory nystagmus). Nystagmus may be caused by a disturbance of each of the pathways contributing to conjugate movements of the eyes. When testing for nystagmus it is important to keep the visual fixation point within the field of binocular vision. The direction of nystagmus is defined by the direction of the fast component. (When severe, nystagmus may be present on looking to the side opposite to the fast component—this is a measure of severity, not an indication of nystagmus to both sides).

Types and Causes of Nystagmus

Voluntary Gaze. Normal people may show fine jerking nystagmus when the eyes are fully deviated to one side. This is more prominent in neurotic individuals, in hysteria and in fatigue. It is usually unsustained if the gaze is maintained. Slow irregular nystagmus is present with supranuclear lesions of the extra-ocular muscles if the patient attempts to look towards the side of the conjugate paralysis of gaze.

Ocular Nystagmus. Blindness is often associated with irregular wandering movements of the eyes. Defective central vision (amblyopia) causes true nystagmus which may be jerking or pendular. (Pendular and oblique nystagmus always have an ocular cause). It may be confined to one eye. Living or working in very dark environments may cause pendular nystagmus (e.g. miner's nystagmus). Ocular nystagmus is due to faulty fixation.

Vestibular Nystagmus. Imbalance between labyrinthine stimuli from the two ears leads to jerking nystagmus of both eyes. With irritative lesions the fast phase of the jerking is to the side of the lesion and with paralytic lesions it is to the opposite side. Nystagmus is greater in amplitude and more rapid on looking in the direction of the quick phase. If the lesion involves the end-organs in the semicircular canals or their central connections, nystagmus is precipitated by sudden movements of the head. Lesions of the otolith organs or their central connections cause nystagmus which occurs when the head is in a particular position.

Disorders of the Labyrinth. Spontaneous nystagmus is present with acute lesions but tends to subside in a few days or months. This tendency to adaptation may be seen during testing as nystagmus, brought on by movement or position of the head or by caloric stimulation, is not maintained. It may become difficult to elicit again if the test is repeated. It is often associated with vertigo (p. 1109) and this too is brief. The patient tends to fall towards the direction of the slow component of the nystagmus. Cochlear function is usually affected, causing tinnitus or deafness. Labyrinthine nystagmus may be caused by inflammatory diseases (serous or purulent labyrinthitis), chronic degenerative middle ear disease, vascular upsets in hypertension, atherosclerosis of the internal auditory artery, head injury and Ménière's syndrome (p. 1110).

Lesions of the Vestibular Nerve. Nystagmus due to lesions of the eighth nerve has the same features. This may be due to an acoustic neuroma or neuronitis (p. 1110). The latter is a short lasting disease.

Lesions of the Central Vestibular Apparatus. Spontaneous nystagmus, or nystagmus induced by head position or head movement, may be found with brain stem lesions affecting the vestibular nuclei. Spontaneous nystagmus unaffected by head position and maximal on looking to the side of the lesion is found with some cerebellar lesions. Central nystagmus often occurs without vertigo, but where it is present it tends to persist and neither the nystagmus nor the vertigo show the adaptation which is a feature of a peripheral lesion. The vertigo tends to make the patient fall to the side of the fast component of the nystagmus. Central nystagmus and vertigo often occur without cochlear symptoms and may be associated with other brain stem symptoms such as diplopia or with asynergia of the limbs or speech if the lesion involves cerebellar connections. The nature of the nystagmus may be like that of peripheral lesions but vertical nystagmus or nystagmus which affects each eye differently is always central in origin. It may be caused by disseminated sclerosis, vascular lesions (e.g. occlusion of the posterior inferior cerebellar artery, p. 1139), pontine and cerebellar tumours, ponto-medullary and cerebellar encephalitis, syringobulbia (p. 1204) or as the result of toxic states of which alcoholism is the most common. Postconcussional vertigo and nystagmus may be peripheral or central in type and they are often precipitated by a particular posture of the head. Indirect disturbance of the vestibular nuclei may occur when the intracranial pressure is raised. Nystagmus is then a 'false localising sign'.

ATAXIC NYSTAGMUS. In lesions of the medial longitudinal bundle the ocular movements are dissociated. On looking to one side the abducting eye shows coarse nystagmus. The other eye fails to adduct fully and nystagmus, if present, is of smaller amplitude. This type of nystagmus is common in disseminated sclerosis.

SPINAL NYSTAGMUS. High spinal cord lesions (traumatic paraplegia or syringomyelia) may cause nystagmus by interfering with the cervical component of gaze control (p. 1100).

NYSTAGMUS DUE TO MUSCLE PARESIS OR FATIGUE. The efferent side of the many reflexes concerned with maintaining the position of the eyes may be responsible for nystagmus. If gaze is held in a strongly deviated position for an uncomfortable period, fatigue leads to jerky nystagmus in normal people. If one or more of the extraocular muscles is weak, the affected eyeball shows jerky nystagmus when the eye is moved by the weak muscle. Examples are partial third nerve palsies and myasthenia gravis.

Disordered function may also be indicated by the failure to evoke nystagmus by stimuli which normally do so. Lesions of one eye or visual pathway or of the posterior temporal lobe may prevent elicitation of optokinetic nystagmus (p. 1100) from the appropriate visual field. Peripheral or central lesions of the vestibular pathway may abolish nystagmus provoked by head rotation or by caloric stimulation. These tests are not part of the routine examination of a patient but are valuable additional investigations for localisation of a lesion in the ear, posterior fossa, or posterior part of the cerebral hemispheres.

The Fifth Cranial Nerve

The trigeminal nerve has an extensive sensory distribution through its three branches, the ophthalmic, maxillary and mandibular divisions. It supplies the skin of the face (excluding the angle of the jaw), the cornea, the sinuses, the mucous membrane of the nose, the teeth, the tympanic membrane and common sensation (but not taste) to the anterior two-thirds of the tongue. The motor division of the nerve innervates the temporal, masseter and pterygoid muscles which are responsible for the closure and opening of the jaw. The nerve fibres and nuclei may be involved within the brain stem by conditions such as syringobulbia and thrombotic lesions, and the peripheral nerve by localised pressure such as occurs in cerebral aneurysms in the region of the cavernous sinus, and by tumours of the cerebellopontine angle. The ganglion of the nerve may also be involved by herpes zoster, giving rise to the characteristic shingles lesion over the skin of the face and causing ulceration of the cornea when the ophthalmic division is involved.

Trigeminal Neuralgia (Tic Douloureux)

This is a condition of unknown aetiology and without recognised histopathology. It is most common in elderly people who are often hypertensive. In rare cases it may be a manifestation of disseminated sclerosis, basilar aneurysm or a cerebral tumour such as a neurofibroma.

Clinical Features. The characteristic feature is the occurrence of brief paroxysms of severe lancinating pain. These usually first involve either the maxillary or mandibular division and spread to the other, but the ophthalmic division is rarely involved and never alone. Each paroxysm lasts for only a few seconds but the stab of pain may be followed by a dull ache, or frequent attacks following one another may make the pain appear to be of longer duration. The pain is precipitated by touching localised 'trigger zones' on the affected side of the face. A cold wind blowing on the face, washing the face, chewing or even talking may be sufficient to bring on an attack. Paroxysms may continue for days or weeks, after which a remission of equal or longer duration may follow, but remissions become shorter and less frequent as the disease progresses. The agonising pain commands the patient's full attention. It may provoke a facial twitch (tic douloureux) and is so severe that the patient avoids washing, shaving and even eating for fear of precipitating an attack, but apart from the signs due to these exclusions nothing abnormal can be detected by the examiner. There is no loss of facial sensation and the corneal reflex is intact in true trigeminal neuralgia.

Diagnosis. Diagnosis is simple from the nature of the pain and the complete absence of sensory loss. Other forms of facial pain such as facial neuralgia, facial migraine, dental and sinus disease, do not cause such brief lancinating pain. Pain due to involvement by organic disease of the trigeminal nerve or its nuclei is always a more continuous and steady pain than tic douloureux and is often accompanied by sensory loss.

Treatment. In view of the possibility of long remissions, medical treatment should be used in the first instance. Carbamazepine, 200 mg. thrice daily, may reduce the frequency of attacks and known precipitants should be avoided. Attacks are treated at this stage with simple analgesics. If pain persists and remissions are rare or of short duration it is necessary to interrupt the central passage of pain impulses by injection of phenol or alcohol into a branch of the nerve, if neuralgia is localised, or into the Gasserian ganglion. Section of the sensory part of the fifth nerve or its descending root in the medulla has the disadvantage of requiring intracranial operation but permits sparing of corneal sensation which is difficult to achieve with injection of the ganglion. This secures permanent relief from pain but the face becomes anaesthetic. Loss of sensibility from the cornea demands that special care must be taken to avoid trauma with its danger of subsequent corneal ulceration.

Prognosis. Remissions are common in the early years but spontaneous recovery is rare. The attacks tend to become more frequent and of longer duration.

The Sixth Cranial Nerve

The abducent nerve supplies the lateral rectus muscle of the eye. A lesion of the nerve causes diplopia due to inability to abduct the eye, and deviation of the eye medially (convergent strabismus) due to the unopposed action of the medial rectus muscle. The methods for determining the cause of diplopia are described on p. 1099. The sixth nerve may be involved by pressure from an aneurysm in the cavernous sinus. Downward displacement of the brain stem due to raised intracranial pressure may stretch it and cause a paralysis without there being local involvement of the nerve. This is then referred to as a false localising sign.

The Seventh Cranial Nerve

The facial nerve innervates the muscles of expression of the face and, through its chorda tympani branch, carries taste fibres from the anterior two-thirds of the tongue. Paralysis of the facial muscles may be due to:—

(1) lesion of the fibres of the upper motor neurones concerned with voluntary movement, (2) lesion of the fibres of the upper motor neurones concerned with emotional movement, (3) lesion of the fibres of the lower motor neurones.

1. Upper motor neurone fibres originating in the lower part of the pre-central gyrus are distributed to the part of the opposite facial nucleus subserving the muscles of the lower part of the face, and to the parts of the facial nuclei on both sides of the pons which supply the upper parts of the face. Accordingly, a lesion of the upper motor neurones affects more severely the voluntary movement of the lower part of the face, contralaterally. Weakness of the upper part (the orbicularis oculi and frontalis muscles) may occur transiently but is often absent because the lower motor neurones to the upper facial muscles are supplied by upper motor neurones from both hemispheres. The patient is unable to retract the angle of the mouth on command, but in smiling and talking the mouth may move well because emotional movement is controlled by upper motor neurones which are not those concerned with voluntary movement of the face.

2. Upper motor neurones concerned with emotional movement of the face take origin further forward in the frontal lobe and so may be damaged by a lesion which spares the fibres for voluntary movement of the face. Involvement of these fibres is revealed by defective movement of the angle of the mouth when the patient smiles and talks, with preservation of the ability to retract the angle of the mouth on command.

3. Since the lower motor neurone is the final common pathway, complete damage to the facial nucleus or nerve abolishes both voluntary and emotional movements equally in upper and lower parts of the face. Lower motor neurone paralysis restricted to part

of the facial muscles can only occur when the lesion is distal to the branching of the nerve e.g. with disease of the parotid gland, through which the nerve passes, or in leprosy.

When the lesion is at the level of the geniculate ganglion, the patient may complain that sounds seem too loud (the hyperacusis is due to paralysis of the stapedius muscle) and there is loss of taste sensation on the anterior two-thirds of the tongue (chorda tympani).

The most common cause of damage to the nerve proximal to its branching in the parotid gland is Bell's palsy but it may be damaged by disease of the brain stem, by an acoustic neuroma, or by inflammation during its passage through the middle ear.

Bell's Palsy

Aetiology. This condition occurs in both sexes at any age. The cause is unknown but is believed to be an inflammatory lesion in the stylomastoid canal, the paralysis being due to compression of the nerve fibres by oedema. A cold draught blowing on the ear may be a precipitating factor. Herpes zoster of the geniculate ganglion is a rare cause which may be recognised when lower motor neurone facial palsy is combined with a vesicular rash on or in the ear (Ramsay Hunt syndrome).

Clinical Features. There may first be a slight aching pain behind the ear for one or two days then unilateral facial paralysis rapidly develops, but pain may be absent. The eye on the affected side cannot be closed and may water. The mouth is drawn over to the opposite side (so that it may appear to the patient to be due to spasm of the normal side), saliva or fluids may run from the angle of the mouth and, during chewing, food may collect between the teeth and the paralysed cheek. The patient often complains that the affected side feels 'numb', as if injected with a local anaesthetic, but there is no objective loss of sensation of the skin. On examination there is paralysis of the upper as well as the lower part of the affected side of the face. The lines of expression are flattened out on the weak side and the patient is unable to wrinkle his brow, whistle or retract the angle of his mouth. He cannot close the eye and on attempting to do so the eyeball rolls up (Bell's sign). The nerve to the stapedius muscle and the chorda tympani leave and join the main trunk before it leaves the stylomastoid foramen so these signs are absent in most cases of Bell's palsy.

Diagnosis. The differential diagnosis of facial palsy due to lesions of the upper and lower motor neurones is discussed above (p. 1106).

Treatment. It is usually sufficient to give aspirin if the ear is painful and to protect the ear from cold but corticosteroids may reduce inflammation and oedema during the first week. A splint may be fitted to prevent over-stretching of the angle of the mouth. When voluntary movement begins to return active facial exercises in front of a mirror should be practised several times a day. Surgical decompression is not widely used. Electrical stimulation does not hasten recovery and may lead to secondary contractures. When recovery does not occur, a nerve anastomosis or a plastic operation should be considered.

Prognosis. Recovery usually starts in three to four weeks and is complete in three to six months but it is sometimes delayed or incomplete. Unfortunately it is difficult to recognise cases with a poor prognosis at a time when surgical treatment might be considered. Recovery is probable if any voluntary contraction of any paralysed muscle can be seen within a month, and the presence of a normal intensity-duration curve on electrical stimulation after the first week is strong evidence that the nerve has not degenerated. Recovery is unlikely if the intensity-duration curve is of the denervation type. Regeneration of the nerve is possible but the cosmetic result may be marred by the presence of inappropriate movements such as closure of the eye when it is intended to move the lips, due to random regeneration of fibres to the wrong muscles. Spontaneous fasciculation or facial spasm may occur as a rare sequel. Recurrence of facial palsy on either side is exceptional but some individuals appear to be unduly susceptible.

The Eighth Nerve

The auditory nerve has two components, the cochlear nerve which is concerned with hearing and the vestibular nerve which is concerned with the appreciation of the position of the head and its movement in space. It is impossible without special tests to differentiate lesions involving these nerves from lesions confined to their end-organs in the inner ear. Irritative lesions of the inner ear or of the cochlear nerve cause tinnitus, and destructive lesions deafness. Thus, tinnitus may be an early symptom of a neuroma of the eighth nerve (acoustic neuroma) but it is often due to aural causes. The most important destructive lesion of the eighth nerve is an acoustic neuroma, but it may also be damaged in meningitis, and by the toxic effects of dihydrostreptomycin and kanamycin.

Irritative lesions of the vestibular part of the eighth nerve cause vertigo.

Vertigo

The term 'vertigo' is used by many people to describe a sensation of 'giddiness' or 'dizziness' but these symptoms are common in patients with an anxiety neurosis or with transient upsets of cerebral function of unlocalised nature as well as in lesions of the vestibular pathways. For this reason it is convenient to restrict the term 'vertigo' to the description of a subjective feeling of movement of the external environment or of the brain within the head. The movement may be rotatory or a feeling of displacement in one direction. Vertigo is always accompanied by a disturbance of balance which usually causes the patient to seek support, and if sudden and severe may throw him to the ground. It often causes a reflex autonomic discharge leading to cold sweating, pallor, nausea, vomiting, and sometimes diarrhoea, bradycardia or even syncope.

The most important causes of vertigo are:

Ocular Lesions. Diplopia may be accompanied by vertigo because the false projection of one image causes confusion regarding position in space.

Cerebellar Lesions. Cerebellar lesions may cause vertigo when the cerebello-vestibular connections are involved but this symptom is not invariable.

Brain-stem Lesions. Lesions such as insufficiency of the basilar artery, medullary infarction or syringobulbia may cause severe vertigo when they involve the vestibular nuclei. The vertigo may be produced by particular positions of the head.

Lesions of the Vestibular Nerve. An acoustic neuroma may damage the nerve and cause vertigo. Vestibular neuronitis is a more common cause. It is a benign short lasting condition of unknown aetiology which may occur in epidemics.

Aural Lesions. Aural lesions of many kinds, including otitis media and Ménière's syndrome, cause vertigo. The labyrinth may be damaged in a head injury and the vertigo may then be most severe when the head is in a certain position, usually backwards and to one side. A similar type of positional vertigo may occur in brief paroxysms. It is a benign condition which may disappear after a few months. The labyrinth may be damaged by mumps and by various toxic drugs such as streptomycin. Quinine and salicylates are also believed to cause vertigo by an action on the middle or inner ear. Hearing is almost invariably affected when the lesion is labyrinthine rather than in the nerve or central connections.

Ménière's Syndrome

Ménière's syndrome is characterised by recurrent paroxysms of vertigo associated with tinnitus and progressive nerve deafness.

Aetiology. The cause is unknown, but the condition is associated with dilatation of the endolymphatic system (hydrops) due to increase in the amount of endolymph. Many patients also give a history of migraine.

Clinical Features. The most common initial symptoms are progressive deafness and tinnitus which are frequently slight at the onset. Sooner or later vertigo occurs and is characterised by suddenness of onset and great severity. It may develop so suddenly that the patient may fall, and at the height of the attack he may be unable to stand. This is usually accompanied by nausea and vomiting and there may be other autonomic symptoms. Deafness and tinnitus may be intensified during the attack which may last for a few minutes to several hours. Examination during an attack shows rotatory nystagmus and ataxia. Between attacks there is only nerve deafness with impaired vestibular function as shown by caloric tests.

Diagnosis. The paroxysmal nature of the attacks, and the association with tinnitus and nerve deafness are characteristic. Other causes of vertigo (p. 1109) are excluded by careful examination.

Treatment. During an attack the patient must lie perfectly still. An anti-emetic drug is valuable (e.g. promethazine 25 mg.) but severe cases require a sedative (phenobarbitone sodium 0·2 g. intramuscularly). For long-term treatment a vasodilator such as nicotinic acid may be helpful. It may be necessary to use 200 mg. or more but as sensitivity varies greatly the initial dose should be 25 mg. and this is increased progressively until flushing of the skin is caused. If these measures are not effective, sedation with phenobarbitone 30 mg. three or four times a day is the best prophylactic. Destruction of the labyrinth by surgery or ultrasonics, or division of the eighth nerve, may be required.

Prognosis. The frequency of attacks tends to decrease as deafness increases but the disease may last many years.

The Ninth, Tenth and Eleventh Cranial Nerves

These nerves are grouped together because isolated lesions of one nerve alone are rarely encountered. The glossopharyngeal nerve (IX) transmits taste and common sensation from the posterior one-third of the tongue and motor fibres to the pharynx; the vagus nerve (X) is the parasympathetic nerve for the viscera of the thorax and upper part of the abdomen and also supplies somatic motor fibres to the soft palate and the larynx; the spinal accessory nerve (XI) supplies the trapezius and sternomastoid muscles. Unilateral lesions disturb their somatic functions but do not appreciably affect visceral function. These nerves or their nuclei may be involved by disease of the medulla such as syringobulbia or in their course across the posterior fossa by neoplasms and basal meningitis. Lesions at the jugular foramen, such as thrombophlebitis of the internal jugular vein following suppuration in the skull or neck, may involve all three nerves as they emerge from the skull.

The Twelfth Nerve

The hypoglossal nerve supplies motor fibres to the muscles of one side of the tongue. Upper motor neurone lesions cause spastic contraction of the muscle fibres. The tongue is small and pointed but not atrophic. Articulation is defective (spastic dysarthria) especially for the lingual sounds. There is rapid recovery of function after a unilateral lesion of upper motor neurone type, but bilateral lesions cause permanent dysarthria. This may occur in motor neurone disease (p. 1199) or in pseudo-bulbar palsy due to bilateral impairment of blood supply in the internal capsules (p. 1137). Lower motor neurone lesions cause wasting and fibrillation of the affected part of the tongue and, when protruded, the tongue deviates to the side of the lesion. The usual cause is motor neurone disease.

The lower cranial nerves may be involved by carcinoma of the nasopharynx spreading to the base of the skull so otolaryngological examination is necessary. All cranial nerves, but particularly those emerging from the base of the skull, may be affected by bone disease in that area, particularly by Paget's disease (p. 718).

The Cervical Sympathetic Fibres

The higher centres for autonomic functions in the hypothalamus are connected with some areas of the cortex, notably the orbital surface of the frontal lobe and the insula. From the hypothalamus sympathetic fibres descend through the brain stem and spinal cord to their lower neurones in the small lateral horn of the thoracic region of the spinal cord from which they pass into the anterior spinal roots from T_1 to L_2. White rami communicantes leave these roots and convey the fibres to the paravertebral sympathetic chain where a relay occurs either immediately or after rising or descending to a ganglion more remote in the chain. Grey rami communicantes then go to peripheral sympathetic plexuses which supply the principal viscera; others rejoin the spinal nerves and are distributed with them to some of the blood vessels and glands in the territory of those nerves. Those destined for the head and neck emerge mainly through the first thoracic anterior root, and ascend in the cervical sympathetic chain, reaching their final destination by means of the plexuses in the walls of blood vessels. Stimulation of the cervical sympathetic fibres causes dilatation of the pupil, protrusion of the eye-ball and elevation of the upper eyelid; conversely paralysis of these fibres results in pupillary constriction, enophthalmos and ptosis (Horner's syndrome). In addition, sweating is impaired on that side of the face. These signs may occur in lesions of the brain stem such as syringobulbia and thrombosis of the posterior inferior cerebellar artery (p. 1139), in lesions of the cervical part of the spinal cord such as syringomyelia, and in conditions at the thoracic outlet such as bronchial carcinoma at the apex of the lung (p. 381).

COMA

The state of consciousness is associated with cortical activity activated by impulses from the thalamus and mid-brain. The reticular formation receives collaaeral axons from the main spinothalamic and special sensory pathways and from the cortex and sends fibres to the cortex which it alerts. The lower part of the reticular formation projects to the spinal cord for regulation of muscle tone (p. 1074). Disorders of the cortical or brain-stem poles of this system, but particularly the latter, are associated with disturbance of consciousness. Loss of consciousness is graded into arbitrary stages of drowsiness, stupor and coma according to the type of stimulus required to cause arousal. In the same way coma can be arbitrarily graded according to the degree of loss of reflex activity. The 'vital' reflexes of coughing, respiration and vasomotor control are the last to disappear with deepening coma and the patient must be protected from the consequences of their loss. Coma may be difficult to differentiate from some *psychotic conditions* of depression or from akinetic mutism in which the patient lies in a stuporous state unresponsive to most stimuli. If he is watched continuously it is seen that the non-comatose patient is not wholly out of touch with his surroundings and his vital reflexes remain intact. Physical examination is negative and a history of psychological abnormality can usually be obtained from a relative or friend. Akinetic mutism may be found in some disorders of the region of the third ventricle but will be associated with signs of cerebral damage. The principal causes of coma are:

Paroxysmal loss of consciousness. Sudden brief loss of consciousness with full recovery but often with recurrences may be found in epilepsy (p. 1116), hysteria (p. 1121) and syncope (p. 182).

Cerebral Disorders. Coma may be associated with acute or chronic disturbance of the upper brain-stem.

HEAD INJURY. There is a history of trauma and there may be signs of external injury. In concussion the face is pale, reflexes diminished or absent, and pupils equal, dilated and sluggish. If there is compression due to intracranial haemorrhage the face may be flushed, breathing is stertorous and the reflexes may be asymmetrical. The pupil on the injured side first contracts and then dilates and the other pupil subsequently reacts similarly. It is well to remember that a patient becoming unconscious or incapable for some reason other than trauma may fall and injure his skull.

Cerebrovascular Accidents (p. 1135). Apoplexy is usually of sudden onset if it causes loss of consciousness. There are signs of a focal cerebral lesion such as a hemiplegia, and of meningism if subarachnoid bleeding has occurred. There may also be evidence of the cause such as hypertension, atherosclerosis, or a cardiac disorder associated with embolism.

Meningitis (p. 1156). Coma is of gradual onset in most types, being preceded by meningeal irritation and fever but in meningococcal meningitis these signs may only have been present for a few hours. The cerebrospinal fluid is turbid and contains polymorphonuclear leucocytes.

Encephalitis. Viral encephalitis as a cause of coma is rare. It is important to bear in mind *cerebral malaria* in the tropics or in any comatose patient who has recently returned from a country in which malaria is prevalent. Early treatment is completely effective (p. 588). Coma also occurs in African trypanosomiasis, but is a late complication (p. 580).

Cerebral Tumour and other causes of raised intracranial pressure. As pressure rises the brain stem becomes displaced and ischaemic. Consciousness is lost slowly and signs of pressure coning and papilloedema develop (p. 1125).

Abnormal Metabolic States

Hypothermia. Coma is associated with body temperature lower than 30° C. (86° F.). A rectal thermometer or special low range thermometer is essential for accurate measurement in this range. It may be due to exposure to severe climatic conditions or from normal loss of body heat if a poorly clad person lies helpless or unconscious in an unheated room for one or more days especially if he is an infant or elderly and thin. Hypothermic coma may occur in the absence of cold if the metabolic rate is depressed by myxoedema (p. 706) or hypopituitarism (p. 685).

Heat Hyperpyrexia. There is a history of heat exposure, a high body temperature and a striking absence of sweating.

Diabetic Ketosis and Hypoglycaemia. The differential diagnosis is fully discussed on p. 762.

Renal Failure (Uraemia). The onset of coma is slow and preceded by signs of toxaemia (p. 820).

Hepatic Failure (Cholaemia). The clinical features of hepatic failure are discussed on p. 1027.

Hypercapnia. Retention of carbon dioxide as a cause of coma is discussed on pp. 312 and 867.

Poisoning

Acute Alcoholism. There may be a history of a drinking bout and the odour of alcohol may be detected in the breath, but the possibility of illness or injury occurring to a patient who has taken a harmless amount of alcohol must be considered or the alcohol may have been administered after the onset of illness. The patient is often stuporous with flushed skin, full pulse, deep respiration and dilated pupils which react sluggishly to light. In severe alcoholic poisoning there may be deep coma with respiratory depression. The pupils then become very small but if the patient is shaken the pupils dilate though he cannot be roused and again constrict when he is left at rest (Macewen's pupil).

Narcotics and Other Substances. There may be a history of the patient having taken some drug, or an empty bottle may be found, or in the case of a caustic, there may be signs of burns around the mouth or in the throat. The pupils are usually dilated and react sluggishly to light; the pulse is rapid and feeble and the breathing shallow. In morphine poisoning the pupils are usually very contracted. Barbiturate poisoning is often a result of attempted suicide. It is so common that it should be considered in every case of coma where the cause is unknown. Treatment must be started without delay (p. 96). In carbon monoxide poisoning the lips and cheeks have a bright pink flush.

Management. The unconscious patient is exposed to special hazards as he is dependent on reflexes to protect his body and maintain respiratory and cardiovascular function and the reflexes are progressively lost as coma deepens. Until full consciousness returns the patient must be protected from these hazards in addition to those of the causative disease.

THE EPILEPSIES

Epilepsy is a brief paroxysmal disorder of cerebral function which recurs periodically.

Aetiology and Pathology. An epileptic fit is associated with sudden paroxysmal discharges from neurones. In some cases the instability is constitutional, and the tendency may be familial, but the factors precipitating the attack are usually obscure. Epilepsy is not a mental disease though it may be associated with cerebral disorders causing mental symptoms. Psychological reactions of resentment and aggression may occur if the patient is deprived of a normal place in school and social life. Emotional disturbances may precipitate an attack in the predisposed. In other cases it is clear that irritative factors are involved, such as cortical scars, ischaemia, infection, toxaemia, alkalaemia, hypoglycaemia, water retention or hypertension. On this basis it is possible to classify epilepsy into two aetiological groups:

1. Idiopathic (cryptogenic) where there is no apparent cause.
2. Symptomatic, where there is an apparent cause.

Fits of identical type may occur in either group and the response to drug treatment tends to be related to type of fit rather than to aetiology. It is therefore desirable to adopt a double classification of the epilepsies, one based on causation and the second on the clinical features of the fit. The latter is based on clinical observation correlated with the findings of electroencephalography (EEG).

Percutaneous recording of the electrical potentials associated with cerebral activity confirms that an epileptic attack is associated with a sudden abnormal electrical discharge from cerebral neurones. Sub-threshold paroxysms may be demonstrable between clinical attacks. The EEG phenomena indicate that the differences in type of seizure are due to the site of the initial abnormal discharge of cerebral neurones and the mode of spread. One group originates in the upper brain stem (p. 1081) (termed the 'centrencephalon' by Penfield) and simultaneously disturbs function in both cerebral hemispheres. The site of discharge is believed to be the upper reticular formation because in grand mal and petit mal suspension of consciousness is invariable. In other seizures the EEG suggests that the discharge originates in another part of the brain, usually in one hemisphere (hence 'local epilepsy' as distinct from 'generalised epilepsy'). The discharge may remain localised, causing one of the various forms of minor epilepsy. Consciousness may not be lost. Where the focus is in or near the cortex, the discharge tends to spread slowly to neighbouring cortex causing a motor or sensory seizure according to the site (Jacksonian seizure). Consciousness is retained. The focal discharge may spread rapidly by neuronal pathways to the upper brain stem from whence a generalised seizure is evoked. This causes a grand mal attack preceded by the symptoms of the local discharge—the so-called 'aura'. The true Jacksonian seizure is most suggestive of symptomatic epilepsy with a local lesion, but this may cause generalised epilepsy without local sign and conversely focal seizures may occur without demonstrable local pathology. Every case of epilepsy therefore must be considered as possibly symptomatic. This is particularly important in 'epilepsy of late onset' (over 30 years of age) when the responsible lesion may be a progressive one. Before starting the specialised investigation required it is necessary to ascertain by close questioning of patient and relatives when the first fit occurred. There may have been an isolated seizure several years before the onset of recurrent attacks of epilepsy. The first seizure, resulting from a cortical scar due to birth injury, need not occur in infancy but may be at any time up to the age of 20. Table 14 lists the most likely causes of epilepsy presenting at different ages. 'Idiopathic' fits commonly start before the age of 20 and there is often a family history of epilepsy. Cerebral tumour is not the most common cause of symptomatic epilepsy except in middle age, but it is obligatory to exclude it in all cases where epilepsy appears to be symptomatic and the cause of the fit is not apparent.

The causes of symptomatic epilepsy may be local or general.

LOCAL. (*a*) Space-occupying lesions, e.g. cerebral tumours, abscess.

(*b*) Vascular lesions, e.g. cerebrovascular disease both acute and chronic, hypertensive encephalopathy, cerebral thrombophlebitis.

(*c*) Brain injury, including birth injuries.

(*d*) Inflammatory lesions, e.g. meningovascular syphilis, general paralysis of the insane, cerebral cysticercosis and occasionally meningitis and encephalitis.

(*e*) Degenerative lesions, e.g. pre-senile dementias.

TABLE 14

RELATIVE FREQUENCY OF CAUSE OF EPILEPSY RELATED TO AGE AT FIRST ATTACK

	Age	*Lesion*
Infancy .	0–2	Birth injury, degeneration, congenital abnormality
Childhood .	2–10	Birth injury, febrile thrombosis, trauma, idiopathic
Adolescence .	10–20	Idiopathic, trauma, birth injury
Youth . .	20–35	Trauma, neoplasm
Middle age .	35–55	Neoplasm, trauma, arteriosclerosis
Senescence .	55–70	Arteriosclerosis, neoplasm

PENFIELD & JASPER (1954). *Epilepsy and the Functional Anatomy of the Human Brain.* London: Churchill.

GENERAL. (*a*) Cerebral anoxia from heart block, asphyxia or carbon monoxide poisoning.

(*b*) Metabolic disturbances such as uraemia, hypoglycaemia, alkalosis and hepatic failure.

(*c*) Poisons such as alcohol, cocaine, lead, ether, cardiazole.

(*d*) Undetermined as occurs in childhood in association with teething and febrile illness.

Clinical Features. Attacks may occur at any time in the 24 hours or may be confined to the night or the day. Precipitating factors such as fatigue, excitement, inadequate food intake or the excessive consumption of alcohol may be apparent. Several attacks may occur in a day or they may be separated by intervals of months or years.

The generalised types of attack show little individual variation. The 'local' types vary according to the exact site of the irritable focus in the brain and the way in which the discharge spreads. The descriptions which follow are characteristic, but individual variation is marked.

Generalised ('Centrencephalic') Seizures

(*a*) *Grand mal* (*Major Epilepsy*). Some patients have warning of an impending attack. There may be a change of mood for many hours or days beforehand and the attack may be ushered in by a psychical sensation or a feeling of a breeze. This is the true *aura*. Other types of subjective experience are part of the content of the fit and indicate local epilepsy even if the seizure rapidly becomes generalised. Most attacks of grand mal epilepsy occur without warning. In many cases the following six stages may be recognised—aura, tonic phase, clonic phase, flaccid coma, post-epileptic automatism, sleep. In others the attack is terminated after the aura or one of the later stages. The patient suddenly loses consciousness and becomes rigid, falling to the ground if standing or sitting. The sudden spasm of respiratory and glottal muscles of this *tonic phase* may cause a cry and the arrested breathing results in cyanosis. This phase lasts about 30 seconds and is succeeded by the *clonic phase* in which a series of short jerks involves the musculature. At this stage the tongue may be bitten because of clonic movements of the jaw, and incontinence of urine may occur. Froth appears at the mouth. The movements persist for about a minute and then give place to a state of *flaccid coma* in which the patient relaxes and breathes deeply and stertorously while remaining unconscious. The corneal reflex is lost, tendon jerks are sluggish and extensor plantar responses may be obtained temporarily. Some patients recover consciousness in a few minutes and are able to continue immediately with their previous activities, but consciousness may not be regained for as long as half an hour, after which the patient has a headache and is often confused and drowsy. He may go into a deep but natural sleep for an hour or two, from which he awakens without recollection of the seizure. Occasionally the attack is followed by *postepileptic automatism* in which the patient carries out complicated actions such as undressing, moving furniture, or making a journey without being aware of having done so. He may on rare occasions be violent during this stage. Exhaustion of the cerebral neurones may lead to a paresis which may persist for as long as 24 hours (Todd's paralysis).

(*b*) *Petit mal*. The main feature of this type of attack is momentary impairment of consciousness. This may be so slight as to pass unnoticed, or the patient may pause in what he is doing or saying ('absence'), only to resume immediately. There is often transient pallor and a vacant expression. Rolling of eyeballs and twitching of eyelids and fingers at a rate of 3/second may occur but there is no generalised convulsion. The patient is usually unaware that he has had an attack, but sometimes a prolonged period of automatism may occur so that he may subsequently deduce that an attack has occurred from the results of his unconscious behaviour. Children may experience many attacks in the course of a day, a condition formerly known as pyknolepsy. Petit mal invariably starts in childhood but may continue into adult life. More usually however it disappears in adolescence or is replaced by grand mal.

Other forms of epileptic fits related to petit mal are characterised by myoclonic jerks or sudden falling to the ground without convulsive movements ('akinetic seizures'). Though classical petit mal is very rarely a symptomatic epilepsy, these related types commonly are.

Local Epilepsy

(*a*) A focal discharge with only local spread is unusual except in the temporal lobe. *Temporal lobe epilepsy* (psychomotor epilepsy) is the name given to a group of seizures commonly associated with a lesion of a temporal lobe or its related structures. It is characterised by subjective awareness of hallucinations or illusions of taste, smell, sight or hearing associated with disorientation and confusion, and with disturbances of memory such as *déjà vu* or failure of recognition, and with alteration but not loss of consciousness. In the 'dreamy state' or automatism resulting from this, the patient may carry out well co-ordinated apparently purposeful actions without any subsequent memory of them. It should therefore be borne in mind that psychotic behaviour may be a manifestation of temporal lobe epilepsy and hence be amenable to treatment. Incomplete temporal lobe seizures are the most commonly found type of minor epilepsy, particularly in adults, and should not be confused with true petit mal, as the treatment is different. An EEG may be required to differentiate them but usually a careful history will reveal that occasional attacks have some of the features just described.

(*b*) *Jacksonian Epilepsy*. This term is sometimes used to describe any seizure which has a focal onset. It is best restricted to those which spread to adjacent parts of the body according to their representation in the cerebral cortex, the 'march' being relatively slow. It may be motor or sensory. The motor seizure is a slow clonic convulsion without preceding tonic phase. The spread may be arrested at any stage, or it may continue until a major attack develops with loss of consciousness, but otherwise consciousness is retained. This type of seizure is strongly indicative of a lesion in or near the cortex but occasionally occurs in idiopathic epilepsy.

(*c*) *Major Epilepsy with focal onset*. Many patients have seizures in all respects like classical grand mal as described above but with an *aura* consisting of a subjective experience or focal twitching produced by the epileptic discharge beginning in a particular part of the brain before spreading to the upper brain stem. Thus a visceral sensation, such as a feeling of discomfort in the epigastrium, may occur, or a smell, taste, sound or visual phenomenon may be experienced. The discharge, which may originate deeply in the white matter of a hemisphere, may result from an irritative lesion or idiopathic epilepsy. A macroscopic lesion should be sought for, particularly if abnormal neurological signs are present between seizures.

Status Epilepticus. In this condition a succession of fits occurs without the patient recovering consciousness between them. It is a most serious state and, unless arrested, is rapidly fatal because of exhaustion of the neurones.

Diagnosis. The first step is to determine whether the attack is epileptic or some other form of paroxysmal incident. The most useful evidence in making this decision is undoubtedly a good description of the attack by a reliable eye-witness; examination of the patient or accessory investigations such as the electroencephalogram are no replacement for this essential requisite. Epilepsy must be considered in any episodic disturbance even if the pattern bears little resemblance to classical descriptions. Syncope is often preceded by a feeling of faintness and is not usually accompanied by convulsions. Heart block may cause sudden loss of consciousness and even precipitate a fit because of cerebral ischaemia, but the very slow pulse rate will make the diagnosis clear. Hysterical convulsions are rare, and are characterised by their bizarre movements, their increasing violence when the patient is restrained and their occurrence only before an audience.

If the attacks are diagnosed as epileptic, the second step is to determine whether they are symptomatic or idiopathic in origin. This is done by taking a careful history and by making a thorough examination which may reveal evidence of the causative lesion in symptomatic epilepsy. A family history or the onset of attacks in childhood favours idiopathic epilepsy. Investigations such as the Wassermann reaction, radiological examination of the skull, chemical and cytological studies of the cerebrospinal fluid, electroencephalography, radioscan and pneumoencephalography (p. 1128) may all be required in some cases before a final decision can be reached. This is especially so when epilepsy appears for the first time in middle age, when the likelihood of its being symptomatic and due to a cerebral neoplasm is much greater.

The EEG is not a short-cut to the diagnosis of epilepsy. It may be diagnostic on the rare occasion when a record is taken during an attack. In these circumstances, however, witnessing the attack may be of equal value, though if the clinical features are ambiguous the presence of an associated electrical discharge is indicative of epilepsy. Between attacks the record may be normal or abnormal. Moreover, abnormal recordings may be found in persons who have never had an epileptic attack. The EEG may, however, be of great value in localising a cerebral cause of symptomatic epilepsy.

Prognosis. A single epileptic attack is seldom fatal except on the rare occasions when it causes an accident to the patient, such as drowning or falling from a height. Status epilepticus is rapidly fatal unless the fits are arrested.

The prognosis in regard to continuance of the fits is hard to determine until the effects of treatment have been observed. In general, however, the more frequent and violent the fits, the less well they respond; a bad family history is not necessarily an adverse factor. In symptomatic epilepsy the prognosis is largely that of the underlying cause, but it should be remembered that even when the cause is removed, as may be done in the case of a meningioma, fits may continue to occur as a result of scarring. Patients with epilepsy are often concerned about the possibility of their children developing epilepsy. If two epileptics marry there is an increased risk of some of their children developing epilepsy, but if an epileptic marries a non-epileptic the risk is not appreciably greater than in the general population.

Treatment. The management of epilepsy is an important social problem as the incidence is about 1 in 200 of the population. In symptomatic epilepsy, treatment is directed to removal of the cause, but anticonvulsant medication must also be employed. It is important that the patient with idiopathic epilepsy should lead as full and normal a life as possible. Children should continue their education at the ordinary school unless the attacks are too frequent, when admission to an epileptic colony where educational facilities are available should be sought. Adults should be found employment that does not involve danger to themselves or others, such as working near fire, water, machinery or at heights or driving vehicles. Such occupations as printing, book binding, light assembly work, packing, store-keeping and clerical work are eminently suitable. They should also undertake normal recreations, but swimming, riding a bicycle and driving a car are prohibited. Precipitating factors, such as lack of sleep, deprivation of food and alcoholic excess should be avoided.

There are various satisfactory anticonvulsant drugs available, but in all cases regular and persistent medication is of the greatest importance. The patient should continue to take the prescribed drug for at least three years after the last attack. The drugs employed are as follows. Phenobarbitone is given in doses of 30-120 mg. t.d.s. It is suitable for the treatment of all forms of epilepsy but has the disadvantage of inducing somnolence in some cases, although this effect decreases if the patient perseveres with the drug. Phenobarbitone may be given in a capsule containing granules of differing solubilities to obtain prolonged effect. Each capsule ('spansule') contains 100 mg. A single morning or evening dose may be adequate. Phenytoin (Epanutin) has little hypnotic effect and is of great value in the treatment of major epilepsy. The average dose is 100 mg. three or four times a day. The drug is frequently combined with phenobarbitone. Toxic symptoms, such as dizziness, fever, ataxia and hyperplasia of the gums may develop and necessitate discontinuance of the drug. Mesontoin (Methoin) is allied to phenytoin and is also of value in the treatment of major epilepsy. The average dose is 100-200 mg. three times a day. Toxic symptoms include skin rashes and, on rare occasions, blood dyscrasias. Primidone (Mysoline) is also of value against major epilepsy, being used in doses of 250 mg. two, three or four times a day. It may give rise to mental confusion and skin rashes.

It is usual to commence treatment with phenobarbitone, and if this is insufficient to control the attacks to supplement it with phenytoin. If this combination fails then primidone or mesontoin alone or in combination with phenobarbitone may be tried. Local epilepsy is treated with the same anticonvulsants. Primidone is probably the drug of choice for temporal lobe epilepsy but sulthiame (Ospolot) may be effective. An average dose is 3-6 tabs. of 200 mg. daily. Its most important side-effect is hyperpnoea.

These drugs are sometimes helpful in petit mal but usually a different range of drugs is necessary. The most effective is ethosuximide (Zarontin, Emeside). It is made up in 250 mg. capsules, 4-6 of which should be taken daily. Troxidone (Tridione) in dosage of 300 mg. two, three or four times a day, is also of great value in the treatment of petit mal, especially when the characteristic pattern is found in the electroencephalogram. The incidence of toxic symptoms is slightly higher than with other drugs, and hence careful watch should be kept for evidence of agranulocytosis, dermatitis or nephrosis. It is ineffective against grand mal, and if a patient has both types of attack, another drug must be combined with troxidone. Should ethosuximide or troxidone fail, phensuximide (Milontin) and acetazolamide (Diamox) are worthy of trial in petit mal.

In cases of temporal lobe epilepsy pathological changes such as scars due to trauma at birth are frequently demonstrated, and surgical excision of these lesions has been undertaken with benefit but it should only be considered if the most vigorous medical treatment has failed and social adaptation is becoming impossible on account of fits or psychotic deterioration.

Treatment of a Major Attack. A padded gag should be placed between the teeth, and the clothing around the neck loosened. It is not necessary to restrain the patient more than is required to prevent him from injuring himself. After the attack, the patient should be turned on to his side and precautions taken to keep the airway clear. He should be observed carefully when he recovers consciousness, in case automatism should develop.

Treatment of Status Epilepticus. Various drugs such as sodium phenobarbitone, 200 mg. intramuscularly, and chloroform anaesthesia or curarisation have been recommended for the treatment of status epilepticus, but paraldehyde given parenterally is undoubtedly the best. The drug should be given by deep intramuscular injection in a dose of 10 ml. and then 5 ml. should be given by the same route every half-hour until the fits stop, when the intervals between the doses should be lengthened. In very severe cases intravenous administration may be more effective, 50 ml. of paraldehyde being added to 500 ml. of normal saline and given by drip. Phenytoin (5 ml.) given intravenously is also valuable. This is also the route of choice when the patient is dehydrated. Adequate long-term anticonvulsant therapy must be started as soon as the patient recovers consciousness.

Narcolepsy

This is characterised by irresistible attacks of sleep from which, however, the patient can be aroused immediately. He may go to sleep at work and several attacks may occur in a day. It is often associated with three other phenomena; *cataplexy*, in which, as a result of a sudden emotion, power is lost from the limbs, though consciousness is preserved; *sleep paralysis*, in which on waking or falling asleep the patient finds himself unable to move though mentally he is wide awake; *hallucinatory states*, in which vivid and terrifying hallucinations occur, often just as the patient is falling asleep. This combination of symptoms may be associated with disease in the region of the hypothalamus. In other cases no abnormality can be demonstrated in the nervous system. Amphetamine sulphate, 5-10 mg. two to four times a day, or one 15 mg. spansule in the morning is of value in reducing the frequency of attacks.

CEREBRAL TUMOURS

Intracranial tumours cause local symptoms by irritation or destruction of cerebral tissue and more diffuse symptoms by raising the intracranial pressure.

Clinical Features. These may be divided into:

1. Symptoms due to local involvement of cerebral structures.
2. Symptoms due to raised intracranial pressure.
3. Symptomatic epilepsy.

Features due to Local Involvement. The development of symptoms due to local damage is progressive but the rate of development varies widely. Encapsulated, non-infiltrating tumours such as meningiomas and acoustic neuromas may cause very slight symptoms for many years and the nervous system adapts so well to slow compression that a very large tumour may be present without causing disabling symptoms. In fact, symptoms may temporarily disappear though physical signs (such as nerve deafness in acoustic neuroma) usually persist. The slow progression may suggest degenerative disease rather than tumour (p. 1066) but an important distinction is that neoplasm is no respecter of tissue barriers. Neurones are progressively involved according to their anatomical contiguity and not according to their functional system as with degeneration. Malignant tumours progress more rapidly and may simulate a vascular lesion at the onset, but the further progressive course is distinctive. Death may occur a few weeks after the first symptom. The particular symptoms and signs due to local damage depend on the site of the tumour. The various cerebral syndromes are outlined on p. 1088. A difficult type of tumour to diagnose is a vascular one (angioma or arteriovenous malformation) since symptoms may then be due to intermittent disturbance of local blood supply causing transient but recurrent symptoms. Auscultation over the skull may reveal a bruit and indicate the site of a vascular tumour.

Features due to Increased Intracranial Pressure. An intracranial tumour or other 'space occupying lesion' increases the pressure as it expands within the non-expansile skull and displaces brain tissue, but the main factors responsible for a rise in intracranial pressure are cerebral oedema due to obstruction of venous drainage and interference with the circulation of cerebrospinal fluid. These factors are more prominent in some sites than others, for example tumours of the posterior fossa or deep in a cerebral hemisphere. In general, pressure effects are more likely with infratentorial than with supratentorial tumours.

The cardinal symptoms and signs of raised intracranial pressure are headache, vomiting and papilloedema. The headache may at first be unilateral and then may have some lateralising value, but it soon becomes diffuse or located round the base of the skull. It is usually throbbing or bursting in quality. Characteristically it is present on first waking in the morning and passes off as the day goes on. It lasts longer each day until eventually it becomes continuous, and may be subject to sudden paroxysms of exacerbation. It is made worse by exertion and lying down, or by straining or coughing, all of which further raise the intracranial pressure. When the headache is severe vomiting occurs. It is classically described as projectile and without preceding nausea, but neither of these features is invariable. Papilloedema (p. 1096) and visual failure also develop, followed soon by drowsiness progressing gradually to coma if pressure is not relieved. In the later stages respiration slows and the pulse rate may decrease too, though this is not significant unless the rise of pressure is rapid (as in subarachnoid haemorrhage). Generalised convulsions may occur and 'false localising signs' may develop such as sixth nerve palsy or bilateral extensor plantar responses, not due to local involvement of the affected structures, but due to raised intracranial pressure. The intracranial contents are shifted by the rise in pressure. As the falx and tentorium form rigid divisions within the skull, a tumour of one cerebral hemisphere displaces the upper brain stem towards the other side and the medial border of the temporal lobe herniates between the edge of the tentorium and the brain stem ('tentorial pressure cone'). Mid-brain pressure causes progressive loss of consciousness and the herniated temporal lobe compresses the third nerve, causing the pupil to dilate on the side of the tumour. As pressure continues to rise and brain stem compression becomes severe coma deepens, plantar reflexes become extensor, and both pupils dilate and fail to respond to light. Cerebellar tumours are particularly liable to cause a rise in pressure and the cerebellar tonsils then tend to herniate through the foramen magnum, compressing the medulla ('foraminal pressure cone') with respiratory or cardiac arrest and death. The pressure often exceeds 300 mm. of cerebrospinal fluid, the upper limit of the normal range being 180-200 mm. It is unwise to do this estimation for purposes of diagnosis since withdrawal of fluid by lumbar puncture may so alter the pressure gradient as to precipitate a pressure cone. Lumbar puncture should only be carried out in the presence of papilloedema if facilities for further intervention are readily available. The patient *must* be observed carefully for early signs of deteriorating level of consciousness. Pupillary changes should not be awaited before starting treatment.

Symptomatic Epilepsy. Generalised fits may occur as a result of raised intracranial pressure, in which case they are of no value in localising the lesion. They may, however, be an early manifestation of a cerebral tumour due to local irritation of neurones by the growing tumour and they may precede all other signs by months or even years. These fits are often focal in type and may be of value in localising the lesion. Fits developing for the first time after the age of 20 should always raise the possibility of a cerebral tumour (p. 1117).

Radiology. Radiological examination of the skull is often negative, but should always be carried out. If the pineal gland is calcified it may be seen to be displaced. Local erosion of the skull or a thickening of bone may be found, especially with meningiomas, and slowly growing tumours and tuberculomas may be calcified. The pituitary fossa may be enlarged or the clinoid processes eroded in the case of pituitary adenomas. Raised intracranial pressure, if of long duration, causes rarefaction of the clinoid processes. In children there may be separation of the sutures and increased convolutional markings on the skull (beaten silver appearance) but it is difficult to distinguish the latter from the normal in childhood. Radiological examination of the lungs is an essential part of the investigation in view of the frequency of cerebral metastases from carcinoma of the bronchus.

Straight X-ray of the skull rarely gives localising information in cerebral tumour such as is necessary for surgical treatment. This usually requires radiography with a contrast medium to outline the tumour but radioscanning with isotopes may provide satisfactory localisation.

Arteriography. This is the method of choice for three reasons. The intracranial vessels, outlined by a radio-opaque dye injected into the carotid or vertebral arteries, may be seen to be displaced in the region of the tumour, and secondly the appearance of the vessels may indicate the pathological nature of the lesion. Thirdly the procedure is relatively safe and does not upset the balance of intracranial pressure as does pneumoencephalography.

Pneumoencephalography. Air injected into the cerebrospinal fluid by lumbar puncture in replacement of an equal volume of fluid (20 to 30 ml.) may be used as a contrast medium which can be manipulated to the various parts of the ventricular and subarachnoid space by suitable positioning of the head, enabling enlargements or displacements of the ventricular system and atrophic dilatations of the cortical sulci to be recognised. In the presence of raised intracranial pressure air is introduced directly into the ventricles through a burr hole in the skull (ventriculography). This diminishes the risk of impacting the brain stem in the foramen magnum but the danger of secondary rise in pressure from expansion of the air is sufficiently great to limit this investigation to a pre-operative procedure. A less risky procedure with special applications is to introduce a radio-opaque medium such as Myodil into the ventricles through a brain cannula.

Electroencephalography. Abnormally slow waves may be detected in the electroencephalogram (EEG) recorded from the scalp over a cerebral tumour. The signs may be obscured by diffuse abnormalities if raised intracranial pressure disturbs consciousness and deep seated hemisphere tumours may be missed in the early stages. Cerebellar tumours may not alter the EEG record. Despite these disadvantages, electroencephalography has the outstanding advantage of being harmless and it can be repeated frequently in early cases when the diagnosis may be in doubt even after the above specialised radiological procedures.

Echo-encephalography. This may also demonstrate a shift of intracranial contents without risk to the patient.

Cerebrospinal Fluid. The dangers of lumbar puncture are discussed above. The risk should never be taken without making sure that the fullest possible information is obtained from a small sample of fluid. The most valuable observation is the pressure of the fluid. This must be measured with a properly fitting manometer. It cannot be judged from the rate of escape of fluid from the needle. The protein content of the CSF is raised if a tumour is near the surface of the brain or involving the ventricles. It is rarely above 100 mg. per 100 ml. but may be 1000 mg. per 100 ml. or more in acoustic neuroma. The cellular content is usually normal but may be raised to 10-20 per c.mm. and some of these cells may be identified as tumour cells by appropriate staining. Sometimes primary, or more often metastatic cerebral tumours may spread over the meninges. (The clinical picture resembles a low grade meningitis.) In these rare cases the cell count may exceed 100 per c.mm. and the glucose content of the fluid is decreased. In all other instances the glucose and chloride content of the fluid is normal and these substances should be omitted from the investigation if only a small sample is available. For purposes of differential diagnosis it is more useful to be assured that the WR and the Lange curve (p. 1151) are normal.

Diagnosis. It is essential that cerebral tumour be diagnosed before signs of raised intracranial pressure appear. This can only be done if the possibility of a tumour being present is considered in every case presenting cerebral symptoms for the first time and if careful examination, continued observation, and if necessary, special investigations are carried out in suspected cases. The differential diagnosis depends largely on the presenting clinical features which may be headache (p. 1131), epilepsy (p. 1116) or manifestations of a focal lesion in a particular area. Other space occupying lesions such abscess a or subdural haematoma must be borne in mind.

Treatment. Meningiomas, acoustic neuromas, some pituitary tumours and favourably sited gliomas should be excised. Other pituitary adenomas and medulloblastomas in children are better treated by radiotherapy. In other types of tumour radiotherapy may produce a temporary remission but the value of the time gained is very doubtful as there are often undesirable side-effects and recurrence is almost certain.

Intracranial pressure may be lowered by dehydration while the nature of the lesion is being investigated or the patient prepared for operation. A retention enema of magnesium sulphate (200 ml. of a 25 per cent. solution) may be valuable. More rapid dehydration is achieved by intravenous injection of urea (1 g. per kg. of body weight as a 30 per cent. solution in 10 per cent. invert sugar) or of 50 ml. of 25 per cent. mannitol, or of 50 per cent. sucrose or glucose. In some cases surgical decompression will have to be undertaken. If a pressure cone develops acutely, recovery is unlikely unless pressure is relieved within half an hour by ventricular cannulation or intravenous dehydration therapy. Relief of headache may often be necessary. Aspirin, phenacetin or codeine may be used but morphine or other respiratory-depressant drugs should not be given until it is established that the tumour is not amenable to surgery. Symptomatic epilepsy is treated with the usual anticonvulsant drugs (p. 1123).

Prognosis. Death is inevitable if a cerebral tumour cannot be removed though it may be postponed by operations designed to lower intracranial pressure by allowing the brain room to expand. Benign tumours can be removed completely if they grow in an accessible part of the brain as can gliomas, or even a solitary metastatic tumour, when they are in a part of the brain such as the frontal lobe or cerebellum which can be sacrificed with relative impunity. Even then recurrence is frequent. In other situations removal is impracticable and even with palliative decompression the average expectation of life is less than six months in the case of the more malignant growths.

HEADACHE

Headache is perhaps the most common symptom a doctor is asked to treat. There is a particular anxiety related to this pain because of its association with the brain, the organ of the mind. The brain itself is insensitive but some intracranial structures have receptors for pain. These are the major venous sinuses, the arteries round the base of the brain and the meningeal arteries and the dura of anterior and posterior fossae (but not the middle fossa). All the extracranial tissues are pain sensitive. The most important mechanisms underlying headache are vasodilatation, muscle spasm, referred pain and psychogenic headache (which is often associated with one of the previous mechanisms). Some common examples are:

Vascular Headaches. Dilatation of intracranial vessels is responsible for the headache in influenza and other systemic infections and acute renal infections, the headache which follows an epileptic fit (p. 1119), post-traumatic headache, and the headache associated with high altitudes, hunger, hypercapnia, anaemia, and the use of vasodilator drugs such as histamine, nitrites and alcohol. Abrupt elevation of blood pressure may cause headache in this way. Vascular headache is typically throbbing in type. The headache of migraine and chronic hypertension on the other hand is due to dilatation of extracranial arteries (p. 1133).

Traction on Intracranial Structures. In addition to distension, traction on the great vessels and dura at the base of the brain causes headache. Pain is momentarily increased by sudden movement of the head. Occasionally pain of this nature indicates the localisation of a cerebral tumour (p. 1126). The value of headache as a localising sign is reduced by the fact that pain may be referred to another part of the head but if unilateral it does help to indicate the side of the tumour.

INFLAMMATION. Meningism, whether due to meningitis, haemorrhage or other cause produces generalised headache which is accentuated by head movement, coughing or straining. Involvement of the roots of the cranial nerves contributes to headache by causing spasm of occipital and nuchal muscles. Neck stiffness is an important sign of meningeal inflammation (p. 1156). Extracranial inflammation usually causes more localised headache. *Temporal arteritis* is a disease of later life characterised by localised throbbing pain in the head, sometimes associated with arteritis in other parts of the body. Tenderness is localised over and around an inflamed artery and if a segment of a vessel is removed for biopsy the pain often disappears.

MUSCLE CONTRACTION. This is one of the most common mechanisms of headache. Contraction is commonly due to emotional tension, producing the most persistent type of headache which varies in intensity from a feeling of tightness to a true aching pain. It may be unilateral but is usually bilateral. Nodular areas and points of tenderness may be palpated in the painful muscles or along the occipital and supraorbital ridges. Secondary muscle spasm may contribute to a prolonged pain referred from other structures. It may also be caused by irritation of cervical nerve roots by cervical spondylosis (p. 1223) though this is probably overestimated as a cause of headache.

REFERRED HEADACHE. Disease of structures in the head may cause pain referred to the cranium. Eye disease such as glaucoma and iritis causes frontal headache. Ciliary spasm induced by some errors of refraction may cause pain but 'eye strain' is certainly not a common cause of headache. Nasal and sinus disease causes pain in the malar, nasal and frontal areas which responds to nasal vasoconstrictors. Dental, aural and temporo-mandibular joint diseases may cause pain spreading far beyond the area of primary pain. Pain may even be referred to the head in angina pectoris.

PSYCHOGENIC HEADACHE. By far the most common cause of headache is emotional upset. It is often vascular or tension in type but may assume peculiar qualities which have features suggesting a mechanism of conversion hysteria (p. 1254). It is often a sense of pressure at the vertex or a tight band round the head, constant day and night, and completely resistant to analgesic drugs though it may respond to non-analgesic sedatives. There is usually an underlying personality defect in this type of 'functional headache' which is much rarer than the vascular or tension types.

Treatment. Headache may disappear on removal of a primary cause such as systemic infection, ocular or sinus disease, or of a simple psychological problem. Otherwise the treatment is symptomatic. Aspirin (300-600 mg.) and other simple analgesics are valuable but opiates should be avoided. Psychogenic headache is resistant to all treatment except psychotherapy. If the mechanism is vascular it may be advisable to use the phenothiazine or ergotamine derivatives recommended for migraine (*vide infra*) and muscle tension headache may respond to tranquillisers such as chlordiazepoxide, meprobamate and barbiturate.

Migraine

Migraine is characterised by periodic headaches which are usually unilateral and are often associated with visual disturbance and vomiting.

Aetiology. The condition is believed to be due to a disturbance in the carotid or vertebro-basilar vascular tree. An initial phase of vasoconstriction causes symptoms of local cortical or brain stem ischaemia and this is followed by vasodilatation. These changes affect both intra- and extracranial arteries and it is dilatation of the extracranial vessels which causes pain by stretching the pain nerve-endings in the arterial wall. Pain may be prolonged by secondary muscular contraction. Heredity plays an important part, migraine and benign essential hypertension being closely linked in the family. The patient with migraine often has an obsessional personality. She sets herself a perfectionist standard and becomes tense and anxious in endeavouring to attain this. In childhood she tends to react to emotional stress with 'biliousness' or 'acidosis', from adolescence to middle life with migraine, and later with a type of Ménière's syndrome (p. 1110). Migraine is a prototype of psychosomatic disease and it is common for 'typical migraine attacks' to be associated with 'tension headache' (p. 1132).

Clinical Features. The condition usually starts after puberty and continues until late middle life. Headache occurs in paroxysms which are often related to emotional stress, particularly during the period of relaxation when the stress is over. Attacks occur at intervals which vary from a few days to several months. The first symptom of an attack is due to vasospasm. This is commonly a sensation of white or coloured lights, scintillating spots, wavy lines, or defects in the visual fields. Paraesthesiae or weakness of one half of the body may be experienced or there may be numbness of both hands and around the mouth. These symptoms may last up to half an hour, and are followed by headache which usually begins in one spot and subsequently involves the whole of one side of the head; this may be the same or the side opposite to the visual or sensory symptoms. The side affected is not constant with each attack and the headache often becomes bilateral. The pain is usually severe and throbbing in character and is associated with vomiting, photophobia, pallor, sweating and prostration which may cause severe loss of muscle tone and necessitate the patient taking to her bed in a darkened room. The attack may last from a few hours to several days and it leaves the patient weak and exhausted. In rare cases the cerebral changes may last for several days, particularly if the motor area is involved (hemiplegic migraine). Permanent cortical damage may result, usually leaving a visual scotoma of cortical type (p. 1095).

Diagnosis. This is based on the periodic nature of the disturbance, the family history and the absence of abnormal physical signs. Rare cases of migraine are caused by a cerebral aneurysm or angioma ('symptomatic migraine'). In these cases migraine is strictly unilateral and usually associated with focal neurological signs.

Treatment. The patient should rest in a quiet dark room. For the occasional attack simple analgesics such as aspirin or tab. codeine co. B.P. may be effective. Phenobarbitone or prochlorperazine (Stemetil) taken regularly may be of prophylactic value and the latter, or related drugs may have some therapeutic value in an attack. If these relatively non-toxic drugs are not effective the acute attack is treated with ergotamine tartrate, which constricts the cranial arteries. This may be given by subcutaneous injection (0·25 to 0·5 mg.) or it may be dissolved under the tongue (2 mg.), being repeated in an hour if necessary. It is most effective when given subcutaneously at the onset of an attack; hence in severe cases it is worthwhile teaching the patient to administer the injection herself. Ergotamine may be combined with caffeine or an anti-emetic drug such as meclozine. Too frequent use of ergotamine may cause peripheral vasoconstriction leading to gangrene of fingers or toes. It is best avoided in patients with hypertension and is contraindicated during pregnancy when the alternative drugs listed above should be used.

The general management of the patient is very important. An attempt should be made to avoid obvious precipitating factors and by means of simple psychotherapy the patient should be encouraged to adopt less exacting standards.

DISORDERS OF THE CEREBRAL BLOOD VESSELS

The blood supply required by the brain does not vary significantly when the brain is active. As it has no means of storing energy or functioning by anaerobic metabolism the brain is particularly vulnerable to disorders of its circulation and so lesions of the cerebral blood vessels are among the most common causes of neurological disease. The brain tissue may be damaged by haemorrhage or rendered ischaemic by an inadequate blood supply. Three factors have to be considered in cerebrovascular disease:

1. *Vascular Disease*. Pathological change must be present in one or more of the arteries supplying the brain. This may be a local abnormality such as aneurysm or arteriovenous malformation or part of more widespread arterial disease (p. 277). The most common vascular disorder is atherosclerosis, which is usually associated with hypertension. Inflammatory disorders such as syphilitic endarteritis, thrombo-angiitis obliterans and polyarteritis nodosa are rare causes of cerebrovascular disturbance but recognition is important as active treatment may be possible. Any of these may be the underlying cause of haemorrhage or thrombosis.

The final accident depends on one or other of the following factors.

2. *Circulatory Dynamics*. Haemorrhage occurs if pressure rises rapidly within a pathological vessel and an existing hypertension makes it more likely that a further rise will exceed the capacity of the damaged vessel to accommodate it. Conversely if pressure falls excessively the flow through a stenosed vessel may be insufficient to enable proper functioning of the brain in its distribution area. Temporary ischaemia causes temporary neurological disturbance but if ischaemia lasts for more than a few minutes infarction of the brain occurs. Hypotension also predisposes to thrombosis within a damaged blood vessel and infarction is then almost inevitable. Infarction may also result if a major vessel is suddenly occluded by impaction of an embolus without any underlying vascular disease in the brain.

3. *Clotting Disorders*. Primary thrombotic diseases (p. 672) rarely cause cerebral arterial thrombosis. Spontaneous thrombosis may, however, occur in the cerebral veins or dural sinuses (p. 1150). Bleeding disorders (p. 660) may cause cerebral purpura and areas of softening may coalesce and lead to more severe haemorrhage as is not uncommon in acute leukaemia of children but cerebral haemorrhage may be the cause of death in idiopathic thrombocytopenic purpura.

Cerebral Atherosclerosis

This is a disease of late middle life and old age affecting the sexes equally.

Pathology. For details of the pathological changes in the blood vessels see p. 278. The progressive obliteration of many cerebral arteries leads to ischaemia which causes degeneration of cells and fibres giving rise to multiple small areas of atrophy, particularly of the grey matter. There is normally an excellent collateral circulation in the brain and this minimises the damage caused by even advanced stenosis, but the compensation becomes inadequate (circulatory insufficiency) if the systemic blood pressure drops appreciably or if narrowing of a collateral vessel occurs. Occlusion of a vessel is followed by necrosis of the cerebral tissue which is replaced by a glial scar, or a cyst may form.

Clinical Features. The onset is usually insidious but may be marked by a minor cerebral infarction (p. 1138). The clinical picture will depend on the area of the brain which is mainly involved but it is commonly a progressive impairment of the higher faculties such as loss of intellectual capacity, impairment of memory for recent events, defective judgement and emotional lability. Selfishness, resistance to change, querulousness and the appearance of paranoid ideas are common features. Impairment of self-control may involve the patient with the authorities because of some public offence.

Physical symptoms may occur with the mental disorder or as the sole abnormality. If caused by brief circulatory insufficiency they may be transient, but recurrent small infarcts lead to a cumulation of minor or major neurological defects which depend on the regions affected. There may be dysphasia, hemiplegia or brain stem symptoms and the signs may be bilateral. A double hemiplegia may leave as a residue a form of pseudobulbar palsy with spasticity of the tongue, dysarthria, emotional lability and bilateral signs of an upper motor neurone lesion. Epilepsy may occur (p. 1118) and a Parkinsonian picture develops when the brunt of the ischaemia falls on the basal ganglia (p. 1187). These lesions may cause their appropriate physical signs but otherwise it is difficult to differentiate the condition from other causes of pre-senile or senile dementia (p. 1269). The CSF usually shows no abnormalities though occasionally there is a slight rise in the protein content. There are no specific radiological or EEG abnormalities though the latter will show the signs of diffuse local brain damage.

Diagnosis. The main problems are to distinguish cerebral atherosclerosis from other causes of dementia and from cerebral tumour. The pre-senile dementias of Pick and Alzheimer occur earlier and physical signs are much less evident. Dementia paralytica usually occurs earlier and gives rise to Argyll Robertson pupils and a positive Wassermann reaction. The diagnosis of chronic alcoholism and chronic subdural haematoma may be an exceedingly difficult problem if these diseases are not borne in mind when taking the history. Cerebral tumour may cause a similar mental state but physical signs are likely to be unilateral. Nevertheless if this possibility cannot be excluded it may be necessary to investigate further with lumbar puncture, arteriography, pneumo-encephalography or isotope encephalography.

Treatment. There is no specific treatment but much can be done to avoid difficulties. Vasodilator drugs are of no value. Epileptic attacks should be controlled by anticonvulsant therapy, and every effort should be made to keep the patient as active as possible. He should not be allowed to undertake matters requiring unimpaired judgement and is best advised to retire from business worries. Confusional states may occur if the patient is moved to an unfamiliar place such as a hospital but this may be required in the later stages.

Prognosis. Degenerative vascular disease is a progressive disorder, the duration of which depends on how soon a major vascular occlusion occurs. This may be postponed by protecting the elderly patient from factors which are likely to cause hypotension. The importance of restoring the blood pressure in elderly people with haematemesis, myocardial infarction, etc., is emphasised. Anaesthetics often make these patients much worse; hypotensive drugs must be used with caution, and even the unnecessary use of hypnotics is to be deprecated.

CEREBRAL INFARCTION

Cerebral Arterial Thrombosis

This may occur at any age according to the cause, in children as a complication of acute fever, in young adults due to meningovascular syphilis and in old people due to atherosclerosis.

Clinical Features. In common with other vascular disorders, arterial thrombosis causes maximum disability within a short time but there is later some recovery. Nevertheless, in comparison with haemorrhage and still more with embolism, the onset of symptoms in thrombosis is comparatively gradual, symptoms continuing to develop over several hours or even one or two days. This mode of onset causes less generalised disturbance of cerebral function. The patient is often dazed and may have an epileptic seizure at the onset, but consciousness is usually retained. The focal signs depend on the area of brain that is involved (p. 1088). Hemiplegia, due to infarction in the territory of the middle cerebral artery, is the most common disability and there may also be hemianaesthesia and hemianopia. These deficits occur on the side of the body opposite to the lesion. The obstruction to blood flow may be in the middle cerebral artery or one of its branches, but a similar picture will result from stenosis or occlusion of the internal carotid artery just beyond its origin from the common carotid artery in the neck, or of the main vessels as they arise from the arch of the aorta. The most common of these sites is the internal carotid artery. This is the probable site if there are recurrent transient episodes of weakness or sensory symptoms on the opposite side ('stuttering hemiplegia') and the localisation is certain if there is a history of one or more brief attacks of blindness or flashing lights in the visual field of the eye on the side of the lesion. This is due to ischaemia of the retina of that eye as the ophthalmic artery which supplies it branches from the internal carotid artery just below its intracranial bifurcation. Visual symptoms are transient because circulation is restored by collateral vessels from the orbit, and the rich intracranial anastomosis accounts for the temporary nature of many of the cerebral symptoms; indeed complete occlusion of the internal carotid artery may occur without causing symptoms. Palpation of the internal carotid artery in the neck may reveal diminished pulsation but a more valuable sign is a bruit. The pressure required to occlude circulation in the retinal arteries may be measured with an ophthalmo-dynamometer. It may be reduced on the side of carotid occlusion during the acute stage until circulatory adjustment takes place.

Similar lesions occur in the vertebro-basilar territory, transient or permanent signs of damage to brain-stem structures and the occipital area of the cerebral cortex being found. The more common symptoms are vertigo (p. 1109), deafness, diplopia, sudden loss of muscle tone causing the patient to fall, loss of consciousness, ataxia and cortical blindness. An attack may resemble migraine. Infarction is commonly limited to the area supplied by a single branch of the basilar or a vertebral artery. One of the most readily diagnosed is infarction of the postero-lateral part of the upper medulla and of the adjacent part of the cerebellum due to occlusion of the posterior inferior cerebellar artery or the vertebral artery from which it arises. (The latter may be distorted by osteophytes of cervical spondylosis as it passes upwards through the foramina of the transverse processes of the cervical vertebrae.) The syndrome of *posterior inferior cerebellar artery thrombosis* is a useful exercise in localisation (Fig. 74). The affected nuclei, cranial nerves, or pathways are indicated after each symptom or sign. There is sudden vertigo (VIII), hiccough or vomiting (X), with dysphagia (IX) at the onset. The palate is paralysed on the side of the lesion (X) and there are usually ipsilateral cerebellar and sympathetic signs (Horner's syndrome, p. 1112). There is often ipsilateral facial pain with loss of pain and temperature sense (V) and, less consistently, hemianalgesia of the other side of the body from the neck down (spinothalamic tract).

It is possible that thrombosis of the carotid or vertebro-basilar vessels may be prevented if stenosis is recognised early. Verification by angiography is justified in these circumstances. The CSF is usually normal but its protein content may be slightly raised.

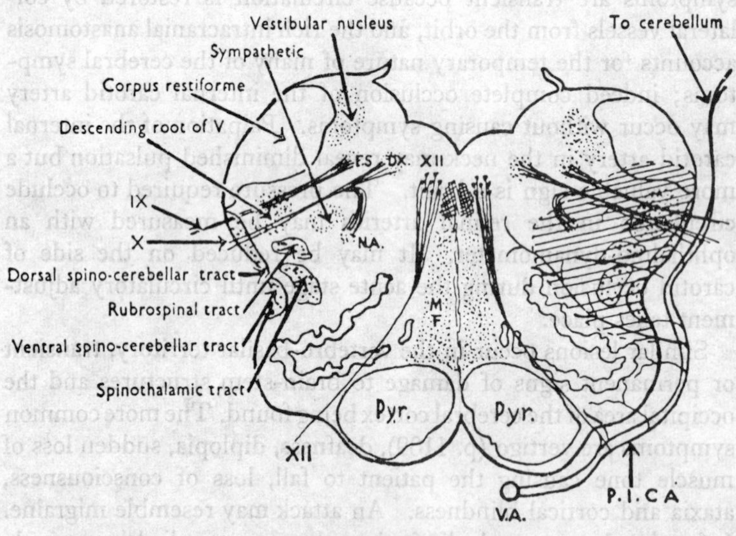

Fig. 74

Thrombosis of the Posterior Inferior Cerebellar Artery
(Lateral Medullary Thrombosis)

A cross section of the medulla at the level of the hypoglossal nucleus. The transverse extent of the thrombosed region in the lateral part of the medulla is cross-hatched. Its vertical extent cannot be represented, but it extends from the middle of the seventh nerve nucleus above to that of the twelfth nerve below. F.S.—Fasciculus solitarius and nucleus gustatorius (IX). D.X.—Dorsal nucleus of Vagus. N.A.—Nucleus ambiguus of the Vagus. Pyr.—Pyramidal tract. M.F.—Mesial fillet. V.A.—Vertebral artery. P.I.C.A.—Posterior inferior cerebellar artery. (Walshe, Sir Francis (1963), *Diseases of the Nervous System*, 10th ed. Edinburgh: Livingstone.)

Treatment. Infarction due to stenosis or thrombosis of intracranial arteries does not benefit from anticoagulant therapy but recurrent transient ischaemic episodes should be treated with anticoagulants on a long-term basis in the hope of preventing a major stroke. If stenosis of the internal carotid or vertebral artery is suspected, it should be confirmed by arteriography and then relieved by surgery, or the patient placed on long term anticoagulant therapy. The management of the stroke is described on p. 1145.

Prognosis. The outlook depends on the site and extent of arterial involvement. If the patient survives the acute stage some recovery of function may be expected during the first one to two months but residual damage is almost certain if infarction has occurred. One thrombosis is often followed sooner or later by another and this sequence might be prevented by the long term use of anticoagulant therapy.

Cerebral Embolism

Unlike other causes of circulatory disturbance, embolism may damage a brain which has previously had healthy blood vessels. An embolus most often lodges in the left middle cerebral artery and arises from sources of thrombus in the arterial side of the circulation. Common causes are atrial fibrillation (especially when it is intermittent or terminated with quinidine), mural thrombus after myocardial infarction, subacute bacterial endocarditis and clot or fragments of heart valve dislodged during cardiac surgery. Thrombosis in peripheral veins rarely causes cerebral embolism except when the embolus can reach the arterial circulation by passing through a patent interventricular septum (paradoxical embolus). Air or fat may enter the arterial circulation after injury to the thoracic cage, long bones or perinephric tissue and the resulting cerebral infarction is similar to that caused by blood clot.

Clinical Features. Of all vascular catastrophes embolism is the most abrupt in onset. This feature should always suggest embolism though the diagnosis can only be tentative unless a source for the embolus can be demonstrated. Loss of consciousness or a seizure may be present but often the patient is only dazed and confused. The signs depend on the site of infarction. The condition may progress due to spread of thrombosis proximal to the embolus, or may regress due to the embolus passing more peripherally. Secondary haemorrhage is common so that red cells may be found in the cerebrospinal fluid, complicating the diagnosis. Frequently the fluid is normal.

Treatment. The treatment during and after the stroke is described on p. 1145. Anticoagulant therapy should be started immediately because of the danger of further emboli. It is not certain how long this should be continued but there is probably only a small risk if treatment is withdrawn after six months. It may also be possible to remove the primary source of emboli.

Prognosis. Embolism is rarely fatal and the prognosis will depend largely on the source of the embolus. The neurological deficit improves to some extent as oedema and neuronal shock subside, but there may be residual symptoms according to the extent of the cerebral damage.

Intracerebral Haemorrhage

This is a common cause of a stroke or apoplexy in people who have both hypertension and atherosclerosis.

Pathology. Bleeding may occur with any disease of the intracranial vessels but most commonly with atherosclerosis and aneurysm. Rupture is usually precipitated by abrupt rise of blood pressure occasioned by physical or emotional stress but sometimes is apparently spontaneous. Coagulation defects are rare causes (p. 660). The effused blood destroys cerebral tissue and later forms a haematoma or a cyst. More often early death occurs as the blood bursts through to the ventricles or to the surface of the brain where it enters the subarachnoid space. Spontaneous intracerebral haemorrhage most often occurs from the lenticulostriate branch of the middle cerebral artery in the external capsule and rapidly involves the internal capsule. The pons is also a frequent site (where bleeding is usually fatal) but haemorrhage may occur from any intracerebral artery.

Clinical Features. The onset is rapid with focal signs according to the site of haemorrhage. About half of the cases lose consciousness within a few minutes. Before consciousness is lost, headache may be complained of and vomiting is common at the onset. Neck stiffness may be found. The rapid displacement of the brain stem causes coma with loss of muscle tone, stertorous breathing and slowing of the pulse and respiration. The face is often congested. Pupils may be unequal. If the haemorrhage is pontine the pupils become pin point in size and temperature rises to 40° C. (104° F.) or higher. The more common external capsular haemorrhage causes contralateral hemiplegia. At first the head and eyes are deviated to the side of the lesion and the loss of tone is greater in the muscles of the contralateral side of the body. The plantar reflex is extensor on the limp side. The naso-labial fold on that side is flattened and the cheek blows in and out on respiration. If the patient survives, the depth of coma lessens in a few days, restless movements appear, and tone returns to the paretic side. The head and eyes now tend to deviate towards the paralysed side and signs of spasticity appear on that side. On recovering consciousness the patient may be dysphasic if the haemorrhage has affected the dominant hemisphere (p. 1090) and contralateral sensory or hemianopic defects may be found. Voluntary movement gradually returns to the proximal muscles of the hemiplegic limbs, but the skilled movements of the hand may be permanently lost. The amount of recovery depends mainly on the extent of the damage. The initial recovery is fairly rapid but the tempo slows down after the second month. The initial improvement is attributed to recovery from 'neuronal shock'. This concept, due to Hughlings Jackson, is applicable to all acute vascular and traumatic lesions of the central nervous system. It is considered that sudden lesions may temporarily suppress the function of neurones which are, however, capable of resuming function at a later date. Neurones damaged beyond the stage of recovery are not capable of regeneration. Some functional recovery is, however, possible by taking advantage of the capacity of the central nervous system to perform functions in different ways. The first order sensory neurones and the lower motor neurones are uniquely necessary and their loss cannot be replaced.

Diagnosis

1. *Cerebral haemorrhage, thrombosis and embolism.* These need to be distinguished from each other. The onset of haemorrhage is

rapid, vomiting frequently occurs and the loss of consciousness is usually deep. It often occurs during the day and during conditions of stress. The blood pressure may be found to be raised above its previous level and there is often retinal and cardiac evidence of pre-existing hypertension. Temporary hypertension may, however, occur as the result of subarachnoid haemorrhage because of disturbance of the vasomotor centres of the brain stem. Thrombosis is usually more gradual in onset, often taking several hours to develop, and often occurs during sleep or after an acute illness which leads to hypotension. Consciousness is frequently preserved. The onset of embolism is very sudden, consciousness may or may not be lost, and usually the source of the embolus can be discovered. After the acute phase of a stroke there is little to distinguish one cause from another. The cerebrospinal fluid contains blood if intracerebral haemorrhage ruptures to the surface of the brain or into the ventricles but may be normal with an intracerebral haematoma. Conversely, bleeding may occur from an area of infarction, particularly after embolism.

2. *Subarachnoid Haemorrhage*. The onset is sudden, signs of meningeal irritation are present and the CSF contains blood.

3. *Cerebral Tumour*. Five per cent. of strokes are due to cerebral tumour but usually the onset of symptoms is gradual. Headache is frequently a prominent feature.

When the history is available the differential diagnosis may be simple but in most cases, especially where coma has occurred, it is not possible to differentiate the types of cerebrovascular disorders with confidence. Where this is essential for treatment it is necessary to investigate the appropriate vascular tree by arteriography.

Treatment. There is no certain method of arresting intracerebral haemorrhage. If the blood pressure remains persistently elevated it should be lowered gradually by hypotensive drugs (p. 239), a careful watch being kept for fresh neurological signs. When consciousness has returned arteriography should be carried out if the history suggests that the cause of the bleeding is a local vascular lesion such as an aneurysm. This may also be desirable if the history, physical findings and EEG record suggest that there is a localised haematoma in a region of the brain which can be explored surgically as it may be possible to aspirate the clot and coagulate the bleeding point. This procedure should be especially considered in the patient who shows signs of a progressive focal lesion after recovering consciousness.

Apart from measures directed at preventing further vascular damage, the management of the patient who has had a stroke is essentially the same irrespective of the cause. The immediate problem is the nursing of an unconscious patient which involves the maintenance of a clear airway, avoidance of respiratory infection, care of the skin, bladder and bowel, and the provision of fluids, and food by an intragastric tube. Passive movements of all limbs should be begun from the outset to prevent the development of contractures, and active movements started as soon as the patient has recovered sufficiently to co-operate. These should be performed against gradually increasing resistance. When power is returning, skilled movements should be re-established by carefully chosen occupational therapy. Early mobilisation and vigorous rehabilitation are essential. The patient should be propped up within 48 hours of recovering consciousness, encouraged to use the limbs and got out of bed as soon as he is able to support himself in a chair. Recovery of postural reflexes is facilitated in this way. Walking should soon be re-established, the optimum method being taught by a physiotherapist. It may be necessary to use aids such as a toe-spring or below-knee caliper. Unfortunately the return of upper limb function after hemiplegia is usually less satisfactory, but the difference between a useful and a useless limb may be determined by the physical treatment given during the first weeks of the illness.

Prognosis. Cerebral haemorrhage is commonly fatal and recovery is unlikely if coma lasts longer than 48 hours. If the patient survives, some functional recovery is probable but it will not be complete. In hemiplegia, the lower limb usually recovers sufficiently for the patient to be able to walk, especially with the aid of such devices as a caliper or a toe-spring. Functional recovery of the upper limb is seldom adequate for useful function and dysphasia due to haemorrhage rarely improves.

Hypertensive Encephalopathy

This is a transient disturbance of cerebral function associated with high blood pressure and is discussed on page 231.

Cerebral Aneurysms

Aetiology and Pathology. Congenital aneurysms are more common within the skull, especially in the vessels comprising the circle of Willis and particularly in its anterior part. Aneurysms, which are frequently multiple, occur at the bifurcation of an artery where there is a congenital defect of the medial coat and often a small anomaly of branching. The medial defect permits local distension of the vessel wall when the blood pressure rises in later life. For this reason clinical manifestations usually occur after the age of 40. They are equally common in both sexes.

Clinical Features. Many cerebral aneurysms cause no symptoms and are found at routine post-mortem. Symptoms may occur in three ways: (*a*) focal pressure symptoms, (*b*) spontaneous subarachnoid haemorrhage, (*c*) intracerebral haemorrhage or infarction. There may be local or generalised headache. This occasionally simulates migraine especially if accompanied by transient focal cerebral symptoms but is distinguished by the fact that it always occurs on the same side and does not vary in successive attacks like true migraine. The most common pressure effect is third nerve palsy (p. 1098) as aneurysms may be in relation to this nerve at several sites in the circle of Willis and in the posterior fossa. Aneurysm of the internal carotid artery within the cavernous sinus presses on the optic nerve or chiasma, the third, fourth or sixth cranial nerves and the first and second divisions of the fifth nerve. Thus, there may be visual failure, ptosis, diplopia or pain and sensory loss on the face. Signs of raised intracranial pressure do not occur as the aneurysms are small in size.

There may be no evidence of intracranial aneurysm until the onset of subarachnoid haemorrhage. Before a major haemorrhage there is often a series of small leaks which cause headache or pain and stiffness in the neck and shoulder. Infraclinoid aneurysms in the cavernous sinus cannot, of course, bleed into the subarachnoid space. Rupture into the cavernous sinus causes unilateral pulsating exophthalmos as the arteriovenous fistula transmits arterial pulsation to the orbit. A loud bruit may be heard over the eye on the affected side. Otherwise a bruit is rare in cerebral aneurysms. Aneurysm rupturing into the brain causes intracerebral haemorrhage which is indistinguishable from that due to other causes and it may be the underlying lesion in transient cerebral ischaemic attacks or infarction by causing arterial spasm or thrombosis.

Diagnosis. Aneurysm presenting as a focal lesion must be distinguished from other causes of visual failure (optic neuritis, neoplasm), other causes of diplopia (disseminated sclerosis, syphilis) and of headache and subarachnoid haemorrhage. Leaking aneurysm may be mistaken for meningitis or 'rheumatism' of the neck and shoulders.

Treatment. The presence and site of the aneurysm must be confirmed by arteriography and surgical treatment undertaken if possible since a second and probably fatal leak commonly occurs.

Prognosis. The aneurysm may remain stationary or may continue to expand, causing progressive focal signs, or may leak causing headache and mild meningeal irritation. Early recognition of the true nature of leaking aneurysm may enable the disaster of severe subarachnoid haemorrhage to be avoided as the danger of frank rupture is ever present.

Subarachnoid Haemorrhage

Aetiology and Pathology. Bleeding into the subarachnoid space is commonly due to rupture of a congenital aneurysm (p. 1146) but it may occur from an arteriovenous or capillary malformation, a ruptured atherosclerotic artery, head injury or rarely from a mycotic aneurysm in subacute bacterial endocarditis. Bleeding from an infarct is rarely serious but subarachnoid haemorrhage may be the presenting symptom of the red infarct caused by cerebral venous thrombosis (p. 1150).

Clinical Features. There may be previous focal signs of pressure due to an aneurysm, especially diplopia (p. 1146) or focal epilepsy from an arteriovenous anomaly. Symptoms of slight leaks from an aneurysm may precede frank rupture by weeks or months (p. 1147). Final rupture is sometimes precipitated by physical strain but is more often spontaneous. There is a sudden onset of severe headache, usually in the occipital region but passing into the neck and shoulders. In severe cases the patient feels as if he had been struck a blow but others may attribute the pain to a local cause in the neck. The patient may vomit at the onset and consciousness may be lost rapidly. Fresh focal signs may appear because of disruption of cerebral tissue by the haemorrhage or from vascular spasm in the vessel bearing the aneurysm and in other branches of the same parent vessel.

The findings on examination are:

Meningeal Irritation. Neck rigidity and Kernig's sign (p. 1157) are usually present but may not be marked with slight haemorrhage. They are the most important clues to the nature of the stroke.

Focal signs. These are only present if an aneurysm has caused local pressure effects or vascular spasm.

Signs of Raised Intracranial Pressure. Coma tends to deepen rapidly and may be accompanied by bilateral extensor plantar responses and the other manifestations of brain stem pressure such as slowing of the pulse and irregular or Cheyne-Stokes breathing (p. 173). There may be a low grade pyrexia. The sudden rise in pressure causes papilloedema in which swelling of the discs is slight but venous congestion and haemorrhage are marked. Haemorrhage is retinal or subhyaloid.

The cerebrospinal fluid is under greatly increased pressure and is uniformly bloodstained. This can be confirmed by comparing the colour of three specimens collected successively from one lumbar puncture. The supernatant fluid of the centrifuged CSF should be xanthochromic if some hours have elapsed since haemorrhage. Blood cells may be seen in the fluid for about three days after a fresh haemorrhage, and xanthochromia may persist for three weeks. Slight albuminuria and glycosuria may be caused by the sudden brain stem compression. These findings should not lead to a conclusion that the stroke is associated with renal disease or diabetes mellitus.

Diagnosis

1. *Coma.* Other causes of loss of consciousness must be considered (p. 1113). Only embolism compares with subarachnoid haemorrhage in rapidity of onset.

2. *Other cerebrovascular accidents.* A previous history compatible with leaking aneurysm is invaluable (p. 1146). Focal signs are

more common and meningeal irritation less prominent in other cerebrovascular accidents. Blood may be found in the CSF in primary intracerebral haemorrhage and in bleeding secondary to infarction but is usually of lesser degree.

3. *Other causes of meningism* (p. 1132). Meningitis has a slower onset and higher fever. The CSF contains leucocytes and organisms but no blood.

Treatment. The diagnosis must be confirmed by lumbar puncture but there is no advantage in repeating the procedure. If consciousness is retained it is sufficient to keep the patient quiet with measures for relief of headache until the source of bleeding can be sought by means of arteriography. The level of consciousness must be watched carefully, especially during the first 48 hours, for evidence that bleeding is continuing. Pre-operative investigation should not be delayed unless the patient is in coma as the risk of interference is then great. The general measures for the care of a comatose patient must be undertaken immediately but the decision to operate is only postponed and should be reconsidered from hour to hour in close collaboration with the surgeon. Surgical treatment may consist of ligature of the neck of an aneurysm or of the main supplying artery proximal to its site or of the common carotid artery in the neck. The danger of a second haemorrhage is greatest during the first 14 days, therefore unnecessary delay must be avoided. Premature surgical intervention may aggravate the condition of the patient by causing vasospasm, but when it is well timed it may reduce the mortality to less than 20 per cent. Recurrence of haemorrhage is improbable after two months and the risks of conservative treatment are then no higher than those of surgery. Conservative treatment is therefore appropriate for the mild case seen for the first time after the period of greatest danger from recurrence or for the case in whom the source of bleeding cannot be identified or in whom surgical intervention is too dangerous. These patients should be kept in bed for a period of about six weeks and then slowly rehabilitated. The choice of treatment requires careful joint consideration by physician and surgeon.

Prognosis. There is a great risk of death from subarachnoid haemorrhage due to ruptured cerebral aneurysm. In the absence of surgical treatment about 40 per cent. of patients die in the initial attack. Of those who survive about one-third have a recurrence of bleeding which frequently develops while the patient is still in hospital for the first attack.

Cerebral Venous Thrombosis

Thrombosis of the intracranial venous sinuses is associated with (*a*) thrombophlebitis spreading from infection of the middle ear, accessory nasal sinuses, face and scalp; (*b*) thrombotic and dehydrated states such as polycythaemia, the puerperium, and in cachectic conditions in infancy and old age; (*c*) head injury without penetration of the skin.

Lateral Sinus Thrombosis. This, the most common type, is usually associated with infection of the middle ear. There may be pain, oedema and venous congestion in the mastoid region from obstruction of the emissary veins which drain into the sinus. Slight facial weakness and sixth nerve palsy on the affected side, and an extensor plantar response on the opposite side are inconstant signs, often absent. Thrombosis commonly extends to the superior longitudinal (sagittal) sinus without evidence of lateral sinus involvement.

Sagittal Sinus Thrombosis. This may be ushered in by fits, especially in children, as thrombosis spreads to cortical veins. As the cortex near the vertex is involved on both sides, signs of an upper motor neurone lesion involving the lower limbs (paraplegia) are commonly found. In other instances, especially in adults, thrombosis on the walls of the upper chamber of the sagittal sinus interferes with absorption of the cerebrospinal fluid causing hydrocephalus. The patient remains alert but complains of headache. Papilloedema may endanger eyesight.

Cavernous Sinus Thrombosis. This is the most dangerous type since it may give rise to septicaemia besides endangering the eye in the orbit which drains into the affected sinus. There is pain behind the eye and oedema of the eyelids. Exophthalmos and papilloedema may also be apparent and ocular palsies due to damage to the third, fourth or sixth nerve in the lateral wall of the sinus may be present.

Treatment of cerebral venous thrombosis is by antibiotics and anticoagulants. The majority of cases recover, but specialist advice should be sought as sight is endangered by prolonged papilloedema.

THE CEREBROSPINAL FLUID

The cerebrospinal fluid is secreted by the choroid plexuses in the lateral, third and fourth ventricles. It leaves the ventricular system through the apertures and flows through the cerebral and spinal subarachnoid spaces. It is returned into the venous sinuses by the arachnoid villi. In health, the fluid is clear and colourless. The pressure at the lumbar theca with the patient lying on his side is 50 to 150 mm. of cerebrospinal fluid. It contains less than 5 lymphocytes per c.mm. and its important chemical constituents are protein 20-45 mg., glucose 50-80 mg., chloride (as sodium chloride) 700-750 mg. all per 100 ml.

The patency of the cerebrospinal fluid pathway is tested by Queckenstedt's test. One or both jugular veins are manually compressed while the CSF pressure is recorded in a manometer (estimations of pressure based on the rate of dripping from the needle are completely fallacious). If there is thrombosis of a jugular vein or obstruction in the cerebrospinal fluid pathway, as by a spinal tumour, the level of fluid in the manometer may not rise, or do so slowly and fail to fall when pressure is released. This result (positive) is found when the pathway for flow of fluid is reduced to a bore comparable with that of the needle; thus a negative result does not indicate that there is no compression of the spinal cord since a positive test does not occur until the block is almost complete.

Alterations in the characteristics of the cerebrospinal fluid are of great help in the diagnosis of neurological disease. The pressure may be raised in the presence of intracranial space-occupying lesions such as tumour and abscess, and also in acute inflammatory lesions such as meningitis. Bleeding into the cerebrospinal fluid (subarachnoid haemorrhage) is shown by blood in the fluid obtained by lumbar puncture. This can be distinguished from blood caused by a traumatic puncture by collecting the fluid in three tubes. In subarachnoid haemorrhage they are all equally blood stained whereas if bleeding is due to trauma by the needle the fluid is progressively less blood stained in each tube. After cessation of a subarachnoid haemorrhage frank blood disappears over the course of a few days, but a yellowish staining (xanthochromia) of the CSF due to altered blood pigments may be present within 24 hours of the haemorrhage and may persist for as long as three weeks.

A rise in the cell count is encountered in infection of the nervous system, lymphocytes being the predominant cell in virus infections, neurosyphilis, tuberculous meningitis and disseminated sclerosis. Polymorphonuclear leucocytes predominate in pyogenic infections. Whether the infection is acute or chronic also influences the type of cell, as acute lesions are more commonly associated with an increase in polymorphonuclear leucocytes, whereas in chronic lesions a lymphocytosis is more usual. A marked increase in the cell count gives a turbid appearance to the CSF. A rise in the protein content of the CSF occurs in many conditions. An increase from the normal figure of 20-45 mg. to several hundred milligrammes per 100 ml. may be present in fluid below the level of a spinal tumour which is causing a block of the CSF pathway, and also in the presence of neurofibromata of the spinal or of the auditory nerves. The rise in protein associated with other cerebro-spinal lesions is of much less degree, not usually exceeding 100 mg. per 100 ml. The glucose content of the CSF is raised in diabetes mellitus. It is reduced in pyogenic meningitis and in tuberculous meningitis, in which diseases it is a valuable diagnostic and prognostic sign. The chloride content of the CSF is reduced in any condition associated with a low blood chloride level (p. 839). The presence of organisms in the CSF can be detected by bacterio-logical examination and is an important part of the investigation of a suspected infection of the nervous system.

The Wassermann reaction of the CSF can be determined and also a precipitation test can be done which gives what is commonly known as the colloidal gold curve (Lange curve). This latter test expresses on a graduated scale from 0 to 5 the degree of precipita-tion of colloidal gold occurring in 10 tubes containing increasing dilutions of CSF. Precipitation in the first four or five tubes (a first zone rise) occurs in general paralysis of the insane, dis-seminated sclerosis and subacute encephalitis, e.g. 5554320000; precipitation which is greatest in the middle tubes in the series (a mid-zone rise) occurs in tabes dorsalis, e.g. 1233210000;

precipitation in the later tubes in the series occurs in meningeal inflammation, e.g. 0012344310. False positive Wassermann and Lange tests may be found if blood is present in the CSF.

INFECTIONS OF THE BRAIN, SPINAL CORD AND MENINGES

Intracerebral Abscess

Aetiology. The causes of cerebral abscess are:

1. Local spread by thrombophlebitis from an infected ear, paranasal sinus or from infection of the scalp or skull (p. 1150). This type is rarer since the introduction of antibiotics.
2. Infected compound fracture of skull, either a penetrating wound of the convexity or a basal fracture involving a sinus.
3. Metastatic spread from bronchopulmonary infection or subacute bacterial endocarditis (p. 213).
4. Bacteraemia is particularly dangerous in the presence of a by-pass of the lungs due to congenital cardiac disease or pulmonary arteriovenous anomalies. These patients now live longer so this cause of cerebral abscess is increasing.

The common organisms are staphylococci, pneumococci and streptococci, but other organisms and fungi such as actinomyces may be involved.

Pathology. The initial thrombophlebitis spreads to surrounding brain causing suppurative encephalitis. The pus is slowly localised by a surrounding wall of gliosis, which in a chronic abscess may form a tough capsule. Multiple abscesses, communicating or discrete, are common particularly with metastatic spread.

Clinical Features. There are three main types of clinical history.

1. ACUTE ENCEPHALITIS. Soon after head injury or otitis media (in which aural discharge may be temporarily suppressed) the patient develops headache, vomiting and drowsiness passing to coma. Focal cerebral signs may be present and the temperature is raised.

2. SUBACUTE OR DELAYED ENCEPHALITIS. Head injury, cranial infection or infected embolism may be followed after weeks or

months of apparent recovery by similar symptoms of encephalitis or of a chronic space-occupying lesion in the brain. During the latent interval there may be minor headache, irritability, general malaise, anorexia and intermittent pyrexia. These symptoms should lead to a search for a focal cerebral lesion in patients with infections such as otitis media, sinusitis or bronchiectasis.

3. Chronic Abscess. This may follow one of the previous types of onset or there may be nothing to suggest that the lesion is infective. The chronic abscess causes focal symptoms of a cerebral lesion (p. 1088) and those of raised intracranial pressure which are indistinguishable from those of cerebral tumour. The temperature is usually normal or even subnormal. The most common sites for abscess secondary to otitis media are the cerebellum and the temporal lobe. Sinusitis and haematogenous spread may cause abscess in any part of the brain but most commonly in the frontal lobes.

Lumbar puncture may help to confirm the diagnosis but should be avoided if the diagnosis is highly likely and especially if localising signs suggest cerebellar abscess. The CSF pressure may be raised and there is usually an increase in cells up to 100 per c.mm. with a predominance of lymphocytes. The protein may be raised up to 200 mg. per 100 ml.; the chloride and glucose content is normal and no organisms are found unless there is also a meningitis. The blood shows a polymorphonuclear leucocytosis and the ESR is often raised (but absence of these findings does not exclude chronic abscess).

Diagnosis. The presence of headache, personality change or unexplained ill-health in a patient with one of the causative diseases should suggest the possibility of cerebral abscess. Chronic abscess is often mistaken for cerebral tumour but this error will be minimised if careful otological and chest examinations are carried out in every case suspected of having an intracranial lesion. The EEG shows certain characteristic changes during the acute stage which may be valuable in diagnosis. As the diffuse encephalitis subsides changes in the EEG may be found which are very valuable for localisation of the abscess cavity or cavities. The radiological signs do not differ from those of cerebral tumour but radiological examination may show a causative lesion in ear, sinuses or chest.

Treatment. Prevention should be the first aim by efficient treatment of otitis media, sinusitis, fractures of the skull and bronchiectasis. Acute suppurative encephalitis is treated by immediate intramuscular injection of benzylpenicillin, 2 million units followed by 1 million units four-hourly. Surgical assistance should be sought early and the abscess, localised by EEG and angiography, tapped with a brain cannula for aspiration of pus and instillation of antibiotics. Myodil, a radio-opaque iodine compound, is also instilled so that progress may be followed by serial radiography. Antibiotic medication is subsequently determined by the bacteriological findings. Measures to reduce intracranial pressure may also be required (p. 1130). Excision of the abscess cavity may require to be undertaken at a later stage. In view of the high incidence of symptomatic epilepsy all patients should be given phenobarbitone prophylactically after the acute stage for a minimum period of two years.

Prognosis. About 15 per cent. of patients with cerebral abscess die despite treatment and half of the survivors develop epilepsy. There may also be residual loss of neurological functions, depending on the site of the abscess. Rupture of the abscess into a ventricle or subarachnoid space causes meningitis which is usually fatal. The possibility of a recurrence of infection must always be borne in mind.

Spinal Epidural Abscess

This condition usually arises as a metastasis from infection elsewhere, often a boil, which may be so trivial as to be easily overlooked. Pain of root distribution is severe. It develops acutely and is followed by progressive loss of sensation and power in the lower limbs with sphincter disturbance. The signs are those of transverse myelitis (p. 1186) but the local root irritation is the clue to the true cause. The temperature may be only slightly raised, but a polymorphonuclear leucocytosis is found in the blood. There may be radiological evidence of localised osteomyelitis of the spine. Paraplegia will become complete and irreversible if treatment is delayed. Large doses of antibiotics such as benzylpenicillin 1 million units four-hourly should be given immediately and the patient transferred to the care of a neurosurgeon without delay.

MENINGITIS

This is an inflammation of the pia and arachnoid membranes.

Aetiology and Pathology. Inflammation of the meninges may be sterile or infective.

Sterile. Blood in the CSF as in subarachnoid haemorrhage causes severe meningeal inflammation (p. 1147). Meningeal irritation ('meningism') without inflammatory reaction occurs in acute specific fevers, otitis media and pneumonia in childhood. Cellular reaction (lymphocytic) may be associated with symptoms and signs of meningeal irritation in poliomyelitis (p. 1173) and acute encephalomyelitis (p. 1186). Carcinomatosis of the meninges is a rare cause.

Infective. Formerly the most common meningeal infections were due to meningococcal infection or infection with pyogenic organisms carried in the blood from a distant focus in the heart or lungs or introduced from without (e.g. a penetrating wound of the skull, an infected ear, a fracture involving an accessory nasal sinus or a lumbar puncture), or from within by rupture of a cerebral abscess (p. 1153). These types of meningitis have become rare since the introduction of the antibiotics has simplified treatment of the primary causes, and for similar reasons, tuberculous meningitis (p. 1159) has become rare. The most common infection is now viral (p. 1162). Rare infections are due to syphilis or to fungi.

The pia-arachnoid is congested and infiltrated with inflammatory cells. A thin layer of pus forms and this may later organise to form adhesions. These may cause obstruction to the free flow of CSF leading to hydrocephalus, or may damage the cranial nerves at the base of the brain. The CSF pressure rises rapidly, the protein content increases and there is a cellular reaction which varies in type and severity according to the nature of the inflammation and the causative organism. The sugar content of the CSF is decreased in bacterial infections and in carcinomatosis of the meninges. If the patient is not kept in electrolyte balance the chloride content may be reduced due to the loss of chloride by sweating and vomiting.

Meningococcal Meningitis

(Cerebrospinal Fever, Spotted Fever)

The meningococcus, spread by droplet infection, enters the body through the nasopharynx and is carried in the blood stream to the choroid plexuses and meninges where it enters the cerebrospinal fluid. This type of meningitis occurs sporadically especially in children, and in epidemics in children and young adults living in crowded conditions such as schools and barracks. Spread of infection may be due to symptomless carriers of the organism.

Clinical Features. The onset is acute, with headache, pyrexia and often rigors. The headache rapidly becomes severe and spreads down the neck. There may be pain in the back and in the limbs. Convulsions are common at the onset in children. Photophobia is usually present; the patient is irritable, resenting interference and lying curled up on his side. He becomes confused and drowsy and later comatose.

SIGNS OF MENINGEAL IRRITATION. These are prominent and present from an early stage:

Neck Rigidity. The patient complains of neck stiffness and the examiner is unable to put the patient's chin on his chest by passive flexion of the neck. When he attempts to do so the muscle spasm evoked makes the neck so rigid that the head and trunk may be lifted from the bed instead of the neck being flexed. Spasm may be so severe, particularly in children, as to cause head retraction.

Kernig's Sign. If the patient's thigh is flexed to 90° from the abdomen, it is then impossible to straighten the knee passively owing to spasm of the hamstring muscles. This manœuvre stretches the roots of the sciatic nerve which are inflamed at their exits from the spinal theca.

Brudzinski's Signs. Passive flexion of a thigh causes spontaneous flexion of the opposite thigh, and flexion of the neck causes flexion of hips and knees on both sides. These signs are probably reflex in nature and so may be valuable indications of meningeal irritation when it is suspected that there may be voluntary rigidity of the neck.

SIGNS OF SEPTICAEMIA. There is often a petechial rash before the third day of the illness. Infection of one or more joints may occur; conjunctivitis is common, and adrenal failure, due to haemorrhage into the adrenal cortex (p. 725), is an occasional complication.

The cerebrospinal fluid is under increased pressure but papilloedema is uncommon. The fluid is turbid and contains a thousand or more cells per c.mm. These are almost entirely polymorphonuclear leucocytes and if a smear is stained with Gram's stain these cells may be seen to contain the Gram-negative diplococci. Failing this the meningococcus can be isolated by culture from the CSF and in the first few days from the blood. The protein content of the CSF is greatly raised and the glucose content markedly lowered. The blood shows a polymorphonuclear leucocytosis.

Diagnosis. The disease must be distinguished from the other causes of meningitis and meningism (p. 1156). The onset of subarachnoid haemorrhage is more acute, the temperature much lower and the CSF is blood stained. In meningism associated with pneumonia or acute infectious disease of children, the CSF pressure is increased but the fluid is clear and without cellular reaction. The exact aetiology of meningitis can only be determined by the results of bacteriological examination.

Treatment. Treatment must be started without waiting for bacteriological confirmation. If the fluid contains excess cells the patient should immediately be given sulphadiazine or sulphadimidine. The initial dose is 6 g. for an adult and 2 g. for an infant, followed by 1 g. four-hourly (or less in proportion to age) until the temperature is normal whereupon half the dose is given for a further six days. This may be administered by mouth, but if the patient is unable to swallow or is vomiting, the intravenous or intramuscular route must be used. Sulphonamides must never be given intrathecally. The CSF should be examined twice in the first 24 hours after starting treatment. If there is no response to sulphadiazine after that interval penicillin may be given parenterally and intrathecally. General measures for the treatment of fever (p. 18) must also be carried out, special attention being paid to the maintenance of hydration and to renal function. Analgesics for the relief of pain and headache may also be required. For the treatment of acute adrenal failure see p. 729.

Acute Pyogenic Meningitis

Infection by staphylococci, streptococci, pneumococci or *Haemophilus influenzae* sometimes occurs primarily in the meninges but it is more commonly secondary to infection in the heart, lungs, bones or elsewhere.

Clinical Features. Signs of meningitis are present (p. 1157) and associated with signs of a local septic focus but there is no rash and other pyaemic signs are rarer than in meningococcal infection. Bacteriological examination of the cerebrospinal fluid establishes the diagnosis and should be performed without delay.

Treatment. Both sulphonamides and penicillin should be started immediately without waiting for bacteriological confirmation as the treatment can later be modified appropriately. Sulphadiazine 6 g. by mouth is given at once followed by 2 g. four-hourly. Benzylpenicillin 10,000 units mixed with 10 ml. of the patient's CSF is injected intrathecally at the start of treatment but thereafter intramuscular injection is usually sufficient if given in large doses (at least 500,000 units every four hours). For an infection with *H. influenzae*, the drugs of choice are chloramphenicol and ampicillin. For an adult 1 to 2 capsules each containing 250 mg. of either drug should be given at six-hourly intervals. Preparations of chloramphenicol but not of ampicillin are available for parenteral administration. In all types of acute pyogenic meningitis treatment must be continued until the CSF has returned to normal and the temperature has been normal for at least two days.

Tuberculous Meningitis

Aetiology. The usual source of infection is a caseous focus in the meninges or brain substance adjacent to the cerebrospinal fluid pathway. The focus arises as a result of spread by the blood stream from a site elsewhere in the body, such as the lungs, lymph glands, bones, joints, alimentary or genito-urinary tract. The condition occurs most commonly shortly after a primary infection in childhood, but people of any age may be affected. The breakdown of the caseous focus may be due to head injury or to any illness causing diminished resistance. Tuberculous meningitis may occur as part of a miliary tuberculous infection.

Pathology. The brain is covered by a greenish, gelatinous exudate especially around the base, and numerous scattered tubercles are found on the meninges.

Clinical Features. Meningitis may be the first overt sign of the infection or the patient may be known to have tuberculosis in another organ. In children the onset of tuberculous meningitis is so insidious that it may be two weeks before the parents realise that the illness is serious. At first there is merely lassitude, loss of interest in toys and in play, unwillingness to talk, anorexia and constipation. Headache, at first slight, gradually becomes worse but meningeal signs may not appear until the third week. In adults the malaise, headache and meningeal signs progress more rapidly though not as quickly as in acute pyogenic meningitis. There may be occasional vomiting. The temperature is intermittently raised to 38° C. (99-100° F.) during the period of ingravescence but remains raised, though rarely to high levels, once meningeal signs appear. The condition then progresses more rapidly, and in untreated cases cranial nerve palsies, hemiparesis or other signs of cerebral damage, hydrocephalus with drowsiness, coma and moderate papilloedema may occur. In miliary tuberculosis choroidal tubercles may be seen in the ocular fundi.

The CSF is under increased pressure. It is usually crystal clear or slightly turbid but, when allowed to stand, a fine clot forms like a cobweb. The fluid contains up to 400 cells per c.mm. predominantly lymphocytes (the count must be made on a fresh specimen before it forms a clot). There is slight rise in protein (60-100 mg. per 100 ml.) and a marked fall in glucose (below 50 mg. per 100 ml.). Detection of the tubercle bacillus in a smear of the centrifuged deposit from the CSF may be difficult, the clot being the most likely place to find it. Inoculation of CSF into a guinea-pig is valuable for confirming the diagnosis if this cannot be done from smears or cultures of the CSF but as the outcome will not be known for six weeks, treatment must be started without waiting for confirmation.

Diagnosis. As the ill effects of delayed treatment are so serious it is extremely important to diagnose tuberculous meningitis early. It should be considered in every child sick without obvious cause, and especially in any patient known to have tuberculosis who develops a persistent headache, perhaps with slight pyrexia in the evening. If there is neck stiffness or choroidal tubercles in the eye grounds there should be no hesitation in performing lumbar puncture and evidence of miliary tuberculosis should be sought by radiography of the chest. The differential diagnosis in the later stage is from other infections of the nervous system and is made largely upon the findings in the cerebrospinal fluid.

Treatment. As soon as the diagnosis is made, treatment should be started with the three standard antituberculosis drugs in the following dosage: streptomycin sulphate intramuscularly, 3 mg. per kg. body weight to a maximum of 1 g. per day; para-aminosalicylic acid (PAS) by mouth, 300 mg. per kg. body weight to a maximum of 15 g. per day, in two divided doses; isoniazid by mouth, 10 mg. per kg. body weight to a maximum of 600 mg. per day in a single dose, along with pyridoxine, 10 mg. per day, to prevent peripheral neuropathy. For the first fortnight of treatment isoniazid should also be given intrathecally in a dose of 0·5 mg. per kg. body weight to a maximum of 50 mg. per day.

If the patient is gravely ill, prednisolone should be given by mouth, or intramuscularly, in a dose of 10 mg. four times per day. If the lumbar puncture findings suggest spinal subarachnoid block, hydrocortisone hemisuccinate should be injected intrathecally every day, along with isoniazid, in a dose of 1 mg. per kg. body weight. If obstructive hydrocephalus develops in spite of treatment with corticosteroids, surgical methods for ensuring continuous ventricular drainage must be adopted. During the acute stage of the illness skilled nursing is essential, and measures must be taken to maintain adequate hydration and nutrition.

When the patient begins to recover, systemic and intrathecal treatment with corticosteroids can be withdrawn gradually and the doses of the three antituberculosis drugs can be reduced to the standard levels (p. 425). Later, when the results of sensitivity tests on the tubercle bacilli isolated from the cerebrospinal fluid are available, one of the three drugs can usually be omitted and treatment continued with the other two. Antituberculosis chemotherapy should be given in every case for at least 18 months. Throughout the treatment great importance is attached to the maintenance of hydration and nutrition.

After treatment has been stopped lumbar puncture should be

carried out every two weeks for three months and less frequently thereafter. The patient should be kept under close supervision in order to detect relapses.

Prognosis. Untreated tuberculous meningitis is fatal in a few weeks but complete recovery is the rule with modern treatment if it is started before the appearance of focal signs or stupor. When treatment is started at a later stage the recovery rate is 60 per cent. or less and the survivors may be mentally deficient, epileptic, deaf, blind or show some other permanent deficit.

Viral Meningitis

Viral infections of the central nervous system are often associated with meningitis (meningo-encephalitis, poliomyelitis, p. 1173) but meningitis without clinical manifestation of parenchymal involvement of the nervous system may also occur. Some recognised clinical types are acute lymphocytic choriomeningitis and infection by ECHO or Coxsackie viruses. Encephalomyelitis or meningitis may occur as a complication of viral infections primarily affecting other organs (mumps, p. 55; measles, p. 51; infectious mononucleosis, p. 645; psittacosis, p. 353; herpes zoster, p. 1178 and infective hepatitis, p. 1007).

In the absence of evidence of viral disease of other organs the various types of viral meningitis can only be differentiated by the virologist. Viral meningitis is the most common type now found in Britain.

Acute Lymphocytic Choriomeningitis

(Benign Lymphocytic Meningitis)

This type of meningitis occurs sporadically or in small epidemics.

Aetiology. The virus is believed to be endemic in house mice. It can sometimes be isolated from the CSF of patients and transmitted to mice. There is probably an initial viraemia, and pneumonitis (p. 353) may be associated with meningitis.

Clinical Features. The condition commonly occurs in children and young adults. The onset is acute and evidence of meningeal irritation develops rapidly. Focal neurological signs are usually absent but diplopia and mild papilloedema may be observed. There may be a high pyrexia which gradually drops to normal in five to seven days. The CSF is under increased pressure. It is usually clear but may be turbid as there is an excess of lymphocytes (100-1500 per c.mm.) which may persist long after clinical cure. There may be a slight increase in the protein but the sugar and chloride levels are normal.

Diagnosis. The diagnosis is from other forms of meningitis.

PYOGENIC MENINGITIS. The turbid CSF contains an excess of polymorphonuclear leucocytes and the causative organism can be isolated.

TUBERCULOUS MENINGITIS. This cause of lymphocytic meningitis may be difficult to diagnose owing to the technical difficulties of isolating the tubercle bacillus. A normal level of sugar in the CSF is in favour of a diagnosis of acute lymphocytic choriomeningitis. If there is any serious doubt as to the diagnosis, it is better to start treatment for tuberculous meningitis while awaiting further bacteriological reports.

OTHER TYPES OF VIRAL MENINGITIS. Non-paralytic poliomyelitis may be impossible to differentiate. Signs of mumps, hepatitis, lymphadenitis, oro-genital ulcers or other causes of viral meningitis may be present but the diagnosis may depend on serological tests.

OTHER TYPES OF MENINGITIS. Canicola fever, secondary syphilis, fungal infections and rarely carcinomatous involvement of the meninges may produce a similar picture of the CSF cytology which is characterised by a mononuclear cell proliferation.

Treatment. There is no specific treatment for the condition. The patient is kept at rest in bed on symptomatic treatment until the temperature has returned to normal.

Prognosis. Complete recovery is the rule in acute lymphocytic choriomeningitis.

NEUROSYPHILIS

The incidence of neurosyphilis, decreasing for many years, is again increasing. The nervous system may be involved in the secondary or tertiary stage.

SECONDARY SYPHILIS. Invasion of the central nervous system in the secondary stage causes a mild lymphocytosis in the cerebrospinal fluid usually without symptoms (*asymptomatic neurosyphilis*) though mild headache and backache may be experienced. The majority of these cases will develop later neurological manifestations if untreated, hence the necessity for repeated lumbar punctures during the first two years after the diagnosis of primary syphilitic infection (p. 62) has been established. Acute syphilitic meningitis is a rare cause of lymphocytic meningitis.

TERTIARY SYPHILIS. Delayed effects of treponemal infection are:

1. Meningovascular syphilis in which the main lesion is an endarteritis obliterans with secondary ischaemic damage to the nervous system or meninges.
2. Parenchymatous neurosyphilis in which the spirochaete involves neurones directly. This includes general paralysis of the insane, tabes dorsalis and primary optic atrophy (p. 1097).

Meningovascular Syphilis

The essential lesion in meningovascular syphilis is an endarteritis obliterans, which may lead to thrombosis, and granuloma formation (gumma). The meninges may be covered with gelatinous exudate which damages the cranial nerves and may obstruct the flow of cerebrospinal fluid. Clinical manifestations which usually occur within five years of infection but may be much later, depend on the site of the lesion. The Argyll Robertson pupil (p. 1168) is a common feature in all types.

CEREBRAL LEPTOMENINGITIS. Basal gummatous meningitis damages the cranial nerves, particularly the second to the seventh inclusive (p. 1095). Meningitis at the vertex causes headaches, fits, mental changes and focal changes such as aphasia and loss of sphincter control.

CEREBRAL ENDARTERITIS. Occlusion of a vessel by endarteritis, especially if thrombosis is added, causes infarction of the brain with characteristic local signs (p. 1138). Infarction in a young patient without signs of degenerative vascular disease should always raise the suspicion of a syphilitic aetiology.

CEREBRAL GUMMA. This is a rare space occupying lesion in the skull.

CERVICAL PACHYMENINGITIS. Gummatous thickening of the dura mater in the cervical region involves the posterior nerve roots causing upper limb pain and the anterior roots causing wasting of muscles, usually in the hands.

MENINGOMYELITIS. This causes girdle pains and signs of progressive transverse myelitis (p. 1186), usually in the dorsal region.

SPINAL ENDARTERITIS. Thrombosis of a branch of the anterior spinal artery gives rise to signs of a lower motor neurone lesion at the level of the affected segments because of damage to the anterior horn cells, and to the loss of sensation of pain, warmth and cold below the level of the lesion. Thrombosis of a posterior spinal artery causes loss of all forms of sensation at the level of the lesion due to damage to the posterior horns, and signs of an upper motor neurone lesion and loss of proprioception below the level of damage to the spinal cord.

The Cerebrospinal Fluid. The CSF contains an excess of lymphocytes (10-100 per c.mm.), and a raised protein content (50-150 mg. per 100 ml.). The Wassermann reaction is positive in the CSF in over 90 per cent. of cases and in the blood in about 70 per cent. The Lange colloidal gold curve is usually of mid-zone type (p. 1152). Adhesions may lead to spinal block with appropriate CSF changes (p. 1209).

Diagnosis. Neurosyphilis may mimic any neurological disease but the main diagnostic problems are (1) isolated cranial nerve palsies, (2) cerebrovascular disease in young people, (3) rapidly progressive myelitis, (4) spinal root irritation which may simulate visceral disease or 'rheumatism'. The presence of Argyll Robertson pupils, a history of infection and serological changes in the blood and CSF should make the diagnosis clear.

Treatment (p. 1170).

Prognosis. If treatment is started early resolution can be expected, but thrombosis of a major vessel may leave residual neurological deficits.

General Paralysis of the Insane
(Dementia Paralytica)

Aetiology. General paralysis of the insane develops five to fifteen years after primary infection. Men are affected four times more frequently than women. Congenital syphilis may rarely give rise to juvenile general paralysis of the insane.

Pathology. The brain is shrunken with cortical atrophy over the anterior two-thirds with compensatory hydrocephalus. The meninges are thickened and the ependyma is granular. Microscopically there is degeneration of cortical neurones, with glial proliferation and infiltration of the meninges and perivascular spaces with lymphocytes.

Clinical Features. The initial symptoms are those of progressive dementia of various types. Delusions of grandeur, once considered characteristic, are uncommon. Usually there is slow, insidious impairment of memory, judgement and intellectual faculties, at first only noticeable to a close relative. Other mental pictures which occur include an anxiety state and a depressive syndrome. As the disease advances the patient becomes careless about his appearance, disregards social conventions and eventually has to be confined to a mental hospital.

Pupillary abnormalities (including Argyll Robertson pupils) are found even at an early stage but other physical signs are delayed. There is a characteristic irregular, wavy tremor of the lips, tongue ('trombone tongue') and hands, and a slow, slurring dysarthria. Extensor plantar reflexes are the first signs of progressive upper motor neurone paralysis. Epileptic attacks and transient hemiplegia, aphasia or hemianopia ('congestive attacks') may occur. Signs of associated cardiovascular syphilis are common.

The cerebrospinal fluid, which may be under pressure, is clear and contains 10-100 lymphocytes per c.mm., 50-100 mg. protein per 100 ml. and a paretic type colloidal gold curve (p. 1152). The Wassermann reaction is always positive in the CSF but may occasionally be negative in the blood.

Diagnosis. Early cases may be considered neurotic but later the differential diagnosis is from other causes of dementia, particularly frontal lobe tumour, presenile dementia or cerebral atherosclerosis. Pupillary abnormalities may suggest the diagnosis which can be confirmed by lumbar puncture. The Wassermann reaction should be done in every unexplained case of organic dementia.

Treatment (p. 1170).

Prognosis. Progression of dementia, paralysis, blindness, incontinence and early death are prevented by early treatment. Acceptable social rehabilitation is possible only if treatment is started before the disease is too far advanced though it may be arrested at any stage.

Tabes Dorsalis

(Locomotor Ataxia)

Aetiology. This late manifestation of syphilis appears 5 to 20 years after infection, usually in middle age, but occasionally in juvenile life it follows congenital syphilis.

Pathology. The lesion is a degeneration of the first order sensory neurones central to the dorsal root ganglion. It usually starts in the lower thoracic and lumbar roots. Only those fibres which do not relay in the posterior horn degenerate in the white columns so wasting is confined to the posterior columns but all modalities of sensation are affected. These changes may be associated with those of other forms of neurosyphilis such as meningovascular syphilis, optic atrophy or general paresis (taboparesis).

Clinical Features. The symptoms can all be explained on the basis of the posterior root lesion which irritates or damages sensory fibres, and interrupts the reflex arcs. The most common presenting symptoms are pain and paraesthesiae. The pains are severe, momentary stabbing pains, which do not run up and down the limb, but feel as though a sharp instrument was being thrust into the skin. They occur in paroxysms and are felt most commonly in the lower limbs and trunk; they are often influenced by weather and this frequently leads to them being labelled as 'rheumatic'. Root pains encircling the thorax (girdle pains) also occur. The paraesthesiae are prominent in the feet, and consist of pins and needles, numbness or feelings of heat and cold.

It is important to remember that tabes may present in many other ways often suggesting disease of some system other than the nervous system. Thus, ataxia may appear, especially if a patient has been confined to bed with an incidental illness, and may be attributed to general weakness. Disturbance of the sphincters, especially retention of urine, may suggest a genito-urinary lesion. Impotence is not infrequently the first symptom causing the patient to seek advice. Diplopia from a cranial nerve lesion or failing vision as a result of optic atrophy may bring the patient to an ophthalmologist. A visceral crisis, in which there is an acute disturbance in the function of a viscus, may bring the affected organ under suspicion rather than its innervation. The most common are gastric crises which are characterised by acute abdominal pain and vomiting lasting for several hours or a few days, but rectal crises with tenesmus, vesical crises with strangury and laryngeal crises with dyspnoea and stridor may also occur.

The signs of tabes are mostly explicable on the basis of the posterior root lesion. Tendon reflexes are lost, due to interruption of the reflex arcs, first at the ankles, then at the knees and later in the upper limbs; hypotonia with resultant hyperextensibility of the joints appears. The pain fibres are affected early with delay in or impairment of the response to pin prick over a characteristic distribution. The classical areas of loss are around the nose, the trunk from the angle of the sternum to the costal margin, the inner border of the forearms and the ring and little fingers, the perineum and the distal part of the lower limbs. Deep pain appreciation is also impaired so that the tendo calcaneus, calf muscles and testes become insensitive to pressure. Vibration and position sense in the feet are also lost early, but light touch is not affected until a later stage. The combination of loss of position sense and hypotonia gives rise to severe ataxia, so that the patient walks on a wide base lifting his feet high and stamping them down in an irregular and forceful manner. As vision compensates to some extent for the loss of proprioception, darkness or closure of the eyes aggravates the ataxia, hence Romberg's test (p. 1082) is positive. Later, unsteadiness of the arms may also appear. The plantar responses remain flexor, but may be absent as a result of sensory loss.

The Argyll Robertson pupil appears in 90 per cent. of cases. The pupils are small, irregular, and do not react to light though the convergence reflex is retained. The iris is pale and atrophic. Bilateral ptosis with compensatory overaction of the frontalis muscle gives rise to the tabetic facies seen in a few cases.

Paralysis of the extra-ocular muscles may be apparent, and examination of the discs may reveal the pallor of primary optic atrophy. A distended painless bladder may be palpable in the abdomen. Trophic changes may also develop; these give rise to painless, perforating ulcers of the soles of the feet and legs, and arthropathies of the knee, hip and other joints (Charcot's joints). The joint is swollen, and radiological examination reveals gross disorganisation with osteoarthritic changes, but the lesion remains painless. Signs of cardiovascular syphilis may also be found.

The cerebrospinal fluid is clear and under normal pressure. There is a mild lymphocytosis (0-50 per c.mm.) and a slight increase in protein up to about 80 mg. per 100 ml. The colloidal gold test usually gives a mid-zone rise. The Wassermann reaction may be positive in the blood or CSF or both, but it should be remembered that in 20 per cent. of cases it is negative in both, even in the presence of active disease.

Diagnosis. With efficient treatment of primary syphilis the fully developed classical picture of tabes is rarely seen nowadays, so that the diagnosis has often to be made from incomplete signs and symptoms. Thus 'rheumatism' may well be lightning pains, and careful examination may enable the true cause of an apparent visceral disturbance to be found. Equally, however, it should be remembered that the development of tabes does not exempt the patient from such conditions as perforation of a peptic ulcer or retention of urine due to enlargement of the prostate gland.

Polyneuritis and subacute combined degeneration of the cord may simulate tabes because of the pain, paraesthesiae, sensory loss and absent reflexes, but muscular wasting and weakness in the former and extensor plantar responses in the latter help in their differentiation. Moreover, both conditions are usually accompanied by muscle tenderness, in contrast to the loss of deep pain sense encountered in tabes. Disseminated sclerosis does not usually present a problem, as nystagmus, dysarthria and intention tremor are not seen in tabes.

Treatment. Treatment (p. 1170) is effective in the early stages, but once irreversible neuronal damage has occurred, restoration of function cannot be expected. The general principles of neurological treatment for disturbed locomotion and bladder function (p. 1211) should be applied.

Prognosis. The natural history of tabes is one of slow progression but arrest of the disease may occur at any stage.

TABOPARESIS

It is not uncommon to find a combination of general paralysis of the insane and tabes dorsalis. Thus, a patient with general paralysis of the insane may suffer from lightning pains or have lost some tendon reflexes, while on the other hand a patient with tabes dorsalis may develop extensor plantar responses and mental impairment. The Lange colloidal gold curve in these cases is usually of the paretic type.

Treatment of Neurosyphilis. The essential part of the treatment of neurosyphilis of all types is the injection of procaine benzylpenicillin, 500,000 units four times a day for at least two weeks, supplemented by bismuth oxychloride (B.P.C.) 200 mg. intramuscularly once each week for 10 weeks. There is some risk of a Herxheimer reaction so this course may be preceded by bismuth given intramuscularly in a dose of 200 mg. weekly for 10 weeks. Such a course is indicated in slowly progressive conditions, e.g. tabes dorsalis, but in rapidly advancing disorders, e.g. meningo-vascular syphilis, penicillin should be started immediately. The aim of treatment is to arrest the disease and restore the blood and CSF to normal. Further courses of penicillin must be given if (*a*) symptoms are not relieved or the picture continues to advance, (*b*) the CSF continues to show signs of active disease. The first abnormality to regress is the increase in cells but these may not return to normal until three months after treatment has been completed. The elevated protein takes longer to subside and the Lange colloidal gold curve may remain abnormal for as long as 12 months. The Wassermann reaction may never revert to normal. Lumbar puncture should be repeated at six-monthly intervals for two years and further courses of penicillin given so long as signs of activity remain. Evidence of clinical progression at any time is an indication for renewed treatment. When there is no further evidence of active disease the clinical examination and blood Wassermann reaction should be repeated annually for five years.

Fever therapy by inoculation with malarial parasites or by intravenous injection of *Esch. coli* vaccine is arduous and dangerous, and is now seldom used except in the rare case of failure to respond to penicillin. It is contraindicated in severe cardiovascular, hepatic, renal or other systemic disease. Symptomatic treatment should not be forgotten. Ataxic patients benefit from Fraenkel's exercises, and tabetic pains may require strong analgesics or even chordotomy. Visceral crises may be terminated by ganglion blocking drugs. The care of the neurogenic bladder is described on p. 1211.

VIRAL INFECTIONS

Some viruses are naturally 'neurotropic' and invade the nervous system causing necrosis of cells with reactive inflammation and perivascular cuffing. The reaction is lymphocytic. Each virus has a predilection for a particular type of nerve cell, e.g. the anterior horn cell in poliomyelitis and the posterior root ganglion in herpes zoster, but may invade other sites. The sites of involvement may be multiple as, for example, in meningo-encephalitis. Other viruses which are usually 'viscerotropic' may occasionally invade the nervous system, e.g. the viruses of mumps and infective hepatitis. A third group of neurological disorders is associated with viral diseases in which the pathological and clinical features may be due to abnormal immunity reactions rather than to invasion of the neurones by the virus. Finally, some disorders such as acute 'infective' polyneuritis are tentatively classified as viral infections without any satisfactory proof.

Encephalitis

Uncritical use of this term has led to some confusion. Non-inflammatory states due to toxic substances, such as arsenic or lead, or to nutritional deficiency, are better termed encephalopathy. In this chapter the disorders following vaccination or acute systemic infections such as measles and chickenpox, and a related sporadic type (acute disseminated encephalomyelitis) are classified with the demyelinating diseases (p. 1186). Suppurative encephalitis is discussed on p. 1153. True viral encephalitis destroys cell bodies rather than myelin.

Viral Encephalitis

Many viruses may cause encephalitis but some are of purely local distribution, depending on the occurrence of an animal carrier (e.g. rabies) and often a vector which is usually an insect such as the mosquito (e.g. yellow fever). Rabies is described on p. 578. Sporadic cases of viral encephalitis occur in Britain; the aetiology of these may be proved in some cases by the finding of antibodies in the patient's serum (e.g. herpes simplex, influenza), but in many cases the diagnosis of the causative agent remains presumptive. Epidemics are rare in this country but since the Second World War there have been several outbreaks of benign myalgic encephalomyelitis.

Pathology. The lesions are widespread throughout the cortex, white matter, basal ganglia and brain stem. The virus destroys the infected nerve cells which are surrounded with inflammatory cells, some packed into the perivascular spaces, and with microglial proliferation.

Clinical Features. The picture varies according to the causative virus, since different viruses appear to have a predilection for particular parts of the brain. For instance, encephalitis of the brain-stem occurs sporadically and in small epidemics. *Encephalitis lethargica*, a condition assumed to be due to a specific virus, affected the mid-brain, basal ganglia and hypothalamus leading to disturbance of ocular movement, failure of convergence, alteration of the sleep rhythm, behavioural disturbance and other hypothalamic manifestations in the acute stage, with Parkinsonism in the acute stage or as a delayed sequela (p. 1189). Most types of encephalitis have a fairly acute onset with headache and pyrexia which may be as high as 39°-40° C. (102°-104° F.). The patient becomes drowsy and confused but, except in the special types just mentioned, focal neurological signs are often absent. Fits may occur and drowsiness may progress to coma, both indicative of a bad prognosis. Other cases have a subacute onset and in still others, notably encephalitis lethargica between epidemics, the onset does not produce a clinically recognisable illness and it is only the late development of post-encephalitic Parkinsonism which betrays that infection has occurred. A *subacute progressive encephalitis* characterised pathologically by the presence of inclusion bodies in the brain or diffuse sclerosis is reported with increasing frequency from all parts of the world. Most patients are children or adolescents. The white matter is more severely damaged than in other types of encephalitis. It appears to be due to measles virus or a closely related virus.

The CSF in viral encephalitis is clear and under increased pressure. There is usually an increase in lymphocytes (50-200 per c.mm.) but this may be transitory. The protein content is often slightly raised but the sugar content is normal. In subacute inclusion-body panencephalitis the Lange colloidal gold curve gradually changes to a paretic type (p. 1152).

Treatment. There is no specific treatment for most viral infections, symptomatic measures being applied as required. Slow intravenous infusion of idoxuride (500 mg. per kg.) should be tried in herpes simplex encephalitis.

Prognosis. This varies according to the virus and its localisation within the nervous system. There is usually full though slow recovery from brain stem encephalitis. Epidemic encephalitis lethargica is often fatal but the sporadic disease has a low immediate mortality. Subacute inclusion-body panencephalitis is always fatal though death may be delayed for 5 to 10 years. Survivors from any form of encephalitis commonly show persisting neurological defects.

Acute Anterior Poliomyelitis

This disease is caused by a group of related viruses which invade the nervous system, and attack the motor neurones of the anterior horns of the spinal cord and of the brain stem.

Aetiology. Infection is mainly transmitted from healthy carriers or, in an epidemic, from infected contacts, by droplet infection when it enters the body through the nasopharynx. It is also spread by food, water and milk and the virus then enters the body through the gastrointestinal tract. Cases occur sporadically throughout the year, with epidemics in the late summer. The severity of the epidemics varies greatly from year to year but they have virtually disappeared from those countries which have a satisfactory proportion of the younger population protected by vaccination. The necessity for vaccination becomes increasingly urgent as there is good evidence that people in hygienically advanced countries have less protection from naturally acquired but sub-clinical infection in infancy. The disease most frequently affects young adults and children and the former term 'infantile paralysis' is now a misnomer.

Pathology. From its site of entry the virus passes into the blood stream. The circulating virus tends to localise in the grey matter of the central nervous system. It is possible, too, that the virus may invade a peripheral nerve at the site of entry and pass centrally along the axons to the cell bodies in the spinal cord or brain stem. They may be demonstrated in the anterior horn cells which rapidly undergo chromatolysis and destruction. The anterior horn as a whole is congested and infiltrated with lymphocytes and polymorphs, and perivascular cuffing with these cells occurs. After the acute stage the irreversibly damaged neurones degenerate and are replaced by neuroglia, while the muscles they supply undergo wasting. Motor neurones which were temporarily damaged by oedema rapidly regain their function.

Clinical Features. Following an incubation period of 7 to 14 days, the viraemia is often accompanied by a mild general reaction in which there is fever, headache, malaise and gastrointestinal disturbances lasting one or two days. This is known as the *minor illness* but its significance cannot be recognised except in an epidemic. Many cases never progress beyond this stage ('abortive poliomyelitis') but others subsequently develop the *major illness* after an interval of three to seven days, with recurrence of fever, producing a 'dromedary temperature chart'. A history of a minor illness can be obtained in about 40 per cent. of those who develop the major illness.

The major illness can be divided into three stages:

1. Pre-paralytic Stage. The temperature rises rapidly again to 39°-40° C. (102-104° F.) with more severe headache and signs of meningeal irritation which prevents flexion of the spine. There is malaise and often vomiting or anorexia and diarrhoea. The

muscles are very tender. A characteristic feature is restlessness which may amount to delirium. In some cases symptoms subside after 24 to 48 hours without further development. This is called *non-paralytic poliomyelitis* and such cases may constitute a high proportion of those affected in an epidemic. The cellular reaction in the CSF (p. 1151) which is present at this stage is evidence that invasion of the nervous system has occurred.

In other cases general symptoms and temperature subside for 24 to 48 hours after which paralysis appears. It is important not to be deceived by the period of temporary improvement which may occur between the two stages, as undue activity at this time aggravates the degree of subsequent paralysis.

2. Paralytic Stage. As paralysis appears the temperature subsides but pain and muscle tenderness persist. Paralysis may appear at any site and is patchy and asymmetrical in distribution. The lower limbs are more often affected than the upper. Spread of paralysis is usually complete within 24 hours but may continue for several days. It is flaccid, with loss of reflexes in the affected muscles, and subsequent atrophy (lower motor neurone paralysis). By the end of the first week signs of returning power may be noted and improvement continues over many months.

The cerebrospinal fluid undergoes characteristic changes in the major illness. There is a rapid increase of cells to 50-250 per c.mm. At first there is an excess of polymorphonuclear cells but by the end of the second day the lymphocyte becomes the preponderant cell and then the cell count begins to fall, whereas the protein content, which was previously normal, rises to 100-200 mg. per 100 ml.

Paralysis of respiration or deglutition endangers life. Respiratory weakness due to paralysis of the intercostal muscles or diaphragm can be recognised by the fact that the respiratory rate rises, speech comes in short bursts, the alae nasi flare and the accessory muscles of respiration are brought into play. The patient becomes restless and anxious and is unable to sleep. Cyanosis is a late sign. The ventilatory capacity can be measured accurately with suitable apparatus but some idea of it can be obtained by seeing how far the patient can count with one deep breath, the normal being a count of 60.

Involvement of the motor nuclei of the lower cranial nerves (bulbar paralysis) impairs swallowing and coughing, makes the voice weak and nasal, and leads to regurgitation of fluids through the nose and a bubbling or rattling in the throat during respiration. Refusal of food may be a sign that a child has difficulty in swallowing. With inability to swallow or cough, secretions accumulate in the pharynx and cause respiratory obstruction. (If this is severe the intercostal muscles and abdomen may be drawn in during inspiration.) This is a grave emergency which must be recognised immediately and treated. A combination of bulbar paralysis and paralysis of the respiratory muscles is particularly dangerous.

3. Stage of Residual Disability. The asymmetrical and patchy distribution of muscular weakness of different degrees leads to deformity and contractures such as scoliosis and talipes equinovarus. A severely affected limb shows the effects of vasomotor abnormalities such as coldness and cyanosis, and there may be retardation of bone growth with resultant shortening.

Diagnosis. Except in an epidemic, diagnosis is difficult before the onset of paralysis, but poliomyelitis should be suspected as the cause of a febrile illness if there is unusual restlessness, meningism or muscular pain. Meningitis has more marked meningeal signs and there is often drowsiness. Other painful conditions which may be confused with poliomyelitis are rhuematic fever, osteomyelitis and scurvy. Acute brachial neuritis (p. 1222) may be extremely difficult to differentiate if the small area of sensory loss is missed. Acute infective polyneuritis also simulates poliomyelitis but there is sensory loss in the former and meningism is not a feature. The diagnosis rests on the CSF findings. If paralysis is minimal it may be overlooked and the disease may then be labelled influenza. In the residual stage of poliomyelitis, the weak wasted muscles may be confused with those of a myopathy or motor neurone disease but the paralysis is static and asymmetric in distribution, and the muscles show no fasciculation.

Prophylaxis. Cases should be isolated for six weeks with the full nursing technique appropriate to enteric fever (p. 32). It is desirable but may be impracticable to isolate contacts for 21 days. Known contacts should avoid undue exertion as exercise during the pre-paralytic phase greatly increases the incidence and severity of paralysis. Subcutaneous and intramuscular injections or operations in the mouth and throat during the pre-paralytic stage may precipitate paralysis, so only urgently necessary prophylactic inoculations, tonsillectomy or dental extraction should be carried out during epidemics.

A high measure of protection can be given by prophylactic vaccination. An oral vaccine containing a mixture of three strains of living attenuated virus is preferable to the parenteral heat-killed vaccine because it prevents colonisation of the gut with naturally occurring virus. The parenteral vaccine does not do this and so does not reduce the incidence of carriers. Persons who have been exposed to the disease and have not been vaccinated may be protected temporarily by gamma-globulin, which should be injected intramuscularly as soon as possible after exposure to infection.

Treatment. The main essential in the pre-paralytic stage is complete rest in bed, with sedatives if required to control restlessness. This must be continued for several days despite an early remission of febrile symptoms as the temperature may be normal for a few days before the appearance of paralysis. In the paralytic stage it is often necessary for the physician to collaborate with a neurologist, orthopaedic surgeon, and an ear, nose and throat surgeon with experience of the special techniques required and this can best be achieved in a hospital equipped for the task.

When paralysis appears the limb should be placed in the optimum position for relaxation of the paralysed muscles but with avoidance of contractures. Gentle passive movements should be carried out in order to maintain mobility and counteract spasm. This is sometimes aided by the use of hot packs. A careful watch must be kept for the development of respiratory difficulties and if paralysis of the respiratory muscles occurs they must be assisted mechanically by the use of a ventilator (p. 320). This should be done sooner rather than later as it may then be tried out before an emergency arises, with less alarm to the patient. The machine will also spare the efforts of the rapidly tiring respiratory muscles.

If respiratory paralysis occurs without difficulty in swallowing the patient may be placed in a cabinet type respirator ('iron lung') but if there is also weakness of bulbar muscles it is necessary to inflate the lungs through a cuffed tracheostomy tube (intermittent positive pressure respiration). A cabinet respirator is extremely dangerous for a patient with bulbar paralysis as the strong negative pressure exerted on the chest wall will draw secretions into the lungs and asphyxiate the patient. This danger may be circumvented by a tracheostomy with surrounding cuff to prevent oesophageal secretions passing into the trachea.

If bulbar paralysis develops rapidly, the patient must be turned on his face immediately and the foot of the bed raised 18 inches so that secretions will drain out of the mouth. This may also be a life-saving measure when respiratory obstruction occurs as an emergency. The same procedure should be used if the patient vomits. He must on no account be allowed to sit up until all vomitus has been removed. Skilful aspiration of the pharynx, combined with postural drainage, is often sufficient to keep the airway clear but, if this proves inadequate, an immediate tracheostomy will be required.

After the acute stage the respiratory muscles may regain power. The patient is gradually weaned from the respirator by progressively increasing the periods of unassisted breathing which he is permitted. The muscles of the limbs are treated by passive and active movements during the recovery stage. At first these are best performed if the limbs are supported in water or by springs or counter weights. Residual disabilities may be treated by orthopaedic procedures.

Prognosis. Epidemics vary widely in their incidence of abortive and non-paralytic cases and in mortality rate. Death occurs from respiratory paralysis. Paralysis is greatest at the end of the first week of the major illness. Gradual recovery may then take place for several months but any muscle showing no signs of recovery by the end of a month will not recover useful function. It is difficult to make a more definite prediction about the extent of permanent disability until three to six months after the onset. Second attacks are very rare.

Herpes Zoster

(Shingles)

Viral invasion of posterior root ganglia causes pain followed by a rash over the cutaneous distribution of the affected nerve root. The virus is the same as that causing varicella (chickenpox), and contacts with one disease may develop the other. In herpes zoster there is a high level of specific antibody in the blood, and this is believed to indicate re-activation of a previous infection by chickenpox virus which has lain dormant in the body. The virus occasionally invades the spinal cord or the brain, giving rise to myelitis or encephalitis. It sometimes involves nerve roots which are the site of another pathological process such as neuroma, metastatic tumours, reticulosis and leukaemia or in certain toxic states (symptomatic herpes).

Clinical Features. The first symptom is usually severe continuous pain in the distribution of the affected nerve root. There is usually little systemic upset but malaise and pyrexia may accompany the pain, especially in old age. After three or four days the skin in the affected area becomes reddened and vesicles appear. The vesicles dry up over the course of five or six days leaving small scars. The affected dermatomes may be permanently anaesthetic. Scarring is more severe if the vesicles are secondarily infected.

Any dorsal root ganglion may be infected, most commonly one supplying the trunk where it usually involves two or three adjacent dermatomes on one side only. If infection of the trigeminal ganglion involves the ophthalmic division, the vesicles appear on the cornea and may lead to corneal ulceration with the danger of resultant scarring and impairment of vision (ophthalmic herpes).

The pain of herpes zoster usually subsides as the eruption fades, but occasionally, especially in old people, it may be followed by a persistent and intractable post-herpetic neuralgia which may last for months or years. Segmental muscle wasting may occur sometimes. It may result from involvement of the motor root in the inflammatory reaction, but it is often delayed until a month after the sensory signs, suggesting a delayed allergic reaction. Facial palsy may be caused by infection of the geniculate ganglion (geniculate herpes) spreading to the trunk of the facial nerve, and occasionally also to the eighth nerve causing deafness or vertigo. Herpetic vesicles may be seen on the auditory meatus and soft palate.

Diagnosis. Herpes zoster is easily diagnosed once the rash has appeared but, in the painful stage before development of the rash, it is frequently misdiagnosed as pleurisy, cholecystitis or a spinal cord lesion. It is important to remember the possibility that herpes may be associated with an underlying lesion of the dorsal root ganglia due often to organic disease (p. 1179).

Treatment. There is no specific antiviral treatment. The vesicles should be kept dry by means of talcum powder or calamine lotion or may be covered with collodion. An ointment containing such local anaesthetic as ung. cinchocain co. BPC applied to the site of the rash gives great relief in the acute stage. Analgesics may also be required. Antibiotics may be needed if secondary infection becomes severe.

The treatment of post-herpetic neuralgia is difficult. Analgesics should be continued, but the more dangerous ones, such as morphine, should be avoided because of the risk of addiction. Radiotherapy to the affected root may be advised if the pain proves intractable. Section of the nerve or nerve root is never successful but in suitable cases section of the spinothalamic tract may be carried out with benefit.

DEMYELINATING DISEASES

Loss of myelin sheaths occurs with many disorders of the central and peripheral nervous systems but there is a particular category with certain clinical and pathological features in common in which loss of myelin is considered to be the primary change and the axis cylinders may be spared or, if affected, are damaged secondarily. The lesions are almost entirely confined to the white matter of the central nervous system. They are initially inflammatory in type but differ from lesions known to be caused by direct viral infection and so they are grouped separately from the 'polioclastic' types of encephalomyelitis (p. 1171). Their nature is uncertain but there are reasons for considering that they may be caused by an 'auto-immune' process which damages the myelin-forming cells, the oligodendrocytes.

Disseminated Sclerosis

(Multiple Sclerosis)

In the Northern Hemisphere this is the most common disease of the nervous system, affecting people from 20 to 50 years of age with maximum incidence in young adults.

Aetiology. The cause is unknown. Six per cent. of patients have affected relatives, suggesting that genetic factors are contributory. The initial attack and later relapses may be precipitated by unusual fatigue, trauma, infection, severe cold and allergic reactions.

Pathology. The acute lesion consists of a circumscribed area in which the myelin sheaths have undergone destruction while the axis cylinders show only irregular swelling. The plaque has a swollen pinkish appearance as blood vessels are dilated but there is little infiltration with inflammatory cells. Reactive gliosis follows, so that the chronic lesion becomes a glial scar with a shrunken greyish appearance. The lesions are widely scattered in the white matter of the brain, especially round the ventricles, in the spinal cord, and in the optic nerves. Despite the disseminated distribution there is a tendency for spinal cord and brain stem lesions to occur in symmetrical situations.

Clinical Features. The most characteristic features are the relapsing and remitting course of the disease and the widespread lesions which result in a multiple symptomatology. These features rather than any combination or pattern of symptoms and signs enable the diagnosis to be made. The clinical features depend on the sites of plaques which may occur in any part of the white matter, but there is a predilection for certain sites which enables some clinical patterns to be distinguished. The acute lesion causes temporary functional interruption of fibres which are not permanently damaged, so the early symptoms often tend to improve. The initial clinical feature develops fairly suddenly and disappears after a few days or weeks. It may be any one of the many associated with this disease but two are particularly common. In young people retrobulbar neuritis is probably the lesion which is produced first most frequently, while over the age of 53 weakness of one or both lower limbs is usually the presenting symptom.

Retrobulbar neuritis causes blurring or loss of the vision of one eye. There may be pain on movement of the eyeball. The optic disc is normal at this stage but there is a large central scotoma in the visual field of the affected eye and direct and consensual light reflexes are reduced when that eye is illuminated (p. 1096). Rarely, when the plaque lies immediately behind the nerve head, ('papillitis'), a mild degree of swelling of the disc may be seen. The vision recovers after two to three weeks, though a partial central scotoma may persist, and pallor of the temporal half of the disc may subsequently appear.

Weakness, heaviness or stiffness of one or both limbs due to corticospinal tract demyelination develops fairly suddenly. It may be so slight as to cause little disability or it may be crippling for a few days or weeks. Spontaneous jerks of the legs while at rest are common in the early stage. Other symptoms which may be the initial ones or occur during relapses are due to plaques in the brain-stem, cerebellum or spinal cord. Common brain-stem symptoms are transient diplopia, often unaccompanied by any observable strabismus, and acute vertigo with vomiting. Cerebellar lesions cause incoordination of an arm (with intention tremor, p. 1077), ataxia of gait or dysarthria (p. 1092.). Transient unsteadiness of an arm or leg may also be due to impaired proprioception. This may render the limb 'useless' though it is not paralysed. Posterior column involvement in the cervical region may cause sudden electric shock-like feelings in the arms or legs when the neck is flexed. Spinothalamic tract lesions cause numbness or paraesthesiae in the face, trunk, or limbs often described as being like a tight band round the limb. Transient disturbances of bladder function such as urgency, precipitancy or hesitancy of micturition (often labelled cystitis) may occur at an early stage, and impotence may be complained of.

Examination usually reveals slight but definite signs of organic disease. Pallor of the temporal half of one or both optic discs is common even though the patient may never have been aware of visual disturbance. Nystagmus of ataxic or cerebellar type (p. 1103), intention tremor, and corticospinal tract signs such as extensor plantar responses, muscle weakness and increase in reflexes and tone are common. Vibration sense is frequently diminished and impairment of the sense of passive movement may also be found. Analgesia or loss of sensation of light touch may be found but rarely persists. Most of these signs recede, but the changes in the optic disc are permanent, and often the abdominal reflexes become fatiguable then disappear permanently.

After the initial attack, there may be an interval of months or years before the second episode occurs which may be characterised by a recurrence of previous clinical features or, more likely, the development of new ones. The later course may be one of relapses and remissions with cumulative neurological defects, or there may be slowly progressive damage of the spinal cord simulating the picture of compression. The progressive course most often occurs when the disease starts in middle age. The course of either type eventually results in permanent disability in which the predominant features may be a spastic paraplegia or tetraplegia with incontinence, gross cerebellar disturbance with an ataxic gait, or mixed signs of widespread lesions. Mental changes may occur such as a failure to appreciate the seriousness of the condition (euphoria) but, although it may be an early feature, it is by no means pathognomonic of disseminated sclerosis.

Abnormalities of the CSF are present in at least half of the cases. A mild lymphocytosis amounting to 10 or 15 cells per c.mm. or a slight rise in protein not exceeding about 80 mg. per 100 ml. may be present. A characteristic feature is a disturbance of the Lange colloidal gold curve (p. 1152). The most common abnormality is a first zone rise, but a mid-zone rise and non-specific changes also occur. The combination of a paretic curve with a negative Wassermann reaction is very suggestive of disseminated sclerosis. The CSF changes do not appear to correlate with the stage or degree of activity of the disease.

Diagnosis. There is no single sign or symptom which is pathognomonic of disseminated sclerosis which may at times simulate almost any affliction of the nervous system. The diagnosis depends on the multiplicity of signs and the natural history of the disease; a history of retrobulbar neuritis, transient paresis or unexplained sensory disturbance is common. Careful examination, even during a period of remission, will often reveal such evidence as definite temporal pallor of the discs, nystagmus, slight ataxia, absent abdominal reflexes or an extensor plantar response. The simultaneous presence of signs indicating multiple lesions in the central nervous system, or a history of previous episodes of neurological disturbance is very suggestive of disseminated sclerosis, particularly if different sites are affected at each relapse. On the other hand, too much insistence must not be placed on the history of relapse and remissions as not all cases pursue this course and, moreover, conditions other than disseminated sclerosis can also remit. The disease must be distinguished from the following disorders:

Cervical Spondylosis is the most common cause of a disorder simulating disseminated sclerosis, especially the progressive spinal type which occurs in older patients. It may give rise to a progressive spastic paraplegia but does not cause nystagmus. There is usually a history of pain, and signs of a root lesion in the arms. Restriction of neck movements and radiological signs of degeneration of the intervertebral discs are usually present, but it must be remembered that they may be present in many diseases including disseminated sclerosis.

Spinal Tumour is also difficult to differentiate from the spinal type of disseminated sclerosis. Both may progress relentlessly and have a horizontal upper level of sensory loss. Pain, however, is rare in disseminated sclerosis, and there may be signs of scattered lesions above the massive cord lesion, for example nystagmus or temporal pallor of an optic disc. Lumbar puncture and myelography are often required to establish the diagnosis of intraspinal tumour and these examinations should never be delayed when there is any doubt.

Meningovascular Syphilis also causes multiple symptoms and signs which may be transient. Pupillary changes, however, may be present, whereas nystagmus and intention tremor are extremely rare. Hesitancy and retention occur rather than urgency and incontinence of micturition. The Wassermann reaction is usually positive in the blood and CSF but may be negative.

Subacute Combined Degeneration of the Cord is accompanied by early and persistent paraesthesiae, and by involvement of the corticospinal tracts and posterior columns, the latter being affected earlier and more frequently than the former. Histamine-fast achlorhydria is almost invariably present and the blood and bone marrow picture of pernicious anaemia is present in a high proportion of cases.

Hereditary Ataxias are distinguished by the family history, the earlier age of onset and the frequent absence of reflexes in the lower limbs. Congenital stigmata such as pes cavus and kyphoscoliosis are often present.

Hysteria (p. 1254) may be distinguished by careful analysis of the symptoms, which have an underlying psychological meaning and purpose, and a thorough physical examination will confirm that the spinal tracts are intact. It should be remembered, however, that hysterical reactions to organic lesions can occur, and may do so in disseminated sclerosis.

Ménière's Syndrome and other causes of acute vertigo (p. 1109) may have to be considered in those cases presenting with vertigo. They are usually associated with tinnitus and deafness and are without other abnormal neurological signs.

Myasthenia Gravis is frequently mistaken for disseminated sclerosis. The remittent history of diplopia, dysarthria, and weakness of limbs may suggest that disease but the sensory and reflex changes of disseminated sclerosis are absent. An edrophonium test may be necessary (p. 1235).

Treatment. There is no specific treatment but a great deal can be done to help the patient. An acute relapse may respond to a high-dosage course of ACTH by injection. During a relapse the patient should be confined to bed but the period of rest must be reduced to a minimum as co-ordination is lost rapidly. A regime of regulated activity is essential, avoiding over-fatigue on the one hand and inactivity on the other. Relapses are often due to urinary or other infections. Successful treatment may result in remission of the neurological symptoms.

Well planned physiotherapy and occupational therapy are of great value. Passive movement will relieve spasticity and exercises to improve co-ordination will help to overcome ataxia. Drugs such as atropine and ephedrine are useful for precipitancy of micturition, and carbachol may be used if there is severe hesitancy or retention of urine. The psychological aspect must not be neglected. An attitude of reasoned optimism and encouragement is helpful and to be preferred to concealment of the true state of affairs or the prescription of useless remedies. Orthopaedic appliances and a wheel-chair may make life quite tolerable for the disabled person.

Prognosis. Recovery from the current attack may reasonably be expected but it is impossible to forecast the next relapse. The time elapsing between the first and second episodes is a useful pointer to the subsequent course. If a second attack occurs in less than a year from the first the course is likely to be progressive. If a considerably longer free period is present the prognosis is so much the better and improves with every year that passes. Some patients have no further attacks, especially if the initial lesion is retrobulbar neuritis, so the picture is not one of unrelieved gloom. The spinal type often progresses extremely slowly and, even at a late stage, is compatible with a wheel-chair life. Brain stem involvement carries a worse prognosis. The most disabling lesion is ataxia. Although some cases progress rapidly, 60 per cent. are without disability five years after the onset of symptoms and 40 per cent. after 10 years. The average duration of life is at least 20 years from the onset. Death is usually caused by urinary infection, pneumonia or pressure sores.

Acute Demyelinating Encephalomyelitis

(Acute Disseminated Encephalomyelitis)

Aetiology. There is a group of related acute disorders occurring without obvious cause or following an upper respiratory infection (acute disseminated encephalomyelitis), shortly after certain infectious diseases such as measles and chickenpox (post-exanthematous encephalomyelitis), or after vaccination. The pathology is probably due to a sensitivity reaction to a viral infection.

Pathology. There are widespread areas of perivenous demyelination throughout the brain and spinal cord. Unlike plaques of disseminated sclerosis they show little tendency to progress.

Clinical Features. The time of onset varies with the different infectious diseases; in measles it is the 4th to the 6th day, and in chickenpox the 5th to the 12th day of the illness. The disease appears on the 10th to the 12th day after vaccination. Headache, vomiting, pyrexia and delirium are common presenting features and signs of meningeal irritation may also be found. Fits or coma may occur. Flaccid paralysis and extensor plantar responses are common but sensory loss is unusual. Cerebellar signs may be present especially when the disorder follows chickenpox. Retention of urine is also a frequent manifestation.

Neuromyelitis Optica is a restricted form of the disease characterised by massive demyelination of the spinal cord and both optic nerves, usually following an upper respiratory infection. Either the optic or the spinal lesion may occur first but they may develop simultaneously.

The CSF may be normal or show a small increase of mononuclear cells and protein. The Lange curve shows no characteristic pattern.

Diagnosis. When the features of an acute encephalitis occur in association with one of the exanthemata or following vaccination the diagnosis should be easy but in cryptogenic cases other causes of 'encephalitis' must be excluded (p. 1171). It may be impossible to distinguish acute disseminated encephalomyelitis (or especially neuromyelitis optica) from acute disseminated sclerosis until the passage of time has shown that remissions and relapses do not occur. Syphilitic myelitis is distinguished by the serological reactions.

Treatment. ACTH 80-120 units by injection or prednisone 60 mg. by mouth daily for several days followed by a maintenance dose for two to three weeks is beneficial. These drugs must be used with caution in chickenpox if encephalitis develops before the rash has subsided as the rash may become confluent and haemorrhagic. The usual care of the paralysed and incontinent patient is required (p. 1211).

Prognosis. The mortality rate is high in neuromyelitis optica and in post-vaccinal encephalomyelitis but is low in the post-exanthematous cases. If the patient survives, the recovery may be remarkably complete and second attacks are very rare.

DISORDERS OF THE EXTRAPYRAMIDAL SYSTEM

In disorders of this system voluntary movement is disturbed involuntary movements appear and muscle tone is altered.

Parkinsonism

This syndrome is characterised by slowness and poverty of emotional and voluntary movement, by rigidity and by tremor.

Aetiology. Parkinsonism is a clinical syndrome resulting from damage to the globus pallidus and substantia nigra which may be caused by several diseases. The main causes are:

Encephalitis Lethargica (p. 1172). This is the usual cause of Parkinsonism occurring before the age of 40 but it is becoming increasingly rare.

Primary Degenerative Disease. The cause of this is unknown. It usually appears between the ages of 50 and 60 and is called paralysis agitans.

Atherosclerosis. The main site of this is the basal ganglia. There is usually evidence of atherosclerosis elsewhere.

Toxic Causes. These are rare, but the basal ganglia may be poisoned by copper in Wilson's disease (p. 1191), manganese or mercury. The latter substances may be ingested during industrial processes. Carbon monoxide poisoning may cause necrosis of the globus pallidus.

Pathology. Post-encephalitic Parkinsonism is due to destruction by a virus of the pigment-bearing cells in the substantia nigra, with lymphocytic infiltration, perivascular cuffing and glial reaction. In paralysis agitans there is degeneration of some of the cells of the basal ganglia, particularly in the globus pallidus, without evidence of inflammatory or vascular changes. In cases due to atherosclerosis the vascular changes are prominent, and secondary degeneration of neurones and cellular necrosis occur. These changes are not confined to extrapyramidal neurones and usually involve the adjacent internal capsule.

Clinical Features. Paralysis agitans may be taken as the prototype of Parkinsonism and the difference between it and the other types is described on pages 1189 and 1190.

Paralysis Agitans. The onset of this disorder is commonly in the 50-60 age group. The first sign is usually tremor of one hand. It is a coarse, regular, rhythmical tremor 4-8 times per second, between opposing groups of muscles such as flexion-extension or pronation-supination at the wrist, or abduction-adduction of the thumb. It is most marked in the distal parts of the limbs. It usually starts in one upper limb, spreading after months or years to the other or to the lower limbs. The tongue and closed eyelids may also be tremulous. The tremor of Parkinsonism is present at rest, disappears during a voluntary movement but may reappear when the limb holds a new posture.

Poverty of movement and rigidity follow soon after tremor. The face loses its movements of expression and the unblinking stare gives a false impression of idiocy. Automatic movements such as swinging the arms when walking are reduced or lost and if the patient trips he does not make the reflex movements necessary to preserve his balance. The gait is composed of small shuffling steps and is often more of a run than a walk. There is no weakness but all movements are infrequent and slow except speech which is rapid and monotonous with slurring of consonants and repetition of syllables. Hand writing is cramped and tends to become progressively smaller. Nevertheless with concentrated effort, movement, speech and writing can often be performed in a normal manner for a few moments, but rapidly return to their former level when attention is relaxed.

Rigidity is of extrapyramidal type. It is usually of the 'cog-wheel' variety (p. 1075), increased by voluntary contraction of the opposite limb. The muscles of the trunk are also rigid, with slight flexion of the trunk and limbs and restricted rotary movement of the spine. The fingers are held flexed at the metacarpo-phalangeal joints but extended at the interphalangeal joints with adduction of the thumb. There is no sensory loss and in general the tendon jerks are not altered. Cramp or muscle pain is quite common.

Post-encephalitic Parkinsonism. This may appear at any age. As there has been little encephalitis lethargica since the epidemic after the First World War the age of onset of new cases is now similar to that of paralysis agitans but long standing cases give a history of onset in early life. Tremor is less prominent than in paralysis agitans but rigidity is a marked feature. Other differences are the disturbances of ocular innervation and the more obvious signs of hypothalamic damage, such as hypersalivation or excess sebaceous secretion. Sleep disturbance and behaviour disorders rarely persist.

Various pupillary abnormalities occur but the most common is failure of the convergence reflex associated with deficient ocular convergence. Oculogyric crises may occur in which there is forced upward deviation of the eyes for minutes or hours.

Atherosclerotic Parkinsonism. The age of onset may be later than paralysis agitans and rigidity is more marked than tremor. Neighbouring tracts are commonly involved in the ischaemic area so that extensor plantar reflexes may be found in this type.

Diagnosis. The CSF is normal in each of these types. Parkinsonism must be differentiated from other causes of rigidity and tremor.

RIGIDITY

Hysterical. Characteristically this is associated with 'paralysis' and both the rigidity and the power exerted by the patient are proportional to the effort made by the examiner in moving the limb.

Arthritic. Stiffness due to multiple arthritis is associated with pain when the affected joint is moved.

Spasticity. The resistance to passive movement in disorders of the upper motor neurone is high during the first part of the movement then collapses suddenly ('clasp-knife'). It involves the flexor muscles of the upper limbs and the extensor muscles of the lower limbs more than their opponents. Extrapyramidal rigidity affects flexors and extensors equally and resistance is maintained throughout the whole range of movement.

TREMOR

Senile Tremor. The common tremor of old people is faster and finer than Parkinsonism and is at first present only during voluntary movement.

Familial Tremor. This may affect several generations. It may be generalised or affect only one limb. It is usually present from early life and does not tend to progress. It is not associated with rigidity.

Hysterical Tremor. This is often coarse and irregular. It is usually absent when the patient's attention is diverted and it is increased by voluntary movement.

Anxiety State. The tremor is fine and affects mainly the hands which usually perspire.

Thyrotoxicosis. The tremor is fine and resembles that of anxiety state, both being most evident when the hands are outstretched. It is associated with other signs of thyrotoxicosis (p. 695).

Toxic Tremor. This may be fine (chronic alcohol or cocaine intoxication) or coarse (hepatic failure, p. 1026; delirium tremens). It is not associated with rigidity.

Disseminated Sclerosis. Tremor is usually 'cerebellar' in type and present only during voluntary movement (intention tremor,

p. 1077), but tremor at rest may appear. It is almost invariably associated with nystagmus and this, and signs of damage to tracts in the spinal cord, differentiate it from Parkinsonism.

Treatment. It is extremely important to keep the patient physically active, so he should remain at work as long as possible. Carrying a newspaper or gloves reduces tremor and thereby may lessen embarrassment. Rigidity is alleviated by warmth and passive movements. Drugs are of great help in the treatment of rigidity but are less effective for tremor. The solanaceous drugs such as atropine and stramonium have largely been replaced by synthetic preparations such as benzhexol hydrochloride (Pipanol, Artane) 2-5 mg; benztropine (Cogentin) 2 mg. and orphenadrine (Disipal), 50 mg. The selected drug is taken orally three times per day then the dose is increased gradually until the patient is beginning to show toxic symptoms, such as dryness of the mouth and blurring of vision. The dose is then reduced slightly and maintained at a level which just fails to produce these symptoms. Adequate dosage is essential if benefit is to be gained.

Destruction of part of the globus pallidus or ventrolateral nucleus of the thalamus by stereotaxic surgical procedures may abolish rigidity and reduce tremor in carefully selected patients, especially those under 60 years with predominantly unilateral signs. Speech disturbances or mental abnormality if present are not alleviated by surgery and indeed form the major contraindication to it. Oculogyric crises are often relieved by surgical treatment of carefully sited lesions.

Prognosis. This depends on the cause. Paralysis agitans and atherosclerotic Parkinsonism tend to progress but the rate may be slow or rapid. Post-encephalitic Parkinsonism does not change much from year to year.

Hepato-lenticular Degeneration

(Wilson's Disease)

Wilson's disease is a rare hereditary disorder of copper metabolism. A brief account is valuable as an illustration of disease due to a biochemical disorder.

Aetiology. Copper is normally absorbed in small amounts from the gut as a loose complex with albumin and carried to the liver. There some of it is re-excreted in the bile but a fraction enters the general circulation. In the liver some of the blood copper is transferred to globulin to which it is more firmly bound, forming caeruloplasmin. This copper-globulin is an oxidase enzyme but its physiological role is unknown.

In Wilson's disease copper is absorbed in excess but the transfer from the albumin-bound to the globulin-bound complex is defective, thus the serum caeruloplasmin level is low. Some of the extra copper absorbed is excreted in the urine while the rest is deposited in the tissues, particularly in the brain, liver, kidney and in Descemet's membrane in the eye. These organs may be damaged either by enzymatic poisoning by the heavy metal or by cellular necrosis followed by fibrosis (or gliosis in the brain).

The metabolic abnormality is inherited as an autosomal recessive characteristic, thus it occurs in either sex but is rare because both parents must carry the abnormal gene. (In practice this is most probable if the parents are related.)

Clinical Features. The biochemical abnormality of Wilson's disease is present from birth, but clinical evidence does not appear until adolescence. There are two main clinical types. Hepatic and cerebral signs may be present in the one case but more often one or the other is most evident.

HEPATIC TYPE. There is progressive hepatic cirrhosis of a coarse nodular type, leading gradually to portal hypertension and eventually to hepatic failure (p. 1020). Juvenile cirrhosis should always suggest the possibility of Wilson's disease. Jaundice may precede it. It is sometimes haemolytic in type.

CEREBRAL TYPE. Necrosis and sclerosis of the corpus striatum cause basal ganglion syndromes in adolescence (p. 1075). Most common is choreo-athetosis, but Parkinsonism may be caused according to the site mainly affected. There is usually cortical involvement leading to progressive dementia in which loss of emotional control is a feature.

Copper deposition in Descemet's membrane of the eye causes a golden-brown, yellow or green ring round the cornea. This Kayser-Fleischer ring, as it is called, appears in both types and is pathognomonic of Wilson's disease.

The urine contains excess copper and often excess amino acids (without any specific pattern). Renal tubular damage by copper may upset excretion of uric acid, sugar, phosphates, etc., but it is not certain whether aminoaciduria is caused in this way or whether it is an independent biochemical defect. Caeruloplasmin (measured as serum copper oxidase) is deficient in the blood.

Differential Diagnosis. The hepatic type must be differentiated from other causes of juvenile cirrhosis (p. 1030). The cerebral type is likely to be confused with congenital disorders of the basal ganglia, kernicterus (p. 1196) or post-encephalitic Parkinsonism (p. 1189). The Kayser-Fleischer ring and the biochemical abnormalities are diagnostic.

Treatment. This disorder was previously progressive and fatal within a few years after the appearance of clinical signs. It can now be arrested by giving copper-binding drugs (chelating agents) which mobilise copper from the tissues and promote its excretion in the urine. The most valuable of these is penicillamine, 300 mg. t.d.s. orally. If it is not available or too expensive, dimercaprol (BAL) or disodium calcium versenate may be given but either is a less satisfactory substitute. Hepatic and cerebral symptoms are treated symptomatically with diet and anti-Parkinsonism drugs.

Siblings should be examined as clinical or biochemical evidence of Wilson's disease may be detected at a stage where treatment, if started promptly and continued throughout life, may prevent the appearance or progression of clinical features.

Sydenham's Chorea

(St. Vitus' Dance)

This is a disease of children characterised by involuntary movements.

Aetiology. Chorea is associated with rheumatic fever though the exact nature of the association is uncertain. Arthritis is absent and only a small percentage of patients with chorea have active carditis. Other manifestations of rheumatism commonly occur but usually not simultaneously with chorea. Chorea generally occurs between the ages of 5 and 15 and girls are affected three times more often than boys. Mental stress may also play a part and is certainly a common precipitating factor. Chorea occurs occasionally during pregnancy in young women (chorea gravidarum).

Pathology. There is generalised oedema and congestion of the brain, most evident in the basal ganglia but also involving the cerebral cortex. Inflammatory cells are few but there is diffuse degeneration of neurones.

Clinical Features. The onset may be insidious, with fidgety movements gradually becoming more violent, or it may be sudden after an emotional disturbance. The movements are irregular, non-repetitive and present at rest but intensified during voluntary movement which is thus made irregular and jerky. They are absent during sleep. The movements may be quasi-purposive or just a series of sudden twitches involving several muscles simultaneously. All limbs and often the face and tongue may be involved. Restless grimacing of the face and inability to maintain the tongue in a protruded position are common features and the tongue movements may interfere with speech and swallowing. Respiration may also be irregular and jerky.

Associated movements are also disturbed by exaggeration or incoordination. Thus if the patient, while grasping the examiner's hand, is asked to protrude his tongue or clench the other fist, irregular contractions of the hand will be felt. Tone is greatly reduced so that hyperextensibility of the joints can be demonstrated. If the hands are held forward, palms down, they assume a typical posture of flexion at the wrist and hyperextension at all the finger joints. There is often hyperpronation of the arms if they are held above the head. The hypotonia also causes the reflexes to be difficult to elicit but when obtained, they show a characteristic sustained contraction. The plantar responses are flexor and there is no sensory loss. The CSF is normal. There is usually no pyrexia and the ESR is normal. If there is fever or a raised ESR it is likely that active carditis is present.

Diagnosis. This is not difficult. In habit spasm (tic) the pattern of involuntary movement is repeated with little variation; in athetosis the movements are more slow and sinuous. Huntington's chorea occurs in middle age in patients with dementia and there is usually a family history to be obtained.

Treatment. Complete bed rest and quiet are essential for at least a month and it may be necessary to remove the child to hospital to obtain this. The sides of the cot or bed should be padded to avoid injury. Skin abrasion must also be prevented. When swallowing is affected, feeding by gastric tube is necessary. There is no specific drug treatment but aspirin gr. 5-15 t.d.s. is commonly given and sedatives such as phenobarbitone or tranquillising drugs may be useful for the control of restlessness.

Prognosis. Death is very rare; most cases recover in 6 to 12 weeks. Second attacks occur in a third of cases and repeated attacks are not uncommon. This increases the possibility of occurrence of rheumatic carditis.

Huntington's Chorea

This is a good example of a human disease inherited as a Mendelian dominant of autosomal type. Sporadic cases may occur. Its incidence is about 6 per 100,000 of the population but because of its familial nature its local incidence may be much greater. The first signs usually appear between the ages of 30 and 45. These are usually choreiform movements which are faster, more jerky and altogether more bizarre than Sydenham's chorea. Subsequently dementia develops and progresses to a state of complete incapacity requiring admission to a mental hospital in 10 to 15 years. Occasionally dementia may precede the involuntary movements. The EEG shows a low voltage, featureless type of record which differs from that found in other types of dementia.

Diagnosis. *Sydenham's chorea* occurs at an earlier age. There is no dementia and usually no family history. The course is not progressive.

Multiple tics occurring in hysterical individuals may be very difficult to differentiate. There is no dementia and no family history.

Pre-senile dementia (p. 1269) of other types may require consideration in the rare cases where dementia precedes chorea.

Cerebral atherosclerosis may cause both dementia and chorea but occurs at a later age and without a family history.

Treatment. There is no specific treatment but thiopropazate (Dartalan) may help to control the involuntary movements.

Athetosis

This is characterised by unilateral or bilateral involuntary movements.

Pathology. The lesion is in the putamen. Most cases are congenital, being due to a primary disorder of myelination of striatal neurones, with glial formation, developing in intrauterine life. It may also be caused by cerebral anoxia at birth or by kernicterus (p. 1196). In childhood it may occur as a result of damage to the basal ganglia during the exanthematous diseases, in adolescence from Wilson's disease (p. 1191) and in the elderly from cerebrovascular disease. The lesions are usually bilateral.

Clinical Features. The slow, sinuous writhing movements ('mobile spasm') affect the distal parts of the limbs more than the proximal. The facial muscles are also affected by grimacing. In congenital cases abnormal movements are seldom noted until several months after birth. Movements persist throughout life but do not get worse. The movements are more slow and writhing than those of chorea, but occasionally the features of both conditions are to be observed, hence the term 'choreo-athetosis.' Similar but slower movements of the proximal parts of the limbs and of the trunk are termed *torsion dystonia.*

Treatment. There is no specific treatment, but pallidotomy and thalamotomy may be of value, particularly for dystonia. Physiotherapy is valuable for securing muscular relaxation.

Kernicterus

Kernicterus is a disorder of the basal ganglia and auditory nuclei occurring in association with neonatal jaundice, particularly in premature infants. It may be caused by icterus gravis neonatorum due to rhesus group incompatibility between the erythrocytes of mother and child (p. 633), but any severe neonatal jaundice may be followed by this complication, and prematurity is more important than Rh incompatibility.

Premature babies have a functional immaturity of the glucuronyl transferase enzyme system of the liver, and as a result of this the indirect-reacting bilirubin formed by haemolysis of any sort is not conjugated to form the direct-reacting type (p. 995). When the infant is born it is deprived of its placental excretion route, and indirect-reacting bilirubin rapidly accumulates in its blood to toxic levels which depress oxidative metabolism of brain cells, and in particular those of the basal ganglia. The danger decreases rapidly about 10 days after the birth in normal full-term infants when the liver enzyme system matures, but the premature baby is in danger for a longer period.

Clinical Features. Convulsions, coma, opisthotonos and rigidity may be early symptoms but athetoid movements or spastic paralysis, deafness of nuclear type, and mental deficiency may not be apparent until the baby is several months old.

Prevention and Treatment. Prevention depends on the early detection of haemolytic jaundice, especially in the premature child, and its prompt treatment by exchange transfusion (p. 635). Since treatment of infants with haemorrhagic disease of the newborn with large doses of some vitamin K substitutes may cause haemolysis and so increase the risk of kernicterus, only natural vitamin K_1 should be used for this disease (p. 667). There is no treatment for the established disorder and the future management is that of the child with cerebral palsy.

Spasmodic Torticollis
(Wry Neck)

This is a condition characterised by involuntary movements affecting many cervical muscles on both sides of the neck. It may occur as the sole manifestation of disease of the extrapyramidal system, or it may be associated with other signs. Torticollis may also occur as a manifestation of hysteria or as a tic (p. 1198). The onset is usually insidious except in hysterical cases when it is often sudden following emotional disturbance. The movements consist of spasmodic rotation, flexion and extension of the cervical spine in the antero-posterior and lateral planes.

Diagnosis. Congenital torticollis due to fibrosis following haematoma of one sternomastoid muscle is present from birth. Local disease of the cervical spine, muscles or lymph glands may also cause torticollis.

Treatment. Spasmodic torticollis is a particularly intractable condition. Physiotherapy and sedation are employed but the results are usually disappointing. Surgical division of the spinal accessory nerves or of the cervical nerves may be tried if the disability is intolerable.

Tic
(Habit Spasm)

Elaborate patterns of movement involving co-ordinated activity of groups of muscles occur at irregular intervals, particularly during emotional stress. The whole pattern of movements is repetitive, unlike the movements of chorea or athetosis. A tic often develops as a neurotic manifestation. It is sometimes a hysterical perpetuation of a movement which has psychological significance to the patient, or one which is involved in his work if this is of a repetitive nature.

Treatment. Early cases may respond to sedation but physiotherapy is usually necessary. It is not always effective.

CONGENITAL AND DEGENERATIVE DISORDERS

There are a number of disorders of the central and peripheral nervous systems which are of unknown cause. It is probable that many of these will prove to be due to a disturbance of biochemical function. A brief consideration of the nature of a 'biochemical lesion' may be helpful. Every cell in the body is derived from one original germ cell which is endowed with a system of enzymes determined by the genes inherited from each parent. In embryological development cells become specialised for various functions by the elimination of unnecessary enzyme systems; thus, one type of specialised cell differs from another in its chemical constitution and, incidentally, in its dependence on other cells. For this reason a biochemical abnormality usually causes disturbance of function of specific cell types. Within the nervous system this may mean that a motor neurone, or a cerebellar neurone may be damaged but not a sensory one.

The enzyme systems within the cell often control chains of chemical reactions such as A—→B—→C—→D. The full chain can only be completed if the necessary enzymes and substrate are present in the cell, but it may also be necessary that essential chemical substances should be supplied from outside the cell and metabolic by-products removed to allow the chain to be completed. There may also be enzymes which limit reaction rates. A biochemical lesion may be determined genetically, as in hereditary ataxias (p. 1203) and in Wilson's disease (p. 1191) or by some factor acquired in later life. Thus the metabolic processes may fail because of deficiency of necessary food factors, as in vitamin deficiency (p. 1215), or because an enzyme is poisoned by some toxic substance, e.g. arsenic (p. 1218). It is possible that genetic peculiarity may predispose cells to poisoning by comparatively small doses of toxic substances.

In many disorders of unknown cause, there is clinical and pathological evidence of damage which is confined to a special type of neurone, e.g. motor neurone disease. Although no causative factors have been identified, it seems probable that many of the following disorders will ultimately be classified together as being due to 'biochemical lesions'. The metabolic functions of the neurone are controlled by its cell body but when any gradual failure of any of these processes occurs the effect is first seen at the end of its axon, so that there occurs a progressive 'dying back' of the neurone from its termination towards the cell-body, associated with loss of nucleoprotein in the cell (chromatolysis). This will be seen to be the typical feature of the pathology of the 'congenital and degenerative' disorders which follow.

Motor Neurone Disease

(Progressive Muscular Atrophy, Amyotrophic Lateral Sclerosis, Progressive Bulbar Palsy)

The cause of this disease is unknown but in occasional cases it may be familial. It is characterised by degeneration of motor neurones only, namely the anterior horn cells of the spinal cord, the motor nuclei of the cranial nerves and the corticospinal tracts.

Clinical Features. The disease begins insidiously, usually appearing between the ages of 50 and 70. The first neurones affected may be in the spinal cord or the brain stem and may be either upper or lower motor neurones predominantly. These differences of distribution have led to the recognition of four main clinical groups.

1. Progressive Muscular Atrophy. In this form lower motor neurone damage in the spinal cord is predominant. Upper motor neurone damage may be recognisable at autopsy but is insufficient to cause clinical signs.

2. Amyotrophic Lateral Sclerosis. Both upper and lower motor neurones are affected causing a mixed picture of spasticity with progressive muscular atrophy.

3. Progressive Bulbar Palsy. Here the brunt of the damage falls on the motor nuclei of the medulla and pons. As in the spinal types the atrophic paralysis may be associated with upper motor neurone signs in the limbs.

4. Pseudo-bulbar Palsy. Rarely the upper motor neurone damage may be dominant and this causes the clinical syndrome of pseudo-bulbar palsy, more commonly produced by cerebrovascular disease (p. 1137).

Though in the early stages the clinical picture may fit into one of these categories, later developments make distinctions superfluous. With the spinal types the early symptoms are weakness and wasting of the affected muscles, usually the small muscles of one hand, followed soon after by the other hand. Weakness gradually spreads proximally and is followed in a few weeks or months by similar weakness in the legs. Painful cramps may be the first symptom and very occasionally the patient may be aware of muscular twitching. Less often the atrophic weakness starts in the shoulder muscles. Sooner or later the bulbar muscles are also involved, the tongue being first affected. On examination there is marked wasting of the weak muscles and this may cause a claw-hand deformity. The muscles to which the disease is extending (usually further up the limbs) show prominent fasciculation at rest. This becomes less evident as these muscles waste in their turn. The reflexes of the wasted muscles become depressed and eventually lost. If there is marked upper motor neurone damage the plantar reflexes are extensor and the tendon reflexes are exaggerated until the lower motor neurones forming their efferent path are destroyed by the advancing disease. Thus the peripheral wasted muscles show no reflex activity while the proximal fasciculating muscles may be spastic in amyotrophic lateral sclerosis. In the lower limbs the upper motor neurone signs are usually most evident and in some cases the patient's first awareness of the disease may be that he notices stiffness and dragging of the lower limbs, especially when he is tired.

In the bulbar types speech is severely disturbed (dysarthria) and swallowing becomes increasingly difficult (dysphagia). The muscles of the lower part of the face may be involved but the extra-ocular muscles are never paralysed. These features are usually due to the lower motor neurone lesions of *progressive bulbar palsy* the signs of which are best seen in the tongue. This first shows fasciculation and fibrillation then progressive atrophy with loss of power. The palate droops, and a pool of saliva may be observed in the pharynx as reflex and voluntary swallowing are impaired. In a late stage bilateral lower motor neurone facial paralysis and paralysis of respiration occur. In *pseudo-bulbar palsy* the tongue is contracted and spastic but not wasted and uncontrollable laughing and crying occur. The jaw-jerk is increased and the plantar reflexes are extensor. (Note that pseudo-bulbar palsy is a clinical syndrome resulting from bilateral damage to pyramidal tracts at a high level, irrespective of the cause of the damage. Cerebrovascular disease is a more common cause.) As with the spinal forms, both types of bulbar palsy may be associated in the one patient. There is no sensory loss in any member of the group comprising motor neurone disease and the CSF is normal.

Diagnosis

SPINAL TYPES. Differentiation is most commonly required from the other causes of wasting of the small muscles of the hand. *Syringomyelia* does not cause such severe wasting, fasciculation is rare and there is sensory loss of dissociated type. A *spinal tumour* may cause wasting of the small muscles of the hand, but sensory loss and pain are early features and examination of the CSF may reveal a block or a rise in the protein content. *Diabetes mellitus*, *lead poisoning* and *carcinomatous neuropathy* occasionally cause a similar cord lesion. *Cervical spondylosis* involving nerve roots usually causes considerable pain, and motor and sensory loss follow a root distribution. The sensory loss extends to all forms of sensation. Signs of an upper motor neurone lesion may be found in the lower limbs when the spinal cord is involved. *Cervical rib* gives rise to pain and sensory loss, and the distribution of the wasting is usually confined to muscles innervated by the first thoracic segment. *Acute brachial neuritis* (p. 1222) may be difficult to distinguish from the proximal type of progressive muscular atrophy but pain is greater, fasciculation is less marked, and it is not progressive. A *peripheral nerve lesion* can be distinguished by the fact that the wasting and weakness are confined to the distribution of the nerve, for example the thenar eminence in the *carpal tunnel syndrome*. *Arthritis* of the hands gives rise to secondary muscular atrophy but the joint involvement is obvious. *Syphilitic amyotrophy*, though rare, is important as it is amenable to therapy. Pain is usually a prominent symptom and the CSF shows the changes of meningovascular syphilis.

In all of these disorders confusion may arise because of the presence of muscular wasting. Fasciculation is absent or confined to the weak muscles. Fasciculation in powerful muscles, particularly in the lower limbs in association with wasting of the upper limb muscles, is very suggestive of motor neurone disease. A common diagnostic problem is presented by '*benign fasciculation*' in which the patient is aware of coarse twitching of muscles. There is no paresis or atrophy and the prognosis is excellent. This condition occurs as a result of debility from illness or overwork. It is usually transient but may be perpetuated by psychological mechanisms. The persistent type is common in doctors and medical students who are alarmed about the possibility of motor neurone disease. In the latter condition the patient is rarely aware of the fasciculation and wasting will always be present by the time fasciculation is noticeable.

BULBAR TYPES. The two conditions most likely to be mistaken for motor neurone disease are atherosclerotic pseudo-bulbar palsy and myasthenia gravis. *Pseudo-bulbar palsy* is more commonly caused by arterial disease, though in these circumstances evidence of such disease is usually readily observable and often there is a history that the symptoms came on suddenly following a stroke. Severe *myasthenia gravis* may occasionally be confused with progressive bulbar palsy, but the absence of fasciculation, the history of variability of the symptoms in the early stages of the condition and the response to neostigmine, all make the diagnosis clear.

Treatment. There is no specific treatment, symptomatic measures being applied as required.

Prognosis. Most cases of motor neurone disease die in two to five years but there is a rare chronic type with a course of 10 to 15 years. Generalised fasciculation and involvement of the brain stem are bad prognostic signs, usually indicating death within a year.

The Hereditary Ataxias

This is a group of related hereditary or familial disorders in which the systems of neurones which 'die back' (p. 1199) are mainly the spinal and brain-stem tracts leading to the cerebellum, the corticospinal tracts, and the optic nerves. Different combinations of these elements form recognisable clinical pictures, which usually 'breed true' in a family, but it may be impossible to differentiate the different types during life. The group forms a link with hereditary disorders of the peripheral nerves such as peroneal muscular atrophy (p. 1218) and with neurofibromatosis (p. 1206) and these may occur in association with the hereditary ataxias either in one individual or in the same family. Congenital deformities of the feet, particularly pes cavus, and of other organs are commonly associated.

Clinical Features. The onset may be any time from infancy to middle life. Symptoms are slowly progressive. Where cerebellar or spinocerebellar neurones are involved there is progressive ataxia of gait, followed by intention tremor of the arms, dysarthria of explosive type and, in some types, nystagmus. Where the main lesion is in corticospinal tracts there is a hereditary spastic paraplegia. Optic atrophy and loss of bladder reflexes may occur. *Friedreich's ataxia* is the most common type, usually familial but occasionally sporadic. Unaffected members of the family as well as the patients may show pes cavus. There is degeneration of the spinocerebellar and corticospinal tracts, and of the posterior columns. There is therefore very severe ataxia.

Tendon jerks are lost at an early stage, the ankle jerks first, then the knee jerks but finally all tendon jerks may be lost due to failure of brain stem facilitation. Muscle tone is decreased. The plantar reflexes are extensor. Muscle-joint and vibration senses are impaired as the posterior column degeneration progresses. Scoliosis and pes cavus are almost invariable and other congenital abnormalities such as spina bifida and conduction defects in the heart, giving rise to ECG abnormalities, are common.

Diagnosis. The familial history, the presence of pes cavus, and the absence of remissions distinguish these diseases from disseminated sclerosis. In Friedreich's ataxia tendon reflexes are absent and there may be electrocardiographic changes.

Onset of cerebellar degeneration in later life is often due to the presence of a neoplasm in a bronchus, ovary or elsewhere (see carcinomatous neuropathy, p. 1216).

Treatment. There is no specific treatment. Co-ordination exercises and occupational therapy will help the patient to overcome his disability in the early stages but a wheel-chair life becomes inevitable. Scoliosis and pes cavus may require appropriate appliances or orthopaedic surgery.

Prognosis. All diseases of this group are progressive but compatible with a long life.

Syringomyelia

This is a disease characterised by cavitation surrounded by gliosis in the spinal cord and brain stem (syringobulbia). The condition probably results from a developmental abnormality of fusion of the lower cervical and upper thoracic cord or the medulla. It usually starts at the base of one posterior horn where it interrupts the second order spinothalamic neurones (p. 1078) and it spreads anteromedially towards the midline of the anterior part of the cord. There it interrupts the same type of fibres crossing from the other side. The cavitation may also extend to invade the anterior horns and may compress the corticospinal tracts in the lateral columns, but the posterior columns are usually spared. The common age of onset is between 25 and 40 years, possibly due to the expansion of a cavity which has hitherto been only a fissure.

Clinical Features. The patient presents most commonly with wasting of the small muscles of the hands, as a result of extension of the cavity into the base of the anterior horn, or he may notice painless burns or injuries of the hands. The onset is insidious and physical signs may be present before the patient notices these abnormalities. Less commonly, when pain fibres are irritated rather than destroyed, pain in the upper limbs is the presenting symptom. Over the areas of the body innervated from the affected segments of the cord there is sensory loss of dissociated type. Sensations dependent on the spinothalamic pathway (pain, warmth and cold) are depressed or lost whereas posterior column sensations (muscle-joint position and vibration sense) are unimpaired. The sense of touch utilises both pathways so it is not lost though it may be impaired. The sensory loss usually starts on the medial border of one forearm, or on the hand, and later spreads to the chest, the lateral side of the arm, and to the neck. It is often bilateral but not necessarily symmetrical. The motor signs if present are of lower motor neurone type at the level of the cavity, due to involvement of the anterior horn, and upper motor neurone type below that level, due to compression of a pyramidal tract. Usually there is wasting of the small muscles of one hand with later involvement of the other. Wasting spreads to involve all the musculature of the upper limbs. Fasciculation is unusual and wasting rarely becomes severe. Tendon reflexes are lost in the arms but increased in the lower limbs and one or both plantar reflexes may be extensor. In advanced cases trophic lesions also occur in the upper limbs and painless ulcers may appear on the soles of the feet if the spreading lesion involves the spinothalamic tracts, causing analgesia below the level of the lesion. Hypertrophy of soft tissues and osteoarthropathy (Charcot's joints) are also seen, usually in upper limbs.

Extension of the cavitation to the brain stem causes dissociated sensory loss (p. 1083) on the face, and paralysis of the palate, larynx and tongue. Rotatory or ataxic nystagmus from involvement of the medial longitudinal bundle (p. 1099) and Horner's syndrome from involvement of the descending fibres in the brain stem destined for the sympathetic system also occur (p. 1112). The sphincters are rarely disturbed. The CSF shows no abnormality. Spina bifida is commonly seen on a radiograph of the lumbo-sacral spine.

Diagnosis. The differential diagnosis of the main conditions with which syringomyelia may be mistaken is discussed on p. 1224. An identical syndrome may develop rapidly after spinal injury and is caused by haematomyelia. The trophic symptoms of Raynaud's disease (p. 295) may simulate syringomyelia but there is no dissociated sensory loss.

Treatment. The patient should be warned of the risks of injury or burning himself and of the need to avoid infection of the hands. Radiotherapy may arrest expansion of the cavity by causing reactive gliosis and may lessen the risk of malignant change. It is valuable in relieving pain when this is a prominent symptom, and may accelerate healing of trophic ulcers.

Prognosis. The condition is slowly progressive over many years. Sometimes neoplastic change occurs (glioma). The outlook is worse when syringobulbia develops, death usually occurring from pneumonia or inanition.

Neurofibromatosis

(von Recklinghausen's Disease)

Aetiology. This is a hereditary disorder occurring in one or many members of a family. It is closely related to other congenital tumours of the nervous system such as tuberous sclerosis (epiloia) and haemangioblastoma of the cerebellum and retina.

Pathology. Neurofibromas are tumours derived from the neurilemmal sheath of peripheral nerves, nerve roots or cranial nerves, especially the fifth (p. 1103) and the eighth (p. 1108). Cutaneous fibromas, which are pedunculated tumours named mollusca fibrosa, are considered to be of similar origin; they are benign but may undergo sarcomatous change. Within the central nervous system the glial and ependymal tissue may also proliferate causing syringomyelia (p. 1204) or tumours such as glioma and ependymoma. Meningiomas are also commonly associated with neurofibromatosis, and secreting tumours of the suprarenal medulla (p. 733) and other chromaffin tissues may be present. Congenital abnormalities such as spina bifida, meningocoele, vascular and lymphatic naevi and ocular and renal malformations also occur.

Clinical Features. A patient may show only one or many of a wide range of cutaneous or of peripheral or central neurological abnormalities. Some of the more common ones are *café-au-lait* coloured patches of skin pigmentation, cutaneous fibromas and benign tumours of peripheral nerves. These are discrete, movable lumps, arranged along lines of nerves. They may be painful or tender on pressure. The nerve trunks may be thickened as in the related condition of hypertrophic polyneuropathy (p. 1218) or there may be a diffuse plexiform growth causing tissue swelling, a type of 'elephantiasis'. The tumours may occur within body cavities and internal organs, in the eyes and within the bones where they cause cystic change or hyperostosis. Kyphoscoliosis and other bony deformities are common.

Solitary neurofibromas may occur on a spinal nerve root (p. 1208) or in a cranial nerve. Acoustic neuroma (p. 1108) is sometimes bilateral. Epilepsy may occur.

Diagnosis. This may be confirmed by biopsy of a tumour but is rarely necessary. With intracranial and intraspinal types the protein level of the CSF is very high, often exceeding 1,000 mg./100 ml. Radiology may show that an internal auditory meatus or intervertebral foramen is widened if it contains a neurofibroma.

Treatment. No treatment is required unless a central type causes cerebral or spinal compression, when operative removal of the tumour is necessary. A tumour, central or peripheral, which becomes sarcomatous must be removed if possible.

Prognosis. New tumours gradually appear throughout life but the progress is slow. Any tumour may become malignant (sarcoma) but the chances of it doing so are small.

COMPRESSION OF THE SPINAL CORD

Aetiology and Pathology. The more important causes of spinal cord compression are:

1. In the vertebral column: crush fracture of a vertebral body; posterior protrusion of an intervertebral disc; secondary carcinoma (from breast, prostate, bronchus or other primary sites); myelomatosis and tuberculous disease of the spine.

2. In relation to the spinal meninges: epidural abscess; tumours (meningioma, neurofibroma, p. 1206); infiltration with Hodgkin's lymphogranuloma and leukaemic deposits; arachnoiditis and syphilitic leptomeningitis (common causes in some tropical countries).

3. In the spinal cord: tumours (gliomas, ependymoma and metastatic deposits).

Tumours, posterior disc protrusions and trauma account for the majority of cases of spinal cord compression. Tuberculosis of the spine (Pott's disease), once so common a cause, is now a rarity in Britain. It is convenient in practice to divide the tumours into those arising outside the spinal cord (extramedullary), which constitute about 80 per cent., and those arising within (intramedullary).

A space-occupying lesion within the spinal canal may involve nerve tissue directly by pressure, or indirectly by interfering with the blood supply. Oedema from venous obstruction impairs the function of the neurones Ischaemia from arterial obstruction leads to necrosis of the spinal cord. The earlier stages are reversible but severely damaged neurones do not recover so it is most important to diagnose and treat spinal compression without delay.

Clinical Features. The onset of symptoms of spinal cord compression is usually slow but it may be acute with trauma or metastases, especially if there is arterial occlusion. Pain localised over the spine or in a root distribution is the most common initial symptom. It may be aggravated by spinal movement or by coughing, sneezing or straining at the toilet which cause temporary increase in the pressure of the spinal fluid. Paraesthesiae and numbness or cold sensations may also develop early, especially in the lower limbs. Motor symptoms, which usually appear later, consist of heaviness, stiffness or weakness of a limb. Urgency or hesitancy of micturition, leading eventually to urinary retention is usually a late manifestation.

The signs found on examination vary according to the structures involved. There may be a gibbus if there is local spinal disease, and local tenderness may be present with vertebral disease or extradural abscess. A bruit may be heard with a stethoscope over the site of a vascular tumour (angioma). Involvement of the posterior roots gives rise to hyperaesthesia and later to sensory loss over the appropriate dermatome. When the anterior roots are affected there are signs of a lower motor neurone lesion at the corresponding level. Interruption of ascending fibres in the spinal cord causes sensory loss below the level of the lesion which may be of superficial sensation or of proprioceptive sense, according to which tracts are mainly involved. Light touch, however, is often affected early. Interruption of descending fibres gives rise to upper motor neurone signs below the level of the lesion and control of the sphincters may be lost. If damage is confined to one side of the cord the *syndrome of Brown-Séquard* results. On the side of the lesion there is a band of hyperaesthesia with below it loss of proprioceptive sense and upper motor neurone signs. On the other side there is loss of spinothalamic sensation (heat, warmth and cold) as fibres of that tract decussate soon after entering the cord.

The distribution of these signs varies with the level of the lesion. Lesions above the fifth cervical segment give signs of an upper motor neurone lesion and sensory loss in upper and lower limbs (tetraplegia); a lesion between the fifth cervical and first thoracic segments gives signs of a lower motor neurone lesion and segmental sensory loss in the upper limbs and signs of an upper motor neuron lesion in the lower limbs; a lesion in the thoracic cord causes a spastic paraplegia with sensory loss having a horizontal upper level on the trunk; a lesion in the lumbosacral cord gives signs of a lower motor neurone lesion in the appropriate segments of the lower limbs and sensory loss. Spinal lesions lower than the first lumbar vertebra cannot damage the spinal cord but may damage the roots of the cauda equina.

Examination of the CSF is of great value but withdrawal of fluid may alter the pressure balance above and below the lesion in the cord and lead to rapid exacerbation of compression. For this reason, if lumbar puncture confirms the diagnosis, the patient should be referred without any delay to a neurosurgeon and if the diagnosis is highly probable on clinical grounds the puncture should be postponed until it is convenient to operate on the patient. Queckenstedt's test may reveal the features of a partial or complete block but a normal result does not exclude the diagnosis (p. 1151). The cell content is normal but there is a great excess of protein (500-3000 mg. per 100 ml.) and xanthochromia is present (Froin's syndrome). Radiological examination of the spine may reveal abnormalities at the site of the lesion but often contrast radiography, after introduction of air or a radio-opaque substance such as Myodil into the spinal canal (myelography), is required.

Diagnosis. Pain, which is so often a presenting symptom of spinal cord compression, may be wrongly attributed to such conditions as pleurisy, cholecystitis or 'fibrositis', but a careful examination will reveal signs of organic nervous disease. It is insufficient to be content with eliciting the tendon reflexes, as motor signs may be delayed long after sensory signs are present. If there is indisputable evidence of spinal cord damage it is essential to decide the site of the primary lesion. A general examination may reveal evidence of disease elsewhere making it likely that the lesion in the cord is secondary to this. A careful search should be made for a primary tumour in another organ, enlargement of lymph glands, the cutaneous signs of neurofibromatosis (p. 1206) and the presence of sepsis which could lead to extradural abscess. (An abscess should always be considered if pain is severe and signs of cord disease develop rapidly as immediate treatment is imperative). If the lesion causing compression arose initially in the spinal cord it is necessary to distinguish it from disseminated sclerosis, syringomyelia, motor neurone disease and subacute combined degeneration. The differential diagnosis from these conditions is considered on pp. 1183 and 1201. Disseminated sclerosis appearing for the first time in middle-aged people may often present as a slowly progressive lesion of the spinal cord. The differentiation from spinal cord compression is, however, so difficult and of such importance that there should be no hesitation in seeking expert advice.

Treatment. Surgical relief of the compression is a matter of great urgency since recovery from severe paralysis is unlikely. A delay of even a few hours may be critical in extradural abscess. Exploration is also often required to ascertain the pathological nature of the lesion. If a benign extramedullary tumour is found, it may be removed. In malignant tumours, leukaemic infiltration, and in most intramedullary lesions decompression helps little if at all. Radiotherapy may halt the course of the disease and may be of help in the relief of pain.

Prognosis. Prognosis depends on the severity and duration of the compression before it is relieved. In addition, the nature of the cause must be taken into account. Thus decompression for a malignant lesion may be undertaken though it will be of only temporary benefit.

Paraplegia

Management. Paraplegia may result from many causes, particularly tumours, trauma and other forms of spinal compression, disseminated sclerosis and subacute combined degeneration of the cord. Treatment must be directed to the cause but management of the paraplegia itself is most important if complications which may in themselves lead to death are to be avoided. Pressure sores, urinary infections, renal calculi, faecal impaction and contractures are complications which can be prevented. Attention must, therefore, be given to the skin, the bladder, the bowel, the paralysed parts and to the rehabilitation of the patient.

SKIN. The skin is very liable to be damaged with the formation of pressure sores because of the loss of sensation, diminished blood supply and the immobility of the patient. The patient must be nursed on a specially made rubber mattress and the skin kept dry and clean. Every two to four hours he should be turned and nursed in such a position as will avoid pressure on bony prominences such as the sacrum and heels. This is most easily done by nursing the patient in a Stryker frame. If a pressure sore forms, the patient must not lie on the affected side and scrupulous asepsis must be observed until healing takes place. Skin grafting may be required. Nutrition must be maintained by a well balanced diet containing adequate amounts of protein, vitamin C and iron. Blood transfusions may be required in individual cases.

BLADDER. If retention occurs, aseptic intermittent catheterisation must be carried out. An indwelling catheter may then be inserted and attached to a water-seal drainage bottle. It should be clipped and allowed to drain at regular intervals to establish reflex emptying of the bladder. As the rhythm becomes established the catheter is withdrawn and the patient trained to micturate reflexly at fixed times. Emptying of the bladder should be assisted by manual compression of the lower abdomen by patient or nurse. It is not advisable to give antibiotics prophylactically but if infection develops then a short course of the appropriate antibiotic should be given. An adequate consumption of fluid should be ensured. Frequent turning and early ambulation where possible are the best measures for reducing the dangers of urinary stagnation and calculus formation.

Bowel. Constipation must be prevented by suitable diet, liquid paraffin and laxatives. If it occurs it must be relieved by enemata, otherwise the faeces will become hard and impacted and may require to be removed manually.

Paralysed Parts. Spasticity readily leads to the development of flexor spasm and contractures in the limbs. This danger can be reduced by regular passive movement of the limbs and by nursing the patient in such positions as will discourage flexion of the joints. The weight of the bedclothes should be taken from the lower limbs by a cradle to reduce reflex stimulation and prevent drop-foot deformity. If there is no hope of recovery, flexor spasms may be abolished by intrathecal injection of phenol in glycerine or by section of anterior nerve roots.

Rehabilitation. When the cause of paraplegia is not progressive, a great deal can be done by rehabilitation. The patient may learn to walk with calipers or to use a wheel-chair. He may thus be able to care for himself and may even follow a suitable occupation.

DEFICIENCY DISEASES

As with the hereditary and degenerative diseases, deficiency diseases affect particular types of cells according to their peculiarities of metabolism (p. 1198). The cell bodies are damaged but the neurones tend to 'die back' from the periphery. The most susceptible neurones appear to be those of the peripheral nerves, the longest fibres usually being the first affected.

Vitamin B_{12} Neuropathy

(Subacute Combined Degeneration of the Cord)

This disease is characterised by peripheral neuropathy together with progressive degeneration of the posterior and lateral columns of the spinal cord. It is associated with Addisonian pernicious anaemia. As a result of earlier diagnosis and the introduction of highly potent remedies it is seen much more rarely than 30 years ago.

Aetiology. The disease is due to deficiency of vitamin B_{12}. It most commonly appears about the age of 50 in patients who are already known to be suffering from pernicious anaemia. Usually the treatment of the pernicious anaemia has been inadequate, though occasionally neuropathy may develop in the presence of an anaemia which is only slight. The condition may be produced by the administration of folic acid to patients with Addisonian pernicious anaemia. Vitamin B_{12} neuropathy is rarely found after gastrectomy or other causes of malabsorption of vitamin B_{12} (p. 626).

Pathology. Degenerative changes develop in the peripheral nerves. Areas of demyelination appear in the lower cervical and upper thoracic regions of the spinal cord, particularly in the posterior columns, the corticospinal tracts and the spino-cerebellar tracts. These tracts then demyelinate and subsequently the axis cylinders break down starting from the termination of the tract and spreading towards the appropriate cells of origin. Areas of degeneration may also appear in the cerebral white matter and in the optic nerves.

Clinical Features. The disease usually develops gradually and almost invariably the presenting symptoms are due to peripheral neuropathy, usually tingling paraesthesiae of the toes, spreading later to the fingers. The patient also complains that the extremities feel cold and numb, and he may notice difficulty in holding small objects. Motor symptoms, such as weakness and ataxia, appear later but become severe as the cord is involved.

The physical signs depend on the relative involvement of the peripheral nerves and the posterior and lateral columns. Objective sensory changes are almost invariably present and consist of impairment of all forms of sensation in the distal parts of the limbs ascending in a 'stocking and glove' fashion. Sensory loss may spread on to the trunk where it may show a horizontal upper border. Tenderness of the muscles, especially of the calves, is commonly found in the early stages of the disease and indicates the presence of peripheral neuropathy. Muscle-joint sense may be impaired by peripheral neuropathy or by posterior column degeneration and either lesion may cause loss of vibration sensation. In the majority of cases ataxia is the outstanding feature. It is of the sensory type with Romberg's sign (p. 1082). In the minority of cases, signs of an upper motor neurone lesion (spasticity, increased tendon reflexes and extensor plantar responses), predominate in the lower limbs. The condition of the tendon reflexes depends on the extent of involvement of peripheral neurones. Most commonly the ankle jerks are lost and later the knee jerks, though increase in these reflexes may be found. Nystagmus may be present. Visual failure due to primary optic atrophy occurs on rare occasions and, in severe cases, mental impairment is not uncommon. The CSF is normal. There is usually a histamine fast achlorhydria though free hydrochloric acid may be found in malabsorption states leading to vitamin B_{12} neuropathy. Examination of the blood and sternal marrow shows a macrocytic anaemia with megaloblastic blood formation (p. 621). The level of cyanocobalamin in the serum is low (under 80 $\mu\mu$g. per ml.), and its uptake from the gastrointestinal tract is impaired.

Diagnosis. The presentation of a patient with symmetrical paraesthesiae in the limbs should always raise the suspicion of vitamin B_{12} neuropathy and evidence of involvement of the posterior and lateral columns of the cord should be sought. The association with glossitis, megaloblastic anaemia and achlorhydria strongly suggests the diagnosis which should be confirmed by estimation of the serum vitamin B_{12} level. Peripheral neuropathy from other causes may present in the same way but without signs of spinal cord involvement. Tabes dorsalis may be confused with vitamin B_{12} neuropathy because of the sensory loss in the distal parts of the limb, absent reflexes and ataxia, but the muscles are less tender than normal, and other signs of syphilitic infection such as the Argyll Robertson pupil and changes in the CSF are commonly found. Disseminated sclerosis and myelopathy due to cervical spondylosis may give rise to damage to the posterolateral columns of the spinal cord but there are no signs of peripheral neuritis. Combined spinal cord and peripheral nerve lesions may be caused by carcinomatous neuropathy (p. 1216).

Prophylaxis. The erythrocyte count must be maintained at 5 million per c.mm. and the haemoglobin at 14·6 g. per 100 ml. It is in the patients whose anaemia is not fully corrected by appropriate treatment that subacute combined degeneration of the cord is liable to develop.

Treatment. The treatment of vitamin B_{12} neuropathy is that of pernicious anaemia (p. 623), but the dose of cyanocobalamin should be two or three times as large as is given in uncomplicated cases of pernicious anaemia and this intensive therapy must be continued as long as there is evidence of neurological improvement. Thereafter, regular maintenance doses sufficient to keep the blood normal must be given for the rest of the patient's life. Temporary increase in dosage is required if the patient develops an infection, especially if it is pyogenic, as this may lead to severe exacerbation.

Prognosis. Untreated subacute combined degeneration of the cord progresses to death within about two years. The response to treatment depends on the stage at which it is initiated. If signs are due only to peripheral neuropathy a complete recovery may be expected. Ataxia may improve remarkably. If, however, there is severe damage to the spinal cord, only limited improvement in signs such as spasticity can be anticipated although the progress of the disease can be arrested.

Wernicke's Encephalopathy

This condition is due to thiamine deficiency (p. 510), and the main pathological lesions are foci of congestion and petechial haemorrhage in the upper part of the mid-brain, the hypothalamus, and the walls of the third ventricle. The corpora mamillaria are always involved and this is believed to account for defects of memory. Vomiting and nystagmus are early symptoms but the patient most commonly presents as an acute psychiatric problem with disorientation, faulty memory, confabulation (p. 1269), delusions and abnormal behaviour. This group of mental symptoms is often called Korsakoff's psychosis. Confusion may progress to stupor or coma. The predominant signs are the loss of pupillary reflexes and of extra-ocular movements. Other signs of deficiency of the B-group vitamins such as polyneuropathy may be present. The possibility of Wernicke's encephalopathy should always be borne in mind in the presence of any acute psychosis, especially when this develops in a patient who is an alcoholic, has chronic gastrointestinal disease or has been restricting his diet severely. It may also complicate hyperemesis gravidarum.

Treatment. Dramatic therapeutic responses have been obtained in early cases by the parenteral administration of thiamine. Thiamine hydrochloride (vitamin B_1) should be given immediately by slow intravenous injection in a dose of 50 mg. and, thereafter, 50 mg. should be given daily by intramuscular injection for several days. Subsequently oral administration will suffice. Thereafter a well balanced mixed diet and a natural supplement of the entire vitamin B complex such as yeast extract or Marmite should be given.

Other Deficiency Diseases

Lesions of the nervous system are also found in pellagra and in nutritional polyneuropathy (pp. 524, 518).

CARCINOMATOUS NEUROPATHY

Carcinoma originating in organs other than the central nervous system may spread metastatically to the brain or spinal cord or to the meninges. The brain, spinal cord or nerve roots may be involved by compression (p. 1207) or by carcinomatosis of the meninges when the clinical features may simulate low-grade meningitis (p. 1156). In addition, however, to their direct effects, neoplasia in other organs particularly in the lung, ovary and breast, occasionally causes remote disorders of a degenerative or 'toxic' type in the central and peripheral nervous system and in the muscles. These manifestations are collectively known as carcinomatous neuropathy. The mechanism by which this effect is produced is unknown and it may precede other manifestations of neoplasia by three years or more. The symptoms may be remittent but do not necessarily resolve on removal of the causative tumour. In addition to carcinoma, similar syndromes occur in patients who have myelomatosis, leukaemia or other types of reticulosis. The various types may occur alone or in association with each other.

Progressive dementia without focal neurological signs is a rare type.

Subacute cerebellar degeneration is one of the common types. It develops rapidly over a period of months, leading to severe dysarthria, gross ataxia of all limbs and nystagmus. There may be involvement of the corticospinal tracts producing upper motor neurone signs.

Degeneration of posterior root ganglia causes severe and persistent pains and painful paraesthesiae of the extremities, followed by gradual development of total sensory loss in the limbs and consequent ataxia. The face and trunk may be included.

Peripheral neuropathy involving sensory and motor fibres is more common. Occasionally only motor fibres may be damaged. The symptoms and signs are those of any peripheral neuropathy (p. 1218).

Carcinomatous myopathy may cause weakness and wasting of the proximal muscles of the limbs and sometimes ptosis, diplopia and bulbar paralysis. Fatiguability of myasthenic type may be striking at first. The response to neostigmine is poorly sustained and soon disappears but guanidine 500 mg./kg. body weight effectively restores strength in carcinomatous myasthenia.

Treatment. Treatment of the primary lesion may arrest these disorders and the peripheral neuropathy and myopathy may improve. Symptomatic treatment is necessary.

DISORDERS OF PERIPHERAL NERVES

The Neuropathies

(Polyneuritis)

In this condition there is impairment of function of many peripheral nerves simultaneously and usually symmetrically. The old term 'polyneuritis' is rarely justified since few of the disorders are inflammatory. There is usually a metabolic disturbance which affects the longest nerve fibres first, then progressively shorter ones irrespective of the nerve they occupy. The result is weakness, impairment or loss of sensation and diminished or absent tendon reflexes especially at the periphery. Inflammatory neuritis on the other hand usually involves the proximal parts of the spinal nerves or individual peripheral nerves (mononeuritis multiplex).

Aetiology. There are numerous causes, the more important of which are:

Hereditary. Peroneal muscular atrophy, hypertrophic interstitial neuropathy and other hereditary neuropathies.

Metabolic. Diabetes mellitus and porphyria.

Deficiency. Vitamin B_{12} neuropathy (p. 1212), beriberi (p. 511), alcoholism and gastrointestinal disease.

Poisons. Lead, arsenic, mercury, triorthocresylphosphate (ginger paralysis). In addition many new substances produced for therapeutic and industrial purposes carry this hazard.

Infectious and Toxic or Allergic Reactions. Leprosy is an infection of peripheral nerves. Diphtheria causes toxic neuropathy. Polyneuritis associated with exanthematous disease and inoculations is probably allergic in nature (p. 1186). Acute infective polyneuritis, for long believed to be due to a virus, may have a similar cause.

Connective Tissue and Vascular Disorders. Polyarteritis nodosa (p. 290) and disorders such as systemic lupus erythematosus cause mononeuritis multiplex.

Malignant Disease. Carcinoma of the bronchus and other tumours may cause polyneuropathy which may be the first manifestation of malignancy (p. 1216).

Pathology. The peripheral nerves show Wallerian degeneration or segmental demyelination. In acute cases little may be found at autopsy since the early changes are biochemical in nature.

Clinical Features. Polyneuropathy presents with paraesthesiae such as tingling, pins and needles and numbness in the periphery of all four limbs, usually starting in the toes and in addition there may be great pain. These symptoms gradually spread proximally as shorter fibres are involved so that the distribution does not follow that of any particular nerve root or peripheral nerve. The patient then has difficulty with fine movements such as fastening buttons because of developing loss of proprioception or he notices that objects feel 'different'. Sensory ataxia may follow and weakness soon becomes apparent. Weakness, too, usually starts peripherally and spreads proximally.

Examination reveals impairment or loss of all forms of sensation, extending from the periphery of the limbs in a 'glove and stocking' fashion. A characteristic feature is that the muscles are often extremely tender to pressure. Damage to the motor fibres causes the signs of a lower motor neurone lesion, especially at the periphery of the limbs, so that wrist-drop and foot-drop may appear. The proximal muscles are later involved and then the trunk and sometimes the face. Respiration may be endangered by paralysis of the intercostal muscles or the diaphragm. Interruption of the reflex arcs causes loss of the tendon reflexes.

There are features peculiar to certain forms of polyneuropathy.

ALCOHOLIC POLYNEUROPATHY. Pain is usually severe and other evidence of alcoholism may be apparent, such as tremor of the hands, mental impairment or signs of liver disease.

LEAD NEUROPATHY. Lead poisoning causes paralysis of muscles, usually within the distribution of the radial or lateral popliteal nerves, but without involving all muscles supplied by these nerves. It is, for instance, common to find paralysis of the extensor muscles of the wrists and fingers with sparing of the brachioradialis and abductor pollicis longus muscles. Some authorities consider that this is due to local poisoning of muscles rather than true neuropathy. There is no loss of sensation. Other clinical features associated with chronic exposure to lead are anaemia with punctate basophilia of red cells (p. 609) and a blue line on the gums if the patient is not edentulous. If the amount of lead ingested is sufficient to cause poisoning there may be colic and headache, chronic nephritis with hypertension (p. 808) and acute or chronic encephalopathy, causing mental changes and epileptic seizures. The clinical picture may resemble that of porphyria.

PORPHYRINURIC POLYNEUROPATHY. This form of neuropathy is often purely motor in type. It is associated with temporary mental disorder and attacks of abdominal pain. The urine contains porphobilinogen and may become the colour of port wine on standing. It may be precipitated by taking barbiturates or sulphonamide drugs or by pregnancy in those who have a hereditary tendency.

DIABETIC POLYNEUROPATHY. This is discussed on p. 772.

DIPHTHERITIC POLYNEURITIS. The initial infection is often mild and unrecognised. Blurring of vision, owing to paralysis of accommodation, and a nasal voice due to paralysis of the soft palate are often the first neuritic signs before manifestations in the limbs become apparent.

ACUTE 'INFECTIVE' POLYNEURITIS (Guillain-Barré syndrome). This condition begins with headache, vomiting, pyrexia and pain in the back and limbs. It is caused by inflammation with oedema of the spinal nerves soon after their formation by junction of the nerve roots. After a variable period of hours or days paralysis appears, beginning usually in all four limbs simultaneously, though sometimes starting in the lower limbs and spreading in ascending fashion. Unlike other types of polyneuropathy, proximal rather than distal muscles in the limbs may be affected. The trunk and respiratory muscles may be involved and also the muscles supplied by the cranial nerves, particularly the seventh. Sensory loss may be confined to the limbs or may spread on to the trunk. Reflexes are lost and sphincter difficulties occur. Death may be caused by respiratory or bulbar paralysis (p. 1175). The CSF shows striking changes, there being a normal cell count but a great increase in protein (100-1000 mg. per 100 ml.). If death from respiratory paralysis is prevented or avoided, the outlook is good, as most cases recover in three to six months. The evidence for an infective aetiology is unsatisfactory. The possibility of an auto-immune mechanism provides a rationale for the use of corticosteroids.

POLYARTERITIS NODOSA (p. 290.) This causes multiple mononeuritis rather than symmetrical polyneuritis. Motor and sensory loss will be distributed according to the nerves involved rather than according to length of fibre so the 'glove and stocking' distribution is absent.

Diagnosis. Pain in the limbs occurs from causes such as ischaemia or arthritis and will be unaccompanied by abnormal neurological signs but neuritis may be associated with each of these conditions. Tabes dorsalis causes lightning pains, absence of the tendon reflexes and sensory loss. The description of the pain however is different, there is decreased rather than increased muscle tenderness and Argyll Robertson pupils are usually present. Acute infective polyneuritis is often mistakenly diagnosed as poliomyelitis but in the latter disease the weakness is asymmetrical, there is no sensory loss and the CSF changes are different (p. 1175). Motor neurone disease should not be confused as no sensory loss occurs in that condition. Nevertheless motor neurone disease and polymyositis (p. 559) may be difficult to differentiate from motor forms of polyneuropathy. If lower motor neurone and sensory signs are restricted to the lower limbs the possibility of a lesion of the cauda equina should be considered.

Treatment. Prevention is very important. Any new drug which is liable to cause neuropathy must be used with care and industrial hazards should be avoided by protective clothing, exhaust ventilation and the other techniques of the industrial medical officer. When polyneuritis has developed as a result of exposure to a toxic substance the first step is to remove the patient from further exposure. When the cause is nutritional or metabolic the appropriate treatment must be initiated without delay. Thus therapy may be required for beriberi, diabetes or pernicious anaemia. Corticosteroids are indicated for acute 'infective' polyneuritis. Chelating agents (p. 1193) are used to eliminate heavy metals such as lead which have been responsible for poisoning.

In severe cases bed rest is essential since the nervous control of the heart may be defective (and cardiomyopathy is sometimes associated). The limbs should be supported in the optimum position, and passive movements carried out several times a day. A cage should protect the feet from the weight of the bed clothes. Respiratory insufficiency may require tracheostomy or institution of intermittent positive pressure respiration (p. 320). When recovery begins, active movements should be carried out under the supervision of a physiotherapist.

PAIN IN THE ARM

(Brachial Neuralgia, Brachial Neuritis, Brachialgia)

There are many causes of pain in the arm, the most common of which are:

1. Herniation of an intervertebral disc and cervical spondylosis.
2. Compression of the nerve roots as they pass through the thoracic outlet.
3. Spinal neoplasm.
4. Acute brachial neuritis (neuralgic amyotrophy).
5. Syringomyelia.
6. Syphilitic cervical pachymeningitis.
7. Pain referred from somatic structures, e.g. shoulder joint and the supraspinatus tendon.
8. Pain referred from viscera, e.g. angina pectoris.

Acute Brachial Neuritis

Aetiology. Most cases of acute brachial neuritis occur in patients in hospital convalescing from an illness resulting from infection, injury or operation. In the last case the onset is usually three or four days after the operation. A few cases occur post-partum. More rarely the illness follows an injection of serum or vaccine, usually, but not invariably, a few days after the occurrence of the symptoms of serum sickness. An allergic mechanism seems probable in the latter group.

Clinical Features. The patient complains of severe pain over one shoulder girdle, sometimes spreading up the neck or down the arm. Simultaneously, or two or three days later, paralysis develops in the painful muscles. These are usually supplied by the fifth and sixth and less commonly the seventh cervical nerves so that the deltoid, spinati, and serratus anterior muscles are usually involved, and frequently also the muscles of the upper arm. The tendon jerks disappear in the affected limb and wasting is rapid. Sensory loss is slight or absent. If present it is usually on the outer aspect of the upper third of the affected arm. The brachial plexus is often tender.

Sometimes paralysis of single nerves of the upper limb occurs and occasionally both shoulder girdles are involved. Constitutional symptoms are mild or absent. The CSF is normal or shows only slight lymphocytosis (10-15 per c.mm.).

Diagnosis. The diagnosis is based on the history of pain and weakness of an arm occurring with a typical latent period after an illness or operation, and on the distribution of neurological signs. A frequent error is to attribute the condition to traction on the arm during operation causing a thoracic outlet syndrome or to the effects of intravenous medication during operation, or to faulty inoculation technique, and this may lead to unfortunate medico-legal difficulties. Cervical disc herniation usually causes more localised pain and paresis. The differential diagnosis from poliomyelitis may be very difficult if there is no sensory loss.

Course and Prognosis. Pain usually subsides in one to two weeks but may last for months. Recovery from paralysis is slow.

It usually takes several months, but eventual complete recovery after two or more years is not exceptional. Recurrent attacks of neuritis in the same or the opposite shoulder may occur after two or three months. For these reasons prognosis should be guarded but optimistic.

Treatment. Corticosteroids should be tried in neuritis believed to be the consequence of an allergic mechanism. Otherwise treatment is symptomatic and the principles are those adopted for poliomyelitis (p. 1177).

Cervical Disc Herniation and Cervical Spondylosis

Introduction. Degenerative changes occur in the cervical intervertebral discs in the same manner as in the lumbar region (p. 1228) and may lead to herniation. The herniation may affect one disc only, most commonly that between the sixth and seventh cervical vertebrae, or there may be involvement of several discs with secondary osteoarthritic changes. The latter changes (cervical spondylosis) are especially liable to interfere with the blood supply to the spinal cord, and thus lead to further damage. Osteoarthritis in any part of the spine is a common degenerative disorder which often causes no symptoms. The clinical syndromes of acute cervical disc protrusion and chronic cervical spondylosis may occur at different times in the same patient, depending on the anatomical relation of disc protrusions and osteophytic outgrowths to the nerve roots and spinal cord, and on secondary postural or traumatic factors. Acute herniation is usually laterally situated and causes compression of a nerve root. The chronic degeneration of discs is frequently associated with mid-line herniation and so spinal cord compression may result.

Acute Protrusion of a Cervical Intervertebral Disc. This may occur at any age, usually without apparent trauma to the neck. The patient complains of attacks of pain in the neck often termed 'cricks' or 'fibrositis'. In severe attacks pain is referred to the skin segmental area of one of the lower cervical nerve roots and to the muscles, bones and joints which it supplies. Hyperaesthesia and hyperalgesia may be found in the affected segment but sensory loss sometimes occurs. Depression of tendon reflexes utilising the affected root is common and lower motor neurone paresis of root distribution is also an occasional finding. The neck is held stiffly, and pain is produced by its movement. The spinal cord is not involved by acute herniation of an intervertebral disc in the cervical region, since this usually occurs in a dorso-lateral direction.

Cervical Spondylosis. This term is usually reserved for the disorder resulting from chronic cervical disc degeneration. The highest incidence is in the decade 60-70. The symptoms are of two types depending on whether the protrusion is lateral or dorso-medial.

(1) Lateral herniation of discs, with secondary calcification and osteophytes encroaching on the intervertebral foramina, causes radicular symptoms like those of the acute disc syndrome just described, but the onset may be subacute or insidious and involvement of more than one root on one or both sides is common.

(2) Dorso-medial herniation of discs which become calcified results in transverse bars which cause pressure on the spinal cord and on the anterior spinal artery which supplies the anterior two-thirds of the cord. The onset is insidious. Upper motor neurone weakness involves one or more limbs and the legs may be spastic before the upper limbs are involved. Sensory loss is most common in the upper limbs where it has a dermatome pattern but involvement of the spinothalamic tracts may cause disturbance of pain and temperature sensation in the lower limbs, and in some cases muscle-joint sense is also defective.

Pain and limitation of movement of the neck are not marked features unless a particular posture causes nipping of a nerve root. Osteophytes on the anterior margin of a cervical disc may cause dysphagia by deflecting the oesophagus.

Diagnosis. The acute disc herniation syndrome must be differentiated from other causes of brachial neuralgia (p. 1221). If the eighth cervical and first thoracic roots are affected by spondylosis the pain may resemble that of coronary artery disease (p. 225). Other causes of acroparaesthesia are listed on p. 1227. Myelopathy due to cervical spondylosis may resemble tumour of the spinal cord, syringomyelia, disseminated sclerosis, motor neurone disease or subacute combined degeneration of the cord. It must be remembered that osteoarthritic changes in the spine are common and may accompany any of these diseases. For this reason it may be necessary to confirm the diagnosis by myelography. Radiological examination shows narrowing of the disc spaces and osteophyte formation with loss of the normal cervical lordosis. Oblique views show encroachment by osteophytes on the intervertebral foramina. Queckenstedt's test (p. 1151) should be performed while the neck is flexed and extended, as a complete or partial block may be present when the head is in one or other of these positions. The fluid is normal unless its circulation is obstructed, when the protein may be raised.

Treatment. The acute syndrome is treated by rest in bed or by intermittent neck traction followed by immobilisation of the neck in a light metal or plastic collar. Some form of immobilisation should be maintained for at least three months. It is important to watch for progressive cervical cord compression. Decompressive surgery is rarely required but is only effective if not too long delayed.

Prognosis. The course of the chronic syndrome is variable. After initial deterioration most cases become stationary, or symptoms and signs may resolve.

Thoracic Outlet Compression Syndrome

In this syndrome, the lower trunk of the brachial plexus and the subclavian artery are either compressed between the clavicle and the first rib, or are stretched as they pass over the first rib behind the point of insertion of the scalenus anterior muscle (Fig. 75). There may be a cervical rib which will aggravate the latter factor; loss of tone in the muscles of the shoulder girdle, with resultant drooping of the upper limbs in an otherwise normal thoracic outlet, may have the same effect. The patient may present with pain in the arm, usually worse at night, and there may be wasting of the small muscles of the hand and sensory loss over the distribution of the eighth cervical and first thoracic nerve roots. There may be impairment of the blood supply to the hand as indicated by pallor or coldness and obliteration of the radial pulse. In most cases symptoms are more prominent than signs. The treatment consists of the removal of aggravating factors, such as the carrying of shopping baskets, and the shoulder girdle muscles should be strengthened by the prescription of graduated exercises. In some

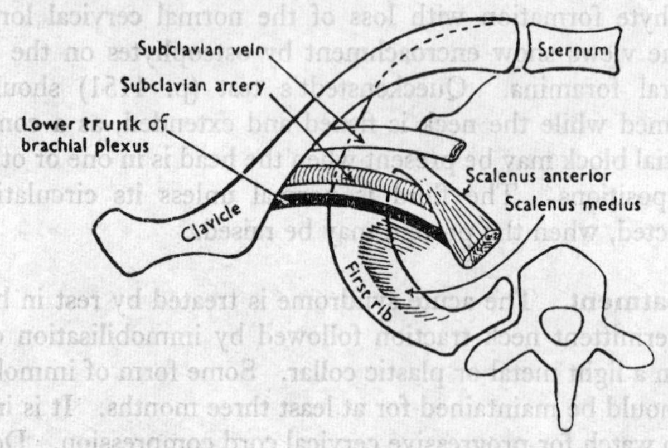

FIG. 75
SITE OF THORACIC OUTLET COMPRESSION

cases an initial period of rest in a sling may be helpful. Occasionally, it is necessary to undertake operative treatment when an anatomical abnormality of the thoracic outlet, such as a cervical rib, has been demonstrated.

Carpal Tunnel Syndrome

A common cause of paraesthesia of the fingers in middle-aged women is compression of the median nerve in the carpal tunnel. It also occurs as a late complication of scaphoid fracture, osteo- or rheumatoid arthritis, and in acromegaly, myxoedema and pregnancy. It sometimes results from intermittent trauma in industry.

The patient complains of pain, numbness, tingling or an 'electric shock' feeling in thumb and fingers supplied by the median nerve, especially after using the hand or in bed at night when it may waken the patient from sleep. There is sometimes objective sensory loss of the radial three and a half digits and there may be weakness and wasting of abductor pollicis brevis and opponens pollicis. The condition is often bilateral. Rest and splinting at night should be tried. Local injection of hydrocortisone is sometimes effective if there is no muscular wasting. Thyroxine therapy relieves the carpal tunnel syndrome in myxoedema. The syndrome occurring in pregnancy usually disappears in the puerperium but may be relieved by the use of diuretics. If these measures are unsuccessful the condition can be rapidly relieved by decompression of the nerve in the carpal tunnel.

Acroparaesthesia

Acroparaesthesia is an unpleasant tingling sensation affecting some or all of the digits of one or both upper limbs. It is a symptom of irritation of sensory nerve fibres, usually due to compression of one or more nerves or their roots. Common causes are: (1) Cervical spondylosis (p. 1223). (2) Thoracic outlet compression syndrome (p). 1225. (3) Carpal tunnel syndrome (p. 1226). (4) Ulnar palsy due to stretching of the ulnar nerve at the elbow if the 'carrying angle' is too acute, or to compression between the two heads of the flexor carpi ulnaris muscle. It may result from previous injury to the elbow region. Symptoms of nerve injury may not occur for a long time ('tardy ulnar palsy'). (5) Raynaud's phenomenon (p. 295).

The sensation of acroparaesthesia usually develops during the night when posture and diminished movement with venous stasis exaggerate the compression in the various sites.

LESIONS OF INDIVIDUAL PERIPHERAL NERVES

The carpal tunnel syndrome (p. 1226) and chronic ulnar palsy (above) are examples of compressive lesions of peripheral nerves. Nerves in other parts of the body may be trapped in similar ways. *Meralgia paraesthetica* is a common painful paraesthesia of the front of the upper part of the thigh due to entrapment of the lateral cutaneous nerve of the thigh. A mechanical explanation of this sort should always be looked for when signs indicate a lesion of a single peripheral nerve (mononeuritis).

Pressure neuropathies develop acutely as the result of trauma, for example, when a person has been sitting with his arm over the back of a chair compressing the radial nerve, or with his legs crossed compressing the lateral popliteal nerve as it passes over the neck of the fibula. The signs of a peripheral nerve lesion are those of a lower motor neurone paralysis and of sensory loss in the territory of the nerve. Impairment of vasomotor function, such as coldness and loss of sweating, may also be apparent.

Mononeuritis may also be caused by ischaemic disease of a limb (p. 284) or by diabetes mellitus, and rarely as the sole manifestation of acute brachial neuritis. Many cases of so called 'neuritis' are in fact due to irritation of a nerve root by a herniated intervertebral disc, and this is the most common cause of 'neuritis' of an arm and of sciatica (pp. 1223 and 1228). The recognition of the nerve involved and the differentiation from a nerve root lesion depend on a knowledge of the anatomy of the peripheral nerves. Pressure palsies almost invariably recover. They are treated by rest with the limb in the position of optimum function, and by physiotherapy and occupational therapy.

The Lumbago-Sciatica Syndrome

Lumbago is pain in the lower part of the back; sciatica is pain in the distribution of the sciatic nerve. They are not, therefore, disease entities but symptoms and they are often associated.

Aetiology and Pathology. The most common cause is herniation of an intervertebral disc. Other causes are much rarer but important to recognise. They include spinal tumour (neurofibroma and meningioma), ankylosing spondylitis (p. 554), malignant disease in the pelvis, and tuberculosis of the vertebral bodies or of the sacro-iliac joint. Degenerative changes in the intervertebral discs may appear as early as 20 years of age, but herniation is often precipitated by trauma such as twisting the spine, lifting heavy weights while the spine is flexed or during childbirth. The nucleus pulposus may bulge or rupture the annulus fibrosus, giving rise to lumbago by pressure on nerve endings in the spinal ligaments and by producing changes in the joints of the vertebral arches, and to sciatica by causing congestion of, or pressure on, the nerve roots (Fig. 76).

Clinical Features. The onset may be sudden or gradual, and may follow closely upon trauma to the back. Attacks of lumbago may precede sciatica by months or years. Lumbago is characterised by sudden severe low back pain when the patient is bending, preventing him from straightening. The sciatic pain is felt in the buttock and radiates down the posterior aspect of the thigh and calf to the outer border of the foot. It is exacerbated by coughing or sneezing which raises the pressure in the spinal subarachnoid space. Paraesthesia and later numbness may be felt over the

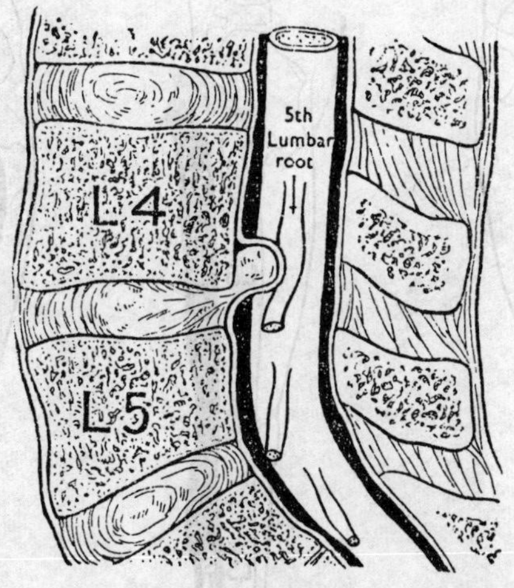

Fig. 76

Posterior Herniation of Intervertebral Disc between Fourth and Fifth Lumbar Vertebrae, showing Compression of Fifth Lumbar Root

distribution of the involved nerve root, most often the first sacral. In severe cases, weakness of the calf muscle or foot-drop may occur, according to which roots are involved. The signs associated with prolapse of an intervertebral disc may be divided into two groups.

Signs due to altered mechanics of the lumbar spine. Spasm of the sacrospinalis muscles causes flattening of the lumbar curve and scoliosis at the level of the prolapsed disc. Scoliosis suddenly increases as pain is felt if the patient tries to touch his toes. He is usually unable to do so as movement of the spine is limited. Tenderness may be found when pressure is applied to the side of the vertebral spines in the region of the affected disc.

Signs due to pressure on the nerve root. These depend on the particular root involved. Involvement of the first sacral root causes loss of the ankle jerk, weakness of eversion and plantar flexion of the foot, and sensory loss over the outer border of the foot (Fig. 77). The glutei may be wasted on the affected side.

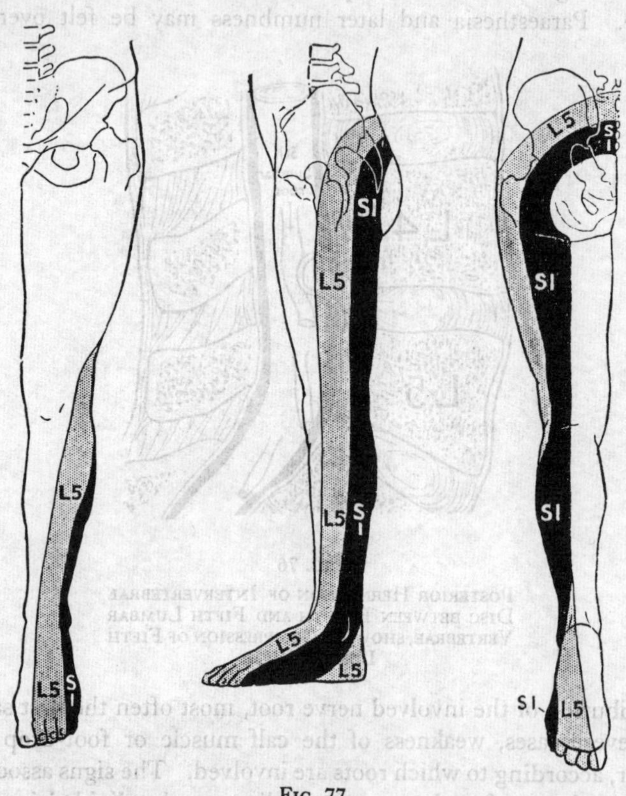

Fig. 77
Areas of Sensory Impairment in Lesions involving Fifth Lumbar and First Sacral Nerve Roots

Involvement of the fifth lumbar root causes weakness of dorsiflexion of the toes and sometimes foot-drop. Sensory loss occurs on the dorsum of the foot and the lateral aspect of the leg over the fifth lumbar dermatome. The ankle jerk is not affected. Involvement of the fourth lumbar root causes weakness of inversion of the foot and of the quadriceps muscle and loss of the knee jerk. Sensory loss is over the medial aspect of the leg. A valuable sign of root pressure is limitation of flexion of the thigh on the affected side if the leg is kept straight at the knee (Lasègue's sign), caused by reflex spasm of the hamstring muscles. The protein content of the CSF may be raised to about 100 mg. per 100 ml.

Diagnosis. The diagnosis is based on the mode of onset of the pain, its aggravation by flexion of the spine, and its relief by immobilisation, as well as on the distribution of the pain and signs of nerve root involvement. Other causes of sciatic pain can be excluded by pelvic examination and by radiological examination of the lumbosacral spine. There may be no apparent radiological change in acute disc herniation, or there may be narrowing of the disc space with osteophyte formation at the margins of the vertebral bodies. Myelography is only required if the diagnosis is in doubt or for purposes of localisation before operation. Intraspinal neoplasm as the cause of the sciatica should be suspected if the CSF protein exceeds 100 mg./100 ml.

Treatment. The initial treatment in all cases is rest in bed on a firm mattress supported by fracture boards. Rest must be absolute with prohibition of the sitting position. Compromise in this respect and permission to leave bed for toilet purposes are the most common reasons for failure of this treatment. The roots most commonly involved are the first sacral and the fifth lumbar. In which case the patient should be kept supine and no rotation of the spine permitted; but in disc protrusion involving the fourth lumbar root the lateral position with flexion of the hips is best suited to relax tension on the affected root and hence to relieve pain. Bed rest is continued for two to four weeks, after which gradual mobilisation with back strengthening exercises is carried out over a further period of 10 to 14 days. For middle-aged or elderly patients with chronic residual backache and a tendency to acute attacks of lumbago, a spinal support may be of great value. Cases which do not respond to rest, or in which there have been several recurrences, may be submitted to surgery.

Prognosis. Pain usually subsides with three to four weeks of adequate bed rest, but in some instances the pain becomes chronic Recurrences are not uncommon.

DISEASES OF MUSCLE
(Myopathies)

Diseases of muscle are not diseases of the nervous system, but as some of their manifestations may be readily confused with neurological conditions, some relevant examples are described here. There are obvious exceptions, but it is a useful generalisation that muscular disease affects mainly the proximal muscles of the limbs whereas neuropathic disease (polyneuritis or motor neurone disease) affects mainly the distal muscles.

Progressive Muscular Dystrophy

This is a group of hereditary disorders characterised by progressive degeneration of groups of muscles without involvement of the nervous system. The wasting and weakness is symmetrical, there is no fasciculation, tendon reflexes are preserved until a late stage and there is no sensory loss. Several clinical types have been described, but from a prognostic viewpoint three major groups can be distinguished.

1. PSEUDO-HYPERTROPHIC TYPE (Duchenne type). This is transmitted by a sex linked recessive gene occurring almost exclusively in males. The disease usually appears within the first three years of life, beginning in the pelvic girdle and lower limbs and later spreading to the shoulder girdle. About 80 per cent. of cases show an initial pseudo-hypertrophy involving the calf muscles, quadriceps, glutei, deltoids and infraspinati. Contractures are common. The affected muscles are larger and firmer than normal, but are nevertheless weak. The weakness gives rise to a characteristic waddling gait, and when rising from the supine position, the child rolls on to his face and then uses his arms to push himself up. Death occurs from inanition or respiratory infection by the middle of the second decade.

2. LIMB GIRDLE TYPE (Juvenile scapulo-humeral type of Erb). The gene carrying this disorder is inherited as an autosomal recessive, affecting both sexes. It usually appears in the second or third decade. It starts in either the shoulder or pelvic girdle and later spreads to involve both. The rate of progression is variable; it may be slow, with long periods of arrest, but severe disablement usually occurs within 20 years and the patient does not survive to middle age.

3. Facio-scapulo-humeral Type (Landouzy-Déjerine). This type is inherited by an autosomal dominant gene so that several siblings of both sexes may be affected. It appears at any age, first in the facial muscles and then in the shoulder girdle. After many years the pelvic girdle may also be involved. The disease progresses very slowly with periods of arrest and is compatible with a long life.

Diagnosis. Hereditary muscular dystrophy must be distinguished from (*a*) acquired myopathies in which treatment is possible or spontaneous remission may occur, and from (*b*) diseases of the lower motor neurone. *Acquired myopathies* occur alone ('polymyositis', p. 559) or as part of dermatomyositis, endocrine disease or carcinomatous myopathy (p. 1217). Spontaneous recovery may occur or there may be improvement with steroid therapy. Myasthenia gravis shows exacerbations of weakness with effort, and responds to injection of edrophonium or neostigmine.

Diseases of the lower motor neurone from which muscular dystrophy must be distinguished are (*a*) motor neurone disease which is associated with fasciculation, (*b*) peripheral neuropathy in which there is distal involvement of muscles and sensory loss, and (*c*) residual poliomyelitis which is commonly mistaken for muscular dystrophy, if the history of the acute illness is not known, but the lesions are asymmetrical and not progressive.

The diagnosis of muscular dystrophy is readily confirmed by electromyography or muscle biopsy. Aldolase, or creatine kinase and other enzymes which are usually intracellular, are increased in the serum, especially in the rapidly advancing Duchenne type. Serum enzyme changes may be found before other clinical signs enabling early detection of the disease in siblings. Less severe changes of the same type are found in women who carry the abnormal gene of the Duchenne type.

Treatment. No effective treatment is known. Deterioration may occur with excessive confinement to bed. Physiotherapeutic and orthopaedic measures may be required to counteract deformities and contractures.

Myotonia

Myotonia consists of prolonged contraction and slow relaxation of muscles due to hyperexcitability of the muscle cell membrane.

In *myotonia congenita* (Thomsen's disease) the myotonia is the sole disability. It is inherited as a Mendelian dominant and appears in early childhood. The only symptom is the slow relaxation of a muscle if it is contracted voluntarily or by mechanical stimulation. The patient may be unable to relax his grasp or to open his eyes if they have been closed tightly. The muscles may be unusually powerful in early life but no dystrophic changes later develop.

Dystrophia Myotonica (myotonia atrophica) is also hereditary and appears between the ages of 20 and 30. There is wasting of the facial and temporal muscles, sternomastoids, shoulder girdle, forearms, quadriceps and leg muscles, and all these and the tongue, show myotonia after voluntary contraction or after percussion of the muscle. Ptosis is prominent. Unlike most muscular diseases, distal muscles are more severely affected than proximal. There is also cataract, frontal baldness in men and gonadal atrophy leading to impotence and sterility in men and amenorrhoea in women.

Treatment. There is no treatment for the muscular dystrophy, but if myotonia is troublesome it can be relieved by procainamide, 0·5-1·0 g. q.i.d. or quinine sulphate gr. 5-10 t.d.s

Myasthenia Gravis

This condition is characterised by undue fatiguability of certain muscle groups, with incapacity to sustain muscular activity.

Aetiology. The cause of the disease is unknown but is in some way related to a disorder of the thymus gland. There is strong evidence for a breakdown of immunological tolerance. A thymoma is present in 15 per cent. of cases and the gland contains an excess of germ centres in the remainder. Myasthenia is sometimes associated with thyrotoxicosis, Hashimoto's disease, rheumatoid arthritis or pernicious anaemia. There are slight histological changes in the muscle fibres and motor nerve terminals, but the typical fatiguability is considered to be due to a failure of transmission at the myoneural junction. The nature of this disorder, which produces an effect resembling curarisation, is unknown.

Clinical Features. The disease usually appears between the ages of 15 and 50 and females are more often affected than males. It tends to run a remitting course. Relapses may be precipitated by emotional disturbance, infections, pregnancy and by severe muscular effort. The cardinal symptom is abnormal fatiguability of muscles so that a muscular movement, though initially strong, rapidly tires. Intensification of symptoms towards the end of the day or following vigorous exercise is characteristic. The first symptoms are usually intermittent ptosis or diplopia but weakness of chewing, swallowing, speaking or of moving the limbs also occurs. Any muscle of a limb may be affected, most commonly the shoulder girdle muscles, so that the patient is unable to undertake work above the level of the shoulder, such as combing the hair, without frequent rests. Respiratory muscles may be involved and respiratory failure is a not uncommon cause of death. Asphyxia occurs readily as the cough may be too weak to clear foreign bodies from the airways. The symptoms fluctuate in intensity, long periods of remission being common during the early years. Muscle atrophy may occur in longstanding cases. There are no signs of involvement of the central nervous system.

The remarkable therapeutic response to an intramuscular injection of neostigmine (1·5 mg.) is a valuable diagnostic aid. Edrophoniume(Tensilon) has a similar action and is invaluable for test purposes as the response is almost immediate, while any unpleasant parasympathomimetic effects are very brief. An initial dose of 2 mg. of edrophonium is injected intravenously and a further 8 mg. half a minute later if no undesirable reactions (fasciculation, sweating, colic) occur. This test also helps in the diagnosis of 'cholinergic crisis' (p. 1236) since weakness due to overdose of anticholinesterase drugs is increased, but only for a few minutes. (It should be noted that some muscle groups may be overdosed while others still require more neostigmine. It is, therefore, important to observe the status of the muscles of respiration and swallowing rather than those of the eyes.)

Diagnosis. Most myasthenic patients are at first considered to be suffering from *hysteria* because the absence of physical signs when the patient is examined after a rest seems incompatible with the description of severe weakness and because attacks are often precipitated by emotional disturbances. *Disseminated sclerosis* may be suggested by the intermittent nature of the symptoms and the frequent occurrence of diplopia and dysarthria. The bulbar type of *motor neurone disease* may also be confused at first, but weakness does not disappear with rest or with edrophonium. *Polymyositis* (p. 559) and *carcinomatous myopathy* (p. 1217) may closely resemble myasthenia gravis because at the onset of these conditions there is often a phase of muscular weakness which responds to neostigmine. *Muscular dystrophy* is progressive and, in the more common types, the extraocular muscles are not involved. The presence of characteristic fatiguability of muscles makes the diagnosis of myasthenia gravis clear.

Treatment. The sheet anchor of medical treatment is neostigmine, but this must be given in adequate dosage (15-45 mg. orally every two to four hours). In severe cases neostigmine may require to be given subcutaneously in doses of 1-3 mg. several times daily. Fifteen minutes before neostigmine is injected, atropine sulphate, 0·6 mg. should be injected subcutaneously to diminish the undesirable side-effects of neostigmine such as bowel colic. Pyridostigmine (Mestinon) gives less prompt relief than neostigmine but has a more prolonged action with fewer side-effects. Hence it gives relief during the sleeping period and is also of value for those patients unable to tolerate adequate amounts of neostigmine. The 60 mg. tablet of pyridostigmine is equipotent with 15 mg. of neostigmine. In some resistant cases it may be necessary to give very large doses of anticholinesterase drugs. This should only be done in hospital as overdosage causes another type of neuromuscular block ('cholinergic'), especially when long-acting preparations which tend to be cumulative are used. Early evidence of a cholinergic crisis is the presence of fasciculation, pallor, sweating, small pupils and excessive salivation. Atropine should be given at once and preparations made to sustain respiration artificially if required. Specific antidotes (oximes) are of little practical value.

The general management of the patient's life is important in order to reduce fatigue and stress. In the severe case the early signs of respiratory embarrassment should be detected so that artificial respiration can be started in time. Spontaneous remission sometimes occurs, but it is rarely of long duration. Thymectomy offers the best prospect of permanent cure or great amelioration of myasthenia. The most suitable cases are young women with myasthenia of less than six years' duration. Older women and men are less often helped, but thymectomy should certainly be considered for all patients who do not respond satisfactorily to drug treatment. Operation is usually unnecessary in a benign type of myasthenia in which the weakness remains confined to the extra-ocular muscles.

Prognosis. The prognosis is very uncertain, particularly in the presence of a thymoma, when it tends to be worse than with simple thymic hyperplasia. If there is radiological evidence of a thymoma it is customary to irradiate it before removing the gland.

Polymyositis Rheumatica

This disorder is discussed on p. 559.

THE PREVENTION OF DISEASES OF THE NERVOUS SYSTEM

The preventive aspect of disease of the nervous system is largely concerned with the infective and deficiency diseases but there is increasing recognition of inherited biochemical disorders which can be influenced by dietary or other means. Kernicterus (p. 1196) may be prevented by the prompt recognition of haemolytic disease in the newborn, followed by immediate exchange transfusion. Excessive doses of vitamin K analogues should be avoided in the newborn infant. As in other systems of the body, the degenerative conditions give little scope for prophylactic treatment, but it is possible that improved obstetrics may lower the later incidence of epilepsy and some types of cerebral palsy. Repeated trauma to the head, as in professional boxing, may lead to dementia and other neurological disorders which can and should be avoidable. Phenylketonuria can be recognised by a simple urine test in infancy before clinical manifestations arise, and these can be prevented by a special diet. Asymptomatic siblings of a known case of hepato-lenticular degeneration (Wilson's disease, p. 1191) can be detected by biochemical tests and further neurological damage minimised by the use of chelating agents such as penicillamine. A major advance in the Duchenne type of muscular dystrophy is the discovery that the female carrier can be detected by serum enzyme studies and advised of the risk of transmitting the disease to any male children which she may bear. Congenital porphyria can also be detected by examination of the blood and urine and the hazard of polyneuropathy (p. 1219) prevented by avoidance of barbiturates. Huntington's chorea is also a hereditary disease but eugenic measures are not possible as the signs do not appear until after the main reproductive period. The development of cerebral abscess and pyogenic meningitis can be avoided by the efficient treatment of primary sources of infection which may arise in the middle ear, fractures of the skull, the accessory nasal sinuses and more distant sites such as the heart and lungs. Outbreaks of meningococcal meningitis can also be controlled by the isolation of cases, the prophylactic treatment of contacts (e.g. with sulphadiazine) and the prevention of factors which favour the spread, such as overcrowding and bad ventilation. The prevention of tuberculous meningitis involves the same factors as the prevention of tuberculosis in general. In addition, the adequate treatment of tuberculous lesions elsewhere in the body will help to reduce the incidence of this condition. Neurosyphilis is preventable by proper treatment of primary infection and by careful follow-up of those infected, to ensure that asymptomatic neurosyphilis (p. 1164) is not overlooked. Poliomyelitis can now be prevented almost completely by suitably repeated vaccination. Demyelinating diseases remain, on the whole, unpreventable, but post-vaccinial encephalomyelitis is extremely rare if primary vaccination against smallpox is carried out during the first two years of life rather than in adult life.

Vitamin B_{12} neuropathy can be eliminated by the early diagnosis and efficient treatment of pernicious anaemia. Peripheral neuropathy due to nutritional causes can also be avoided by ensuring an adequate diet. Early recognition and treatment of diabetes mellitus and alcoholism may prevent peripheral neuropathy. Polyneuropathy due to toxic causes may also be prevented by the careful use of therapeutic substances which are known to have a tendency to cause this condition, and also by the avoidance of industrial hazards.

The scope of preventative treatment in the vascular diseases is not great. The recognition and surgical treatment of cerebral aneurysms before rupture occurs may, however, prevent the more devastating effects associated with subarachnoid haemorrhage. The value of anticoagulants in ischaemic cerebral disease is debatable, but during periods of a few months when embolism is a hazard or the blood-flow through the carotid and vertebral arteries is undergoing adjustment, their use may prevent cerebral infarction.

In many other conditions where the primary lesion is not as yet preventable, a great deal can, nevertheless, be done to minimise its effects. Efficient treatment in the early stage of conditions such as disseminated sclerosis greatly reduces the incidence of the more distressing complications such as massive bed sores, contractures, painful flexor spasms and ascending urinary infection.

J. A. SIMPSON.

Book recommended:

Brain, Lord (1962). *Diseases of the Nervous System*, 6th ed. London: Oxford University Press.

PSYCHOLOGICAL MEDICINE

A SECTION on psychological disorders in a textbook for students and doctors needs no apology, for psychological illness is so common that it is encountered daily in the practice of medicine. Nor is psychological medicine the preserve of the specialist; not only must the initial diagnosis be made by the general practitioner but treatment of minor degrees of mental ill-health must be undertaken by him since reference of all such patients to a psychiatrist is both unnecessary and impracticable. What is more, the effectiveness of modern drugs in controlling the symptoms of schizophrenia and of depression has made it possible for general practitioners to treat many psychotic patients who formerly would have had to be admitted to a psychiatric ward.

Psychiatry deals with three large groups of patients: the mentally retarded, the psychotic and the non-psychotic. Mental retardation is a congenital handicap, present from birth or an early age; mental disorders supervene after a more or less normal mental development. When the illness interferes with a patient's perceptions, thinking and feelings so profoundly that what he says to his fellow-men no longer makes any sense to them, he is regarded as insane, or in medical language psychotic. There are, however, many patients who remain in touch with their surroundings, and whose symptoms are recognisable as something we have all experienced at some time, but not with the same painful intensity; these are the neurotics. The distinction between the psychotic and the neurotic has been summed up by saying that a psychotic believes that two and two make five, whereas a neurotic knows that two and two make four—but worries about it.

Before discussing the more important psychiatric illnesses in some detail, it may be helpful to present a brief classification of mental disorders, in order to familiarise the reader with their names. A useful categorisation has been provided in the International Classification of Disease published by the World Health Organization, which distinguishes the following conditions.

MENTAL RETARDATION. In England, two categories are distinguished, termed mental subnormality and severe subnormality respectively; in Scotland, the term 'mental deficiency' is still used, with the subdivisions high-grade defective, imbecile and idiot. The categories severe subnormality, imbecile or idiot refer to patients who are so severely handicapped that they require very considerable attention and support and are incapable of leading an independent existence. The most common single cause of mental retardation at the imbecile level is Down's syndrome, or mongolism, due to a chromosomal abnormality. Most imbeciles and all idiots have gross abnormalities in their brains, due either to early trauma or to congenital anomalies of development. Patients who are mentally retarded may also suffer from the other mental illnesses listed below. They may, for example, become depressed, or schizophrenic or psychopathic, but when this happens the symptoms of their mental illness will be modified by their basic handicap of mental backwardness.

Organic Brain Syndromes. In these conditions the functioning of the brain is impaired either by a physical lesion (trauma, tumour or infection) or by a toxic process (as in intoxication with alcohol, barbiturates or amphetamines, or in the delirium associated with fever or with cerebral anoxia). Organic brain syndromes may be acute, as in febrile delirium, or chronic, where an irreversible brain lesion has occurred. The most common instances of chronic brain lesions are those associated with advancing years—cerebral arteriosclerosis and senile psychoses. Mild degrees of interference with brain function may make the patient forgetful, easily confused, irritable and emotional; more severe disturbances can give rise to delusions, hallucinations and a loss of contact with reality of a psychotic degree.

Functional Psychoses. The two most common forms of severe mental illness have so far eluded all attempts at explanation in terms of physical or biochemical pathology. These are *manic-depressive psychosis*, in which the principal symptom is a profound disturbance of the patient's mood, and the *schizophrenias* in which the patient's thoughts become bizarre and strange, so that he loses contact with his fellows, and with his surroundings.

The Neuroses. These represent by far the most common forms of psychiatric illness encountered in general medical practice. They are conveniently subdivided into *anxiety states*, *hysteria* and *obsessive-compulsive neurosis*.

PSYCHOSOMATIC ILLNESSES. These are also extremely common. Some physicians find this a misleading term, pointing out that there is a mutual interplay of psychological factors in many physical illnesses, and of physical factors in many psychiatric illnesses. The term 'psychosomatic' has, however, come to be used for those illnesses (such as some cases of asthma, peptic ulcer, dermatitis or 'rheumatism') in which emotional factors have been shown to be clearly related to the onset or exacerbation of the symptoms.

PERSONALITY DISORDERS. This term is used to describe patients whose personality and behaviour differ markedly from those of the normal population. The category includes *sexual deviation*, *alcoholism* and *drug addiction* and the various forms of *psychopathy*. Many of these individuals do not regard themselves as sick, and have no wish to be 'cured'; they most often consult (or are brought to) their doctor only when their abnormality has become seriously disturbing to their relatives or has brought them into conflict with the law. Some, however, are themselves distressed by their inability to conform to prevailing norms, and these offer the best prospects for treatment.

Incidence of Psychiatric Morbidity. Serious mental illness is relatively infrequent: about 1 : 200 of a practitioner's adult patients is likely to suffer from severe depression in the course of a year; the incidence of schizophrenia is much less, but since this illness runs a long course the cases tend to accumulate. Nearly 1 : 100 will suffer from schizophrenia at some stage in his life. As people grow older the occurrence of mental illness due to disease of the brain becomes increasingly common. The frequency of minor forms of emotional illness, such as neurosis, hysteria and psychosomatic disorders is very much greater. Careful counts have shown that minor psychiatric illness occurs every year in no less than 14 per cent. of the patients on a general practitioner's list: if one includes cases in which psychological factors significantly influence co-existing physical complaints, the count rises to over 40 per cent.

Patients with emotional disorders tend to consult their doctors more often than patients with physical diseases and complain of a wide variety of symptoms. As a result, they are often referred to a succession of clinics for specialist investigation, and commonly undergo minor or major surgery without avail. This involves a waste of both the doctors' and the patients' time, which could be avoided if the psychological disorder had been recognised and treated at an earlier stage. It is therefore necessary for every practitioner to include a psychological appraisal as part of the clinical examination of his patients. This is a skill which has tended to be neglected in the past, but now, prompted by the General Medical Council, an increasing number of medical schools provide clerkships in psychological medicine; and where this has been done, medical students have shown themselves able to acquire the technique quite rapidly.

The Psychological Examination. It should be emphasised that attention should be paid to the patient's emotional state not only when a frank psychiatric illness is suspected, but in the course of *every* thorough clinical examination. Psychological disturbances can be elicited (*a*) while taking the history, and (*b*) while examining the patient's mental state.

Before discussing these two aspects of the psychological examination, it is necessary to draw attention to certain ways in which functional nervous illnesses differ from other illnesses. From the beginning of our clinical studies, most of us have been taught to think in terms of *disease entities*; that is, we assume that our patient is suffering from a particular disease with its specific aetiology, pathology, signs and symptoms. Our clinical examination is therefore so organised as to make sure that we do not overlook indications of pathology in any of the major bodily systems, and our history-taking consists largely of a form of cross-examining of the patient in order to elicit further clues. The whole exercise is a sort of detective-work with the aim of unmasking the disease which is causing our patient's symptoms. The disease entity model serves admirably in certain pathological conditions, notably in the case of sudden acute infections caused by identifiable micro-organisms such as acute lobar pneumonia or virus hepatitis or the exanthemata of childhood. It can be adapted, although less neatly, to chronic and degenerative conditions, but here one may have to take into account a number of contributory factors both in the host and in the environment, and also a wider range of manifestations of the disease.

Only a few psychiatric illnesses conform to the classical disease tenity model. These are described in American psychiatric terminology as 'acute brain syndromes' because they are due to infection, toxins or direct trauma affecting the brain; instances are febrile delirium, amphetamine psychosis, acute porphyria, post-traumatic confusional state. Here, just as in an acute infection, there is one all-important aetiological factor, and effective treatment depends upon its being recognised in the course of the clinical examination.

With a few exceptions, most of the major psychiatric illnesses (such as schizophrenia, manic-depressive psychosis, many forms of congenital subnormality and the senile psychoses) correspond to the category of chronic and degenerative diseases: that is, they are variable both in severity and in the particular pattern of symptoms which they present, and they appear to be due to multiple causal factors in which heredity usually plays a significant part.

This still leaves the majority of minor emotional and psychosomatic disorders unaccounted for: and here it is open to question whether they really constitute illnesses at all. Because they are usually associated with bodily discomfort, patients naturally consult their doctors about these complaints; doctors have given them medical-sounding names, like anorexia nervosa or globus hystericus or cardiac neurosis, and as a result it is easy to assume that each such diagnostic term refers to a separate disease process. Here, however, the 'disease entity' model can be quite misleading. These conditions are not diseases, but patterns of behaviour. Because they recur with great regularity, we can learn to recognise these patterns, and to investigate their causes; and when we do so, we find that they are simply habits of maladaptive behaviour. Like all human behaviour, these habits have been learned by life-experience: only, the life of the neurotic or psychosomatic patient has included some painful, frustrating or damaging experiences which still disturb his peace of mind and interfere with his performance.

When we operate with the 'disease entity' model in mind, our business is to identify the particular disease as quickly and as economically as possible; when we operate with the 'faulty learning' model in mind, our business is to elicit our patient's worries, his sensitivities, his irrational fears—and then to try to reconstruct the stage or stages in his emotional development where things went wrong. The medical history-taking is 'disease-oriented', the psychiatric history-taking is 'person-oriented' and employs a somewhat different technique: both techniques are relevant for their respective purposes, and both can be employed in different stages of the investigation of any given patient.

The Psychiatric History. The first essential in taking a good psychiatric history is to help the patient to express what is really troubling him. When a medical student 'sits in' on his first few psychiatric interviews, he is apt to be struck by the psychiatrist's apparent inactivity. In fact, the more skilled the interviewer, the less he needs to say. He prompts the patient with an occasional, quite general remark, such as: 'Can you tell me what caused you to consult your doctor?', and then 'Tell me more about those attacks of breathlessness (or headaches, or fits of depression)'. Often an inarticulate, encouraging murmur is enough to help the patient to bring out more relevant information. Although he holds his tongue, the interviewer is far from inactive: he must convey a real interest in what the patient has to say, and above all he must let the patient feel that he will not be shocked, angry or disdainful, no matter how embarrassing or unpleasant may be the content of what is uttered. Really painful feelings are never easy to communicate. Sometimes a patient will back away from such feelings and start talking about trivialities, or try to engage the interviewer in a social conversation; as soon as this happens, one can sense a drop in the emotional tension of the interview, and it is necessary to take him back to the sensitive topic, by simply repeating some of his words: 'You said a moment ago . . .' and let him take it on again from there. Some interviewers are better than others at being alert to their patient's feelings, but everyone can heighten their sensitivity in this respect with practice. In so doing, one learns to use one's own personal response to the patient as an instrument of investigation—less accurate, no doubt, than a blood-sugar estimation, but just as important in its proper context.

This open-ended interview may yield important clues within 10 or 20 minutes; by now some of the patient's current sources of anxiety, and the types of social situation in which they occur, should become apparent; it is time for the interviewer to become more active, asking questions about the patient's family setting, his early years, his relationship with his parents and other figures in his household. This is done because in the great majority of cases of emotional disorder the faulty learning which finds expression in symptoms dates back to painful childhood experiences.

Following this, one asks about his schooling and his occupational career. By this stage in the interview, one should have gained the patient's confidence sufficiently to be able to broach the sometimes embarrassing, but often crucially important topic of his sexual development and his emotional involvements with other people. It is essential that the interviewer should be able to show that he is not shocked or disturbed by whatever the patient has to tell him. This is not easy at first, because unpractised interviewers may find themselves reacting with strong personal feelings of sympathy, disgust or anger; but it is precisely in acquiring control over one's own responses, while still maintaining a lively interest in the patient, that one becomes a skilled interviewer.

The interesting thing about an interview of this kind is that it often begins with a purely physical complaint, such as constipation, back-ache or dyspepsia; then, as the patient is able to unburden himself of painful feelings and memories the initial complaint appears to be forgotten: but of course, it must not be ignored. Dyspepsia may be provoked by painful relations with one's boss, and these in turn may recall painful relations with one's father, and the investigation of a particular patient's dyspepsia may be incomplete unless these factors have been elicited and further explored; but at the same time, it is necessary, before the end of the interview, to look into the details of his present symptoms, to give him a careful physical examination and to decide whether a barium meal or other special investigations are required.

Examining the mental state

As the interview proceeds, the interviewer will want to observe the patient's current mental functioning, just as, in the physical examination, he will want to satisfy himself that he has not ignored pathology in the cardiovascular, respiratory or other systems. It helps to do this in a systematic manner, paying attention in turn to the patient's *behaviour*, *mood* and *thought processes*.

The patient's behaviour during the interview is partly verbal, partly non-verbal. While listening to what he tells us, we can at the same time pick up clues about his intellectual level from his choice of words and from the ease or difficulty with which he expresses himself. If there is reason to suspect that he may be mentally backward, one can test his general information by posing simple questions, such as asking him to name the Prime Minister, the capitals of the larger countries in Europe, or to perform simple sums of mental arithmetic. The best cue to mental retardation, however, is given by the patient's scholastic record and by the type of job which he has been able to perform in adult life.

Some patients talk rapidly, jumping from subject to subject, some frequently lose the thread of what they are saying and need to be prompted, while others talk slowly, in dull flat tones which reveal melancholy. At the same time, the patient's non-verbal behaviour should be noted, i.e. whether his attitude and gestures are tense and restless or heavy and slow. In some cases we may be struck from the very start by something unusual about a male patient's dress or a woman's make-up; the writer recalls a war-time sick parade in which an aircraftsman caught his eye because he wore his forage cap at a different angle to all the others. This man proved to be a schizophrenic. Before jumping to hasty conclusions, however, especially where young people are concerned, one has to make sure that the oddity is indeed an individual one, and not merely the latest twist of teenage fashion.

During the interview, it is necessary to learn about the patient's mood, that is whether he feels cheerful or depressed, confident or fearful, suspicious or bewildered. In ordinary social encounters, we do this all the time, but we observe the restraint of good manners, in that if a companion does not wish to reveal his feelings, we respect his reticence, even though we may suspect that he is, as we say, only 'putting a brave face on it'. In the clinical situation, these rules do not apply: we must make it our business to find out how he is really feeling. Many patients need some help before they can unburden themselves of fears, anxieties or feelings of intense unhappiness. Once these painful feelings are revealed, they are readily recognisable; but a greater effort of attention has to be made in order to recognise the *lack* of emotional involvement of any kind, which is characteristic of the schizophrenic. Sometimes these patients will make our task easier by themselves complaining of their inability to experience emotions in the way they used to do; at other times one is simply aware of an inability to elicit any real warmth, any sense of human contact with the patient and this failure of rapport should alert one to the possibility that he may be schizophrenic.

The third task in the examination of the mental state is to observe any abnormalities in the patient's intellectual functions. We note whether he knows the date and time of day, and recognises where he is and to whom he is talking: this tests his *orientation* for time, place and person. Impairment of mental function is commonly shown by inability to concentrate, to 'take things in', and hence to remember recent events. This may become apparent during the interview or it may be elicited by asking the patient to remember a name and address or a telephone number and then asking him to repeat it after an interval of one or two minutes. Some patients, however, may have a perfectly good memory and yet show profound mental disturbances such as *hallucinations* (that is, they have perceptions of sight, sound or touch with all the vividness of reality in the absence of any external stimulus) and *delusions* (that is, they express bizarre, illogical beliefs which are not shared by other people in their surroundings, and hold to these beliefs in spite of assurances and demonstrations of their falsity). Finally, an assessment is made of the patient's degree of insight into his condition; that is, does he recognise that he is ill or is he convinced that it is his environment and his fellows that are at fault?

THE PSYCHONEUROSES

In describing some of the particular syndromes of psychiatric illness we shall give priority to those which are most frequently met with in general medical practice, namely the psychoneuroses and psychosomatic disorders. The former category includes the *anxiety states* in which disturbance of mood is the most prominent feature, *hysteria* and the less common *obsessive-compulsive* neuroses.

ANXIETY NEUROSIS

Anxiety may be defined as a state of anticipation of something unpleasant about to happen, accompanied by a feeling of inner tension, and somatic manifestations such as tense muscles, sweating, tremor and tachycardia.

Although anxiety is a symptom of many psychological disorders, there is a state in which it dominates the picture, and other symptoms are but minor features of the total illness; this is known as anxiety neurosis or anxiety state, and is the most common form of psychoneurosis.

Aetiology. Research has shown that hereditary factors play a part, although a relatively small part, in the genesis of anxiety neuroses; manifestations of anxiety being found a little more frequently in the patients' parents than in the population as a whole.

This is not surprising, because not only laboratory workers but also breeders of dogs and of racehorses know that nervous excitability is a recognisable genetic trait. In human subjects, however, it appears that encounters with emotionally disturbing experiences during the early formative years play an even more important aetiological role. These traumatic experiences need not be dramatic, single events; a sudden severe fright may cause a child to become timid and to have nightmares and other symptoms for weeks or months, but if he has the support of a stable, affectionate home life, he will outgrow such an isolated trauma. On the other hand, if a child's early years are attended by prolonged insecurity, for example, when one or both parents are so burdened by their own problems that they let their child feel unloved, if not unwanted, or where a brother or sister seems to receive preferential treatment, or where a mother's own exaggerated anxieties impart an excessive timidity to her child, than there may be a profound undermining of the child's self-confidence.

This may not be apparent for several years, particularly if the experiences of school life and early adolescence have been free of alarming or painful incidents: but in early adult life any one of the 'slings and arrows of outrageous fortune' may reveal the weakness of the patient's defences against adversity. Painful events, which most of us encounter at some time or another—such as bereavements, reverses in a love affair, disappointments in one's career, being obliged to contend with disagreeable or frankly hostile people at work, or being involved in prolonged domestic strife—may cause a vulnerable individual to succumb to feelings of anxiety, interfering materially with his or her ability to cope with their day-to-day routine.

Clinical Features. The illness may take many forms; it may be an acute anxiety state, often severe in intensity, appearing against a relatively normal background, or a chronic anxiety state, present since adolescence in mild degree, but subject to periodic exacerbations according to the tide of life's fortunes.

The outstanding feature of the illness is the anxiety, with its accompanying feeling of inner tension and unpleasant anticipation. Sometimes the anxiety is referred to a potential happening, but often it is a diffuse feeling unrelated to any particular event. It may be aggravated by a specific form of activity such as travelling in a bus or train, and so much may this be dreaded, that the patient is eventually unable to travel at all. The anxiety fluctuates in intensity, being sometimes a mild feeling of tension or nervousness, but at other times a state of panic, in which the patient may be overwhelmed by a feeling of terror, which is no less disturbing because he is unable to say just what it is that makes him so afraid.

This state of anxiety gives rise to other symptoms. The ability to concentrate is impaired, and constant fears make decisions difficult. There may be a continuous state of restlessness and excitement of varying degree, or extreme irritability. Fear of insanity or of committing suicide commonly afflicts these patients though, in fact, both are extremely rare. Pre-occupation with bodily functions and fear of serious illness are frequently manifested. The continued stress exhausts them so that they lack energy and perseverance, and feel that they can no longer carry on with their work.

Somatic symptoms are also prominent. There is a general tenseness of the musculature, with hyperactivity, especially of the fingers and hands, shown in such movements as screwing up a handkerchief or constantly intertwining the fingers. A fine tremor of the fingers is present, and profuse perspiration, especially of the palms and forehead, is common. The pulse rate is raised, the blood pressure labile and overactivity of plain muscle is commonly manifest by frequency of micturition or of calls to stool. Breathing is often rapid and feelings of nausea and flatulence occur; headache of tension type, dizziness and unsteadiness are frequently mentioned. The patient sleeps badly, finding it difficult to get off to sleep, and being easily disturbed. Appetite is poor, and loss of weight may be a pronounced feature. Disturbances of menstruation are common.

Diagnosis. It may be quite difficult to distinguish an acute anxiety neurosis from an acute thyrotoxicosis, in which one also finds anxiety, restlessness, sympathetic over-activity and feelings of exhaustion, unless the eye signs and the bruit heard on auscultation over the thyroid are present to support the latter diagnosis. In an anxiety state, the tachycardia diminishes quite markedly when the patient is sleeping, a change which is not found in thyrotoxicosis. Thyroid function tests are helpful only when their findings are clearly outwith the normal range (p. 699).

The patient's hypochondriacal fears often raise the question of co-existing physical disease, and it may prove necessary to supplement a thorough physical examination with appropriate ancillary investigations. It is scarcely surprising that some patients who know that they suffer from diabetes, angina, haematemesis, renal failure or other forms of chronic disease undergo episodes of severe anxiety which is in part at least related to a real threat to their lives. These patients have to be distinguished from those, no less painfully anxious, who are crippled by the fear that they have just such diseases; the differential diagnosis is prompted by a negative physical examination, but clinched only when the patient has been helped to give free expression to his fears, and in so doing has shown that they are prompted by earlier sources of distress.

Differentiation from other forms of psychological illness is less difficult. Though hysterical, obsessive or depressive symptoms may be present in an anxiety state, the diagnosis can usually be made on the totality of the picture, anxiety and its accompanying manifestations dominating the scene. It may, however, be quite difficult to distinguish an acute anxiety state from a case of depressive psychosis with severe agitation and restlessness. A carefully taken history will reveal the underlying severe depression, with feelings of unworthiness, guilt and failure, and frequently delusions about impending, and merited, punishment. This form of depression is so intensely distressing to the patient that the risk of suicide is especially high, so it is particularly important to start antidepressant treatment without delay. If the diagnosis remains in doubt, a course of amitryptiline can be given, in the knowledge that it will help both conditions.

HYSTERIA

It is important to remember that hysteria is a term which is used in one sense by lay people, and in a different sense in medical parlance. In popular speech, to be hysterical means to lose control of one's feelings, and to behave in an extravagant, socially embarrassing manner. Psychiatrists, on the other hand, distinguish between *hysterical personality traits* and *hysterical symptoms*. The *hysterical personality* is emotionally immature, self-centred, attention-seeking and child-like; but we all know people who show these attributes to a certain extent but still manage to function reasonably well, even if they remain rather dependent on other persons' attention and support.

Hysterical symptoms consist of the reproduction of the symptoms or signs of an illness by a patient for some advantageous purpose without his being fully aware of his motive in doing so. Familiar examples are sudden 'blackouts' or 'loss of memory' which enable a patient to forget a particularly painful or embarrassing occurrence, and the dramatic intensification of symptoms after relatively minor injury in an accident where compensation payments may be awarded—in contrast with accidents on the sports field or in the home, which are seldom complicated by psychological reactions. The unawareness of his motive distinguishes the hysteric from the malingerer who deliberately and consciously simulates illness for some purpose. The differentiation of the two can usually be made in practice as the malingerer is unable to maintain the fiction under questioning and examination; at times, however, it may be very difficult to say where hysteria ends and malingering begins.

Aetiology. Heredity is even less important in the development of hysteria than it is in anxiety neurosis, and plays but a minor role in its aetiology. Environment, by contrast, is of great moment not only in producing the hysterical type of personality, but also in providing those situational factors which precipitate the development of hysterical symptoms. Excessive 'babying' in the early years can encourage, and prolong a state of childlike dependency. Such persons, denied the experience of tackling practical difficulties by themselves, tend to continue to rely on infantile devices, such as denial, magical thinking and looking to others to solve their problems.

The hysterical personality appears to arise largely from unwise psychological management by parents in the formative years of life. Its features are in essence the normal manifestations of childhood exaggerated and prolonged into adult life. The dividing line in childhood between reality and the world of make-believe is a tenuous one, and the child finds no difficulty in being an Indian chief whilst carrying out some mundane task in obedience to his mother's commands. If the demands of reality are too unpleasant, there is an exaggeration of this tendency to escape into the world of simulation and imagination, and especially is this so when the child learns that advantage may be gained. Thus feeling sick at the beginning of the new school term is a common hysterical symptom, and is not incompatible with the eating of hearty meals. As the child grows older, however, the realities of life can be accepted more easily, and the world of imagination recedes; but if the environment is too harsh and the management of the child injudicious, this normal development is arrested and the tendency to escape from reality by subconscious simulation becomes the lifetime habit of the hysterical personality.

The hysterical personality is characterised by a great tendency to react excessively to situations and surroundings; the patient responds to his environment in an extravagant manner like an actor playing a part upon the stage. This becomes so habitual that the patient finds nothing amiss in behaviour which is manifestly illogical or inappropriate. This constant change of pose leads to a lability of emotional response so that his reaction to joy and sorrow is excessive but short lived, and the extravagance of the emotional demonstration is not matched by its depth. In the sexual sphere this is manifest by a flirtatious attitude; the female hysteric indulges in much sexual stimulation and excitement, but when faced with the logical conclusion of coitus, becomes frigid and develops dyspareunia.

This over-reaction to situations is the basis of the undue suggestibility so characteristic of the hysteric. Suggestions, deliberately or inadvertently given, are subconsciously accepted by the patient and are consequently acted upon without his being aware of their origin. Hence it is that hysterics are so easily hypnotised, or, when put in a ward with other patients, so readily develop the symptoms of their neighbours. All this excessive responsiveness to situations and suggestions is not the result of conscious, deliberate activity, but takes place with a greater or lesser degree of unawareness on the part of the patient of his real motives.

This marked degree of suggestibility and emotional immaturity can sometimes be found in people who are quite intelligent and even sophisticated (at least in some respects) but it occurs most frequently in association with intellectual and educational retardation. This is also true of the manifestation of gross hysterical symptoms.

During the First World War, hysterical symptoms occurred much more frequently among 'other ranks' than among officers, who were subject to anxiety neurosis; during the second World War, as a result of the general increase in the standard of education and sophistication, anxiety states were much commoner than hysterical symptoms in all ranks of our military forces. Frank hysteria was, however, still commonly found among members of the British Pioneer Corps, which was a repository for able-bodied but intellectually retarded citizens, and also among the hardy, but simple and untutored peasants who fought in General Tito's army of Jugoslav partisans.

The term '*conversion symptoms*' is used to describe illnesses in which the patient presents with a mimic physical lesion, such as sudden blindness, or paralysis of one or more limbs, or total loss of sensation in a part of the body. Careful neurological examination will often reveal that the disability does not correspond to the anatomical areas served by motor or sensory nerves: instead, the lesion illustrates the patient's often naïve idea of what it is like to lose the power of his right hand, or to be unable to walk. In many cases, the patient has acquired a concept of a particular affliction as a result of seeing someone who was dramatically handicapped—perhaps a case of poliomyelitis, of angina, or of epilepsy. The mimicry is the result of auto-suggestion, the patient becoming suddenly overwhelmed by the conviction that he is similarly afflicted. A striking feature of conversion hysteria is that although the patient may be quite severely incapacitated by his symptoms, he appears remarkably unconcerned about them. This is because the incapacity has in fact intervened to remove a cause of anxiety, so that the patient feels strangely relieved, although he is not aware of the reason for his being so calm.

The precipitating cause of a hysterical illness is usually an emotionally charged situation, the inexorable and unpleasant consequences of which the patient cannot face, and so he excludes it from consciousness, and escapes from the situation (or makes himself the object of solicitous attention) by means of his symptoms. Thus the soldier who found the strain of battle too great and developed 'shell-shock' was able to persuade himself, and his comrades, that his retirement from the fray was not voluntary, but imposed upon him by his disability.

The form the symptom takes may be symbolical, as when the attitude of crucifixion is adopted in a hysterical fit, or it may be determined by identification with another person, as when the daughter, after her mother's death, develops the symptoms of her mother's last illness.

The grosser forms of conversion symptoms are not so common today as they were a generation ago, but instances of involuntary mimicry of physical ailments are still frequently encountered in cardiac, gastro-intestinal and orthopaedic clinics, and are a particularly common complication of injuries where a compensation award enters the picture.

Clinical Features. The list of hysterical symptoms and signs is coextensive with that of physical illness, for there is no clinical feature which may not be woven into the hysterical pattern. Some features, however, occur more commonly than others and may be arbitrarily divided into three groups, sensory, motor and psychological. Sensory symptoms may be of the special senses such as blindness and deafness, or in the somatic sphere, when cutaneous and deep sensibility in their various forms are lost. The sensory loss does not obey anatomical or physiological laws, but follows the patient's concept of the disability. Cutaneous sensory loss may have a sharp horizontal upper margin on the limb. In monocular blindness, the use of coloured letters and glasses may reveal that the patient is seeing with his 'blind' eye. There may also be positive sensory symptoms such as headache, pain, tinnitus and so on.

Motor symptoms consist of aphonia, mutism and paralysis and rigidity of movements. These again are not anatomical in distribution, and often a muscle seemingly paralysed when employed as an agonist, is found to be acting when used as a synergist or antagonist. Positive clinical features in the motor sphere consist of tremors, tics and explosive utterances, spasm of ocular muscles, abnormal gaits and fits. These fits may vary from simply falling to the ground as in syncope, to bizarre attacks with wild movements of arms and legs. They can usually be distinguished from epileptic attacks by the absence of cyanosis or pallor, the increased violence of the movements when restraint is applied, the absence of incontinence and the preservation of reflexes such as the corneal. Carpopedal spasm and other manifestations of tetany may result from hysterical hyperventilation.

The major psychological symptoms consist of fugues in which the memory is lost, twilight states in which consciousness appears impaired, stupor in which the patient lies motionless showing no reaction to the environment and pseudo-dementia in which the patient behaves as though insane.

It is also possible for patients to mimic symptoms of psychiatric illness just as they may do those of a somatic complaint. Because depression is itself so frequent, the symptoms of depression may be reproduced in this way. At first sight the hysterical patient, with tears coursing down her cheeks, may appear severely depressed; but the observer soon finds that there is little depth of feeling behind the histrionic display of misery. These patients respond with animation to an attentive audience, and, unlike a true depressive, can readily be distracted from their grief.

Diagnosis. The diagnosis of hysteria can be the most difficult in medicine. Two steps are required: the first is to demonstrate that there is no organic disease which can account for the symptoms and signs, a demonstration which demands a wide knowledge of medicine. Not infrequently a symptom may be labelled hysterical which a greater experience would have recognised as due to an organic lesion. Error would be less frequent, however, if the diagnosis were not made until the second step was also taken: this consists of discovering what situation the patient subconsciously seeks to avoid, and showing how the development of symptoms has achieved this object. If in addition to this evidence of a hysterical personality, or of previous hysterical breakdowns can be uncovered, the diagnosis is more secure. It should always be remembered, however, that the stress of organic disease may provoke a superadded hysterical reaction in a person so disposed. An axiom worth remembering is that alleged hysteria, appearing for the first time in a stable person in middle life, has almost always an organic basis.

OBSESSIVE-COMPULSIVE NEUROSIS

Definition. An *obsession* is a constantly recurring thought which the patient recognises as his own, but resists because it is foolish or repugnant. In spite of his efforts to dismiss the thought, it persists in returning so that in the end he becomes tormented by it. A *compulsion* is a similarly insistent urge to perform, or to repeat, some act which the patient consciously repudiates as meaningless or troublesome; he struggles against the urge, but finds himself experiencing very acute anxiety, which is only allayed by his giving in and performing the compulsive act.

Obsessive-compulsive traits commonly occur to some degree in normal individuals—Dr. Samuel Johnson, for example, experienced spells of 'the touching mania'—and they may become aggravated during an episode of psychological illness (as Dr. Johnson's compulsions were, during his accesses of melancholia). Sometimes obsessions and/or compulsions are the outstanding, if not the only, symptoms of which a patient complains. This condition, in which the patient, although perfectly lucid and in contact with his environment, may be quite severely handicapped by the unrelenting pressure of his unwelcome thoughts and impulses, is termed an obsessive-compulsive neurosis.

Aetiology. Obsessive-compulsive neurosis is often found in the children of parents who are similarly affected, but it is not clear whether this is due to transmission of a hereditary predisposition to the disorder. Many observers believe that the meticulous, rigid routine imposed by such parents is more conducive to obsessional neurosis in the child than the hereditary endowment itself. Psychoanalytic studies have suggested that obsessional traits have their origin in a pathological over-concern with the achievement of bowel control, imposed by parents who in their turn were similarly treated in their infancy. However that may be, such children usually grow up with typical personalities: they are excessively neat and tidy and are conscientious to a fault. They are sticklers for precision and detail; this does not necessarily lead to a higher standard of work, for so lost do they become in attention to detail, that there is interference with the main stream of activity. So long and finely do they weight the pros and cons of every situation that conclusions and decisions are never reached. These characteristics make the obsessional neurotic rigid in outlook, stubborn in character and morose in temperament.

Extrinsic factors, other than the influence of obsessive parents during the formative years, appear to contribute little to the causation of obsessional neurosis.

Clinical Features. Obsessions may be arbitrarily divided into (*a*) ideas; (*b*) impulses; (*c*) phobias; and (*d*) ruminations.

The *ideas* consist of thoughts, images (often obscene) and strings of words and phrases, which constantly recur to the patient despite his resistance to them, and his recognition that they are absurd and meaningless. The *impulses* are urges to some act such as killing offspring, or jumping under a train, or to less fearsome activities like laughing at sorrow or arranging objects in a certain manner. The *phobias* are fears of some act, and are often indistinguishable from impulses. They may, however, be separate, as when a phobia of knives develops for fear of an impulse to use them for murderous ends. Likewise, a patient may not be troubled by obscene thoughts, but rather by the fear that he may have such thoughts; he fills his mind with neutral thoughts lest obscenity should intrude. Obsessive phobias are distinguished from the phobic fears encountered in anxiety states by the fact that phobic anxiety can be allayed by simply avoiding the object, or place, which provokes it, whereas the idea representing an obsessive phobia keeps on invading the patient's consciousness. *Ruminations* comprise the practice of constantly turning over problems in the mind, seeking an answer to a question. Religious scruples are of this order, when the patient has to repeatedly examine and re-examine his conscience, uncertain as to whether he has offended or not.

These symptoms are often intermingled one with another, and may be of all degrees of intensity. Sometimes they are merely a nuisance, not interfering seriously with life, but preventing easy, enjoyable activity. In other cases they become so severe as to arrest all activity, and make the ordinary daily round an impossible task. Thus a patient, who was a house painter, stood for three hours, unable to paint over a crack on the wall until he had the 'right' thoughts in his mind. Another patient, a housewife, spent all her time washing her hands for fear they should be contaminated, and so was unable to do her housework.

When the obsessions are severe they cause great anxiety and tension, the patients becoming increasingly agitated as they fight against the compulsion. In addition, they frequently become depressed, since life becomes so difficult and escape from the obsessions seems to be impossible. Suicide is, however, relatively uncommon.

Diagnosis. The diagnosis of obsessional neurosis does not present great difficulty providing there is adherence to the exact criteria of the definition given at the beginning of this section. There must be the feeling of compulsion and, most important, the patient must recognise it as senseless or absurd and resist it. Delusions must be distinguished from obsessions; the patient does not feel his delusions are silly, but firmly believes in their truth. Similarly, such schizophrenic symptoms as feelings of compulsion or direction by some unknown force should not be confused with those of the obsessive-compulsive, who knows that the thoughts and impulses, however unwelcome, are *his own* thoughts and impulses. When the severity of such symptoms shows very marked fluctuation, a co-existing recurrent depressive illness should be suspected.

PSYCHOSOMATIC DISEASES

It has long been an axiom in medicine that not only the disease must be treated but also the patient. There are patients whose symptoms are limited to the mental sphere and who have an obvious neurotic or psychotic disorder, and there are patients whose illness appears to be the result solely of physical disease, such as neoplasm or infection. Between these two extremes there are however many patients who show not only physical symptoms and signs but psychological disturbances as well In some cases a recognisable physical disease is responsible for the psychological changes, as for instance the depression and hopelessness which may be seen in a patient who realises he is dying from an incurable new growth, but in others emotional disturbances and physical symptoms and signs occur together without any primary physical disease to account for them. Examples of such conditions are peptic ulcer, hyperthyroidism, bronchial asthma, various forms of dermatitis, migraine and ulcerative colitis, and these are sometimes called psychosomatic disorders. The implication of this term is that tension arising from a long-standing emotional conflict can induce changes in bodily function (e.g. excessive secretion of gastric juice, spasm of bronchiolar musculature, spasm of blood vessels, etc.) which, when repeated over a period of time, can in turn lead to actual tissue damage. In this way a distinction is sometimes made between psychosomatic disorders in which objective physical changes appear as a result of emotional conflict, and the neuroses in which symptoms are predominantly subjective and psychological. It is arguable, however, whether this distinction is really justified or indeed possible. It is easy to see, for instance, in the case of peptic ulcer, where there is destruction of part of the mucosa, and in hyperthyroidism, where there is hypertrophy of the glandular epithelium and in many cases exophthalmos, that there are definite structural changes which accompany the emotional disturbance. In asthma, on the other hand, there are repeated attacks of bronchial spasm which are at first completely reversible but which may, with the passage of time, lead to structural changes in the lung, such as emphysema, and predispose the lungs to chronic infection. In this case it is clear that a disturbance which was purely functional at the outset ends by producing structural changes, but it is less easy to recognise the exact point at which the disorder, which may at first have been purely psychological, becomes a psychosomatic disease. At the other end of the scale the effort syndrome, known also as disorderly action of the heart, or da Costa's syndrome, which is regarded by some authorities as a psychosomatic disorder, has as its main symptoms inframammary pain, palpitations, breathlessness, and fatigue on effort, together with undue elevation of the pulse rate and blood pressure with exercise. These same symptoms and signs, however, occur as a normal physiological response accompanying the emotion of fright produced by any dangerous situation and the effort syndrome may therefore more justifiably be regarded as a form of anxiety neurosis, especially since the symptoms and signs are all reversible and do not lead to permanent structural changes. It is inevitable therefore that the borderline between neurosis and psychosomatic disease is very indistinct. Nevertheless, the idea of a psychosomatic relationship is valuable in drawing attention to the influence which the patient's emotional state may have on his physical symptoms and signs. On the experimental side it has been possible to demonstrate the production of tissue damage by purely emotional stimuli, as when a blister appears on the skin of a person under hypnosis to whom the suggestion has been made that he has been burnt, although in fact no trauma has been applied to the skin. Wolff and Wolf have directly observed the changes which occur in the gastric mucosa as a result of emotional disturbance, and have seen these changes proceed to actual ulceration.

For many years, attempts have been made to delineate particular personality patterns associated with particular forms of psychosomatic illness, such as peptic ulcer, asthma, ulcerative colitis. A review of this literature, however, reveals the recurrence in very diverse contexts, of relatively few emotional elements, the chief of which are dependency, anger, fear, which appear to be most harmful when they are denied conscious expression. Repressed dependency needs have been particularly associated with peptic ulcer and colitis, repressed anger with asthma and hypertension. Individual cases, however, when studied in depth, are not easily fitted into any common mould. Modern psychosomatic theory has, therefore, retreated to the more general observation that all psychosomatic patients have long-standing problems in the control of their own internal emotional homeostasis, and in the conduct of their relationships with people who matter in their private lives.

The physiological processes which accompany emotional experiences continue to be the subject of a great deal of research, which tends to reveal ever-increasing complexity in the neurohumoral, metabolic and biochemical transactions underlying changing emotional states. Attention has been paid especially to the pituitary-adrenal system which mobilises one type of response when a threat can be countered by vigorous activity, another when a threat is apparent, but the subject is unable to do anything about it, and yet another, with deleterious effects on certain bodily tissues, when the stress becomes prolonged. For example, studies of athletes engaged in boxing, ice-hockey and water-polo have shown sharp increases in the internal secretion of noradrenaline during particularly violent episodes, while reserves waiting on the side-lines (and the team coach) showed increases in their secretion of adrenaline. This is, however, only one example of a system in which *every* response to the challenges of living is the end-product of an extremely complex series of interactions.

Each individual is equipped with the memory-store of a lifetime of previous experiences and emotionally-charged perceptions of things, events and especially people in his environment. Stresses, both physical and emotional, are encountered by all of us. Our ability to surmount them depends partly on our inheritance and partly on our several life-histories. Traumatic experiences during crucial stages of early development leave us predisposed both to neurosis and to psychosomatic illness; it is probable that genetic factors, which have endowed some of us with a particularly vulnerable organ or organ system, will dictate both the occurrence of a psychosomatic illness (which often indeed co-exists with neurotic symptoms) and the choice of the organ which is affected.

Treatment of the emotional disturbance and disregard of the local physical factors or vice versa, will seldom lead to benefit for the patient, and an assessment must be made in each case of the relative importance of these two factors, so that whichever appears to have the greater aetiological significance can be the main target for therapy. The general practitioner is often in the best position to know the unrealised ambitions, the frustrations at work or at home, or the marital unhappiness which may form the background to the patient's illness. A knowledge of the family history may also reveal important hereditary predisposition, as in migraine for example, which plays a part in determining the physical aspect of the illness.

PERSONALITY DISORDERS

In every large community there are a number of people who do not conform to the prevailing norm. Statistically speaking, exceptionally gifted individuals are no less abnormal than the eccentric and the social misfits; but it is the latter who are more likely to come to medical attention. These include sexual deviants, alcoholics and drug addicts; but as is well known, persons belonging to each of these categories may be quite content to remain as they are. The sexual deviant and the addict may seek help only when they are in danger of getting into trouble with the police or have already done so. Alcoholics are often brought reluctantly to their doctor by close relatives who can see more clearly than the patient how seriously his life is being interfered with by his addiction. These unwilling patients are particularly difficult to treat; but the prospect is very different when the patient himself is distressed by his abnormality, and is anxious for change.

Addiction to drugs or to alcohol represents a form of psychological dependence and indicates that the patient has been unable to attain adequate satisfactions or self-esteem in his personal life. If untreated, both of these conditions are associated with a high risk of suicide. The underlying lack of self-confidence is often so deep-seated that prolonged treatment and rehabilitation is necessary, once the anodyne of drug or alcohol has been taken away. Alcoholism is a serious health problem in Britain, and more especially in Scotland. In 1965 mental disorders due to alcoholism were responsible for nearly 20 per cent. of all admissions to Scottish mental hospitals. It is an insidious condition, because the enjoyment of alcohol is socially accepted and even encouraged. The process by which an occasional drinker becomes an habitual drinker, and finally dependent on drink can be gradual; acquaintances, and even friends, are reluctant to draw attention to a man's excessive drinking because the alcoholic is notoriously liable to take offence. Here, however, doctors have a clear responsibility because often an intercurrent illness, a chronic dyspepsia or haematemesis, or even a street accident will bring the patient to medical care, and a carefully taken history (especially if supplemented by information from others in the patient's family) will reveal the increasing dependence upon alcohol. Sometimes an unexpected hospital admission, interrupting a sustained high intake of spirits, results in the onset of delirium which compels attention to the seriousness of the drinking problem. It is often forgotten, however, that alcohol is not the only common drug of addiction in Western society; another, of more recent origin, is dependence upon barbiturates. Many middle-aged or elderly women come to rely upon a nightly dose of sleeping tablets and some of these find that if they take one or two during the day, this helps to calm their nerves. Gradually, they begin to show the signs of chronic barbiturate over-dosage: slight ataxia, absent-mindedness amounting at times to confusion as to time and place, slurred speech and tremor of the fingers. A sudden cessation of alcohol or of barbiturates can be followed by a major epileptic seizure or by delirium tremens, characterised by gross peripheral tremors, great restlessness, confusion, misidentification of people and places and delusional ideas. These delusions may be agreeable (as in the case of an alcoholic who sat cheerfully at the edge of his bed, convinced that he was engaged in trout fishing) but much more often they are threatening or even terrifying, especially when accompanied by hallucinatory visions. Fortunately, the delirium can usually be promptly controlled by intramuscular injections of chlorpromazine; but it is essential to use the occasion to try to impress on the convalescent patient the importance of seeking help in order to relieve his state of drug dependence, and the serious consequences which may follow if he resumes his excessive drinking.

DEPRESSIVE ILLNESS

Depression is a state which all of us experience from time to time, usually as a result of some distressing circumstance. There are however many patients who attend their doctors seeking relief for a large number of symptoms loosely grouped under the term 'depression'. Some may complain of feeling unduly depressed following some unhappy experience, while others are clearly neurotics of long-standing. Many patients are unaware of being depressed, but report feelings of exhaustion or vague aches and pains, and attribute their low spirits to these physical ailments. Yet others, although looking a picture of misery, do not complain of being depressed, but seem anxious only to impress the doctor with their own wickedness and unworthiness.

Clinical Features. From the many patients suffering from 'depression' it is important to separate a group who have certain features in common—important because these patients can often be cured quite rapidly and because, if left untreated, they are the most likely to commit suicide. The clinical features shown by this group, in addition to a mood varying from mild depression to black despair are: *insomnia* of a type characterised by early waking after two to three hours sleep; *diurnal variation of mood*, in which the depression often lifts considerably towards evening; *slowness of thought*, and inability to make decisions; *ideas of guilt*, unworthiness and self-blame which are often delusional in intensity, i.e. they are impervious to reasoned argument or demonstration of their falsity; and various somatic manifestations such as loss of appetite, loss of weight, amenorrhoea, occipital pressure headache, backache, constipation, retardation of physical activity (more rarely aimless over-activity or agitation), and hypochondriacal delusions. Such a patient may sit bowed and immobile on the edge of a chair obviously in the depths of misery, weeping silently, wringing his hands and answering questions in slow monosyllables; but in the earlier stages the physical appearance is less striking and the diagnosis depends on the doctor's ability to elicit the symptoms described above.

Such patients are suffering from endogenous depression, known in earlier times as melancholia or 'the spleen'. They are often people who have been subject previously to mood changes (cyclothymia) or people who have over-scrupulous, rigid personalities following too strict upbringing and who develop depression particularly in later middle age (involutional melancholia). Endogenous depression may be precipitated by physical diseases such as influenza, pyelonephritis and infective hepatitis, and may sometimes be the first symptom of cerebral disease, such as general paralysis of the insane or cerebral atherosclerosis, but more often, as its name suggests, it arises without detectable external influences.

Endogenous depression is seen particularly in patients of middle-age or older. Other forms of depression, sometimes called reactive depression, may be seen in younger or middle-aged people, many of whom show concomitant symptoms of anxiety neurosis rather than the symptoms described above. When there is insomnia it usually takes the form of inability to get to sleep without the early waking characteristic of endogenous depression, and such patients often feel better in company in contrast to the sufferer from endogenous depression, who finds meeting people a painful ordeal and prefers to suffer alone. It must be remembered that both profound, endogenous depression and relatively superficial depressive moods may be precipitated by external events, particularly those which impart a sense of loss, separation or disappointment. The difference in their manifestations is largely a matter of the intensity of the suffering involved, but some very depressed patients are prevented, by the illness itself, from revealing the full extent of their suffering. Their self-deprecation and sense of unworthiness may make them believe that they deserve to suffer and their feelings of guilt may make them reluctant to disclose the full intensity of their feelings. Many severely depressed patients are afraid that they are 'going mad', and many are frightened, as well as ashamed, at their own suicidal thoughts. Some doctors, out of a mistaken fear of adding to their distress, may connive in these patients' attempt to avoid mentioning these painful topics; but in fact, so far from harming the very depressed patient, it often brings a measure of solace if he is helped to give expression to these deep-seated fears. One should not, therefore, hesitate to help him put them into words. The fear of insanity can often be relieved by a frank discussion of the illness, accepting its severity but indicating its likely favourable outcome; thoughts of suicide have to be evaluated differently according to whether they have been fleeting and resisted, or constant and insistent. In the latter case, and especially when the patient states that his mind has been dwelling upon a particular method of killing himself, admission to hospital for psychiatric care is urgently indicated.

SCHIZOPHRENIA

Schizophrenia is the illness whose symptoms correspond most closely to the popular conception of the madman. These patients are likely, at least during the acute phase of their illness, to experience hallucinations (most commonly, in the form of threatening or unfriendly voices) and to express bizarre delusions with little or no appreciation of why it is that their ideas are unacceptable to those around them. Both delusions and hallucinations may occur in other forms of mental illness, such as severe depression, mania or delirium, but certain features are especially suggestive of schizophrenia. These include (1) *passivity feelings*, in which the patient is convinced that his actions are controlled by some alien power, (2) *thought insertion* and *thought broadcasting*, in which he feels that other people put thoughts into his mind, and are able to read his thoughts and (3) *paranoid delusions* in which he believes that he is surrounded by hostile forces which watch him and secretly intervene to do him harm. Depressed patients may also develop paranoid ideas, but these are coloured by their all-pervading feelings of guilt. For example, a depressed patient may believe that he is being watched by secret police because they have found out that he has committed a terrible crime. The paranoid schizophrenic, on the other hand, is quite sure that it is his unseen enemies who are the villains of the piece, and he their innocent victim. These patients, unfortunately, tend to have little insight into the fact that they are ill and in need of treatment. As a result, when their behaviour is becoming alarming or threatening towards their neighbours, it may be necessary to consult a psychiatrist and arrange for them to be admitted for treatment by means of an emergency order (signed by one doctor) or a formal certificate (signed by a psychiatrist and by the patient's own physician). In England and Wales this certificate is itself sufficient authority for the compulsory treatment of a mentally ill patient; in Scotland, the authority for such treatment is given by a Sheriff, after reading the two doctors' reports. In both countries, the patient's state must be reviewed after 28 days, and in many cases it is found no longer necessary to detain him 'on order'.

These are the more florid manifestations of schizophrenia. Milder signs are less easy to recognise, because they merge into the peculiarities of everyday living. These include instances of unexpected rudeness or tactlessness, abrupt and inexplicable behaviour and a marked withdrawal from ordinary social contacts. Such persons may be considered awkward or unsociable and it is only when they reveal quite bizarre ideas, shout back at their hallucinatory voices, or otherwise behave in a conspicuously strange manner, that one realises that they are not merely eccentric, but mentally ill.

In former years the treatment of schizophrenia was the concern only of psychiatrists but now, because of the remarkable degree to which the phenothiazine drugs help to control hallucinations and delusions, many schizophrenics are able to return to work and to live in the community. The ability to do so is often dependent on their continuing to take the drug prescribed, responsibility for which is taken by their general practitioner. When the episode of schizophrenic illness has been prolonged for more than six months, complete recovery is unusual. It has been found that chronic schizophrenics fare best in their subsequent careers if they are able to come to terms with their affliction and accept work of a relatively undemanding, routine nature. Their relatives, too, will be well advised to bear in mind that, as Dr. Johnson once said of a hypersensitive youth: 'Creatures such as this should be nurtured in the shade'. A former schizophrenic should not be expected to be affectionate or demonstrative of his feelings or even particularly sociable; if allowed to go his own way, and to participate inconspicuously on the fringe of group activities he will not only be much happier, but will be more likely to avoid a relapse into psychosis.

ORGANIC MENTAL SYNDROMES

Psychiatric symptoms may arise in the course of physical illnesses which either primarily or secondarily affect the brain. The occurrence of delirium during the course of febrile illnesses or the mental symptoms of general paralysis of the insane are two well-known examples. It is important to recognise certain mental symptoms which occur in organic mental syndromes, since their presence should lead to the search for physical factors which may not otherwise have declared themselves. The organic mental syndromes can be divided into two groups: *delirium*, which is an acute disorder, and *dementia*, which is a chronic disorder. Generally speaking the acute form is potentially recoverable, being the result of temporary effects on the brain from toxic processes or disorders of metabolism, while the chronic form is the expression of more severe and progressive tissue changes in the brain and is thus less amenable to treatment. The mental symptoms of each of these organic syndromes are not specific to the causative disease and will be the same whatever may be the underlying physical disorder producing the delirium or dementia.

Delirium

This acute syndrome may be produced by such varied conditions as drug intoxication (alcoholism, bromism), infections (encephalitis, smallpox, typhoid fever), trauma to the brain, electrolyte imbalance and metabolic disorders (hepatic failure, uraemia), vitamin deficiency (Wernicke's encephalopathy), and cerebral hypoxia (congestive heart failure). In addition to the physical symptoms appropriate to the disorder in question there are often found slurred speech, tremor, nystagmus, diplopia and sluggish pupillary reactions. The characteristic mental symptoms are: insomnia and restlessness; disorientation; impairment of memory and of ability to grasp the significance of a situation;

hallucinations, particularly in the visual sphere; ideas of persecution (paranoid ideas); and a feeling of fear or terror. All the symptoms and particularly the level of consciousness are variable. The patient when undisturbed may appear deeply asleep, but quite weak stimuli may rouse him to a state of restlessness varying from simple tossing and turning to such activities as aimless searching in the bedclothes or repeated carrying out of motions associated with his occupation. He may appear orientated for time and space and be able to recognise visitors at one moment, only to be quite confused soon after. The patient will often give the easiest answer to a question without regard to the truth and may supplement his faulty memory and perception by invention (confabulation), as when he describes in detail a large meal which he says he has just had, when in fact he has eaten nothing. Visual hallucinations are characteristic of delirium, and are usually vivid and may be terrifying. Many are based on illusional misinterpretations of objects seen in the room; thus patterns on the wallpaper may become an advancing army of hideous and menacing reptiles. Hallucinations of other senses may occur. Doubt and suspicion are readily induced by the impaired mentality leading to misinterpretations, and may blossom for a short time into transient and rather ill-defined delusions of persecution. Such an acute organic syndrome is commonly precipitated by withdrawal of alcohol or of barbiturates, from patients who have become habituated to taking them in substantial amounts. When the syndrome is due to alcoholism it is known as *delirium tremens*, but its features do not greatly differ from those of delirium from other causes.

The course and prognosis of delirium depend, of course, on the underlying physical disease, and treatment of this in most cases clears up the mental symptoms completely. Sometimes, however, delirium may be an episode in a progressive organic dementia or the herald of a serious psychosis.

Dementia

This chronic organic syndrome may be caused by a wide number of diseases of the brain. The most common of these is cerebral atherosclerosis, and other important causes include cerebral trauma, inflammations (neurosyphilis, encephalitis), disseminated sclerosis, intoxications and deficiency disorders (chronic alcoholism, pellagra, vitamin B_{12} deficiency), prolonged hypoglycaemia, carbon monoxide poisoning, cerebral neoplasm, and a group of degenerative disorders including Huntington's chorea and senile dementia. It will be seen that some of these conditions (encephalitis, alcoholism, vitamin deficiencies) may also cause delirium. The cerebral changes brought about at first by these factors result in delirium and can be reversed by treatment, but if they are allowed to continue unchecked too long, permanent cerebral damage occurs, giving rise to dementia. The clinical picture of dementia varies to some extent with the cause, the previous personality of the patient, the age of onset, and the rate of progression, but in all cases the mental symptoms are seen to involve the intellect, memory, emotions and behaviour, although the actual degree of impairment depends on the factors mentioned above. Insomnia is often an early symptom and may lead to nocturnal restlessness and confusion as the disease advances. Judgement and reasoning are early involved, and the disability caused by this will depend on the extent to which these faculties are utilised in the patient's daily life and work; it will be more noticeable in a barrister than in an unskilled labourer. Memory is impaired, particularly in relation to recent events, and in the later stages this may combine with defective perception to produce disorientation in space and time. Impairment of higher control leads to emotional instability and outbursts of violence or sexual aberrations at variance with the patient's previous character. There may be wide fluctuations of mood with euphoria or depression but finally, with all passion spent, the patient sinks into apathy. Delusions are common, and may be either centred on the patient himself, when they are grandiose or self-condemnatory and hypochondriacal according to the mood, or centred on others, when they tend to be paranoid. As the structure of the personality disintegrates, the patient neglects his appearance, becomes lax in personal cleanliness, and careless incontinence occurs. Focal neurological signs may be found, e.g. dysphasia, apraxia, agnosia, hemiplegia, and epileptic attacks, either focal or generalised.

TREATMENT

Psychological treatment begins the moment that the patient and doctor meet, for the latter's personality and attitude to the patient and his illness are powerful therapeutic factors which operate immediately. The first therapeutic step is the taking of the history. If this is done patiently, thoroughly and objectively the patient feels interest in his case is being taken, and that his problem is being understood. A spontaneous account of the illness by the patient should be first encouraged, further details being filled in later. Too systematic an approach to the history often results in a mass of facts being obtained, but the nature of the problem, from the patient's point of view, being entirely overlooked.

When the history has been completed, a thorough physical examination should be undertaken and following this, appropriate investigations when required. This part needs to be handled well. Investigations which are necessary must be carefully planned, and quickly executed, and then a halt must be called. The pernicious habit of 'just having one more test' must be avoided as it undermines the confidence of the patient in the certainty of the diagnosis; the practitioner must be able to decide how much evidence is required to elucidate the nature and the cause of the disorder, and having obtained it, he must act upon it.

The doctor is now in a position to draw up what may be described as the formulation of the case, which is a brief assessment of the nature of the disturbance, and the part that particular intrinsic and extrinsic factors have played in its development. It is often difficult to decide upon a formal diagnosis, but the attempt should be made if only because it helps to clarify one's own thinking and also helps one to set about the next task which consists in drawing up a plan of treatment. This will have a somewhat different emphasis, depending upon whether the patient's illness falls in the general class of neurosis, functional psychosis or organic mental illness, but in each case psychiatric treatment (like all good medical treatment) should start with the attempt to understand both the disorder and the person who is suffering from it. The advent of new and powerful drugs has tempted some doctors to forget that their patients are not merely 'biological preparations' on which interesting pharmacological experiments can be carried out; they are themselves active participants in the processes of cure and recovery. This has been shown again and again, in demonstrations of the 'placebo effect', and it is particularly important in all forms of psychiatric illness, where a patient's confidence in his therapist contributes so largely to his peace of mind.

The treatment of the individual psychological disorders will now be discussed.

Neuroses and Psychosomatic Disorders. When the formulation of the case indicates that emotional factors are prominent, some form of psychotherapy is required; simply informing the patient that there is nothing wrong with him, or that he must pull himself together, is useless. Even telling the patient that his difficulties are psychological and indicating the emotional problems in his life is unlikely to be of benefit, because although he may acquiesce verbally, his emotional tension will not be thereby lessened; he needs an opportunity for emotional catharsis, and gaining greater insight into the nature of his difficulties.

Such insight may be gained by a series of discussions, for which periods of at least half an hour or longer should be set aside, in which the patient is encouraged to talk about his difficulties. Initially, the discussions should be allowed to proceed in any direction the patient desires; subsequently, aspects of his problems which seem relevant may be suggested by the doctor as themes for discussion. The error that is commonly made with this form of psychotherapy is for the doctor to talk too much by lecturing the patient and giving advice. In order that the patient may achieve a better knowledge of himself, it is essential that he should do most of the talking, the doctor saying little, but maintaining an attitude of interest and expectation. If the patient's flow of talk is arrested, encouragement can often be given, without diverting him from his present theme, by repeating his last phrase in a query form. Thus, if he says, 'I found the job far too much for me,' and then becomes silent, after giving him ample time to resume spontaneously, the doctor may say, 'You found the job far too much for you?', which starts the patient off again. The effect of this approach is first that the patient feels better for having talked to someone about his troubles; a second effect is that frequently the patient comes to realise the true nature of his problems, and will, at that stage, often accept suggestions and interpretations which, if given earlier, would have been rejected.

When somatic symptoms, and fear of bodily disease are prominent, it is not sufficient simply to tell the patient that there is on evidence of organic pathology; he will at once suspect that he is being accused of malingering, if not of being 'mental'. It is necessary to let him know that his distress and his symptoms are recognised as genuine and in need of explanation. It is often possible to use events in the patient's own experience to illustrate the influence of emotion on bodily functions. Many people can recognise what it feels like to be sick with excitement, to be aware of a pounding of the heart in moments of fear or to experience frequency of micturition when keyed up before an examination. At a general level, however, this understanding becomes much more meaningful when, in the course of an emotionally-charged interview, the patient has been able to see for himself that his physical symptoms are related to particular aspects of his own private life. Patients are seldom convinced about this until they have been helped to go one stage further, to confront the painful situation, and to master it. When this is done, there is commonly an immediate, even if only temporary, relief from the distressing symptom, together with a sense of accomplishment which encourages the patient to persevere with further efforts of self-discovery.

It is important, at the same time, not to overlook physical factors, such as anaemia or faulty nutrition, which can be rectified. A poor physical condition in itself gives rise to symptoms which further aggravate the anxiety of the patient. Adequate food, exercise and rest are, therefore, essential. Should drugs be employed as an adjunct, their specific purpose should be made abundantly clear, so that no possibility will arise of the patient feeling that their prescription indicates that he is suffering from an organic disease. Measures such as these are often adequate for a mild anxiety state with somatic symptoms, when the emotional problems are not too great.

The treatment of hysteria is a more difficult problem, as often the hysterical pattern of reaction is ingrained and the extrinsic, precipitating factors not susceptible to adjustment. Removal of a symptom can often be achieved by a prolonged session, in which intense persuasion is used, but, if the precipitating situation is unaltered, relapse is certain. The method may be justified, however, in certain circumstances as when aphonia prevents discussion, or paralysis is leading to contracture. The management of a hysterical patient has much in common with that of a frightened or petulant child. It consists in convincing her that you are on her side, even while refusing to comply with some of her requests. Treating a hysterical patient is often a test of nerve;

in the face of dramatic protestations and apparently alarming symptoms, one must quietly but firmly insist upon facing the painful realities from which the hysteric has taken flight. If one has succeeded in gaining her confidence, long-established symptoms will sometimes disappear with dramatic suddenness, but all too often they are replaced by others. The hysterical patient finds it difficult to abandon the defences against alarming feelings which she has been using since her early adolescence. In addition these patients are especially prone to develop an emotional dependence upon their therapist, which must be recognised and brought to their attention kindly but firmly. The family doctor can give helpful advice to other people in the patient's immediate environment, warning them that hysterical symptoms only become aggravated if too much attention is paid to them, and encouraging them to avoid entering into the hysteric's pattern of self-deception. It is usually much easier for the onlookers than for the patient herself to see the real motivation of her symptoms, but of course, it is no use simply *telling* her—she has to discover for herself why she behaves in the way she does.

The achievement of a long-term cure of an hysterical illness is a formidable task since it requires the emotional maturation of the patient. Not surprisingly, both patients and their doctors often tacitly agree not to attempt it. Instead, the doctor may concentrate upon dealing with the most pressing difficulties of the patient's immediate predicament and may settle for her remaining a somewhat demanding and dependent patient.

The obsessional neurotic does not respond well to treatment but often the condition is self-limiting, at least in its acute phases. The patient should be encouraged not to endeavour to overcome the obsessions by will-power; he should be assured that his doctor knows that his irrational, obscene or murderous thoughts are not indicative of his true nature. He should be encouraged to avoid situations which foster the development of the obsessions, and should diversify his interests as much as possible. The best antidote for obsessive ruminations is to keep the patient busy with practical tasks which demand his attention.

In the treatment of all forms of neurotic illness it is important to decide what can best be done, within the limitations of resources for treatment and in the circumstances of each individual patient. For example, one may recognise that a patient has shown a lifelong pattern of minor phobias and proneness to worry, but that recent events in her personal life have caused one particular phobia (such as the fear of going into crowded places) seriously to interfere with her normal activities. Here, the principal aim of treatment should be limited to helping her to master the presenting symptom. It is inevitable that in doing so, she will have to take stock of her relationships with people close to her and she may even have to modify some of her habitual pattern of behaviour towards them, but no attempt need be made to effect any radical change in her personality.

The same is true of many hysterical symptoms and of exacerbations of psychosomatic disorders. By focussing upon recent events in the patient's personal experience and exploring their emotional significance for him, many patients can be helped to reconstitute that *modus vivendi* between personal quirks and practical necessities which, for most of us, represents normal mental health.

Depression. Depression is a very common symptom in all forms of psychiatric disorder. This is not surprising, because mild depression of spirits is indistinguishable from unhappiness, a state which naturally accompanies any condition which makes one feel physically or mentally 'out of sorts'. The first task in treating depression, therefore, is to consider whether it is the consequence of the patient's painful circumstances or of some other illness, in which case it is the life-situation or the illness which must receive attention. In true 'endogenous depression', however, the depression of mood, sleeplessness, loss of energy and loss of weight are out of proportion to any precipitating factors which may be elicited. In such cases it is best to proceed without delay to treat the patient with one of the potent antidepressant drugs (p. 1281). One has to bear in mind, however, that these drugs do not take effect until after some 6 to 14 days.

Severe depression, especially when associated with restlessness and agitation, with delusions of unworthiness and preoccupation with thoughts of death, is an extremely distressing condition and fraught with risks of suicide. Such cases should be admitted to psychiatric care in hospital, where electric shock therapy, administered under intravenous anaesthesia and modified by muscle-relaxant drugs, is often still indicated, because this is the speediest way to relieve the patient's suffering.

As a general rule, it is wise to postpone any practical decisions about business, change of work or domestic matters until the patient has regained his normal frame of mind. Once the patient's mood has responded to physical methods of treatment, it is essential to review his personal circumstances with him and to help him make plans to cope with the difficulties which may have precipitated his illness.

Schizophrenia. The advent of the phenothiazine drugs (p. 1280) has very significantly changed the prognosis of schizophrenia but it should be remembered that even before there was any specific drug treatment for this illness, many cases made a spontaneous recovery from the acute stage of the psychosis in the course of three to nine months. Even now, the new drugs offer symptomatic relief of the patient's delusions, hallucinations and alienation from reality, rather than a radical cure of this little-understood disease. There is abundant evidence that the way in which the patient is treated, both in hospital and in the community, will influence both his degree of recovery and the probability of a subsequent relapse.

Putting it briefly, it may be said that schizophrenic patients do badly if they are allowed to withdraw too completely from social contacts and practical activities; but they also do badly if they are involved in emotionally demanding relationships, to which they are unable to respond. Many, if not most, schizophrenics must be regarded as having particularly vulnerable personalities and many emerge from the acute stage of their illness with some residual defects. They are best able to cope with their handicap if they can be helped to come to terms with their limitations. These patients are not necessarily intellectually impaired—they may be highly intelligent—but they are seldom able to cope with positions of responsibility, particularly when they are required to supervise, or interact with other people. Hence, they do best in tasks in which they can work on their own, with only rather formal contacts with their fellows.

In recent years, the psychiatric hospitals have treated their schizophrenic patients with phenothiazines, together with an active regime of occupational and industrial therapy and have been able to discharge the great majority back to the community and to the care of their general practitioners. The latter can best help them by ensuring that the patients take their prescribed course of drugs for at least the first year or two after discharge. In addition the doctor should be ready to enlist the help of a Mental Health Officer or a social worker if his patients appear to be having difficulties either at work or in their domestic relationships.

Organic Mental Illness. Acute episodes of delirium, paranoid or hallucinatory psychosis are encountered from time to time in general medical and surgical practice. These are particularly common in two circumstances.

1. When there is impairment of brain function due to trauma or anoxia; this is especially the case with the elderly, whose brains may already be showing some degenerative changes. Not uncommonly elderly patients will become temporarily deluded or confused after a coronary thrombosis, a mild stroke, or a chest infection.

2. As a sequel to events which have greatly alarmed the patient (for example, conjuring up fears of death by cancer or heart failure) and in circumstances which make it difficult for him to find reassurance from familiar sights, sounds and persons. For example, some patients have catastrophic reactions following operations on the eyes, when they must submit to being blindfolded for some time, and others have reacted adversely to the accoutrements of cardiac resuscitation or renal dialysis. These reactive psychoses contain an element of panic.

The use of intramuscular injections of chlorpromazine has transformed the management of acute deliria, enabling the majority of patients to be cared for in a side-room of the medical or surgical ward where their primary disease is being treated. In all these conditions the patient can be helped by allowing him to express his fears; patients who are frightened and bewildered tend to regress to a state of childlike dependency and welcome a firm reassurance from someone whom they are willing to trust. They cannot, however, be effectively reassured until they have had an opportunity of unburdening themselves of their fears. Elderly patients often find it particularly difficult to adapt to sudden changes of scene and bewildering happenings. It is helpful for them if they can be visited by only a few nurses and doctors who take pains to identify themselves; their sick-room should be well lit and they should be encouraged to keep a few treasured possessions on their bed-side table. Since patients with even very slight clouding of consciousness are prone to misunderstand what is happening round about them, any changes of routine or new procedures should be explained to them in advance, in simple terms and if necessary more than once.

In today's medical practice, the care of the elderly is playing an increasingly large part. Geriatricians and family doctors have learned to cope with the multiple minor ailments and chronic handicaps which beset old age. In the realm of psychiatry, too, it has been increasingly realised that old people do not merely suffer from progressive loss of memory and intellectual powers. Even those who show signs of cerebral atherosclerosis, with a succession of minor cerebrovascular accidents, often show fluctuations in their mental capabilities and at times they are themselves acutely aware of the reduction in their mental and physical powers and become correspondingly depressed. Severe depression is by no means uncommon in the elderly and this responds well to active antidepressant treatment. What is not so widely appreciated, however, is the fact that episodes of neurotic illness, with anxiety states, phobias, hysterical symptoms or compulsions are also encountered in this age group, and are no less amenable to simple psychotherapy than at other ages. In the after-care of these older patients it is important to remember that *social isolation* is an important threat to their mental well-being. This becomes even more important when physical disability or deafness further restricts their opportunities of making contact with other people. Here voluntary agencies as well as local authority welfare and preventive services can do useful prophylactic work, but the family doctor is often in the best position to recognise when an ageing (and perhaps recently bereaved) patient is in especial need of such help.

THE USES AND MISUSES OF PSYCHOTROPIC DRUGS

The consideration of drug treatment in psychological medicine is kept to the end of this chapter in order to guard against the misleading idea (which pharmaceutical advertising literature is only too ready to convey) that for every psychiatric syndrome there is a specific medicinal remedy. Used wisely, the new psychotropic drugs can do a great deal to reduce the distress of psychiatrically disturbed patients, but it has to be remembered that they are almost without exception palliative and not curative remedies, and also that they can be dangerous if misused. During the past 20 years, one of the most striking changes in morbidity in Britain as in other advanced societies, has been a conspicuous increase in the incidence of attempted suicide, particularly in the form of 'taking an overdose'. In 1966, cases of self-poisoning or self-injury amounted to no less than 10 per cent. of all admissions to acute medical wards in Britain. More than 80 per cent. of these patients had swallowed overdoses of medicines prescribed by a doctor, the most common class of drug being the barbiturates, followed closely by the tranquillisers and antidepressants. These figures can be variously interpreted, but they demonstrate very clearly the danger of relying upon drugs alone to solve the problems of emotionally disturbed patients.

The drugs which are most commonly misused are barbiturate sleeping tablets. It is not generally recognised that barbiturates very quickly create a physiological adaptation in the central nervous system, which gives rise to withdrawal symptoms, and even epileptic fits, when the drug is withheld. Recent EEG studies have shown that when normal subjects take as little as 200 mg. of sodium amylobarbitone nightly for one week and then stop, their sleep pattern remains disturbed for several nights before reverting to normal. Patients who have become dependent on sleeping tablets have some justification for being reluctant to do without them, because they will be very likely to experience broken sleep and troubled dreams for up to two weeks before they can re-establish a natural sleep routine. Unfortunately, few drugs provide as effective sedation as do the barbiturates. Chloral hydrate is of particular value for elderly patients. The new sedative nitrazepam has the merit of being remarkably safe. The best policy is probably to regard insomnia as the symptom of some underlying disturbance and to restrict its treatment to short courses, emphasising to the patient that it is preferable, in the long run, to tolerate a number of sleepless nights rather than to become dependent on a habit-forming drug.

Another class of drugs whose disadvantages have come to outweigh their therapeutic usefulness is the amphetamines. These drugs have been used to counteract sensations of lassitude and vague depression. They very readily give rise to psychological dependency because they provide a rapid subjective lifting of the spirits and a feeling of euphoria. As is well recognised, teenagers have frequently used or abused amphetamines (including the mixture of barbiturate and amphetamine popularly known as 'purple hearts') for this purpose. It is less well known, however, that many older men and women renew their prescriptions for amphetamines month after month. Amphetamines not only create dependency but can also give rise to an acute psychotic reaction, with auditory and visual hallucinations and delusions of persecution. These features can be clinically indistinguishable from those of paranoid schizophrenia, but they clear up in about three weeks' time after withdrawal of the drug. Because of these adverse effects, psychiatrists no longer employ amphetamines for their adult patients, although they still have a place in the treatment of enuretic children.

Tranquillisers and Antidepressants. The new psychotropic drugs fall into two main groups, the *tranquillisers* and the psychic energisers, or *antidepressants*. These drugs have emerged only during the last 10 to 15 years, and as a result some doctors are still apt to be confused about their proper uses. It is not uncommon to find a tranquilliser, such as chlorpromazine, prescribed for a deeply depressed patient, or an antidepressant offered in homeopathic doses to a patient who is only a little depressed, but in neither case is the medication appropriate.

Tranquillisers. Tranquillisers are drugs which allay a variety of symptoms, such as acute anxiety, restlessness, agitation, without sedating the patient, who remains alert and in touch with his surroundings but is no longer oppressed by his symptoms. There are three main categories of tranquillisers:

1. *Rauwolfia derivatives*, containing the alkaloid reserpine, and the *phenothiazines* (chlorpromazine, thioridazine, etc.). These drugs are principally used in the treatment of schizophrenia. Reserpine has the advantage of being cheaper, but the disadvantages that it may provoke a severe depression and like many of the phenothiazines, it may give rise to the symptoms of Parkinsonism. Chlorpromazine and thioridazine are in general use, 150 mg. to 1,000 mg. being given each day in divided doses during the acute

stage of the illness. A suitable maintenance dose for a schizophrenic in remission is 100 mg. three times a day. Chlorpromazine is also given by intramuscular injections (50-100 mg.) in order to control states of delirium or over-excitement. An important side-effect to remember is its tendency to lower the blood-pressure; patients should be warned against the occurrence of moments of dizziness when they get up quickly from a sitting position. Because this tendency is more marked with elderly patients, they should be given smaller doses.

2. The *diazepines*, particularly diazepam and chlordiazepoxide which relieve the distress of acute anxiety, and *meprobamate* which was one of the first of the class of milder tension-relaxing drugs, and can be used to give symptomatic relief to patients whose anxiety is accompanied by feeling 'keyed up' and unable to relax.

Drugs of the two latter groups can be particularly helpful in tiding a neurotic patient over an especially difficult period of subjective distress. They do not, however, do anything to resolve the causes of the patient's symptoms, and unless this is altered either through psychotherapy or through a significant change in his personal circumstances, the symptoms will tend to recur and the patient may find himself becoming dependent on his palliative drug.

Antidepressants. There are two principal groups of antidepressant drugs:

1. Imipramine and Amitriptyline.
2. The monoamine oxidase inhibitors (phenelzine, isoniazid, iproniazid, etc.).

1. The former drugs are indicated for the treatment of severe depression of the endogenous type, with symptoms indicating a disturbance of sleep, appetite and energy. In order to be effective, they have to be given in sufficient dosage, which may be from 50 to 75 mg. three times a day. Both drugs give rise to some disagreeable side-effects. Imipramine may make the patient feel even more on edge and restless during the first few days, and it may also cause some difficulty in micturition. Both drugs have an atropine-like effect on the eyes, causing difficulty in focussing. Amitryptilline tends to make some patients feel uncomfortably

drowsy, and causes dryness of the mouth. These side-effects usually recede with continued use and become quite easily tolerated once the patient begins to experience a lifting of his mood and a return of his former energy, which usually becomes apparent after six to ten days. A course of either of these drugs should be taken for three to six months, because if they are stopped too soon the symptoms of depression may again assert themselves.

2. Psychiatrists are themselves in dispute over the effectiveness of the mono-amine oxidase inhibitor (MAOI) drugs. Controlled trials have shown them to be much less effective than either imipramine or amitryptilline in the treatment of severe depression, but some workers have claimed that they are especially helpful in the treatment of milder 'atypical' depressions or prolonged phobic symptoms, occurring in patients with good previous personalities. The action of MAOI drugs is associated with an accumulation of catecholamines in the brain and other tissues of the body; hence patients should be warned not to partake of substances rich in tyramine (such as cheese, chianti and some types of beer) because these may interact with the drug to provoke a hypertensive crisis, with splitting headaches and a risk of subarachnoid haemorrhage. The MAOI drugs also potentiate other drugs, including pethidine, opiates, barbiturates, phenothiazines, amphetamine and alcohol, all of which should be avoided while a patient is taking this form of antidepressant.

No attempt has been made in this chapter to discuss all the psychotropic drugs, of which new variants are being introduced every year. However, Table 15 gives the pharmacopoeial and trade names and usual doses of drugs in the principal categories which have been frequently recommended.

G. M. Carstairs

References:

Curran, D. & Partridge, M. (1965). *Psychological Medicine: a Short Introduction to Psychiatry*. Edinburgh: Livingstone.

Henderson, D. K. & Batchelor, I. R. C., (1962). *Textbook of Psychiatry*. London: Oxford University Press.

World Health Organization (1967). *International Classification of Disease*, 8th revision. Geneva: WHO.

TABLE 15.

Summary of Psychotropic Drugs

Designation	Dose Range (in 24 hours)	Trade Name
SEDATIVES		
Chloral hydrate preparations		
Dichloralphenazone	650 mg. tabs.—one or two at night	Welldorm
Barbiturates		
Amylobarbitone sodium	60-400 mg. at night	Sodium Amytal
Butobarbitone	100 mg. tabs.—one or two at night	Soneryl
Quinalbarbitone sodium	50 mg. tabs.—one or two at night	Seconal
Pentobarbitone sodium	50 mg.capsules—one or two at night	Nembutal Gardenal
Benzodiazepine derivative		
Nitrazepam	5-20 mg. at night	Mogadon
TRANQUILLISERS		
Rauwolfia preparations	50 mg. tabs.—up to 400 mg.	Raudixin
Rauwolfia serpentina (whole root)		
Reserpine	Up to 1 mg.	Serpasil
Phenothiazines		
Chlorpromazine	150-900 mg.	Largactil
Thioridazine	150-900 mg.	Melleril
Promazine	50-250 mg.	Sparine
Perphenazine	6-24 mg.	Fentazin
Trifluoperazine	10-30 mg.	Stelazine
Prochlorperazine	10-30 mg.	Stemetil
Diazepines		
Chlordiazepoxide	10-30 mg.	Librium
Diazepam	6-40 mg.	Valium
Meprobamate	400-1,200 mg.	Equanil, Miltown
ANTIDEPRESSANTS		
Imipramine	75-225 mg.	Tofranil
Amitriptyline	75-225 mg.	Tryptizol Elavel
Monoamine Oxidase Inhibitors		
Phenelzine	45-90 mg.	Nardil
Nialamide	50-150 mg.	Niamid
Ipromiazid	150-300 mg.	Marsilid
Isocarboxazid	30-60 mg.	Marplan

DIETS[1]

The diet sheets that follow have been constructed to illustrate the quantitative and qualitative aspects of diets required for the treatment of various diseases. The quantities given in a standard diet sheet will obviously require some modification in relation to the size, age, sex and occupation of the patient. In the dietetic treatment of most diseases it is unnecessary to weigh accurately the amounts of the different foods eaten. Under these circumstances sufficient accuracy will be secured by the use of the terms 'small', 'medium' or 'large' helping. A small helping weighs approximately 1 to 2 oz. (30-60 g.), a medium helping 2 to 3 oz. (60-90 g.) and a large helping 4 oz. (120 g.) or more.

DIET 1

SEMI-FLUID LOW-ROUGHAGE DIET

suitable for patients who have

DIFFICULTY IN CHEWING OR SWALLOWING OR WHO ARE SEVERELY ILL WITH ULCERATIVE OR MALIGNANT DISEASE OF THE ALIMENTARY TRACT

Approximately: Protein 90 g., Carbohydrate 270 g., Fat 120 g., Cal. 2500

Early morning Fruit juice with sugar.

8 a.m. Strained porridge with milk or cream from allowance.* Coffee with fortified milk or cream and sugar from allowance.

10 a.m. Fortified milk *or* some proprietary preparation of milk, e.g. Bengers Food, Horlicks *or* Ovaltine.

12 noon Strained cream soup.
Savoury custard—using cheese, very finely minced chicken, ham, pounded white or smoked fish, *or* scrambled eggs *or* omelette.

2 p.m. Sweet made with puréed fruit, cream and sugar, *or* small helping of mousse or cold soufflé, *or* ice-cream with fruit, chocolate or butterscotch sauce, *or* jelly made with fruit juice, gelatine and sugar--served with cream.

4 p.m. Coffee made with fortified milk or cream and sugar from allowance, or fortified milk flavoured with yeast or vegetable extract.

6 p.m. Milk pudding with puréed fruit *or* sweet as at 2 p.m.

8 p.m. Savoury custard as at lunch *or* scrambled or poached egg *or* omelette. Coffee with milk or cream and sugar from allowance.

10 p.m. Proprietary preparation of milk *or* cocoa, *or* chocolate and fortified milk.
Fruit juice with sugar *or* glucose to drink as desired.

* *Allowance for day:* 1 pint (0·5 *l.*) of whole milk.
1 pint (0·5 *l.*) of whole milk fortified with 2 oz. (60 g.) of full cream dried milk powder.
3 oz. (90 g.) sugar, or more if desired.

Management: When necessary, the calories can be increased by adding more cream, butter or sugar.

[1] Diets constructed by Miss K. Rose, formerly Senior Dietitian, Royal Infirmary, Edinburgh

DIET 2

BLAND DIET, LOW IN ROUGHAGE

suitable for patients who have

PEPTIC ULCER OR ANY INFLAMMATORY, IRRITATIVE OR MALIGNANT DISEASE OF THE ALIMENTARY TRACT WITH SYMPTOMS OF MODERATE SEVERITY

On waking Glass of milk *or* weak tea—milk and sugar if desired.
Biscuit *or* ½ slice of crisp toast, buttered when cold.

Breakfast Strained porridge with milk from allowance* *or* small helping of crisp cereal (avoiding those containing bran, nuts or fruit) with purée fruit *or* fruit juice *or* milk from allowance.
1 egg *or* small piece of white or smoked fish.
Crisp toast buttered when cold *or* buttered bread at least 24 hours old.
Jelly marmalade, run honey *or* golden syrup.
Weak fresh tea or coffee with milk and sugar if desired.

Mid-morning Glass of milk or milk drink.
Smooth biscuit.

Mid-day meal Strained cream soup, if desired
Small helping of lean and tender meat *or* fish.
Sieved vegetables.
Potatoes, mashed or creamed, *or* crisp toast.
Milk pudding with sieved fruit *or* jelly made with fresh fruit juice *or* fruit fool *or* soufflé, *or* mousse with cream.

Tea Crisp toast, buttered when cold, *or* bread (not new)—may be made into sandwiches using sieved hard-boiled egg, *or* scrambled egg, *or* finely minced chicken or ham or cream cheese.
Jelly *or* run honey, if desired.
Plain sponge *or* madeira cake *or* biscuits.
Weak fresh tea with milk and sugar as desired.

Supper Egg *or* creamed or grated cheese *or* meat *or* fish, as at dinner
Sieved vegetable, if desired.
Small helping of milk pudding with puréed fruit *or* puréed fruit with smooth biscuits *or* sweet as at dinner.
Bread and butter *or* crisp toast may be substituted for sweet.
Weak fresh tea *or* coffee with milk and sugar, if desired.

Bedtime Milk drink and biscuits.

* *Allowance for day:* 2 pints (1 *l.*) milk.

Instructions for a Patient with Dyspepsia

1. Take four meals a day.
2. Take your meals at regular times daily.
3. Eat your meals slowly; chew your food carefully.
4. Avoid rush and hurry before and after meals. If possible rest for a few minutes before and after eating.
5. See that you get sufficient sleep at night.
6. Remember that anxiety and worry can upset digestion.
7. Avoid large, heavy meals, fried foods and any article of food which you find disagrees with you.
8. Avoid foods which are mechanically irritating or chemically stimulating (see list below) and very hot or very cold foods.
9. Do not smoke or drink alcohol before meals, when the stomach is empty.
10. Drink only sparingly at meals for this will help to ensure proper mastication, but drink plenty of water between meals.
11. Consult your dentist at regular intervals.

The following foods should be avoided during the acute stage of dyspepsia and taken sparingly during intermissions by those liable to frequent attacks of dyspepsia. For those who suffer from dyspepsia only occasionally, no special restrictions may be necessary; by trial and error the patient can find out which of the articles listed below should be avoided:—

1. Alcohol, strong tea and coffee, gravies and soups made from meat extracts.
2. Raw vegetables, celery, cucumber, onions, radishes, watercress, tomatoes, mushrooms.
3. Raw unripe fruit and dried fruit (e.g. currants, raisins and figs), nuts, and the pips, skins and peel of all fruits, whether cooked or in puddings, cakes or jam.
4. Pickles, spices and condiments.
5. Tough, twice-cooked, or highly seasoned meats, including sausages, bacon and pork.
6. Fried fish and fatty fish such as herring, kipper, mackerel, salmon and sardines.
7. Rich and heavy puddings.
8. All fried foods.
9. New bread and scones, hot buttered toast, wholemeal bread or biscuits, rye or wheat crispbread, coarse cereals, pastry, cakes containing dried fruit or peel.

The following foods are permitted:—

1. Weak tea or coffee.
2. Dairy products, i.e. milk, cream, butter, cream cheese, eggs (not fried).
3. Fish—white fish, steamed, baked or boiled.
4. Meat—sweetbreads, brains, tripe, chicken, rabbit, lean ham, tender beef, mutton or lamb.
5. Crisp toast (buttered cold), rusks and white bread (not new).
6. Plain biscuits and cakes, e.g. sponge cake. Honey, golden syrup, jellies.
7. Cereals—refined and well cooked, e.g. cornflour, semolina, ground rice and oatflour porridge.
8. Puddings—junket, jellies, custards, blancmange, soufflé, mousse.
9. Vegetables—potatoes, boiled and baked, and green and yellow vegetables finely sieved and puréed with butter.
10. Fruits—stewed and finely sieved, and served as purées or fools, and fruit juices strained, sweetened and diluted with water, or used in jellies.

DIET 3

LOW CALORIE DIET

suitable for the treatment of

OBESITY

Approximately: Protein 60 g., Carbohydrate 100 g., Fat 40 g., Cal. 1000

Breakfast Piece of fruit (fresh or stewed, no sugar) *or* small glass of fruit juice.
1 egg *or* 2 rashers of lean bacon (grilled and drained of fat) *or* small piece of white or smoked fish.
1 thin slice (1 oz.) bread.*
Butter and milk from allowance.**
Tea *or* coffee (no sugar).

Mid-morning Tea *or* coffee, milk from allowance (no sugar).

Mid-day meal Clear soup made from meat, vegetable or yeast extract.
Medium helping (2 oz.) of lean meat, poultry, game, lean ham, tongue, liver, kidney, tripe or white or smoked fish.
Large helping of any kind of vegetables except potatoes, peas, beans, lentils and sweet corn.
Piece of fruit (fresh or stewed, no sugar).
Tea *or* coffee—milk from allowance if desired.

Tea 1 thin slice (1 oz.) bread.
Salad vegetables *or* tomatoes if desired.
Butter and milk from allowance.
Tea.

Supper Small helping (1 oz.) of white fish *or* 1 egg *or* small piece of cheese *or* small helping of very lean meat.
Salad *or* other vegetables as desired.
1 thin slice (1 oz.) bread.
Piece of fruit (fresh or stewed, no sugar).
Butter and milk from allowance.
Tea *or* coffee.

** *Allowance for day:*
½ pint (0·25 *l.*) skimmed milk (use of whole milk increases diet to 1100 Cal.)
¾ oz. (22 g.) butter or margarine (to include any fat used in cooking).

* *Instead of* 1 *thin slice of bread the following may be taken:*
2 crispbreads,
or 2 plain biscuits, e.g. rich tea,
or 3 water or cream cracker biscuits,
or 2 oatcakes.

Foods to be avoided: Sugar, sweets, chocolate, jam, marmalade, honey, cakes, buns, scones, potatoes, pastry, pies, porridge, puddings, thickened gravy, sauces, cream, ice cream, tinned and dried fruit, thickened tinned or packet soups, fried food and food cooked with flour or sugar, beer, stout, heavy wines and spirits.

Management:

If it is desired to increase or decrease the value of the diet in respect of proteins, carbohydrates, fats or calories, the exchange list given for diabetic diets (p. 1300) may be used.

Saccharine may be used for sweetening.

Meals may be rearranged to suit the patient's preferences.

DIET 4

LOW CALORIE DIET

with restricted salt regime suitable for patients with
Severe Cardiac Failure

Approximately: Cal. 900, Sodium content 1 g.

Breakfast	1 thin slice of very crisp toast. Butter and milk from allowance.* Weak freshly made tea.
Mid-morning	Small glass of fruit juice.
Mid-day meal	Small helping of white fish, chicken, sweetbreads *or* rabbit. 1 tablespoonful of sieved vegetable. Small helping of milk pudding made with milk from allowance
Tea	1 thin slice of very crisp toast. Butter and milk from allowance. Weak freshly made tea.
Supper	Egg custard made with milk from allowance. Small helping of sieved fruit.
Bedtime	Milk drink made with remainder of milk from allowance

* *Allowance for day:* ¾ pint (0·45 *l.*) of milk.
½ oz. (15 g.) of butter.

No salt to be used in cooking or at table.

DIET 5

VERY LOW FAT, HIGH CARBOHYDRATE DIET

suitable for patients who have

ACUTE PARENCHYMAL DISEASE OF THE LIVER DUE TO TOXIC OR INFECTIVE AGENTS
SEVERE OBSTRUCTIVE JAUNDICE

Approximately: Protein 80 g., Carbohydrate 400 g., Fat 20 g. Cal. 2100

Early morning Glass of fruit juice, with glucose *or* sugar.

Breakfast Strained porridge *or* breakfast cereal with milk from allowance.*
1 slice of bread—may be toasted.
Jelly marmalade *or* honey.
Tea with milk and sugar from allowance.

Mid-morning Glass of fruit juice with sugar *or* coffee made with milk from allowance.

Mid-day meal Small helping of very lean tender meat, poultry, liver, sweetbreads, tripe, lean ham *or* white or smoked fish.
Small helping of sieved vegetables.
Helping of mashed potato.
Cereal pudding made with milk from allowance.
Fruit—fresh, stewed or tinned.

Tea 2 thin slices of bread *or* plain biscuits.
Jam, jelly *or* honey.
Tea with milk and sugar.

Supper 2 thin slices of bread *or* plain biscuits.
Jam, jelly *or* honey.
Cereal pudding made with milk from allowance.
Fruit—fresh, stewed or tinned.
Tea *or* coffee with milk and sugar.

Bedtime Milk drink *or* fruit juice with sugar.

Allowance for day: ½ pint (0·25 *l.*) of skimmed milk—for use in tea.
1 pint (0·5 *l.*) of skimmed milk with 2 oz. dried skimmed milk powder.
2 oz. (60 g.) sugar, or more if desired.

Management:
Take liberally fruit juice with sugar or glucose throughout day.

Avoid: Butter, margarine, dripping, cooking fat, lard and any foods including them. Fat of meat, fatty meat such as goose, duck, pork, or bacon or tinned meat. Fatty fish such as herring, kippers, bloaters, mackerel, sardines, pilchards and salmon. Oils, cream, egg yolk, salad cream, ice-cream, sauces made with fat. Pastry, pies, puddings other than milk pudding. Cakes, chocolates, sweets containing fat such as toffee, fudge or tablet. Fried foods and the use of fat in cooking.

DIET 6

HIGH PROTEIN, LOW FAT DIET

suitable for patients who have

SUBACUTE OR CHRONIC PANCREATIC DISEASE[1]
SUBACUTE PARENCHYMAL LIVER DISEASE WITH JAUNDICE
SEVERE OBSTRUCTIVE JAUNDICE (RECOVERING)
TROPICAL SPRUE[1]
IDIOPATHIC STEATORRHOEA[2]

Approximately: Protein 120 g., Carbohydrate 350 g., Fat 45 g., Cal. 2300

Breakfast Helping of crisp breakfast cereal with fresh or stewed fruit with milk from allowance* *or* fruit juice.
1 egg *or* 2 rashers of lean bacon, grilled and drained of fat, *or* piece of white fish.
Crisp toast *or* bread.
Jelly marmalade, honey *or* syrup.
Tea *or* coffee with milk and sugar from allowance.

Mid-morning Cup of coffee *or* milk drink with milk and sugar from allowance.

Mid-day meal Tomato or fruit juice *or* extracts of yeast, meat or vegetables.
Large helping very lean meat *or* fish.
Helping of sieved vegetables.
Potatoes, boiled, mashed or baked.
Fruit, fresh, tinned or stewed, made into jelly or whipped with egg white.
Milk pudding with milk from allowance.
Tea *or* coffee with milk and sugar, if desired.

Tea Sandwiches with filling of egg, chicken, lean ham, cheese or very lean meat.
Tea with milk and sugar from allowance.

Supper Large helping of very lean meat or fish.
Vegetables, if desired.
Potato, if desired.
Helping of milk pudding with fruit *or* bread with jam, honey or syrup.
Tea *or* coffee with milk from allowance

Bedtime Proprietary milk drink with milk from allowance.
1 plain biscuit.

* *Allowance for day:* 2 pints (1 *l.*) of skimmed milk.
2 oz. (60 g.) sugar, more if desired to increase calories.

Management. See p. 1291.

[1] In those cases of the sprue syndrome and subacute and chronic pancreatic disease in which acid frothy stools indicate an intolerance to starch, the amount of starchy foods (porridge, bread, cereal products and potatoes) in this diet should be reduced.

[2] Idiopathic steatorrhoea does not include coeliac disease since the latter is known to be due to an idiosyncrasy to gluten. In this disease bread or other wheaten or rye products should be avoided entirely.

Management:

Foods to be avoided—Butter, margarine, lard, dripping, cooking fat, fat of meat, tinned meat or fish; foods incorporating fat in cooking, e.g. pastry, suet puddings, cakes, sauces, soups, fried food; cream, ice-cream, nuts, chocolate, caramels, toffee.

Foods suitable—Sugar, boiled sweets, fruit, jam, marmalade, honey, syrup, jelly. Very lean meat—except pork; poultry—except goose and duck; liver, kidney, tripe, heart, rabbit, hare, very lean ham, white or smoked fish. Egg—boiled, poached or baked, or made into custard with skimmed milk. Cheese—not cream cheese. Sieved vegetables, flower of cauliflower, tomato without skins or pips, asparagus tips. Sauce may be made for meat, fish or vegetables with skimmed milk, flour, and grated cheese, hard-boiled egg or parsley. No fat to be used.

DIET 7

HIGH-PROTEIN, MODERATE FAT DIET

suitable for patients who have

SUBACUTE PARENCHYMAL LIVER DISEASE (RECOVERING)
CIRRHOSIS OF THE LIVER WITHOUT JAUNDICE AND ASCITES
THE NEPHROTIC SYNDROME

Approximately: Protein 120 g., Carbohydrate 360 g., Fat 105 g., Cal. 2900

Early morning Tea with milk from allowance*—sugar if desired—*or* fruit juice with glucose.

Breakfast Porridge *or* cereal *or* stewed fruit with milk from allowance *or* fruit juice.
Lean bacon—grilled and drained of fat—*or* egg—poached, boiled or scrambled—*or* a piece of fish.
Bread—may be toasted.
Marmalade *or* honey, if desired.
Butter and milk from allowance.
Tea *or* coffee.

Mid-morning Coffee or milk drink made with milk from allowance.
Plain biscuit.

Mid-day meal Large helping of any kind of lean meat, poultry, game, liver, kidney, tripe, sweetbreads, lean ham, white or smoked fish.
Helping of vegetables.
Helping of potato—boiled, mashed or baked.
Light sweet, incorporating egg if possible.
Fruit—fresh, stewed, or tinned as desired.
2 plain biscuits with cheese.

Tea Sandwiches with filling of scrambled or sieved hard-boiled egg, cheese, minced meat, chicken or ham.
Small piece of plain cake *or* plain biscuits.
Butter and milk from allowance.
Tea—sugar if desired.

Supper Average helping of meat as at mid-day meal *or* egg with lean bacon, or cheese *or* 2 eggs scrambled.
Vegetables if desired.
Bread with butter from allowance.
Jam, jelly or honey.
Or milk pudding with fruit.
Tea *or* coffee with milk from allowance.

Bedtime Milk drink.
Plain biscuit.

* *Allowance for day:* 1 pint (0·5 *l.*) of milk.
1 oz. (30 g.) of butter or margarine.

Management:

1. Hepatic Disease. Avoid fried food, fat in excess of allowance, pastry, pies, puddings including much fat, such as suet puddings and dumpling.

In severe cases of acute hepatitis and in the terminal phases of chronic hepatitis a careful watch should be kept for signs of hepatic failure and impending coma. When these are present the protein intake must be severely restricted or even totally forbidden until improvement occurs.

2. The Nephrotic Syndrome. The intake of salt must be restricted by not adding salt at table, by using minimal amounts in cooking, and by avoiding salt-rich foods.

DIET 8

LOW SODIUM DIET

suitable for patients who have

MEMBRANEOUS GLOMERULONEPHRITIS
CONGESTIVE HEART FAILURE WITH OEDEMA
NEPHROTIC SYNDROME WITH MARKED OEDEMA[1]
CIRRHOSIS OF THE LIVER WITH ASCITES AND OEDEMA[1]

Approximately: Sodium 0·5 g., Protein 60 g., Carbohydrate 250 g., Fat 60 g., Cal. 1800

Breakfast
Fruit *or* fruit juice, sweetened as desired.
1 egg *or* small helping of white fish.
1½ thin slices of 'salt-free' bread,[2] which may be toasted.
Marmalade or honey.
'Salt-free' butter and milk from allowance.*
Tea *or* coffee, with sugar if desired.

Mid-morning
Tea *or* coffee with milk from allowance *or* fruit *or* fruit juice.

Mid-day meal
No soup.
Small helping of tender meat, chicken, tripe, liver, sweetbread or white fish.
Helping of sieved vegetables.
Helping of mashed or creamed potato.
Fruit (fresh, stewed or tinned) *or* jelly *or* whip made with egg white.

Tea
1½ thin slices of 'salt-free' bread, which may be made into sandwiches using tomato, apple, banana, jam, jelly or honey.
Home-made biscuit to which no bicarbonate of soda, salt baking powder or salt butter has been added.
'Salt-free' butter and milk from allowance.
Tea with sugar if desired.

Supper
1 egg *or* small helping of meat *or* fish as at dinner.
Fruit—fresh, stewed or tinned.
1½ thin slices of 'salt-free' bread.
Jam, jelly or honey.
'Salt-free' butter and milk from allowance.
Tea *or* coffee with sugar, if desired.

* *Allowance for day:* ½ pint (0·25 *l.*) of milk.
1 oz. (30 g.) 'salt-free' butter or margarine.

Management: See p. 1294.

[1] In the nephrotic syndrome and cirrhosis of the liver a high protein intake (120 g.) is usually required. This is most easily obtained, without increasing the sodium intake significantly, by adding to the diet 60 g. of a preparation of milk protein (e.g. Casilan, Glaxo or Lonolac, Mead-Johnson).

[2] Use only bread which has been made without salt, and butter or margarine to which no salt has been added. Do not exceed the amounts of bread, milk or butter allowed, as the so-called 'salt free' bread and butter do contain a certain amount of sodium. 'Salt free' bread contains 50-100 mg. Na/100 g. compared with 400 mg. Na/100 g. (average) in ordinary bread.

Management:

No salt to be used in cooking or at table.

Avoid all cured meat and fish, e.g. bacon, ham, tongue, pickled brisket and silverside, finnan haddock, kippers, sardines, pilchards, smoked salmon; all tinned foods except fruit; bottled sauces, pickles, sausages and all foods made with bicarbonate of soda or baking powder.

To increase the calories the following may be added: sugar, fruit, jam, marmalade and boiled sweets and pastilles.

A limit must be put on the time during which a patient may be expected to remain on this *low sodium diet.* This is usually about three to six weeks. By this time if there is no clinical improvement perseverance is useless and other therapeutic measures must be tried.

DIET 9

LOW PROTEIN DIET

suitable for patients who have

SEVERE ACUTE GLOMERULONEPHRITIS (RECOVERING)
CHRONIC RENAL DISEASE WITH MARKED NITROGEN RETENTION

Approximately: Protein 40 g., Carbohydrate 250 g., Fat 60 g., Cal. 1700

Breakfast Fruit (fresh or stewed) *or* small glass of fruit juice.
1½ thin slices of bread, which may be toasted.
Marmalade or honey.
Butter and milk from allowance.*
Tea with sugar.

Mid-morning 1 cup of tea *or* coffee with milk and sugar from allowance.
1 biscuit.

Mid-day meal Small helping of meat *or* poultry *or* fish *or* 2 eggs scrambled or baked.
Small helping of vegetables.
1 medium-size potato.
Milk pudding, using milk from allowance and sugar.
Fruit (fresh, stewed or tinned).

Tea 2 thin slices of bread with jam, jelly or honey, or may be made into sandwiches, using tomato, lettuce, cucumber, dates or banana.
Butter and milk from allowance.
1 cup of tea.

Supper 1 thin slice of bread *or* 2 plain biscuits.
Jam, jelly or honey.
Fruit (fresh, stewed or tinned).
Butter and milk from allowance.
Tea *or* coffee with milk from allowance and sugar.

* *Allowance for day:* ½ pint (0·25 *l.*) of milk.
1¼ oz. (37 g.) butter or margarine.

For patients with acute glomerulonephritis some restriction of fluid is necessary. No more than one cup of tea should be allowed on each occasion. Salt should not be used in cooking, nor should table salt be allowed.

For patients with renal failure and nitrogen retention but without oedema, restriction of fluid intake is strongly contraindicated.

DIET 10

RESTRICTED PROTEIN DIET

suitable for patients who have

MILD ACUTE PROLIFERATIVE GLOMERULONEPHRITIS
ACUTE FOCAL NEPHRITIS
CHRONIC RENAL FAILURE OF MODERATE SEVERITY

Approximately: Protein 60 g., Carbohydrate 280 g., Fat 100 g., Cal. 2300

Breakfast
Cornflakes or similar cereal with fruit and milk from allowance.*
1 egg, poached, boiled or scrambled, *or* 2 rashers of bacon *or* small helping of fish.
1½ thin slices of bread, which may be toasted.
Marmalade or honey.
Butter and milk from allowance.
Tea *or* coffee with milk from allowance and sugar.

Mid-morning
Tea *or* coffee with milk from allowance and sugar, *or* fruit juice with glucose.
1 plain biscuit.

Mid-day meal
Small helping of any kind of meat, poultry, game or fish.
Helping of vegetables.
Helping of potato.
Milk pudding with milk from allowance.
Fruit (fresh, stewed or tinned).

Tea
2 thin slices of bread which may be made into sandwiches, using tomato, cucumber, lettuce, dates or banana, jam, jelly or honey.
Butter and milk from allowance.
Tea.

Supper
1 egg, poached, boiled, scrambled or as omelette with filling of tomato, asparagus or spinach, *or* baked egg with tomato or asparagus, *or* small helping of macaroni cheese *or* fish kedgeree *or* fish cake.
Vegetables if desired.
Milk pudding with milk from allowance, *or* fruit (fresh, stewed, or tinned).
1½ slices thin of bread.
Jam, jelly or honey.
Butter and milk from allowance.
Tea *or* coffee.

Allowance for day: ¾ pint (0·45 *l.*) of milk
2 oz. (60 g.) butter or margarine.

No salt to be added at table and the minimum used in cooking if hypertension or œdema is present.

DIET 11

HIGH ROUGHAGE, HIGH FAT DIET

suitable for patients who have

ATONIC CONSTIPATION AND WHO ARE NORMAL OR LESS THAN NORMAL IN WEIGHT

Early morning	Glass of hot water.
Breakfast	Porridge with cream or milk, *or* bran cereal with stewed fruit, dried or fresh.
	Egg, bacon, sausage, liver *or* fish—may be served with tomato or potatoes.
	Wholemeal bread, may be toasted, *or* oatcakes *or* bran scone—buttered liberally.
	Thick marmalade *or* jam.
	Tea *or* coffee with milk and sugar as desired.
Mid-morning	Yeast, meat or vegetable extract, *or* glass of milk, tea *or* coffee.
Mid-day meal	Vegetable soup, including plenty of chopped fresh vegetables, dried peas and beans, lentils and barley.
	Helping of any kind of meat *or* fish.
	Large helping of vegetables; include raw salads frequently.
	Potatoes.
	Fresh or stewed fruit *or* pudding made with dried fruit or nuts *or* suet pudding *or* tarts—may be served with cream.
	Oatcakes with cheese.
	Tea *or* coffee.
Tea	Sandwiches made with wholemeal bread and filling of dates date and walnut, apple and walnut, cheese and apple, lettuce, tomato, cucumber or cress, *or* wholemeal bread, liberally buttered, with thick jam or comb honey.
	Gingerbread, fruit cakes or other cakes and biscuits incorporating dried fruit, nuts or coconut.
	Tea.
Supper	Helping of any kind of meat *or* fish.
	Large helping of vegetable *or* salad.
	Wholemeal bread *or* oatcake *or* wholemeal scone—liberally buttered—cheese *or* jam if desired.
	Fruit, fresh or stewed.
	Tea *or* coffee.
Bedtime	Glass of hot water.
Take liberally	Vegetables—particularly raw salads and coarse green vegetables.
	Fruit, fresh or raw, and nuts.
	Water.

METHOD OF CONSTRUCTING A DIET RESTRICTED IN CARBOHYDRATE CONTAINING APPROXIMATELY 2,000 CALORIES WITH 180 g. CARBOHYDRATE, 100 g. PROTEIN, 100 g. FAT (Diet 12, p. 1302).

suitable for an adult who has

DIABETES MELLITUS

EXCHANGES

Each *carbohydrate* exchange contains approximately 10 g. carbohydrate, 2 g. protein and ⅔ g. fat. Calorie value is about 54 (equivalent to ⅔ oz. of bread)

Each *protein* exchange contains approximately 8 g. protein and 5 g. fat. Calorie value is about 80 (equivalent to 1 oz. of meat).

Each *fat* exchange contains approximately 12 g. fat and almost no carbohydrate or protein. Calorie value is about 110 (equivalent to ½ oz. of butter).

One pint of milk is equivalent approximately to 3 exchanges of carbohydrate 2 of protein and 1 of fat.

A list of sample exchanges is shown on pp. 1300 and 1301.

The table below shows the number of exchanges prescribed. These were calculated in the following manner.

1. The daily allowance of milk is decided usually on the basis of the patient's food habits. In this example it is 1 pint which contains 3 carbohydrate exchanges.

2. The number of carbohydrate exchanges which the daily intake of carbohydrate (180 g.) represents is calculated by dividing the latter by 10. Thus in this diet 18 carbohydrate exchanges are needed. As 3 carbohydrate exchanges are already allocated in 1 pint of milk, 15 remain for distribution throughout the day.

3. The daily allowance of protein is then decided. The 18 carbohydrate exchanges already allotted will provide 36 g. and the 2 protein exchanges in the milk a further 16 g. Another 6 protein exchanges will provide 48 g., making a total of 100 g.

4. The Calories allocated so far amount to 1710 (see table). A further 290 Calories are needed to bring the total up to 2000 Cal. daily. This must be provided by fat. As one fat exchange provides 110 Cal., 3 are needed.

5. Finally the exchanges (15 carbohydrate, 6 protein and 3 fat) are distributed throughout the day according to the eating habits and daily routine of the patient. Diet 12, p. 1302 shows a specimen menu.

Exchanges	Carbohydrate	Protein	Fat	Calories
	g.	g.	g.	
1 pint milk which contains				
3 carbohydrate exchanges .	30	6	2	160
2 protein exchanges . .	...	16	10	160
1 fat exchange . . .	...	...	12	110
15 carbohydrate exchanges	150	30	10	800
6 protein exchanges . .	...	48	30	480
Total .	180	100	64	1,710
3 fat exchanges . .	...	...	36	330
GRAND TOTAL .	180	100	100	2,040

A Sample of

A MENU SHOWING DISTRIBUTION OF EXCHANGES FOR A DIET RESTRICTED IN CARBOHYDRATE

suitable for an adult who has

Diabetes Mellitus

Approximately: Protein 100 g., Carbohydrate 180 g., Fat 100 g., Cal. 2000.

Breakfast	1 protein exchange.* 4 carbohydrate exchanges.* Butter and milk from allowance.** Tea *or* coffee (no sugar).
Mid-morning	2 carbohydrate exchanges. Butter and milk from allowance. Tea *or* coffee (no sugar).
Mid-day meal	Clear soup, if desired. 2 protein exchanges. 3 carbohydrate exchanges (1 to be taken as fruit). Vegetables from Group 2 (see following Table). Butter and milk from allowance.
Tea	1 protein exchange. 3 carbohydrate exchanges. Butter and milk from allowance. Tea (no sugar).
Supper	2 protein exchanges. 3 carbohydrate exchanges. Vegetables from Group 2 (see following Table) Butter and milk from allowance. Tea *or* coffee (no sugar).

Allowance for day: 1 pint (0·5 *l.*) whole milk.
2 oz. (60 g.) butter *or* 4 fat exchanges.

* A list of suitable exchanges is given in the following Table.

DIETARY EXCHANGES FOR DIABETICS

	Amount		Remarks
	oz.	g.	
1. Carbohydrate Exchanges			
Each exchange contains approximately 10 g. of carbohydrate, 2 g. of protein and ⅔ g. of fat. Caloric value is about 54			
Cereals—			
Bread	⅔	20	
Toast	½	15	
Rice, oatmeal, wheatflour, cornflour, arrowroot, sago, tapioca, breakfast cereals	½	15	All in dry state
Rice, macaroni, spaghetti	1½	45	Boiled
Porridge	4	120	Cooked
Biscuits and scones—			
Water, cream cracker, rich tea or digestive biscuits, crispbreads	½	15	
Oatcakes	⅔	20	
Scones and baps	½	15	
Sponge cake, gingerbread	½	15	No icing or filling
Miscellaneous—			
Marmalade, jam	½	15	
White sauce (savoury)	3	90	
Soup (creamed, tinned or packet)	10	300	Prepared
Fruit—			
Brambles (blackberries), blackcurrants, redcurrants, raspberries	7	200	Raw or stewed
Grapefruit, melon, strawberries	7	200	Raw
Apricots, apples, cherries, gooseberries, pears, plums	7	200	Stewed
Apples, cherries, gooseberries, oranges, pears, pineapple, plums, peaches	3	90	Raw
Bananas	2	60	Without skin
Grapes	2	60	
Prunes	2	60	Stewed without sugar
Apricots, currants, dates, figs, peaches, prunes, raisins, sultanas	⅔	20	All in dry state
Vegetables (*Group* 1)—			
Dried peas, beans and lentils	⅔	20	
Potatoes—chip or roast	1	30	
Potatoes boiled, tinned peas, baked beans, sweet corn	2	60	
Parsnip, beetroot, fresh or frozen peas	3	90	Fresh and boiled
Vegetables (*Group* 2)—unrestricted—			
The following vegetables can be eaten in unrestricted amounts: artichokes, asparagus, french beans, runner beans, brussels sprouts, cabbage, cauliflower, celery, cucumber, lettuce, marrow, mustard and cress, radish, spinach, tomatoes, turnips, watercress, carrots, leeks, onions, mushrooms, rhubarb.			

DIETARY EXCHANGES FOR DIABETICS—*continued*

	Amount		Remarks
	oz.	g.	
2. Protein Exchanges			
Each exchange contains almost no carbohydrate, and approximately 8 g. of protein and 5 g. of fat. Caloric value is about 80			
Lean beef, mutton, pork, bacon, ham, poultry, game or offal	1	30	Cooked weight
Corned beef, tinned meats . .	1	30	
Meat paste, pate . . .	1½	45	
Egg (1)	2	60	
Cheese . . .	1	30	
Fish (white, smoked or tinned), shellfish	1½	45	Cooked weight
Peas, beans, lentils (include 1 carbohydrate exchange) . .	1	30	In dry state
Sausage (includes ½ carbohydrate exchange)	2	60	Cooked
3. Fat Exchanges			
Each exchange contains approximately 12 g. of fat and almost no carbohydrate or protein. Caloric value is about 110			
Butter, margarine, lard, dripping, cooking fat, olive oil or vegetable oil .	½	15	
Cream—'single'	1	30	
Cream—'double'	¾	22	
Salad cream, mayonnaise	¾	22	
Nuts	¾	22	Shelled

DIET 12

A Sample of

A MENU RESTRICTED IN CARBOHYDRATE, BASED ON DISTRIBUTION OF EXCHANGES

Shown on p. 1299

suitable for a patient in Britain who has

Diabetes Mellitus

Approximately: Protein 100 g., Carbohydrate 180 g., Fat 100 g., Cal. 2000

Breakfast
Porridge 6 oz. with milk from allowance.
1 egg.
Bread 2 oz. with butter from allowance.*
Tea *or* coffee with milk from allowance.

Mid-morning
Biscuits ¾ oz.
Tea *or* coffee with milk from allowance.

Mid-day meal
Clear soup with shredded vegetables.
Lean meat 2 oz.
Boiled potatoes 3 oz.
Generous helping of vegetables (Group 2) either cooked or as salad.
Orange 4 oz.
Milk from allowance taken with coffee or as curds.

Tea
Sandwiches containing meat, egg or cheese (1 protein exchange), using 2 oz. bread and butter from allowance.
Tea with milk from allowance.

Supper
Fish 3 oz.
Tomato *or* other Group 2 vegetables.
Bread 2 oz.
Tea *or* coffee with milk from allowance.

* *Allowance for day:* 1 pint milk (0·5 *l.*).
1½ oz. (45 g.) butter or margarine.

Management:

Avoid (unless expressly permitted): sugar, sweets, honey, jam, jelly, marmalade, preserves, syrup, molasses, fruit pies, cake, cookies, sweet condensed milk, soft drinks, alcoholic drinks.

UNWEIGHED DIET

Patients who are unable to weigh their diet or for whom this is unnec essary are given a list of foods which are grouped into three categories.

The following list of foods is used in the Dietetic Department of the Royal Infirmary, Edinburgh.

I. *Foods to be avoided altogether.*

1. Sugar, glucose, jam, marmalade, honey, syrup, treacle, tinned fruits, sweets, chocolate, lemonade, glucose drinks, Ovaltine, Horlicks, Benger's Food and similar foods which are sweetened with sugar.
2. Cakes, sweet biscuits, chocolate biscuits, pastries, pies, puddings, thick sauces.
3. Alcoholic drinks unless permission has been given by the doctor.

II. *Foods to be eaten in moderation only.*

1. Breads of all kinds (including so-called 'slimming' and 'starch-reduced' breads, brown or white, plain or toasted).
2. Rolls, scones, biscuits and crispbreads.
3. Potatoes, peas and baked beans.
4. Breakfast cereals and porridge.
5. All fresh or dried fruit.
6. Macaroni, spaghetti, custard and foods with much flour.
7. Thick soups.
8. Diabetic foods.
9. Milk.

III. *Foods to be eaten as desired.*

1. All meats, fish, eggs.
2. Cheese.
3. Clear soups or meat extracts, tomato or lemon juice.
4. Tea or coffee.
5. Cabbage, Brussels sprouts, broccoli, cauliflower, spinach, turnip, runner or French beans, onions, leeks or mushrooms. Lettuce, cucumber, tomatoes, spring onions, radishes, mustard and cress, asparagus, parsley, rhubarb.
6. Herbs, spices, salt, pepper and mustard.
7. Saccharine or Saxin for sweetening.

For overweight diabetics butter, margarine, fatty and dried foods must be restricted.

Table 16. Average Weights for Men and Women According to Height and Age

Height (in shoes)*	Weight in pounds (in indoor clothing) Ages 20–24	Ages 25–29	Ages 30–39	Ages 40–49	Ages 50–59	Ages 60–69
			Men			
5 ft. 2 in.	128	134	137	140	142	139
5 ft. 3 in.	132	138	141	144	145	142
5 ft. 4 in.	136	141	145	148	149	146
5 ft. 5 in.	139	144	149	152	153	150
5 ft. 6 in.	142	148	153	156	157	154
5 ft. 7 in.	145	151	157	161	162	159
5 ft. 8 in.	149	155	161	165	166	163
5 ft. 9 in.	153	159	165	169	170	168
5 ft. 10 in.	157	163	170	174	175	173
5 ft. 11 in.	161	167	174	178	180	178
6 ft. 0 in.	166	172	179	183	185	183
6 ft. 1 in.	170	177	183	187	189	188
6 ft. 2 in.	174	182	188	192	194	193
6 ft. 3 in.	178	186	193	197	199	198
6 ft. 4 in.	181	190	199	203	205	204
			Women			
4 ft. 10 in.	102	107	115	122	125	127
4 ft. 11 in.	105	110	117	124	127	129
5 ft. 0 in.	108	113	120	127	130	131
5 ft. 1 in.	112	116	123	130	133	134
5 ft. 2 in.	115	119	126	133	136	137
5 ft. 3 in.	118	122	129	136	140	141
5 ft. 4 in.	121	125	132	140	144	145
5 ft. 5 in.	125	129	135	143	148	149
5 ft. 6 in.	129	133	139	147	152	153
5 ft. 7 in.	132	136	142	151	156	157
5 ft. 8 in.	136	140	146	155	160	161
5 ft. 9 in.	140	144	150	159	164	165
5 ft. 10 in.	144	148	154	164	169	†
5 ft. 11 in.	149	153	159	169	174	†
6 ft. 0 in.	154	158	164	174	180	†

* 1 in. heels for men and 2 in. heels for women.
† Average weights not determined because of insufficient data.
Source: Metropolitan Life Insurance Company.

Table 16 gives figures for *average* height and weight at various ages for adults. The figures were obtained as a result of an investigation called 'The Build and Blood Pressure Study, 1959'. This study combines the experiences of 26 large life insurance companies in the United States and Canada between 1935 and 1954. It involved the observation of nearly five million insured persons over periods up to 20 years. Measurements were made with the subjects wearing *indoor clothing and shoes*. The clothing was estimated to weigh 7 to 9 lb. for men and 4 to 6 lb. for women. Heels added about 1 in. to the height of men and 2 in. to the height of women.

TABLE 17. DESIRABLE WEIGHTS FOR MEN AND WOMEN ACCORDING TO HEIGHT AND FRAME. AGES 25 AND OVER

Height (in shoes)*	Weight in pounds (in indoor clothing)		
	Small frame	Medium frame	Large frame
	MEN		
5 ft. 2 in.	112–120	118–129	126–141
5 ft. 3 in.	115–123	121–133	129–144
5 ft. 4 in.	118–126	124–136	132–148
5 ft. 5 in.	121–129	127–139	135–152
5 ft. 6 in.	124–133	130–143	138–156
5 ft. 7 in.	128–137	134–147	142–161
5 ft. 8 in.	132–141	138–152	147–166
5 ft. 9 in.	136–145	142–156	151–170
5 ft. 10 in.	140–150	146–160	155–174
5 ft. 11 in.	144–154	150–165	159–179
6 ft. 0 in.	148–158	154–170	164–184
6 ft. 1 in.	152–162	158–175	168–189
6 ft. 2 in.	156–167	162–180	173–194
6 ft. 3 in.	160–171	167–185	178–199
6 ft. 4 in.	164–175	172–190	182–204
	WOMEN		
4 ft 10 in	92–98	96–107	104–119
4 ft 11 in	94–101	98–110	106–122
5 ft 0 in.	96–104	101–113	109–124
5 ft. 1 in.	99–107	104–116	112–128
5 ft. 2 in.	102–110	107–119	115–131
5 ft. 3 in.	105–113	110–122	118–134
5 ft. 4 in.	108–116	113–126	121–138
5 ft. 5 in.	111–119	116–130	125–142
5 ft. 6 in.	114–123	120–135	129–146
5 ft. 7 in.	118–127	124–139	133–150
5 ft. 8 in.	122–131	128–143	137–154
5 ft. 9 in.	126–135	132–147	141–158
5 ft. 10 in.	130–140	136–151	145–163
5 ft. 11 in.	134–144	140–155	149–168
6 ft. 0 in.	138–148	144–159	153–174

* 1 in. heels for men and 2 in. heels for women.

Table 17 has been constructed by the Metropolitan Life Insurance Company (1959). The *desirable* weights are those which have been found to be associated with the lowest mortality. The death rate in overweight persons is higher than in those of *average* weight and the death rate in persons of *average* weight is higher than those of *desirable* weight. Hence in clinical practice the aim should be to see that as far as possible patients should not exceed *desirable* weight.

This table differs from the table for *average* weight in that there is no correction for increasing age. *Desirable* weights are subdivided into those for persons with small, medium and large frames This division is based on various anthropometric studies including width and depth of chest and hip width, but the exact criteria used have not been published. It is stated that 'as a rule of thumb', if persons of any particular build kept their weight down to the *average* in the early 20's, it would be fairly close to the *desirable* weight at ages over 25.

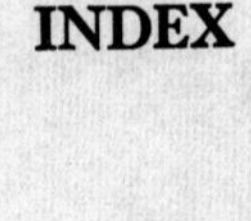

INDEX

D

H

I

J

K

L

M

P

T

V

USEFUL DATA

Abbreviations

(According to the *British Pharmacopoeia*, 1958, pp. 973-975)

Microgram = μg.	Micron = μ	Grain = gr.	Minim = min.
Milligram = mg.	Millimetre = mm.	Ounce = oz.	Fluid drachm = fl. dr.
*Gramme = g.	Centimetre = cm.	Pound = lb.	Fluid ounce = fl. oz.
Kilogram = kg.	Metre = m.		
Millilitre = ml.			
Litre = l.			

Inch = in. Foot = ft. Yard = yd.

Note : 1 microgram = 1,000th part of 1 milligram
1 micron = 1,000th part of 1 millimetre

Equivalents

Grains & oz.	*Grams*	*Approximate equivalent suitable for most clinical purposes (Grams)*
Oz. (av.)		
1	28·35	30
½	14·18	15
Grains		
15	0·97	1
12	0·78	0·75
10	0·65	0·6
8	0·52	0·5
6	0·39	0·4
5	0·32	0·3
4	0·26	0·25
3	0·19	0·2
1½	0·097	0·1

* For the purpose of writing prescriptions as distinct from analytical procedures, the symbol ' G.' should be used as the contraction for ' gramme ' ; this divergence from international practice is recommended in order to avoid the possibility of confusion between ' gramme ' and ' grain.' (Extract from *British Pharmacopoeia*, 1958, p. 973.)

Grains	Milligrams	Approximate equivalent suitable for most clinical purposes (Milligrams)
1	64·8	60
$\frac{1}{2}$	32·4	30
$\frac{1}{3}$	21·6	20
$\frac{1}{4}$	16·2	15
$\frac{1}{6}$	10·8	10
$\frac{1}{8}$	8·1	8
$\frac{1}{12}$	5·4	5
$\frac{1}{50}$	1·3	1·3
$\frac{1}{60}$	1·1	1
$\frac{1}{100}$	0·65	0·6
$\frac{1}{120}$	0·54	0·5

Fluid measure	Millilitres	Approximate equivalent suitable for most clinical purposes (Millilitres)
1$\frac{3}{4}$ pints	994·4	1000
1 pint	568·2	600
1 fl. oz.	28·41	30
1 fl. dr.	3·55	4
30 minims	1·78	2
15	0·89	1
10	0·59	0·6
8	0·47	0·5
5	0·30	0·3
3	0·18	0·2
1$\frac{1}{2}$	0·09	0·1

Miscellaneous

11 stones = 70 kg.

2·2 lb. = 1 kg.

1 teaspoonful = 1 fl. dr. = 4 ml.

1 dessertspoonful = 2 fl. dr. = 8 ml.

1 tablespoonful = $\frac{1}{2}$ fl. oz. = 15 ml.

Normal Values for some Blood Constituents

The values are expressed per unit of plasma or serum, whichever is appropriate, with the exception of the values for glucose which are expressed per unit of blood.

Amylase	80–200 Somogyi units/100 ml.	
	< 10 Wohlgemuth units/ml.	
Bicarbonate	22–28 m.Eq/litre	
Bilirubin	0·2–0·8 mg./100 ml.	
Calcium	4·25–5·25 m.Eq/litre	
	8·5–10·5 mg./100 ml.	
Cephalin cholesterol flocculation	No reaction	
Chloride	100–108 m.Eq/litre	
Cholesterol	125–260 mg./100 ml.	
Copper	75–140 μg./100 ml.	
Copper oxidase	> 25 mg./100 ml.	
Creatinine	0·6–1·2 mg./100 ml.	
Fibrinogen	0·2–0·4 g./100 ml.	
Glucose (fasting)	60–100 mg./100 ml.	
Hydroxybutyrate dehydrogenase	100–240 units/ml.	
Iron	Males 80–180 μg./100 ml.	
	Females 60–160 μg./100 ml.	
Iron binding capacity (total)	250–400 μg./100 ml.	
Lactic Acid dehydrogenase	100–400 units/ml.	
Oxygen saturation	Not less than 94%	
P_{CO_2} (arterial blood)	36–44 mm. Hg.	
pH (arterial blood)	7·37–7·44	
Phosphatase, acid	1–3·5 King Armstrong units/100 ml.	
Phosphatase, alkaline	3–12 King Armstrong units/100 ml.	
Phosphate	2·5–4·5 mg./100 ml. (as P)	
Potassium	3·6–5·3 m.Eq/litre	
Proteins :		
Total	5·6–8·0 g./100 ml.	
Albumin	3·8–5·0 g./100 ml.;	52–68% of total protein
α_1 globulin	0·15–0·45 g./100 ml.;	2–6% of total protein
α_2 globulin	0·4–0·8 g./100 ml.;	5–11% of total protein
β globulin	0·65–1·15 g./100 ml.;	8–16% of total protein
γ globulin	0·8–1·6 g./100 ml.;	10–22% of total protein
Protein-bound iodine	4·0–7·5 μg./100 ml.	
Sodium	135–150 m.Eq/litre	
Thymol turbidity	1–4 units	
Aspartate aminotransferase (GOT)	10–40 units/ml.	
Alanine aminotransferase (GPT)	10–35 units/ml.	
Urea	15–40 mg./100 ml. (up to 50 years)	
Uric acid	2–7 mg./100 ml.	
Zinc turbidity	1–5 units	

The amounts of some substances dissolved in the body fluids have customarily been expressed by weight. The significance of their relative concentrations is more easily appreciated by expressing the latter in terms of chemical equivalence. Inorganic ions are expressed as milliequivalents per litre, and this figure is obtained by dividing milligrams per litre by the equivalent weight. Non-electrolytes are sometimes expressed as millimoles per litre by dividing milligrams per litre by molecular weight.